18th Edition

HARRISON'S™
MANUAL OF
MEDICINE

EDITORS

Dan L. Longo, MD
Professor of Medicine, Harvard Medical School;
Senior Physician, Brigham and Women's Hospital;
Deputy Editor, *New England Journal of Medicine*,
Boston, Massachusetts; Adjunct Investigator,
National Institute on Aging, National Institutes of Health,
Bethesda, Maryland

Anthony S. Fauci, MD, ScD(HON)
Chief, Laboratory of Immunoregulation;
Director, National Institute of Allergy and Infectious Diseases,
National Institutes of Health, Bethesda, Maryland

Dennis L. Kasper, MD, MA(HON)
William Ellery Channing Professor of Medicine, Professor of
Microbiology and Molecular Genetics, Harvard Medical School;
Director, Channing Laboratory, Department of Medicine, Brigham
and Women's Hospital, Boston, Massachusetts

Stephen L. Hauser, MD
Robert A. Fishman Distinguished Professor and Chairman,
Department of Neurology, University of California, San Francisco,
San Francisco, California

J. Larry Jameson, MD, PhD
Robert G. Dunlop Professor of Medicine; Dean, University
of Pennsylvania Perelman School of Medicine; Executive
Vice-President, University of Pennsylvania Health System,
Philadelphia, Pennsylvania

Joseph Loscalzo, MD, PhD
Hersey Professor of the Theory and Practice of Medicine, Harvard
Medical School; Chairman, Department of Medicine;
Physician-in-Chief, Brigham and Women's Hospital, Boston,
Massachusetts

18th Edition

HARRISON'S™
MANUAL OF
MEDICINE

EDITORS

Dan L. Longo, MD

Anthony S. Fauci, MD

Dennis L. Kasper, MD

Stephen L. Hauser, MD

J. Larry Jameson, MD, PhD

Joseph Loscalzo, MD, PhD

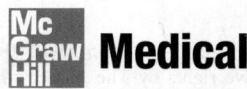

New York   Chicago   San Francisco   Lisbon   London   Madrid   Mexico City
Milan   New Delhi   San Juan   Seoul   Singapore   Sydney   Toronto

NOTE: Dr. Fauci's work as editor and author was performed outsid
his employment as a U.S. government employee. This work repre
sonal and professional views and not necessarily those of the U.S.

Harrison's
PRINCIPLES OF INTERNAL MEDICINE
Eighteenth Edition
MANUAL OF MEDICINE

Copyright © 2013, 2009, 2005, 2002, 1998, 1995, 1991, 1988 by The McGraw-Hill
Companies, Inc. All rights reserved. Printed in the United States of America. Except
as permitted under the United States Copyright Act of 1976, no part of this publication may be reproduced or distributed in any form or by any means, or stored in a
data base or retrieval system, without the prior written consent of the author.

1 2 3 4 5 6 7 8 9 0   DOC/DOC   17 16 15 14 13 12

ISBN 978-0-07-174519-2
MHID 0-07-174519-X

This book was set in Minion Pro by Cenveo Publisher Services. The editors were
James F. Shanahan and Kim J. Davis. The production supervisor was Catherine
H. Saggese; project management was provided by Vastavikta Sharma, Cenveo
Publisher Services. The designer was Alan Barnett; the cover designer was
Anthony Landi. RR Donnelly was printer and binder.

Library of Congress Cataloging-in-Publication Data

Harrison's manual of medicine / editors, Dan L. Longo ... [et al.].—18th ed.
    p. ; cm.
    Manual of medicine
    Includes index.
    ISBN 978-0-07-174519-2 (pbk. : alk. paper)—ISBN 0-07-174519-X (pbk. :
alk. paper)
    I. Harrison, Tinsley Randolph, 1900-1978.   II. Longo, Dan L. (Dan Louis),
1949-   III. Harrison's principles of internal medicine.   IV. Title: Manual of
medicine.
    [DNLM: 1. Clinical   Medicine—Handbooks.   2. Internal   Medicin—
Handbooks. WB 39]
    616—dc23

                                                              2012008873

International Edition ISBN 978-0-07-179290-5; MHID 0-07-179290-2.
Copyright © 2013. Exclusive rights by The McGraw-Hill Companies, Inc., for
manufacture and export. This book cannot be re-exported from the country to
which it is consigned by McGraw-Hill. The International Edition is not available
in North America.

CONTENTS

SECTION 3	Common Patient Presentations

SECTION 4   Ophthalmology and Otolaryngology

SECTION 5   Dermatology

SECTION 6   Hematology and Oncology

SECTION 13   Endocrinology and Metabolism

SECTION 14   Neurology

CONTRIBUTORS

ASSOCIATE EDITORS

GERHARD P. BAUMANN, MD
Professor of Medicine Emeritus
Division of Endocrinology, Metabolism, and Molecular Medicine
Northwestern University Feinberg School of Medicine
Chicago, Illinois

S. ANDREW JOSEPHSON, MD
Assistant Professor of Neurology, Director, Neurohospitalist Program
University of California, San Francisco
San Francisco, California

CAROL A. LANGFORD, MD, MHS
Director, Center for Vasculitis Care and Research
Department of Rheumatic and Immunologic Diseases
Cleveland Clinic
Cleveland, Ohio

LEONARD S. LILLY, MD
Professor of Medicine
Harvard Medical School
Chief, Brigham and Women's/Faulkner Cardiology
Brigham and Women's Hospital
Boston, Massachusetts

DAVID B. MOUNT, MD
Assistant Professor of Medicine
Harvard Medical School
Associate Physician, Renal Division, Brigham and Women's Hospital
Staff Physician, Renal Division, VA Boston Healthcare System
Boston, Massachusetts

EDWIN K. SILVERMAN, MD, PhD
Associate Professor of Medicine
Chief, Channing Division of Network Medicine
Department of Medicine, Brigham and Women's Hospital
Harvard Medical School
Boston, Massachusetts

NEERAJ K. SURANA, MD, PhD
Instructor in Pediatrics
Harvard Medical School
Assistant in Medicine
Boston Children's Hospital
Boston, Massachusetts

Numbers indicate the chapters written or co-written by the contributor.

GERHARD P. BAUMANN, MD
1, 3, 4, 7, 8, 24, 25, 30, 32, 35, 36, 127, 179–190, 210, 213, 218, 220

ANTHONY S. FAUCI, MD
28, 33, 48, 49, 53, 65, 66, 114, 161–178

STEPHEN L. HAUSER, MD
6, 17–23, 54–63, 84, 191–209, 211, 212, 217

J. LARRY JAMESON, MD, PhD
1, 3, 4, 7, 8, 24, 25, 30, 32, 35, 36, 127, 179–190, 210, 213, 218, 220

S. ANDREW JOSEPHSON, MD
6, 17–23, 54–63, 84, 191–209, 211, 212, 217

DENNIS L. KASPER, MD
13, 26, 29, 31, 34, 64, 85–113, 115–118, 141, 154, 214

CAROL A. LANGFORD, MD
28, 33, 48, 49, 53, 65, 66, 114, 161–178

LEONARD S. LILLY, MD
11, 12, 14, 37, 38, 40, 119–126, 128–136, 215

DAN L. LONGO, MD
9, 10, 27, 43–47, 50, 51, 67–83, 158–160, 216

JOSEPH LOSCALZO, MD, PhD
5, 11, 12, 14–16, 37–42, 52, 119–126, 128–153, 155–157, 215

DAVID B. MOUNT, MD
42, 52, 147–153, 155–157

EDWIN K. SILVERMAN, MD, PhD
5, 15, 16, 39, 41, 137–146

NEERAJ K. SURANA, MD
13, 26, 29, 31, 34, 64, 85–113, 115–118, 141, 154, 214

PREFACE

Harrison's Principles of Internal Medicine (HPIM) provides a comprehensive body of information important to an understanding of the biological and clinical aspects of quality patient care. It remains the premier medical text-book for students and clinicians. With the rapidly expanding base of medical knowledge and the time constraints associated with heavy patient-care responsibilities in modern health care settings, it is not always possible to read a comprehensive account of diseases and their presentations, clinical manifestations, and treatments before or even immediately after encountering the patient. It was for these reasons, among others, that in 1988 the Editors first condensed the clinical portions of *HPIM* into a pocket-sized volume, *Harrison's Manual of Medicine.* Similar to the prior seven editions, this new edition of the *Manual,* drawn from the 18th edition of *HPIM,* presents the key features of the diagnosis, clinical manifestations, and treatment of the major diseases that are likely to be encountered on a medical service.

The Editors stress that the *Manual* should not substitute for in-depth analysis of the clinical problem, but should serve as a ready source of well-crafted and informative summaries that will be useful "on-the-spot" and that will prepare the reader for a more in-depth analysis drawn from more extensive reading at a later time. The *Manual* has met with increasing popularity over the years; its popularity and value relate in part to its abbreviated format, which has proven to be extremely useful for initial diagnosis, brief description of pathogenesis, and outline of management in time-restricted clinical settings. The book's full-color format will increase the speed with which readers can locate and use information within its chapters. The *Manual* has been written for easy and seamless reference to the full text of the 18th edition of *HPIM,* and the Editors recommend that the full textbook—or *Harrison's Online*—be consulted as soon as time allows. As with previous editions, this latest edition of the *Manual* attempts to keep up with the continual and sometimes rapid evolution of internal medicine practices. In this regard, every chapter has received a close review and has been updated from the prior edition, with substantial revisions and new chapters provided where appropriate. The format of the book has been further streamlined to reflect more use of abbreviated text, with use of numerous tables and graphics to help guide understanding and decisions at the point of care. In full recognition of the important role of digital information delivery in alleviating the increasing time demands put on clinicians, the 18th edition of the *Manual* has also been made available in portable format for the smartphone and tablet.

We would like to thank our friend and colleague Eugene Braunwald, MD for his many contributions and years of wise advice in shaping the *Manual* and indeed all the publications in the Harrison's family.

ACKNOWLEDGMENTS

The Editors and McGraw-Hill wish to thank their editorial staff whose assistance and patience made this edition come out in a timely manner:

From the Editors' offices: Pat Duffey; Gregory K. Folkers; Julie B. McCoy; Elizabeth Robbins, MD; Marie E. Scurti; Kristine Shontz; and Stephanie Tribuna.

From McGraw-Hill: James F. Shanahan, Kim J. Davis, and Catherine H. Saggese.

The Editors also wish to acknowledge contributors to past editions of this Manual, whose work formed the basis for many of the chapters herein: Eugene Braunwald, MD; Joseph B. Martin, MD, PhD; Kurt Isselbacher, MD; Jean Wilson, MD; Tamar F. Barlam, MD; Daryl R. Gress, MD; Michael Sneller, MD; John W. Engstrom, MD; Kenneth Tyler, MD; Sophia Vinogradov, MD; Dan B. Evans, MD; Punit Chadha, MD; Glenn Chertow, MD; and James Woodrow Weiss, MD.

NOTICE

Medicine is an ever-changing science. As new research and clinical experience broaden our knowledge, changes in treatment and drug therapy are required. The authors and the publisher of this work have checked with sources believed to be reliable in their efforts to provide information that is complete and generally in accord with the standards accepted at the time of publication. However, in view of the possibility of human error or changes in medical sciences, neither the authors nor the publisher nor any other party who has been involved in the preparation or publication of this work warrants that the information contained herein is in every respect accurate or complete, and they disclaim all responsibility for any errors or omissions or for the results obtained from use of the information contained in this work. Readers are encouraged to confirm the information contained herein with other sources. For example and in particular, readers are advised to check the product information sheet included in the package of each drug they plan to administer to be certain that the information contained in this work is accurate and that changes have not been made in the recommended dose or in the contraindications for administration. This recommendation is of particular importance in connection with new or infrequently used drugs.

CHAPTER **1**
Initial Evaluation and Admission Orders for the General Medicine Patient

Pts are admitted to the hospital when (1) they present the physician with a complex diagnostic challenge that cannot be safely or efficiently performed in the outpatient setting; or (2) they are acutely ill and require inpatient diagnostic tests, interventions, and treatments. The decision to admit a pt includes identifying the optimal clinical service (e.g., medicine, urology, neurology), the level of care (observation, general floor, telemetry, ICU), and necessary consultants. Admission should always be accompanied by clear communication with the pt and family, both to obtain information and to outline the anticipated events in the hospital. Pts often have multiple physicians, and based on the nature of the clinical problems, they should be contacted to procure relevant medical history and to assist with clinical care during or after admission. Electronic health records promise to facilitate the communication of medical information among physicians, hospitals, and other medical care providers.

The scope of illnesses cared for by internists is enormous. During a single day on a typical general medical service, it is not unusual for physicians, especially residents in training, to admit ten pts with ten different diagnoses affecting ten different organ systems. Given this diversity of disease, it is important to be systematic and consistent in the approach to any new admission.

Physicians are often concerned about making errors of commission. Examples would include prescribing an improper antibiotic for a pt with pneumonia or miscalculating the dose of heparin for a pt with new deep venous thrombosis (DVT). However, errors of omission are also common and can result in pts being denied life-saving interventions. Simple examples include: not checking a lipid panel for a pt with coronary heart disease, not prescribing an angiotensin-converting enzyme (ACE) inhibitor to a diabetic with documented albuminuria, or forgetting to give a pt with an osteoporotic hip fracture calcium, vitamin D, and an oral bisphosphonate.

Inpatient medicine typically focuses on the diagnosis and treatment of acute medical problems. However, most pts have multiple medical problems affecting different organ systems, and it is equally important to prevent nosocomial complications. Prevention of common hospital complications, such as DVT, peptic ulcers, line infections, falls, delirium, and pressure ulcers, is an important aspect of the care of all general medicine pts.

A consistent approach to the admission process helps to ensure comprehensive and clear orders that can be written and implemented in a timely manner. Several mnemonics serve as useful reminders when writing admission orders. A suggested checklist for admission orders is shown below; it

1

includes several interventions targeted to prevent common nosocomial complications. Computerized order entry systems are also useful when designed to prompt structured sets of admission orders. However, these should not be used to the exclusion of orders tailored for the needs of an individual pt.

Checklist mnemonic: ADMIT VITALS AND PHYSICAL EXAM

- *A*dmit to: service (Medicine, Oncology, ICU); provide status (acute or observation).
- *D*iagnosis: state the working diagnosis prompting this particular hospitalization.
- *M*D: name the attending, resident, intern, student, primary care MD, and consultants.
- *I*solation requirements: state respiratory or contact isolation and reason for order.
- *T*elemetry: state indications for telemetry and specify monitor parameters.
- *V*ital signs (VS): frequency of VS; also specify need for pulse oximetry and orthostatic VS.
- *I*V access and IV fluid or TPN orders (Chap. 2).
- *T*herapists: respiratory, speech, physical, and/or occupational therapy needs.
- *A*llergies: also specify type of adverse reaction.
- *L*abs: blood count, chemistries, coagulation tests, type & screen, UA, special tests.
- *S*tudies: CT scans (also order contrast), ultrasounds, angiograms, endoscopies, etc.
- *A*ctivity: weight bear/ambulating instructions, fall/seizure precautions and restraints.
- *N*ursing Orders: call intern if ($x/y/z$), also order I/Os, daily weights, and blood glucose.
- *D*iet: include NPO orders and tube feeding. State whether to resume diet after tests.
- *P*eptic ulcer prevention: proton-pump inhibitor or misoprostol for high-risk pts.
- *H*eparin or other modality (warfarin, compression boots, support hose) for DVT prophylaxis.
- *Y*ank all Foley catheters and nonessential central lines to prevent iatrogenic infections.
- *S*kin care: prevent pressure sores with heel guards, air mattresses, and RN wound care.
- *I*ncentive spirometry: prevent atelectasis and hospital-acquired pneumonia.
- *C*alcium, vitamin D, and bisphosphonates if steroid use, bone fracture, or osteoporosis.
- *A*CE inhibitor and aspirin: use for nearly all pts with coronary disease or diabetes.
- *L*ipid panel: assess and treat all cardiac and vascular pts for hyperlipidemia.
- *E*CG: for nearly every pt >50 years at the time of admission.
- *X*-rays: chest x-ray, abdominal series; evaluate central lines and endotracheal tubes.
- *A*dvance directives: Full code or DNR; specify whether to rescind for any procedures.
- *M*edications: be specific with your medication orders.

It may be helpful to remember the medication mnemonic "Stat DRIP" for different routes of administration (*s*tat, *d*aily, *r*ound-the-clock, *I*V, and *p*rn medications). For the sake of cross-covering colleagues, provide relevant prn orders for acetaminophen, diphenhydramine, stool softeners or laxatives, and sleeping pills. Specify any stat medications since routine medication orders entered as "once daily" may not be dispensed until the following day unless ordered as stat or "first dose now."

CHAPTER **2**
Electrolytes/Acid-Base Balance

SODIUM

Disturbances of sodium concentration [Na^+] result in most cases from abnormalities of H_2O homeostasis, which change the relative ratio of Na^+ to H_2O. Disorders of Na^+ balance per se are, in contrast, associated with changes in extracellular fluid volume, either hypo- or hypervolemia. Maintenance of the "effective circulating volume" is achieved in large part by changes in urinary sodium excretion, whereas H_2O balance is achieved by changes in both H_2O intake and urinary H_2O excretion (Table 2-1). Confusion can result from the coexistence of defects in both H_2O and Na^+ balance. For example, a hypovolemic pt may have an appropriately low urinary Na^+ due to increased renal tubular reabsorption of filtered NaCl; a concomitant increase in circulating arginine vasopressin (AVP)—part of the defense of effective circulating volume (Table 2-1)—will cause the renal retention of ingested H_2O and the development of hyponatremia.

■ HYPONATREMIA

This is defined as a serum [Na^+] <135 mmol/L and is among the most common electrolyte abnormalities encountered in hospitalized pts. Symptoms include nausea, vomiting, confusion, lethargy, and disorientation; if severe (<120 mmol/L) and/or abrupt, seizures, central herniation, coma, or death may result (see Acute Symptomatic Hyponatremia, below). Hyponatremia is almost always the result of an increase in circulating AVP and/or increased renal sensitivity to AVP; a notable exception is in the setting of low solute intake ("beer potomania"), wherein a markedly reduced urinary solute excretion is inadequate to support the excretion of sufficient free H_2O. The serum [Na^+] by itself does not yield diagnostic information regarding total-body Na^+ content; hyponatremia is primarily a disorder of H_2O homeostasis. Pts with hyponatremia are thus categorized diagnostically into three groups, depending on their clinical volume status: hypovolemic, euvolemic, and hypervolemic hyponatremia (Fig. 2-1). All three forms of hyponatremia share an exaggerated, "nonosmotic" increase in circulating AVP, in the setting of reduced serum osmolality. Notably, hyponatremia is often multifactorial; clinically important nonosmotic stimuli that can cause a release of AVP and increase the risk of hyponatremia include drugs, pain, nausea, and strenuous exercise.

TABLE 2-1 OSMOREGULATION VERSUS VOLUME REGULATION

	Osmoregulation	Volume Regulation
What is sensed	Plasma osmolality	"Effective" circulating volume
Sensors	Hypothalamic osmoreceptors	Carotid sinus
		Afferent arteriole
		Atria
Effectors	AVP	Sympathetic nervous system
	Thirst	Renin-angiotensin-aldosterone system
		ANP/BNP
		AVP
What is affected	Urine osmolality	Urinary sodium excretion
	H_2O intake	Vascular tone

Note: See text for details.
Abbreviations: ANP, atrial natriuretic peptide; AVP, arginine vasopressin; BNP, brain natriuretic peptide.
Source: Adapted from Rose BD, Black RM (eds): *Manual of Clinical Problems in Nephrology*. Boston, Little Brown, 1988; with permission.

Laboratory investigation of a pt with hyponatremia should include a measurement of serum osmolality to exclude "pseudohyponatremia" due to hyperlipidemia or hyperproteinemia. Serum glucose also should be measured; serum Na^+ falls by 1.4 mM for every 100-mg/dL increase in glucose, due to glucose-induced H_2O efflux from cells. Hyperkalemia may suggest adrenal insufficiency or hypoaldosteronism; increased blood urea nitrogen (BUN) and creatinine may suggest a renal cause. Urine electrolytes and osmolality are also critical tests in the initial evaluation of hyponatremia. In particular, a urine Na^+ <20 meq/L is consistent with hypovolemic hyponatremia in the clinical absence of a "hypervolemic," Na^+-avid syndrome such as congestive heart failure (CHF) (Fig. 2-1). Urine osmolality <100 mosmol/kg is suggestive of polydipsia or, in rare cases, of decreased solute intake; urine osmolality >400 mosmol/kg suggests that AVP excess is playing a more dominant role, whereas intermediate values are more consistent with multifactorial pathophysiology (e.g., AVP excess with a component of polydipsia). Finally, in the right clinical setting, thyroid, adrenal, and pituitary function should also be tested.

Hypovolemic Hyponatremia

Hypovolemia from both renal and extrarenal causes is associated with hyponatremia. Renal causes of hypovolemia include primary adrenal insufficiency and hypoaldosteronism, salt-losing nephropathies (e.g., reflux nephropathy, nonoliguric acute tubular necrosis), diuretics, and osmotic diuresis. Random "spot" urine Na^+ is typically >20 meq/L in these cases but may be <20 meq/L in diuretic-associated hyponatremia if tested long after

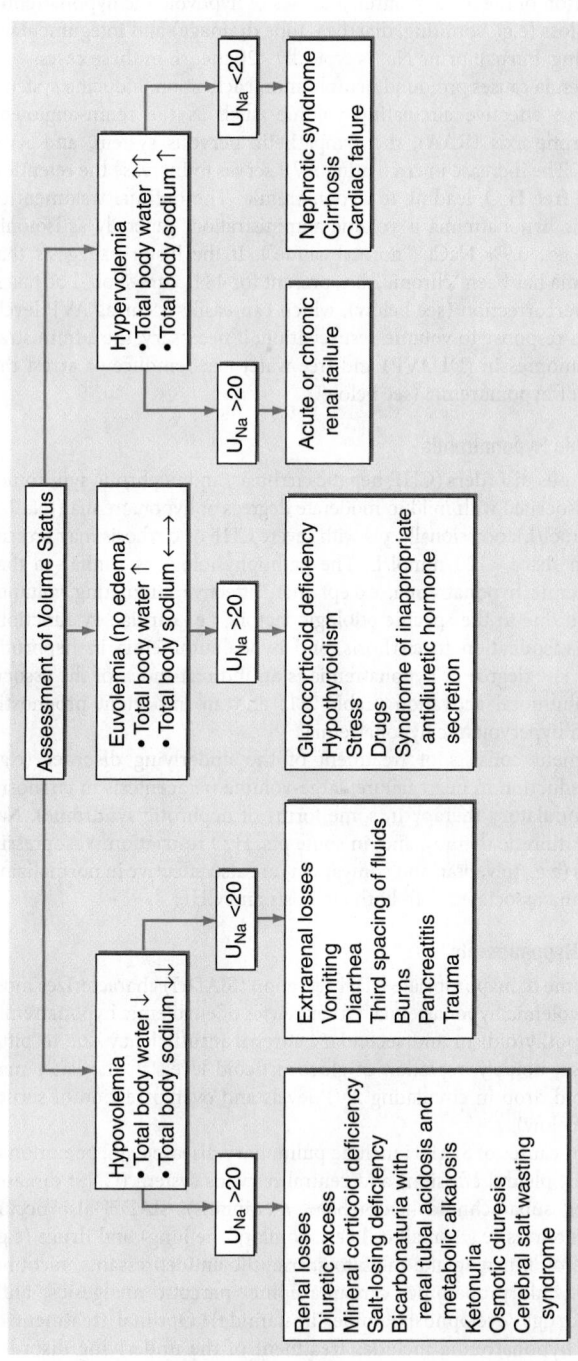

FIGURE 2-1 The diagnostic approach to hyponatremia. See text for details. [*From S Kumar, T Berl: Diseases of water metabolism, in Atlas of Diseases of the Kidney, RW Schrier (ed). Philadelphia, Current Medicine, Inc, 1999; with permission.*]

Assessment of Volume Status

Hypovolemia
• Total body water ↓
• Total body sodium ↓↓

$U_{Na} >20$

Renal losses
Diuretic excess
Mineral corticoid deficiency
Salt-losing deficiency
Bicarbonaturia with
renal tubal acidosis and
metabolic alkalosis
Ketonuria
Osmotic diuresis
Cerebral salt wasting
syndrome

$U_{Na} <20$

Extrarenal losses
Vomiting
Diarrhea
Third spacing of fluids
Burns
Pancreatitis
Trauma

Euvolemia (no edema)
• Total body water ↑
• Total body sodium ←→

$U_{Na} >20$

Glucocorticoid deficiency
Hypothyroidism
Stress
Drugs
Syndrome of inappropriate
antidiuretic hormone
secretion

Hypervolemia
• Total body water ↑↑
• Total body sodium ↑

$U_{Na} >20$

Acute or chronic
renal failure

$U_{Na} <20$

Nephrotic syndrome
Cirrhosis
Cardiac failure

administration of the drug. Nonrenal causes of hypovolemic hyponatremia include GI loss (e.g., vomiting, diarrhea, tube drainage) and integumentary loss (sweating, burns); urine Na^+ is typically <20 meq/L in these cases.

Hypovolemia causes profound neurohumoral activation, inducing systems that preserve effective circulating volume, such as the renin-angiotensin-aldosterone axis (RAA), the sympathetic nervous system, and AVP (Table 2-1). The increase in circulating AVP serves to increase the retention of ingested free H_2O, leading to hyponatremia. The optimal treatment of hypovolemic hyponatremia is volume administration, generally as isotonic crystalloid, i.e., 0.9% NaCl ("normal saline"). If the history suggests that hyponatremia has been "chronic," i.e., present for 48 h, care should be taken to avoid overcorrection (see below), which can easily occur as AVP levels plummet in response to volume-resuscitation; if necessary, the administration of desmopressin (DDAVP) and free water can reinduce or arrest the correction of hyponatremia (see below).

Hypervolemic Hyponatremia

The edematous disorders (CHF, hepatic cirrhosis, and nephrotic syndrome) are often associated with mild to moderate degrees of hyponatremia ([Na^+] = 125–135 mmol/L); occasionally, pts with severe CHF or cirrhosis may present with serum [Na^+] <120 mmol/L. The pathophysiology is similar to that in hypovolemic hyponatremia, except that "effective circulating volume" is decreased due to the specific etiologic factors, i.e., cardiac dysfunction, peripheral vasodilation in cirrhosis, and hypoalbuminemia in nephrotic syndrome. The degree of hyponatremia is an indirect index of the associated neurohumoral activation (Table 2-1) and an important prognostic indicator in hypervolemic hyponatremia.

Management consists of treatment of the underlying disorder (e.g., afterload reduction in heart failure, large-volume paracentesis in cirrhosis, immunomodulatory therapy in some forms of nephrotic syndrome), Na^+ restriction, diuretic therapy, and, in some pts, H_2O restriction. Vasopressin antagonists (e.g., tolvaptan and conivaptan) are also effective in normalizing hyponatremia associated with both cirrhosis and CHF.

Euvolemic Hyponatremia

The syndrome of inappropriate ADH secretion (SIADH) characterizes most cases of euvolemic hyponatremia. Other causes of euvolemic hyponatremia include hypothyroidism and secondary adrenal insufficiency due to pituitary disease; notably, repletion of glucocorticoid levels in the latter may cause a rapid drop in circulating AVP levels and overcorrection of serum [Na^+] (see below).

Common causes of SIADH include pulmonary disease (e.g., pneumonia, tuberculosis, pleural effusion) and central nervous system (CNS) diseases (e.g., tumor, subarachnoid hemorrhage, meningitis); SIADH also occurs with malignancies (e.g., small cell carcinoma of the lung) and drugs (e.g., selective serotonin reuptake inhibitors, tricyclic antidepressants, nicotine, vincristine, chlorpropamide, carbamazepine, narcotic analgesics, antipsychotic drugs, cyclophosphamide, ifosfamide). Optimal treatment of euvolemic hyponatremia includes treatment of the underlying disorder.

H_2O restriction to <1 L/d is a cornerstone of therapy, but may be ineffective or poorly tolerated. However, vasopressin antagonists are predictably effective in normalizing serum [Na^+] in SIADH. Alternatives include the coadministration of loop diuretics to inhibit the countercurrent mechanism and reduce urinary concentration, combined with oral salt tablets to abrogate diuretic-induced salt loss and attendant hypovolemia.

Acute Symptomatic Hyponatremia

Acute symptomatic hyponatremia is a medical emergency; a sudden drop in serum [Na^+] can overwhelm the capacity of the brain to regulate cell volume, leading to cerebral edema, seizures, and death. Women, particularly premenopausal women, are particularly prone to such sequelae; neurologic consequences are comparatively rare in male pts. Many of these pts develop hyponatremia from iatrogenic causes, including hypotonic fluids in the postoperative period, prescription of a thiazide diuretic, colonoscopy preparation, or intraoperative use of glycine irrigants. Polydipsia with an associated cause of increased AVP may also cause acute hyponatremia, as can increased H_2O intake in the setting of strenuous exercise, e.g., a marathon. The recreational drug Ecstasy [methylenedioxymethamphetamine (MDMA)] can cause acute hyponatremia, rapidly inducing both AVP release and increased thirst.

Severe symptoms may occur at relatively modest levels of serum [Na^+], e.g., in the mid-120s. Nausea and vomiting are common premonitory symptoms of more severe sequelae. An important concomitant is respiratory failure, which may be hypercapnic due to CNS depression or normocapnic due to neurogenic, noncardiogenic pulmonary edema; the attendant hypoxia amplifies the impact of hyponatremic encephalopathy.

TREATMENT ▶ Hyponatremia

Three considerations are critical in the therapy of hyponatremia. First, the presence, absence, and/or severity of symptoms determine the urgency of therapy (see above for acute symptomatic hyponatremia). Second, pts with hyponatremia that has been present for >48 h ("chronic hyponatremia") are at risk for osmotic demyelination syndrome, typically central pontine myelinolysis, if serum Na^+ is corrected by >10–12 mM within the first 24 h and/or by >18 mM within the first 48 h. Third, the response to interventions, such as hypertonic saline or vasopressin antagonists, can be highly unpredictable, such that frequent monitoring of serum Na^+ (every 2–4 h) is imperative.

Treatment of acute symptomatic hyponatremia should include hypertonic saline to acutely increase serum Na^+ by 1–2 mM/h to a total increase of 4–6 mM; this increase is typically sufficient to alleviate acute symptoms, after which corrective guidelines for "chronic" hyponatremia are appropriate (see below). A number of equations and algorithms have been developed to estimate the required rate of hypertonic solution; one popular approach is to calculate a "Na^+ deficit," where the Na^+ deficit = 0.6 × body weight × (target [Na^+] – starting [Na^+]). Regardless of the method used to determine the rate of administered hypertonic saline, the increase in serum $[Na^+]$ can be highly unpredictable, as the underlying physiology rapidly changes; serum $[Na^+]$ should be monitored every 2–4 h during and after treatment with hypertonic saline. The administration of supplemental O_2 and ventilatory support can also be critical in acute hyponatremia, if pts develop acute pulmonary edema or hypercapnic respiratory failure. IV loop diuretics will help treat acute pulmonary edema and will also increase free H_2O excretion by interfering with the renal countercurrent multiplier system. It is noteworthy that vasopressin antagonists do not have a role in the management of acute hyponatremia.

The rate of correction should be comparatively slow in *chronic* hyponatremia (<10–12 m*M* in the first 24 h and <18 m*M* in the first 48 h), so as to avoid osmotic demyelination syndrome. Vasopressin antagonists are highly effective in SIADH and in hypervolemic hyponatremia due to heart failure or cirrhosis. Should pts overcorrect serum $[Na^+]$ in response to vasopressin antagonists, hypertonic saline, or isotonic saline (in chronic hypovolemic hyponatremia), hyponatremia can be safely reinduced or stabilized by the administration of the vasopressin *agonist* DDAVP and the administration of free H_2O, typically IV D_5W; again, close monitoring of the response of serum $[Na^+]$ is essential to adjust therapy.

■ HYPERNATREMIA

This is rarely associated with hypervolemia, where the association is typically iatrogenic, e.g., administration of hypertonic sodium bicarbonate. More commonly, hypernatremia is the result of a combined H_2O and volume deficit, with losses of H_2O in excess of Na^+. Elderly individuals with reduced thirst and/or diminished access to fluids are at the highest risk of hypernatremia due to decreased free H_2O intake. Common causes of renal H_2O loss are osmotic diuresis secondary to hyperglycemia, postobstructive diuresis, or drugs (radiocontrast, mannitol, etc.); H_2O diuresis occurs in central or nephrogenic diabetes insipidus (DI) (Chap. 51). In pts with hypernatremia due to renal loss of H_2O, it is critical to quantify *ongoing* daily losses in addition to calculation of the baseline H_2O deficit (Table 2-2).

TREATMENT	Hypernatremia

The approach to correction of hypernatremia is outlined in Table 2-2. As with hyponatremia, it is advisable to correct the H_2O deficit slowly to avoid neurologic compromise, decreasing the serum $[Na^+]$ over 48–72 h. Depending on the blood pressure or clinical volume status, it may be appropriate to initially treat with hypotonic saline solutions (1/4 or 1/2 normal saline); blood glucose should be monitored in pts treated with large volumes of D_5W, should hyperglycemia ensue. Calculation of urinary electrolyte-free H_2O clearance is helpful to estimate daily, ongoing loss of free H_2O in pts with nephrogenic or central DI (Table 2-2). Other forms of therapy may be helpful in

TABLE 2-2 CORRECTION OF HYPERNATREMIA

H_2O Deficit

1. Estimate total-body water (TBW): 50–60% body weight (kg) depending on body composition
2. Calculate free-water deficit: $[(Na^+ 140)/140] \times TBW$
3. Administer deficit over 48–72 h

Ongoing H_2O Losses

4. Calculate free-water clearance, C_eH_2O:

$$C_eH_2O = V\left(1 - \frac{U_{Na} + U_K}{S_{Na}}\right)$$

where V is urinary volume, U_{Na} is urinary $[Na^+]$, U_K is urinary $[K^+]$, and SNa is serum $[Na^+]$.

Insensible Losses

5. ~10 mL/kg per day: less if ventilated, more if febrile

Total

6. Add components to determine H_2O deficit and ongoing H_2O loss; correct the H_2O deficit over 48–72 h and replace daily H_2O loss.

selected cases of hypernatremia. Pts with central DI may respond to the administration of intranasal DDAVP. Stable pts with nephrogenic DI due to lithium may reduce their polyuria with amiloride (2.5–10 mg/d) or hydrochlorothiazide (12.5–50 mg/d) or both in combination. These diuretics are thought to increase proximal H_2O reabsorption and decrease distal solute delivery, thus reducing polyuria; amiloride may also decrease entry of lithium into principal cells in the distal nephron by inhibiting the amiloride-sensitive epithelial sodium channel (ENaC). Notably, however, most pts with lithium-induced nephrogenic DI can adequately accommodate by increasing their H_2O intake. Occasionally, nonsteroidal anti-inflammatory drugs (NSAIDs) have also been used to treat polyuria associated with nephrogenic DI, reducing the negative effect of local prostaglandins on urinary concentration; however, the nephrotoxic potential of NSAIDs typically makes them a less attractive therapeutic option.

POTASSIUM

Since potassium (K^+) is the major intracellular cation, discussion of disorders of K^+ balance must take into consideration changes in the exchange of intra- and extracellular K^+ stores. (Extracellular K^+ constitutes <2% of total-body K^+ content.) Insulin, β_2-adrenergic agonists, and alkalosis tend to promote K^+ uptake by cells; acidosis, insulinopenia, or acute hyperosmolality (e.g., after treatment with mannitol or D50W) promote the efflux or reduced uptake of K^+. A corollary is that tissue necrosis and the attendant release of K^+ can cause severe hyperkalemia, particularly in the setting of acute kidney injury. Hyperkalemia due to rhabdomyolysis is thus particularly common, due to the enormous store of K^+ in muscle; hyperkalemia may also be prominent in tumor lysis syndrome.

The kidney plays a dominant role in K^+ excretion. Although K^+ is transported along the entire nephron, it is the principal cells of the connecting segment and cortical collecting duct that play a dominant role in K^+ excretion. Apical Na^+ entry into principal cells via the amiloride-sensitive epithelial Na^+ channel (ENaC) generates a lumen-negative potential difference, which drives passive K^+ exit through apical K^+ channels. *This relationship is key to the bedside understanding of potassium disorders.* For example, decreased distal delivery of Na^+ tends to blunt the ability to excrete K^+, leading to hyperkalemia. Abnormalities in the RAA can cause both hypo- and hyperkalemia; aldosterone has a major influence on potassium excretion, increasing the activity of ENaC channels and thus amplifying the driving force for K^+ secretion across the luminal membrane of principal cells.

■ HYPOKALEMIA

Major causes of hypokalemia are outlined in Table 2-3. Atrial and ventricular arrhythmias are the most serious health consequences of hypokalemia. Pts with concurrent Mg deficit and/or digoxin therapy are at a particularly increased risk of arrhythmias. Other clinical manifestations include muscle weakness, which may be profound at serum $[K^+]$ <2.5 mmol/L, and, if hypokalemia is sustained, hypertension, ileus, polyuria, renal cysts, and even renal failure.

The cause of hypokalemia is usually obvious from history, physical examination, and/or basic laboratory tests. However, persistent hypokalemia may require a more thorough, systematic evaluation (Fig. 2-2). Initial laboratory evaluation should include electrolytes, BUN, creatinine, serum osmolality, Mg^{2+}, and Ca^{2+}, a complete blood count, and urinary pH, osmolality, creatinine, and electrolytes. Serum and urine osmolality are required for

---

TABLE 2-3 CAUSES OF HYPOKALEMIA

I. Decreased intake

  A. Starvation

  B. Clay ingestion

II. Redistribution into cells

  A. Acid-base

    1. Metabolic alkalosis

  B. Hormonal

    1. Insulin

    2. Increased β_2-adrenergic sympathetic activity: post–myocardial infarction, head injury

TABLE 2-3 CAUSES OF HYPOKALEMIA (CONTINUED)

    3. β_2-Adrenergic agonists: bronchodilators, tocolytics

    4. α-Adrenergic antagonists

    5. Thyrotoxic periodic paralysis

    6. Downstream stimulation of Na^+/K^+-ATPase: theophylline, caffeine

C. Anabolic state

    1. Vitamin B_{12} or folic acid administration (red blood cell production)

    2. Granulocyte-macrophage colony-stimulating factor (white blood cell production)

    3. Total parenteral nutrition

D. Other

    1. Pseudohypokalemia

    2. Hypothermia

    3. Familial hypokalemic periodic paralysis

    4. Barium toxicity: systemic inhibition of "leak" K^+ channels

III. Increased loss

A. Nonrenal

    1. Gastrointestinal loss (diarrhea)

    2. Integumentary loss (sweat)

B. Renal

    1. Increased distal flow and distal Na^+ delivery: diuretics, osmotic diuresis, salt-wasting nephropathies

    2. Increased secretion of potassium

        a. Mineralocorticoid excess: primary hyperaldosteronism [aldosterone-producing adenomas (APAs)], primary or unilateral adrenal hyperplasia (PAH or UAH), idiopathic hyperaldosteronism (IHA) due to bilateral adrenal hyperplasia and adrenal carcinoma, familial hyperaldosteronism (FH-I, FH-II, congenital adrenal hyperplasias), secondary hyperaldosteronism (malignant hypertension, renin-secreting tumors, renal artery stenosis, hypovolemia), Cushing's syndrome, Bartter's syndrome, Gitelman's syndrome

        b. Apparent mineralocorticoid excess: genetic deficiency of 11β-dehydrogenase-2 (syndrome of apparent mineralocorticoid excess), inhibition of 11β-dehydrogenase-2 (glycyrrhetinic/glycyrrhizinic acid and/or carbenoxolone; licorice, food products, drugs), Liddle's syndrome [genetic activation of epithelial Na^+ channels (ENaC)]

        c. Distal delivery of nonreabsorbed anions: vomiting, nasogastric suction, proximal renal tubular acidosis, diabetic ketoacidosis, glue sniffing (toluene abuse), penicillin derivatives (penicillin, nafcillin, dicloxacillin, ticarcillin, oxacillin, and carbenicillin)

    3. Magnesium deficiency, amphotericin B, Liddle's syndrome

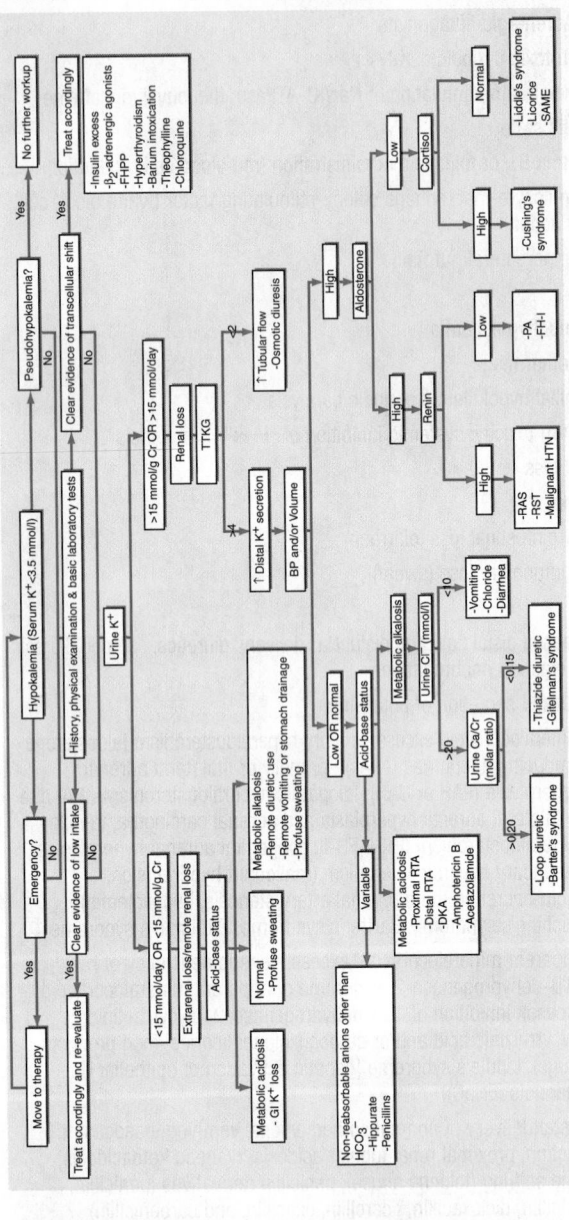

FIGURE 2-2 The diagnostic approach to hypokalemia. See text for details. BP, blood pressure; DKA, diabetic ketoacidosis; FHPP, familial hypokalemic periodic paralysis; FH-I, familial hyperaldosteronism type 1; GI, gastrointestinal; HTN, hypertension; PA, primary aldosteronism; RAS, renal artery stenosis; RST, renin-secreting tumor; RTA, renal tubular acidosis; SAME, syndrome of apparent mineralocorticoid excess; TTKG, transtubular potassium gradient. [*From Mount DB, Zandi-Nejad K: Disorders of potassium balance, in The Kidney, 8th ed, BM Brenner (ed). Philadelphia, Saunders, 2008; with permission.*]

calculation of the transtubular K^+ gradient (TTKG), which should be <3 in the presence of hypokalemia (see also Hyperkalemia). Further tests such as urinary Mg^{2+} and Ca^{2+} and/or plasma renin and aldosterone levels may be necessary in specific cases.

| **TREATMENT** | Hypokalemia |

Hypokalemia can generally be managed by correction of the underlying disease process (e.g., diarrhea) or withdrawal of an offending medication (e.g., loop or thiazide diuretic), combined with oral KCl supplementation. However, hypokalemia is refractory to correction in the presence of Mg deficiency, which also should be corrected when present; renal wasting of both cations may be particularly prominent after renal tubular injury, e.g., from cisplatin nephrotoxicity. If loop or thiazide diuretic therapy cannot be discontinued, a distal tubular K-sparing agent, such as amiloride or spironolactone, can be added to the regimen. Angiotensin-converting enzyme (ACE) inhibition in pts with CHF attenuates diuretic-induced hypokalemia and protects against cardiac arrhythmia. If hypokalemia is severe (<2.5 mmol/L) and/or if oral supplementation is not feasible or tolerated, IV KCl can be administered through a central vein with cardiac monitoring in an intensive care setting, at rates that should not exceed 20 mmol/h. KCl should always be administered in saline solutions, rather than dextrose; the dextrose-induced increase in insulin can acutely exacerbate hypokalemia.

■ HYPERKALEMIA

Causes are outlined in Table 2-4; in most cases, hyperkalemia is due to decreased renal K^+ excretion. However, increases in dietary K^+ intake can have a major effect in susceptible pts, e.g., diabetics with hyporeninemic hypoaldosteronism and chronic kidney disease. Drugs that impact on the renin-angiotensin-aldosterone axis are also a major cause of hyperkalemia, particularly given recent trends to coadminister these agents, e.g., spironolactone or angiotensin receptor blockers with an ACE inhibitor in cardiac and/or renal disease.

The first priority in the management of hyperkalemia is to assess the need for emergency treatment (ECG changes and/or K^+ ≥6.0 mM). This should be followed by a comprehensive workup to determine the cause (Fig. 2-3). History and physical examination should focus on medications (e.g., ACE inhibitors, NSAIDs, trimethoprim/sulfamethoxazole), diet and dietary supplements (e.g., salt substitute), risk factors for acute kidney failure, reduction in urine output, blood pressure, and volume status. Initial laboratory tests should include electrolytes, BUN, creatinine, serum osmolality, Mg^{2+}, and Ca^{2+}, a complete blood count, and urinary pH, osmolality, creatinine, and electrolytes. A urine [Na^+] <20 meq/L suggests that distal Na^+ delivery is a limiting factor in K^+ excretion; volume repletion with 0.9% saline or treatment with furosemide may then be effective in reducing serum [K^+] by increasing distal Na^+ delivery. Serum and urine osmolality are required for calculation of

TABLE 2-4 CAUSES OF HYPERKALEMIA

I. "Pseudo" hyperkalemia

   A. Cellular efflux: thrombocytosis, erythrocytosis, leukocytosis, in vitro hemolysis

   B. Hereditary defects in red cell membrane transport

II. Intra- to extracellular shift

   A. Acidosis

   B. Hyperosmolality; radiocontrast, hypertonic dextrose, mannitol

   C. β-adrenergic antagonists (noncardioselective agents)

   D. Digoxin and related glycosides (yellow oleander, foxglove, bufadienolide)

   E. Hyperkalemic periodic paralysis

   F. Lysine, arginine, and ε-aminocaproic acid (structurally similar, positively charged)

   G. Succinylcholine; thermal trauma, neuromuscular injury, disuse atrophy, mucositis, or prolonged immobilization

   H. Rapid tumor lysis

III. Inadequate excretion

   A. Inhibition of the renin-angiotensin-aldosterone axis; ↑ risk of hyperkalemia when used in combination

      1. Angiotensin-converting enzyme (ACE) inhibitors

      2. Renin inhibitors: aliskiren [in combination with ACE inhibitors or angiotensin receptor blockers (ARBs)]

      3. ARBs

      4. Blockade of the mineralocorticoid receptor: spironolactone, eplerenone, drospirenone

      5. Blockade of ENaC: amiloride, triamterene, trimethoprim, pentamidine, nafamostat

   B. Decreased distal delivery

      1. Congestive heart failure

      2. Volume depletion

   C. Hyporeninemic hypoaldosteronism

      1. Tubulointerstitial diseases: systemic lupus erythematosus (SLE), sickle cell anemia, obstructive uropathy

      2. Diabetes, diabetic nephropathy

      3. Drugs: nonsteroidal anti-inflammatory drugs, cyclooxygenase 2 (COX-2) inhibitors, beta blockers, cyclosporine, tacrolimus

      4. Chronic kidney disease, advanced age

      5. Pseudohypoaldosteronism type II: defects in WNK1 or WNK4 kinases

TABLE 2-4 CAUSES OF HYPERKALEMIA (CONTINUED)

  D. Renal resistance to mineralocorticoid

    1. Tubulointerstitial diseases: SLE, amyloidosis, sickle cell anemia, obstructive uropathy, post-acute tubular necrosis

    2. Hereditary: pseudohypoaldosteronism type I: defects in the mineralocorticoid receptor or ENaC

  E. Advanced renal insufficiency with low GFR

    1. Chronic kidney disease

    2. End-stage renal disease

    3. Acute oliguric kidney injury

  F. Primary adrenal insufficiency

    1. Autoimmune: Addison's disease, polyglandular endocrinopathy

    2. Infectious: HIV, cytomegalovirus, tuberculosis, disseminated fungal infection

    3. Infiltrative: amyloidosis, malignancy, metastatic cancer

    4. Drug-associated: heparin, low-molecular-weight heparin

    5. Hereditary: adrenal hypoplasia congenita, congenital lipoid adrenal hyperplasia, aldosterone synthase deficiency

    6. Adrenal hemorrhage or infarction, including in antiphospholipid syndrome

the TTKG. The expected values of the TTKG are largely based on historic data: <3 in the presence of hypokalemia and >7–8 in the presence of hyperkalemia.

$$\text{TTKG} = \frac{[\text{K}^+]_{\text{urine}} \times \text{OSM}_{\text{serum}}}{[\text{K}^+]_{\text{serum}} \times \text{OSM}_{\text{urine}}}$$

TREATMENT Hyperkalemia

The most important consequence of hyperkalemia is altered cardiac conduction, with the risk of bradycardic cardiac arrest. Figure 2-4 shows serial ECG patterns of hyperkalemia; ECG manifestations of hyperkalemia should be considered a true medical emergency and treated urgently. However, ECG changes of hyperkalemia are notoriously insensitive, particularly in pts with chronic kidney disease; given these limitations, pts with significant hyperkalemia (K$^+$ ≥6–6.5 mmol/L) in the absence of ECG changes should also be aggressively managed.

Urgent management of hyperkalemia constitutes a 12-lead ECG, admission to the hospital, continuous cardiac monitoring, and immediate treatment. Treatment of hyperkalemia is divided into three categories:

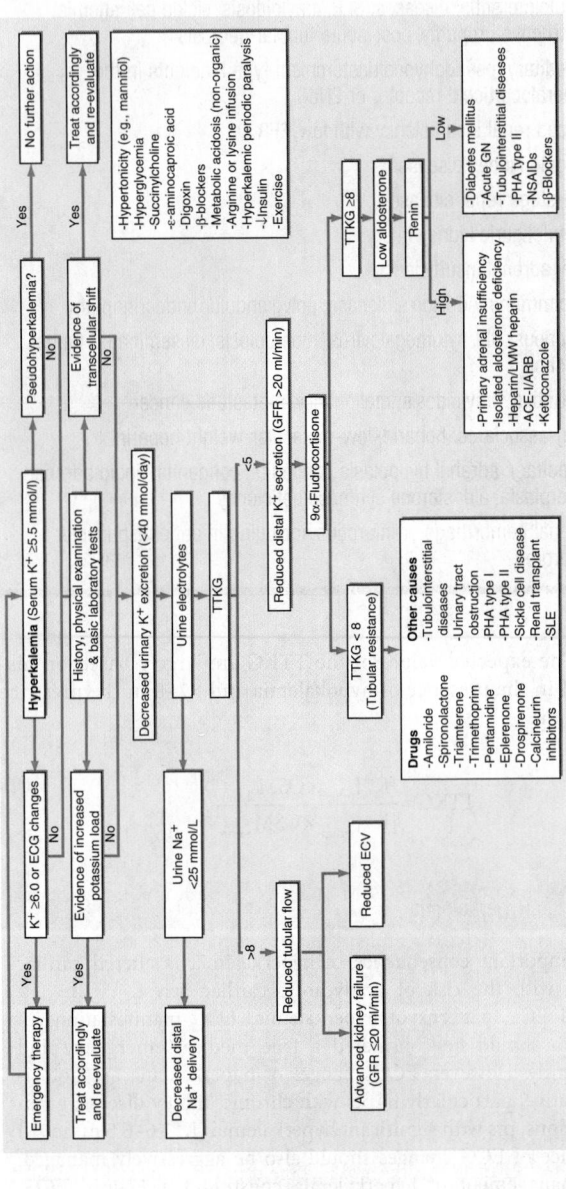

FIGURE 2-3 The diagnostic approach to hyperkalemia. See text for details. ACE-I, angiotensin converting enzyme inhibitor; ARB, angiotensin II receptor blocker; ECG, electrocardiogram; ECV, effective circulatory volume; GFR, glomerular filtration rate; LMW heparin, low-molecular-weight heparin; NSAIDs, nonsteroidal anti-inflammatory drugs; PHA, pseudohypoaldosteronism; SLE, systemic lupus erythematosus; TTKG, transtubular potassium gradient. [*From Mount DB, Zandi-Nejad K: Disorders of potassium balance, in The Kidney, 8th ed, BM Brenner (ed). Philadelphia, Saunders, 2008; with permission.*]

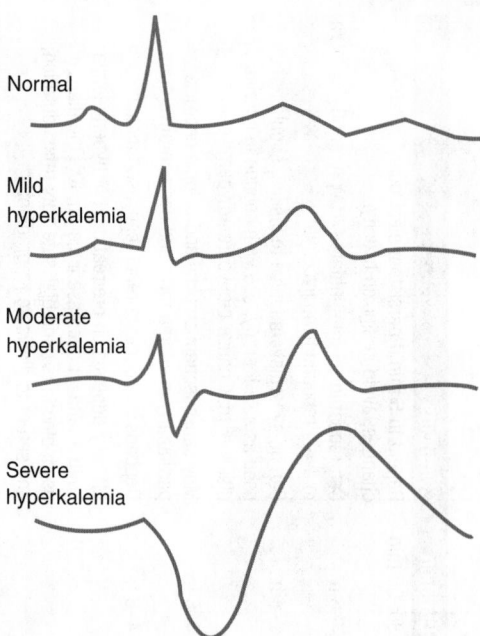

Normal

Mild
hyperkalemia

Moderate
hyperkalemia

Severe
hyperkalemia

FIGURE 2-4 Diagrammatic ECGs at normal and high serum K. Peaked T waves (precordial leads) are followed by diminished R wave, wide QRS, prolonged P-R, loss of P wave, and ultimately a sine wave.

(1) antagonism of the cardiac effects of hyperkalemia, (2) rapid reduction in [K⁺] by redistribution into cells, and (3) removal of K⁺ from the body. Treatment of hyperkalemia is summarized in Table 2-5.

ACID-BASE DISORDERS (FIG. 2-5)

Regulation of normal pH (7.35–7.45) depends on both the lungs and kidneys. By the Henderson-Hasselbalch equation, pH is a function of the ratio of HCO_3^- (regulated by the kidney) to P_{CO_2} (regulated by the lungs). The HCO_3/P_{CO_2} relationship is useful in classifying disorders of acid-base balance. Acidosis is due to gain of acid or loss of alkali; causes may be metabolic (fall in serum HCO_3^-) or respiratory (rise in P_{CO_2}). Alkalosis is due to loss of acid or addition of base and is either metabolic (↑ serum [HCO_3^-]) or respiratory (↓ P_{CO_2}).

To limit the change in pH, metabolic disorders evoke an immediate compensatory response in ventilation; full renal compensation for respiratory disorders is a slower process, such that "acute" compensations are of lesser magnitude than "chronic" compensations. Simple acid-base disorders consist of one primary disturbance and its compensatory response. In mixed disorders, a combination of primary disturbances is present.

TABLE 2-5 TREATMENT OF HYPERKALEMIA

Mechanism	Therapy	Dose	Onset	Duration	Comments
Stabilize membrane potential	Calcium	10% Ca gluconate, 10 mL over 10 min	1–3 min	30–60 min	Repeat in 5 min if persistent electrocardiographic changes; avoid in digoxin toxicity.
Cellular K+ uptake	Insulin	10 U R with 50 mL of D50, if blood sugar <250	30 min	4–6 h	Can repeat in 15 min; initiate D10W IV at 50–75 mL/h to avoid rebound hypoglycemia.
	β₂-agonist	Nebulized albuterol, 10–20 mg in 4 mL saline	30 min	2–4 h	Can be synergistic/additive to insulin; should not be used as sole therapy; use with caution in cardiac disease; may cause tachycardia/hyperglycemia.
K+ removal	Kayexalate	30–60 g PO in 20% sorbitol	1–2 h	4–6 h	May cause ischemic colitis and colonic necrosis, particularly in enema form and postoperative state.
	Furosemide	20–250 mg IV	15 min	4–6 h	Depends on adequate renal response/function.
	Hemodialysis		Immediate		Efficacy depends on pretreatment of hyperkalemia (with attendant decrease in serum K+); the dialyzer used, blood flow and dialysate flow rates, duration, and serum to dialysate K+ gradient.

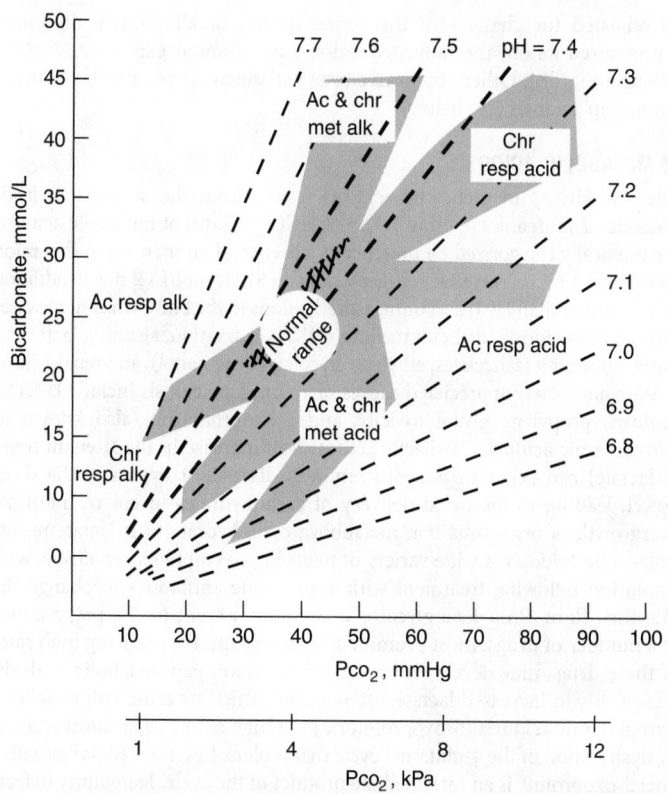

FIGURE 2-5 Nomogram showing bands for uncomplicated respiratory or metabolic acid-base disturbances in intact subjects. Each confidence band represents the mean ±2 SD for the compensatory response of normal subjects or pts to a given primary disorder. Ac, acute; chr, chronic; resp, respiratory; met, metabolic; acid, acidosis; alk, alkalosis. (*From Levinsky NG: HPIM-12, p. 290; modified from Arbus GS: Can Med Assoc J 109:291, 1973.*)

The cause of simple acid-base disorders is usually obvious from history, physical examination, and/or basic laboratory tests. Initial laboratory evaluation depends on the dominant acid-base disorder, but for metabolic acidosis and alkalosis this should include electrolytes, BUN, creatinine, albumin, urinary pH, and urinary electrolytes. An arterial blood gas (ABG) is not always required for pts with a simple acid-base disorder, e.g., mild metabolic acidosis in the context of chronic renal failure. However, concomitant ABG and serum electrolytes are necessary to fully evaluate more complex acid-base disorders. The compensatory response should be estimated from the ABG; Winter's formula $[P_{aCO_2} = (1.5 \times [HCO_3^-]) + 8 \pm 2]$ is particularly useful for assessing the respiratory response to metabolic acidosis. The anion gap should also be calculated; the anion gap = $[Na^+] - ([HCO_3^-] + [Cl^-])$ = unmeasured anions – unmeasured cations. The anion gap should be adjusted for changes in the concentration of albumin, a dominant unmeasured anion; the "adjusted anion gap" = anion gap + ~2.5 × (4 – albumin mg/dL). Other supportive tests will elucidate the specific form of anion-gap acidosis (see below).

■ METABOLIC ACIDOSIS

The low HCO_3^- in metabolic acidosis results from the addition of acids (organic or inorganic) or from a loss of HCO_3^-; causes of metabolic acidosis are classically categorized by presence or absence of an increase in the anion gap (Table 2-6). Increased anion-gap acidosis (>12 mmol/L) is due to addition of acid (other than HCl) and unmeasured anions to the body. Common causes include ketoacidosis [diabetes mellitus (DKA), starvation, alcohol], lactic acidosis, poisoning (salicylates, ethylene glycol, and methanol), and renal failure.

Rare and newly appreciated causes of anion-gap acidosis include D-lactic acidosis, propylene glycol toxicity, and 5-oxoprolinuria (also known as pyroglutamic aciduria). D-Lactic acidosis (an increase in the D-enantiomer of lactate) can occur in pts with removal, disease, or bypass of the short bowel, leading to increased delivery of carbohydrates to colon. Intestinal overgrowth of organisms that metabolize carbohydrate to D-lactate results in D-lactic acidosis; a wide variety of neurologic symptoms can ensue, with resolution following treatment with appropriate antibiotics to change the intestinal flora. Propylene glycol is a common solvent for IV preparations of a number of drugs, most prominently lorazepam. Pts receiving high rates of these drugs may develop a hyperosmolar anion-gap metabolic acidosis, due mostly to increased lactate, often accompanied by acute kidney failure. Pyroglutamic aciduria (5-oxoprolinuria) is a high anion-gap acidosis caused by dysfunction of the γ-glutamyl cycle that replenishes intracellular glutathione; 5-oxoproline is an intermediate product of the cycle. Hereditary defects in the γ-glutamyl cycle are associated with 5-oxoprolinuria; acquired defects occur in the context of acetaminophen therapy, due to derepression of the cycle by reduced glutathione and overproduction of 5-oxoproline. Resolution occurs after withdrawal of acetaminophen; treatment with N-acetyl cysteine to replenish glutathione stores may hasten recovery.

The differentiation of the various anion-gap acidoses depends on the clinical scenario and routine laboratory tests (Table 2-6) in conjunction with measurement of serum lactate, ketones, toxicology screens (if ethylene glycol or methanol ingestion are suspected), and serum osmolality. D-Lactic acidosis can be diagnosed by a specific assay for the D-enantiomer; 5-oxoprolinuria can be diagnosed by the clinical scenario and confirmed by gas chromatographic/mass spectroscopic (GC/MS) analysis of urine, a widely available pediatric screening test for inborn errors of metabolism (typically "urine for organic acids").

Pts with ethylene glycol, methanol, or propylene glycol toxicity may have an "osmolar gap," defined as a >10-mosm/kg difference between calculated and measured serum osmolality. Calculated osmolality = 2 × Na^+ + glucose/18 + BUN/2.8. Of note, pts with alcoholic ketoacidosis and lactic acidosis may also exhibit a modest elevation in the osmolar gap; pts may alternatively metabolize ethylene glycol or methanol to completion by presentation, with an increased anion gap and no increase in the osmolar gap. However, the rapid

TABLE 2-6 METABOLIC ACIDOSIS

Non-Anion-Gap Acidosis		Anion-Gap Acidosis	
Cause	Clue	Cause	Clue
Diarrhea enterostomy	Hx; ↑ K⁺ Drainage	DKA	Hyperglycemia, ketones
RF	Early chronic kidney disease	RF	Late chronic kidney disease
RTA		Lactic acidosis (L-lactate)	Clinical setting + ↑ serum lactate
Proximal	↓ K⁺, presence of other proximal tubular defects (Fanconi Syndrome)	Alcoholic ketoacidosis	Hx; weak + ketones; + osm gap
Distal—hypokalemic	↓ K⁺; hypercalciuria; UpH >5.5	Starvation	Hx; mild acidosis; + ketones
Distal—hyperkalemic	↑ K⁺; nl PRA/aldo; UpH >5.5	Salicylates	Hx; tinnitus; high serum level; + ketones
Distal—hyporeninemic hypoaldosteronism	↑ K⁺; ↓ PRA/aldo; UpH <5.5	Methanol	Large AG; concomitant respiratory alkalosis; retinitis; + toxic screen; + osm gap
Dilutional	Massive volume expansion with saline	Ethylene glycol	RF; CNS symptoms; + toxic screen; crystalluria; + osm gap
Ureterosigmoidostomy	Obstructed ileal loop	D-lactic acidosis	Small-bowel disease; prominent neuro symptoms
Hyperalimentation	Amino acid infusion	Propylene glycol	IV infusions, e.g., lorazepam; + osm gap; RF
Acetazolamide, NH₄Cl, lysine HCl, arginine HCl, sevelamer-HCl	Hx of administration of these agents	Pyroglutamic aciduria, 5-oxoprolinuria	Large AG; chronic acetaminophen

Abbreviations: AG, anion gap; CNS, central nervous system; DKA, diabetic ketoacidosis; osm gap, osmolar gap; PRA, plasma renin activity; RF, renal failure; RTA, renal tubular acidosis; UpH, urinary pH.

availability of a measured serum osmolality may aid in the urgent assessment and management of pts with these medical emergencies.

Normal anion-gap acidosis can result from HCO_3^- loss from the GI tract. Diarrhea is by far the most common cause, but other GI conditions associated with external losses of bicarbonate-rich fluids may lead to large alkali losses—e.g., in ileus secondary to intestinal obstruction, in which liters of alkaline fluid may accumulate within the intestinal lumen. Various forms of kidney disease are associated with non-anion-gap acidosis due to reduced tubular reabsorption of filtered bicarbonate and/or reduced excretion of ammonium (NH_4^+). The early stages of progressive renal disease are frequently associated with a non-anion-gap acidosis, with development of an anion-gap component in more advanced renal failure. Non-anion-gap acidosis is also seen in renal tubular acidosis or in the context of tubulointerstitial injury, e.g., after acute tubular necrosis, allergic interstitial nephritis, or urinary tract obstruction. Finally, non-anion-gap acidosis due to exogenous acid loads may occur after rapid volume expansion with saline-containing solutions, the administration of NH_4Cl (a component of cough syrup), lysine HCl, or treatment with the phosphate binder sevelamer hydrochloride.

Calculation of the urinary anion gap may be helpful in the evaluation of hyperchloremic metabolic acidosis, along with a measurement of urine pH. The urinary anion gap is defined as urinary $([Na^+] + [K^+]) - [Cl^-] =$ [unmeasured anions] – [unmeasured cations]); the NH_4^+ ion is the major unmeasured urinary cation in metabolic acidosis, wherein the urinary anion gap should be strongly negative. A negative anion gap thus suggests GI losses of bicarbonate, with appropriate renal response and increased NH_4^+ excretion; a positive anion gap suggests altered urinary acidification, as seen in renal failure or distal renal tubular acidoses. An important caveat is that the rapid renal excretion of unmeasured anions in anion-gap acidosis, classically seen in DKA, may reduce the serum anion gap and generate a positive value for the urinary anion gap, despite the adequate excretion of urinary NH_4^+; this may lead to misdiagnosis as a renal tubular acidosis.

TREATMENT   Metabolic Acidosis

Treatment of metabolic acidosis depends on the cause and severity. DKA responds to insulin therapy and aggressive hydration; close attention to serum $[K^+]$ and administration of KCl is essential, given that the correction of insulinopenia can cause profound hypokalemia. The administration of alkali in anion-gap acidoses is controversial and is rarely appropriate in DKA. It is reasonable to treat severe lactic acidosis with IV HCO_3^- at a rate sufficient to maintain a pH >7.20; treatment of moderate lactic acidosis with HCO_3^- is controversial. IV HCO_3^- is however appropriate to reduce acidosis in D-lactic acidosis, ethylene glycol and methanol toxicity, and 5-oxoprolinuria.

Chronic metabolic acidosis should be treated when HCO_3^- is <18–20 mmol/L. In pts with chronic kidney disease, there is some evidence that acidosis promotes protein catabolism and may worsen bone disease. Sodium citrate may be more palatable than oral $NaHCO_3$, although the former should be avoided in pts with advanced renal insufficiency, as it augments aluminum absorption. Oral therapy with $NaHCO_3$ usually begins with 650 mg tid and is titrated upward to maintain serum $[HCO_3^-]$.

■ METABOLIC ALKALOSIS

Metabolic alkalosis is due to a primary increase in serum $[HCO_3^-]$, distinguished from chronic respiratory acidosis—with a compensatory increase in renal HCO_3^- reabsorption—by the associated increase in arterial pH (normal or decreased in chronic respiratory acidosis). Administered, exogenous alkali (HCO_3^-, acetate, citrate, or lactate) may cause alkalosis if the normal capacity to excrete HCO_3^- is reduced or if renal HCO_3^- reabsorption is enhanced. A recently resurgent problem is "milk alkali syndrome," a triad of hypercalcemia, metabolic alkalosis, and acute renal failure due to ingested calcium carbonate, typically taken for the treatment or prevention of osteoporosis.

Metabolic alkalosis is primarily caused by renal retention of HCO_3^- and is due to a variety of underlying mechanisms. Pts are typically separated into two major subtypes: Cl⁻-responsive and Cl⁻-resistant. Measurement of urine Cl⁻ affords this separation in the clinical setting (Fig. 2-6). The quintessential causes of Cl⁻-responsive alkalosis are GI-induced from

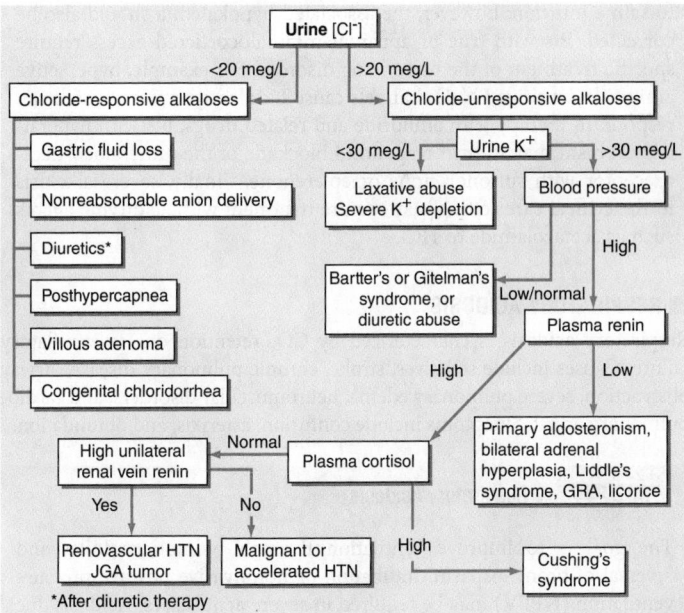

FIGURE 2-6 The diagnostic approach to metabolic alkalosis. See text for details. GRA, glucocorticoid-remediable aldosteronism; HTN, hypertension; JGA, juxtaglomerular apparatus. [*Modified from Dubose TD: Disorders of acid-base balance, in The Kidney, 8th ed, BM Brenner (ed). Philadelphia, Saunders, 2008; with permission.*]

vomiting or gastric aspiration through a nasogastric tube, and renal-induced from diuretic therapy. Hypovolemia, chloride deficiency, activation of the renin-angiotensin-aldosterone axis, and hypokalemia play interrelated roles in the maintenance of this hypochloremic or "contraction" alkalosis. The various syndromes of true or apparent mineralocorticoid excess cause Cl^--resistant metabolic alkalosis (Fig. 2-6); most of these pts are hypokalemic, volume-expanded, and/or hypertensive.

Common forms of metabolic alkalosis are generally diagnosed from the history, physical examination, and/or basic laboratory tests. ABGs will help determine whether an elevated $[HCO_3^-]$ is reflective of metabolic alkalosis or chronic respiratory acidosis; ABGs are required for the diagnosis of mixed acid-base disorders. Measurement of urinary electrolytes will aid in separating Cl^--responsive and Cl^--resistant forms. Urinary $[Na^+]$ may thus be >20 meq/L in Cl^--responsive alkalosis despite the presence of hypovolemia; however, urinary $[Cl^-]$ will be very low. Notably, urinary $[Cl^-]$ may be variable in pts with diuretic-associated alkalosis, depending on the temporal relationship to diuretic administration. Other diagnostic tests—e.g., plasma renin, aldosterone, cortisol—may be appropriate in Cl^--resistant forms with high urinary $[Cl^-]$ (Fig. 2-6).

TREATMENT Metabolic Alkalosis

The acid-base disorder in Cl^--responsive alkalosis will typically respond to saline infusion; however, the associated hypokalemia should also be corrected. Pts with true or apparent mineralocorticoid excess require specific treatment of the underlying disorder. For example, hyperactive amiloride-sensitive ENaC channels cause Liddle's syndrome, which can respond to therapy with amiloride and related drugs; pts with hyperaldosteronism may in turn respond to blockade of the mineralocorticoidreceptor with spironolactone or eplerenone. Finally, severe alkalosis in the critical care setting may require treatment with acidifying agents such as acetazolamide or HCl.

■ RESPIRATORY ACIDOSIS

Respiratory acidosis is characterized by CO_2 retention due to ventilatory failure. Causes include sedatives, stroke, chronic pulmonary disease, airway obstruction, severe pulmonary edema, neuromuscular disorders, and cardiopulmonary arrest. Symptoms include confusion, asterixis, and obtundation.

TREATMENT Respiratory Acidosis

The goal is to improve ventilation through pulmonary toilet and reversal of bronchospasm. Intubation or noninvasive positive pressure ventilation (NPPV) may be required in severe acute cases. Acidosis due to hypercapnia is usually mild; however, combined respiratory and metabolic acidosis may cause a profound reduction in pH. Respiratory acidosis may accompany low tidal volume ventilation in ICU pts and may require metabolic "overcorrection" to maintain a neutral pH.

■ RESPIRATORY ALKALOSIS

Excessive ventilation causes a primary reduction in CO_2 and ↑ pH in pneumonia, pulmonary edema, interstitial lung disease, and asthma. Pain and psychogenic causes are common; other etiologies include fever, hypoxemia, sepsis, delirium tremens, salicylates, hepatic failure, mechanical overventilation, and CNS lesions. Pregnancy is associated with a mild respiratory alkalosis. Severe respiratory alkalosis may acutely cause seizures, tetany, cardiac arrhythmias, or loss of consciousness.

> **TREATMENT**   Respiratory Alkalosis
>
> Treatment should be directed at the underlying disorders. In psychogenic cases, sedation or a rebreathing bag may be required.

■ "MIXED" DISORDERS

In many circumstances, more than a single acid-base disturbance exists. Examples include combined metabolic and respiratory acidosis with cardiogenic shock; metabolic alkalosis and anion-gap acidosis in pts with vomiting and diabetic ketoacidosis; and anion-gap metabolic acidosis with respiratory alkalosis in pts with salicylate toxicity. The diagnosis may be clinically evident and/or suggested by relationships between the PCO_2 and $[HCO_3^-]$ that diverge from those found in simple disorders. For example, the PCO_2 in a pt with metabolic acidosis and respiratory alkalosis will be considerably less than that predicted from the $[HCO_3^-]$ and Winter's formula $[P_aCO_2 = (1.5 \times [HCO_3^-]) + 8 + 2]$.

In "simple" anion-gap acidosis, the anion gap increases in proportion to the fall in $[HCO_3^-]$. A lesser drop in serum $[HCO_3^-]$ than in the anion gap suggests a coexisting metabolic alkalosis. Conversely, a proportionately *larger* drop in $[HCO_3^-]$ than in the anion gap suggests the presence of a mixed anion-gap and non-anion-gap metabolic acidosis. Notably, however, these interpretations assume 1:1 relationships between unmeasured anions and the fall in $[HCO_3^-]$, which are not uniformly present in individual pts or as acidoses evolve. For example, volume resuscitation of pts with DKA will typically increase glomerular filtration and the urinary excretion of ketones, resulting in a decrease in the anion gap in the absence of a supervening non-anion-gap acidosis.

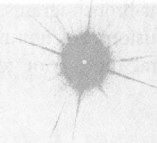

For a more detailed discussion, see Mount DB: Fluid and Electrolyte Disturbances, Chap. 45, p. 341; and DuBose TD Jr: Acidosis and Alkalosis, Chap. 47, p. 363, in HPIM-18. See also Mount DB, Zandi-Nejad K: Disorders of potassium balance, in *The Kidney*, 9th ed, BM Brenner (ed). Philadelphia, Saunders, 2011; and Ellison DH, Berl T: Clinical practice. The syndrome of inappropriate antidiuresis. N Engl J Med 356:2064, 2007.

CHAPTER **3**
Diagnostic Imaging in Internal Medicine

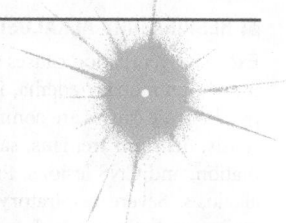

Clinicians have a wide array of radiologic modalities at their disposal to aid them in noninvasive diagnosis. Despite the introduction of highly specialized imaging modalities, radiologic tests such as chest radiographs and ultrasound continue to serve a vital role in the diagnostic approach to pt care. At most institutions, CT is available on an emergent basis and is invaluable for initial evaluation of pts with trauma, stroke, suspected CNS hemorrhage, or ischemic stroke. MRI and related techniques (MR angiography, functional MRI, MR spectroscopy) provide remarkable resolution of many tissues including the brain, vascular system, joints, and most large organs. Radionuclide scans including PET (positron emission tomography) can provide functional assessment of organs or specific regions within organs. Combination of PET with MRI or CT scanning provides highly informative images of the location and configuration of metabolically active lesions, such as cancers.

This chapter will review the indications and utility of the most commonly utilized radiologic studies used by internists.

■ CHEST RADIOGRAPHY (FIG. 3-1)
- Can be obtained quickly and should be part of the standard evaluation for pts with cardiopulmonary complaints.
- Is able to identify life-threatening conditions such as pneumothorax, intra-peritoneal air, pulmonary edema, pneumonia, and aortic dissection.
- Is most often normal in a pt with an acute pulmonary embolus.
- Should be repeated in 4–6 weeks in a pt with an acute pneumonic process to document resolution of the radiographic infiltrate.
- Is used in conjunction with the physical exam to support the diagnosis of congestive heart failure. Radiographic findings supporting the diagnosis of heart failure include cardiomegaly, cephalization, Kerley B lines, and pleural effusions.
- Should be obtained daily in intubated pts to examine endotracheal tube position and the possibility of barotrauma.
- Helps to identify alveolar or airspace disease. Radiographic features of such diseases include inhomogeneous, patchy opacities and air-bronchograms.
- Helps to document the free-flowing nature of pleural effusions. Decubitus views should be obtained to exclude loculated pleural fluid prior to attempts to extract such fluid.

■ ABDOMINAL RADIOGRAPHY
- Should be the initial imaging modality in a pt with suspected bowel obstruction. Signs of small-bowel obstruction on plain radiographs include multiple air-fluid levels, absence of colonic distention, and a "stepladder" appearance of small-bowel loops.

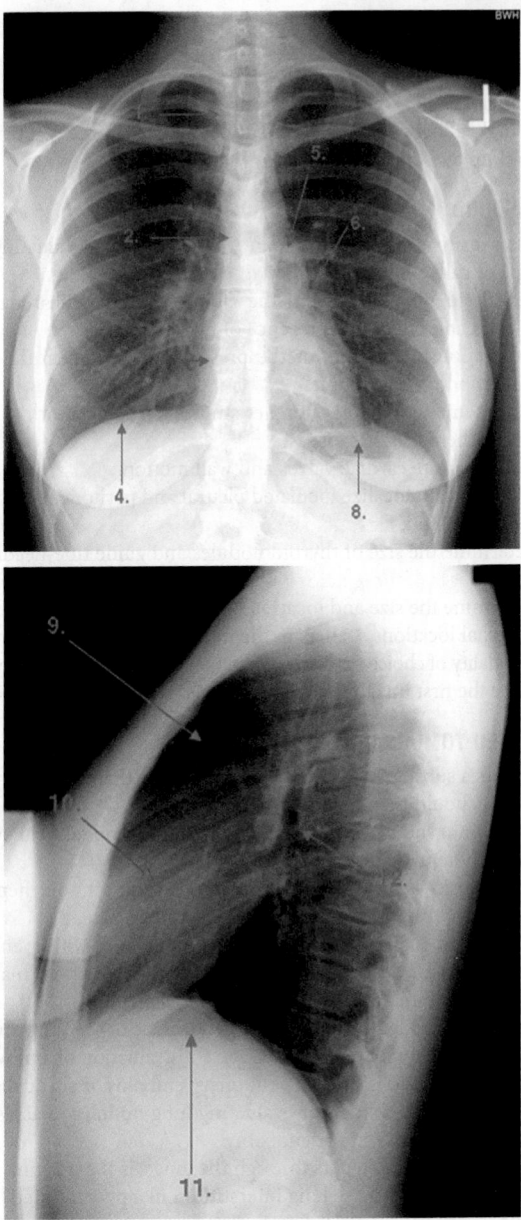

FIGURE 3-1 Normal chest radiograph-review of anatomy. **1.** Trachea. **2.** Carina. **3.** Right atrium. **4.** Right hemi-diaphragm. **5.** Aortic knob. **6.** Left hilum. **7.** Left ventricle. **8.** Left hemi-diaphragm (with stomach bubble). **9.** Retrosternal clear space. **10.** Right ventricle. **11.** Left hemi-diaphragm (with stomach bubble). **12.** Left upper lobe bronchus.

- Should not be performed with barium enhancement when perforated bowel, portal venous gas, or toxic megacolon is suspected.
- Is used to evaluate the size of bowel:
  1. Normal small bowel is <3 cm in diameter.
  2. Normal caliber of the cecum is up to 9 cm, with the rest of the large bowel up to 6 cm in diameter.

■ ULTRASOUND

- Is more sensitive and specific than CT scanning in evaluating for the presence of gallstone disease.
- Can readily identify the size of the kidneys in a pt with renal insufficiency and can exclude the presence of hydronephrosis.
- Can expeditiously evaluate for the presence of peritoneal fluid in a pt with blunt abdominal trauma.
- Is used in conjunction with Doppler studies to evaluate for the presence of arterial atherosclerotic disease.
- Is used to evaluate cardiac valves and wall motion.
- Should be used to localize loculated pleural and peritoneal fluid prior to draining such fluid.
- Can determine the size of thyroid nodules and guide fine-needle aspiration biopsy.
- Can determine the size and location of enlarged lymph nodes, especially in superficial locations such as in the neck.
- Is the modality of choice for assessing known or suspected scrotal pathology.
- Should be the first imaging modality utilized when evaluating the ovaries.

■ COMPUTED TOMOGRAPHY

- CT delivers a substantially higher radiation dose than conventional radiography; it should therefore be used judiciously.
- CT of the brain should be the initial radiographic modality in evaluating a pt with a potential stroke.
- Is highly sensitive for diagnosing an acute subarachnoid hemorrhage and, in the acute setting, is more sensitive than MRI.
- CT of the brain is an essential test in evaluating a pt with mental status changes to exclude entities such as intracranial bleeding, mass effect, subdural or epidural hematomas, and hydrocephalus.
- Is better than MRI for evaluating osseous lesions of the skull and spine.
- CT of the chest should be considered in the evaluation of a pt with chest pain to rule out entities such as pulmonary embolus or aortic dissection.
- CT of the chest is essential for evaluating lung nodules to assess for the presence of thoracic lymphadenopathy.
- CT, with high-resolution cuts through the lungs, is the imaging modality of choice for evaluating the lung interstitium in a pt with interstitial lung disease.
- Can be used to evaluate for presence of pleural and pericardial fluid and to localize loculated effusions.
- Is useful in a pt with unexplained abdominal pain to evaluate for conditions such as appendicitis, mesenteric ischemia or infarction, diverticulitis, or pancreatitis.

- CT of the abdomen is also the test of choice for evaluating for nephrolithiasis in a pt with renal colic.
- Is the test of choice for evaluating for the presence of an abscess in the chest or abdomen.
- In conjunction with abdominal radiography, CT can help identify the cause of bowel obstruction.
- Can identify abdominal conditions such as intussusception and volvulus in a pt with abdominal pain.
- Is the imaging modality of choice for evaluating the retroperitoneum.
- Should be obtained expeditiously in a pt with abdominal trauma to evaluate for the presence of intraabdominal hemorrhage and to assess injury to abdominal organs.

■ MAGNETIC RESONANCE IMAGING

- Is more useful than CT in the evaluation of ischemic infarction, dementia, mass lesions, demyelinating diseases, and most nonosseous spinal disorders.
- Provides excellent imaging of large joints including the knee, hip, and shoulder.
- Can be used, often with CT or angiography, to assess possible dissecting aortic aneurysms and congenital anomalies of the cardiovascular system.
- Cardiac MRI is proving useful to evaluate cardiac wall motion and for assessing cardiac muscle viability in ischemic heart disease.
- Is preferable to CT for evaluating adrenal masses such as pheochromocytoma and for helping to distinguish benign and malignant adrenal masses.
- Is preferable to CT for evaluating pituitary lesions and parasellar pathology.

■ RADIONUCLIDE IMAGING

- Radionuclides can be used in the form of radioactive ions (iodide, gallium, thallium) or radiolabeled substances with affinity for specific tissues (radiopharmaceuticals, e.g., bisphosphonates, sestamibi, octreotide, metaiodobenzylguanidine [MIBG], iodocholesterol, etc.), or in the form of fluorodeoxyglucose for PET scanning.
- Radionuclide scintigraphy can be combined/merged with CT or MRI for precise anatomic localization of the radionuclide-imaged tissue.
- Tomographic radionuclide scintigraphy (single photon emission computed tomography, SPECT) is analogous to CT, using radionuclide emissions instead of x-rays. It permits visualization of sequential slices that can be computer-manipulated to yield a three-dimensional reconstruction.
- PET is very useful for detection of metabolically active tissues, such as cancers and their metastases, and has largely supplanted older modalities of radionuclide scanning (e.g., gallium scintigraphy).
- Radionuclide scans frequently ordered by the general internist are:
  1. Bone scan to identify metastatic disease in bone or osteomyelitis
  2. Sestamibi scans for preoperative localization of parathyroid adenomas
  3. Thyroid scans (technetium or iodine) to identify hot or cold thyroid nodules

- Specialized radionuclide scans include thallium or sestamibi myocardial perfusion scans, pulmonary ventilation/perfusion scans, octreotide scans for neuroendocrine tumors, MIBG scans for pheochromocytoma, iodocholesterol scans for adrenocortical adenomas, and whole-body radioiodine scans for disseminated thyroid cancer.
- Radioiodine scanning of the thyroid can be used to obtain quantitative information on iodine uptake by the thyroid, which is useful to differentiate subacute thyroiditis from Graves' disease.

CHAPTER 4
Procedures Commonly Performed by Internists

Internists perform a wide range of medical procedures, although practices vary widely among institutions and by specialty. Internists, nurses, or other ancillary health care professionals perform venipuncture for blood testing, arterial puncture for blood gases, endotracheal intubation, and flexible sigmoidoscopy, and insert IV lines, nasogastric (NG) tubes, and urinary catheters. These procedures are not covered here, but require skill and practice to minimize pt discomfort and potential complications. Here, we review more invasive diagnostic and therapeutic procedures performed by internists—thoracentesis, lumbar puncture, and paracentesis. Many additional procedures are performed by specialists and require additional training and credentialing, including the following:

- Allergy—skin testing, rhinoscopy
- Cardiology—stress testing, echocardiograms, coronary catheterization, angioplasty, stent insertion, pacemakers, electrophysiology testing and ablation, implantable defibrillators, cardioversion
- Endocrinology—thyroid biopsy, dynamic hormone testing, bone densitometry
- Gastroenterology—upper and lower endoscopy, esophageal manometry, endoscopic retrograde cholangiopancreatography, stent insertion, endoscopic ultrasound, liver biopsy
- Hematology/Oncology—bone marrow biopsy, stem cell transplant, lymph node biopsy, plasmapheresis
- Pulmonary—intubation and ventilator management, bronchoscopy
- Renal—kidney biopsy, dialysis
- Rheumatology—joint aspiration

Increasingly, ultrasound, CT, and MRI are being used to guide invasive procedures, and flexible fiberoptic instruments are extending the reach into the body. For most invasive medical procedures, including those reviewed below, informed consent should be obtained in writing before beginning the procedure.

THORACENTESIS

Drainage of the pleural space can be performed at the bedside. Indications for this procedure include diagnostic evaluation of pleural fluid, removal of pleural fluid for symptomatic relief, and instillation of sclerosing agents in pts with recurrent, usually malignant pleural effusions.

◼ PREPARATORY WORK

Familiarity with the components of a thoracentesis tray is a prerequisite to performing a thoracentesis successfully. Recent PA and lateral chest radiographs with bilateral decubitus views should be obtained to document the free-flowing nature of the pleural effusion. Loculated pleural effusions should be localized by ultrasound or CT prior to drainage.

◼ TECHNIQUE

A posterior approach is the preferred means of accessing pleural fluid. Comfortable positioning is a key to success for both pt and physician. The pt should sit on the edge of the bed, leaning forward with the arms abducted onto a pillow on a bedside stand. Pts undergoing thoracentesis frequently have severe dyspnea, and it is important to assess if they can maintain this positioning for at least 10 min. The entry site for the thoracentesis is based on the physical exam and radiographic findings. Percussion of dullness is utilized to ascertain the extent of the pleural effusion with the site of entry being the first or second highest interspace in this area. The entry site for the thoracentesis is at the superior aspect of the rib, thus avoiding the inter-costal nerve, artery, and vein, which run along the inferior aspect of the rib (Fig. 4-1).

The site of entry should be marked with a pen to guide the thoracentesis. The skin is then prepped and draped in a sterile fashion with the operator

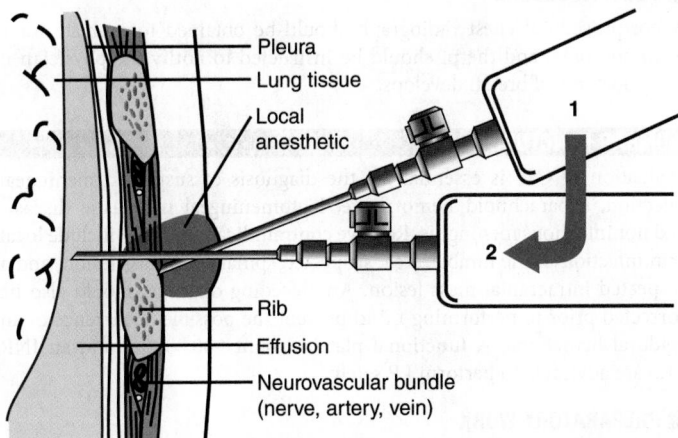

Pleura
Lung tissue
Local anesthetic
1
2
Rib
Effusion
Neurovascular bundle (nerve, artery, vein)

FIGURE 4-1 In thoracentesis, the needle is passed over the top of the rib to avoid the neurovascular bundle. (*From LG Gomella, SA Haist: Clinician's Pocket Reference, 11th ed. New York, McGraw-Hill, 2007.*)

observing sterile technique at all times. A small-gauge needle is used to anesthetize the skin, and a larger-gauge needle is used to anesthetize down to the superior aspect of the rib. The needle should then be directed over the upper margin of the rib to anesthetize down to the parietal pleura. The pleural space should be entered with the anesthetizing needle, all the while using liberal amounts of lidocaine.

A dedicated thoracentesis needle with an attached syringe should next be utilized to penetrate the skin. This needle should be advanced to the superior aspect of the rib. While maintaining gentle negative pressure, the needle should be slowly advanced into the pleural space. If a diagnostic tap is being performed, aspiration of only 30–50 mL of fluid is necessary before termination of the procedure. If a therapeutic thoracentesis is being performed, a three-way stopcock is utilized to direct the aspirated pleural fluid into collection bottles or bags. No more than 1 L of pleural fluid should be withdrawn at any given time, as quantities >1–1.5 L can result in re-expansion pulmonary edema.

After all specimens have been collected, the thoracentesis needle should be withdrawn and the needle site occluded for at least 1 min.

■ SPECIMEN COLLECTION

The diagnostic evaluation of pleural fluid depends on the clinical situation. All pleural fluid samples should be sent for cell count and differential, Gram stain, and bacterial cultures. LDH and protein determinations should also be made to differentiate between exudative and transudative pleural effusions. The pH should be determined if empyema is a diagnostic consideration. Other studies on pleural fluid include mycobacterial and fungal cultures, glucose, triglyceride level, amylase, and cytologic determination.

■ POSTPROCEDURE

A postprocedural chest radiograph should be obtained to evaluate for a pneumothorax, and the pt should be instructed to notify the physician if new shortness of breath develops.

LUMBAR PUNCTURE

Evaluation of CSF is essential for the diagnosis of suspected meningeal infection, subarachnoid hemorrhage, leptomeningeal neoplastic disease, and noninfectious meningitis. Relative contraindications to LP include local skin infection in the lumbar area, suspected spinal cord mass lesion, and a suspected intracranial mass lesion. Any bleeding diathesis should also be corrected prior to performing LP to prevent the possible occurrence of an epidural hematoma. A functional platelet count >50,000/μL and an INR <1.5 are advisable to perform LP safely.

■ PREPARATORY WORK

Familiarity with the components of a lumbar puncture tray is a prerequisite to performing LP successfully. In pts with focal neurologic deficits or with evidence of papilledema on physical exam, a CT scan of the head should be obtained prior to performing LP.

■ TECHNIQUE

Proper positioning of the pt is important to ensure a successful LP. Two different pt positions can be used: the lateral decubitus position and the sitting position. Most routine LPs should be performed using the lateral decubitus position (Fig. 4-2). The sitting position may be preferable in obese pts. With either position, the pt should be instructed to flex the spine as much as possible. In the lateral decubitus position, the pt is instructed to assume the fetal position with the knees flexed toward the abdomen. In the sitting position, the pt should bend over a bedside table with the head resting on folded arms.

The entry site for an LP is below the level of the conus medullaris, which extends to L1-L2 in most adults. Thus, either the L3-L4 or L4-L5 interspace can be utilized as the entry site. The posterior superior iliac crest should be identified and the spine palpated at this level. This represents the L3-L4 interspace, with the other interspaces referenced from this landmark. The midpoint of the interspace between the spinous processes represents the entry point for the thoracentesis needle. This entry site should be marked with a pen to guide the LP. The skin is then prepped and draped in a sterile fashion with the operator observing sterile technique at all times. A small-gauge needle is then used to anesthetize the skin and subcutaneous tissue. The spinal needle should be introduced perpendicular to the skin in the midline and should be advanced slowly. The needle stylette should be withdrawn frequently as the spinal needle is advanced. As the needle enters the subarachnoid space, a "popping" sensation can sometimes be felt. If bone is encountered, the needle should be withdrawn to just below the skin and then redirected more caudally. Once CSF begins to flow, the opening pressure can be measured. This should be measured in the lateral decubitus position with the pt shifted to this position if the procedure was begun with the pt in the sitting position. After the opening pressure is measured, the CSF should be collected in a series of specimen tubes for various tests. At a minimum, a total of 10–15 mL of CSF should be collected in the different specimen tubes.

Once the required spinal fluid is collected, the stylette should be replaced and the spinal needle removed.

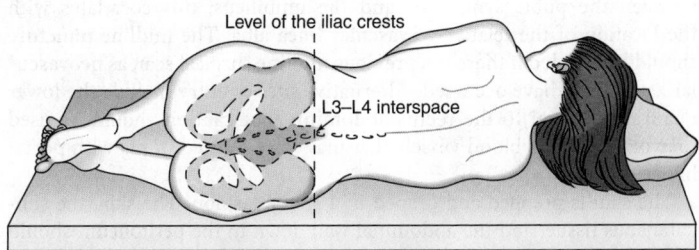

FIGURE 4-2 Proper positioning of a pt in the lateral decubitus position. Note that the shoulders and hips are in a vertical plane; the torso is perpendicular to the bed. *[From RP Simon et al (eds):* Clinical Neurology, *7th ed. New York, McGraw-Hill, 2009.]*

■ **SPECIMEN COLLECTION**

Diagnostic evaluation of CSF is based on the clinical scenario. In general, spinal fluid should always be sent for cell count with differential, protein, glucose, and bacterial cultures. Other specialized studies that can be obtained on CSF include viral cultures, fungal and mycobacterial cultures, VDRL, cryptococcal antigen, oligoclonal bands, and cytology.

■ **POSTPROCEDURE**

To reduce the chance of a post-LP headache, the pt should be instructed to lie prone for at least 3 h. If a headache does develop, bedrest, hydration, and oral analgesics are often helpful. If an intractable post-LP headache ensues, the pt may have a persistent CSF leak. In this case, consultation with an anesthesiologist should be considered for the placement of a blood patch.

PARACENTESIS

Removal and analysis of peritoneal fluid is invaluable in evaluating pts with new-onset ascites or ascites of unknown etiology. It is also requisite in pts with known ascites who have a decompensation in their clinical status. Relative contraindications include bleeding diathesis, prior abdominal surgery, distended bowel, or known loculated ascites.

■ **PREPARATORY WORK**

Prior to performing a paracentesis, any severe bleeding diathesis should be corrected. Bowel distention should also be relieved by placement of a nasogastric tube, and the bladder should also be emptied before beginning the procedure. If a large-volume paracentesis is being performed, large vacuum bottles with the appropriate connecting tubing should be obtained.

■ **TECHNIQUE**

Proper pt positioning greatly improves the ease with which a paracentesis can be performed. The pt should be instructed to lie supine with the head of the bed elevated to 45°. This position should be maintained for ~15 min to allow ascitic fluid to accumulate in the dependent portion of the abdomen.

The preferred entry site for paracentesis is a midline puncture halfway between the pubic symphysis and the umbilicus; this correlates with the location of the relatively avascular linea alba. The midline puncture should be avoided if there is a previous midline surgical scar, as neovascularization may have occurred. Alternative sites of entry include the lower quadrants, lateral to the rectus abdominis, but caution should be used to avoid collateral blood vessels that may have formed in pts with portal hypertension.

The skin is prepped and draped in a sterile fashion. The skin, the subcutaneous tissue, and the abdominal wall down to the peritoneum should be infiltrated with an anesthetic agent. The paracentesis needle with an attached syringe is then introduced in the midline perpendicular to the skin. To prevent leaking of ascitic fluid, "Z-tracking" can sometimes be helpful: after penetrating the skin, the needle is inserted 1–2 cm before advancing further. The needle is then advanced slowly while continuous aspiration is performed. As the peritoneum is pierced, the needle will "give" noticeably. Fluid should flow freely into the syringe soon thereafter. For a diagnostic paracentesis, removal of 50 mL of ascitic fluid is adequate. For a large-volume paracentesis, direct drainage into large vacuum containers using connecting tubing is a commonly utilized option.

After all samples have been collected, the paracentesis needle should be removed and firm pressure applied to the puncture site.

■ SPECIMEN COLLECTION

Peritoneal fluid should be sent for cell count with differential, Gram stain, and bacterial cultures. Albumin measurement of ascitic fluid is also necessary for calculating the serum–ascitic albumin gradient. Depending on the clinical scenario, other studies that can be obtained include mycobacterial cultures, amylase, adenosine deaminase, triglycerides, and cytology.

■ POSTPROCEDURE

The pt should be monitored carefully after paracentesis and should be instructed to lie supine in bed for several hours. If persistent fluid leakage occurs, continued bedrest with pressure dressings at the puncture site can be helpful. For pts with hepatic dysfunction undergoing large-volume paracentesis, the sudden reduction in intravascular volume can precipitate hepatorenal syndrome. Administration of 25 g IV albumin following large-volume paracentesis has been shown to decrease the incidence of postprocedure renal failure. Finally, if the ascites fluid analysis shows evidence of spontaneous bacterial peritonitis, then antibiotics (directed toward gram-negative gut bacteria) and IV albumin should be administered as soon as possible.

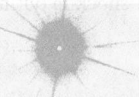

For a more detailed discussion, see Robbins E, Hauser SL: Technique of Lumbar Puncture, Chap. e46, and the Clinical Procedure Tutorial videos in Chaps. e54–e57 in HPIM-18.

CHAPTER **5**
Principles of Critical Care Medicine

■ INITIAL EVALUATION OF THE CRITICALLY ILL PATIENT

Initial care of critically ill pts must often be performed rapidly and before a thorough medical history has been obtained. Physiologic stabilization begins with the principles of advanced cardiovascular life support and frequently involves invasive techniques such as mechanical ventilation and renal replacement therapy to support organ systems that are failing. A variety of severity-of-illness scoring systems, such as APACHE (acute physiology and chronic health evaluation), have been developed. Although these tools are useful for ensuring similarity among groups of pts involved in clinical trials or in quality assurance monitoring, their relevance to individual pts is less clear. These scoring systems are not typically used to guide clinical management.

■ SHOCK

Shock, which is characterized by multisystem end-organ hypoperfusion and tissue hypoxia, is a frequent problem requiring ICU admission. A variety of clinical indicators of shock exist, including reduced mean arterial pressure, tachycardia, tachypnea, cool extremities, altered mental status, oliguria, and lactic acidosis. Although hypotension is usually observed in shock, there is not a specific blood pressure threshold that is used to define it. Shock can result from decreased cardiac output, decreased systemic vascular resistance, or both. The three main categories of shock are hypovolemic, cardiogenic, and high cardiac output/low systemic vascular resistance. Clinical evaluation can be useful to assess the adequacy of cardiac output, with narrow pulse pressure, cool extremities, and delayed capillary refill suggestive of reduced cardiac output. Indicators of high cardiac output (e.g., widened pulse pressure, warm extremities, and rapid capillary refill) associated with shock suggest reduced systemic vascular resistance. Reduced cardiac output can be due to intravascular volume depletion (e.g., hemorrhage) or cardiac dysfunction. Intravascular volume depletion can be assessed through the jugular venous pressure, changes in right atrial pressure with spontaneous respirations, or changes in pulse pressure during positive pressure mechanical ventilation. Reduced systemic vascular resistance is often caused by sepsis, but high cardiac output hypotension is also seen in pancreatitis, liver failure, burns, anaphylaxis, peripheral arteriovenous shunts, and thyrotoxicosis. Early resuscitation of septic and cardiogenic shock may improve survival; objective assessments such as echocardiography and/or invasive vascular monitoring should be used to complement clinical evaluation and minimize end-organ damage. The approach to the pt in shock is outlined in Fig. 5-1.

■ MECHANICAL VENTILATORY SUPPORT

Critically ill pts often require mechanical ventilation. During initial resuscitation, standard principles of advanced cardiovascular life support should be followed. Mechanical ventilation should be considered for acute hypoxemic respiratory failure, which may occur with cardiogenic shock, pulmonary edema (cardiogenic or noncardiogenic), or pneumonia. Mechanical ventilation should also be considered for treatment of ventilatory failure, which can result from an increased load on the respiratory system—often manifested by lactic acidosis or decreased lung compliance. Mechanical ventilation may decrease respiratory work, improve arterial oxygenation with improved tissue O_2 delivery, and reduce acidosis. Reduction in mean arterial pressure after institution of mechanical ventilation commonly occurs due to reduced venous return from positive pressure ventilation, reduced endogenous catecholamine secretion, and administration of drugs used to facilitate intubation. Since hypovolemia often contributes to postintubation hypotension, IV volume administration should be considered. The major types of respiratory failure are discussed in Chap. 16.

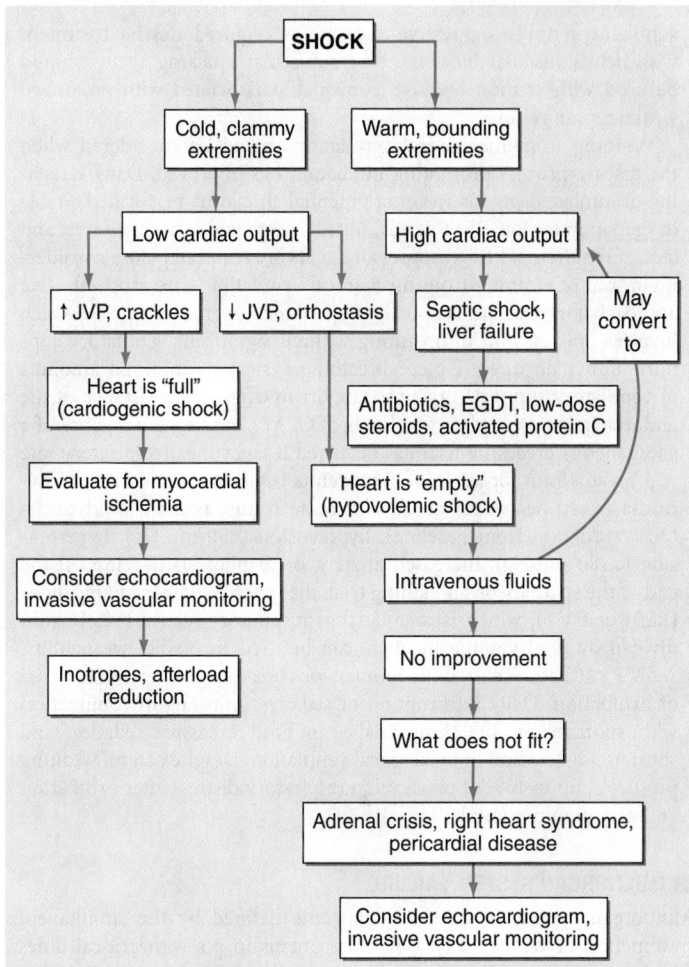

FIGURE 5-1 Approach to pt in shock. EGDT, early goal directed therapy; JVP, jugular venous pulse.

Many pts receiving mechanical ventilation require treatment for pain (typically with opiates) and for anxiety (typically with benzodiazepines, which also have the benefit of providing amnesia). Less commonly, neuromuscular blocking agents are required to facilitate ventilation when there is extreme dyssynchrony between the pt's respiratory efforts and the ventilator that cannot be corrected with manipulation of the ventilator settings; aggressive sedation is required during treatment with neuromuscular blockers. Neuromuscular blocking agents should be used with caution because a myopathy associated with prolonged weakness can result.

Weaning from mechanical ventilation should be considered when the disease process prompting intubation has improved. Daily screening of intubated pts for weaning potential should be performed. Stable oxygenation (at low PEEP levels), intact cough and airway reflexes, and lack of requirement for vasopressor agents are required before considering a trial of weaning from mechanical ventilation. The most effective approach for weaning is usually a spontaneous breathing trial, which involves 30–120 min of breathing without significant ventilatory support. Either an open T-piece breathing system or minimal amounts of ventilatory support (pressure support to overcome resistance of the endotracheal tube and/or low levels of CPAP) can be used. Failure of a spontaneous breathing trial has occurred if tachypnea (respiratory rate >35 breaths/min for >5 min), hypoxemia (O_2 saturation <90%), tachycardia (>140 beats/min or 20% increase from baseline), bradycardia (20% reduction from baseline), hypotension (<90 mmHg), hypertension (>180 mmHg), increased anxiety, or diaphoresis develop. At the end of the spontaneous breathing trial, the *rapid shallow breathing index* (RSBI or f/VT), which is calculated as respiratory rate in breaths/min divided by tidal volume in liters, can be used to predict weanability. A f/VT <105 at the end of the spontaneous breathing test warrants a trial of extubation. Daily interruption of sedative infusions in conjunction with spontaneous breathing trials can limit excessive sedation and shorten the duration of mechanical ventilation. Despite careful weaning protocols, up to 10% of pts develop respiratory distress after extubation and may require reintubation.

◼ MULTIORGAN SYSTEM FAILURE

Multiorgan system failure is a syndrome defined by the simultaneous dysfunction or failure of two or more organs in pts with critical illness. Multiorgan system failure is a common consequence of systemic inflammatory conditions (e.g., sepsis, pancreatitis, and trauma). To meet the criteria for multiorgan system failure, organ failure must persist for >24 h. Prognosis worsens with increased duration of organ failure and increased number of organ systems involved.

◼ MONITORING IN THE ICU

With critical illness, close and often continuous monitoring of multiple organ systems is required. In addition to pulse oximetry, frequent arterial blood gas analysis can reveal evolving acid-base disturbances and assess the adequacy of ventilation. Intra-arterial pressure monitoring is frequently performed to follow blood pressure and to provide arterial blood gases and other blood samples. Pulmonary artery (Swan-Ganz) catheters can provide pulmonary artery pressure, cardiac output, systemic vascular resistance, and oxygen delivery measurements. However, no morbidity or mortality benefit from pulmonary artery catheter use has been demonstrated, and rare but significant complications from placement of central venous access (e.g., pneumothorax, infection) or the pulmonary artery catheter (e.g., cardiac arrhythmias, pulmonary artery rupture) can result. Thus, routine pulmonary artery catheterization in critically ill pts is not recommended.

For intubated pts receiving volume-controlled modes of mechanical ventilation, respiratory mechanics can be followed easily. The peak airway pressure is regularly measured by mechanical ventilators, and the plateau pressure can be assessed by including an end-inspiratory pause. The inspiratory airway resistance is calculated as the difference between the peak and plateau airway pressures (with adjustment for flow rate). Increased airway resistance can result from bronchospasm, respiratory secretions, or a kinked endotracheal tube. Static compliance of the respiratory system is calculated as the tidal volume divided by the gradient in airway pressure (plateau pressure minus PEEP). Reduced respiratory system compliance can result from pleural effusions, pneumothorax, pneumonia, pulmonary edema, or auto-PEEP (elevated end-expiratory pressure related to insufficient time for alveolar emptying before the next inspiration).

■ PREVENTION OF CRITICAL ILLNESS COMPLICATIONS

Critically ill pts are prone to a number of complications, including the following:

- Sepsis—Often related to the invasive monitoring performed of critically ill pts.
- Anemia—Usually due to chronic inflammation as well as iatrogenic blood loss. A conservative approach to providing blood transfusions is recommended unless pts have active hemorrhage.
- Deep-vein thrombosis—May occur despite standard prophylaxis with SC heparin or lower extremity sequential compression devices and may occur at the site of central venous catheters. Low-molecular-weight heparins (e.g., enoxaparin) are more effective for high-risk pts than is unfractionated heparin.
- GI bleeding—Stress ulcers of the gastric mucosa frequently develop in pts with bleeding diatheses, shock, or respiratory failure, necessitating prophylactic acid neutralization in such pts.
- Acute renal failure—A frequent occurrence in ICU pts, exacerbated by nephrotoxic medications and hypoperfusion. The most common etiology is acute tubular necrosis. Low-dose dopamine treatment does not protect against the development of acute renal failure.
- Inadequate nutrition and hyperglycemia—Enteral feeding, when possible, is preferred over parenteral nutrition, since the parenteral route is associated with multiple complications including hyperglycemia, cholestasis, and sepsis. The utility of tight glucose control in the ICU is controversial.
- ICU-acquired weakness—Neuropathies and myopathies have been described—typically after at least one week of ICU care. These complications are especially common in sepsis.

■ NEUROLOGIC DYSFUNCTION IN CRITICALLY ILL PATIENTS

A variety of neurologic problems can develop in critically ill pts. Most ICU pts develop delirium, which is characterized by acute changes in mental status, inattention, disorganized thinking, and an altered level of consciousness. Use of dexmedetomidine was associated with less ICU delirium than midazolam, one of the conventional sedatives. Less common but important neurologic complications include anoxic brain injury, stroke, and status epilepticus.

■ LIMITATION OR WITHDRAWAL OF CARE

Withholding or withdrawing care commonly occurs in the ICU. Technological advances have allowed many pts to be maintained in the ICU with little or no chance of recovery. Increasingly, pts, families, and caregivers have acknowledged the ethical validity to withhold or withdraw care when the pt or surrogate decision-maker determines that the pt's goals for care are no longer achievable with the clinical situation.

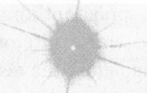

> For a more detailed discussion, see Kress JP, Hall JB:
> Approach to the Patient With Critical Illness, Chap. 267,
> p. 2196, in HPIM-18.

CHAPTER **6**
Pain and Its Management

APPROACH TO THE PATIENT	Pain

Pain is the most common symptom that brings a pt to a physician's attention. Management depends on determining its cause, alleviating triggering and potentiating factors, and providing rapid relief whenever possible. Pain may be of somatic (skin, joints, muscles), visceral, or neuropathic (injury to nerves, spinal cord pathways, or thalamus) origin. Characteristics of each are summarized in Table 6-1.

NEUROPATHIC PAIN Definitions: *neuralgia*: pain in the distribution of a single nerve, as in trigeminal neuralgia; *dysesthesia*: spontaneous, unpleasant, abnormal sensations; *hyperalgesia* and *hyperesthesia*: exaggerated responses to nociceptive or touch stimulus, respectively; *allodynia*: perception of light mechanical stimuli as painful, as when vibration evokes painful sensation. Reduced pain perception is called *hypalgesia* or, when absent, *analgesia*. *Causalgia* is continuous severe burning pain with indistinct boundaries and accompanying sympathetic nervous system dysfunction (sweating; vascular, skin, and hair changes—sympathetic dystrophy) that occurs after injury to a peripheral nerve.

   Sensitization refers to a lowered threshold for activating primary nociceptors following repeated stimulation in damaged or inflamed tissues;

TABLE 6-1 CHARACTERISTICS OF SOMATIC AND NEUROPATHIC PAIN

Somatic pain
  Nociceptive stimulus usually evident
  Usually well localized
  Similar to other somatic pains in pt's experience
  Relieved by anti-inflammatory or narcotic analgesics

Visceral pain
  Most commonly activated by inflammation
  Pain poorly localized and usually referred
  Associated with diffuse discomfort, e.g., nausea, bloating
  Relieved by narcotic analgesics

Neuropathic pain
  No obvious nociceptive stimulus
  Associated evidence of nerve damage, e.g., sensory impairment, weakness
  Unusual, dissimilar from somatic pain, often shooting or electrical quality
  Only partially relieved by narcotic analgesics, may respond to antidepressants
  or anticonvulsants

inflammatory mediators play a role. Sensitization contributes to tenderness, soreness, and hyperalgesia (as in sunburn).

Referred pain results from the convergence of sensory inputs from skin and viscera on single spinal neurons that transmit pain signals to the brain. Because of this convergence, input from deep structures is mislocalized to a region of skin innervated by the same spinal segment.

CHRONIC PAIN The problem is often difficult to diagnose, and pts may appear emotionally distraught. Several factors can cause, perpetuate, or exacerbate chronic pain: (1) painful disease for which there is no cure (e.g., arthritis, cancer, migraine headaches, diabetic neuropathy); (2) neural factors initiated by a bodily disease that persist after the disease has resolved (e.g., damaged sensory or sympathetic nerves); (3) psychological conditions. Pay special attention to the medical history and to depression. Major depression is common, treatable, and potentially fatal (suicide).

■ **PATHOPHYSIOLOGY: ORGANIZATION OF PAIN PATHWAYS**

Pain-producing (nociceptive) sensory stimuli in skin and viscera activate peripheral nerve endings of primary afferent neurons, which synapse on second-order neurons in spinal cord or medulla (Fig. 6-1). These second-order neurons form crossed ascending pathways that reach the thalamus and are projected to the somatosensory cortex. Parallel ascending neurons

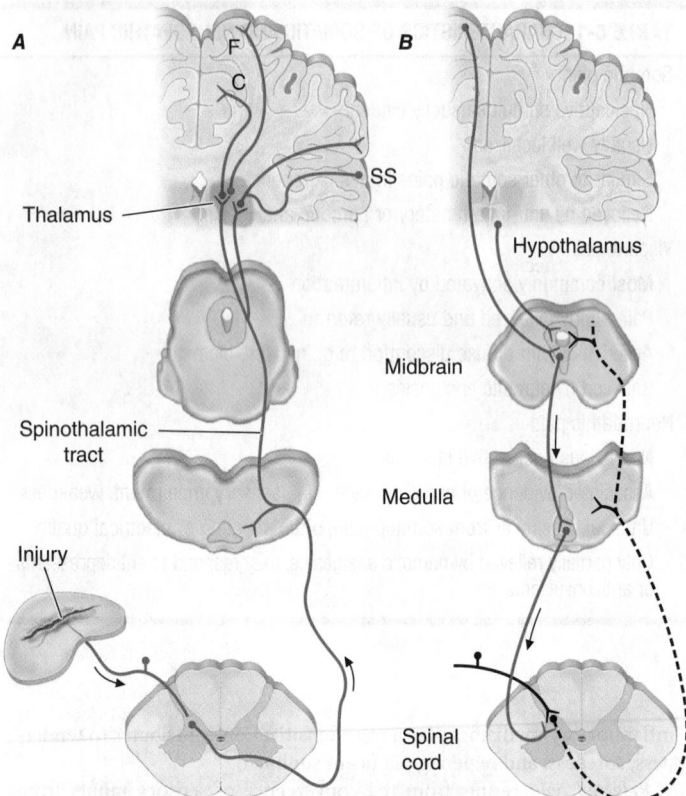

FIGURE 6-1 Pain transmission and modulatory pathways. **A.** Transmission system for nociceptive messages. Noxious stimuli activate the sensitive peripheral ending of the primary afferent nociceptor by the process of transduction. The message is then transmitted over the peripheral nerve to the spinal cord, where it synapses with cells of origin of the major ascending pain pathway, the spinothalamic tract. The message is relayed in the thalamus to the anterior cingulate (C), frontal insular (F), and somatosensory cortex (SS). **B.** Pain-modulation network. Inputs from frontal cortex and hypothalamus activate cells in the midbrain that control spinal pain-transmission cells via cells in the medulla.

connect with brainstem nuclei and ventrocaudal and medial thalamic nuclei. These parallel pathways project to the limbic system and underlie the emotional aspect of pain. Pain transmission is regulated at the dorsal horn level by descending bulbospinal pathways that contain serotonin, norepinephrine, and several neuropeptides.

Agents that modify pain perception may act by reducing tissue inflammation (NSAIDs, prostaglandin synthesis inhibitors), interfering with pain transmission (narcotics), or enhancing descending modulation (narcotics and antidepressants). Anticonvulsants (gabapentin, carbamazepine) may be effective for aberrant pain sensations arising from peripheral nerve injury.

TREATMENT Pain (Table 6-2)

ACUTE SOMATIC PAIN

- Moderate pain: usually treated effectively with nonnarcotic analgesics, e.g., aspirin, acetaminophen, and NSAIDs, which inhibit cyclooxygenase (COX) and, except for acetaminophen, have anti-inflammatory actions, especially at high dosages. Particularly effective for headache and musculoskeletal pain.
- Parenteral ketorolac is sufficiently potent and rapid in onset to supplant opioids for many pts with acute severe pain.
- Narcotic analgesics in oral or parenteral form can be used for more severe pain. These are the most effective drugs available; the opioid antagonist naloxone should be readily available when narcotics are used in high doses or in unstable pts.
- Pt-controlled analgesia (PCA) permits infusion of a baseline dose plus self-administered boluses (activated by press of a button) as needed to control pain.

CHRONIC PAIN

- Develop an explicit treatment plan including specific and realistic goals for therapy, e.g., getting a good night's sleep, being able to go shopping, or returning to work.
- A multidisciplinary approach that utilizes medications, counseling, physical therapy, nerve blocks, and even surgery may be required to improve quality of life.
- Psychological evaluation is key; behaviorally based treatment paradigms are frequently helpful.
- Some pts may require referral to a pain clinic; for others, pharmacologic management alone can provide significant help.
- Tricyclic antidepressants are useful in management of chronic pain from many causes, including headache, diabetic neuropathy, postherpetic neuralgia, chronic low back pain, and central post-stroke pain.
- Anticonvulsants or antiarrhythmics benefit pts with neuropathic pain and little or no evidence of sympathetic dysfunction (e.g., diabetic neuropathy, trigeminal neuralgia).
- The long-term use of opioids is accepted for pain due to malignant disease, but is controversial for chronic pain of nonmalignant origin. When other approaches fail, long-acting opioid compounds such as levorphanol, methadone, sustained-release morphine, or transdermal fentanyl may be considered for these pts.

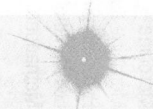

For a more detailed discussion, see Rathmell HP, Fields HL: Pain: Pathophysiology and Management, Chap. 11, p. 93, in HPIM-18.

TABLE 6-2 DRUGS FOR RELIEF OF PAIN

Generic Name	Dose, mg	Interval	Comments
Nonnarcotic analgesics: usual doses and intervals			
Acetylsalicylic acid	650 PO	q4h	Enteric-coated preparations available
Acetaminophen	650 PO	q4h	Side effects uncommon
Ibuprofen	400 PO	q4–6h	Available without prescription
Naproxen	250–500 PO	q12h	Delayed effects may be due to long half-life
Fenoprofen	200 PO	q4–6h	Contraindicated in renal disease
Indomethacin	25–50 PO	q8h	Gastrointestinal side effects common
Ketorolac	15–60 IM/IV	q4–6h	Available for parenteral use
Celecoxib	100–200 PO	q12–24h	Useful for arthritis
Valdecoxib	10–20 PO	q12–24h	Removed from U.S. market in 2005

Generic Name	Parenteral Dose, mg	PO Dose, mg	Comments
Narcotic analgesics: usual doses and intervals			
Codeine	30–60 q4h	30–60 q4h	Nausea common
Oxycodone	—	5–10 q4–6h	Usually available with acetaminophen or aspirin
Morphine	5 q4h	30 q4h	
Morphine sustained release	—	15–60 bid to tid	Oral slow-release preparation
Hydromorphone	1–2 q4h	2–4 q4h	Shorter acting than morphine sulfate
Levorphanol	2 q6–8h	4 q6–8h	Longer acting than morphine sulfate; absorbed well PO
Methadone	5–10 q6–8h	5–20 q6–8h	Delayed sedation due to long half-life; therapy should not be initiated with >40 mg/day and dose escalation should be made no more frequently than every 3 days

44

Generic Name			
Meperidine	50–100 q3–4h	300 q4h	Poorly absorbed PO; normeperidine a toxic metabolite; routine use of this agent is not recommended
Butorphanol	—	1–2 q4h	Intranasal spray
Fentanyl	25–100 µg/h	—	72-h transdermal patch
Tramadol	—	50–100 q4–6h	Mixed opioid/adrenergic action

Antidepressants[a]

Generic Name	Uptake Blockade 5-HT	Uptake Blockade NE	Sedative Potency	Anticholinergic Potency	Orthostatic Hypotension	Cardiac Arrhythmia	Ave. Dose, mg/d	Range, mg/d
Doxepin	++	+	High	Moderate	Moderate	Less	200	75–400
Amitriptyline	++++	++	High	Highest	Moderate	Yes	150	25–300
Imipramine	++++	++	Moderate	Moderate	High	Yes	200	75–400
Nortriptyline	+++	++	Moderate	Moderate	Low	Yes	100	40–150
Desipramine	+++	++++	Low	Low	Low	Yes	150	50–300
Venlafaxine	+++	++	Low	None	None	No	150	75–400
Duloxetine	+++	+++	Low	None	None	No	40	30–60

Anticonvulsants and antiarrhythmics[a]

Generic Name	PO Dose, mg	Interval	Generic Name	PO Dose, mg	Interval
Phenytoin	300	Daily/qhs	Clonazepam	1	q6h
Carbamazepine	200–300	q6h	Gabapentin[b]	600–1200	q8h
Oxcarbazepine	300	bid	Pregabalin	150–600	bid

[a]Antidepressants, anticonvulsants, and antiarrhythmics have not been approved by the U.S. Food and Drug Administration (FDA) for the treatment of pain.

[b]Gabapentin in doses up to 1800 mg/d is FDA approved for postherpetic neuralgia.

Abbreviations: 5-HT, serotonin; NE, norepinephrine.

CHAPTER **7**
Assessment of Nutritional Status

Stability of body weight requires that energy intake and expenditures are balanced over time. The major categories of energy output are resting energy expenditure (REE) and physical activity; minor sources include the energy cost of metabolizing food (thermic effect of food or specific dynamic action) and shivering thermogenesis. The average energy intake is about 2800 kcal/d for men and about 1800 kcal/d for women, though these estimates vary with age, body size, and activity level. Basal energy expenditure (BEE), measured in kcal/d, may be estimated by the Harris and Benedict formula (Fig. 7-1).

Dietary reference intakes (DRI) and recommended dietary allowances (RDA) have been defined for many nutrients, including 9 essential amino acids, 4 fat-soluble and 10 water-soluble vitamins, several minerals, fatty acids, choline, and water (Tables 73-1 and 73-2, pp. 590 and 591, in HPIM-18). The usual water requirements are 1.0–1.5 mL/kcal energy expenditure in adults, with adjustments for excessive losses. The RDA for protein is 0.6 g/kg ideal body weight, representing 15% of total caloric intake. Fat should constitute ≤30% of calories, and saturated fat should be <10% of calories. At least 55% of calories should be derived from carbohydrates.

■ MALNUTRITION

Malnutrition results from inadequate intake or abnormal gastrointestinal assimilation of dietary calories, excessive energy expenditure, or altered metabolism of energy supplies by an intrinsic disease process.

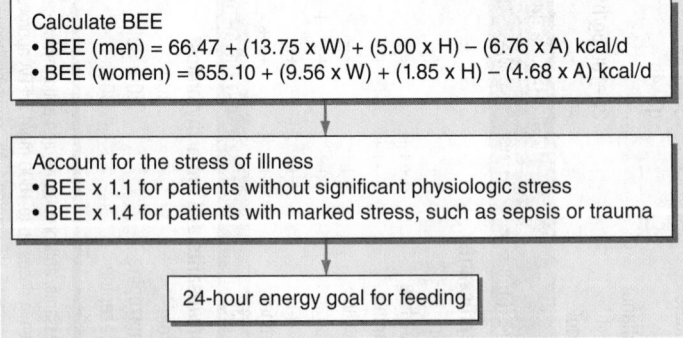

FIGURE 7-1 Basal energy expenditure (BEE) calculation in kcal/d, estimated by the Harris and Benedict formula. A, age in years; H, height in cm; W, Weight in kg.

Both outpatients and inpatients are at risk for malnutrition if they meet one or more of the following criteria:

• Unintentional loss of >10% of usual body weight in the preceding 3 months
• Body weight <90% of ideal for height (Table 7-1)
• Body mass index (BMI: weight/height^2 in kg/m^2) <18.5

Two forms of severe malnutrition can be seen: *marasmus*, which refers to generalized starvation that occurs in the setting of chronically decreased energy intake, and *kwashiorkor*, which refers to selective protein malnutrition due to decreased protein intake and catabolism in the setting of acute, life-threatening illnesses or chronic inflammatory disorders. Aggressive

TABLE 7-1 IDEAL WEIGHT FOR HEIGHT

Men				Women			
Height[a]	Weight[a]	Height	Weight	Height	Weight	Height	Weight
145	51.9	166	64.0	140	44.9	161	56.9
146	52.4	167	64.6	141	45.4	162	57.6
147	52.9	168	65.2	142	45.9	163	58.3
148	53.5	169	65.9	143	46.4	164	58.9
149	54.0	170	66.6	144	47.0	165	59.5
150	54.5	171	67.3	145	47.5	166	60.1
151	55.0	172	68.0	146	48.0	167	60.7
152	55.6	173	68.7	147	48.6	168	61.4
153	56.1	174	69.4	148	49.2	169	62.1
154	56.6	175	70.1	149	49.8		
155	57.2	176	70.8	150	50.4		
156	57.9	177	71.6	151	51.0		
157	58.6	178	72.4	152	51.5		
158	59.3	179	73.3	153	52.0		
159	59.9	180	74.2	154	52.5		
160	60.5	181	75.0	155	53.1		
161	61.1	182	75.8	156	53.7		
162	61.7	183	76.5	157	54.3		
163	62.3	184	77.3	158	54.9		
164	62.9	185	78.1	159	55.5		
165	63.5	186	78.9	160	56.2		

[a]Values are expressed in cm for height and kg for weight. To obtain height in inches, divide by 2.54. To obtain weight in pounds, multiply by 2.2.
Source: Adapted from GL Blackburn et al.: Nutritional and metabolic assessment of the hospitalized patient. *J Parenter Enteral Nutr* 1:11, 1977; with permission.

nutritional support is indicated in kwashiorkor to prevent infectious complications and poor wound healing.

Etiology

The major etiologies of malnutrition are starvation, stress from surgery or severe illness, and mixed mechanisms. Starvation results from decreased dietary intake (from poverty, chronic alcoholism, anorexia nervosa, fad diets, severe depression, neurodegenerative disorders, dementia, or strict vegetarianism; abdominal pain from intestinal ischemia or pancreatitis; or anorexia associated with AIDS, disseminated cancer, heart failure, or renal failure) or decreased assimilation of the diet (from pancreatic insufficiency; short bowel syndrome; celiac disease; or esophageal, gastric, or intestinal obstruction). Contributors to physical stress include fever, acute trauma, major surgery, burns, acute sepsis, hyperthyroidism, and inflammation as occurs in pancreatitis, collagen vascular diseases, and chronic infectious diseases such as tuberculosis or AIDS opportunistic infections. Mixed mechanisms occur in AIDS, disseminated cancer, chronic obstructive pulmonary disease, chronic liver disease, Crohn's disease, ulcerative colitis, and renal failure.

Clinical Features

- *General*—weight loss, temporal and proximal muscle wasting, decreased skin-fold thickness
- *Skin, hair, and nails*—easily plucked hair (protein); sparse hair (protein, biotin, zinc); coiled hair, easy bruising, petechiae, and perifollicular hemorrhages (vit. C); "flaky paint" rash of lower extremities (zinc); hyperpigmentation of skin in exposed areas (niacin, tryptophan); spooning of nails (iron)
- *Eyes*—conjunctival pallor (anemia); night blindness, dryness, and Bitot spots (vit. A); ophthalmoplegia (thiamine)
- *Mouth and mucous membranes*—glossitis and/or cheilosis (riboflavin, niacin, vit. B_{12}, pyridoxine, folate), diminished taste (zinc), inflamed and bleeding gums (vit. C)
- *Neurologic*—disorientation (niacin, phosphorus); confabulation, cerebellar gait, or past pointing (thiamine); peripheral neuropathy (thiamine, pyridoxine, vit. E); lost vibratory and position sense (vit. B_{12})
- *Other*—edema (protein, thiamine), heart failure (thiamine, phosphorus), hepatomegaly (protein)

Laboratory findings in protein malnutrition include a low serum albumin, low total iron-binding capacity, and anergy to skin testing. Specific vitamin deficiencies also may be present.

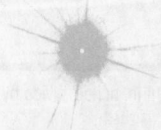

For a more detailed discussion, see Dwyer J: Nutritional Requirements and Dietary Assessment, Chap. 73, p. 588; Russell RM and Suter PM: Vitamin and Trace Mineral Deficiency and Excess, Chap. 74, p. 594; and Heimberger DC: Malnutrition and Nutritional Assessment, Chap. 75, p. 605 in HPIM-18.

CHAPTER 8
Enteral and Parenteral Nutrition

Nutritional support should be initiated in pts with malnutrition or in those at risk for malnutrition (e.g., conditions that preclude adequate oral feeding or pts in catabolic states, such as sepsis, burns, or trauma). An approach for deciding when to use various types of specialized nutrition support (SNS) is summarized in Fig. 8-1.

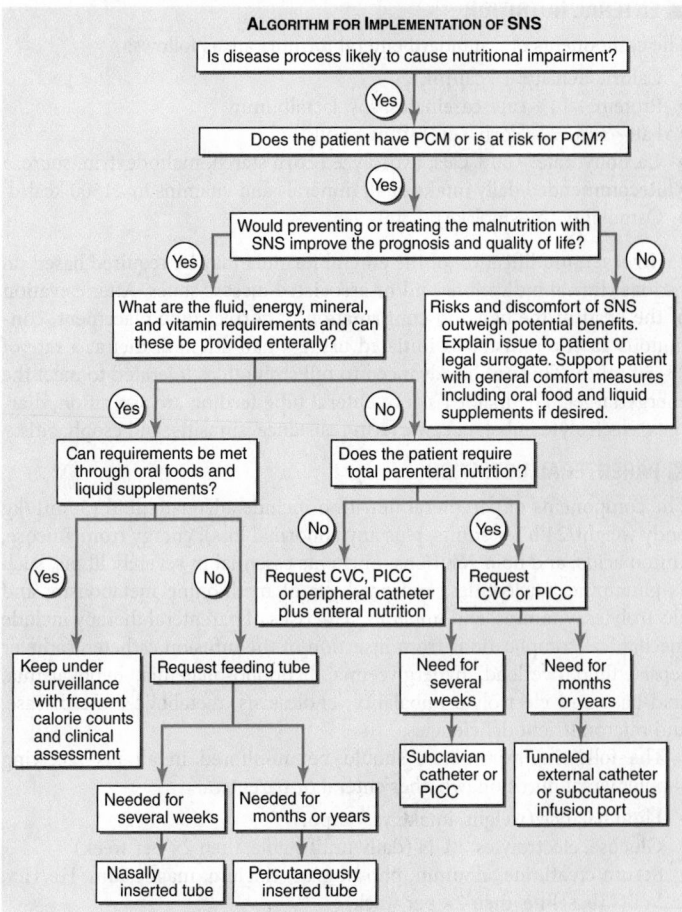

FIGURE 8-1 Decision-making for the implementation of specialized nutrition support (SNS). CVC, central venous catheter; PCM, protein-calorie malnutrition; PICC, peripherally inserted central catheter. *(Adapted from chapter in* Harrison's Principles of Internal Medicine, *16e, by Lyn Howard, MD.)*

Enteral therapy refers to feeding via the gut, using oral supplements or infusion of formulas via various feeding tubes (nasogastric, nasoduodenal, gastrostomy, jejunostomy, or combined gastrojejunostomy). *Parenteral therapy* refers to the infusion of nutrient solutions into the bloodstream via a peripherally inserted central catheter (PICC), a centrally inserted externalized catheter, or a centrally inserted tunneled catheter or subcutaneous port. When feasible, enteral nutrition is the preferred route because it sustains the digestive, absorptive, and immunologic functions of the GI tract, and because it minimizes the risk of fluid and electrolyte imbalance. Parenteral nutrition is often indicated in severe pancreatitis, necrotizing enterocolitis, prolonged ileus, and distal bowel obstruction.

■ **ENTERAL NUTRITION**

The components of a standard enteral formula are as follows:

- Caloric density: 1 kcal/mL
- Protein: ~14% cals; caseinates, soy, lactalbumin
- Fat: ~30% cals; corn, soy, safflower oils
- Carbohydrate: ~60% cals; hydrolyzed corn starch, maltodextrin, sucrose
- Recommended daily intake of all minerals and vitamins in ≥1500 kcal/d
- Osmolality (mosmol/kg): ~300

However, modification of the enteral formula may be required based on various clinical indications and/or associated disease states. After elevation of the head of the bed and confirmation of correct tube placement, continuous gastric infusion is initiated using a half-strength diet at a rate of 25–50 mL/h. This can be advanced to full strength as tolerated to meet the energy target. The major risks of enteral tube feeding are aspiration, diarrhea, electrolyte imbalance, warfarin resistance, sinusitis, and esophagitis.

■ **PARENTERAL NUTRITION**

The components of parenteral nutrition include adequate fluid (30 mL/kg body weight/24 h for adults, plus any abnormal loss); energy from glucose, amino acids, and lipid solutions; nutrients essential in severely ill pts, such as glutamine, nucleotides, and products of methionine metabolism; and electrolytes, vitamins, and minerals. The risks of parenteral therapy include mechanical complications from insertion of the infusion catheter, catheter sepsis, fluid overload, hyperglycemia, hypophosphatemia, hypokalemia, acid-base and electrolyte imbalance, cholestasis, metabolic bone disease, and micronutrient deficiencies.

The following parameters should be monitored in all pts receiving supplemental nutrition, whether enteral or parenteral:

- Fluid balance (weight, intake vs. output)
- Glucose, electrolytes, BUN (daily until stable, then 2× per week)
- Serum creatinine, albumin, phosphorus, calcium, magnesium, Hb/Hct, WBC (baseline, then 2× per week)
- INR (baseline, then weekly)
- Micronutrient tests as indicated

■ **SPECIFIC MICRONUTRIENT DEFICIENCY**

Appropriate therapies for micronutrient deficiencies are outlined in Table 8-1.

TABLE 8-1 THERAPY FOR COMMON VITAMIN AND MINERAL DEFICIENCIES

Nutrient	Therapy
Vitamin A[a,b,c]	60 mg PO, repeated 1 and 14 days later if ocular changes; 30 mg for ages 6–11 months
	15 mg PO qd × 1 month if chronic malabsorption
Vitamin C	200 mg PO qd
Vitamin D[a,d]	Encourage sun exposure if possible
	50,000 units PO once weekly for 4–8 weeks, then 400–800 units PO qd
	Substantially higher dose may be required in chronic malabsorption
Vitamin E[a]	800–1200 mg PO qd
Vitamin K[a]	10 mg IV × 1
	1–2 mg PO qd or 1–2 mg IV weekly in chronic malabsorption
Thiamine[b]	100 mg IV qd × 7 days, followed by 10 mg PO qd
Niacin	100–200 mg PO tid for 5 days
Pyridoxine	50 mg PO qd, 100–200 mg PO qd if deficiency related to medication
Zinc[b,c]	60 mg PO bid

[a]Associated with fat malabsorption.
[b]Associated with chronic alcoholism; always replete thiamine before carbohydrates in alcoholics to avoid precipitation of acute thiamine deficiency.
[c]Associated with protein-calorie malnutrition.
[d]Therapy must be monitored by serum calcium measurements.

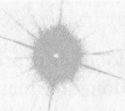

For a more detailed discussion, see Russell RM and Suter PM: Vitamin and Trace Mineral Deficiency and Excess, Chap. 74, p. 594; and Bistrian BR and Driscoll DF: Enteral and Parenteral Nutrition Therapy, Chap. 76, p. 612, HPIM-18.

CHAPTER 9
Transfusion and Pheresis Therapy

TRANSFUSIONS

WHOLE BLOOD TRANSFUSION

Indicated when acute blood loss is sufficient to produce hypovolemia, whole blood provides both oxygen-carrying capacity and volume expansion. In acute blood loss, hematocrit may not accurately reflect degree of blood loss for 48 h until fluid shifts occur.

■ RED BLOOD CELL TRANSFUSION

Indicated for symptomatic anemia unresponsive to specific therapy or requiring urgent correction. Packed red blood cell (RBC) transfusions may be indicated in pts who are symptomatic from cardiovascular or pulmonary disease when Hb is between 70 and 90 g/L (7 and 9 g/dL). Transfusion is usually necessary when Hb is <70 g/L (<7 g/dL). One unit of packed RBCs raises the Hb by approximately 10 g/L (1 g/dL). In the setting of acute hemorrhage, packed RBCs, fresh-frozen plasma (FFP), and platelets in an approximate ratio of 3:1:10 units are an adequate replacement for whole blood. Removal of leukocytes reduces risk of alloimmunization and transmission of cytomegalovirus. Washing to remove donor plasma reduces risk of allergic reactions. Irradiation prevents graft-versus-host disease in immunocompromised recipients by killing alloreactive donor lymphocytes. Avoid related donors.

Other Indications

(1) *Hypertransfusion therapy* to block production of defective cells, e.g., thalassemia, sickle cell anemia; (2) *exchange transfusion*—hemolytic disease of newborn, sickle cell crisis; (3) *transplant recipients*—decreases rejection of cadaveric kidney transplants.

Complications (See Table 9-1)

(1) *Transfusion reaction*—immediate or delayed, seen in 1–4% of transfusions; IgA-deficient pts at particular risk for severe reaction; (2) *infection*—bacterial (rare); hepatitis C, 1 in 1,800,000 transfusions; HIV transmission, 1 in 2,300,000; (3) *circulatory overload*; (4) *iron overload*—each unit contains 200–250 mg iron; hemochromatosis may develop after 100 U of RBCs (less in children), in absence of blood loss; iron chelation therapy with deferoxamine indicated; (5) *graft-versus-host disease*; (6) *alloimmunization*.

■ AUTOLOGOUS TRANSFUSION

Use of pt's own stored blood avoids hazards of donor blood; also useful in pts with multiple RBC antibodies. Pace of autologous donation may be accelerated using erythropoietin (50–150 U/kg SC three times a week) in the setting of normal iron stores.

■ RED CELL EXCHANGE

The main goal of red cell exchange transfusions is to remove sickle cells and replace them with normal red cells to interrupt the vicious cycle of sickling, stasis, vasoocclusion, and hypoxia that propagate sickle cell crises. The usual target is 70% hemoglobin A.

■ PLATELET TRANSFUSION

Prophylactic transfusions usually reserved for platelet count <10,000/μL (<20,000/μL in acute leukemia). One unit elevates the count by about 10,000/μL if no platelet antibodies are present as a result of prior transfusions. Efficacy assessed by 1-h and 24-h posttransfusion platelet counts. HLA-matched single-donor platelets may be required in pts with platelet alloantibodies.

TABLE 9-1 RISKS OF TRANSFUSION COMPLICATIONS

	Frequency, Episodes: Unit
Reactions	
Febrile (FNHTR)	1–4:100
Allergic	1–4:100
Delayed hemolytic	1:1000
TRALI	1:5000
Acute hemolytic	1:12,000
Fatal hemolytic	1:100,000
Anaphylactic	1:150,000
Infections[a]	
Hepatitis B	1:220,000
Hepatitis C	1:1,800,000
HIV-1, HIV-2	1:2,300,000
HTLV-I, HTLV-II	1:2,993,000
Malaria	1:4,000,000
Other complications	
RBC allosensitization	1:100
HLA allosensitization	1:10
Graft-versus-host disease	Rare

[a]Infectious agents rarely associated with transfusion, theoretically possible, or of unknown risk include West Nile virus, hepatitis A virus, parvovirus B-19, *Babesia microti* (babesiosis), *Borrelia burgdorferi* (Lyme disease), *Anaplasma phagocytophilum* (human granulocytic ehrlichiosis), *Trypanosoma cruzi* (Chagas' disease), *Treponema pallidum*, and human herpesvirus 8. **Abbreviations:** FNHTR, febrile nonhemolytic transfusion reaction; HTLV, human T lymphotropic virus; RBC, red blood cell; TRALI, transfusion-related acute lung injury.

■ TRANSFUSION OF PLASMA COMPONENTS

Fresh frozen plasma (FFP) is a source of coagulation factors, fibrinogen, antithrombin, and proteins C and S. It is used to correct coagulation factor deficiencies, rapidly reverse warfarin effects, and treat thrombotic thrombocytopenic purpura (TTP). Cryoprecipitate is a source of fibrinogen, factor VIII, and von Willebrand factor; it may be used when recombinant factor VIII or factor VIII concentrates are not available.

THERAPEUTIC HEMAPHERESIS

Hemapheresis is removal of a cellular or plasma constituent of blood; the specific procedure is referred to by the blood fraction removed.

■ LEUKAPHERESIS

Removal of WBCs; most often used in acute leukemia, esp. acute myeloid leukemia (AML) in cases complicated by marked elevation (>100,000/μL) of the peripheral blast count, to lower risk of leukostasis (blast-mediated vasoocclusive events resulting in central nervous system or pulmonary infarction, hemorrhage). Leukapheresis is replacing bone marrow aspiration to obtain hematopoietic stem cells. After treatment with a chemotherapeutic agent and granulocyte-macrophage colony-stimulating factor, hematopoietic stem cells are mobilized from marrow to the peripheral blood; such cells are leukapheresed and then used for hematopoietic reconstitution after high-dose myeloablative therapy. A third emerging medical use of leukapheresis is to harvest lymphocytes to use as adoptive immunotherapy.

■ PLATELETPHERESIS

Used in some pts with thrombocytosis associated with myeloproliferative disorders with bleeding and/or thrombotic complications. Other treatments are generally used first. Plateletpheresis also enhances platelet yield from blood donors.

■ PLASMAPHERESIS

Indications

(1) *Hyperviscosity states*—e.g., Waldenström's macroglobulinemia; (2) *TTP*; (3) *immune-complex* and *autoantibody disorders*—e.g., Goodpasture's syndrome, rapidly progressive glomerulonephritis, myasthenia gravis; possibly Guillain-Barré, systemic lupus erythematosus, idiopathic thrombocytopenic purpura; (4) cold agglutinin disease, cryoglobulinemia. In plasma exchange, abnormal proteins are removed and normal plasma or plasma components are replaced; useful in TTP to remove anti-ADAMTS13 antibody and provide normal ADAMTS13 levels.

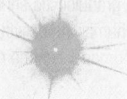

> For a more detailed discussion, see Dzieczkowski JS, Anderson KC: Transfusion Biology and Therapy, Chap. 113, p. 951, in HPIM-18.

CHAPTER **10**
Palliative and End-of-Life Care

In 2008, 2,473,000 people died in the United States; death rates are declining. Heart disease and cancer are the two leading causes of death and together account for nearly half of all deaths. About 70% of deaths occur in people who have a condition that is known to be leading to their death; thus, planning for terminal care is relevant and important. An increasing fraction of deaths are occurring in hospices or at home rather than in the hospital.

Optimal care depends on a comprehensive assessment of pt needs in all four domains affected by illness: physical, psychological, social, and spiritual. A variety of assessment tools are available to assist in the process.

Communication and continuous assessment of management goals are key components to addressing end-of-life care. Physicians must be clear about the likely outcome of the illness(es) and provide an anticipated schedule with goals and landmarks in the care process. When the goals of care have changed from cure to palliation, that transition must be clearly explained and defended. Seven steps are involved in establishing goals:

1. Ensure that the medical information is as complete as possible and understood by all relevant parties.
2. Explore the pt's goals while making sure the goals are achievable.
3. Explain the options.
4. Show empathy as the pt and the family adjust to changing expectations.
5. Make a plan with realistic goals.
6. Follow through with the plan.
7. Review and revise the plan periodically as the pt's situation changes.

■ ADVANCE DIRECTIVES

About 70% of pts lack decision-making capacity in their final days. Advance directives define ahead of time the level of intervention the pt is willing to accept. Two types of legal documents can be used: the advance directive, in which specific instructions from the pt may be made known; and the durable attorney for health care, in which a person is designated as having the pt's authority to make health decisions on the pt's behalf. Forms are available free of charge from the National Hospice and Palliative Care Organization (www.nhpco.org). Physicians also should complete these forms for themselves.

■ PHYSICAL SYMPTOMS AND THEIR MANAGEMENT

The most common physical and psychological symptoms among terminally ill pts are shown in Table 10-1. Studies of pts with advanced cancer have shown that pts experience an average of 11.5 symptoms.

Pain

Pain is noted in 36–90% of terminally ill pts. The various types of pain and their management are discussed in Chap. 6.

Constipation

Constipation is noted in up to 87% of terminally ill pts. Medications that commonly contribute to constipation include opioids used to manage pain and dyspnea and tricyclic antidepressants with their anticholinergic effects. Inactivity, poor diet, and hypercalcemia may contribute. GI tract obstruction also may play a role in some settings.

Interventions Improved physical activity (if possible), adequate hydration; opioid effects can be antagonized by the μ-opioid receptor blocker methyln-altrexone (8–12 mg SC daily); rule out surgically correctable obstruction; laxatives and stool softeners (Table 10-2).

TABLE 10-1 COMMON PHYSICAL AND PSYCHOLOGICAL SYMPTOMS OF TERMINALLY ILL PATIENTS

Physical Symptoms	Psychological Symptoms
Pain	Anxiety
Fatigue and weakness	Depression
Dyspnea	Hopelessness
Insomnia	Meaninglessness
Dry mouth	Irritability
Anorexia	Impaired concentration
Nausea and vomiting	Confusion
Constipation	Delirium
Cough	Loss of libido
Swelling of arms or legs	
Itching	
Diarrhea	
Dysphagia	
Dizziness	
Fecal and urinary incontinence	
Numbness/tingling in hands/feet	

Nausea

Up to 70% of pts with advanced cancer have nausea. Nausea may result from uremia, liver failure, hypercalcemia, bowel obstruction, severe constipation, infection, gastroesophageal reflux disease, vestibular disease, brain metastases, medications (cancer chemotherapy, antibiotics, nonsteroidal anti-inflammatory drugs, opioids, proton pump inhibitors), and radiation therapy.

Interventions Treatment should be tailored to the cause. Offending medications should be stopped. Underlying conditions should be alleviated, if possible. If decreased bowel motility is suspected, metoclopramide may help. Nausea from cancer chemotherapy agents can generally be prevented with glucocorticoids and serotonin receptor blockers like ondansetron or dolasetron. Aprepitant is useful in controlling nausea from highly emetogenic agents like cisplatin. Vestibular nausea may respond to antihistamines (meclizine) or anticholinergics (scopolamine). Anticipatory nausea may be prevented with a benzodiazepine such as lorazepam. Haloperidol is sometimes useful when the nausea does not have a single specific cause.

Dyspnea

Up to 75% of dying pts experience dyspnea. Dyspnea exerts perhaps the greatest adverse effect on the pt, often even more distressing than pain.

TABLE 10-2 MEDICATIONS FOR THE MANAGEMENT OF CONSTIPATION

Intervention	Dose	Comment
Stimulant laxatives		These agents directly stimulate peristalsis and may reduce colonic absorption of water.
Prune juice	120–240 mL/d	
Senna (Senokot)	2–8 tablets PO bid	Work in 6–12 h.
Bisacodyl	5–15 mg/d PO, PR	
Osmotic laxatives		These agents are not absorbed. They attract and retain water in the gastrointestinal tract.
Lactulose	15–30 mL PO q4–8h	Lactulose may cause flatulence and bloating.
Magnesium hydroxide (Milk of Magnesia)	15–30 mL/d PO	Lactulose works in 1 day, magnesium products in 6 h.
Magnesium citrate	125–250 mL/d PO	
Stool softeners		These agents work by increasing water secretion and as detergents, increasing water penetration into the stool.
Sodium docusate (Colace)	300–600 mg/d PO	
Calcium docusate	300–600 mg/d PO	
		Work in 1–3 days.
Suppositories and enemas		
Bisacodyl	10–15 PR qd	
Sodium phosphate enema	PR qd	Fixed dose, 4.5 oz, Fleet's.

It may be caused by parenchymal lung disease, infection, effusions, pulmonary emboli, pulmonary edema, asthma, or compressed airway. While many of the causes may be treated, often the underlying cause cannot be reversed.

Interventions Underlying causes should be reversed, where possible, as long as the intervention is not more unpleasant (e.g., repeated thoracenteses) than the dyspnea. Most often the treatment is symptomatic (Table 10-3).

Fatigue

Fatigue is nearly a universal symptom in terminally ill pts. It is often a direct consequence of the disease process (and the cytokines produced in response to that process) and may be complicated by inanition, dehydration, anemia, infection, hypothyroidism, and drug effects. Depression may also contribute to fatigue. Functional assessments include the Karnofsky performance

TABLE 10-3 MEDICATIONS FOR THE MANAGEMENT OF DYSPNEA

Intervention	Dose	Comments
Weak opioids		For pts with mild dyspnea
Codeine (or codeine with 325 mg acetaminophen)	30 mg PO q4h	For opioid-naïve pts
Hydrocodone	5 mg PO q4h	
Strong opioids		For opioid-naïve pts with moderate to severe dyspnea
Morphine	5–10 mg PO q4h	For pts already taking opioids for pain or other symptoms
	30–50% of baseline opioid dose q4h	
Oxycodone	5–10 mg PO q4h	
Hydromorphone	1–2 mg PO q4h	
Anxiolytics		Give a dose every hour until the pt is relaxed, then provide a dose for maintenance
Lorazepam	0.5–2.0 mg PO/SL/IV qh then q4–6h	
Clonazepam	0.25–2.0 mg PO q12h	
Midazolam	0.5 mg IV q15min	

status or the Eastern Cooperative Oncology Group system based on how much time the pt spends in bed each day: 0, normal activity; 1, symptomatic without being bedridden; 2, in bed <50% of the day; 3, in bed >50% of the day; 4, bedbound.

Interventions Modest exercise and physical therapy may reduce muscle wasting and depression and improve mood; discontinue medications that worsen fatigue, if possible; glucocorticoids may increase energy and enhance mood; dextroamphetamine (5–10 mg/d) or methylphenidate (2.5–5 mg/d) in the morning may enhance energy levels but should be avoided at night because they may produce insomnia; modafinil and L-carnitine have shown some early promise.

Depression

Up to 75% of terminally ill pts experience depression. The inexperienced physician may feel that depression is an appropriate response to terminal illness; however, in a substantial fraction of pts the depression is more intense and disabling than usual. Pts with a previous history of depression are at greater risk. A number of treatable conditions can cause depression-like symptoms including hypothyroidism, Cushing's syndrome, electrolyte abnormalities (e.g., hypercalcemia), and drugs including dopamine blockers, interferon, tamoxifen, interleukin 2, vincristine, and glucocorticoids.

Interventions Dextroamphetamine or methylphenidate (see above); serotonin reuptake inhibitors such as fluoxetine, paroxetine, and citalopram; modafinil 100 mg/d; pemoline 18.75 mg in the A.M. and at noon.

Delirium

Delirium is a global cerebral dysfunction associated with altered cognition and consciousness; it is frequently preceded by anxiety. Unlike dementia, it is of sudden onset, is characterized by fluctuating consciousness and inattention, and may be reversible. It is generally manifested in the hours before death. It may be caused by metabolic encephalopathy in renal or liver failure, hypoxemia, infection, hypercalcemia, paraneoplastic syndromes, dehydration, constipation, urinary retention, and central nervous system spread of cancer. It is also a common medication side effect; offending agents include those commonly used in dying pts including opioids, glucocorticoids, anticholinergics, antihistamines, antiemetics, and benzodiazepines. Early recognition is key because the pt should be encouraged to use the periods of lucidity for final communication with loved ones. Day-night reversal with changes in mentation may be an early sign.

Interventions Stop any and all unnecessary medications that may have this side effect; provide a calendar, clock, newspaper, or other orienting signals; gently correct hallucinations or cognitive mistakes; pharmacologic interventions are shown in Table 10-4.

■ CARE DURING THE LAST HOURS

The clinical course of a dying pt may largely be predictable. Figure 10-1 shows common and uncommon changes during the last days of life.

TABLE 10-4 MEDICATIONS FOR THE MANAGEMENT OF DELIRIUM

Interventions	Dose
Neuroleptics	
Haloperidol	0.5–5 mg q2–12h, PO/IV/SC/IM
Thioridazine	10–75 mg q4–8h, PO
Chlorpromazine	12.5–50 mg q4–12h, PO/IV/IM
Atypical neuroleptics	
Olanzapine	2.5–5 mg qd or bid, PO
Risperidone	1–3 mg q12h, PO
Anxiolytics	
Lorazepam	0.5–2 mg q1–4h, PO/IV/IM
Midazolam	1–5 mg/h continuous infusion, IV/SC
Anesthetics	
Propofol	0.3–2.0 mg/h continuous infusion, IV

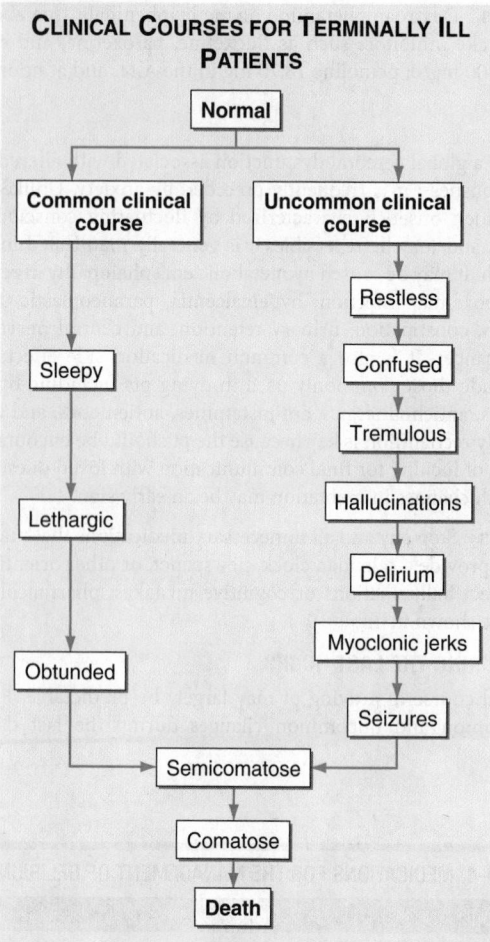

CLINICAL COURSES FOR TERMINALLY ILL PATIENTS

```
                    Normal
                      │
        ┌─────────────┴─────────────┐
        │                           │
 Common clinical            Uncommon clinical
    course                      course
        │                           │
        │                        Restless
        │                           │
     Sleepy                      Confused
        │                           │
        │                        Tremulous
        │                           │
    Lethargic                  Hallucinations
        │                           │
        │                        Delirium
        │                           │
     Obtunded                Myoclonic jerks
        │                           │
        │                         Seizures
        │                           │
        └────► Semicomatose ◄───────┘
                      │
                  Comatose
                      │
                    Death
```

FIGURE 10-1 Common and uncommon clinical courses in the last days of terminally ill pts. (*Adapted from FD Ferris et al: Module 4: Palliative care, in Comprehensive Guide for the Care of Persons with HIV Disease. Toronto: Mt. Sinai Hospital and Casey Hospice, 1995, www.cpsonline.info/content/resources/hivmodule/module4complete.pdf.*)

Informing families that these changes might occur can help minimize the distress that they cause. In particular, the physician needs to be sensitive to the sense of guilt and helplessness that family members feel. They should be reassured that the illness is taking its course and their care of the pt is not at fault in any way. The pt stops eating because they are dying; they are not dying because they have stopped eating. Families and caregivers should be encouraged to communicate directly with the dying pt whether or not the pt is unconscious. Holding the pt's hand may be a source of comfort to both the pt and the family member/caregiver. Table 10-5 provides a listing

TABLE 10-5 MANAGING CHANGES IN THE PATIENT'S CONDITION DURING THE FINAL DAYS AND HOURS

Changes in the Patient's Condition	Potential Complication	Family's Possible Reaction and Concern	Advice and Intervention
Profound fatigue	Bedbound with development of pressure ulcers that are prone to infection, malodor, and pain, and joint pain	Pt is lazy and giving up.	Reassure family and caregivers that terminal fatigue will not respond to interventions and should not be resisted. Use an air mattress if necessary.
Anorexia	None	Pt is giving up; pt will suffer from hunger and will starve to death.	Reassure family and caregivers that the pt is not eating because he or she is dying; not eating at the end of life does not cause suffering or death. Forced feeding, whether oral, parenteral, or enteral, does not reduce symptoms or prolong life.
Dehydration	Dry mucosal membranes (see below)	Pt will suffer from thirst and die of dehydration.	Reassure family and caregivers that dehydration at the end of life does not cause suffering because pts lose consciousness before any symptom distress. IV hydration can worsen symptoms of dyspnea by pulmonary edema and peripheral edema as well as prolong dying process.
Dysphagia	Inability to swallow oral medications needed for palliative care		Do not force oral intake. Discontinue unnecessary medications that may have been continued, including antibiotics, diuretics, antidepressants, and laxatives. If swallowing pills is difficult, convert essential medications (analgesics, antiemetics, anxiolytics, and psychotropics) to oral solutions, buccal, sublingual, or rectal administration.

(continued)

TABLE 10-5 MANAGING CHANGES IN THE PATIENT'S CONDITION DURING THE FINAL DAYS AND HOURS (CONTINUED)

Changes in the Patient's Condition	Potential Complication	Family's Possible Reaction and Concern	Advice and Intervention
"Death rattle"—noisy breathing		Pt is choking and suffocating.	Reassure the family and caregivers that this is caused by secretions in the oropharynx and the pt is not choking.
			Reduce secretions with scopolamine (0.2–0.4 mg SC q4h or 1–3 patches q3d).
			Reposition pt to permit drainage of secretions.
			Do not suction. Suction can cause pt and family discomfort and is usually ineffective.
Apnea, Cheyne-Stokes respirations, dyspnea		Pt is suffocating.	Reassure family and caregivers that unconscious pts do not experience suffocation or air hunger.
			Apneic episodes are frequently a premorbid change.
			Opioids or anxiolytics may be used for dyspnea.
			Oxygen is unlikely to relieve dyspneic symptoms and may prolong the dying process.
Urinary or fecal incontinence	Skin breakdown if days until death	Pt is dirty, malodorous, and physically repellent.	Remind family and caregivers to use universal precautions.
	Potential transmission of infectious agents to caregivers		Frequent changes of bedclothes and bedding.
			Use diapers, urinary catheter, or rectal tube if diarrhea or high urine output.

TABLE 10-5 MANAGING CHANGES IN THE PATIENT'S CONDITION DURING THE FINAL DAYS AND HOURS (CONTINUED)

Changes in the Patient's Condition	Potential Complication	Family's Possible Reaction and Concern	Advice and Intervention
Agitation or delirium	Day/night reversal	Pt is in horrible pain and going to have a horrible death.	Reassure family and caregivers that agitation and delirium do not necessarily connote physical pain.
	Hurt self or caregivers		Depending on the prognosis and goals of treatment, consider evaluating for causes of delirium and modify medications.
			Manage symptoms with haloperidol, chlorpromazine, diazepam, or midazolam.
Dry mucosal membranes	Cracked lips, mouth sores, and candidiasis can also cause pain.	Pt may be malodorous, physically repellent.	Use baking soda mouthwash or saliva preparation q15–30min.
	Odor		Use topical nystatin for candidiasis.
			Coat lips and nasal mucosa with petroleum jelly q60–90min.
			Use ophthalmic lubricants q4h or artificial tears q30min.

of some changes in the pt's condition in the final hours and advice on how to manage the changes.

Additional resources for managing terminally ill pts may be found at the following websites: www.epec.net, www.eperc.mcw.edu, www.capc.org, and www.nhpco.org.

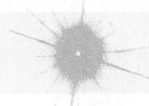

For a more detailed discussion, see Emanuel EJ: Palliative and End-of-Life Care, Chap. 9, p. 67, in HPIM-18.

CHAPTER 11
Cardiovascular Collapse and Sudden Death

Unexpected cardiovascular collapse and death most often result from ventricular fibrillation in pts with acute or chronic atherosclerotic coronary artery disease. Other common etiologies are listed in Table 11-1. Arrhythmic causes may be provoked by electrolyte disorders (primarily hypokalemia), hypoxemia, acidosis, or massive sympathetic discharge, as may occur in CNS injury. Immediate institution of cardiopulmonary resuscitation (CPR) followed by advanced life support measures (see below) is mandatory. Ventricular fibrillation, or asystole, without institution of CPR within 4–6 min is usually fatal.

TABLE 11-1 CARDIAC ARREST AND SUDDEN CARDIAC DEATH

Structural Associations and Causes

I. Coronary heart disease (chronic, or acute coronary syndromes)

II. Myocardial hypertrophy (e.g., hypertrophic cardiomyopathy)

III. Dilated cardiomyopathy

IV. Inflammatory (e.g., myocarditis) and infiltrative disorders

V. Valvular heart diseases

VI. Electrophysiologic abnormalities (e.g., Wolff-Parkinson-White syndrome)

VII. Inherited disorders associated with electrophysiological abnormalities (e.g., congenital long QT syndromes, right ventricular dysplasia, Brugada syndrome, catecholaminergic polymorphic ventricular tachycardia)

Functional Contributing Factors

I. Transient ischemia

II. Low cardiac output states (heart failure, shock)

III. Systemic metabolic abnormalities

    A. Electrolyte imbalance (e.g., hypokalemia)

    B. Hypoxemia, acidosis

IV. Neurologic disturbances (e.g., CNS injury)

V. Toxic responses

    A. Proarrhythmic drug effects

    B. Cardiac toxins (e.g., cocaine, digitalis intoxication)

■ MANAGEMENT OF CARDIAC ARREST

Basic life support (BLS) must commence immediately (Fig. 11-1):

1. Phone emergency line (e.g., 911); retrieve automated external defibrillator (AED) if quickly available.
2. If respiratory stridor is present, assess for aspiration of a foreign body and perform Heimlich maneuver.
3. Perform chest compressions (depressing sternum 4–5 cm) at rate of 100 per min without interruption. A second rescuer should attach and utilize AED if available.

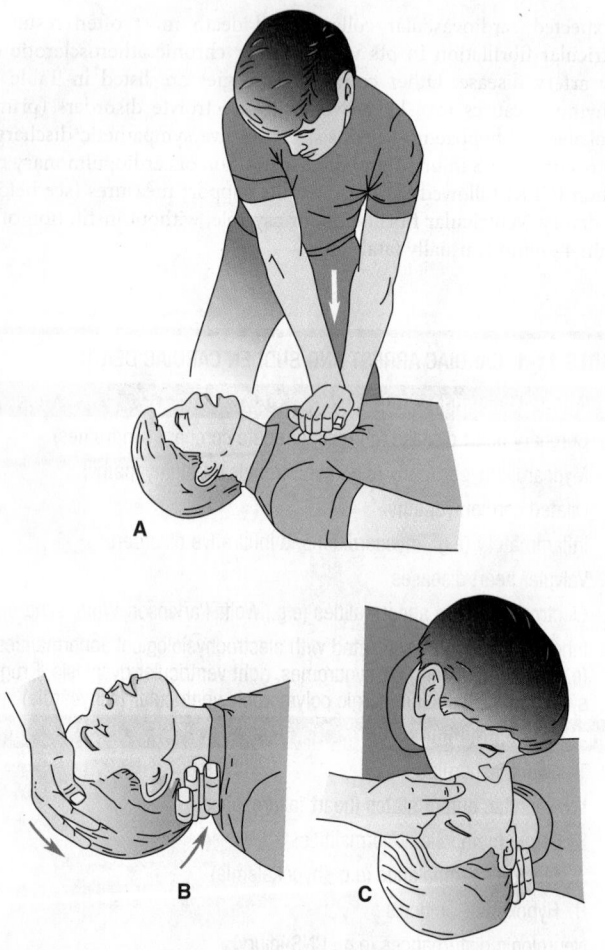

FIGURE 11-1 Major steps in cardiopulmonary resuscitation. **A.** Begin cardiac compressions at 100 compressions/min. **B.** Confirm that victim has an open airway. **C.** Trained rescuers begin mouth-to-mouth resuscitation if advanced life support equipment is not available. (*Modified from J Henderson,* Emergency Medical Guide, *4th ed, New York, McGraw-Hill, 1978.*)

4. If second trained rescuer available, tilt pt's head backward, lift chin, and begin mouth-to-mouth respiration (pocket mask is preferable to prevent transmission of infection), while chest compressions continue. The lungs should be inflated twice in rapid succession for every 30 chest compressions. For untrained lay rescuers, chest compression only, without ventilation, is recommended until advanced life support capability arrives.

5. As soon as resuscitation equipment is available, begin **advanced life support** with continued chest compressions and ventilation. Although performed as simultaneously as possible, defibrillation (≥300 J monophasic, or 120–150 J biphasic) takes highest priority (Fig. 11-2), followed by placement of IV access and intubation. 100% O_2 should be administered

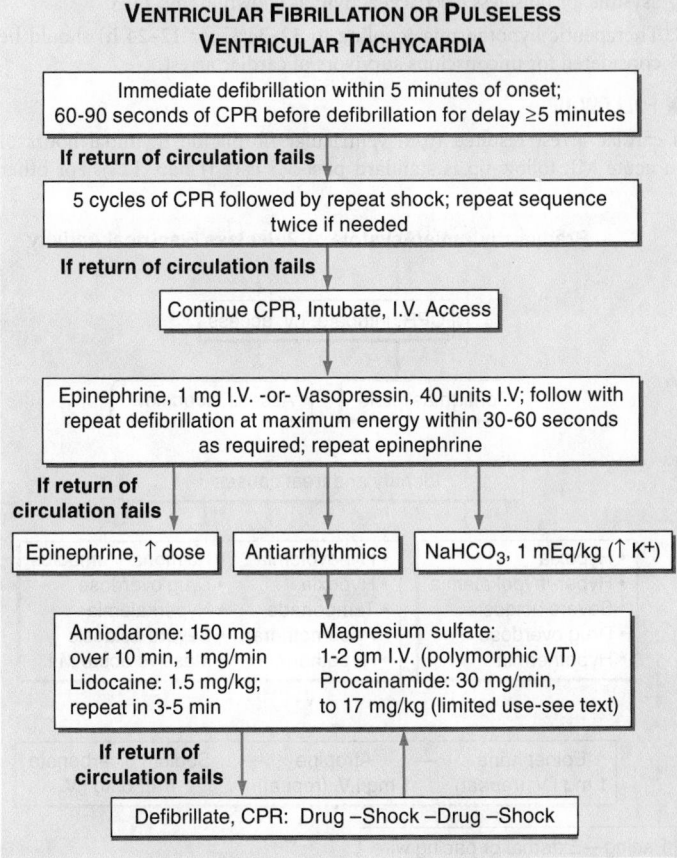

FIGURE 11-2 Management of cardiac arrest. The algorithm of ventricular fibrillation or hypotensive ventricular tachycardia begins with defibrillation attempts. If that fails, it is followed by epinephrine or vasopressin and then antiarrhythmic drugs. CPR, cardiopulmonary resuscitation. *[Modified from Myerburg R. and Castellanos A. Chap. 23, HPIM-18.]*

by endotracheal tube or, if rapid intubation cannot be accomplished, by bag-valve-mask device; respirations should not be interrupted for more than 30 s while attempting to intubate.

6. Initial IV access should be through the antecubital vein, but if drug administration is ineffective, a central line (internal jugular or subclavian) should be placed. IV NaHCO$_3$ should be administered only if there is persistent severe acidosis (pH <7.15) despite adequate ventilation. Calcium is not routinely administered but should be given to pts with known hypocalcemia, those who have received toxic doses of calcium channel antagonists, or if acute hyperkalemia is thought to be the triggering event for resistant ventricular fibrillation.

7. The approach to cardiovascular collapse caused by bradyarrhythmias, asystole, or pulseless electrical activity is shown in Fig. 11-3.

8. Therapeutic hypothermia (cooling to 32–34°C for 12–24 h) should be considered for unconscious survivors of cardiac arrest.

■ FOLLOW-UP

If cardiac arrest resulted from ventricular fibrillation in initial hours of an acute MI, follow-up is standard post-MI care (Chap. 128). For other

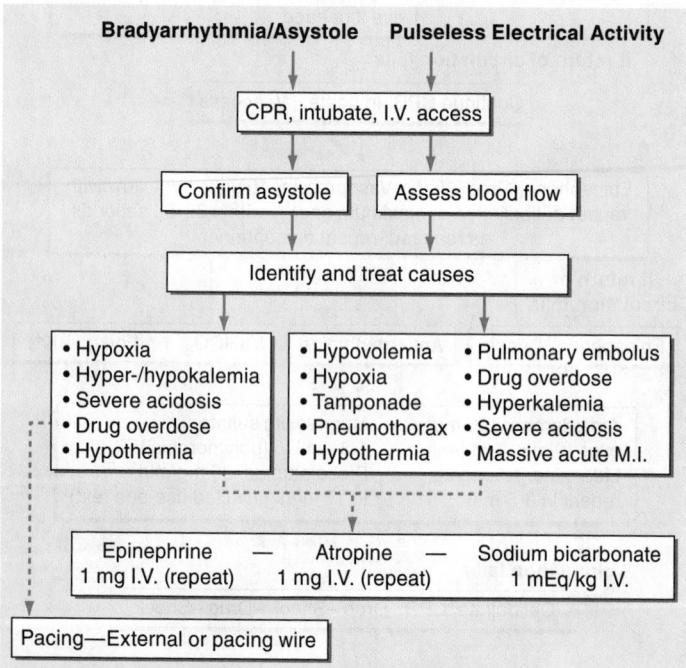

FIGURE 11-3 The algorithms for bradyarrhythmia/asystole (left) or pulseless electrical activity (right) are dominated first by continued life support and a search for reversible causes. CPR, cardiopulmonary resuscitation; MI, myocardial infarction. [Modified from Myerburg R. and Castellanos A. Chap. 23, HPIM-18.]

survivors of a ventricular fibrillation arrest, further assessment, including evaluation of coronary anatomy, and left ventricular function, is typically recommended. In absence of a transient or reversible cause, placement of an implantable cardioverter defibrillator is usually indicated.

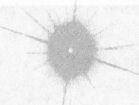

> For a more detailed discussion, see Myerburg RJ, Castellanos A: Cardiovascular Collapse, Cardiac Arrest, and Sudden Cardiac Death, Chap. 273, p. 2238, in HPIM-18.

CHAPTER **12**
Shock

■ DEFINITION
Condition of severe impairment of tissue perfusion leading to cellular injury and dysfunction. Rapid recognition and treatment are essential to prevent irreversible organ damage and death. Common causes are listed in Table 12-1.

■ CLINICAL MANIFESTATIONS
- Hypotension (mean arterial bp <60 mmHg), tachycardia, tachypnea, pallor, restlessness, and altered sensorium.
- Signs of intense peripheral vasoconstriction, with weak pulses and cold clammy extremities. In distributive (e.g., septic) shock, vasodilatation predominates and extremities are warm.
- Oliguria (<20 mL/h) and metabolic acidosis common.
- Acute lung injury and acute respiratory distress syndrome (ARDS; see Chap. 15) with noncardiogenic pulmonary edema, hypoxemia, and diffuse pulmonary infiltrates.

APPROACH TO THE PATIENT | Shock

Obtain history for underlying causes, including cardiac disease (coronary disease, heart failure, pericardial disease), recent fever or infection leading to sepsis, drug effects (e.g., excess diuretics or antihypertensives), conditions leading to pulmonary embolism (Chap. 142), potential sources of bleeding.

■ PHYSICAL EXAMINATION
Jugular veins are flat in oligemic or distributive (septic) shock; jugular venous distention (JVD) suggests cardiogenic shock; JVD in presence of paradoxical pulse (Chap. 119) may reflect cardiac tamponade (Chap. 125). Check for asymmetry of pulses (aortic dissection—Chap. 134). Assess for evidence of

TABLE 12-1 COMMON FORMS OF SHOCK

Oligemic shock
  Hemorrhage
  Volume depletion (e.g., vomiting, diarrhea, diuretic overusage, ketoacidosis)
  Internal sequestration (ascites, pancreatitis, intestinal obstruction)
Cardiogenic shock
  Myopathic (acute MI, dilated cardiomyopathy)
  Mechanical (acute mitral regurgitation, ventricular septal defect, severe aortic stenosis)
  Arrhythmic
Extracardiac obstructive shock
  Pericardial tamponade
  Massive pulmonary embolism
  Tension pneumothorax
Distributive shock (profound decrease in systemic vascular tone)
  Sepsis
  Toxic overdoses
  Anaphylaxis
  Neurogenic (e.g., spinal cord injury)
  Endocrinologic (Addison's disease, myxedema)

heart failure (Chap. 133), murmurs of aortic stenosis, acute mitral or aortic regurgitation, ventricular septal defect. Tenderness or rebound in abdomen may indicate peritonitis or pancreatitis; high-pitched bowel sounds suggest intestinal obstruction. Perform stool guaiac to rule out GI bleeding.

Fever and chills typically accompany septic shock. Sepsis may not cause fever in elderly, uremic, or alcoholic pts. Skin lesions may suggest specific pathogens in septic shock: petechiae or purpura (*Neisseria meningitidis* or *Haemophilus influenzae*), ecthyma gangrenosum (*Pseudomonas aeruginosa*), generalized erythroderma (toxic shock due to *Staphylococcus aureus* or *Streptococcus pyogenes*).

■ **LABORATORY**

Obtain hematocrit, WBC, electrolytes, platelet count, PT, PTT, DIC screen, electrolytes. Arterial blood gas usually shows metabolic acidosis (in septic shock, respiratory alkalosis precedes metabolic acidosis). If sepsis suspected, draw blood cultures, perform urinalysis, and obtain Gram stain and cultures of sputum, urine, and other suspected sites.

Obtain ECG (myocardial ischemia or acute arrhythmia), chest x-ray (heart failure, tension pneumothorax, pneumonia). Echocardiogram is often helpful (cardiac tamponade, left/right ventricular dysfunction, aortic dissection).

TABLE 12-2 PHYSIOLOGIC CHARACTERISTICS OF FORMS OF SHOCK

Type of Shock	CVP and PCWP	Cardiac Output	Systemic Vascular Resistance	Venous O_2 Saturation
Hypovolemic	↓	↓	↑	↓
Cardiogenic	↑	↓	↑	↓
Septic				
Hyperdynamic	↓↑	↑	↓	↑
Hypodynamic	↓↑	↓	↓	↑↓
Traumatic	↓	↓↑	↑↓	↓
Neurogenic	↓	↓	↓	↓
Hypoadrenal	↓↑	↓	=↓	↓

Abbreviations: CVP, central venous pressure; PCWP, pulmonary capillary wedge pressure.

Central venous pressure or pulmonary capillary wedge (PCW) pressure measurements may be necessary to distinguish between different categories of shock (Table 12-2): Mean PCW <6 mmHg suggests oligemic or distributive shock; PCW >20 mmHg suggests left ventricular failure. Cardiac output (thermodilution) is decreased in cardiogenic and oligemic shock, and usually increased initially in septic shock.

TREATMENT Shock (See Fig. 12-1).

Aimed at rapid improvement of tissue hypoperfusion and respiratory impairment:

- Serial measurements of bp (intraarterial line preferred), heart rate, continuous ECG monitor, urine output, pulse oximetry, blood studies: Hct, electrolytes, creatinine, BUN, ABGs, pH, calcium, phosphate, lactate, urine Na concentration (<20 mmol/L suggests volume depletion). Consider monitoring of CVP and/or pulmonary artery pressure/ PCW pressures in pts with ongoing blood loss or suspected cardiac dysfunction.
- Insert Foley catheter to monitor urine flow.
- Assess mental status frequently.
- Augment systolic bp to >100 mmHg: (1) place in reverse Trendelenburg position; (2) IV volume infusion (500- to 1000-mL bolus), unless cardiogenic shock suspected (begin with normal saline or Ringer's lactate, then whole blood, or packed RBCs, if anemic); continue volume replacement as needed to restore vascular volume.
- Add vasoactive drugs after intravascular volume is optimized; administer vasopressors (Table 12-3) if systemic vascular resistance (SVR) is decreased (begin with norepinephrine [preferred] or dopamine; for persistent hypotension add phenylephrine or vasopressin).

- If CHF present, add inotropic agents (usually dobutamine) (Table 12-3); aim to maintain cardiac index >2.2(L/m²)/min [>4.0(L/m²)/min in septic shock].
- Administer 100% O_2; intubate with mechanical ventilation if Po_2 <70 mmHg.
- If severe metabolic acidosis present (pH <7.15), administer $NaHCO_3$.
- Identify and treat underlying cause of shock. Cardiogenic shock in acute MI is discussed in Chap. 128. Emergent coronary revascularization may be lifesaving if persistent ischemia is present.

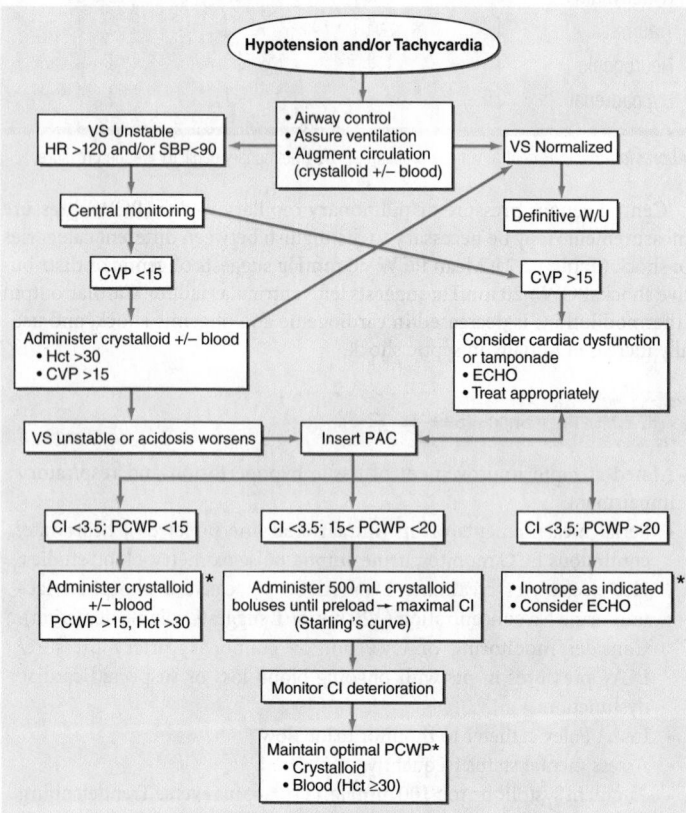

FIGURE 12-1 An algorithm for the resuscitation of the pt in shock. *Monitor Svo_2, SVRI, and RVEDVI as additional markers of correction for perfusion and hypovolemia. Consider age-adjusted CI. Svo_2, saturation of hemoglobin with O_2 in venous blood; SVRI, systemic vascular resistance index; RVEDVI, right-ventricular end-diastolic volume index. CI, cardiac index in (L/min) per m²; CVP, central venous pressure; ECHO, echocardiogram; Hct, hematocrit; HR, heart rate; PAC, pulmonary artery catheter; PCWP, pulmonary capillary wedge pressure in mmHg; SBP, systolic blood pressure; VS, vital signs; W/U, work up.

TABLE 12-3 VASOPRESSORS USED IN SHOCK STATES[a]

Drug	Dose	Notes
Dopamine	1–2 µg/kg per min	Facilitates diuresis
	2–10 µg/kg per min	Positive inotropic and chronotropic effects; may increase O_2 consumption as well as O_2 delivery; use may be limited by tachycardia
	10–20 µg/kg per min	Generalized vasoconstriction (decrease renal perfusion)
Norepinephrine	0.5–30 µg/min	Potent vasoconstrictor; moderate inotropic effect; in septic shock is thought to increase tissue O_2 consumption as well as O_2 delivery; may be chosen over dopamine in sepsis due to less chronotropic and adverse effects; may be useful in cardiogenic shock with reduced SVR but should generally be reserved for refractory hypotension
Dobutamine	2–20 µg/kg per min	Primarily for cardiogenic shock (Chap. 128): positive inotrope; lacks vasoconstrictor activity; most useful when only mild hypotension present and avoidance of tachycardia desired
Phenylephrine	40–180 µg/min	Potent vasoconstrictor without inotropic effect; may be useful in distributive (septic) shock
Vasopressin	0.01–0.04 U/min	Occasionally used in refractory septic (distributive) shock; restores vascular tone in vasopressin-deficient states (e.g., sepsis)

[a]Isoproterenol not recommended in shock states because of potential hypotension and arrhythmogenic effects.

Abbreviation: SVR, systemic vascular resistance.

SEPTIC SHOCK (SEE CHAP. 13)

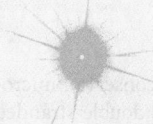

For a more detailed discussion, see Maier RV: Approach to the Patient With Shock, Chap. 270, p. 2215, and Hochman JS, Ingbar DH: Cardiogenic Shock and Pulmonary Edema, Chap. 272, p. 2232, in HPIM-18.

CHAPTER **13**
Sepsis and Septic Shock

■ DEFINITIONS

- *Systemic inflammatory response syndrome (SIRS)*—Two or more of the following:
  - Fever (oral temperature >38°C) or hypothermia (oral temperature <36°C)
  - Tachypnea (>24 breaths/min)
  - Tachycardia (>90 beats/min)
  - Leukocytosis (>12,000/μL), leukopenia (<4000/μL), or >10% bands; may have a noninfectious etiology
- *Sepsis*—SIRS with a proven or suspected microbial etiology
- *Severe sepsis*—Sepsis with one or more signs of organ dysfunction
- *Septic shock*—Sepsis with hypotension (arterial blood pressure <90 mmHg or 40 mmHg below pt's normal blood pressure for at least 1 h despite fluid resuscitation) or need for vasopressors to maintain systolic blood pressure ≥90 mmHg or mean arterial pressure ≥70 mmHg

■ ETIOLOGY

- Blood cultures are positive in 20–40% of sepsis cases and in 40–70% of septic shock cases.
- A single bacterial species accounts for ~70% of isolates in positive blood cultures; the remainder are fungal or polymicrobial.

■ EPIDEMIOLOGY

- The incidence of severe sepsis and septic shock in the United States continues to increase, with >700,000 cases each year contributing to >200,000 deaths.
- Invasive bacterial infections are a prominent cause of death around the world, especially among young children.
- Sepsis-related incidence and mortality rates increase with age and preexisting comorbidity, with two-thirds of cases occurring in pts with significant underlying disease.
- The increasing incidence of sepsis is attributable to the aging of the population, longer survival of pts with chronic diseases, a relatively high frequency of sepsis among AIDS pts, and medical treatments that circumvent host defenses (e.g., immunosuppressive agents, indwelling catheters, and mechanical devices).

■ PATHOPHYSIOLOGY

Local and Systemic Host Responses

- Hosts have numerous receptors that recognize highly conserved microbial molecules (e.g., lipopolysaccharide, lipoproteins, double-stranded RNA), triggering the release of cytokines and other host molecules

that increase blood flow and neutrophil migration to the infected site, enhance local vascular permeability, and elicit pain.
- Many local and systemic control mechanisms diminish cellular responses to microbial molecules, including intravascular thrombosis (which prevents spread of infection and inflammation) and an increase in anti-inflammatory cytokines (e.g., IL-4 and IL-10).

Organ Dysfunction and Shock

- Widespread vascular endothelial injury is believed to be the major mechanism for multiorgan dysfunction.
- Septic shock is characterized by compromised oxygen delivery to tissues followed by a vasodilatory phase (a decrease in peripheral vascular resistance despite increased levels of vasopressor catecholamines).

■ CLINICAL FEATURES

- Hyperventilation
- Encephalopathy (disorientation, confusion)
- Acrocyanosis and ischemic necrosis of peripheral tissues (e.g., digits) due to hypotension and DIC
- Skin: hemorrhagic lesions, bullae, cellulitis, pustules. Skin lesions may suggest specific pathogens—e.g., petechiae and purpura suggest *Neisseria meningitidis*, and ecthyma gangrenosum suggests *Pseudomonas aeruginosa*.
- Gastrointestinal: nausea, vomiting, diarrhea, ileus, cholestatic jaundice

Major Complications

- *Cardiopulmonary manifestations*
  - Ventilation-perfusion mismatch, increased alveolar capillary permeability, increased pulmonary water content, and decreased pulmonary compliance impede oxygen exchange and lead to acute respiratory distress syndrome (progressive diffuse pulmonary infiltrates and arterial hypoxemia) in ~50% of pts.
  - Hypotension: Normal or increased cardiac output and decreased systemic vascular resistance distinguish septic shock from cardiogenic and hypovolemic shock.
  - The ejection fraction is decreased, but ventricular dilatation allows maintenance of a normal stroke volume.
- *Adrenal insufficiency:* May be difficult to diagnose in critically ill pts.
- *Renal manifestations*: oliguria or polyuria, azotemia, proteinuria, and renal failure due to acute tubular necrosis
- *Coagulopathy*: thrombocytopenia
- *Neurologic manifestations*: polyneuropathy with distal motor weakness in prolonged sepsis
- *Immunosuppression*: Pts may have reactivation of HSV, CMV, or VZV.

Laboratory Findings

- *CBC:* leukocytosis with a left shift, thrombocytopenia
- *Coagulation*: prolonged thrombin time, decreased fibrinogen, presence of D-dimers, suggestive of DIC. With DIC, platelet counts usually fall below 50,000/μL.

- *Chemistries:* metabolic acidosis, elevated anion gap, elevated lactate levels
- *LFTs:* transaminitis, hyperbilirubinemia, azotemia, hypoalbuminemia

■ DIAGNOSIS

Definitive diagnosis requires isolation of the microorganism from blood or a local site of infection. Culture of infected cutaneous lesions may help establish the diagnosis.

TREATMENT Sepsis and Septic Shock

Pts in whom sepsis is suspected must be managed expeditiously, if possible within 1 h of presentation.

1. Antibiotic treatment: See Table 13-1.
2. Removal or drainage of a focal source of infection
   a. Remove indwelling intravascular catheters; replace Foley and other drainage catheters; drain local sources of infection.
   b. Rule out sinusitis in pts with nasal intubation.
   c. Image the chest, abdomen, and/or pelvis to evaluate for abscess.
3. Hemodynamic, respiratory, and metabolic support
   a. Initiate treatment with 1–2 L of normal saline administered over 1–2 h, keeping the central venous pressure at 8–12 cmH$_2$O, urine output at >0.5 mL/kg per hour, and mean arterial blood pressure at >65 mmHg. Add vasopressor therapy if needed.
   b. If hypotension does not respond to fluid replacement therapy, hydrocortisone (50 mg IV q6h) should be given. If clinical improvement results within 24–48 h, most experts would continue hydrocortisone treatment for 5–7 days.
   c. Maintain oxygenation with ventilator support as indicated. Recent studies favor the use of low tidal volumes—typically 6 mL/kg of ideal body weight—provided the plateau pressure is ≤30 cmH$_2$O.
   d. Erythrocyte transfusion is recommended when the blood hemoglobin level decreases to ≤7 g/dL, with a target level of 9 g/dL.
4. Recombinant activated protein C (aPC) has been approved for treatment of severe sepsis or septic shock in pts with APACHE II scores of ≥25 prior to aPC infusion; however, given the increased risk of severe bleeding and uncertain performance in clinical practice, many experts are awaiting the results of additional trials before recommending further use of aPC.
5. General support: Nutritional supplementation should be given to pts with prolonged sepsis (i.e., that lasting >2–3 days), with available evidence suggesting an enteral delivery route. Prophylactic heparin should be administered to prevent deep-venous thrombosis if no active bleeding or coagulopathy is present. Insulin should be used to maintain the blood glucose concentration below ~150 mg/dL.

TABLE 13-1 INITIAL ANTIMICROBIAL THERAPY FOR SEVERE SEPSIS WITH NO OBVIOUS SOURCE IN ADULTS WITH NORMAL RENAL FUNCTION

Clinical Condition	Antimicrobial Regimens (IV Therapy)
Immunocompetent adult	The many acceptable regimens include (1) piperacillin-tazobactam (3.375 g q4–6h); (2) imipenem-cilastatin (0.5 g q6h) or meropenem (1 g q8h); or (3) cefepime (2 g q12h). If the pt is allergic to β-lactam agents, use ciprofloxacin (400 mg q12h) or levofloxacin (500–750 mg q12h) plus clindamycin (600 mg q8h). Vancomycin (15 mg/kg q12h) should be added to each of the above regimens.
Neutropenia (<500 neutrophils/μL)	Regimens include (1) imipenem-cilastatin (0.5 g q6h) or meropenem (1 g q8h) or cefepime (2 g q8h); (2) piperacillin-tazobactam (3.375 g q4h) plus tobramycin (5–7 mg/kg q24h). Vancomycin (15 mg/kg q12h) should be added if the pt has an indwelling vascular catheter, has received quinolone prophylaxis, or has received intensive chemotherapy that produces mucosal damage; if staphylococci are suspected; if the institution has a high incidence of MRSA infections; or if there is a high prevalence of MRSA isolates in the community. Empirical antifungal therapy with an echinocandin (for caspofungin: a 70-mg loading dose, then 50 mg daily) or a lipid formulation of amphotericin B should be added if the pt is hypotensive or has been receiving broad-spectrum antibacterial drugs.
Splenectomy	Cefotaxime (2 g q6–8h) or ceftriaxone (2 g q12h) should be used. If the local prevalence of cephalosporin-resistant pneumococci is high, add vancomycin. If the pt is allergic to β-lactam drugs, vancomycin (15 mg/kg q12h) plus either moxifloxacin (400 mg q24h) or levofloxacin (750 mg q24h) or aztreonam (2 g q8h) should be used.
IV drug user	Vancomycin (15 mg/kg q12h)
AIDS	Cefepime (2 g q8h) or piperacillin-tazobactam (3.375 g q4h) plus tobramycin (5–7 mg/kg q24h) should be used. If the pt is allergic to β-lactam drugs, ciprofloxacin (400 mg q12h) or levofloxacin (750 mg q12h) plus vancomycin (15 mg/kg q12h) plus tobramycin should be used.

Abbreviation: MRSA, methicillin-resistant *Staphylococcus aureus*.
Sources: Adapted in part from WT Hughes et al: Clin Infect Dis 25:551, 1997; and DN Gilbert et al: The Sanford Guide to Antimicrobial Therapy, 2009.

■ PROGNOSIS

In all, 20–35% of pts with severe sepsis and 40–60% of pts with septic shock die within 30 days, and further deaths occur within 6 months. Prognostic stratification systems (e.g., APACHE II) can estimate the risk of dying of severe sepsis.

■ PREVENTION

Nosocomial infections cause most episodes of severe sepsis and septic shock in the United States. Measures to reduce those infections could reduce the incidence of sepsis.

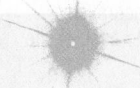

> For a more detailed discussion, see Munford RS: Severe Sepsis and Septic Shock, Chap. 271, p. 2223, in HPIM-18.

CHAPTER **14**
Acute Pulmonary Edema

Life-threatening, acute development of alveolar lung edema due to one or more of the following:

1. Elevation of hydrostatic pressure in the pulmonary capillaries (left heart failure, mitral stenosis)
2. Specific precipitants (Table 14-1), resulting in cardiogenic pulmonary edema in pts with previously compensated heart failure or without previous cardiac history
3. Increased permeability of pulmonary alveolar-capillary membrane (noncardiogenic pulmonary edema). For common causes, see Table 14-2.

TABLE 14-1 PRECIPITANTS OF ACUTE PULMONARY EDEMA

Acute tachy- or bradyarrhythmia

Infection, fever

Acute MI

Severe hypertension

Acute mitral or aortic regurgitation

Increased circulating volume (Na+ ingestion, blood transfusion, pregnancy)

Increased metabolic demands (exercise, hyperthyroidism)

Pulmonary embolism

Noncompliance (sudden discontinuation) of chronic CHF medications

TABLE 14-2 COMMON CAUSES OF NONCARDIOGENIC PULMONARY EDEMA

Direct Injury to Lung	
Chest trauma, pulmonary contusion	Pneumonia
Aspiration	Oxygen toxicity
Smoke inhalation	Pulmonary embolism, reperfusion
Hematogenous Injury to Lung	
Sepsis	Multiple transfusions
Pancreatitis	IV drug use, e.g., heroin
Nonthoracic trauma	Cardiopulmonary bypass
Possible Lung Injury Plus Elevated Hydrostatic Pressures	
High altitude pulmonary edema	Reexpansion pulmonary edema
Neurogenic pulmonary edema	

■ PHYSICAL FINDINGS

Pt appears severely ill, often diaphoretic, sitting bolt upright, tachypneic, cyanosis may be present. Bilateral pulmonary rales; third heart sound may be present. Frothy, blood-tinged sputum may occur.

■ LABORATORY

Early arterial blood gases show reductions of both Pao_2 and $Paco_2$. With progressive respiratory failure, hypercapnia develops with acidemia. CXR shows pulmonary vascular redistribution, diffuse haziness in lung fields with perihilar "butterfly" appearance.

> **TREATMENT** Acute Pulmonary Edema

Immediate, aggressive therapy is mandatory for survival. The following measures should be instituted as simultaneously as possible for cardiogenic pulmonary edema:

1. Administer 100% O_2 by mask to achieve Pao_2 >60 mmHg; if inadequate, use positive-pressure ventilation by face or nasal mask, and if necessary, proceed to endotracheal intubation.
2. Reduce preload:
   a. Seat pt upright to reduce venous return, if not hypotensive.
   b. Intravenous loop diuretic (e.g., furosemide, initially 0.5–1.0 mg/kg); use lower dose if pt does not take diuretics chronically.
   c. Nitroglycerin (sublingual 0.4 mg × 3 q5min) followed by 5–10 μg/min IV if needed.
   d. Morphine 2–4 mg IV (repetitively); assess frequently for hypotension or respiratory depression; naloxone should be available to reverse effects of morphine if necessary.
   e. Consider ACE inhibitor if pt is hypertensive, or in setting of acute MI with heart failure.

 f. Consider nesiritide (2-μg/kg bolus IV followed by 0.01 μg/kg per min) for refractory symptoms—do not use in acute MI or cardiogenic shock.

3. Inotropic agents are indicated in cardiogenic pulmonary edema and severe LV dysfunction: dopamine, dobutamine, milrinone (see Chap. 12).

4. The precipitating cause of cardiogenic pulmonary edema (Table 14-1) should be sought and treated, particularly acute arrhythmias or infection. For refractory pulmonary edema associated with persistent cardiac ischemia, early coronary revascularization may be life-saving. For noncardiac pulmonary edema, identify and treat/remove cause (Table 14-2).

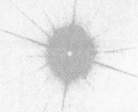

> For a more detailed discussion, see Schwartzstein RM: Dyspnea, Chap. 33, p. 277; and Hochman JS, Ingbar D: Cardiogenic Shock and Pulmonary Edema, Chap. 272, p. 2232, in HPIM-18.

CHAPTER **15**
Acute Respiratory Distress Syndrome

■ DEFINITION AND ETIOLOGY

Acute respiratory distress syndrome (ARDS) develops rapidly and includes severe dyspnea, diffuse pulmonary infiltrates, and hypoxemia; it typically causes respiratory failure. Key diagnostic criteria for ARDS include (1) diffuse bilateral pulmonary infiltrates on chest x-ray (CXR); (2) Pao_2 (arterial partial pressure of oxygen in mmHg)/Fio_2 (inspired O_2 fraction) ≤200 mmHg; and (3) absence of elevated left atrial pressure (pulmonary capillary wedge pressure ≤18 mmHg). Acute lung injury is a related but milder syndrome, with less profound hypoxemia (Pao_2/Fio_2 ≤300 mmHg), that can develop into ARDS. Although many medical and surgical conditions can cause ARDS, most cases (>80%) result from sepsis, bacterial pneumonia, trauma, multiple transfusions, gastric acid aspiration, and drug overdose. Individuals with more than one predisposing factor have a greater risk of developing ARDS. Other risk factors include older age, chronic alcohol abuse, metabolic acidosis, and overall severity of critical illness.

■ CLINICAL COURSE AND PATHOPHYSIOLOGY

There are three phases in the natural history of ARDS:

1. *Exudative phase*—Characterized by alveolar edema and leukocytic inflammation, with subsequent development of hyaline membranes from

diffuse alveolar damage. The alveolar edema is most prominent in the dependent portions of the lung; this causes atelectasis and reduced lung compliance. Hypoxemia, tachypnea, and progressive dyspnea develop, and increased pulmonary dead space can also lead to hypercarbia. CXR reveals bilateral, diffuse alveolar and interstitial opacities. The differential diagnosis is broad, but common alternative etiologies to consider are cardiogenic pulmonary edema, pneumonia, and alveolar hemorrhage. Unlike cardiogenic pulmonary edema, the CXR in ARDS rarely shows cardiomegaly, pleural effusions, or pulmonary vascular redistribution. The exudative phase duration is typically up to 7 days in length and usually begins within 12–36 h after the inciting insult.

2. *Proliferative phase*—This phase typically lasts from approximately days 7 to 21 after the inciting insult. Although most pts recover, some will develop progressive lung injury and evidence of pulmonary fibrosis. Even among pts who show rapid improvement, dyspnea and hypoxemia often persist during this phase.

3. *Fibrotic phase*—Although the majority of pts recover within 3–4 weeks of the initial pulmonary injury, some experience progressive fibrosis, necessitating prolonged ventilatory support and/or supplemental O_2. Increased risk of pneumothorax, reductions in lung compliance, and increased pulmonary dead space are observed during this phase.

TREATMENT   ARDS

Progress in recent therapy has emphasized the importance of general critical care of pts with ARDS in addition to lung protective ventilator strategies. General care requires treatment of the underlying medical or surgical problem that caused lung injury, minimizing iatrogenic complications (e.g., procedure-related), prophylaxis to prevent venous thromboembolism and GI hemorrhage, prompt treatment of infections, and adequate nutritional support. An algorithm for the initial management of ARDS is presented in Fig. 15-1.

MECHANICAL VENTILATORY SUPPORT Pts with ARDS typically require mechanical ventilatory support due to hypoxemia and increased work of breathing. A substantial improvement in outcomes from ARDS occurred with the recognition that mechanical ventilator–related over-distention of normal lung units with positive pressure can produce or exacerbate lung injury, causing or worsening ARDS. Currently recommended ventilator strategies limit alveolar distention but maintain adequate tissue oxygenation.

It has been clearly shown that low tidal volumes (≤6 mL/kg predicted body weight) provide reduced mortality compared with higher tidal volumes (12 mL/kg predicted body weight). In ARDS, alveolar collapse can occur due to alveolar/interstitial fluid accumulation and loss of surfactant, thus worsening hypoxemia. Therefore, low tidal volumes are combined with the use of positive end-expiratory pressure (PEEP) at levels that strive to minimize alveolar collapse and achieve adequate

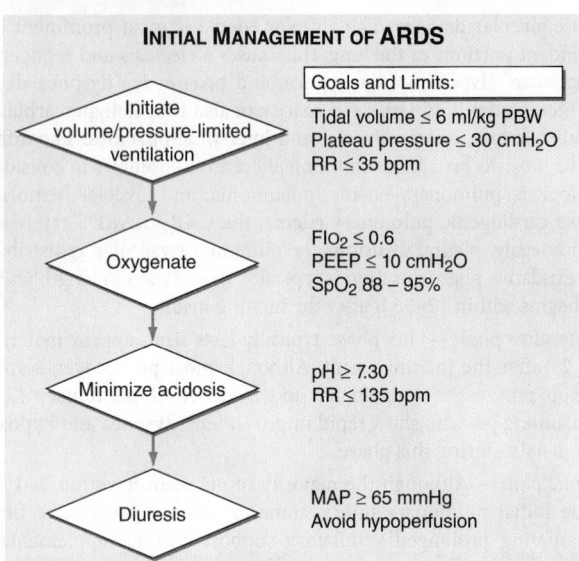

FIGURE 15-1 Algorithm for the initial management of ARDS. Clinical trials have provided evidence-based therapeutic goals for a step-wise approach to the early mechanical ventilation, oxygenation, correction of acidosis and diuresis of critically ill pts with ARDS.

oxygenation with the lowest FIO_2. Use of PEEP levels higher than required to optimize oxygenation has not been proven to be of benefit. Measurement of esophageal pressures to estimate transpulmonary pressure may help to identify an optimal level of PEEP. Other techniques that may improve oxygenation while limiting alveolar distention include extending the time of inspiration on the ventilator (inverse ratio ventilation) and placing the pt in the prone position. However, these approaches are not of proven benefit in reducing mortality from ARDS.

ANCILLARY THERAPIES Pts with ARDS have increased pulmonary vascular permeability leading to interstitial and alveolar edema. Therefore, they should receive IV fluids only as needed to achieve adequate cardiac output and tissue O_2 delivery as assessed by urine output, acid-base status, and arterial pressure. There is not convincing evidence currently to support the use of glucocorticoids or nitric oxide in ARDS.

▉ OUTCOMES

Mortality from ARDS has declined with improvements in general critical care treatment and with the introduction of low tidal volume ventilation. Current mortality from ARDS is 26–44%, with most deaths due to sepsis and nonpulmonary organ failure. Increased risk of mortality from ARDS is associated with advanced age, preexisting organ dysfunction (e.g., chronic liver disease, chronic alcohol abuse, chronic immunosuppression, and chronic renal disease), and direct lung injury (e.g., pneumonia, pulmonary contusion, and aspiration) compared with indirect lung injury (e.g., sepsis, trauma, and pancreatitis). Most surviving ARDS pts do not have significant long-term pulmonary disability.

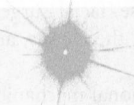

> For a more detailed discussion, see Levy BD, Choi AMK: Acute Respiratory Distress Syndrome, Chap. 268, p. 2205, in HPIM-18.

CHAPTER **16**
Respiratory Failure

■ DEFINITION AND CLASSIFICATION OF RESPIRATORY FAILURE

Respiratory failure is defined as inadequate gas exchange due to malfunction of one or more components of the respiratory system.

There are two main types of acute respiratory failure: hypoxemic and hypercarbic. Hypoxemic respiratory failure is defined by arterial O_2 saturation <90% while receiving an inspired O_2 fraction >0.6. Acute hypoxemic respiratory failure can result from pneumonia, pulmonary edema (cardiogenic or noncardiogenic), and alveolar hemorrhage. Hypoxemia results from ventilation-perfusion mismatch and intrapulmonary shunting.

Hypercarbic respiratory failure is characterized by respiratory acidosis with pH <7.30. Hypercarbic respiratory failure results from decreased minute ventilation and/or increased physiologic dead space. Common conditions associated with hypercarbic respiratory failure include neuromuscular diseases, such as myasthenia gravis, and respiratory diseases associated with respiratory muscle fatigue, such as asthma and chronic obstructive pulmonary disease (COPD). In acute hypercarbic respiratory failure, $Paco_2$ is typically >50 mmHg. With acute-on-chronic respiratory failure, as is often seen with COPD exacerbations, considerably higher $Paco_2$ values may be observed. The degree of respiratory acidosis, the pt's mental status, and the pt's degree of respiratory distress are better indicators of the need for mechanical ventilation than a specific $Paco_2$ level in acute-on-chronic respiratory failure. Two other types of respiratory failure are commonly considered: (1) perioperative respiratory failure related to atelectasis; and (2) hypoperfusion of respiratory muscles related to shock.

■ MODES OF MECHANICAL VENTILATION

Respiratory failure often requires treatment with mechanical ventilation. There are two general classes of mechanical ventilation: noninvasive ventilation (NIV) and conventional mechanical ventilation. NIV, administered through a tightly fitting nasal or full-face mask, is widely used in acute-on-chronic respiratory failure related to COPD exacerbations. NIV typically involves a preset positive pressure applied during inspiration and a lower pressure applied during expiration; it is associated with fewer complications such as nosocomial pneumonia than conventional mechanical ventilation through an endotracheal tube. However, NIV is contraindicated in cardiopulmonary arrest, severe encephalopathy, severe GI hemorrhage, hemodynamic instability, unstable coronary artery disease, facial surgery or trauma, upper airway obstruction, inability to protect the airway, and inability to clear secretions.

Most pts with acute respiratory failure require conventional mechanical ventilation via a cuffed endotracheal tube. The goal of mechanical ventilation is to optimize oxygenation while avoiding ventilator-induced lung injury. Various modes of conventional mechanical ventilation are commonly used; different modes are characterized by a trigger (what the ventilator senses to initiate a machine-delivered breath), a cycle (what determines the end of inspiration), and limiting factors (operator-specified values for key parameters that are monitored by the ventilator and not allowed to be exceeded). Three of the common modes of mechanical ventilation are described below; additional information is provided in Table 16-1.

- Assist-control ventilation: The trigger for a machine delivered breath is the pt's inspiratory effort, which causes a synchronized breath to be delivered. If no effort is detected over a prespecified time interval, a timer-triggered machine breath is delivered. Assist control is volume-cycled with an operator-determined tidal volume. Limiting factors include the minimum respiratory rate, which is specified by the operator; pt efforts can lead to higher respiratory rates. Other limiting factors include the airway pressure limit, which is also set by the operator. Because the pt will receive a full tidal breath with each inspiratory effort, tachypnea due to nonrespiratory drive (such as pain) can lead to respiratory alkalosis. In pts with airflow obstruction (e.g., asthma or COPD), auto-PEEP can develop.
- Synchronized intermittent mandatory ventilation (SIMV): As with assist-control, SIMV is volume-cycled, with similar limiting factors. As with assist-control, the trigger for a machine-delivered breath can be either pt effort or a specified time interval. However, if the pt's next inspiratory effort occurs before the time interval for another mandatory breath has elapsed, only their spontaneous respiratory effort (without machine support) is delivered. Thus, the number of machine-delivered breaths is limited in SIMV, allowing pts to exercise their inspiratory muscles between assisted breaths.
- Pressure-support ventilation (PSV): PSV is triggered by the pt's inspiratory effort. The cycle of PSV is determined by the inspiratory flow rate. Because a specific respiratory rate is not provided, this mode of ventilation may be combined with SIMV to ensure that an adequate respiratory rate is achieved in pts with respiratory depression.

Other modes of ventilation may be appropriate in specific clinical situations; for example, pressure-control ventilation is helpful to regulate airway pressures in pts with barotrauma or in the postoperative period from thoracic surgery.

TABLE 16-1 CLINICAL CHARACTERISTICS OF COMMONLY USED MODES OF MECHANICAL VENTILATION

Ventilator Mode	Independent Variables (Set by User)	Dependent Variables (Monitored by User)	Trigger/Cycle Limit	Advantages	Disadvantages
ACMV (assist-control mandatory ventilation)	FIo_2 Tidal volume Ventilator rate Level of PEEP Inspiratory flow pattern Peak inspiratory flow Pressure limit	Peak airway pressure ABG Minute Ventilation Plateau pressure Mean airway pressure I/E ratio	Pt/timer Pressure limit	Timer backup Pt-vent synchrony Pt controls minute ventilation	Not useful for weaning Potential for dangerous respiratory alkalosis
SIMV (synchronized intermittent mandatory ventilation)	Same as for ACMV	Same as for ACMV	Same as for ACMV	Timer backup is useful for weaning Comfort for spontaneous breaths	Potential dyssynchrony
PSV (pressure-support ventilation)	FIo_2 Inspiratory pressure level PEEP Pressure limit	Tidal volume Respiratory Rate Minute Ventilation	Inspiratory flow Pressure limit	Assures synchrony Good for weaning	No timer backup; may result in hypoventilation
NIV (noninvasive ventilation)	Inspiratory and expiratory pressure levels FIo_2	Tidal Volume Respiratory Rate I/E Ratio Minute Ventilation	Pressure limit Inspiratory flow	Pt control	Discomfort and bruising from mask Leaks are common Hypoventilation

Abbreviations: I/E, inspiration/expiration; FIo_2, inspired O_2; PEEP, positive end-expiratory pressure.

■ MANAGEMENT OF MECHANICALLY VENTILATED PATIENTS

General care of mechanically ventilated pts is reviewed in Chap. 5, along with weaning from mechanical ventilation. A cuffed endotracheal tube is often used to provide positive pressure ventilation with conditioned gas. A protective ventilation approach is generally recommended, including the following elements: (1) target tidal volume of approximately 6 mL/kg of ideal body weight; (2) avoid plateau pressures >30 cm H_2O; (3) use the lowest fraction of inspired oxygen (FIo_2) to maintain arterial oxygen saturation ≥90%; and (4) apply PEEP to maintain alveolar patency while avoiding overdistention. After an endotracheal tube has been in place for an extended period of time, tracheostomy should be considered, primarily to improve pt comfort and management of respiratory secretions. No absolute time frame for tracheostomy placement exists, but pts who are likely to require mechanical ventilatory support for >2 weeks should be considered for a tracheostomy.

A variety of complications can result from mechanical ventilation. Barotrauma—overdistention and damage of lung tissue—typically occurs at high airway pressures (>50 cm H_2O). Barotrauma can cause pneumomediastinum, subcutaneous emphysema, and pneumothorax; pneumothorax typically requires treatment with tube thoracostomy. Ventilator-associated pneumonia is a major complication in intubated pts; common pathogens include *Pseudomonas aeruginosa* and other gram-negative bacilli, as well as *Staphylococcus aureus*.

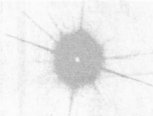

> For a more detailed discussion, see Celli BR: Mechanical Ventilatory Support, Chap. 269, p. 2210; and Kress JP and Hall JB: Approach to the Patient With Critical Illness, Chap. 267, p. 2196, in HPIM-18.

CHAPTER **17**
Confusion, Stupor, and Coma

APPROACH TO THE PATIENT   **Disorders of Consciousness**

Disorders of consciousness are common; these always signify a disorder of the nervous system. Assessment should determine whether there is a change in level of consciousness (drowsy, stuporous, comatose) and/or content of consciousness (confusion, perseveration, hallucinations). *Confusion* is a lack of clarity in thinking with inattentiveness; *delirium* is used to describe an acute confusional state; *stupor*, a state in which vigorous stimuli are needed to elicit a response; *coma*, a condition of unresponsiveness. Pts in such states are usually seriously ill, and etiologic factors must be assessed (Tables 17-1 and 17-2).

TABLE 17-1 COMMON ETIOLOGIES OF DELIRIUM

Toxins

    Prescription medications: especially those with anticholinergic properties, narcotics, and benzodiazepines

    Drugs of abuse: alcohol intoxication and alcohol withdrawal, opiates, ecstasy, LSD, GHB, PCP, ketamine, cocaine

    Poisons: inhalants, carbon monoxide, ethylene glycol, pesticides

Metabolic conditions

    Electrolyte disturbances: hypoglycemia, hyperglycemia, hyponatremia, hypernatremia, hypercalcemia, hypocalcemia, hypomagnesemia

    Hypothermia and hyperthermia

    Pulmonary failure: hypoxemia and hypercarbia

    Liver failure/hepatic encephalopathy

    Renal failure/uremia

    Cardiac failure

    Vitamin deficiencies: B_{12}, thiamine, folate, niacin

    Dehydration and malnutrition

    Anemia

Infections

    Systemic infections: urinary tract infections, pneumonia, skin and soft tissue infections, sepsis

    CNS infections: meningitis, encephalitis, brain abscess

Endocrinologic conditions

    Hyperthyroidism, hypothyroidism

    Hyperparathyroidism

    Adrenal insufficiency

Cerebrovascular disorders

    Global hypoperfusion states

    Hypertensive encephalopathy

    Focal ischemic strokes and hemorrhages: especially nondominant parietal and thalamic lesions

Autoimmune disorders

    CNS vasculitis

    Cerebral lupus

Seizure-related disorders

    Nonconvulsive status epilepticus

    Intermittent seizures with prolonged postictal states

Neoplastic disorders

    Diffuse metastases to the brain

(*continued*)

TABLE 17-1 COMMON ETIOLOGIES OF DELIRIUM (CONTINUED)

Gliomatosis cerebri
Carcinomatous meningitis
Hospitalization
Terminal end-of-life delirium

Abbreviations: CNS, central nervous system; GHB, γ-hydroxybutyrate; LSD, lysergic acid diethylamide; PCP, phencyclidine.

■ DELIRIUM

Delirium is a clinical diagnosis made at the bedside; a careful history and physical exam are necessary, focusing on common etiologies of delirium, especially toxins and metabolic conditions. Observation will usually reveal an altered level of consciousness or a deficit of attention. Attention can be assessed through a simple bedside test of digits forward—pts are asked to repeat successively longer random strings of digits beginning with two digits in a row; a digit span of four digits or less usually indicates an attentional deficit unless hearing or language barriers are present. Delirium is vastly underrecognized, especially in pts presenting with a quiet, hypoactive state.

A cost-effective approach to the evaluation of delirium allows the history and physical exam to guide tests. No single algorithm will fit all pts due to the large number of potential etiologies, but one step-wise approach is shown in Table 17-2.

Management of the delirious pt begins with treatment of the underlying inciting factor (e.g., pts with systemic infections should be given appropriate antibiotics, and electrolyte disturbances judiciously corrected). Relatively simple methods of supportive care can be quite effective, such as frequent reorientation by staff, preservation of sleep-wake cycles, and attempting to mimic the home environment as much as possible. Chemical restraints exacerbate delirium and should be used only when necessary to protect pt or staff from possible injury; antipsychotics at low dose are usually the treatment of choice.

■ COMA (SEE TABLE 17-3)

Because coma demands immediate attention, the physician must employ an organized approach. Almost all instances of coma can be traced to widespread abnormalities of the bilateral cerebral hemispheres or to reduced activity of the reticular activating system in the brainstem.

History

Pt should be aroused, if possible, and questioned regarding use of insulin, narcotics, anticoagulants, other prescription drugs, suicidal intent, recent trauma, headache, epilepsy, significant medical problems, and preceding symptoms. Witnesses and family members should be interviewed, often by phone. History of sudden headache followed by loss of consciousness suggests intracranial hemorrhage; preceding vertigo, nausea, diplopia, ataxia, hemisensory disorder suggest basilar insufficiency; chest pain, palpitations, and faintness suggest a cardiovascular cause.

TABLE 17-2 STEPWISE EVALUATION OF A PATIENT WITH DELIRIUM

Initial evaluation

    History with special attention to medications (including over-the-counter and herbals)

    General physical examination and neurologic examination

    Complete blood count

    Electrolyte panel including calcium, magnesium, phosphorus

    Liver function tests, including albumin

    Renal function tests

First-tier further evaluation guided by initial evaluation

    Systemic infection screen

        Urinalysis and culture

        Chest radiograph

        Blood cultures

    Electrocardiogram

    Arterial blood gas

    Serum and/or urine toxicology screen (perform earlier in young persons)

    Brain imaging with MRI with diffusion and gadolinium (preferred) or CT

    Suspected CNS infection: lumbar puncture after brain imaging

    Suspected seizure-related etiology: electroencephalogram (EEG) (if high suspicion, should be performed immediately)

Second-tier further evaluation

    Vitamin levels: B_{12}, folate, thiamine

    Endocrinologic laboratories: thyroid-stimulating hormone (TSH) and free T_4; cortisol

    Serum ammonia

    Sedimentation rate

    Autoimmune serologies: antinuclear antibodies (ANA), complement levels; p-ANCA, c-ANCA

    Infectious serologies: rapid plasmin reagin (RPR); fungal and viral serologies if high suspicion; HIV antibody

    Lumbar puncture (if not already performed)

    Brain MRI with and without gadolinium (if not already performed)

Abbreviations: c-ANCA, cytoplasmic antineutrophil cytoplasmic antibody; p-ANCA, perinuclear antineutrophil cytoplasmic antibody.

Immediate Assessment

Acute respiratory and cardiovascular problems should be attended to prior to the neurologic assessment. Vital signs should be evaluated, and appropriate support initiated. Thiamine, glucose, and naloxone should be administered if the etiology of coma is not immediately apparent. Blood

TABLE 17-3 DIFFERENTIAL DIAGNOSIS OF COMA

1. Diseases that cause no focal or lateralizing neurologic signs, usually with normal brainstem functions; CT scan and cellular content of the CSF are normal

   a. Intoxications: alcohol, sedative drugs, opiates, etc.

   b. Metabolic disturbances: anoxia, hyponatremia, hypernatremia, hypercalcemia, diabetic acidosis, nonketotic hyperosmolar hyperglycemia, hypoglycemia, uremia, hepatic coma, hypercarbia, Addisonian crisis, hypo- and hyperthyroid states, profound nutritional deficiency

   c. Severe systemic infections: pneumonia, septicemia, typhoid fever, malaria, Waterhouse-Friderichsen syndrome

   d. Shock from any cause

   e. Postseizure states, status epilepticus, subclinical epilepsy

   f. Hypertensive encephalopathy, eclampsia

   g. Severe hyperthermia, hypothermia

   h. Concussion

   i. Acute hydrocephalus

2. Diseases that cause meningeal irritation with or without fever, and with an excess of WBCs or RBCs in the CSF, usually without focal or lateralizing cerebral or brainstem signs; CT or MRI shows no mass lesion

   a. Subarachnoid hemorrhage from ruptured aneurysm, arteriovenous malformation, trauma

   b. Acute bacterial meningitis

   c. Viral encephalitis

   d. Miscellaneous: fat embolism, cholesterol embolism, carcinomatous and lymphomatous meningitis, etc.

3. Diseases that cause focal brainstem or lateralizing cerebral signs, with or without changes in the CSF; CT and MRI are abnormal

   a. Hemispheral hemorrhage (basal ganglionic, thalamic) or infarction (large middle cerebral artery territory) with secondary brainstem compression

   b. Brainstem infarction due to basilar artery thrombosis or embolism

   c. Brain abscess, subdural empyema

   d. Epidural and subdural hemorrhage, brain contusion

   e. Brain tumor with surrounding edema

   f. Cerebellar and pontine hemorrhage and infarction

   g. Widespread traumatic brain injury

   h. Metabolic coma (see above) with preexisting focal damage

   i. Miscellaneous: Cortical vein thrombosis, herpes simplex encephalitis, multiple cerebral emboli due to bacterial endocarditis, acute hemorrhagic leukoencephalitis, acute disseminated (postinfectious) encephalomyelitis, thrombotic thrombocytopenic purpura, cerebral vasculitis, gliomatosis cerebri, pituitary apoplexy, intravascular lymphoma, etc.

Abbreviations: CSF, cerebrospinal fluid; RBCs, red blood cells; WBCs, white blood cells.

should be drawn for glucose, electrolytes, calcium, and renal (BUN, creatinine) and hepatic (ammonia, transaminases) function; also screen for presence of alcohol and other toxins, and obtain blood cultures if infection is suspected. Arterial blood-gas analysis is helpful in pts with lung disease and acid-base disorders. Fever, especially with petechial rash, suggests meningitis. Examination of CSF is essential in diagnosis of meningitis and encephalitis; lumbar puncture should not be deferred if meningitis is a possibility, but CT scan should be obtained first to exclude a mass lesion. Empirical antibiotic and glucocorticoid coverage for meningitis may be instituted until CSF results are available. Fever with dry skin suggests heat shock or intoxication with anticholinergics. Hypothermia suggests myxedema, intoxication, sepsis, exposure, or hypoglycemia. Marked hypertension occurs with increased intracranial pressure (ICP) and hypertensive encephalopathy.

Neurologic Examination

Focus on establishing pt's best level of function and uncovering signs that enable a specific diagnosis. Comatose pt's best motor and sensory function should be assessed by testing reflex responses to noxious stimuli; carefully note any asymmetric responses, which suggest a focal lesion. Multifocal myoclonus indicates that a metabolic disorder is likely; intermittent twitching may be the only sign of a seizure.

Responsiveness

Stimuli of increasing intensity are applied to gauge the degree of unresponsiveness and any asymmetry in sensory or motor function. Motor responses may be purposeful or reflexive. Spontaneous flexion of elbows with leg extension, termed *decortication*, accompanies severe damage to contralateral hemisphere above midbrain. Internal rotation of the arms with extension of elbows, wrists, and legs, termed *decerebration*, suggests damage to midbrain or diencephalon. These postural reflexes occur in profound encephalopathic states.

Pupillary Signs

In comatose pts, equal, round, reactive pupils exclude mid-brain damage as cause and suggest a metabolic abnormality. Pinpoint pupils occur in narcotic overdose (except meperidine, which can cause midsize pupils), pontine damage, hydrocephalus, or thalamic hemorrhage; the response to naloxone and presence of reflex eye movements (usually intact with drug overdose) can distinguish these. A unilateral, enlarged, often oval, poorly reactive pupil is caused by midbrain lesions or compression of third cranial nerve, as occurs in transtentorial herniation. Bilaterally dilated, unreactive pupils indicate severe bilateral midbrain damage, anticholinergic overdose, or ocular trauma.

Ocular Movements

Examine spontaneous and reflex eye movements. Intermittent horizontal divergence is common in drowsiness. Slow, to-and-fro horizontal movements suggest bihemispheric dysfunction. Conjugate eye deviation to one side indicates damage to the pons on the opposite side or a lesion in the frontal lobe on the same side ("*The eyes look toward a hemispheral lesion and away from a brainstem lesion*"). An adducted eye at rest with impaired ability to turn eye laterally indicates an abducens (VI) nerve palsy, common in raised ICP or pontine damage. The eye with a dilated, unreactive pupil is often abducted at rest and cannot adduct fully due to third nerve dysfunction, as occurs with transtentorial herniation. Vertical separation of ocular axes (skew deviation) occurs in pontine or cerebellar lesions. Doll's head maneuver (oculocephalic reflex) and cold caloric–induced eye movements allow diagnosis of gaze or cranial nerve palsies in pts who do not move their eyes purposefully. Doll's head maneuver is tested by observing eye movements in response to lateral rotation of head (this should not be performed in pts with possible neck injury); full conjugate movement of eyes occurs in bihemispheric dysfunction. In comatose pts with intact brainstem function, raising head to 60° above the horizontal and irrigating external auditory canal with cool water causes tonic deviation of gaze to side of irrigated ear ("cold calorics"). In conscious pts, it causes nystagmus, vertigo, and emesis.

Respiratory Patterns

Respiratory pattern may suggest site of neurologic damage. Cheyne-Stokes (periodic) breathing occurs in bihemispheric dysfunction and is common in metabolic encephalopathies. Respiratory patterns composed of gasps or other irregular breathing patterns are indicative of lower brainstem damage; such pts usually require intubation and ventilatory assistance.

Radiologic Examination

Lesions causing raised ICP commonly cause impaired consciousness. CT or MRI scan of the brain is often abnormal in coma but may not be diagnostic; appropriate therapy should not be postponed while awaiting a CT or MRI scan. Pts with disordered consciousness due to high ICP can deteriorate rapidly; emergent CT study is necessary to confirm presence of mass effect and to guide surgical decompression. CT scan is normal in some pts with subarachnoid hemorrhage; the diagnosis then rests on clinical history combined with RBCs or xanthochromia in spinal fluid. CT, MR, or conventional angiography may be necessary to establish basilar artery stroke as cause of coma in pts with brainstem signs. The EEG is useful in metabolic or drug-induced states but is rarely diagnostic; exceptions are coma due to seizures or herpesvirus encephalitis.

◼ BRAIN DEATH

This results from total cessation of cerebral function while somatic function is maintained by artificial means and the heart continues to pump. It is legally and ethically equivalent to cardiorespiratory death. The pt is unresponsive to all forms of stimulation (widespread cortical destruction), brainstem reflexes are absent (global brainstem damage), and there is complete apnea (destruction of the medulla). Demonstration of apnea requires that the P_{CO_2} be high enough to stimulate respiration, while Po$_2$ and bp are maintained. EEG is isoelectric at high gain. The absence of deep tendon reflexes is not required because the spinal cord may remain functional. Special care must be taken to exclude drug toxicity and hypothermia prior to making a diagnosis of brain death. Diagnosis should be made only if the state persists for some agreed-upon period, usually 6–24 h.

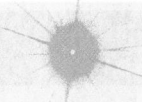

For a more detailed discussion, see Josephson SA, Miller BL: Confusion and Delirium, Chap. 25, p. 196, in HPIM-18. and Ropper AH: Coma, Chap. 274, p. 2247, in HPIM-18.

CHAPTER **18**
Stroke

Sudden onset of a neurologic deficit from a vascular mechanism: 85% are ischemic; 15% are primary hemorrhages [subarachnoid (Chap. 19) and intraparenchymal]. An ischemic deficit that resolves rapidly is termed a *transient ischemic attack* (TIA); 24 h is a commonly used boundary between TIA and stroke whether or not a new infarction has occurred, although most TIAs last between 5 and 15 min. Recently proposed new definitions classify all brain infarctions as strokes regardless of duration of symptoms. Stroke is the leading cause of neurologic disability in adults; 200,000 deaths annually in the United States. Much can be done to limit morbidity and mortality through prevention and acute intervention.

■ PATHOPHYSIOLOGY

Ischemic stroke is most often due to embolic occlusion of large cerebral vessels; source of emboli may be heart, aortic arch, or other arterial lesions such as the carotid arteries. Small, deep ischemic lesions are most often related to intrinsic small-vessel disease (lacunar strokes). Low-flow strokes are seen with severe proximal stenosis and inadequate collaterals challenged by systemic hypotensive episodes. Hemorrhages most frequently result from rupture of aneurysms or small vessels within brain tissue. Variability in stroke recovery is influenced by collateral vessels, blood pressure, and the specific site and mechanism of vessel occlusion; if blood flow is restored prior to significant cell death, the pt may experience only transient symptoms, i.e., a TIA.

■ CLINICAL FEATURES

Ischemic Stroke

Abrupt and dramatic onset of focal neurologic symptoms is typical of ischemic stroke. Pts may not seek assistance on their own because they are rarely in pain and may lose appreciation that something is wrong (*anosognosia*). Symptoms reflect the vascular territory involved (Table 18-1). Transient monocular blindness (amaurosis fugax) is a particular form of TIA due to retinal ischemia; pts describe a shade descending over the visual field.

TABLE 18-1 ANATOMIC LOCALIZATION IN STROKE

Signs and Symptoms
Cerebral Hemisphere, Lateral Aspect (Middle Cerebral A.)
Hemiparesis
Hemisensory deficit
Motor aphasia (Broca's)—hesitant speech with word-finding difficulty and preserved comprehension
Sensory aphasia (Wernicke's)—anomia, poor comprehension, jargon speech
Unilateral neglect, apraxias
Homonymous hemianopia or quadrantanopia
Gaze preference with eyes deviated toward side of lesion
Cerebral Hemisphere, Medial Aspect (Anterior Cerebral A.)
Paralysis of foot and leg with or without paresis of arm
Cortical sensory loss over leg
Grasp and sucking reflexes
Urinary incontinence
Gait apraxia
Cerebral Hemisphere, Posterior Aspect (Posterior Cerebral A.)
Homonymous hemianopia
Cortical blindness
Memory deficit
Dense sensory loss, spontaneous pain, dysesthesias, choreoathetosis
Brainstem, Midbrain (Posterior Cerebral A.)
Third nerve palsy and contralateral hemiplegia
Paralysis/paresis of vertical eye movement
Convergence nystagmus, disorientation
Brainstem, Pontomedullary Junction (Basilar A.)
Facial paralysis
Paresis of abduction of eye
Paresis of conjugate gaze
Hemifacial sensory deficit

TABLE 18-1 ANATOMIC LOCALIZATION IN STROKE (CONTINUED)

Brainstem, Pontomedullary Junction (Basilar A.)
Horner's syndrome
Diminished pain and thermal sense over half body (with or without face)
Ataxia

Brainstem, Lateral Medulla (Vertebral A.)
Vertigo, nystagmus
Horner's syndrome (miosis, ptosis, decreased sweating)
Ataxia, falling toward side of lesion
Impaired pain and thermal sense over half body with or without face

Lacunar Syndromes (Small-Vessel Strokes)

Most common are:
- Pure motor hemiparesis of face, arm, and leg (internal capsule or pons)
- Pure sensory stroke (ventral thalamus)
- Ataxic hemiparesis (pons or internal capsule)
- Dysarthria—clumsy hand (pons or genu of internal capsule).

Intracranial Hemorrhage

Vomiting and drowsiness occur in some cases, and headache in about one-half. Signs and symptoms are often not confined to a single vascular territory. Etiologies are diverse but hypertension-related is the most common (Table 18-2). Hypertensive hemorrhages typically occur in the following locations:

- Putamen: Contralateral hemiparesis often with homonymous hemianopia.
- Thalamus: Hemiparesis with prominent sensory deficit.
- Pons: Quadriplegic, "pinpoint" pupils, impaired horizontal eye movements.
- Cerebellum: Headache, vomiting, gait ataxia.

A neurologic deficit that evolves gradually over 5–30 min strongly suggests intracerebral bleeding.

TREATMENT Stroke

Principles of management are outlined in Fig. 18-1. Stroke needs to be distinguished from potential mimics, including seizure, migraine, tumor, and metabolic derangements.

- Imaging. After initial stabilization, an emergency noncontrast head CT scan is necessary to differentiate ischemic from hemorrhagic stroke. With large ischemic strokes, CT abnormalities are usually evident within the first few hours, but small infarcts can be difficult to visualize by CT. CT or MR angiography (CTA/MRA) and perfusion

TABLE 18-2 CAUSES OF INTRACRANIAL HEMORRHAGE

Cause	Location	Comments
Head trauma	Intraparenchymal: frontal lobes, anterior temporal lobes; subarachnoid	Coup and contrecoup injury during brain deceleration
Hypertensive hemorrhage	Putamen, globus pallidus, thalamus, cerebellar hemisphere, pons	Chronic hypertension produces hemorrhage from small (~100 μm) vessels in these regions
Transformation of prior ischemic infarction	Basal ganglion, subcortical regions, lobar	Occurs in 1–6% of ischemic strokes with predilection for large hemispheric infarctions
Metastatic brain tumor	Lobar	Lung, choriocarcinoma, melanoma, renal cell carcinoma, thyroid, atrial myxoma
Coagulopathy	Any	Uncommon cause; often associated with prior stroke or underlying vascular anomaly
Drug	Lobar, subarachnoid	Cocaine, amphetamine, phenylpropanolamine
Arteriovenous malformation	Lobar, intraventricular, subarachnoid	Risk is ~2–4% per year for bleeding
Aneurysm	Subarachnoid, intraparenchymal, rarely subdural	Mycotic and nonmycotic forms of aneurysms
Amyloid angiopathy	Lobar	Degenerative disease of intracranial vessels; linkage to Alzheimer's disease, rare in pts <60 years
Cavernous angioma	Intraparenchymal	Multiple cavernous angiomas linked to mutations in *KRIT1*, *CCM2*, and *PDCD10* genes
Dural arteriovenous fistula	Lobar, subarachnoid	Produces bleeding by venous hypertension
Capillary telangiectasias	Usually brainstem	Rare cause of hemorrhage

may help reveal vascular occlusions and tissue at risk for infarction. Diffusion-weighted MRI has a high sensitivity for identifying ischemic stroke even minutes after onset.

ACUTE ISCHEMIC STROKE Treatments designed to reverse or lessen tissue infarction include: (1) medical support, (2) thrombolysis and endovascular techniques, (3) antiplatelet agents, (4) anticoagulation, and (5) neuroprotection.

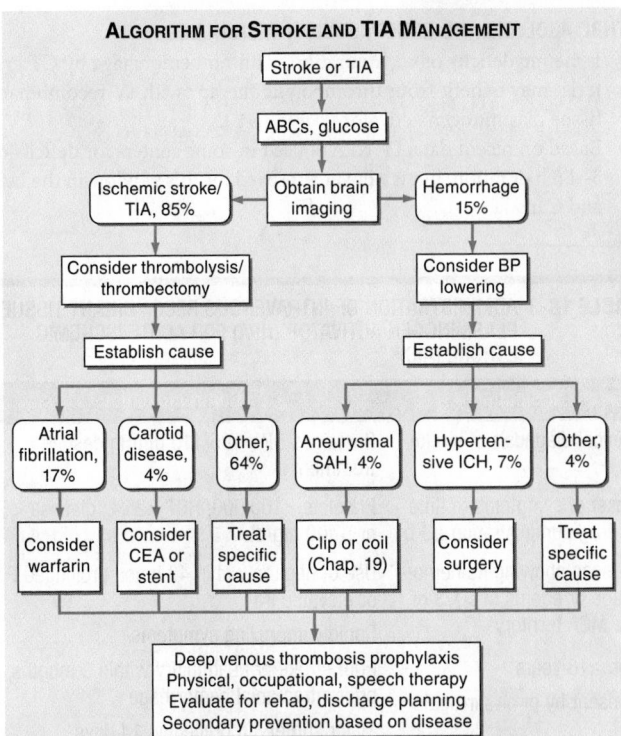

FIGURE 18-1 Medical management of stroke and TIA. Rounded boxes are diagnoses; rectangles are interventions. Numbers are percentages of stroke overall. ABCs, airway, breathing, circulation; BP, blood pressure; CEA, carotid endarterectomy; ICH, intracerebral hemorrhage; SAH, subarachnoid hemorrhage; TIA, transient ischemic attack.

MEDICAL SUPPORT Optimize perfusion in ischemic penumbra surrounding the infarct.

- Blood pressure should never be lowered precipitously (exacerbates the underlying ischemia), and only in the most extreme situations should gradual lowering be undertaken (e.g., malignant hypertension with bp > 220/120 or, if thrombolysis planned, bp > 185/110 mmHg).
- Intravascular volume should be maintained with isotonic fluids as volume restriction is rarely helpful. Osmotic therapy with mannitol may be necessary to control edema in large infarcts, but isotonic volume must be replaced to avoid hypovolemia.
- In cerebellar infarction (or hemorrhage), rapid deterioration can occur from brainstem compression and hydrocephalus, requiring neurosurgical intervention.

THROMBOLYSIS AND ENDOVASCULAR TECHNIQUES

- Ischemic deficits of <3 h duration, with no hemorrhage by CT criteria, may benefit from thrombolytic therapy with IV recombinant tissue plasminogen activator (Table 18-3).
- Based on recent data, IV rtPA is used in some centers for deficits of 3–4.5 h duration, but is not yet approved for this window in the U.S. and Canada.

TABLE 18-3 ADMINISTRATION OF INTRAVENOUS RECOMBINANT TISSUE PLASMINOGEN ACTIVATOR (rtPA) FOR ACUTE ISCHEMIC STROKE (AIS)[a]

Indication	Contraindication
Clinical diagnosis of stroke	Sustained BP >185/110 mmHg despite treatment
Onset of symptoms to time of drug administration ≤3 h	Platelets <100,000; HCT <25%; glucose <50 or >400 mg/dL
CT scan showing no hemorrhage or edema of >1/3 of the MCA territory	Use of heparin within 48 h and prolonged PTT, or elevated INR
	Rapidly improving symptoms
Age ≥18 years	Prior stroke or head injury within 3 months; prior intracranial hemorrhage
Consent by pt or surrogate	
	Major surgery in preceding 14 days
	Minor stroke symptoms
	Gastrointestinal bleeding in preceding 21 days
	Recent myocardial infarction
	Coma or stupor

Administration of rtPA
Intravenous access with two peripheral IV lines (avoid arterial or central line placement)
Review eligibility for rtPA
Administer 0.9 mg/kg IV (maximum 90 mg) IV as 10% of total dose by bolus, followed by remainder of total dose over 1 h
Frequent cuff blood pressure monitoring
No other antithrombotic treatment for 24 h
For decline in neurologic status or uncontrolled blood pressure, stop infusion, give cryoprecipitate, and reimage brain emergently
Avoid urethral catheterization for ≥2 h

[a]See Activase (tissue plasminogen activator) package insert for complete list of contraindications and dosing.
Abbreviations: BP, blood pressure; HCT, hematocrit; INR, international normalized ratio; MCA, middle cerebral artery; PTT, partial thromboplastin time.

- Ischemic stroke from large-vessel intracranial occlusion results in high rates of morbidity and mortality; pts with such occlusions may benefit from intraarterial thrombolysis (<6 h duration) or embolectomy (<8 h duration) administered at the time of an urgent cerebral angiogram at specialized centers.

ANTIPLATELET AGENTS

- Aspirin (up to 325 mg/d) is safe and has a small but definite benefit in acute ischemic stroke.

ANTICOAGULATION

- Trials do not support the use of heparin or other anticoagulants acutely for pts with acute stroke.

NEUROPROTECTION

- Hypothermia is effective in coma following cardiac arrest but has not been adequately studied in pts with stroke. Other neuroprotective agents have shown no benefit in human trials despite promising animal data.

STROKE CENTERS AND REHABILITATION

- Pt care in comprehensive stroke units followed by rehabilitation services improves neurologic outcomes and reduces mortality.

ACUTE INTRACEREBRAL HEMORRHAGE

- Noncontrast head CT will confirm diagnosis.
- Rapidly identify and correct any coagulopathy.
- Nearly 50% of pts die; prognosis is determined by volume and location of hematoma.
- Stuporous or comatose pts generally are treated presumptively for elevated ICP. Treatment for edema and mass effect with osmotic agents may be necessary; glucocorticoids not helpful.
- Neurosurgical consultation should be sought for possible urgent evacuation of cerebellar hematoma; in other locations, data do not support surgical intervention.

■ EVALUATION: DETERMINING THE CAUSE OF STROKE

Although initial management of acute ischemic stroke or TIA does not depend on the etiology, establishing a cause is essential to reduce risk of recurrence (Table 18-4); particular attention should be on atrial fibrillation and carotid atherosclerosis as these etiologies have proven secondary prevention strategies. Nearly 30% of strokes remain unexplained despite extensive evaluation.

Clinical examination should be focused on the peripheral and cervical vascular system. Routine studies include CXR and ECG, urinalysis, CBC/platelets, electrolytes, glucose, ESR, lipid profile, PT, PTT, and serologic tests for syphilis. If a hypercoagulable state is suspected, further studies of coagulation are indicated.

Imaging evaluation may include brain MRI (compared with CT, increased sensitivity for small infarcts of cortex and brainstem); MR or

TABLE 18-4 CAUSES OF ISCHEMIC STROKE

Common Causes	Uncommon Causes
Thrombosis	Hypercoagulable disorders
Lacunar stroke (small vessel)	Protein C deficiency
Large vessel thrombosis	Protein S deficiency
Dehydration	Antithrombin III deficiency
Embolic occlusion	Antiphospholipid syndrome
Artery-to-artery	Factor V Leiden mutation[a]
Carotid bifurcation	Prothrombin G20210 mutation[a]
Aortic arch	Systemic malignancy
Arterial dissection	Sickle cell anemia
Cardioembolic	β-Thalassemia
Atrial fibrillation	Polycythemia vera
Mural thrombus	Systemic lupus erythematosus
Myocardial infarction	Homocysteinemia
Dilated cardiomyopathy	Thrombotic thrombocytopenic purpura
Valvular lesions	Disseminated intravascular coagulation
Mitral stenosis	Dysproteinemias
Mechanical valve	Nephrotic syndrome
Bacterial endocarditis	Inflammatory bowel disease
Paradoxical embolus	Oral contraceptives
Atrial septal defect	Venous sinus thrombosis[b]
Patent foramen ovale	Fibromuscular dysplasia
Atrial septal aneurysm	Vasculitis
Spontaneous echo contrast	Systemic vasculitis [PAN, granulomatosis with polyangiitis (Wegener's), Takayasu's, giant cell arteritis]
	Primary CNS vasculitis
	Meningitis (syphilis, tuberculosis, fungal, bacterial, zoster)
	Cardiogenic
	Mitral valve calcification
	Atrial myxoma
	Intracardiac tumor
	Marantic endocarditis
	Libman-Sacks endocarditis
	Subarachnoid hemorrhage vasospasm
	Drugs: cocaine, amphetamine
	Moyamoya disease
	Eclampsia

[a]Chiefly cause venous sinus thrombosis.
[b]May be associated with any hypercoagulable disorder.
Abbreviations: CNS, central nervous system; PAN, polyarteritis nodosa.

CT angiography (evaluate patency of intracranial vessels and extracranial carotid and vertebral vessels); noninvasive carotid tests ("duplex" studies, combine ultrasound imaging of the vessel with Doppler evaluation of blood flow characteristics); or cerebral angiography ("gold standard" for evaluation of intracranial and extracranial vascular disease). For suspected cardiogenic source, cardiac echocardiogram with attention to right-to-left shunts, and 24-h Holter or long-term cardiac event monitoring indicated.

■ PRIMARY AND SECONDARY PREVENTION OF STROKE

Risk Factors

Atherosclerosis is a systemic disease affecting arteries throughout the body. Multiple factors including hypertension, diabetes, hyperlipidemia, and family history influence stroke and TIA risk (Table 18-5). Cardioembolic risk factors include atrial fibrillation, MI, valvular heart disease, and cardiomyopathy. Hypertension and diabetes are also specific risk factors for lacunar stroke and intraparenchymal hemorrhage. Smoking is a potent risk factor for all vascular mechanisms of stroke. *Identification of modifiable risk factors and prophylactic interventions to lower risk is probably the best approach to stroke overall.*

TABLE 18-5 RISK FACTORS FOR STROKE

Risk Factor	Relative Risk	Relative Risk Reduction with Treatment	Number Needed to Treat[a]	
			Primary Prevention	Secondary Prevention
Hypertension	2–5	38%	100–300	50–100
Atrial fibrillation	1.8–2.9	68% warfarin, 21% aspirin	20–83	13
Diabetes	1.8–6	No proven effect		
Smoking	1.8	50% at 1 year, baseline risk at 5 years post cessation		
Hyperlipidemia	1.8–2.6	16–30%	560	230
Asymptomatic carotid stenosis	2.0	53%	85	N/A
Symptomatic carotid stenosis (70–99%)		65% at 2 years	N/A	12
Symptomatic carotid stenosis (50–69%)		29% at 5 years	N/A	77

[a]Number needed to treat to prevent one stroke annually. Prevention of other cardiovascular outcomes is not considered here.
Abbreviations: N/A, not applicable.

TABLE 18-6 CONSENSUS RECOMMENDATION FOR ANTITHROMBOTIC PROPHYLAXIS IN ATRIAL FIBRILLATION

CHADS2 Score[a]	Recommendation
0	Aspirin or no antithrombotic
1	Aspirin or warfarin INR 2.5
>1	Warfarin INR 2.5

[a]CHADS2 score calculated as follows: 1 point for age > 75 years, 1 point for hypertension, 1 point for congestive heart failure, 1 point for diabetes, and 2 points for stroke or TIA; sum of points is the total CHADS2 score.
Source: Modified from DE Singer et al: Chest 133:546S, 2008; with permission.

Antiplatelet Agents

Platelet antiaggregation agents can prevent atherothrombotic events, including TIA and stroke, by inhibiting the formation of intraarterial platelet aggregates. Aspirin (50–325 mg/d) inhibits thromboxane A_2, a platelet aggregating and vasoconstricting prostaglandin. Aspirin, clopidogrel (blocks the platelet ADP receptor), and the combination of aspirin plus extended-release dipyridamole (inhibits platelet uptake of adenosine) are the antiplatelet agents most commonly used. In general, antiplatelet agents reduce new stroke events by 25–30%. Every pt who has experienced an atherothrombotic stroke or TIA and has no contraindication should take an antiplatelet agent regularly because the average annual risk of another stroke is 8–10%. The choice of aspirin, clopidogrel, or dipyridamole plus aspirin must balance the fact that the latter are more effective than aspirin but the cost is higher.

Embolic Stroke

In pts with atrial fibrillation, the choice between anticoagulant or aspirin prophylaxis is determined by age and risk factors; the presence of any risk factor tips the balance in favor of anticoagulation (Table 18-6).

Anticoagulation Therapy for Noncardiogenic Stroke

Data do not support the use of long-term warfarin for preventing atherothrombotic stroke for either intracranial or extracranial cerebrovascular disease.

Carotid Revascularization

Carotid endarterectomy benefits many pts with *symptomatic* severe (>70%) *carotid stenosis*; the relative risk reduction is ~65%. However, if the perioperative stroke rate is >6% for any surgeon, the benefit is lost. Endovascular stenting is an emerging option; there remains controversy as to who should receive a stent or undergo endarterectomy. Surgical results in pts with *asymptomatic carotid stenosis* are less robust, and medical therapy for reduction of atherosclerosis risk factors plus antiplatelet medications is generally recommended in this group.

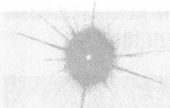

For a more detailed discussion, see Smith WS, English JD, Johnston SC: Cerebrovascular Diseases, Chap. 370, p. 3270, in HPIM-18.

CHAPTER **19**
Subarachnoid Hemorrhage

Excluding head trauma, the most common cause of subarachnoid hemorrhage (SAH) is rupture of an intracranial (saccular) aneurysm; other etiologies include bleeding from a vascular malformation (arteriovenous malformation or dural arterial-venous fistula), infective (mycotic) aneurysms, and extension into the subarachnoid space from a primary intracerebral hemorrhage. Approximately 2% of the population harbor aneurysms, and 25,000–30,000 cases of aneurysmal rupture producing SAH occur each year in the United States; rupture risk for aneurysms <10 mm in size is 0.1% per year; for unruptured aneurysms, the surgical morbidity risk far exceeds the percentage.

■ CLINICAL PRESENTATION

Sudden, severe headache, often with transient loss of consciousness at onset; vomiting is common. Bleeding may injure adjacent brain tissue and produce focal neurologic deficits. A progressive third nerve palsy, usually involving the pupil, along with headache suggests posterior communicating artery aneurysm. In addition to dramatic presentations, aneurysms can undergo small ruptures with leaks of blood into the subarachnoid space (sentinel bleeds). The initial clinical manifestations of SAH can be graded using established scales (Table 19-1); prognosis for good outcome falls as the grade increases.

■ INITIAL EVALUATION

- Noncontrast CT is the initial study of choice and usually demonstrates the hemorrhage if obtained within 72 h. LP is required for diagnosis of suspected SAH if the CT is nondiagnostic; xanthochromia of the spinal fluid is seen within 6–12 h after rupture and lasts for 1–4 weeks.
- Cerebral angiography is necessary to localize and define the anatomic details of the aneurysm and to determine if other unruptured aneurysms exist; angiography should be performed as soon as possible after the diagnosis of SAH is made.
- ECG may reveal ST-segment and T-wave changes similar to those associated with cardiac ischemia; caused by circulating catecholamines and excessive discharge of sympathetic neurons. A reversible cardiomyopathy producing shock or congestive heart failure may result.
- Studies of coagulation and platelet count should be obtained, and rapid correction should ensue if SAH is documented.

TABLE 19-1 GRADING SCALES FOR SUBARACHNOID HEMORRHAGE

Grade	Hunt-Hess Scale	World Federation of Neurosurgical Societies (WFNS) Scale
1	Mild headache, normal mental status, no cranial nerve or motor findings	GCS[a] score 15, no motor deficits
2	Severe headache, normal mental status, may have cranial nerve deficit	GCS score 13–14, no motor deficits
3	Somnolent, confused, may have cranial nerve or mild motor deficit	GCS score 13–14, with motor deficits
4	Stupor, moderate to severe motor deficit, may have intermittent reflex posturing	GCS score 7–12, with or without motor deficits
5	Coma, reflex posturing or flaccid	GCS score 3–6, with or without motor deficits

[a]Glasgow Coma Scale: See Table 20-2.

TREATMENT   Subarachnoid Hemorrhage

ANEURYSM REPAIR
- Early aneurysm repair prevents rerupture.
- The International Subarachnoid Aneurysm Trial (ISAT) demonstrated improved outcomes with endovascular therapy compared to surgery; however, some aneurysms have a morphology not amenable to endovascular treatment, and therefore surgery is still an important treatment option for some pts.

MEDICAL MANAGEMENT
- Closely follow serum electrolytes and osmolality; hyponatremia ("cerebral salt wasting") frequently develops several days after SAH, and supplemental oral salt plus IV normal saline or hypertonic saline may be used to overcome renal losses.
- Anticonvulsants may be begun until the aneurysm is treated, although most experts reserve this therapy only for pts in whom a seizure has occurred.
- Blood pressure should be carefully controlled, while preserving cerebral blood flow, in order to decrease the risk of rerupture until the aneurysm is repaired.
- All pts should have pneumatic compression stockings applied to prevent pulmonary embolism; unfractionated heparin administered subcutaneously for deep-vein thrombosis prophylaxis can be initiated immediately following endovascular treatment and within days following craniotomy and surgical clipping.

HYDROCEPHALUS

- Severe hydrocephalus may require urgent placement of a ventricular catheter for external CSF drainage; some pts will require permanent shunt placement.
- Deterioration of a SAH pt in the first hours to days should prompt repeat CT scanning to evaluate ventricular size.

VASOSPASM

- The leading cause of mortality and morbidity following initial rupture; may develop by day 4 and continue through day 14, leading to focal ischemia and possibly stroke.
- Medical treatment with the calcium channel antagonist nimodipine (60 mg PO q4h) improves outcome, probably by preventing ischemic injury rather than reducing the risk of vasospasm.
- Cerebral perfusion can be improved in symptomatic vasospasm by increasing mean arterial pressure with vasopressor agents such as phenylephrine or norepinephrine, and intravascular volume can be expanded with crystalloid, augmenting cardiac output and reducing blood viscosity by reducing the hematocrit; this so-called "triple-H" (hypertension, hemodilution, and hypervolemic) therapy is widely used.
- If symptomatic vasospasm persists despite optimal medical therapy, intra-arterial vasodilators and angioplasty of the cerebral vessels can be effective.

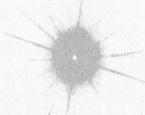

For a more detailed discussion, see Hemphill JC III, Smith WS, and Gress DR: Neurologic Critical Care, Including Hypoxic-Ischemic Encephalopathy and Subarachnoid Hemorrhage. Chap. 275, p. 2254, in HPIM-18.

CHAPTER **20**
Increased Intracranial Pressure and Head Trauma

INCREASED INTRACRANIAL PRESSURE

A limited volume of extra tissue, blood, CSF, or edema can be added to the intracranial contents without raising the intracranial pressure (ICP). Clinical deterioration or death may follow increases in ICP that shift intracranial contents, distort vital brainstem centers, or compromise cerebral perfusion. Cerebral perfusion pressure (CPP), defined as the mean arterial pressure (MAP) minus the ICP, is the driving force for circulation across capillary beds of the brain; decreased CPP is a fundamental mechanism of secondary ischemic brain injury and constitutes an emergency that requires immediate attention. In general, ICP should be maintained at <20 mmHg and CPP should be maintained at ≥60 mmHg.

■ CLINICAL FEATURES

Elevated ICP may occur in a wide range of disorders including head trauma, intracerebral hemorrhage, subarachnoid hemorrhage (SAH) with hydrocephalus, and fulminant hepatic failure.

Symptoms of high ICP include drowsiness, headache (especially a constant ache that is worse upon awakening), nausea, emesis, diplopia, and blurred vision. Papilledema and sixth nerve palsies are common. If not controlled, then cerebral hypoperfusion, pupillary dilation, coma, focal neurologic deficits, posturing, abnormal respirations, systemic hypertension, and bradycardia may result.

Masses that cause raised ICP also distort midbrain and diencephalic anatomy, leading to stupor and coma. Brain tissue is pushed away from the mass against fixed intracranial structures and into spaces not normally occupied. Posterior fossa masses, which may initially cause ataxia, stiff neck, and nausea, are especially dangerous because they can both compress vital brainstem structures and cause obstructive hydrocephalus.

Herniation syndromes (Fig. 20-1) include:

- *Uncal:* Medial temporal lobe displaced through the tentorium, compressing the third cranial nerve and pushing the cerebral peduncle against the tentorium, leading to ipsilateral pupillary dilation, contralateral hemiparesis, and posterior cerebral artery compression.

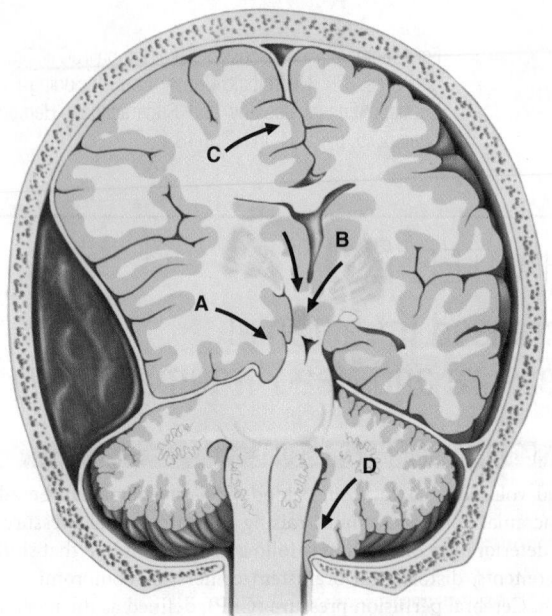

FIGURE 20-1 Types of cerebral herniation. **A**. uncal; **B**. central; **C**. transfalcial; **D**. foraminal.

- *Central:* Downward displacement of the thalamus through the tentorium; miotic pupils and drowsiness are early signs.
- *Transfalcial:* Cingulate gyrus displaced under the midline falx, leading to anterior cerebral artery compression.
- *Foraminal:* Cerebellar tonsils displaced into the foramen magnum, causing medullary compression and respiratory arrest.

TREATMENT   Increased Intracranial Pressure

- A number of different interventions may lower ICP, and ideally the selection of treatment will be based on the underlying mechanism responsible for the elevated ICP (Table 20-1).
- With hydrocephalus, the principal cause of elevated ICP is impaired CSF drainage; in this setting, ventricular drainage of CSF is likely to be sufficient.

TABLE 20-1 STEPWISE APPROACH TO TREATMENT OF ELEVATED INTRACRANIAL PRESSURE*

Insert ICP monitor—ventriculostomy versus parenchymal device general goals: maintain ICP <20 mmHg and CPP ≥60 mmHg For ICP >20–25 mmHg for >5 min:

1. Drain CSF via ventriculostomy (if in place)
2. Elevate head of the bed; midline head position
3. Osmotherapy—mannitol 25–100 g q4h as needed (maintain serum osmolality <320 mosmol) or hypertonic saline (30 mL, 23.4% NaCl bolus)
4. Glucocorticoids—dexamethasone 4 mg q6h for vasogenic edema from tumor, abscess (avoid glucocorticoids in head trauma, ischemic and hemorrhagic stroke)
5. Sedation (e.g., morphine, propofol, or midazolam); add neuromuscular paralysis if necessary (pt will require endotracheal intubation and mechanical ventilation at this point, if not before)
6. Hyperventilation—to $Paco_2$ 30–35 mmHg
7. Pressor therapy—phenylephrine, dopamine, or norepinephrine to maintain adequate MAP to ensure CPP ≥ 60 mmHg (maintain euvolemia to minimize deleterious systemic effects of pressors)
8. Consider second-tier therapies for refractory elevated ICP
   a. High-dose barbiturate therapy ("pentobarb coma")
   b. Aggressive hyperventilation to $Paco_2$ <30 mmHg
   c. Hypothermia
   d. Hemicraniectomy

*Throughout ICP treatment algorithm, consider repeat head CT to identify mass lesions amenable to surgical evacuation.
Abbreviations: CPP, cerebral perfusion pressure; CSF, cerebrospinal fluid; MAP, mean arterial pressure; $Paco_2$, arterial partial pressure of carbon dioxide.

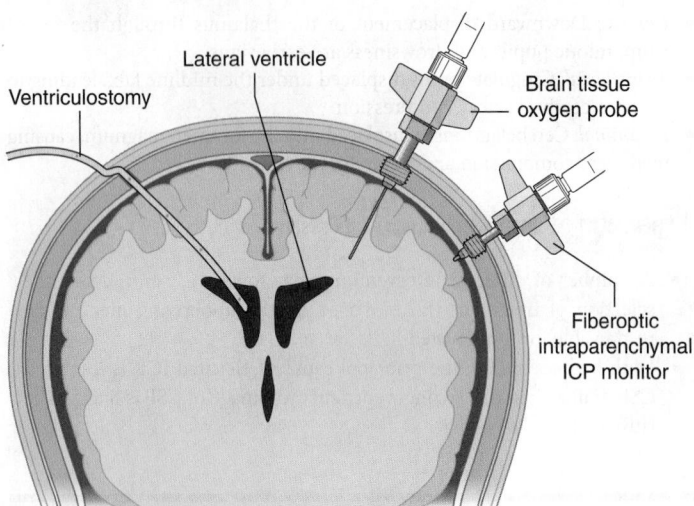

FIGURE 20-2 Intracranial pressure and brain tissue oxygen monitoring. A ventriculostomy allows for drainage of cerebrospinal fluid to treat elevated intracranial pressure (ICP). Fiberoptic ICP and brain tissue oxygen monitors are usually secured using a screwlike skull bolt. Cerebral blood flow and microdialysis probes (not shown) may be placed in a manner similar to the brain tissue oxygen probe.

- If cytotoxic edema is responsible, as in head trauma or stroke, use of osmotic diuretics such as mannitol or hypertonic saline is an appropriate early step.
- Elevated ICP may cause tissue ischemia; resulting vasodilatation can lead to a cycle of worsening ischemia. Paradoxically, administration of vasopressor agents to increase mean arterial pressure may actually lower ICP by increasing perfusion; therefore, hypertension should be treated carefully, if at all.
- Free water should be restricted.
- Fever should be treated aggressively.
- Hyperventilation is best used for only short periods of time until a more definitive treatment can be instituted.
- ICP monitoring is an important tool to guide medical and surgical decisions in selected pts with cerebral edema (Fig. 20-2).

After stabilization and initiation of the above therapies, a CT scan (or MRI, if feasible) is performed to delineate the cause of the elevated ICP. Emergency surgery is sometimes necessary to decompress the intracranial contents in cerebellar stroke with edema, surgically accessible tumor, and subdural or epidural hemorrhage.

HEAD TRAUMA

Almost 10 million head injuries occur annually in the United States, about 20% of which are serious enough to cause brain damage.

TABLE 20-2 GLASGOW COMA SCALE FOR HEAD INJURY

Eye opening (E)		Verbal response (V)	
Spontaneous	4	Oriented	5
To loud voice	3	Confused, disoriented	4
To pain	2	Inappropriate words	3
Nil	1	Incomprehensible sounds	2
		Nil	1
Best motor response (M)			
Obeys	6		
Localizes	5		
Withdraws (flexion)	4		
Abnormal flexion posturing	3		
Extension posturing	2		
Nil	1		

Note: Coma score = E + M + V. Pts scoring 3 or 4 have an 85% chance of dying or remaining vegetative, while scores >11 indicate only a 5–10% likelihood of death or vegetative state and 85% chance of moderate disability or good recovery. Intermediate scores correlate with proportional chances of recovery.

■ CLINICAL FEATURES

Head trauma can cause immediate loss of consciousness. If transient and accompanied by a short period of amnesia, it is called *concussion*. Prolonged alterations in consciousness may be due to parenchymal, subdural, or epidural hematoma or to diffuse shearing of axons in the white matter. Skull fracture should be suspected in pts with CSF rhinorrhea, hemotympanum, and periorbital or mastoid ecchymoses. Glasgow Coma Scale (Table 20-2) useful for grading severity of brain injury.

APPROACH TO THE PATIENT — **Head Injury**

Medical personnel caring for head injury pts should be aware that:

- Spinal injury often accompanies head injury and care must be taken to prevent compression of the spinal cord due to instability of the spinal column.
- Intoxication is a frequent accompaniment of traumatic brain injury; when appropriate, testing should be carried out for drugs and alcohol.
- Accompanying systemic injuries, including ruptures of abdominal organs, may produce vascular collapse or respiratory compromise requiring immediate attention.

MINOR CONCUSSIVE INJURY The pt with minor head injury who is alert and attentive after a short period of unconsciousness (<1 min) may have headache, dizziness, faintness, nausea, a single episode of emesis, difficulty with concentration, or slight blurring of vision. Such pts have usually sustained a concussion and are expected to have a brief amnestic period.

TABLE 20-3 GUIDELINES FOR MANAGEMENT OF CONCUSSION IN SPORTS

Severity of Concussion

Grade 1: Transient confusion, no loss of consciousness (LOC), all symptoms resolve within 15 min.

Grade 2: Transient confusion, no LOC, but concussive symptoms or mental status abnormalities persist longer than 15 min.

Grade 3: Any LOC, either brief (seconds) or prolonged (minutes).

On-Site evaluation

1. Mental status testing
    a. Orientation—time, place, person, circumstances of injury
    b. Concentration—digits backward, months of year in reverse order
    c. Memory—names of teams, details of contest, recent events, recall of three words and objects at 0 and 5 min
2. Finger-to-nose with eyes open and closed
3. Pupillary symmetry and reaction
4. Romberg and tandem gait
5. Provocative testing—40-yard sprint, 5 push ups, 5 sit ups, 5 knee bends (development of dizziness, headaches, or other symptoms is abnormal)

Management guidelines

Grade 1: Remove from contest. Examine immediately and at 5-min intervals. May return to contest if exam clears within 15 min. A second grade 1 concussion eliminates player for 1 week, with return contingent upon normal neurologic assessment at rest and with exertion.

Grade 2: Remove from contest, cannot return for at least 1 week. Examine at frequent intervals on sideline. Formal neurologic exam the next day. If headache or other symptoms persist for 1 week or longer, CT or MRI scan is indicated. After 1 full asymptomatic week, repeat neurologic assessment at rest and with exercise before cleared to resume play. A second grade 2 concussion eliminates player for at least 2 weeks following complete resolution of symptoms at rest or with exertion. If imaging shows abnormality, player is removed from play for the season.

Grade 3: Transport by ambulance to emergency department if still unconscious or worrisome signs are present; cervical spine stabilization may be indicated. Neurologic exam and, when indicated, CT or MRI scan will guide subsequent management. Hospital admission indicated when signs of pathology are present or if mental status remains abnormal. If findings are normal at the time of the initial medical evaluation, the athlete may be sent home, but daily exams as an outpatient are indicated. A brief (LOC for seconds) grade 3 concussion eliminates player for 1 week, and a prolonged (LOC for minutes) grade 3 concussion for 2 weeks, following complete resolution of symptoms. A second grade 3 concussion should eliminate player from sports for at least 1 month following resolution of symptoms. Any abnormality on CT or MRI scans should result in termination of the season for the athlete, and return to play at any future time should be discouraged.

Source: Modified from Quality Standards Subcommittee of the American Academy of Neurology: *The American Academy of Neurology Practice Handbook.* The American Academy of Neurology, St. Paul, MN, 1997.

After several hours of observation, these pts can be accompanied home and observed for a day by family or friends. Persistent severe headache and repeated vomiting are usually benign if the neurologic exam remains normal, but in such situations radiologic studies should be obtained and hospitalization is justified.

Timing of return to contact sports depends on the severity of concussion and examination; this common sense approach is not guided by adequate data (Table 20-3).

Older age, two or more episodes of vomiting, >30 min of retrograde or persistent anterograde amnesia, seizure, and concurrent drug or alcohol intoxication are sensitive (but not specific) indicators of intracranial hemorrhage that justify CT scanning; it is appropriate to be more liberal in obtaining CT scans in children.

INJURY OF INTERMEDIATE SEVERITY Pts who are not comatose but who have persistent confusion, behavioral changes, subnormal alertness, extreme dizziness, or focal neurologic signs such as hemiparesis should be hospitalized and have a CT scan. A cerebral contusion or subdural hematoma is often found. Pts with intermediate head injury require medical observation to detect increasing drowsiness, respiratory dysfunction, pupillary enlargement, or other changes in the neurologic exam. Abnormalities of attention, intellect, spontaneity, and memory tend to return to normal weeks or months after the injury, although some cognitive deficits may be persistent.

SEVERE INJURY Pts who are comatose from onset require immediate neurologic attention and often resuscitation. After intubation (with care taken to avoid deforming the cervical spine), the depth of coma, pupillary size and reactivity, limb movements, and Babinski responses are assessed. As soon as vital functions permit and cervical spine x-rays and a CT scan have been obtained, the pt should be transported to a critical care unit. CT scan may be normal in comatose pts with axonal shearing lesions in cerebral white matter.

The finding of an epidural or subdural hematoma or large intracerebral hemorrhage requires prompt decompressive surgery in otherwise salvageable pts. Subsequent treatment is probably best guided by direct measurement of ICP. The use of prophylactic anticonvulsants has been recommended but supportive data is limited.

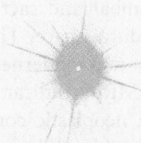

For a more detailed discussion, see Hemphill JC Smith WS Gress DR: Neurologic Critical Care, Including Hypoxic-Ischemic Encephalopathy and Subarachnoid Hemorrhage, Chap. 275, p. 2254; Ropper AH: Concussion and Other Head Injuries, Chap. 378, p. 3377; and Ropper AH: Coma, Chap. 274, p. 2247; in HPIM-18.

CHAPTER **21**
Spinal Cord Compression

| APPROACH TO THE PATIENT | Spinal Cord Compression |

Initial symptoms, focal neck or back pain, may evolve over days to weeks. These are followed by various combinations of paresthesias, sensory loss, motor weakness, and sphincter disturbance evolving over hours to several days. Partial lesions may selectively involve one or more tracts and may be limited to one side of the cord. In severe or abrupt cases, areflexia reflecting spinal shock may be present, but hyperreflexia supervenes over days to weeks. With thoracic lesions, a sensory level to pain may be present on the trunk, indicating localization to the cord at that dermatomal level.

In any pt who presents with spinal cord symptoms, the first priority is to exclude treatable compression by a mass. Compression is more likely to be preceded by warning signs of neck or back pain, bladder disturbances, and sensory symptoms prior to development of weakness; noncompressive etiologies such as infarction and hemorrhage are more likely to produce myelopathy without antecedent symptoms.

MRI with gadolinium, centered on the clinically suspected level, is the initial diagnostic procedure. (CT myelography may be helpful in pts who have contraindications to MRI.) It is often useful to image the entire spine to search for additional clinically silent lesions. Infectious etiologies, unlike tumor, often cross the disc space to involve adjacent vertebral bodies.

◼ NEOPLASTIC SPINAL CORD COMPRESSION

Occurs in 3–5% of pts with cancer; epidural tumor may be the initial manifestation of malignancy. Most neoplasms are epidural in origin and result from metastases to the adjacent spinal bones. Almost any malignant tumor can metastasize to the spinal column with lung, breast, prostate, kidney, lymphoma, and plasma cell dyscrasia being particularly frequent. The thoracic cord is most commonly involved; exceptions include prostate and ovarian tumors, which preferentially involve the lumbar and sacral segments from spread through veins in the anterior epidural space. The most common presenting symptom is localized back pain and tenderness followed by symptoms of neurologic compromise. Urgent MRI is indicated when the diagnosis is suspected; up to 40% of pts with neoplastic cord compression at one level are found to have asymptomatic epidural disease elsewhere, so the entire spine should be imaged. Plain radiographs will miss 15–20% of metastatic vertebral lesions.

TREATMENT	Neoplastic Spinal Cord Compression

- Glucocorticoids to reduce edema (dexamethasone, up to 40 mg daily) can be administered before the imaging study if the clinical suspicion is high, and continued at a lower dose until radiotherapy (generally 3000 cGy administered in 15 daily fractions) is completed.
- Early surgery, either decompression by laminectomy or vertebral body resection, should be considered as a recent clinical trial indicated that surgery followed by radiotherapy is more effective than radiotherapy alone for pts with a single area of spinal cord compression by extradural tumor.
- Time is of the essence in treatment; fixed motor deficits (paraplegia or quadriplegia) once established for >12 h do not usually improve, and beyond 48 h the prognosis for substantial motor recovery is poor.
- Biopsy is needed if there is no history of underlying malignancy; a simple systemic workup including chest imaging, mammography, measurement of prostate-specific antigen (PSA), and abdominal CT may reveal the diagnosis.

■ SPINAL EPIDURAL ABSCESS

Presents as a triad of pain, fever, and progressive limb weakness. Aching pain is almost always present, either over the spine or in a radicular pattern. The duration of pain prior to presentation is generally <2 weeks but may be several months or longer. Fever is usually present along with elevated white blood cell count, sedimentation rate, and C-reactive protein. Risk factors include an impaired immune status (diabetes mellitus, HIV, renal failure, alcoholism, malignancy), intravenous drug abuse, and infections of the skin or other soft tissues. Most cases are due to *Staphylococcus aureus*; other important causes include gram-negative bacilli, *Streptococcus*, anaerobes, fungi, and tuberculosis (Pott's disease).

MRI localizes the abscess. Lumbar puncture (LP) is required only if encephalopathy or other clinical signs raise the question of associated meningitis, a feature found in <25% of cases. The level of the LP should be planned to minimize risk of meningitis due to passage of the needle through infected tissue.

TREATMENT	Spinal Epidural Abscess

- Decompressive laminectomy with debridement combined with long-term antibiotic treatment.
- Surgical evacuation is unlikely to improve deficits of more than several days' duration.
- Broad-spectrum antibiotics should be started empirically before surgery and then modified on the basis of culture results and continued for at least 4 weeks.
- With prompt diagnosis and treatment, up to two-thirds of pts experience significant recovery.

■ SPINAL EPIDURAL HEMATOMA

Hemorrhage into the epidural (or subdural) space causes acute focal or radicular pain followed by variable signs of a spinal cord disorder. Therapeutic anticoagulation, trauma, tumor, or blood dyscrasia are predisposing conditions; rarely complication of LP or epidural anesthesia. Treatment consists of prompt reversal of any underlying bleeding disorder and surgical decompression.

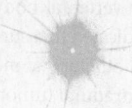

> For a more detailed discussion, see Gucalp R and Dutcher J: Oncologic Emergencies, Chap. 276, p. 2266; and Hauser SL and Ropper AH: Diseases of the Spinal Cord, Chap. 377, p. 3366, in HPIM-18.

CHAPTER **22**
Hypoxic-Ischemic Encephalopathy

Results from lack of delivery of oxygen to the brain because of hypotension or respiratory failure. Most common causes are MI, cardiac arrest, shock, asphyxiation, paralysis of respiration, and carbon monoxide or cyanide poisoning. In some circumstances, hypoxia may predominate. Carbon monoxide and cyanide poisoning are termed *histotoxic hypoxia* since they cause a direct impairment of the respiratory chain.

■ CLINICAL MANIFESTATIONS

Mild degrees of pure hypoxia (e.g., at high altitude) cause impaired judgment, inattentiveness, motor incoordination, and, at times, euphoria. However, with hypoxia-ischemia, such as occurs with circulatory arrest, consciousness is lost within seconds. If circulation is restored within 3–5 min, full recovery may occur, but with longer periods permanent cerebral damage usually results. It may be difficult to judge the precise degree of hypoxia-ischemia, and some pts make a relatively full recovery even after 8–10 min of global ischemia. The distinction between pure hypoxia and hypoxia-ischemia is important, since a Pao_2 as low as 2.7 kPa (20 mmHg) can be well tolerated if it develops gradually and normal blood pressure is maintained, but short durations of very low or absent cerebral circulation may result in permanent impairment.

Clinical examination at different time points after an insult (especially cardiac arrest) helps to assess prognosis (Fig. 22-1). The prognosis is better for pts with intact brainstem function, as indicated by normal pupillary light responses, intact oculocephalic (doll's eyes) reflexes, and oculovestibular (caloric) and corneal reflexes. Absence of these reflexes and the presence of persistently dilated pupils that do not react to light are grave prognostic signs. A uniformly dismal prognosis is conveyed by the absence of a pupillary light reflex or absence of a motor response to pain on day 3 following the injury. Bilateral absence of the cortical somatosensory evoked

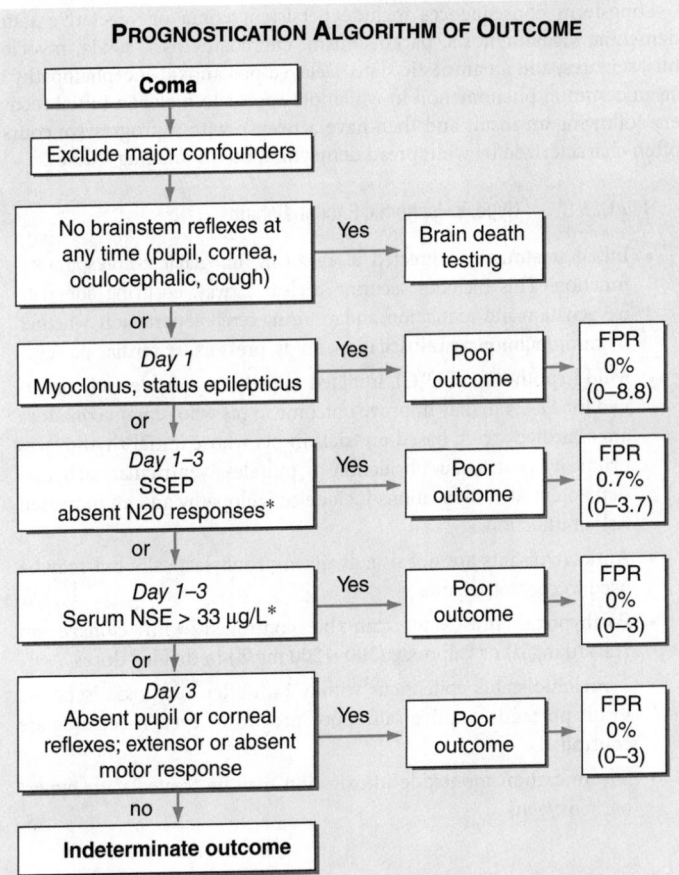

PROGNOSTICATION ALGORITHM OF OUTCOME

Coma

Exclude major confounders

No brainstem reflexes at any time (pupil, cornea, oculocephalic, cough) — Yes → Brain death testing

or

Day 1 Myoclonus, status epilepticus — Yes → Poor outcome → FPR 0% (0–8.8)

or

Day 1–3 SSEP absent N20 responses* — Yes → Poor outcome → FPR 0.7% (0–3.7)

or

Day 1–3 Serum NSE > 33 µg/L* — Yes → Poor outcome → FPR 0% (0–3)

or

Day 3 Absent pupil or corneal reflexes; extensor or absent motor response — Yes → Poor outcome → FPR 0% (0–3)

no ↓

Indeterminate outcome

FIGURE 22-1 Prognostication of outcome in comatose survivors of cardiopulmonary resuscitation. Numbers in parentheses are 95% confidence intervals. Confounders could include use of sedatives or neuromuscular blocking agents, hypothermia therapy, organ failure, or shock. Tests denoted with an asterisk (*) may not be available in a timely and standardized manner. SSEP, somatosensory evoked potentials; NSE, neuron-specific enolase; FPR, false-positive rate. *[From EFM Wijdicks et al: Practice parameter: Prediction of outcome in comatose survivors after cardiopulmonary resuscitation (an evidence-based review). Neurology 67:203, 2006; with permission.]*

potentials (SSEP) in the first several days also conveys a poor prognosis, as does a very elevated serum level (>33 µg/L) of the biochemical marker neuron-specific enolase (NSE). Usefulness of SSEP and NSE often limited: difficult to obtain in a timely fashion; need for expert interpretation (SSEP); and lack of standardization (NSE measurements). Whether administration of mild hypothermia after cardiac arrest will alter the usefulness of these clinical and electrophysiologic predictors is unknown.

Long-term consequences include persistent coma or vegetative state, dementia, visual agnosia, parkinsonism, choreoathetosis, ataxia, myoclonus, seizures, and an amnestic state. Delayed postanoxic encephalopathy is an uncommon phenomenon in which pts appear to make an initial recovery following an insult and then have a relapse with a progressive course often characterized by widespread demeylination on imaging studies.

TREATMENT Hypoxic-Ischemic Encephalopathy

- Initial treatment is directed at restoring normal cardiorespiratory function. This includes securing a clear airway, ensuring adequate oxygenation and ventilation, and restoring cerebral perfusion, whether by cardiopulmonary resuscitation, fluids, pressors, or cardiac pacing.

- Mild hypothermia (33°C), initiated as early as possible and continued for 12–24 h, may improve outcome in pts who remain comatose after cardiac arrest, based on trials in pts whose initial rhythm was primarily ventricular fibrillation or pulseless ventricular tachycardia. Potential complications include coagulopathy and an increased risk of infection.

- Anticonvulsants are not usually given prophylactically but may be used to control seizures.

- Posthypoxic myoclonus can be controlled with clonazepam (1.5–10 mg/d) or valproate (300–1200 mg/d) in divided doses.

- Myoclonic status epilepticus within 24 h after a hypoxic-ischemic insult portends a universally poor prognosis, even if seizures are controlled.

- Severe carbon monoxide intoxication may be treated with hyperbaric oxygen.

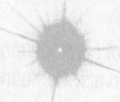

For a more detailed discussion, see Hemphill JC III, Smith WS, Gress DR: Neurologic Critical Care, Including Hypoxic-Ischemic Encephalopathy and Subarachnoid Hemorrhage, Chap. 275, p. 2254, in HPIM-18.

CHAPTER **23**
Status Epilepticus

Defined as continuous seizures or repetitive, discrete seizures with impaired consciousness in the interictal period. The duration of seizure activity to meet the definition has traditionally been 15–30 min. A more practical definition is any situation requiring the acute use of anticonvulsants; in generalized convulsive status epilepticus (GCSE), this is typically when seizures last >5 min.

■ CLINICAL FEATURES

Has numerous subtypes: GCSE (e.g., persistent, generalized electrographic seizures, coma, and tonic-clonic movements), and nonconvulsive status epilepticus (e.g., persistent absence seizures or focal seizures, confusion, or partially impaired consciousness, and minimal motor abnormalities). GCSE is obvious when overt convulsions are present, but after 30–45 min of uninterrupted seizures, the signs may become increasingly subtle (mild clonic movements of the fingers; fine, rapid movements of the eyes; or paroxysmal episodes of tachycardia, pupillary dilatation, and hypertension). EEG may be the only method of diagnosis with these subtle signs; therefore, if a pt remains comatose after a seizure, EEG should be performed to exclude ongoing status epilepticus. GCSE is life-threatening when accompanied by cardiorespiratory dysfunction, hyperthermia, and metabolic derangements such as acidosis (from prolonged muscle activity). Irreversible neuronal injury may occur from persistent seizures, even when a pt is paralyzed from neuromuscular blockade.

■ ETIOLOGY

Principal causes of GCSE are antiepileptic drug withdrawal or noncompliance, metabolic disturbances, drug toxicity, CNS infections, CNS tumors, refractory epilepsy, and head trauma.

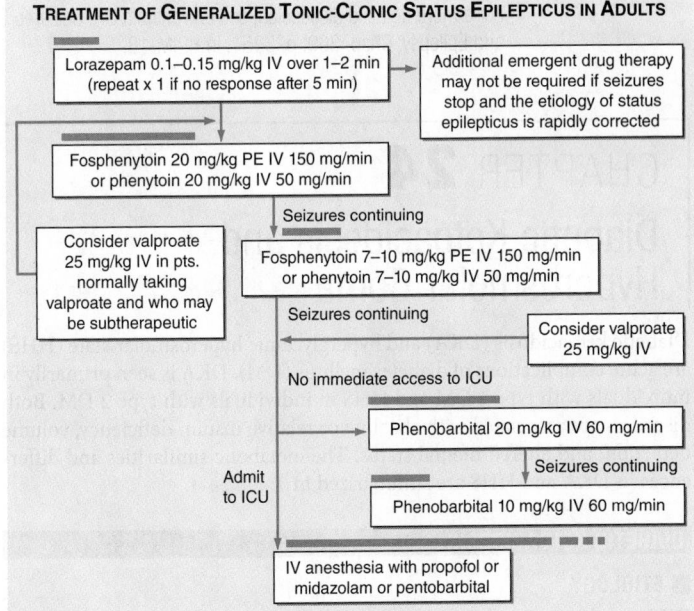

TREATMENT OF GENERALIZED TONIC-CLONIC STATUS EPILEPTICUS IN ADULTS

Lorazepam 0.1–0.15 mg/kg IV over 1–2 min (repeat x 1 if no response after 5 min)

Additional emergent drug therapy may not be required if seizures stop and the etiology of status epilepticus is rapidly corrected

Fosphenytoin 20 mg/kg PE IV 150 mg/min or phenytoin 20 mg/kg IV 50 mg/min

Seizures continuing

Consider valproate 25 mg/kg IV in pts. normally taking valproate and who may be subtherapeutic

Fosphenytoin 7–10 mg/kg PE IV 150 mg/min or phenytoin 7–10 mg/kg IV 50 mg/min

Seizures continuing

Consider valproate 25 mg/kg IV

No immediate access to ICU

Phenobarbital 20 mg/kg IV 60 mg/min

Seizures continuing

Phenobarbital 10 mg/kg IV 60 mg/min

Admit to ICU

IV anesthesia with propofol or midazolam or pentobarbital

FIGURE 23-1 Pharmacologic treatment of generalized tonic-clonic status epilepticus in adults. The horizontal gray bars indicate the approximate duration of drug infusions. IV, intravenous; PE, phenytoin equivalents.

> **TREATMENT**   Status Epilepticus
>
> GCSE is a medical emergency and must be treated immediately.
> - First attend to any acute cardiorespiratory problems or hyperthermia.
> - Perform a brief medical and neurologic exam, establish venous access, and send labs to screen for metabolic abnormalities including anticonvulsant levels if pt has a history of epilepsy.
> - Anticonvulsant therapy should then begin without delay (Fig. 23-1)
> - In parallel, it is essential to determine the cause of the seizures to prevent recurrence and treat any underlying abnormalities.
>
> The treatment of nonconvulsive status epilepticus is somewhat less urgent since the ongoing seizures are not accompanied by the severe metabolic disturbances of GCSE; however, evidence points to local cellular injury in the region of the seizure focus, so the condition should be treated as promptly as possible using the general approach for GCSE.

■ PROGNOSIS

The mortality rate is 20% in GCSE, and the incidence of permanent neurologic sequelae is 10–50%.

> For a more detailed discussion, see Lowenstein DH: Seizures and Epilepsy, Chap. 369, p. 3251, in HPIM-18.

CHAPTER **24**
Diabetic Ketoacidosis and Hyperosmolar Coma

Diabetic ketoacidosis (DKA) and hyperglycemic hyperosmolar state (HHS) are acute complications of diabetes mellitus (DM). DKA is seen primarily in individuals with type 1 DM and HHS in individuals with type 2 DM. Both disorders are associated with absolute or relative insulin deficiency, volume depletion, and altered mental status. The metabolic similarities and differences in DKA and HHS are summarized in Table 24-1.

DIABETIC KETOACIDOSIS

■ ETIOLOGY

DKA results from insulin deficiency with a relative or absolute increase in glucagon and may be caused by inadequate insulin administration, infection (pneumonia, urinary tract infection, gastroenteritis, sepsis), infarction (cerebral, coronary, mesenteric, peripheral), surgery, trauma,

TABLE 24-1 LABORATORY VALUES IN DIABETIC KETOACIDOSIS (DKA) AND HYPERGLYCEMIC HYPEROSMOLAR STATE (HHS) (REPRESENTATIVE RANGES AT PRESENTATION)

	DKA	HHS
Glucose,[a] mmol/L (mg/dL)	13.9–33.3 (250–600)	33.3–66.6 (600–1200)[c]
Sodium, meq/L	125–135	135–145
Potassium,[a] meq/L	Normal to ↑[b]	Normal
Magnesium[a]	Normal[b]	Normal
Chloride[a]	Normal	Normal
Phosphate[a]	Normal to ↓[b]	Normal
Creatinine, μmol/L (mg/dL)	Slightly ↑	Moderately ↑
Osmolality (mOsm/mL)	300–320	330–380
Plasma ketones[a]	++++	±
Serum bicarbonate,[a] meq/L	<15 meq/L	Normal to slightly ↓
Arterial pH	6.8–7.3	>7.3
Arterial P_{CO_2},[a] mmHg	20–30	Normal
Anion gap[a] [Na − (Cl + HCO₃)], meq/L	↑	Normal to slightly ↑

[a]Large changes occur during treatment of DKA.
[b]Although plasma levels may be normal or high at presentation, total-body stores are usually depleted.
[c]Large changes occur during treatment

drugs (cocaine), or pregnancy. A common precipitating scenario is the pt with type 1 DM who erroneously stops administering insulin because of anorexia/lack of food intake caused by a minor illness, followed by lipolysis and progressive ketosis leading to DKA.

CLINICAL FEATURES

The initial symptoms of DKA include anorexia, nausea, vomiting, polyuria, and thirst. Abdominal pain, altered mental function, or frank coma may ensue. Classic signs of DKA include Kussmaul respirations and an acetone odor on the pt's breath. Volume depletion can lead to dry mucous membranes, tachycardia, and hypotension. Fever and abdominal tenderness may also be present. Laboratory evaluation reveals hyperglycemia, ketosis (β-hydroxybutyrate > acetoacetate), and metabolic acidosis (arterial pH 6.8–7.3) with an increased anion gap (Table 24-1). The fluid deficit is often 3–5 L and can be greater. Despite a total-body potassium deficit, the serum potassium at presentation may be normal or mildly high as a result of acidosis. Similarly, phosphate may be normal at presentation despite total body phosphate depletion. Leukocytosis, hypertriglyceridemia, and hyperlipoproteinemia are common. Hyperamylasemia is usually of salivary origin but may suggest a diagnosis of pancreatitis. The measured sodium is reduced as a consequence of osmotic fluid shifts due to hyperglycemia [1.6-meq reduction for each 5.6-mmol/L (100-mg/dL) rise in the serum glucose].

The management of DKA is outlined in Table 24-2.

TABLE 24-2 MANAGEMENT OF DIABETIC KETOACIDOSIS

1. Confirm diagnosis (plasma glucose, positive serum ketones, metabolic acidosis).

2. Admit to hospital; intensive-care setting may be necessary for frequent monitoring or if pH <7.00 or unconscious.

3. Assess: Serum electrolytes (K^+, Na^+, Mg^{2+}, Cl^-, bicarbonate, phosphate) Acid-base status—pH, HCO_3^-, P_{CO_2}, β-hydroxybutyrate Renal function (creatinine, urine output)

4. Replace fluids: 2–3 L of 0.9% saline over first 1–3 h (10–15 mL/kg per hour); subsequently, 0.45% saline at 150–300 mL/h; change to 5% glucose and 0.45% saline at 100–200 mL/h when plasma glucose reaches 14 mmol/L (250 mg/dL).

5. Administer short-acting insulin: IV (0.1 units/kg) or IM (0.3 units/kg), then 0.1 units/kg per hour by continuous IV infusion; increase 2- to 3-fold if no response by 2–4 h. If initial serum potassium is <3.3 meq/L, do not administer insulin until the potassium is corrected to >3.3 meq/L. If the initial serum potassium is >5.2 meq/L, do not supplement K^+ until the potassium is corrected.

6. Assess pt: What precipitated the episode (noncompliance, infection, trauma, infarction, cocaine)? Initiate appropriate workup for precipitating event (cultures, chest x-ray, ECG).

7. Measure capillary glucose every 1–2 h; measure electrolytes (especially K^+, bicarbonate, phosphate) and anion gap every 4 h for first 24 h.

8. Monitor blood pressure, pulse, respirations, mental status, fluid intake and output every 1–4 h.

9. Replace K^+: 10 meq/h when plasma K^+ <5.0–5.2 meq/L, ECG normal, urine flow and normal creatinine documented; administer 40–80 meq/h when plasma K^+ <3.5 meq/L or if bicarbonate is given.

10. Continue above until pt is stable, glucose goal is 150–250 mg/dL, and acidosis is resolved. Insulin infusion may be decreased to 0.05–0.1 units/kg per hour.

11. Administer intermediate or long-acting insulin as soon as pt is eating. Allow for overlap in insulin infusion and SC insulin injection.

Abbreviations: ECG, electrocardiogram.
Source: Adapted from M Sperling, in *Therapy for Diabetes Mellitus and Related Disorders*, American Diabetes Association, Alexandria, VA, 1998; and AE Kitabchi et al: Diabetes Care 29:2739, 2006.

HYPERGLYCEMIC HYPEROSMOLAR STATE

■ ETIOLOGY

Relative insulin deficiency and inadequate fluid intake are the underlying causes of HHS. Hyperglycemia induces an osmotic diuresis that leads to profound intravascular volume depletion. HHS is often precipitated by a serious, concurrent illness such as myocardial infarction or sepsis and compounded by conditions that impede access to water.

■ CLINICAL FEATURES

Presenting symptoms include polyuria, thirst, and altered mental state, ranging from lethargy to coma. Notably absent are symptoms of nausea, vomiting, and abdominal pain and the Kussmaul respirations characteristic of DKA. The prototypical pt is an elderly individual with a several week history of polyuria, weight loss, and diminished oral intake. The laboratory features are summarized in Table 24-1. In contrast to DKA, acidosis and ketonemia are usually not found; however, a small anion gap may be due to lactic acidosis, and moderate ketonuria may occur from starvation. Prerenal azotemia is typically present. Although the measured serum sodium may be normal or slightly low, the corrected serum sodium is usually increased [add 1.6 meq to measured sodium for each 5.6-mmol/L (100-mg/dL) rise in the serum glucose]. HHS, even when adequately treated, has a significant mortality rate (up to 15%), which is in part explained by comorbidities and pt age.

> **TREATMENT** Hyperglycemic Hyperosmolar State
>
> The precipitating problem should be sought and treated. Sufficient IV fluids (1–3 L of 0.9% normal saline over the first 2–3 h) must be given to stabilize the hemodynamic status. The calculated free water deficit (usually 9–10 L) should be reversed over the next 1–2 days, using 0.45% saline initially then 5% dextrose in water. Overly rapid fluid replacement should be avoided to prevent worsening of neurologic status. Potassium repletion is usually necessary. The plasma glucose may drop precipitously with hydration alone, though insulin therapy with an IV bolus of 0.1 units/kg followed by a constant infusion rate (0.1 units/kg per hour) is usually required. If the serum glucose does not fall, the insulin infusion rate should be doubled. Glucose should be added to IV fluid and the insulin infusion rate decreased when the plasma glucose falls to 13.9 mmol/L (250 mg/dL). The insulin infusion should be continued until the pt has resumed eating and can be transitioned to a subcutaneous insulin regimen.

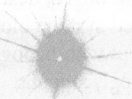

For a more detailed discussion, see Powers AC: Diabetes Mellitus, Chap. 344, p. 2968, in HPIM-18.

CHAPTER **25**
Hypoglycemia

Glucose is an obligate metabolic fuel for the brain. Hypoglycemia should be considered in any pt with confusion, altered level of consciousness, or seizures. Counterregulatory responses to hypoglycemia include insulin suppression and the release of catecholamines, glucagon, growth hormone, and cortisol.

The laboratory diagnosis of hypoglycemia is usually defined as a plasma glucose level <2.5–2.8 mmol/L (<45–50 mg/dL), although the absolute glucose level at which symptoms occur varies among individuals. For this reason, *Whipple's triad* should be present: (1) symptoms consistent with hypoglycemia, (2) a low plasma glucose concentration measured by a method capable of accurately measuring low glucose levels (not a glucose monitor), and (3) relief of symptoms after the plasma glucose level is raised.

■ ETIOLOGY

Hypoglycemia occurs most commonly as a result of treating pts with diabetes mellitus. Additional factors to be considered in any pt with hypoglycemia are listed below.

1. Drugs: insulin, insulin secretagogues (especially chlorpropamide, repaglinide, nateglinide), alcohol, high doses of salicylates, sulfonamides, pentamidine, quinine, quinolones
2. Critical illness: hepatic, renal, or cardiac failure; sepsis; prolonged starvation
3. Hormone deficiencies: adrenal insufficiency, hypopituitarism (particularly in young children)
4. Insulinoma (pancreatic β cell tumor), β cell hyperplasia (nesidioblastosis; congenital or after gastric or bariatric surgery)
5. Other rare etiologies: Non–β cell tumors (large mesenchymal or epithelial tumors producing an incompletely processed IGF-II, other nonpancreatic tumors), antibodies to insulin or the insulin receptor, inherited enzymatic defects such as hereditary fructose intolerance and galactosemia.

■ CLINICAL FEATURES

Symptoms of hypoglycemia can be divided into autonomic (adrenergic: palpitations, tremor, and anxiety; cholinergic: sweating, hunger, and paresthesia) and neuroglycopenic (behavioral changes, confusion, fatigue, seizure, loss of consciousness, and, if hypoglycemia is severe and prolonged, death). Signs of autonomic discharge, such as tachycardia, elevated systolic blood pressure, pallor, and diaphoresis are typically present in a pt with hypoglycemia awareness but may be absent in a pt with pure neuroglycopenia.

Recurrent hypoglycemia shifts thresholds for the autonomic symptoms and counterregulatory responses to lower glucose levels, leading to hypoglycemic unawareness. Under these circumstances, the first manifestation of hypoglycemia is neuroglycopenia, placing pts at risk of being unable to treat themselves.

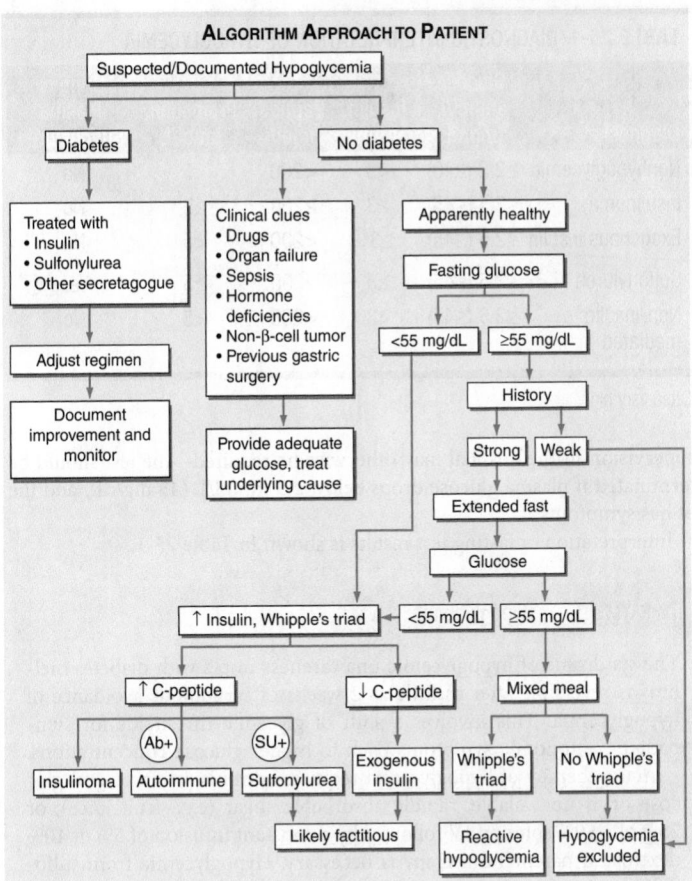

FIGURE 25-1 Diagnostic approach to a pt with suspected hypoglycemia based on a history of symptoms, a low plasma glucose concentration, or both. AB+, positive for antibodies against insulin or the insulin receptor; SU+, positive for sulfonylurea.

■ DIAGNOSIS

Diagnosis of the hypoglycemic mechanism is critical for choosing a treatment that prevents recurrent hypoglycemia (Fig. 25-1). Urgent treatment is often necessary in pts with suspected hypoglycemia. Nevertheless, blood should be drawn at the time of symptoms, whenever possible before the administration of glucose, to allow documentation of the glucose level. If the glucose level is low and the cause of hypoglycemia is unknown, additional assays should be performed on blood obtained at the time of a low plasma glucose. These should include insulin, proinsulin, C-peptide, sulfonylurea levels, cortisol, and ethanol. In the absence of documented spontaneous hypoglycemia, overnight fasting or food deprivation during observation in the outpatient setting will sometimes elicit hypoglycemia and allow diagnostic evaluation. An extended (up to 72 h) fast under careful

TABLE 25-1 DIAGNOSTIC INTERPRETATION OF HYPOGLYCEMIA

Diagnosis	Glucose, mmol/L (mg/dL)	Insulin, μU/mL	C-Peptide, pmol/L	Proinsulin, pmol/L	Urine or Plasma Sulfonylurea
Nonhypoglycemic	≥2.2 (≥40)	<3	<200	<5	No
Insulinoma	≤2.5 (≤45)	≥3	≥200	≥5	No
Exogenous insulin	≤2.5 (≤45)	≥3[a]	<200	<5	No
Sulfonylurea	≤2.5 (≤45)	≥3	≥200	≥5	Yes
Non-insulin mediated	≤2.5 (≤45)	<3	<200	<5	No

[a]Often very high.

supervision in the hospital may otherwise be required—the test should be terminated if plasma glucose drops below 2.5 mmol/L (45 mg/dL) and the pt has symptoms.

Interpretation of fasting test results is shown in Table 25-1.

TREATMENT   Hypoglycemia

The syndrome of hypoglycemic unawareness in pts with diabetes mellitus is reversible after as little as 2 weeks of scrupulous avoidance of hypoglycemia. This involves a shift of glycemic thresholds for sympathetic autonomic symptoms back to higher glucose concentrations.

Acute therapy of hypoglycemia requires administration of oral glucose or, if unavailable, rapidly absorbable sugar (e.g., fruit juice), or 25 g of a 50% solution IV followed by a constant infusion of 5% or 10% dextrose if parenteral therapy is necessary. Hypoglycemia from sulfonylureas is often prolonged, requiring treatment and monitoring for 24 h or more. SC or IM glucagon can be used in diabetics. Prevention of recurrent hypoglycemia requires treatment of the underlying cause of hypoglycemia, including discontinuation or dose reduction of offending drugs, treatment of critical illnesses, replacement of hormonal deficiencies, and surgery of insulinomas or other tumors. Diazoxide or octreotide therapy can be used to control hypoglycemia in inoperable metastatic insulinoma or nesidioblastosis. Treatment of other forms of hypoglycemia is dietary, with avoidance of fasting and ingestion of frequent small meals.

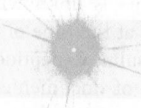

For a more detailed discussion, see Cryer PE, Davis SN: Hypoglycemia, Chap. 345, p. 3003, in HPIM-18.

CHAPTER **26**
Infectious Disease Emergencies

APPROACH TO THE PATIENT   Infectious Disease Emergencies

- Acutely ill febrile pts require emergent attention and must be appropriately evaluated and treated at presentation to improve outcome. A quick assessment of general appearance provides a subjective sense of whether the pt is septic or toxic.
- *History*: Although presenting symptoms are frequently nonspecific, the physician should elicit the following elements of a directed history to help identify risk factors for particular infections:
  - Onset and duration of symptoms, changes in severity or rate of progression over time
  - Host factors (e.g., alcoholism, IV drug use) and comorbid conditions (e.g., asplenia, diabetes, HIV infection)
  - Potential nidus for invasive infection (e.g., recent URI or influenza, trauma, burn, surgery, foreign body)
  - Exposure history (e.g., travel, pets, diet, medication use, vaccination history, sick contacts, menstruation history, sexual contacts)
- *Physical examination*: A complete physical examination should be performed, with particular attention to general appearance, vital signs, skin and soft tissue exam, and neurologic evaluation (including mental status).
- *Diagnostic workup*: should be initiated rapidly, preferably before antibiotics are given
  - Bloodwork: cultures, CBC with differential, electrolytes, BUN, creatinine, LFTs, blood smear examination (for parasitic or tick-borne diseases), buffy coat
  - CSF cultures if meningitis is possible. If focal neurologic signs, papilledema, or abnormal mental status is noted, administer antibiotics after blood culture samples are obtained, perform brain imaging, and then consider LP.
  - CT or MRI to evaluate focal abscesses; cultures of wounds or scraping of skin lesions as indicated
  - No diagnostic procedure should delay treatment for more than minutes.
- *Treatment*: Empirical antibiotic therapy (Table 26-1) is critical.
  - Adjunctive therapy (e.g., glucocorticoids or IV immunoglobulin) may reduce morbidity and mortality rates for specific conditions. Dexamethasone for bacterial meningitis must be given before or with the first dose of antibiotic.

TABLE 26-1 COMMON INFECTIOUS DISEASE EMERGENCIES

Clinical Syndrome	Possible Etiologies	Treatment	Comments
Sepsis without a clear focus			
Septic shock	*Pseudomonas* spp., gram-negative enteric bacilli, *Staphylococcus* spp., *Streptococcus* spp.	Vancomycin (1 g q12h) *plus* Gentamicin (5 mg/kg per day) *plus either* Piperacillin/tazobactam (3.375 g q4h) *or* Cefepime (2 g q12h)	Adjust treatment when culture data become available. Drotrecogin alfa (activated)[a] or low-dose hydrocortisone and fludrocortisone[b] may improve outcome in pts with septic shock.
Overwhelming post-splenectomy sepsis	*Streptococcus pneumoniae, Haemophilus influenzae, Neisseria meningitidis*	Ceftriaxone (2 g q12h) *plus* Vancomycin (1 g q12h)	If a β-lactam–sensitive strain is identified, vancomycin can be discontinued.
Babesiosis	*Babesia microti* (U.S.), *B. divergens* (Europe)	*Either:* Clindamycin (600 mg tid) *plus* Quinine (650 mg tid) *or:* Atovaquone (750 mg q12h) *plus* Azithromycin (500-mg loading dose, then 250 mg/d)	Atovaquone and azithromycin are as effective as clindamycin and quinine and are associated with fewer side effects. Treatment with doxycycline (100 mg bid[c]) for potential co-infection with *Borrelia burgdorferi* or *Anaplasma* spp. may be prudent.

Sepsis with Skin Findings

Condition	Pathogens	Treatment	Notes
Meningococcemia	*N. meningitidis*	Penicillin (4 mU q4h) *or* Ceftriaxone (2 g q12h)	Consider protein C replacement in fulminant meningococcemia.
Rocky Mountain spotted fever (RMSF)	*Rickettsia rickettsii*	Doxycycline (100 mg bid)	If both meningococcemia and RMSF are being considered, use ceftriaxone (2 g q12h) *plus* doxycycline (100 mg bid) *or* chloramphenicol alone (50–75 mg/kg per day in four divided doses). If RMSF is diagnosed, doxycycline is the proven superior agent.
Purpura fulminans	*S. pneumoniae, H. influenzae, N. meningitidis*	Ceftriaxone (2 g q12h) *plus* Vancomycin (1 g q12h)	If a β-lactam–sensitive strain is identified, vancomycin can be discontinued.
Erythroderma: toxic shock syndrome	Group A *Streptococcus, Staphylococcus aureus*	Vancomycin (1 g q12h) *plus* Clindamycin (600 mg q8h)	If a penicillin- or oxacillin–sensitive strain is isolated, these agents are superior to vancomycin (penicillin, 2 mU q4h; or oxacillin, 2 g q4h). The site of toxigenic bacteria should be debrided; IV immunoglobulin can be used in severe cases.[d]

Sepsis with Soft Tissue Findings

Condition	Pathogens	Treatment	Notes
Necrotizing fasciitis	Group A *Streptococcus*, mixed aerobic/anaerobic flora, CA-MRSA[e]	Vancomycin (1 g q12h) *plus* Clindamycin (600 mg q8h) *plus* Gentamicin (5 mg/kg per day)	Urgent surgical evaluation is critical. If a penicillin- or oxacillin–sensitive strain is isolated, these agents are superior to vancomycin (penicillin, 2 mU q4h; or oxacillin, 2 g q4h).

(*continued*)

127

TABLE 26-1 COMMON INFECTIOUS DISEASE EMERGENCIES (CONTINUED)

Clinical Syndrome	Possible Etiologies	Treatment	Comments
Sepsis with soft tissue findings			
Clostridial myonecrosis	*Clostridium perfringens*	Penicillin (2 mU q4h) *plus* Clindamycin (600 mg q8h)	Urgent surgical evaluation is critical.
Neurologic infections			
Bacterial meningitis	*S. pneumoniae, N. meningitidis*	Ceftriaxone (2 g q12h) *plus* Vancomycin (1 g q12h)	If a β-lactam–sensitive strain is identified, vancomycin can be discontinued. If the pt is >50 years old or has comorbid disease, add ampicillin (2 g q4h) for *Listeria* coverage. Dexamethasone (10 mg q6h × 4 days) improves outcome in adult pts with meningitis (especially pneumococcal) and cloudy CSF, positive CSF Gram's stain, or a CSF leukocyte count >1000/mL.
Brain abscess, suppurative intracranial infections	*Streptococcus* spp., *Staphylococcus* spp., anaerobes, gram-negative bacilli	Vancomycin (1 g q12h) *plus* Metronidazole (500 mg q8h) *plus* Ceftriaxone (2 g q12h)	Urgent surgical evaluation is critical. If a penicillin- or oxacillin-sensitive strain is isolated, these agents are superior to vancomycin (penicillin, 4 mU q4h; or oxacillin, 2 g q4h).
Cerebral malaria	*Plasmodium falciparum*	Artesunate (2.4 mg/kg IV at 0, 12, and 24 h; then once daily)ʳ *or* Quinine (IV loading dose of 20 mg salt/kg; then 10 mg/kg q8h) *plus* Doxycycline (100 mg IV q12h)	Do not use glucocorticoids. Use IV quinidine if IV quinine is not available. During IV quinidine treatment, blood pressure and cardiac function should be monitored continuously and blood glucose monitored periodically.

| Spinal epidural abscess | *Staphylococcus* spp., gram-negative bacilli | Vancomycin (1 g q12h) *plus* Ceftriaxone (2 g q24h) | Surgical evaluation is essential. If a penicillin- or oxacillin-sensitive strain is isolated, these agents are superior to vancomycin (penicillin, 4 mU q4h; or oxacillin, 2 g q4h). |

Focal infections

| Acute bacterial endocarditis | *S. aureus*, β-hemolytic streptococci, HACEK group,[g] *Neisseria* spp., *S. pneumoniae* | Ceftriaxone (2 g q12h) *plus* Vancomycin (1 g q12h) | Adjust treatment when culture data become available. Surgical evaluation is essential. |

[a]Drotrecogin alfa (activated) is administered at a dose of 24 μg/kg per hour for 96 h. It has been approved for use in pts with severe sepsis and a high risk of death as defined by an Acute Physiology and Chronic Health Evaluation II (APACHE II) score of ≥25 and/or multiorgan failure.

[b]Hydrocortisone (50-mg IV bolus q6h) with fludrocortisone (50-μg tablet daily for 7 days) may improve outcomes of severe sepsis, particularly in the setting of relative adrenal insufficiency.

[c]Tetracyclines can be antagonistic in action to β-lactam agents. Adjust treatment as soon as the diagnosis is confirmed.

[d]The optimal dose of IV immunoglobulin has not been determined, but the median dose in observational studies is 2 g/kg (total dose administered over 1–5 days).

[e]Community-acquired methicillin-resistant *S. aureus*.

[f]In the United States, artesunate must be obtained by the Centers for Disease Control and Prevention. For pts diagnosed with severe malaria, full doses of parenteral antimalarial treatment should be started with whichever recommended antimalarial agent is first available.

[g]*Haemophilus aphrophilus, H. paraphrophilus, H. parainfluenzae, Aggregatibacter* (formerly *Actinobacillus*) *actinomycetemcomitans, Cardiobacterium hominis, Eikenella corrodens,* and *Kingella kingae.*

■ SPECIFIC PRESENTATIONS (TABLE 26-1)

Sepsis without an Obvious Focus of Primary Infection

1. Septic shock: A primary site of infection may not be evident initially.
2. Overwhelming infection in asplenic pts
   a. Most infections occur within 2 years after splenectomy, with ~50% mortality.
   b. Encapsulated organisms cause the majority of infections; *Streptococcus pneumoniae* is the most common isolate.
3. Babesiosis: A history of recent travel to endemic areas raises the possibility of this diagnosis.
   a. Nonspecific symptoms occur 1–4 weeks after a tick bite and can progress to renal failure, acute respiratory failure, and DIC.
   b. Asplenia, age >60 years, underlying immunosuppressive conditions, infection with the European strain *Babesia divergens*, and co-infection with *Borrelia burgdorferi* (Lyme disease) or *Anaplasma phagocytophilum* are risk factors for severe disease.
4. Tularemia and plague can produce typhoidal or septic syndromes with mortality rates ~30% and should be considered in the appropriate epidemiologic setting.
5. Viral hemorrhagic fevers: zoonotic viral illness from animal reservoirs or arthropod vectors (e.g., Lassa fever in Africa, hantavirus hemorrhagic fever with renal syndrome in Asia, Ebola and Marburg virus infections in Africa, and yellow fever in Africa and South America). Dengue is the most common arboviral disease worldwide; dengue hemorrhagic fever is the more severe form, with a triad of hemorrhagic manifestations, plasma leakage, and platelet counts <100,000/μL. Mortality is 10–20% but approaches 40% if dengue shock syndrome develops. Supportive care and volume replacement therapy are life-saving.

Sepsis with Skin Manifestations

1. Maculopapular rashes: usually not emergent but can occur in early meningococcemia or rickettsial disease
2. Petechiae: warrant urgent attention when accompanied by hypotension or a toxic appearance
   a. Meningococcemia: Young children and their household contacts are at greatest risk; outbreaks occur in schools, day-care centers, and military barracks.
      i. Petechiae begin at ankles, wrists, axillae, and mucosal surfaces and progress to purpura and DIC.
      ii. Other symptoms include headache, nausea, myalgias, altered mental status, and meningismus.
      iii. Mortality rates are 50–60%; early treatment initiation may be life-saving.
   b. Rocky Mountain spotted fever: A history of a tick bite and/or travel or outdoor activity can often be ascertained.
      i. Rash appears by day 3 (but never develops in 10–15% of pts). Blanching macules become hemorrhagic, starting at wrists and ankles and spreading to legs and trunk (centripetal spread), then palms and soles.

ii. Other symptoms include headache, malaise, myalgias, nausea, vomiting, and anorexia. In severe cases, hypotension, encephalitis, and coma can ensue.

c. Other rickettsial diseases: Mediterranean spotted fever (Africa, southwestern and south-central Asia, southern Europe) is characterized by an inoculation eschar at the site of the tick bite and has a mortality rate of ~50%. Epidemic typhus occurs in louse-infested areas, usually in a setting of poverty, war, or natural disaster; mortality rates are 10–15%. In scrub typhus (southeastern Asia and western Pacific), the etiologic organism is found in areas of heavy scrub vegetation (e.g., riverbanks); 1–35% of pts die.

3 Purpura fulminans: cutaneous manifestation of DIC with large ecchymotic areas and hemorrhagic bullae. It is associated primarily with *Neisseria meningitidis* but can also be associated with *S. pneumoniae* and *Haemophilus influenzae* in asplenic pts.

4. Ecthyma gangrenosum: hemorrhagic vesicles with central necrosis and ulceration and a rim of erythema seen in pts with septic shock due to *Pseudomonas aeruginosa* or *Aeromonas hydrophila*

5. Bullous or hemorrhagic lesions: can be caused by *Escherichia coli* and organisms in the genus *Vibrio* (*V. vulnificus* and other noncholera vibrios from seawater or contaminated raw shellfish), *Aeromonas*, and *Klebsiella*, particularly in pts with liver disease

6. Erythroderma: diffuse sunburn-like rash, often associated with toxic shock syndrome (TSS, defined by clinical criteria of hypotension, multiorgan failure, fever, and rash) in acutely ill pts; more common in staphylococcal TSS than streptococcal TSS

Sepsis with a Soft Tissue/Muscle Primary Focus

1. Necrotizing fasciitis: characterized by extensive necrosis of the SC tissue and fascia; typically caused by group A streptococci

   a. Exam is notable for high fever and pain out of proportion to physical findings; the infected area is red, hot, shiny, and exquisitely tender. Lessening of pain in the absence of treatment is an ominous sign that represents destruction of peripheral nerves.

   b. Risk factors: trauma, varicella, childbirth, and comorbid conditions (e.g., diabetes, peripheral vascular disease, IV drug use)

   c. Mortality rates are ~100% without surgery, >70% in the setting of TSS, and 15–34% overall.

2. Clostridial myonecrosis: often associated with trauma or surgery, with massive necrotizing gangrene developing within hours of onset

   a. Spontaneous cases are associated with *Clostridium septicum* infection and underlying malignancy.

   b. Pain and toxic appearance are out of proportion to physical findings. Pts are apathetic and may have a sense of impending doom.

   c. Skin overlying the affected area is mottled, bronze-brown in color, and edematous. Crepitus may be present. Bullous lesions may drain serosanguineous fluid with a mousy or sweet odor.

   d. Mortality rates are 12% for myonecrosis of extremities, 63% for myonecrosis of the trunk, and >65% for spontaneous myonecrosis.

Neurologic Infections with or without Septic Shock

1. Bacterial meningitis: Most cases in adults are caused by *S. pneumoniae* (30–50%) or *N. meningitidis* (10–35%).
   a. Classic triad of headache, meningismus, and fever in only one-half to two-thirds of pts
   b. Blood cultures positive in 50–70% of pts
   c. Predictors of a poor outcome include meningitis due to *S. pneumoniae*, coma, respiratory distress, hypotension, CSF protein >2.5 g/L, CSF glucose <10 mg/dL, peripheral WBC count <5000/µL, and serum Na⁺ <135 mmol/L.

2. Brain abscess: often present without systemic signs. Presentations are more consistent with a space-occupying lesion in the brain.
   a. 70% of pts have headache and/or altered mental status, 50% have focal neurologic signs, and 25% have papilledema.
   b. Lesions arise from contiguous foci (e.g., sinusitis or otitis) or hematogenous infection (e.g., endocarditis).
   c. >50% of cases are polymicrobial, involving both aerobic (primarily streptococcal) and anaerobic organisms.
   d. Mortality is low, but morbidity is high (30–55%).

3. Intracranial and spinal epidural abscesses (ICEAs and SEAs): ICEAs are rare in the United States, but SEAs are on the rise. Both are more common in areas with limited access to health care.
   a. ICEAs are typically polymicrobial and present as fever, mental status changes, and neck pain.
   b. SEAs are typically due to hematogenous seeding (with staphylococci most commonly isolated) and present as fever, localized spinal tenderness, and back pain.

4. Cerebral malaria: should be urgently considered in pts who have recently traveled to endemic areas and present with a febrile illness and neurologic signs
   a. Fulminant *Plasmodium falciparum* infection is associated with fever >40°C, hypotension, jaundice, ARDS, and bleeding. Nuchal rigidity and photophobia are rare.
   b. Unrecognized infection results in a 20–30% mortality rate.

Focal Syndromes with a Fulminant Course

1. Rhinocerebral mucormycosis: presents as low-grade fever, dull sinus pain, diplopia, impaired mental status, chemosis, proptosis, hard-palate lesions that respect the midline, and dusky or necrotic nasal turbinates; generally occurs in pts with immunocompromising conditions

2. Acute bacterial endocarditis: presents as fever, fatigue, and malaise within 2 weeks of infection and is associated with rapid valvular destruction, pulmonary edema, and myocardial abscesses
   a. Etiologies include *Staphylococcus aureus, S. pneumoniae, Listeria monocytogenes, Haemophilus* spp., and streptococci of group A, B, or G.
   b. Although Janeway lesions (hemorrhagic macules on the palms or soles) can be seen, other embolic phenomena (e.g., petechiae, Roth's spots, splinter hemorrhages) are less common.

c. Features can include rapid valvular destruction, pulmonary edema, hypotension, myocardial abscesses, conduction abnormalities and arrhythmias, large friable vegetations, and major arterial emboli with tissue infarction.

d. Mortality rates are 10–40%.

3. Inhalational anthrax: of increasing concern, given the potential of *Bacillus anthracis* as a bioterrorism agent

a. Clinical symptoms are nonspecific, but chest x-rays show mediastinal widening, pulmonary infiltrates, and pleural effusions.

b. Hemorrhagic meningitis occurs in 38% of pts.

c. Urgent antimicrobial therapy is needed, ideally with a multidrug regimen in the prodromal period.

4. Avian influenza (H5N1): occurs primarily in Southeast Asia after exposure to poultry. Pts can rapidly develop bilateral pneumonia, ARDS, and multiorgan failure, culminating in death. Human-to-human transmission is rare.

5. Hantavirus pulmonary syndrome: occurs primarily following rodent exposure in rural areas of the southwestern United States, Canada, and South America.

a. A nonspecific viral prodrome can rapidly progress to pulmonary edema, respiratory failure, myocardial depression, and death.

b. In an appropriate epidemiologic setting, the early onset of thrombocytopenia may distinguish this syndrome from other febrile illnesses.

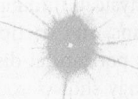

For a more detailed discussion, see Barlam TF, Kasper DL: Approach to the Acutely Ill Infected Febrile Patient, Chap. 121, p. 1023, in HPIM-18.

CHAPTER **27**
Oncologic Emergencies

Emergencies in the cancer pt may be classified into three categories: effects from tumor expansion, metabolic or hormonal effects mediated by tumor products, and treatment complications.

STRUCTURAL/OBSTRUCTIVE ONCOLOGIC EMERGENCIES

The most common problems are superior vena cava syndrome; pericardial effusion/tamponade; spinal cord compression; seizures (Chap. 193) and/or increased intracranial pressure; and intestinal, urinary, or biliary obstruction. The last three conditions are discussed in Chap. 276 in HPIM-18.

■ **SUPERIOR VENA CAVA SYNDROME**

Obstruction of the superior vena cava reduces venous return from the head, neck, and upper extremities. About 85% of cases are due to lung cancer; lymphoma and thrombosis of central venous catheters are also causes. Pts often present with facial swelling, dyspnea, and cough. In severe cases, the mediastinal mass lesion may cause tracheal obstruction. Dilated neck veins and increased collateral veins on anterior chest wall are noted on physical exam. Chest x-ray (CXR) documents widening of the superior mediastinum; 25% of pts have a right-sided pleural effusion.

TREATMENT	Superior Vena Cava Syndrome

Radiation therapy is the treatment of choice for non-small cell lung cancer; addition of chemotherapy to radiation therapy is effective in small cell lung cancer and lymphoma. Symptoms recur in 10–30% and can be palliated by venous stenting. Clotted central catheters producing this syndrome should be removed and anticoagulation therapy initiated.

■ **PERICARDIAL EFFUSION/TAMPONADE**

Accumulation of fluid in the pericardium impairs filling of the heart and decreases cardiac output. Most commonly seen in pts with lung or breast cancers, leukemias, or lymphomas, pericardial tamponade may also develop as a late complication of mediastinal radiation therapy (constrictive pericarditis). Common symptoms are dyspnea, cough, chest pain, orthopnea, and weakness. Pleural effusion, sinus tachycardia, jugular venous distention, hepatomegaly, and cyanosis are frequent physical findings. Paradoxical pulse, decreased heart sounds, pulsus alternans, and friction rub are less common with malignant than nonmalignant pericardial disease. Echocardiography is diagnostic; pericardiocentesis may show serous or bloody exudate, and cytology usually shows malignant cells.

TREATMENT	Pericardial Effusion/Tamponade

Drainage of fluid from the pericardial sac may be lifesaving until a definitive surgical procedure (pericardial stripping or window) can be performed.

■ **SPINAL CORD COMPRESSION**

Primary spinal cord tumors occur rarely, and cord compression is most commonly due to epidural metastases from vertebral bodies involved with tumor, especially from prostate, lung, breast, lymphoma, and myeloma primaries. Pts present with back pain, worse when recumbent, with local tenderness. Loss of bowel and bladder control may occur. On physical exam, pts have a loss of sensation below a horizontal line on the trunk, called a *sensory level*, which usually corresponds to one or two vertebrae below the site of compression. Weakness and spasticity of the legs and hyperactive reflexes with upgoing toes on Babinski testing are often noted. Spine radiographs may reveal erosion of the pedicles (winking owl sign), lytic or sclerotic vertebral body lesions, and vertebral collapse. Collapse alone is not

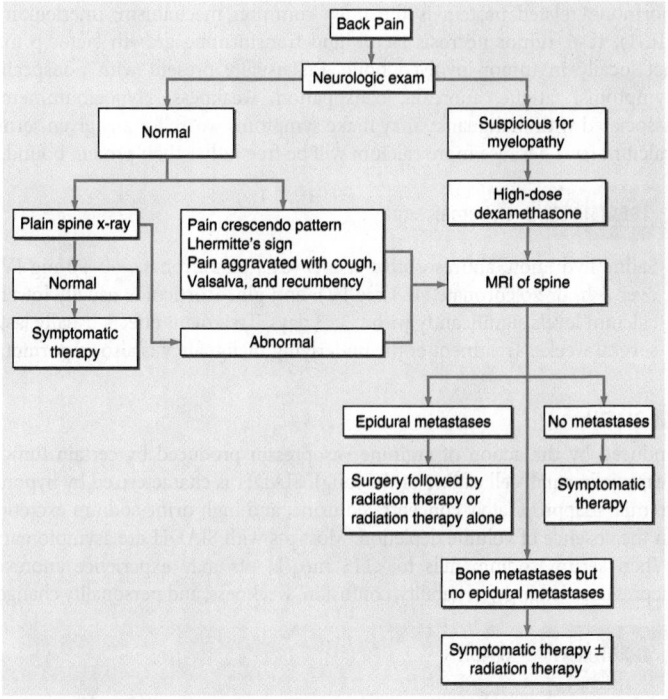

FIGURE 27-1 Management of cancer pts with back pain.

a reliable indicator of tumor; it is a common manifestation of a more common disease, osteoporosis. MRI can visualize the cord throughout its length and define the extent of tumor involvement.

TREATMENT Spinal Cord Compression (See Fig. 27-1)

Radiation therapy plus dexamethasone, 4 mg IV or PO q4h, is successful in arresting and reversing symptoms in about 75% of pts who are diagnosed while still ambulatory. Surgery results in better recovery rates but may be extensive (vertebral body resection with spine stabilization). Only 10% of pts made paraplegic by the tumor recover the ability to ambulate.

EMERGENT PARANEOPLASTIC SYNDROMES

Most paraneoplastic syndromes have an insidious onset (Chap. 83). Hypercalcemia, syndrome of inappropriate antidiuretic hormone secretion (SIADH), and adrenal insufficiency may present as emergencies.

■ HYPERCALCEMIA

The most common paraneoplastic syndrome, hypercalcemia occurs in about 10% of cancer pts, particularly those with lung, breast, head and neck, and kidney cancer and myeloma. Bone resorption mediated by parathyroid hormone–related protein is the most common mechanism; interleukin 1 (IL-1), IL-6, tumor necrosis factor, and transforming growth factor β may act locally in tumor-involved bone. Pts usually present with nonspecific symptoms: fatigue, anorexia, constipation, weakness. Hypoalbuminemia associated with malignancy may make symptoms worse for any given serum calcium level because more calcium will be free rather than protein bound.

TREATMENT   Hypercalcemia

Saline hydration, antiresorptive agents (e.g., pamidronate, 60–90 mg IV over 4 h, or zoledronate, 4–8 mg IV), and glucocorticoids usually lower calcium levels significantly within 1–3 days. Treatment effects usually last several weeks. Treatment of the underlying malignancy is also important.

■ SIADH

Induced by the action of arginine vasopressin produced by certain tumors (especially small cell cancer of the lung), SIADH is characterized by hyponatremia, inappropriately concentrated urine, and high urine sodium excretion in the absence of volume depletion. Most pts with SIADH are asymptomatic. When serum sodium falls to <115 meq/L, pts may experience anorexia, depression, lethargy, irritability, confusion, weakness, and personality changes.

TREATMENT   SIADH

Water restriction controls mild forms. Demeclocycline (150–300 mg PO tid or qid) inhibits the effects of vasopressin on the renal tubule but has a slow onset of action (1 week). Treatment of the underlying malignancy is also important. If the pt has mental status changes with sodium levels <115 meq/L, normal saline infusion plus furosemide to increase free water clearance may provide more rapid improvement. Rate of correction should not exceed 0.5–1 meq/L per h. More rapid change can produce fluid shifts that lead to brain damage.

■ ADRENAL INSUFFICIENCY

The infiltration of the adrenals by tumor and their destruction by hemorrhage are the two most common causes. Symptoms such as nausea, vomiting, anorexia, and orthostatic hypotension may be attributed to progressive cancer or to treatment side effects. Certain treatments (e.g., ketoconazole, aminoglutethimide) may directly interfere with steroid synthesis in the adrenal.

TREATMENT   Adrenal Insufficiency

In emergencies, a bolus of 100 mg IV hydrocortisone is followed by a continuous infusion of 10 mg/h. In nonemergent but stressful circumstances, 100–200 mg/d oral hydrocortisone is the beginning dose, tapered to maintenance of 15–37.5 mg/d. Fludrocortisone (0.1 mg/d) may be required in the presence of hyperkalemia.

TREATMENT COMPLICATIONS

Complications from treatment may occur acutely or emerge only many years after treatment. Toxicity may be either related to the agents used to treat the cancer or from the response of the cancer to the treatment (e.g., leaving a perforation in a hollow viscus or causing metabolic complications such as tumor lysis syndrome). Several treatment complications present as emergencies. Fever and neutropenia and tumor lysis syndrome will be discussed here; others are discussed in Chap. 276 in HPIM-18.

◼ FEVER AND NEUTROPENIA

Many cancer pts are treated with myelotoxic agents. When peripheral blood granulocyte counts are <1000/µL, the risk of infection is substantially increased (48 infections/100 pts). A neutropenic pt who develops a fever (>38°C) should undergo physical exam with special attention to skin lesions, mucous membranes, IV catheter sites, and perirectal area. Two sets of blood cultures from different sites should be drawn and a CXR performed, and any additional tests should be guided by findings from the history and physical exam. Any fluid collections should be tapped, and urine and/or fluids should be examined under the microscope for evidence of infection.

> **TREATMENT** Fever and Neutropenia
>
> After cultures are obtained, all pts should receive IV broad-spectrum antibiotics (e.g., ceftazidime, 1 g q8h). If an obvious infectious site is found, the antibiotic regimen is designed to cover organisms that may cause the infection. Usually therapy should be started with an agent or agents that cover both gram-positive and -negative organisms. If the fever resolves, treatment should continue until neutropenia resolves. Persistence of febrile neutropenia after 7 days should lead to addition of amphotericin B (or another broad spectrum antifungal agent) to the antibiotic regimen.

◼ TUMOR LYSIS SYNDROME

When rapidly growing tumors are treated with effective chemotherapy regimens, the dying tumor cells can release large amounts of nucleic acid breakdown products (chiefly uric acid), potassium, phosphate, and lactic acid. The phosphate elevations can lead to hypocalcemia. The increased uric acid, especially in the setting of acidosis, can precipitate in the renal tubules and lead to renal failure. The renal failure can exacerbate the hyperkalemia.

> **TREATMENT** Tumor Lysis Syndrome
>
> Prevention is the best approach. Maintain hydration with 3 L/d of saline, keep urine pH > 7.0 with bicarbonate administration, and start allopurinol, 300 mg/m^2 per day, 24 h before starting chemotherapy. Once chemotherapy is given, monitor serum electrolytes every 6 h. If after 24 h, uric acid (>8 mg/dL) and serum creatinine (>1.6 mg/dL) are elevated,

rasburicase (recombinant urate oxidase), 0.2 mg/kg IV daily, may lower uric acid levels. If serum potassium is >6.0 meq/L and renal failure ensues, hemodialysis may be required. Maintain normal calcium levels.

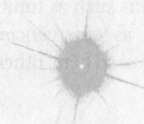

For a more detailed discussion, see Finberg R: Infections in Patients With Cancer, Chap. 86, p. 712; Jameson JL, Longo DL: Paraneoplastic Syndromes: Endocrinologic/Hematologic, Chap. 100, p. 826, and Gucalp R, Dutcher J: Oncologic Emergencies, Chap. 276, p. 2266, in HPIM-18.

CHAPTER 28
Anaphylaxis

■ DEFINITION

A life-threatening systemic hypersensitivity reaction to contact with an allergen; it may appear within minutes of exposure to the offending substance. Manifestations include respiratory distress, pruritus, urticaria, mucous membrane swelling, gastrointestinal disturbances (including nausea, vomiting, abdominal pain, and diarrhea), and vascular collapse. Virtually any allergen may trigger an anaphylactic reaction, but among the more common agents are proteins such as antisera, hormones, pollen extracts, Hymenoptera venom, and foods; drugs (especially antibiotics); and diagnostic agents such as IV contrast material. Atopy does not seem to predispose to anaphylaxis from penicillin or venom exposures. Anaphylactic transfusion reactions are covered in Chap. 9.

■ CLINICAL PRESENTATION

Time to onset is variable, but symptoms usually occur within seconds to minutes of exposure to the offending antigen:

- Respiratory: mucous membrane swelling, hoarseness, stridor, wheezing
- Cardiovascular: tachycardia, hypotension
- Cutaneous: pruritus, urticaria, angioedema

■ DIAGNOSIS

Made by obtaining history of exposure to offending substance with subsequent development of characteristic complex of symptoms.

TREATMENT Anaphylaxis

Mild symptoms such as pruritus and urticaria can be controlled by administration of 0.3–0.5 mL of 1:1000 (1.0 mg/mL) epinephrine SC or IM, with repeated doses as required at 5- to 20-min intervals for a severe reaction.

An IV infusion should be initiated for administration of 2.5 mL of 1:10,000 epinephrine solution at 5- to 10-min intervals, and volume expanders such as normal saline, and vasopressor agents, e.g., dopamine, if intractable hypotension occurs.

Epinephrine provides both α- and β-adrenergic effects, resulting in vasoconstriction and bronchial smooth-muscle relaxation. Beta blockers are relatively contraindicated in persons at risk for anaphylactic reactions.

The following should also be used as necessary:

- Antihistamines such as diphenhydramine 50–100 mg IM or IV
- Nebulized albuterol or aminophylline 0.25–0.5 g IV for bronchospasm
- Oxygen
- Glucocorticoids (medrol 0.5–1.0 mg/kg IV); not useful for acute manifestations but may help alleviate later recurrence of hypotension, bronchospasm, or urticaria.
- For antigenic material injected into an extremity consider: use of a tourniquet proximal to the site, 0.2 mL of 1:1000 epinephrine into the site, removal of an insect stinger if present.

■ PREVENTION

Avoidance of offending antigen, where possible; skin testing and desensitization to materials such as penicillin and Hymenoptera venom, if necessary. Individuals should wear an informational bracelet and have immediate access to an unexpired epinephrine kit.

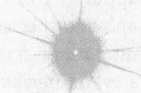

For a more detailed discussion, see Austen KF: Allergies, Anaphylaxis, and Systemic Mastocytosis, Chap. 317, p. 2707, in HPIM-18.

CHAPTER **29**
Bites, Venoms, Stings, and Marine Poisonings

MAMMALIAN BITES

- Each year, there are ~300 dog and cat bites per 100,000 population in the United States, with most bites inflicted by pet animals.
- The microflora of bite wounds typically reflects the oral flora of the biting animal.
- Bites from many different animals can transmit rabies and tularemia.

■ DOG BITES

- **Epidemiology:** Dogs bite ≥4.7 million people per year, causing 80% of all animal bites; 15–20% of dog bites become infected.
- **Bacteriology:** includes aerobic and anaerobic organisms, such as β-hemolytic streptococci; *Eikenella corrodens; Capnocytophaga canimorsus;* and *Pasteurella, Staphylococcus, Actinomyces,* and *Fusobacterium* species

- **Clinical Features:** typically manifest within 8–24 h after the bite as local cellulitis with purulent, sometimes foul-smelling discharge. Systemic spread (e.g., bacteremia, endocarditis, brain abscess) can occur. *C. canimorsus* infection can present as sepsis syndrome, DIC, and renal failure, particularly in pts who are splenectomized, have hepatic dysfunction, or are otherwise immunosuppressed.

■ CAT BITES

- **Epidemiology:** Cat bites and scratches result in infection in >50% of cases.
- **Bacteriology:** includes organisms similar to those involved in dog bites. *Pasteurella multocida* and *Bartonella henselae*, the agent of cat-scratch disease, are important cat-associated pathogens.
- **Clinical Features:** *P. multocida* infections can cause rapidly advancing inflammation and purulent discharge within a few hours after the bite. Dissemination (e.g., bacteremia, pneumonia) may occur. Because of deep tissue penetration by narrow, sharp feline incisors, cat bites are more likely than dog bites to cause septic arthritis or osteomyelitis.

■ OTHER NONHUMAN MAMMALIAN BITES

- Old World monkeys (*Macaca* species): Bites may transmit herpes B virus (*Herpesvirus simiae*), which can cause CNS infections with high mortality rates.
- Seals, walruses, polar bears: Bites may cause a chronic suppurative infection known as *seal finger*, which is probably due to *Mycoplasma* species.
- Small rodents (and their predators): Bites may transmit *rat-bite fever*, caused by *Streptobacillus moniliformis* (in the United States) or *Spirillum minor* (in Asia).
  - Rat-bite fever occurs after the initial wound has healed, a feature distinguishing it from an acute bite-wound infection.
- *S. moniliformis* infections manifest 3–10 days after the bite as fever, chills, myalgias, headache, and severe migratory arthralgias followed by a maculopapular rash involving the palms and soles. Disease can progress to metastatic abscesses, endocarditis, meningitis, and pneumonia.
  - Haverhill fever is an *S. moniliformis* infection acquired from contaminated milk or drinking water and has manifestations similar to those described above.
    - *S. minor* infections cause local pain, purple swelling at the bite site, and associated lymphangitis and regional lymphadenopathy 1–4 weeks after the bite, with evolution into a nonspecific systemic illness.

■ HUMAN BITES

- **Epidemiology:** Human bites become infected 10–15% of the time.
  - *Occlusional* injuries are inflicted by actual biting; *clenched-fist* injuries result when the fist of one individual strikes the teeth of another and are particularly prone to serious infection.
  - Clenched-fist injuries are more common and typically result in more serious infections (e.g., septic arthritis, tenosynovitis).
- **Bacteriology:** See Table 29-1.

TABLE 29-1 MANAGEMENT OF WOUND INFECTIONS FOLLOWING ANIMAL AND HUMAN BITES

Biting Species	Commonly Isolated Pathogens	Preferred Antibiotic(s)[a]	Alternative in Penicillin-Allergic Pt	Prophylaxis Advised for Early Uninfected Wounds[b]	Other Considerations
Dog	Staphylococcus aureus, Pasteurella multocida, anaerobes, Capnocytophaga canimorsus	Amoxicillin/clavulanate (250–500 mg PO tid) or ampicillin/sulbactam (1.5–3.0 g IV q6h)	Clindamycin (150–300 mg PO qid) plus either TMP-SMX (1 DS tablet PO bid) or ciprofloxacin (500 mg PO bid)	Sometimes	Consider rabies prophylaxis.
Cat	P. multocida, S. aureus, anaerobes	Amoxicillin/clavulanate or ampicillin/sulbactam as above	Clindamycin plus TMP-SMX as above or a fluoroquinolone	Usually	Consider rabies prophylaxis. Carefully evaluate for joint/bone penetration.
Human, occlusional	Viridans streptococci, S. aureus, Haemophilus influenzae, anaerobes	Amoxicillin/clavulanate or ampicillin/sulbactam as above	Erythromycin (500 mg PO qid) or a fluoroquinolone	Always	Examine for tendon, nerve, or joint involvement.
Human, clenched-fist	As for occlusional plus Eikenella corrodens	Ampicillin/sulbactam as above or imipenem (500 mg q6h)	Cefoxitin[c]	Always	Examine for tendon, nerve, or joint involvement.
Monkey	As for human bite	As for human bite	As for human bite	Always	For macaque monkeys, consider B virus prophylaxis with acyclovir.

(continued)

141

TABLE 29-1 MANAGEMENT OF WOUND INFECTIONS FOLLOWING ANIMAL AND HUMAN BITES (CONTINUED)

Biting Species	Commonly Isolated Pathogens	Preferred Antibiotic(s)[a]	Alternative in Penicillin-Allergic Pt	Prophylaxis Advised for Early Uninfected Wounds	Other Considerations
Snake	*Pseudomonas aeruginosa, Proteus* spp., *Bacteroides fragilis, Clostridium* spp.	Ampicillin/sulbactam as above	Clindamycin plus TMP-SMX as above *or* a fluoroquinolone	Sometimes, especially with venomous snakes	Antivenin for venomous snake bite
Rodent	*Streptobacillus moniliformis, Leptospira* spp., *P. multocida*	Penicillin VK (500 mg PO qid)	Doxycycline (100 mg PO bid)	Sometimes	—

[a]Antibiotic choices should be based on culture data when available. These suggestions for empirical therapy need to be tailored to individual circumstances and local conditions. IV regimens should be used for hospitalized pts. A single IV dose of antibiotics may be given to pts who will be discharged after initial management.

[b]Prophylactic antibiotics are suggested for severe or extensive wounds, facial wounds, and crush injuries; when bone or joint may be involved; and when comorbidity is present (see text).

[c]May be hazardous in pts with immediate-type hypersensitivity reaction to penicillin.

Abbreviations: DS, double-strength; TMP-SMX, trimethoprim-sulfamethoxazole.

TREATMENT Mammalian Bites

- *Wound management:* Wound closure is controversial in bite injuries. After thorough cleansing, facial wounds are usually sutured for cosmetic reasons and because the abundant facial blood supply lessens the risk of infection. For wounds elsewhere on the body, many authorities do not attempt primary closure, preferring instead to irrigate the wound copiously, debride devitalized tissue, remove foreign bodies, and approximate the margins. Delayed primary closure may be undertaken after the risk of infection has passed. Puncture wounds due to cat bites should be left unsutured because of the high rate at which they become infected.
- *Antibiotic therapy:* See Table 29-1. Antibiotics are typically given for 3–5 days as prophylaxis or for 10–14 days as treatment for established infections.
- *Other prophylaxis:* Rabies prophylaxis (passive immunization with rabies immune globulin and active immunization with rabies vaccine) should be given in consultation with local and regional public health authorities. A tetanus booster for pts immunized previously but not boosted within 5 years should be considered, as should primary immunization and tetanus immune globulin administration for pts not previously immunized against tetanus.

VENOMOUS SNAKEBITES

- **Epidemiology:** Worldwide, 1.2–5.5 million snakebites are sustained each year, with 421,000–1,841,000 envenomations and 20,000–94,000 deaths.
  - Bite rates are highest in temperate and tropical climates where populations subsist by manual agriculture.
  - Differentiation of venomous from nonvenomous snake species can be difficult; color pattern is notoriously misleading.
- **Clinical Features:** Snake venoms are complex mixtures of enzymes and other substances that promote vascular leaking, cause tissue necrosis, affect the coagulation cascade, inhibit peripheral nerve impulses, and impair organ function.
  - Specific presentations differ somewhat with the particular snake species.
  - Systemic symptoms may include hypotension, pulmonary edema, hemorrhage, altered mental status, or paralysis (including muscles of respiration).
- **Prognosis:** The overall mortality rate for venomous snakebite is <1% among U.S. victims who receive antivenom; most U.S. snakebite-related deaths are caused by eastern and western diamondback rattlesnakes.

TREATMENT Venomous Snakebites

FIELD MANAGEMENT
- Get the victim to definitive care as soon as possible.
- Splint a bitten extremity and keep it at heart level to lessen bleeding and discomfort.

- *Avoid* incisions into the bite wound, cooling, consultation with traditional healers, tourniquets, and electric shock.
- If the offending snake is reliably identified and known to be primarily neurotoxic, pressure immobilization (wrapping of the entire limb in a bandage at a pressure of 40–70 mmHg for upper limbs or 55–70 mmHg for lower limbs) may be used. The victim must be carried to medical care, as walking will disperse venom from the bite site regardless of its anatomic location.

HOSPITAL MANAGEMENT

- Monitor vital signs, cardiac rhythm, urine output, and O_2 saturation closely, and watch for evidence of cranial nerve dysfunction (e.g., ptosis), which may precede difficulty swallowing or respiratory insufficiency.
- Note the level of swelling and the circumference of the affected limb every 15 min until swelling has stabilized.
- Treat shock initially with isotonic saline (20–40 mL/kg IV); if hypotension persists, try 5% albumin (10–20 mL/kg IV) and vasopressors.
- Begin the search for appropriate, specific antivenom early in all cases of known venomous snakebite. In the United States, round-the-clock assistance is available from regional poison control centers.
  1. Any evidence of systemic envenomation (systemic symptoms or signs, laboratory abnormalities) and significant, progressive local findings (e.g., swelling that crosses a joint or involves more than half of the bitten limb) are indications for antivenom administration.
  2. Treating physicians should seek advice from snakebite experts regarding indications and dosing of antivenom. The duration of antivenom administration depends on the offending snake species, but multiple doses are not effective in reversing bite responses that have already been established (e.g., renal failure, established paralysis, necrosis).
  3. Worldwide, antivenom quality varies; rates of anaphylactoid reaction can exceed 50%, prompting some authorities to recommend pretreatment with IV antihistamines (diphenhydramine, 1 mg/kg to a maximum of 100 mg; and cimetidine, 5–10 mg/kg to a maximum of 300 mg) or even a prophylactic SC or IM dose of epinephrine (0.01 mg/kg, up to 0.3 mg). CroFab, an antivenom used in the United States against North American pit viper species, poses a low risk of allergy elicitation.
  4. A trial of acetylcholinesterase inhibitors should be undertaken for pts with objective evidence of neurologic dysfunction, as this treatment may cause neurologic improvement in pts bitten by snakes with postsynaptic neurotoxins.
- Elevate the bitten extremity once antivenom administration has been initiated.
- Update tetanus immunization.
- Observe pts for muscle-compartment syndrome.

- Observe pts with signs of envenomation in the hospital for at least 24 h. Pts with "dry" bites should be watched for at least 8 h because symptoms are commonly delayed.

MARINE ENVENOMATIONS

- Much of the management of envenomation by marine creatures is supportive in nature. Specific marine antivenom can be used when appropriate.

■ INVERTEBRATES

- **Etiology:** Injuries from cnidocysts (stinging cells) of hydroids, fire coral, jellyfish, Portuguese man-of-wars, and sea anemones cause similar clinical symptoms that differ in severity. Other invertebrates (e.g., sea sponges, annelid worms, sea urchins) have spines that can inflict painful stings.
- **Clinical Features:** Pain (prickling, burning, and throbbing), pruritus, and paresthesia develop immediately at the site of the bite. Neurologic, GI, renal, cardiovascular, respiratory, rheumatologic, and ocular symptoms have been described.

TREATMENT	Marine Invertebrate Envenomations

- Decontaminate the skin immediately with vinegar (5% acetic acid). Rubbing alcohol (40–70% isopropanol), baking soda, papain (unseasoned meat tenderizer), lemon or lime juice, household ammonia, olive oil, or sugar may be effective, depending on the species of the stinging creature.
- Shaving the skin may help remove remaining nematocysts.
- After decontamination, topical anesthetics, antihistamines, or steroid lotions may be helpful.
- Narcotics may be necessary for persistent pain.
- Muscle spasms may respond to diazepam (2–5 mg titrated upward as needed) or IV 10% calcium gluconate (5–10 mL).

■ VERTEBRATES

- **Etiology:** Many marine vertebrates, including stingrays, scorpionfish (e.g., lionfish and stonefish), marine catfish, and horned venomous sharks are capable of envenomating humans.
- **Clinical Features:** depend on the offending fish
  - Stingrays: represent both an envenomation and a traumatic wound. The venom causes immediate, intense pain that may last up to 48 h. The wound often becomes ischemic and heals poorly. Systemic effects can include weakness, dysrhythmias, hypotension, paralysis, and rare deaths.
  - Stonefish: Because of the neuromuscular toxicity of the venom, stings may be life-threatening, and death may occur within 6–8 h. Local pain is immediate and intense and may last for days. Systemic effects are similar to those of stingray envenomations.

TREATMENT > Marine Vertebrate Envenomations

- Immerse the affected part immediately in nonscalding hot water (113°F/45°C) for 30–90 min or until there is significant pain relief. Repeated hot-water therapy may help with recurrent pain.
- Explore, debride, and vigorously irrigate the wound after local/regional anesthetics are given.
- Antivenom is available for stonefish and serious scorpionfish envenomations. In the United States, contact the nearest regional poison control center for assistance.
- Leave wounds to heal by secondary intention or to be treated by delayed primary closure.
- Update tetanus immunization.
- Consider empirical antibiotics to cover *Staphylococcus* and *Streptococcus* species for serious wounds or envenomations in immunocompromised hosts. Coverage should be broadened to include *Vibrio* species if the wound is primarily closed.

MARINE POISONINGS

■ CIGUATERA

- **Epidemiology:** the most common fish-associated nonbacterial food poisoning in the United States, with most cases occurring in Florida and Hawaii
    - Almost exclusively involves tropical and semitropical marine coral fish common in the Indian Ocean, the South Pacific, and the Caribbean Sea
    - 75% of non-Hawaiian cases involve barracuda, snapper, jack, or grouper.
- **Pathogenesis:** Ciguatera syndrome is associated with at least five toxins that originate in photosynthetic dinoflagellates and accumulate in the food chain. Three major ciguatoxins—CTX-1, -2, and -3—are found in the flesh and viscera of ciguateric fish, are typically unaffected by external factors (e.g., heat, cold, freeze-drying, gastric acid), and do not generally affect the fish (e.g., odor, color, or taste).
- **Clinical Features:** Virtually all pts are affected within 24 h; most experience symptoms within 2–6 h. The diagnosis is made on clinical grounds.
    - Symptoms can be numerous (>150 reported) and include diarrhea, vomiting, abdominal pain, neurologic signs (e.g., paresthesias, weakness, fasciculations, ataxia), maculopapular or vesicular rash, and hemodynamic instability.
    - A pathognomonic symptom—reversal of hot and cold tactile perception—develops within 3–5 days and can last for months.
    - Death is rare.

> **TREATMENT** Ciguatera Poisoning
>
> - Therapy is supportive and based on symptoms.
> - Cool showers, hydroxyzine (25 mg PO q6–8h), or amitriptyline (25 mg PO bid) may ameliorate pruritus and dysesthesias.
> - During recovery, the pt should avoid ingestion of fish, shellfish, fish oils, fish or shellfish sauces, alcohol, nuts, and nut oils.

■ PARALYTIC SHELLFISH POISONING

- **Etiology:** induced by ingestion of contaminated filter-feeding organisms (e.g., clams, oysters, scallops, mussels) that concentrate water-soluble, heat- and acid-stable chemical toxins
  - The best-characterized and most frequently identified paralytic shellfish toxin is saxitoxin.
  - Paralytic shellfish toxins cannot be destroyed by ordinary cooking.
- **Clinical Features:** Oral paresthesias (initially tingling and burning, later numbness) develop within minutes to hours after ingestion of contaminated shellfish and progress to involve the neck and distal extremities. Flaccid paralysis and respiratory insufficiency may follow 2–12 h later.

> **TREATMENT** Paralytic Shellfish Poisoning
>
> - If pts present within hours of ingestion, gastric lavage and stomach irrigation with 2 L of a 2% sodium bicarbonate solution may be of benefit, as may administration of activated charcoal (50–100 g) and non-magnesium-based cathartics (e.g., sorbitol, 20–50 g).
> - The pt should be monitored for respiratory paralysis for at least 24 h.

■ SCOMBROID

- **Etiology:** histamine intoxication due to bacterial decomposition of inadequately preserved or refrigerated scombroid fish (e.g., tuna, mackerel, saury, needlefish, wahoo, skipjack, and bonito)
  - This syndrome can also occur with nonscombroid fish (e.g., sardines, herring, dolphinfish, amberjack, and bluefish).
  - Affected fish typically have a sharply metallic or peppery taste but may be normal in appearance and flavor.
  - Because of uneven distribution of decay within the fish, not all people who eat an affected fish will become ill.
- **Clinical Features:** Within 15–90 min of ingestion, pts present with flushing (exacerbated by ultraviolet exposure), pruritus, urticaria, angioneurotic edema, bronchospasm, GI symptoms, and hypotension.
  - Symptoms generally resolve within 8–12 h.
  - May be worse in pts concurrently taking isoniazid because of inhibition of GI tract histaminase

---

TREATMENT Scombroid Poisoning

- Treatment consists of antihistamine (H_1 or H_2) administration.
- If bronchospasm is severe, an inhaled bronchodilator or injected epinephrine may be used.

ARTHROPOD BITES AND STINGS

■ TICK BITES AND TICK PARALYSIS

- **Epidemiology:** Ticks are important carriers of vector-borne diseases (e.g., Lyme disease, babesiosis, anaplasmosis, ehrlichiosis) in the United States.
- **Etiology:** While ticks feed on blood from their hosts, their secretions may produce local reactions, transmit diverse pathogens, induce a febrile illness, or cause paralysis. Soft ticks attach for <1 h; hard ticks can feed for >1 week.
- **Clinical Features:** Except for tick-borne diseases, most manifestations of tick bites are self-limited following tick removal.
  - Tick-induced fever, associated with headache, nausea, and malaise, usually resolves ≤36 h after the tick is removed.
  - Tick paralysis is an ascending flaccid paralysis due to a toxin in tick saliva that causes neuromuscular block and decreased nerve conduction.
    - Weakness begins in the lower extremities ≤6 days after the tick's attachment and ascends symmetrically, causing complete paralysis of the extremities and cranial nerves.
    - Deep tendon reflexes are decreased or absent, but sensory examination and LP yield normal findings.
    - Tick removal results in improvement within hours; failure to remove the tick may lead ultimately to respiratory paralysis and death.

TREATMENT Tick Bites and Tick Paralysis

- Ticks should be removed with forceps applied close to the point of attachment.
- The site of attachment should be disinfected.
- Tick removal within 36 h of attachment usually prevents transmission of the agents of Lyme disease, babesiosis, anaplasmosis, and ehrlichiosis.

■ SPIDER BITES

Recluse Spider Bites

Epidemiology: Brown recluse spiders occur mainly in the southern and midwestern United States, and their close relatives are found in the Americas, Africa, and the Middle East. These spiders only infrequently bite humans, typically if threatened or pressed against the skin.

Clinical Features

- Most bites by the brown recluse spider result in only minor injury with edema and erythema, although severe necrosis of the skin and SC tissue and systemic hemolysis may occur.
- Within hours, the site of the bite becomes painful and pruritic, with central induration surrounded by zones of ischemia and erythema.
- Fever and other nonspecific systemic symptoms may develop within 3 days of the bite.
- Lesions typically resolve within 2–3 days, but severe cases can leave a large ulcer and a depressed scar that take months or years to heal.
- Deaths are rare and are due to hemolysis and renal failure.

TREATMENT   Recluse Spider Bites

- Initial management includes RICE (rest, ice, compression, elevation); administration of analgesics, antihistamines, antibiotics, and tetanus prophylaxis should be undertaken as indicated.
- Immediate surgical excision of the wound is detrimental and should be avoided.

Widow Spider Bites

Epidemiology: Black widow spiders, recognized by a red hourglass marking on a shiny black ventral abdomen, are most abundant in the southeastern United States. Other *Latrodectus* species are present in other temperate and subtropical parts of the world.

Pathogenesis: Female widow spiders produce a potent neurotoxin that binds irreversibly to nerves and causes release and depletion of acetylcholine and other neurotransmitters from presynaptic terminals.

Clinical Features

- Within 60 min, painful cramps spread from the bite site to large muscles of the extremities and trunk.
- Extreme abdominal muscular rigidity and pain may mimic peritonitis, but the abdomen is nontender.
- Other features are similar to that of acetylcholine overdose (e.g., excessive salivation, lacrimation, urination, and defecation; GI upset; and emesis).
- Although pain may subside within the first 12 h, it can recur for weeks.
- Respiratory arrest, cerebral hemorrhage, or cardiac failure may occur.

TREATMENT   Widow Spider Bites

- Treatment consists of RICE and tetanus prophylaxis.
- Because of questionable efficacy and the risk of anaphylaxis and serum sickness, antivenom use should be reserved for severe cases involving respiratory arrest, refractory hypertension, seizures, or pregnancy.

SCORPION STINGS

Epidemiology: Only ~30 of the ~1000 species of scorpions produce potentially lethal venoms, causing >5000 deaths worldwide each year. Among scorpions in the United States, only the bark scorpion (*Centruroides sculpturatus* or *C. exilicauda*) produces a potentially lethal venom.

Clinical Features: The severity of symptoms depends on the particular scorpion species. For the U.S. bark scorpion, symptoms progress to maximal severity in ~5 h and typically subside within 1–2 days.

- Bark scorpion: Swelling generally is not apparent, and tapping on the affected area (the tap test) can accentuate pain, paresthesia, and hyperesthesia. Cranial nerve dysfunction and skeletal muscle hyperexcitability develop within hours. Complications include tachycardia, arrhythmias, hypertension, hyperthermia, rhabdomyolysis, acidosis, and occasional fatal respiratory arrests.
- Outside the United States, scorpion envenomations can cause massive release of endogenous catecholamines with hypertensive crises, arrhythmias, pulmonary edema, and myocardial damage.

TREATMENT   Scorpion Stings

- Stings of nonlethal species require at most ice packs, analgesics, or antihistamines.
- In severe envenomations, aggressive supportive care should include pressure dressings and cold packs to decrease the absorption of venom.
- A continuous IV infusion of midazolam helps control agitation and involuntary muscle movements.
- *C. sculpturatus* antivenom is available as an investigational drug only in Arizona and has not been approved by the FDA. The benefit of scorpion antivenom has not been established in controlled trials.

HYMENOPTERA STINGS

Epidemiology: The hymenoptera include bees, wasps, hornets, yellow jackets, and ants. About 100 deaths from hymenoptera stings occur annually in the United States, nearly all due to allergic reactions to venoms. An estimated 0.4–4.0% of the U.S. population exhibits immediate-type hypersensitivity to insect stings.

Clinical Features
- Uncomplicated stings cause pain, a wheal-and-flare reaction, and local edema that subside within hours.
- Multiple stings (e.g., from wasps, hornets, ants) can lead to vomiting, diarrhea, generalized edema, dyspnea, hypotension, rhabdomyolysis, renal failure, and death.
- Large (>10-cm) local reactions progressing over 1–2 days are not uncommon; while they resemble cellulitis, they are in fact hypersensitivity reactions. Such reactions recur on subsequent exposure but are seldom accompanied by anaphylaxis.

- Serious reactions occur within 10 min (and rarely >5 h) after the sting and include upper airway edema, bronchospasm, hypotension, shock, and death.

TREATMENT   Hymenoptera Stings

- Stingers embedded in skin should be removed promptly by grasping with forceps or scraping with a blade or fingernail.
- The site should be disinfected and ice packs applied to slow the spread of venom.
- Elevation of the bite site and administration of analgesics, oral antihistamines, and topical calamine lotion may ease symptoms.
- Large local reactions may require a short course of glucocorticoids.
- Anaphylaxis is treated with epinephrine hydrochloride (0.3–0.5 mL of a 1:1000 solution, given SC q20–30min as needed). For profound shock, epinephrine (2–5 mL of a 1:10,000 solution by slow IV push) is indicated. Pts should be observed for 24 h for recurrent anaphylaxis.
- Pts with a history of allergy to insect stings should carry a sting kit and seek medical attention immediately after the kit is used. Adults with a history of anaphylaxis should undergo desensitization.

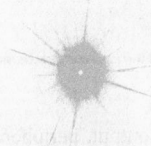

For a more detailed discussion, see Madoff LC, Pereyra F: Infectious Complications of Bites, Chap. e24 in HPIM-18; and Auerbach PS, Norris RL: Disorders Caused by Venomous Snakebites and Marine Animal Exposures, Chap. 396, p. 3566; and Pollack RJ: Ectoparasite Infestations and Arthropod Bites and Stings, Chap. 397, p. 3576, in HPIM-18.

CHAPTER **30**
Hypothermia and Frostbite

HYPOTHERMIA

Hypothermia is defined as a core body temperature of ≤35°C and is classified as mild (32.2°–35°C), moderate (28°–32.2°C), or severe (<28°C).

■ ETIOLOGY

Most cases occur during the winter in cold climates, but hypothermia may occur in mild climates and is usually multifactorial. Heat is generated in most tissues of the body and is lost by radiation, conduction, convection, evaporation, and respiration. Factors that impede heat generation and/or increase heat loss lead to hypothermia (Table 30-1).

TABLE 30-1 RISK FACTORS FOR HYPOTHERMIA

Age extremes	Endocrine
Elderly	Diabetes mellitus
Neonates	Hypoglycemia
Environmental exposure	Hypothyroidism
Occupational	Adrenal insufficiency
Sports-related	Hypopituitarism
Inadequate clothing	Neurologic
Immersion	Cerebrovascular accident
Toxicologic and pharmacologic	Hypothalamic disorders
Ethanol	Parkinson's disease
Phenothiazines	Spinal cord injury
Barbiturates	Multisystem
Anesthetics	Trauma
Neuromuscular blockers	Sepsis
Antidepressants	Shock
Insufficient fuel	Hepatic or renal failure
Malnutrition	Burns and exfoliative dermatologic disorders
Marasmus	Immobility or debilitation
Kwashiorkor	

■ CLINICAL FEATURES

Acute cold exposure causes tachycardia, increased cardiac output, peripheral vasoconstriction, and increased peripheral vascular resistance, tachypnea, increased skeletal muscle tone, shivering, and dysarthria. As body temperature drops below 32°C, cardiac conduction becomes impaired, the heart rate slows, and cardiac output decreases. Atrial fibrillation with slow ventricular response is common. Other ECG changes include Osborn (J) waves. Additional manifestations of hypothermia include volume depletion, hypotension, increased blood viscosity (which can lead to thrombosis), coagulopathy, thrombocytopenia, DIC, acid-base disturbances, and bronchospasm. CNS abnormalities are diverse and can include ataxia, amnesia, hallucinations, hyporeflexia, and (in severe hypothermia) an isoelectric EEG. Hypothermia may mask other concurrent disorders, such as an acute abdomen, drug toxicity, or spinal cord injury. Hypothermia in the ICU setting (sepsis, etc.) is a poor prognostic sign.

■ DIAGNOSIS

Hypothermia is confirmed by measuring the core temperature, preferably at two sites. Since oral thermometers are usually calibrated only as low as 34.4°C, the exact temperature of a pt whose initial reading is <35°C should be determined with a rectal thermocouple probe inserted to ≥15 cm and not adjacent to cold feces. Simultaneously, an esophageal probe should be placed 24 cm below the larynx.

TREATMENT   Hypothermia

Cardiac monitoring and supplemental oxygen should be instituted, along with attempts to limit further heat loss. Mild hypothermia is managed by passive external rewarming and insulation. The pt should be placed in a warm environment and covered with blankets to allow endogenous heat production to restore normal body temperature. With the head also covered, the rate of rewarming is usually 0.5°–2.0°C/h. Active rewarming is necessary for moderate to severe hypothermia, cardiovascular instability, age extremes, CNS dysfunction, endocrine insufficiency, or hypothermia due to complications from systemic disorders. Active rewarming may be external (forced-air heating blankets, radiant heat sources, and hot packs) or internal (by inspiration of heated, humidified oxygen warmed to 40°–45°C, by administration of IV fluids warmed to 40°–42°C, or by peritoneal or pleural lavage with dialysate or saline warmed to 40°–45°C). The most efficient active internal rewarming techniques are extracorporeal rewarming by hemodialysis and cardiopulmonary bypass. External rewarming may cause a fall in blood pressure by relieving peripheral vasoconstriction. Volume should be repleted with warmed isotonic solutions; lactated Ringer's solution should be avoided because of impaired lactate metabolism in hypothermia. If sepsis is a possibility, empirical broad-spectrum antibiotics should be administered after sending blood cultures. Atrial arrhythmias usually require no specific treatment. Ventricular fibrillation is often refractory. Only a single sequence of 3 defibrillation attempts (2 J/kg) should be attempted when the temperature is <30°C; defibrillation can be reattempted after the temperature has risen above 30°C. Since it is sometimes difficult to distinguish profound hypothermia from death, cardiopulmonary resuscitation efforts and active internal rewarming should continue until the core temperature is >32°C or cardiovascular status has been stabilized.

FROSTBITE

Frostbite occurs when the tissue temperature drops below 0°C. Clinically, it is most practical to classify frostbite as superficial (involves skin only) or deep (involves deep tissues, muscle, and bone). Classically, frostbite is retrospectively graded like a burn (first- to fourth-degree) once the resultant pathology is demarcated over time.

■ CLINICAL FEATURES

The initial presentation of frostbite can be deceptively benign. The symptoms always include a sensory deficit affecting light touch, pain, and temperature perception. Deep frostbitten tissue can appear waxy, mottled, yellow, or violaceous-white. Favorable presenting signs include some warmth or sensation with normal color. Hemorrhagic vesicles reflect a serious injury to the microvasculature and indicate third-degree frostbite. Differential diagnosis of frostbite includes frostnip (superficial freezing of skin without tissue destruction) as well as chilblain (pernio) and immersion (trench) foot, both of which occur at temperatures above freezing.

TABLE 30-2 TREATMENT FOR FROSTBITE

Before Thawing	During Thawing	After Thawing
Remove from environment	Consider parenteral analgesia and ketorolac	Gently dry and protect part; elevate; pledgets between toes, if macerated
Prevent partial thawing and refreezing	Administer ibuprofen, 400 mg PO	If clear vesicles are intact, aspirate sterilely; if broken, debride and dress with antibiotic or sterile aloe vera ointment
Stabilize core temperature and treat hypothermia	Immerse part in 37°–40°C (99°–104°F) (thermometer-monitored) circulating water containing an antiseptic soap until distal flush (10–45 min)	Leave hemorrhagic vesicles intact to prevent desiccation and infection
Protect frozen part—no friction or massage	Encourage pt to gently move part	Continue ibuprofen 400 mg PO (12 mg/kg per day) q8–12h
Address medical or surgical conditions	If pain is refractory, reduce water temperature to 35°–37°C (95°–99°F) and administer parenteral narcotics	Consider tetanus and streptococcal prophylaxis; elevate part
		Hydrotherapy at 37°C (99°F)
		Consider phenoxybenzamine or thrombolysis in severe cases

TREATMENT   Frostbite

A treatment protocol for frostbite is summarized in Table 30-2. Frozen tissue should be rapidly and completely thawed by immersion in circulating water at 37°–40°C. Thawing should not be terminated prematurely due to pain from reperfusion; ibuprofen, 400 mg, should be given, and parenteral narcotics are often required. If cyanosis persists after rewarming, the tissue compartment pressures should be monitored carefully. Pts with parts showing no flow on ^{99m}Tc scintiscan may be candidates for tissue plasminogen activator (tPA).

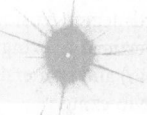

For a more detailed discussion, see Danzl DF: Hypothermia and Frostbite, Chap. 19, p. 165, in HPIM-18.

CHAPTER **31**
Altitude Illness

■ EPIDEMIOLOGY

- Altitude illness is likely to occur at >2500 m and has occurred even at 1500–2500 m.
- 100 million persons travel to high-altitude locations each year.

■ CLINICAL SYNDROMES

Acute Mountain Sickness (AMS), Including HACE

AMS represents a clinical continuum of neurologic disease, of which high-altitude cerebral edema (HACE) is the most severe form.

- **Risk factors:** rate of ascent, history of high-altitude illness, exertion
  - Lack of physical fitness is not a risk factor.
  - Exposure to high altitude within the preceding 2 months may be protective.
  - Pts >50 years old may be less likely to develop AMS than younger pts.
- **Pathophysiology:** Although the exact mechanisms remain unknown, hypoxic cerebral vasodilatation and altered permeability of the blood-brain barrier contribute to cerebral edema in AMS.
- **Clinical manifestations**
  - Nonspecific symptoms (headache, nausea, fatigue, and dizziness) with a paucity of physical findings, developing 6–12 h after ascent to a high altitude
  - HACE: encephalopathy whose hallmarks are ataxia and altered consciousness with diffuse cerebral involvement but generally without focal neurologic deficits
    - Retinal hemorrhages and, less commonly, papilledema may be seen.
    - Retinal hemorrhages occur frequently at ≥5000 m irrespective of the presence of symptoms of AMS or HACE.
- **Prevention:** Gradual ascent with acclimation is the best measure to prevent AMS.
  - At >3000 m, a graded ascent of ≤300 m each day is recommended.
  - Taking an extra day for acclimation after 3 days of gain in sleeping altitude is helpful.
  - Pharmacologic prophylaxis is warranted when the pt has a history of AMS or when flight to a high-altitude location is required.
    - Acetazolamide (125–250 mg PO bid) or dexamethasone (8 mg/d in divided doses), administered 1 day before ascent and continued for 2–3 days, is effective.
    - *Gingko biloba* is ineffective for prevention of AMS.

TREATMENT	Acute Mountain Sickness

See Table 31-1.

- **Prognosis:** With AMS, the pt may reascend gradually to a higher altitude after symptoms abate. In HACE, reascent after a few days is not advisable.

TABLE 31-1 MANAGEMENT OF ALTITUDE ILLNESS

Condition	Management
Acute mountain sickness (AMS), mild[a]	Discontinuation of ascent
	Treatment with acetazolamide (250 mg q12h)
	Descent[b]
AMS, moderate[a]	Immediate descent for worsening symptoms
	Use of low-flow oxygen if available
	Treatment with acetazolamide (250 mg q12h) and/or dexamethasone (4 mg q6h)[c]
	Hyperbaric therapy[d]
High-altitude cerebral edema (HACE)	Immediate descent or evacuation
	Administration of oxygen (2–4 L/min)
	Treatment with dexamethasone (8 mg PO/IM/IV; then 4 mg q6h)
	Hyperbaric therapy if descent is not possible
High-altitude pulmonary edema (HAPE)	Immediate descent or evacuation
	Minimization of exertion while pt is kept warm
	Administration of oxygen (4–6 L/min) to bring O_2 saturation to >90%
	Adjunctive therapy with nifedipine[e] (30 mg, extended-release, q12h)
	Hyperbaric therapy if descent is not possible

[a]Categorization of cases as mild or moderate is a subjective judgment based on the severity of headache and the presence and severity of other manifestations (nausea, fatigue, dizziness, insomnia).

[b]No fixed altitude is specified; the pt should descend to a point below that at which symptoms developed.

[c]Acetazolamide treats and dexamethasone masks symptoms. For prevention (as opposed to treatment), acetazolamide (125–250 mg q12h) or—when acetazolamide is contraindicated, as in sulfa allergy—dexamethasone (4 mg q12h) may be used.

[d]In hyperbaric therapy, the pt is placed in a portable altitude chamber or bag to simulate descent.

[e]Nifedipine (30 mg, extended-release, q12h) is also effective for the prevention of HAPE, as is salmeterol (125 mg inhaled bid), tadalafil (10 mg bid), or dexamethasone (8 mg bid).

High-Altitude Pulmonary Edema (HAPE)

HAPE is primarily a pulmonary problem and not necessarily preceded by AMS.

- **Risk factors:** rapid rate of ascent, history of HAPE, respiratory tract infections, cold environmental temperatures, male sex, abnormalities of the cardiopulmonary circulation leading to pulmonary hypertension (e.g., patent foramen ovale, mitral stenosis, 1° pulmonary hypertension)
- **Pathophysiology:** noncardiogenic pulmonary edema characterized by patchy pulmonary vasoconstriction that leads to overperfusion in some areas. Hypoxia-induced impairment of nitric oxide release may play a role in vasoconstriction.
- **Clinical manifestations:** reduction in exercise tolerance greater than that expected at the given altitude; dry, persistent cough with blood-tinged sputum; tachypnea and tachycardia at rest
    - Chest x-rays may reveal patchy or localized opacities or streaky interstitial edema.
    - Kerley B lines or a bat-wing appearance typically is not seen.
- **Prevention**
    - Gradual ascent with acclimation is the best measure to prevent HAPE.
    - Pharmacologic prophylaxis with sustained-release nifedipine (30 mg PO qd or bid) is effective for pts who have a history of HAPE or who must ascend rapidly.

TREATMENT High-Altitude Pulmonary Edema

See Table 31-1.

- **Prognosis:** Pts may reascend slowly a few days after symptoms resolve. The architecture of the lung is well preserved, with rapid reversibility of abnormalities.

Other High-Altitude Problems

- **Sleep impairment**
    - Increased periodic breathing and changes in sleep architecture (e.g., increased time in lighter sleep stages) lead to poor-quality sleep.
    - Acetazolamide (125 mg PO qhs) decreases hypoxemic episodes and alleviates sleeping disruptions caused by excessive periodic breathing.
- **GI issues:** abdominal bloating, distension, and excessive flatus can result from decreased atmospheric pressure. Diarrhea is not associated with high altitude but may indicate bacterial or parasitic infection, which is common in many high-altitude locations in the developing world.
- **High-altitude cough:** Hypoxia and bronchoconstriction (due to cold and exercise) lead to a debilitating cough that is sometimes severe enough to cause rib fractures, especially above 5000 m.
- **High-altitude neurologic events unrelated to "altitude illness":** Even without other symptoms of AMS, transient ischemic attacks, strokes, subarachnoid hemorrhage, transient global amnesia, delirium, and cranial nerve palsies can occur, particularly in pts with few traditional risk factors for these conditions.

■ **PREEXISTING MEDICAL CONDITIONS**

Few medical conditions influence susceptibility to altitude illness, and no evidence-based guidelines exist regarding the advisability of high-altitude travel by pts with these conditions.

- **Cardiac disease:** Pts with ischemic heart disease, previous myocardial infarction, angioplasty, and/or bypass surgery should have an exercise treadmill test. A strongly positive treadmill test is a contraindication for high-altitude trips. Pts with poorly controlled arrhythmias also should avoid high-altitude travel.
- **Asthma:** Severely asthmatic pts should be cautioned against ascending to high altitudes.
- **Pregnancy:** Although there are no relevant data, it is unadvisable for pregnant women to travel to altitudes >3000 m, given the steep drops in oxygen saturation at these altitudes.
- **Sickle cell disease:** High altitude is one of the rare environmental exposures that occasionally provoke a crisis in persons with the sickle cell trait, even at 2500 m.
- **Diabetes mellitus:** Trekking at high altitudes may enhance sugar uptake. Pts taking insulin may require lower doses on trekking/climbing days than on rest days.
- **Chronic lung disease:** Pts with preexisting pulmonary hypertension should be discouraged from ascending to high altitudes. If such travel is necessary, treatment with sustained-release nifedipine (20 mg PO bid) should be considered.
- **Chronic kidney disease:** Acetazolamide should be avoided by pts with preexisting metabolic acidosis and by pts with a glomerular filtration rate (GFR) ≤10 mL/min; the dose of acetazolamide should be adjusted if the GFR is ≤50 mL/min.

DECOMPRESSION SICKNESS (DCS)

DCS is caused by the formation of bubbles from dissolved inert gas (usually nitrogen) during or after ascent (decompression) from a compressed gas dive.

- **Incidence:** 1:10,000 recreational dives. Risk factors are deeper and longer dives and too rapid of an ascent.
- **Pathophysiology:** Bubbles may form within tissues themselves, leading to symptoms by mechanical distraction of pain-sensitive or functionally-important structures. Bubbles also appear in the venous circulation where they can incite inflammatory and coagulation cascades, damage endothelium, activate formed elements of blood such as platelets, and cause symptomatic vascular obstruction (also in arterial beds when a patent foramen ovale is present).
- **Clinical manifestations:** Most cases present with mild symptoms of pain, fatigue, and minor neurologic illnesses such as patchy paresthesias. Pulmonary and cardiovascular manifestations can be life-threatening including dyspnea, chest pain, arrhythmia, coagulopathy, and hypotension.
- **Diagnosis**
  - Based on integration of findings and examination of the dive profile while correlating relationship of symptoms temporally to the dive.

Decompression Sickness

Horizontal positioning to prevent bubble entry into the cerebral circulation, IV fluids, and 100% oxygen. Definitive treatment with hyperbaric oxygen administered in a compression chamber with stepwise decompression over variable periods adjusted to treatment response. If recovery is complete, diving can be resumed after a period of at least 1 month; if residual symptoms exist, diving is discouraged.

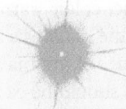

For a more detailed discussion, see Basnyat B, Tabin G: Altitude Illness, Chap. e51; and Bennett MH, Mitchell SJ: Hyperbaric and Diving Medicine, Chap. e52 in HPIM-18.

CHAPTER **32**
Poisoning and Drug Overdose

Poisoning refers to the development of dose-related harmful effects following exposure to chemicals, drugs, or other xenobiotics. *Overdosage* is exposure to excessive amounts of a substance normally intended for consumption (a pharmaceutical) or an illicit drug. Chemical exposures result in an estimated 5 million requests in the United States for medical advice or treatment each year, and about 5% of victims require hospitalization. Overall mortality is low (<1% of exposures); suicide attempts account for most serious or fatal poisonings (1–2% mortality). Up to 30% of psychiatric admissions are prompted by attempted suicide via overdosage.

Carbon monoxide is the leading cause of death from poisoning. Acetaminophen toxicity is the most common pharmaceutical agent causing fatalities. Other drug-related fatalities are commonly due to analgesics, antidepressants, sedative-hypnotics, neuroleptics, stimulants and street drugs, cardiovascular drugs, anticonvulsants, antihistamines, and asthma therapies. Nonpharmaceutical agents implicated in fatal poisoning include alcohols and glycols, gases and fumes, cleaning substances, pesticides, and automotive products. The diagnosis of poisoning or drug overdose must be considered in any pt who presents with coma, seizure, or acute renal, hepatic, or bone marrow failure.

DIAGNOSIS

The correct diagnosis can usually be reached by history, physical exam, and routine and toxicologic laboratory evaluation. All available sources should be used to determine the exact nature of the ingestion or exposure. The *history* should include the time, route, duration, and circumstances (location, surrounding events, and intent) of exposure; name of chemical(s) involved, time of onset, nature, and severity of symptoms; relevant past medical and psychiatric history. The Physicians Desk Reference, regional poison control centers, and local/hospital pharmacies may be useful for identification of ingredients and potential effects of toxins.

The diagnosis of poisoning in cases of unknown etiology primarily relies on pattern recognition. The first step is a *physical exam* with initial focus on the pulse, blood pressure, respiratory rate, temperature, and neurologic status and then characterization of the overall physiologic state as stimulated, depressed, discordant, or normal (Table 32-1).

Examination of the eyes (for nystagmus, pupil size, and reactivity), neuromuscular status (for tremors, dyskinesia, rigidity, dystonia), abdomen (for bowel activity and bladder size), and skin (for burns, bullae, color, warmth, moisture, pressure sores, and puncture marks) may narrow the diagnosis to a particular disorder. The pt should also be examined for evidence of trauma and underlying illnesses. When the history is unclear, all orifices should be examined for the presence of chemical burns and drug packets. The odor of breath or vomitus and the color of nails, skin, or urine may provide diagnostic clues.

Initial laboratory studies should include glucose, serum electrolytes, serum osmolality, BUN/creatinine, LFTs, PT/PTT, and ABGs. An increased anion-gap metabolic acidosis is characteristic of advanced methanol, ethylene glycol, and salicylate intoxication, but can occur with other agents and in any poisoning that results in hepatic, renal, or respiratory failure; seizures; or shock. An increased osmolal gap—the difference between the measured serum osmolality (determined by freezing point depression) and that calculated from the serum sodium, glucose, and BUN of >10 mmol/L—suggests the presence of a low-molecular-weight solute such as an alcohol, glycol, ketone, unmeasured electrolyte, or sugar. Ketosis suggests acetone, isopropyl alcohol, or salicylate poisoning. Hypoglycemia may be due to poisoning with β-adrenergic blockers, ethanol, insulin, oral hypoglycemic agents, quinine, and salicylates, whereas hyperglycemia can occur in poisoning with acetone, β-adrenergic agonists, calcium channel blockers, iron, theophylline, or the rodenticide Vacor.

Radiologic studies should include a chest x-ray to exclude aspiration or ARDS. Radiopaque densities may be visible on abdominal x-rays. Head CT or MRI is indicated in stuporous or comatose pts to exclude structural lesions or subarachnoid hemorrhage, and LP should be performed when CNS infection is suspected. The ECG can be helpful in pointing to a poisoning agent: Bradycardia and A–V block may occur with poisoning by α-adrenergic agonists, antiarrhythmic agents, beta blockers, calcium channel blockers, cholinergic agents (carbamate and organophosphate insecticides), cardiac glycosides, lithium, or tricyclic antidepressants. QRS- and QT-interval prolongation may be seen with antidepressant and other membrane-active drug exposure. Ventricular tachyarrhythmias may be observed with exposure to cardiac glycosides, fluoride, methylxanthines, sympathomimetics, antidepressants, and agents that cause hyperkalemia or potentiate the effects of endogenous catecholamines (e.g., chloral hydrate, aliphatic and halogenated hydrocarbons).

Toxicologic analysis of urine and blood (and occasionally of gastric contents and chemical samples) may be useful to confirm or rule out suspected poisoning. Although rapid screening tests for a limited number of drugs of abuse are available, comprehensive screening tests require 2–6 h for completion, and immediate management must be based on the history, circumstantial evidence,

TABLE 32-1 DIFFERENTIAL DIAGNOSIS OF POISONING BASED ON PHYSIOLOGIC STATE

Stimulated	Depressed	Discordant	Normal
Sympathetics Sympathomimetics	Sympatholytics	Asphyxiants	Nontoxic exposure
Ergot alkaloids	α_1-Adrenergic antagonists	Cytochrome oxidase inhibitors	Psychogenic illness
Methylxanthines	α_2-Adrenergic agonists	Inert gases	Toxic time bombs
Monoamine oxidase inhibitors	ACE inhibitors	Irritant gases	Slow absorption
Thyroid hormones	Angiotensin receptor blockers	Methemoglobin inducers	Anticholinergics
Anticholinergics	Antipsychotics	Oxidative phosphorylation	Carbamazepine
Antihistamines	β-Adrenergic blockers	inhibitors	Concretion formers
Antiparkinsonian agents	Calcium channel blockers	AGMA inducers	Extended-release phenytoin
Antipsychotics	Cardiac glycosides	Alcohol (ketoacidosis)	sodium capsules (Dilantin
Antispasmodics	Cyclic antidepressants	Ethylene glycol	Kapseals)
Belladonna alkaloids	Cholinergics	Iron	Drug packets
Cyclic antidepressants	Acetylcholinesterase inhibitors	Methanol	Enteric-coated pills
Muscle relaxants	Muscarinic agonists	Salicylate	Diphenoxylate-atropine (Lomotil)
Mushrooms and plants	Nicotinic agonists	Toluene	Opioids
Hallucinogens	Opioids	CNS syndromes	Salicylates
Cannabinoids (marijuana)	Analgesics	Extrapyramidal reactions	Sustained-release pills
LSD and analogues	GI antispasmodics	Hydrocarbon inhalation	Valproate
Mescaline and analogues	Heroin	Isoniazid	Slow distribution
Mushrooms	Sedative-hypnotics	Lithium	Cardiac glycosides
Phencyclidine and analogues	Alcohols	Neuroleptic malignant syndrome	Lithium
Withdrawal syndromes	Anticonvulsants	Serotonin syndrome	Heavy metals
Barbiturates	Barbiturates	Strychnine	Salicylate

(continued)

161

TABLE 32-1 DIFFERENTIAL DIAGNOSIS OF POISONING BASED ON PHYSIOLOGIC STATE (CONTINUED)

Stimulated	Depressed	Discordant	Normal
Benzodiazepines	Benzodiazepines	Membrane-active agents	Valproate
Ethanol	GABA precursors	Amantadine	Toxic metabolite
Opioids	Muscle relaxants	Antiarrhythmics	Acetaminophen
Sedative-hypnotics	Other agents	Antihistamines	Carbon tetrachloride
Sympatholytics	GHB products	Antipsychotics	Cyanogenic glycosides
		Carbamazepine	Ethylene glycol
		Cyclic antidepressants	Methanol
		Local anesthetics	Methemoglobin inducers
		Opioids (some)	Mushroom toxins
		Orphenadrine	Organophosphate insecticides
		Quinoline antimalarials	Paraquat
			Metabolism disruptors
			Antineoplastic agents
			Antiviral agents
			Colchicine
			Hypoglycemic agents
			Immunosuppressive agents
			MAO inhibitors
			Heavy metals
			Salicylate
			Warfarin

Abbreviations: ACE, angiotensin-converting enzyme; AGMA, anion-gap metabolic acidosis; CNS, central nervous system; GABA, γ-aminobutyric acid; GHB, γ-hydroxybutyrate; GI, gastrointestinal; LSD, lysergic acid diethylamide; MAO, monoamine oxidase.

physical exam, and routine ancillary tests. Quantitative analysis is useful for poisoning with acetaminophen, acetone, alcohols (including ethylene glycol), antiarrhythmics, anticonvulsants, barbiturates, digoxin, heavy metals, lithium, salicylate, and theophylline, as well as for carboxyhemoglobin and methemoglobin. Results can often be available within an hour.

The response to antidotes may be useful for diagnostic purposes. Resolution of altered mental status and abnormal vital signs within minutes of IV administration of dextrose, naloxone, or flumazenil is virtually diagnostic of hypoglycemia, narcotic poisoning, and benzodiazepine intoxication, respectively. The prompt reversal of acute dystonic (extrapyramidal) symptoms following an IV dose of benztropine or diphenhydramine confirms a drug etiology. Although physostigmine reversal of both central and peripheral manifestations of anticholinergic poisoning is diagnostic, it may cause arousal in pts with CNS depression of any etiology.

TREATMENT   Poisoning and Drug Overdose

Goals of therapy include support of vital signs, prevention of further absorption, enhancement of elimination, administration of specific antidotes, and prevention of reexposure. Fundamentals of poisoning management are listed in Table 32-2. When the type of poison is unknown or uncertain, blood and urine specimens for toxicologic studies should be obtained if possible before treatment is started. Treatment is usually initiated before routine and toxicologic data are known. All symptomatic pts need large-bore IV access, supplemental O_2, cardiac monitoring, continuous observation, and, if mental status is altered, 100 mg thiamine (IM or IV), 1 ampule of 50% dextrose in water, and 4 mg of naloxone along with specific antidotes as indicated. Unconscious pts should be intubated. Activated charcoal may be given PO or via a large-bore gastric tube; gastric lavage requires an orogastric tube. Severity of poisoning determines the management. Admission to an ICU is indicated for pts with severe poisoning (coma, respiratory depression, hypotension, cardiac conduction abnormalities, arrhythmias, hypothermia or hyperthermia, seizures); those needing close monitoring, antidotes, or enhanced elimination therapy; and those with progressive clinical deterioration or significant underlying medical problems. Suicidal pts require constant observation by qualified personnel.

SUPPORTIVE CARE   Airway protection is mandatory. Gag reflex alone is not a reliable indicator of the need for intubation. Intubation is required in all pts with CNS depression or seizures to prevent aspiration of gastric contents. Need for O_2 supplementation and ventilatory support can be assessed by measurement of ABGs. Drug-induced pulmonary edema is usually secondary to hypoxia, but myocardial depression may contribute. Measurement of pulmonary artery pressure may be necessary to establish etiology. Electrolyte imbalances should be corrected as soon as possible.

Adequate cardiovascular function and organ perfusion is necessary for elimination of toxin and pt recovery. If hypotension is unresponsive to volume expansion, pressors such as norepinephrine, epinephrine or dopamine may be required. In severe cases, intra-aortic balloon pump or

TABLE 32-2 FUNDAMENTALS OF POISONING MANAGEMENT

Supportive Care	
Airway protection	Treatment of seizures
Oxygenation/ventilation	Correction of temperature abnormalities
Treatment of arrhythmias	Correction of metabolic derangements
Hemodynamic support	Prevention of secondary complications
Prevention of Further Poison Absorption	
Gastrointestinal decontamination	Decontamination of other sites
Gastric lavage	Eye decontamination
Activated charcoal	Skin decontamination
Whole-bowel irrigation	Body cavity evacuation
Dilution	
Endoscopic/surgical removal	
Enhancement of Poison Elimination	
Multiple-dose activated charcoal	Extracorporeal removal
Diuresis	Hemodialysis
Alteration of urinary pH	Hemoperfusion
Chelation	Hemofiltration
	Plasmapheresis
	Exchange transfusion
	Hyperbaric oxygenation
Administration of Antidotes	
Neutralization by antibodies	Metabolic antagonism
Neutralization by chemical binding	Physiologic antagonism
Prevention of Reexposure	
Adult education	Notification of regulatory agencies
Child-proofing	Psychiatric referral

other mechanical perfusion assists may be considered. Supraventricular tachycardia (SVT) with hypertension and CNS excitation is almost always due to sympathetic, anticholinergic, or hallucinogenic stimulation or to drug withdrawal. Treatment is indicated if associated with hemodynamic instability, chest pain, or ischemia on ECG. Treatment with combined α and β blockers or combinations of β blocker and vasodilator is indicated in severe sympathetic hyperactivity. Physostigmine is useful for hyperactivity due to an anticholinergic overdose. SVT without hypertension usually responds to fluid administration.

Ventricular tachycardia (VT) can be caused by sympathetic stimulation, myocardial membrane destabilization, or metabolic derangements. Lidocaine and phenytoin are generally safe. Sodium bicarbonate should be the agent given first for VT of toxicologic origin. Drugs that prolong the QT interval (quinidine, procainamide) should not be used in VT due to tricyclic antidepressant overdose. Magnesium sulfate and overdrive pacing (by isoproterenol or a pacemaker) may be useful for torsades de pointes. Arrhythmias may be resistant to therapy until underlying acid-base and electrolyte derangements, hypoxia, and hypothermia are corrected. It is acceptable to observe hemodynamically stable pts without pharmacologic intervention.

Seizures are best treated with γ-aminobutyric acid agonists such as benzodiazepines or barbiturates. Barbiturates should be given only after intubation. Seizures caused by isoniazid overdose may respond only to large doses of pyridoxine IV. Seizures from beta blockers or tricyclic antidepressants may require phenytoin and benzodiazepines.

PREVENTION OF POISON ABSORPTION Whether to perform GI decontamination, and which procedure to use, depends on the time since ingestion; the existing and predicted toxicity of the ingestant; the availability, efficacy, and contraindications of the procedure; and the nature, severity, and risk of complications. The efficacy of activated charcoal and gastric lavage decreases with time, and there are insufficient data to support or exclude a beneficial effect when they are used >1 h after ingestion. Activated charcoal has comparable or greater efficacy, fewer contraindications and complications, and is less invasive than gastric lavage and is the preferred method of GI decontamination in most situations.

Activated charcoal is prepared as a suspension in water, either alone or with a cathartic. It is given orally via a nippled bottle (for infants), or via a cup, straw, or small-bore nasogastric tube. The recommended dose is 1 g/kg body weight, using 8 mL of diluent per gram of charcoal if a premixed formulation is not available. Charcoal may inhibit absorption of other orally administered agents and is contraindicated in pts with corrosive ingestion.

When indicated, gastric lavage is performed using a 28F orogastric tube in children and a 40F orogastric tube in adults. Saline or tap water may be used in adults or children. (Use saline in infants.) Place pt in Trendelenburg and left lateral decubitus position to minimize aspiration (occurs in 10% of pts). Repeated administration of fluid (5 mL/kg) followed by aspiration results in progressive removal of gastric content. Lavage is contraindicated in pts resisting the procedure, and with ingested corrosives and petroleum distillate hydrocarbons because of risk of aspiration-induced pneumonia and gastroesophageal perforation.

Syrup of ipecac, once the most commonly used decontamination procedure, has no role in the hospital setting and is no longer recommended for the management of poisoning.

TABLE 32-3 PATHOPHYSIOLOGIC FEATURES AND TREATMENT OF SPECIFIC TOXIC SYNDROMES AND POISONINGS

Physiologic Condition, Causes	Examples	Mechanism of Action	Clinical Features	Specific Treatments
Stimulated				
Sympathetics (see also HPIM-18 Chap. 394)				
Sympathomimetics	α_1-Adrenergic agonists (decongestants); phenylephrine, phenylpropanolamine β_2-Adrenergic agonists (bronchodilators): albuterol, terbutaline Nonspecific adrenergic agonists: amphetamines, cocaine, ephedrine	Stimulation of central and peripheral sympathetic receptors directly or indirectly (by promoting the release or inhibiting the reuptake of norepinephrine and sometimes dopamine)	Physiologic stimulation (HPIM-18 Table e50-2); reflex bradycardia can occur with selective α_1 agonists; β agonists can cause hypotension and hypokalemia.	Phentolamine, a nonselective α_1-adrenergic receptor antagonist, for severe hypertension due to α_1-adrenergic agonists; propranolol, a nonselective β blocker, for hypotension and tachycardia due to β_2 agonists; labetalol, a β blocker with α-blocking activity, or phentolamine with esmolol, metoprolol, or other cardioselective β blocker for hypertension with tachycardia due to nonselective agents (β blockers, if used alone, can exacerbate hypertension and vasospasm due to unopposed α stimulation); benzodiazepines; propofol.
Ergot alkaloids	Ergotamine, methysergide, bromocriptine, pergolide	Stimulation and inhibition of serotonergic and α-adrenergic receptors; stimulation of dopamine receptors	Physiologic stimulation (HPIM-18 Table e50-2); formication; vasospasm with limb (isolated or generalized), myocardial, and cerebral ischemia progressing to gangrene or infarction; hypotension, bradycardia, and involuntary movements can also occur.	Nitroprusside or nitroglycerine for severe vasospasm; prazosin (an α_1 blocker), captopril, nifedipine, and cyproheptadine (a serotonin receptor antagonist) for mild to moderate limb ischemia; dopamine receptor antagonists (antipsychotics) for hallucinations and movement disorders.

Methylxanthines	Caffeine, theophylline	Inhibition of adenosine synthesis and adenosine receptor antagonism; stimulation of epinephrine and norepinephrine release; inhibition of phosphodiesterase resulting in increased intracellular cyclic adenosine and guanosine monophosphate	Physiologic stimulation (HPIM-18 Table e50-2); pronounced gastrointestinal symptoms and β agonist effects (see above). Toxicity occurs at lower drug levels in chronic poisoning than in acute poisoning.	Propranolol, a nonselective β blocker, for tachycardia with hypotension; any β blocker for supraventricular or ventricular tachycardia without hypotension; elimination enhanced by multiple-dose charcoal, hemoperfusion, and hemodialysis; indications for hemoperfusion or hemodialysis include unstable vital signs, seizures, and a theophylline level of 80–100 μg/mL after acute overdose and 40–60 μg/mL with chronic exposure.
Monoamine oxidase inhibitors	Phenelzine, tranylcypromine, selegiline	Inhibition of monoamine oxidase resulting in impaired metabolism of endogenous catecholamines and exogenous sympathomimetic agents	Delayed or slowly progressive physiologic stimulation (HPIM-18 Table e50-2); terminal hypotension and bradycardia in severe cases.	Short-acting agents (e.g., nitroprusside, esmolol) for severe hypertension and tachycardia; direct-acting sympathomimetics (e.g., norepinephrine, epinephrine) for hypotension and bradycardia.

(*continued*)

TABLE 32-3 PATHOPHYSIOLOGIC FEATURES AND TREATMENT OF SPECIFIC TOXIC SYNDROMES AND POISONINGS (CONTINUED)

Physiologic Condition, Causes	Examples	Mechanism of Action	Clinical Features	Specific Treatments
Anticholinergics				
Antihistamines	Diphenhydramine, doxylamine, pyrilamine	Inhibition of central and postganglionic parasympathetic muscarinic cholinergic receptors. At high doses, amantadine, diphenhydramine, orphenadrine, phenothiazines, and tricyclic antidepressants have additional nonanticholinergic activity (see below).	Physiologic stimulation (HPIM-18 Table e50-2); dry skin and mucous membranes, decreased bowel sounds, flushing, and urinary retention; myoclonus and picking activity. Central effects may occur without significant autonomic dysfunction.	Physostigmine, an acetylcholinesterase inhibitor (see below) for delirium, hallucinations, and neuromuscular hyperactivity. Contraindications include nonanticholinergic cardiovascular toxicity (e.g., cardiac conduction abnormalities, hypotension, and ventricular arrhythmias).
Antiparkinsonian agents	Amantadine, trihexyphenidyl			
Antipsychotics	Chlorpromazine, olanzapine, quetiapine, thioridazine			
Antispasmotics	Clidinium, dicyclomine			
Belladonna alkaloids	Atropine, hyoscyamine, scopolamine			
Cyclic antidepressants	Amitriptyline, doxepin, imipramine			
Muscle relaxants	Cyclobenzaprine, orphenadrine			
Mushrooms and plants	*Amanita muscaria* and *A. pantherina*, henbane, jimson weed, nightshade			

Depressed

Sympatholytics

α_2-Adrenergic agonists	Clonidine, guanabenz, tetrahydrozoline and other imidazoline decongestants, tizanidine and other imidazoline muscle relaxants	Stimulation of α_2-adrenergic receptors leading to inhibition of CNS sympathetic outflow; activity at non-adrenergic imidazoline binding sites also contributes to CNS effects.	Physiologic depression (HPIM-18 Table e50-2), miosis. Transient initial hypertension may be seen.	Dopamine and norepinephrine for hypotension. Atropine for symptomatic bradycardia. Naloxone for CNS depression (inconsistently effective).
Antipsychotics	Chlorpromazine, clozapine, haloperidol, risperidone, thioridazine	Inhibition of α-adrenergic, dopaminergic, histaminergic, muscarinic, and serotonergic receptors. Some agents also inhibit sodium, potassium, and calcium channels.	Physiologic depression (HPIM-18 Table e50-2), miosis, anticholinergic effects (see above), extrapyramidal reactions (see below). Cardiac tachycardia. Cardiac conduction delays (increased PR, QRS, JT, and QT intervals) with ventricular tachydysrhythmias, including torsades des pointes, can sometimes develop.	Sodium bicarbonate and lidocaine for ventricular tachydysrhythmias associated with QRS prolongation. Magnesium, isoproterenol, and overdrive pacing for torsades de pointes. Avoid class IA, IC, and III antiarrhythmics. IV lipid emulsion therapy may be beneficial in some cases.

(continued)

TABLE 32-3 PATHOPHYSIOLOGIC FEATURES AND TREATMENT OF SPECIFIC TOXIC SYNDROMES AND POISONINGS (CONTINUED)

Physiologic Condition, Causes	Examples	Mechanism of Action	Clinical Features	Specific Treatments
Depressed				
β-Adrenergic blockers	Cardioselective (β₁) blockers: atenolol, esmolol, metoprolol Nonselective (β₁ and β₂) blockers: nadolol, propranolol, timolol Partial β agonists: acebutolol, pindolol α₁ Antagonists: carvedilol, labetalol Membrane-active agents: acebutolol, propranolol, sotalol	Inhibition of β-adrenergic receptors (class II antiarrhythmic effect). Some agents have activity at additional receptors or have membrane effects (see below).	Physiologic depression (HPIM-18 Table e50-2), atrioventricular block, hypoglycemia, hyperkalemia, seizures. Partial agonists can cause hypertension and tachycardia. Sotalol can cause increased QT interval and ventricular tachydysrhythmias. Onset may be delayed after sotalol and sustained-release formulation overdose.	Glucagon and calcium for hypotension and symptomatic bradycardia. Atropine, isoproterenol, amrinone, dopamine, dobutamine, epinephrine, and norepinephrine may sometimes be effective. High-dose insulin (with glucose and potassium to maintain euglycemia and normokalemia), electrical pacing, and mechanical cardiovascular support for refractory cases.
Calcium channel blockers	Diltiazem, nifedipine and other dihydropyridine derivatives, verapamil	Inhibition of slow (type L) cardiovascular calcium channels (class IV antiarrhythmic effect).	Physiologic depression (HPIM-18 Table e50-2), atrioventricular block, organ ischemia and infarction, hyperglycemia, seizures.	Calcium and glucagon for hypotension and symptomatic bradycardia. Dopamine, epinephrine, norepinephrine, atropine, and isoproterenol are less often effective but can be used adjunctively. Amrinone, high-dose insulin (with glucose and

		Hypotension is usually due to decreased vascular resistance rather than to decreased cardiac output. Onset may be delayed for ≥12 h after overdose of sustained-release formulations.	potassium to maintain euglycemia and normokalemia), IV lipid emulsion therapy, electrical pacing, and mechanical cardiovascular support for refractory cases.
Cardiac glycosides	Digoxin, endogenous cardioactive steroids, foxglove and other plants, toad skin secretions (*Bufonidae* sp.)	Inhibition of cardiac Na$^+$, K$^+$-ATPase membrane pump.	Physiologic depression (HPIM-18 Table e50-2); gastrointestinal, psychiatric, and visual symptoms; atrioventricular block with or without concomitant supraventricular tachyarrhythmia; ventricular tachyarrhythmias. Hyperkalemia in acute poisoning. Toxicity occurs at lower drug levels in chronic poisoning than in acute poisoning.	Digoxin-specific antibody fragments for hemodynamically compromising dysrhythmias, Mobitz II or third-degree atrioventricular block, hyperkalemia (>5.5 meq/L; in acute poisoning only). Temporizing measures include atropine, dopamine, epinephrine, phenytoin, and external cardiac pacing for bradydysrhythmias and magnesium, lidocaine, or phenytoin for ventricular tachydysrhythmias. Internal cardiac pacing and cardioversion can increase ventricular irritability and should be reserved for refractory cases.

(*continued*)

TABLE 32-3 PATHOPHYSIOLOGIC FEATURES AND TREATMENT OF SPECIFIC TOXIC SYNDROMES AND POISONINGS (CONTINUED)

Physiologic Condition, Causes	Examples	Mechanism of Action	Clinical Features	Specific Treatments
Depressed				
Cyclic antidepressants	Amitriptyline, doxepin, imipramine	Inhibition of α-adrenergic dopaminergic, GABA-ergic, histaminergic, muscarinic, and serotonergic receptors; inhibition of sodium channels (see membrane-active agents); inhibition of norepinephrine and serotonin reuptake.	Physiologic depression (HPIM-18 Table e50-2), seizures, tachycardia, cardiac conduction delays (increased PR, QRS, JT, and QT intervals; terminal QRS right axis deviation) with aberrancy and ventricular tachydysrhythmias. Anticholinergic toxidrome (see above).	Hypertonic sodium bicarbonate (or hypertonic saline) and lidocaine for ventricular tachydysrhythmias associated with QRS prolongation. Use of phenytoin is controversial. Avoid class IA, IC, and III antiarrhythmics.
Cholinergics				
Acetylcholinesterase inhibitors	Carbamate insecticides (aldicarb, carbaryl, propoxur) and medicinals (neostigmine, physostigmine, tacrine); nerve gases (sarin, soman, tabun, VX) organophosphate insecticides (diazinon, chlorpyrifos-ethyl, malathion)	Inhibition of acetylcholinesterase leading to increased synaptic acetylcholine at muscarinic and nicotinic cholinergic receptor sites	Physiologic depression (HPIM-18 Table e50-2). Muscarinic signs and symptoms: seizures, excessive secretions (lacrimation, salivation, bronchorrhea and wheezing, diaphoresis), and increased bowel and bladder activity with nausea, vomiting, diarrhea, abdominal cramps, and incontinence	Atropine for muscarinic signs and symptoms. Pralidoxime (2-PAM), a cholinesterase reactivator, for nicotinic signs and symptoms due to organophosphates, nerve gases, or an unknown anticholinesterase.

Muscarinic agonists	Bethanecol, mushrooms (*Boletus, Clitocybe, Inocybe* spp.), pilocarpine	Stimulation of CNS and postganglionic parasympathetic cholinergic (muscarinic) receptors	of feces and urine. Nicotinic signs and symptoms: hypertension, tachycardia, muscle cramps, fasciculations, weakness, and paralysis. Death is usually due to respiratory failure. Cholinesterase activity in plasma and red cells <50% of normal in acetylcholinesterase inhibitor poisoning.
Nicotinic agonists	Lobeline, nicotine (tobacco)	Stimulation of preganglionic sympathetic and parasympathetic and striated muscle (neuromuscular junction) cholinergic (nicotine) receptors	
Sedative-hypnotics (see also HPIM-18 Chap. 393)			
Anticonvulsants	Carbamazepine, ethosuximide, felbamate, gabapentin, lamotrigine, levetiracetam, oxcarbazepine, phenytoin, tiagabine, topiramate, valproate, zonisamide	Potentiation of the inhibitory effects of GABA by binding to the neuronal GABA-A chloride channel receptor complex and increasing the frequency or duration of chloride channel opening in response to GABA stimulation. Baclofen and, to	Physiologic depression (HPIM-18 Table e50-2), nystagmus. Delayed absorption can occur with carbamazepine, phenytoin, and valproate. Myoclonus, seizures, hypertension, and tachyarrhythmias can occur with baclofen, carbamazepine, and orphenadrine.	Benzodiazepines, barbiturates or propofol for seizures. Elimination of phenobarbital and possibly other long-acting agents enhanced by multiple-dose charcoal.

Hemodialysis and hemoperfusion may be indicated for severe poisoning by some agents (see Extracorporeal Removal, in text). |

(continued)

173

TABLE 32-3 PATHOPHYSIOLOGIC FEATURES AND TREATMENT OF SPECIFIC TOXIC SYNDROMES AND POISONINGS (CONTINUED)

Physiologic Condition, Causes	Examples	Mechanism of Action	Clinical Features	Specific Treatments
Cholinergics				
Barbiturates	Short-acting: butabarbital, pentobarbital, secobarbital Long-acting: phenobarbital, primidone	some extent, GHB act at the GABA-B rector complex; meprobamate, its metabolite carisoprodol, felbamate, and orphenadrine antagonize N-methyl-D-aspartate NMDA excitatory receptors; ethosuximide, valproate, and zonisamide decrease		See above and below for treatment of anticholinergic and sodium channel (membrane) blocking effects.
Benzodiazepines	Ultrashort-acting: estazolam, midazolam, temazepam, triazolam Short-acting: alprazolam, flunitrazepam, lorazepam, oxazepam Long-acting: chlordiazepoxide, clonazepam, diazepam, flurazepam	conduction through T-type calcium channels; valproate decreases GABA degradation, and tiagabine blocks GABA reuptake; carbamazepine, lamotrigine, oxcarbazepine, phenytoin, topiramate, valproate, and zonisamide slow the	Tachyarrhythmias can also occur with chloral hydrate. AGMA, hypernatremia, hyperosmolality, hyperammonemia, chemical hepatitis, and hypoglycemia can be seen in valproate poisoning. Carbamazepine and oxcarbazepine may produce hyponatremia from SIADH.	

	Pharmacologically related agents: zaleplon, zolpidem	rate of recovery of inactivated sodium channels. Some agents also have α_2 agonist, anticholinergic, and sodium channel-blocking activity (see above and below).	
GABA precursors	γ-Hydroxybutyrate (sodium oxybate; GHB); γ-butyrolactone (GBL), 1,4-butanediol.		Some agents can cause anticholinergic and sodium channel (membrane) blocking effects (see above and below).
Muscle relaxants	Baclofen, carisoprodol, cyclobenzaprine, etomidate, metaxalone, methocarbamol, orphenadrine, propofol, tizanidine and other imidazoline muscle relaxants.		
Other agents	Chloral hydrate, ethchlorvynol, glutethimide, meprobamate, methaqualone, methyprylon.		

(continued)

TABLE 32-3 PATHOPHYSIOLOGIC FEATURES AND TREATMENT OF SPECIFIC TOXIC SYNDROMES AND POISONINGS (CONTINUED)

Physiologic Condition, Causes	Examples	Mechanism of Action	Clinical Features	Specific Treatments
Discordant				
Asphyxiants				
Cytochrome oxidase inhibitors	Carbon monoxide, cyanide, hydrogen sulfide	Inhibition of mitochondrial cytochrome oxidase, thereby blocking electron transport and oxidative metabolism. Carbon monoxide also binds to hemoglobin and myoglobin and prevents oxygen binding, transport, and tissue uptake (binding to hemoglobin shifts the oxygen dissociation curve to the left).	Signs and symptoms of hypoxia with initial physiologic stimulation and subsequent depression (HPIM-18 Table e50-2); lactic acidosis; normal Po_2 and calculated oxygen saturation but decreased oxygen saturation by pulse oximetry is falsely elevated but is less than normal and less than the calculated value). Headache and nausea are common with carbon monoxide. Sudden collapse may occur with cyanide and hydrogen sulfide exposure. A bitter almond breath odor may be noted with cyanide ingestion, and hydrogen sulfide smells like rotten eggs.	High-dose oxygen. Inhaled amyl nitrite and IV sodium nitrite and sodium thiosulfate (Lilly cyanide antidote kit) for coma, metabolic acidosis, and cardiovascular dysfunction in cyanide poisoning. Amyl and sodium nitrite (without thiosulfate) for similar toxicity in hydrogen sulfide poisoning. Hyperbaric oxygen for moderate to severe carbon monoxide poisoning and for cyanide or hydrogen sulfide poisoning unresponsive to other measures.

| Methemoglobin inducers | Aniline derivatives, dapsone, local anesthetics, nitrates, nitrites, nitrogen oxides, nitro- and nitroso hydrocarbons, phenazopyridine, primaquine-type antimalarials, sulfonamides. | Oxidation of hemoglobin iron from ferrous (Fe^{2+}) to ferric (Fe^{3+}) state prevents oxygen binding, transport, and tissue uptake (methemoglobinemia shifts oxygen dissociation curve to the left). Oxidation of hemoglobin protein causes hemoglobin precipitation and hemolytic anemia (manifest as Heinz bodies and "bite cells" on peripheral blood smear). | Signs and symptoms of hypoxia with initial physiologic stimulation and subsequent depression (HPIM-18 Table e50-2), gray-brown cyanosis unresponsive to oxygen at methemoglobin fractions >15–20%, headache, lactic acidosis (at methemoglobin fractions >45%), normal P_{O_2} and calculated oxygen saturation but decreased oxygen saturation and increased methemoglobin fraction by co-oximetry (oxygen saturation by pulse oximetry may be falsely increased or decreased but is less than the normal and less than the calculated value). | High-dose oxygen. Intravenous methylene blue for methemoglobin fraction >30%, symptomatic hypoxia, or ischemia (contraindicated in G6PD deficiency). Exchange transfusion and hyperbaric oxygen for severe or refractory cases. |

(continued)

TABLE 32-3 PATHOPHYSIOLOGIC FEATURES AND TREATMENT OF SPECIFIC TOXIC SYNDROMES AND POISONINGS (CONTINUED)

Physiologic Condition, Causes	Examples	Mechanism of Action	Clinical Features	Specific Treatments
Discordant				
AGMA inducers	Ethylene glycol	Ethylene glycol causes CNS depression and increased serum osmolality. Metabolites (primarily glycolic acid) cause AGMA, CNS depression, and renal failure. Precipitation of oxalic acid metabolite as calcium salt in tissues and urine results in hypocalcemia, tissue edema, and crystalluria.	Initial ethanol-like intoxication, nausea, vomiting, increased osmolar gap, calcium oxalate crystalluria. Delayed AGMA, back pain, renal failure. Coma, seizures, hypotension, ARDS in severe cases.	Gastric aspiration for recent ingestions. Sodium bicarbonate to correct acidemia. Thiamine, folinic acid, magnesium, and high-dose pyridoxine to facilitate metabolism. Ethanol or fomepizole for AGMA, crystalluria or renal dysfunction, ethylene glycol level >3 mmol/L (>20 mg/dL), and for ethanol-like intoxication or increased osmolal gap if level not readily obtainable. Hemodialysis for persistent AGMA, lack of clinical improvement, and renal dysfunction. Hemodialysis also useful for enhancing ethylene glycol elimination and shortening duration of treatment when ethylene glycol level >8 mmol/L (>50 mg/dL).
AGMA inducers	Iron	Hydration of ferric (Fe^{3+}) ion generates H^+. Non-transferrin-bound iron catalyzes formation of free radicals that cause mitochondrial injury, lipid peroxidation, increased capillary permeability, vasodilation, and organ toxicity.	Initial nausea, vomiting, abdominal pain, diarrhea. AGMA, cardiovascular and CNS depression, hepatitis, coagulopathy, and seizures in severe cases. Radiopaque iron tablets may be seen on abdominal x-ray.	Whole-bowel irrigation for large ingestions. Endoscopy and gastrostomy if clinical toxicity and large number of tablets still visible on x-ray. IV hydration. Sodium bicarbonate for acidemia. IV deferoxamine for systemic toxicity, iron level >90 μmol/L (>500 g/dL).

Methanol	Methanol causes ethanol-like CNS depression and increased serum osmolality. Formic acid metabolite causes AGMA and retinal toxicity.	Initial ethanol-like intoxication, nausea, vomiting, increased osmolar gap. Delayed AGMA, visual (clouding, spots, blindness) and retinal (edema, hyperemia) abnormalities. Coma, seizures, cardiovascular depression in severe cases. Possible pancreatitis.	Gastric aspiration for recent ingestions. Sodium bicarbonate to correct acidemia. High-dose folinic acid or folate to facilitate metabolism. Ethanol or fomepizole for AGMA, visual symptoms, methanol level >6 mmol/L (>20 mg/dL), and for ethanol-like intoxication or increased osmolal gap if level not readily obtainable. Hemodialysis for persistent AGMA, lack of clinical improvement, and renal dysfunction. Hemodialysis also useful for enhancing methanol elimination and shortening duration of treatment when methanol level >15 mmol/L (>50 mg/dL).
Salicylate	Increased sensitivity of CNS respiratory center to changes in P_{O_2} and P_{CO_2} stimulates respiration. Uncoupling of oxidative phosphorylation, inhibition of Krebs cycle enzymes, and stimulation of carbohydrate and lipid metabolism generate unmeasured endogenous anions and cause AGMA.	Initial nausea, vomiting, hyperventilation, alkalemia, alkaluria. Subsequent alkalemia with both respiratory alkalosis and AGMA, and paradoxical aciduria. Late acidemia with CNS and respiratory depression. Cerebral and pulmonary edema in severe cases. Hypoglycemia, hypocalcemia, hypokalemia, and seizures can occur.	IV hydration and supplemental glucose. Sodium bicarbonate to correct acidemia. Alkaline diuresis for systemic toxicity. Hemodialysis for coma, cerebral edema, seizures, pulmonary edema, renal failure, progressive acid-base disturbances or clinical toxicity, salicylate level >7 mmol/L (>100 mg/dL) following acute overdose.

(continued)

179

TABLE 32-3 PATHOPHYSIOLOGIC FEATURES AND TREATMENT OF SPECIFIC TOXIC SYNDROMES AND POISONINGS (CONTINUED)

Physiologic Condition, Causes	Examples	Mechanism of Action	Clinical Features	Specific Treatments
Discordant				
CNS syndromes				
Extrapyramidal reactions	Antipsychotics (see above), some cyclic antidepressants and antihistamines.	Decreased CNS dopaminergic activity with relative excess of cholinergic activity.	Akathisia, dystonia, parkinsonism	Oral or parenteral anticholinergic agent such as benztropine or diphenhydramine.
Isoniazid		Interference with activation and supply of pyridoxal-5-phosphate, a cofactor for glutamic acid decarboxylase, which converts glutamic acid to GABA, results in decreased levels of this inhibitory CNS neurotransmitter; complexation with and depletion of pyridoxine itself; inhibition of nicotine-adenine dinucleotide dependent lactate and	Nausea, vomiting, agitation, confusion; coma, respiratory depression, seizures, lactic and ketoacidosis in severe cases.	High-dose IV pyridoxine (vitamin B₆) for agitation, confusion, coma, and seizures. Diazepam or barbiturates for seizures.

	hydroxybutyrate dehydrogenases resulting in substrate accumulation.		
Lithium	Interference with cell membrane ion transport, adenylate cyclase and Na$^+$, K$^+$-ATPase activity, and neurotransmitter release.	Nausea, vomiting, diarrhea, ataxia, choreoathetosis, encephalopathy, hyperreflexia, myoclonus, nystagmus, nephrogenic diabetes insipidus, falsely elevated serum chloride with low anion gap, tachycardia. Coma, seizures, arrhythmias, hyperthermia, and prolonged or permanent encephalopathy and movement disorders in severe cases. Delayed onset after acute overdose, particularly with delayed-release formations. Toxicity occurs at lower drug levels in chronic poisoning than in acute poisoning.	Whole-bowel irrigation for large ingestions. IV hydration. Hemodialysis for coma, seizures, severe, progressive, or persistent encephalopathy or neuromuscular dysfunction, peak lithium level >8 meq/L following acute overdose.

(continued)

TABLE 32-3 PATHOPHYSIOLOGIC FEATURES AND TREATMENT OF SPECIFIC TOXIC SYNDROMES AND POISONINGS (CONTINUED)

Physiologic Condition, Causes	Examples	Mechanism of Action	Clinical Features	Specific Treatments
Discordant				
Serotonin syndrome	Amphetamines, cocaine, dextromethorphan, meperidine, MAO inhibitors, selective serotonin (5HT) reuptake inhibitors, tricyclic antidepressants, tramadol, triptans, tryptophan.	Promotion of serotonin release, inhibition of serotonin reuptake, or direct stimulation of CNS and peripheral serotonin receptors (primarily 5HT-1a and 5HT-2), alone or in combination.	Altered mental status (agitation, confusion, mutism, coma, seizures), neuromuscular hyperactivity (hyperreflexia, myoclonus, rigidity, tremors), and autonomic dysfunction (abdominal pain, diarrhea, diaphoresis, fever, flushing, labile hypertension, mydriasis, tearing, salivation, tachycardia). Complications include hyperthermia, lactic acidosis, rhabdomyolysis, and multisystem organ failure.	Serotonin receptor antagonists such as cyproheptadine, discontinue offending agent(s).
Membrane-active agents	Amantadine, antiarrhythmics (class I and III agents; some β blockers), antipsychotics (see above), antihistamines (particularly	Blockade of fast sodium membrane channels prolongs phase 0 (depolarization) of the cardiac action potential, which prolongs the QRS duration	QRS and JT prolongation (or both) with hypotension, ventricular tachyarrhythmias, CNS depression, seizures. Anti-cholinergic effects with amantadine, antihistamines,	Hypertonic sodium bicarbonate (or hypertonic saline) for cardiac conduction delays and monomorphic ventricular tachycardia. Lidocaine for monomorphic ventricular tachycardia (except when due to class Ib antiarrhythmics). Magnesium, isoproterenol, and overdrive pacing

diphenhydramine), carbamazepine, local anesthetics (including cocaine), opioids (meperidine, propoxyphene, orphenadrine, quinoline antimalarials (chloroquine, hydroxychloroquine, quinine), cyclic antidepressants (see above).

and promotes reentrant (monomorphic) ventricular tachycardia. Class Ia, Ic, and III antiarrhythmics also block potassium channels during phases 2 and 3 (repolarization) of the action potential, prolonging the JT interval and promoting early after-depolarizations and polymorphic (torsades des pointes) ventricular tachycardia. Similar effects on neuronal membrane channels cause CNS dysfunction. Some agents also block α-adrenergic and cholinergic receptors or have opioid effects (see above and HPIM-18 Chap. 393).

carbamazepine, disopyramide, antipsychotics, and cyclic antidepressants (see above). Opioid effects with meperidine and propoxyphene (see HPIM-18 Chap. 393). Cinchonism (hearing loss, tinnitus, nausea, vomiting, vertigo, ataxia, headache, flushing, diaphoresis) and blindness with quinoline antimalarials.

for polymorphic ventricular tachycardia. Physostigmine for anticholinergic effects (see above). Naloxone for opioid effects (see HPIM-18 Chap. 393). Extracorporeal removal for some agents (see text).

Abbreviations: AGMA, anion-gap metabolic acidosis; ARDS, adult respiratory distress syndrome; ATPase, adenosine triphosphatase; CNS, central nervous system; 5-HT, 5-hydroxytryptamine (serotonin); GABA, γ-aminobutyric acid; G6PD, glucose-6-phosphate dehydrogenase; MAO, monoamine oxidase; SIADH, syndrome of inappropriate antidiuretic hormone secretion; VX, extremely toxic persistent nerve agent (no common chemical name).

TABLE 32-4 HEAVY METALS

Main Sources	Metabolism	Toxicity	Diagnosis	Treatment
Arsenic				
Smelting and micro-electronics industries; wood preservatives, pesticides, herbicides, fungicides; contaminant of deep-water wells; folk remedies; and coal; incineration of these products	Organic arsenic (arseno-betaine, arsenocholine) is ingested in seafood and fish, but is nontoxic; inorganic arsenic is readily absorbed (lung and GI); sequesters in liver, spleen, kidneys, lungs, and GI tract; residues persist in skin, hair, and nails; biomethylation results in detoxification, but this process saturates.	Acute arsenic poisoning results in necrosis of intestinal mucosa with hemorrhagic gastroenteritis, fluid loss, hypotension, delayed cardiomyopathy, acute tubular necrosis, and hemolysis. Chronic arsenic exposure causes diabetes, vasospasm, peripheral vascular insufficiency and gangrene, peripheral neuropathy, and cancer of skin, lung, liver (angiosarcoma), bladder, and kidney. Lethal dose: 120–200 mg (adults); 2 mg/kg (children).	Nausea, vomiting, diarrhea, abdominal pain, delirium, coma, seizures; garlicky odor on breath; hyperkeratosis, hyperpigmentation, exfoliative dermatitis, and Mees' lines (transverse white striae of the fingernails); sensory and motor polyneuritis, distal weakness. Radiopaque sign on abdominal x-ray; ECG–QRS broadening, QT prolongation, ST depression, T-wave flattening; 24-h urinary arsenic >67 μmol/d or 50 μg/d; (no seafood for 24 h); if recent exposure, serum arsenic >0.9 μmol/L (7 μg/dL). High arsenic in hair or nails.	If acute ingestion, gastric lavage, activated charcoal with a cathartic. Supportive care in ICU. Dimercaprol 3–5 mg/kg IM q4h × 2 days; q6h × 1 day, then q12h × 10 days; alternative: oral succimer.

Cadmium

Metal-plating, pigment, smelting, battery, and plastics industries; tobacco; incineration of these products; ingestion of food that concentrates cadmium (grains, cereals).	Absorbed through ingestion or inhalation; bound by metallothionein, filtered at the glomerulus, but reabsorbed by proximal tubules (thus, poorly excreted). Biologic half-life: 10–30 y. Binds cellular sulfhydryl groups, competes with zinc, calcium for binding sites. Concentrates in liver and kidneys.	Acute cadmium inhalation causes pneumonitis after 4–24 h; acute ingestion causes gastroenteritis. Chronic exposure causes anosmia, yellowing of teeth, emphysema, minor LFT elevations, microcytic hypochromic anemia unresponsive to iron therapy, proteinuria, increased urinary β_2-microglobulin, calciuria, leading to chronic renal failure, osteomalacia, and fractures.	With inhalation: pleuritic chest pain, dyspnea, cyanosis, fever, tachycardia, nausea, noncardiogenic pulmonary edema. With ingestion: nausea, vomiting, cramps, diarrhea. Bone pain, fractures with osteomalacia. If recent exposure, serum cadmium >500 nmol/L (5 μg/dL). Urinary cadmium >100 nmol/L (10 μg/g creatinine) and/or urinary β_2-microglobulin >750 μg/g creatinine (but urinary β_2-microglobulin also increased in other renal diseases such as pyelonephritis).	There is no effective treatment for cadmium poisoning (chelation not useful; dimercaprol can exacerbate nephrotoxicity). Avoidance of further exposure, supportive therapy, vitamin D for osteomalacia.

Lead

Manufacturing of auto batteries, lead crystal, ceramics, fishing weights, etc.; demolition or sanding of lead-painted houses; stained glass making, plumbing, soldering, bridges;	Absorbed through ingestion or inhalation; organic lead (e.g., tetraethyl lead) absorbed dermally. In blood, 95–99% sequestered in RBCs—thus, must measure lead in whole blood (not serum). Distributed widely in soft tissue, with half-life	Acute exposure with blood lead levels (BPb) of >60–80 μg/dL can cause impaired neurotransmission and neuronal cell death (with central and peripheral nervous system effects); impaired hematopoiesis and renal tubular dysfunction.	Abdominal pain, irritability, lethargy, anorexia, anemia, Fanconi's syndrome, pyuria, azotemia in children with blood lead level (BPb) >80 μg/dL; may also see epiphyseal plate "lead lines" on long bone x-rays. Convulsions, coma at BPb >120 μg/dL.	Identification and correction of exposure sources is critical. In some U.S. states, screening and reporting to local health boards of children with BPb >10 μg/dL and workers with BPb >40 μg/dL is required. In the highly exposed individual with symptoms, chelation

(continued)

TABLE 32-4 HEAVY METALS (CONTINUED)

Main Sources	Metabolism	Toxicity	Diagnosis	Treatment
Lead				
environmental exposure to paint chips, house dust (in homes built before 1975), firing ranges (from bullet dust), food or water from improperly glazed ceramics, lead pipes; contaminated herbal remedies, candies; exposure to the combustion of leaded fuels.	~30 days; 15% of dose sequestered in bone with half-life of >20 years. Excreted mostly in urine, but also appears in other fluids including breast milk. Interferes with mitochondrial oxidative phosphorylation, ATPases, calcium-dependent messengers; enhances oxidation and cell apoptosis.	At higher levels of exposure (e.g., BPb >80–120 µg/dL), acute encephalopathy with convulsions, coma, and death may occur. Subclinical exposures in children (BPb 25–60 µg/dL) are associated with anemia; mental retardation; and deficits in language, motor function, balance, hearing, behavior, and school performance. Impairment of IQ appears to occur at even lower levels of exposure with no measurable threshold above the limit of detection in most assays of 1 µg/dL. In adults, chronic subclinical exposures (BPb >40 µg/dL) are associated with an	Noticeable neurodevelopmental delays at BPb of 40–80 µg/dL; may also see symptoms associated with higher BPb levels. In the U.S., screening of all children when they begin to crawl (~6 months) is recommended by the CDC; source identification and intervention is begun if the BPb >10 µg/dL. In adults, acute exposure causes similar symptoms as in children as well as headaches, arthralgias, myalgias, depression, impaired short-term memory, loss of libido. Physical exam may reveal a "lead line" at the gingiva-tooth border, pallor, wrist drop, and cognitive dysfunction (e.g., declines on the	is recommended with oral DMSA (succimer); if acutely toxic, hospitalization and IV or IM chelation with edetate calcium disodium (CaEDTA) may be required, with the addition of dimercaprol to prevent worsening of encephalopathy. It is uncertain whether children with asymptomatic lead exposure (e.g., BPb 20–40 µg/dL) benefit from chelation. Correction of dietary deficiencies in iron, calcium, magnesium, and zinc will lower lead absorption and may also improve toxicity. Vitamin C is a weak but natural chelating agent. Calcium supplements

| | | (1200 mg at bedtime) have been shown to lower blood lead levels in pregnant women. |
| | increased risk of anemia, demyelinating peripheral neuropathy (mainly motor), impairments of reaction time, hypertension, ECG conduction delays, interstitial nephritis and chronic renal failure, diminished sperm counts, spontaneous abortions. | mini-mental status exam); lab tests may reveal a normocytic, normochromic anemia, basophilic stippling, an elevated blood protoporphyrin level (free erythrocyte or zinc), and motor delays on nerve conduction. In the U.S., OSHA requires regular testing of lead-exposed workers with removal if BPb >40 µg/ dL. New guidelines have been proposed recommending monitoring of cumulative exposure parameters (Kosnett, 2007). | |

Mercury

| Metallic, mercurous, and mercuric mercury (Hg, Hg^+, Hg^{2+}) exposures occur in some chemical, metal-processing, electrical-equipment, automotive industries; they are also in thermometers, dental amalgams, batteries. | Elemental mercury (Hg) is not well absorbed; however, it will volatilize into highly absorbable vapor. Inorganic mercury is absorbed through the gut and skin. Organic mercury is well absorbed through inhalation and ingestion. Elemental and organic mercury cross | Acute inhalation of Hg vapor causes pneumonitis and noncardiogenic pulmonary edema leading to death, CNS symptoms, and polyneuropathy.

Chronic high exposure causes CNS toxicity (mercurial erethism, see Diagnosis); | Chronic exposure to metallic mercury vapor produces a characteristic intention tremor and mercurial *erethism*: excitability, memory loss, insomnia, timidity, and delirium ("mad as a hatter" —hat makers used mercury in the manufacturing process). On neurobehavioral tests: decreased motor speed, visual | Treat acute ingestion of mercuric salts with induced emesis or gastric lavage and polythiol resins (to bind mercury in the GI tract). Chelate with dimercaprol (up to 24 mg/kg per day IM in divided doses), DMSA (succimer), or penicillamine, with 5-day courses separated |

(continued)

187

TABLE 32–4 HEAVY METALS (CONTINUED)

Main Sources	Metabolism	Toxicity	Diagnosis	Treatment
Mercury				
Mercury is dispersed by waste incineration. Environmental bacteria convert inorganic to organic mercury, which then bioconcentrates up the aquatic food chain to contaminate tuna, swordfish, and other pelagic fish.	the blood-brain barrier and placenta. Mercury is excreted in urine and feces and has a half-life in blood of ~60 days; however, deposits will remain in the kidney and brain for years. Exposure to mercury stimulates the kidney to produce metallothionein, which provides some detoxification benefit. Mercury binds sulfhydryl groups and interferes with a wide variety of critical enzymatic processes.	lower exposures impair renal function, motor speed, memory, coordination. Acute ingestion of inorganic mercury causes gastroenteritis, the nephritic syndrome, or acute renal failure, hypertension, tachycardia, and cardiovascular collapse, with death at a dose of 10–42 mg/kg. Ingestion of organic mercury causes gastroenteritis, arrhythmias, and lesions in the basal ganglia, gray matter, and cerebellum at doses >1.7 mg/kg.	scanning, verbal and visual memory, visuomotor coordination. Children exposed to mercury in any form may develop *acro dynia* ("pink disease"): flushing, itching, swelling, tachycardia, hypertension, excessive salivation or perspiration, irritability, weakness, morbilliform rashes, desquamation of palms and soles. Toxicity from elemental or inorganic mercury exposure begins when blood levels are >180 nmol/L (3.6 µg/dL) and urine levels >0.7 µmol/L (15 µg/dL).	by several days of rest. If renal failure occurs, treat with peritoneal dialysis, hemodialysis, or extra-corporeal regional complexing hemodialysis and succimer. Chronic inorganic mercury poisoning is best treated with N-acetyl penicillamine.

High exposure during pregnancy causes derangement of fetal neuronal migration resulting in severe mental retardation.

Mild exposures during pregnancy (from fish consumption) are associated with declines in neurobehavioral performance in offspring.

Dimethylmercury, a compound only found in research labs, is "supertoxic"—a few drops of exposure via skin absorption or inhaled vapor can cause severe cerebellar degeneration and death.

Exposures that ended years ago may result in a >20-μg increase in 24-h urine after a 2-g dose of succimer.

Organic mercury exposure is best measured by levels in blood (if recent) or hair (if chronic); CNS toxicity in children may derive from fetal exposures associated with maternal hair Hg > 30 nmol/g (6 μg/g).

Abbreviations: ATPase, adenosine triphosphatase; CDC, Centers for Disease Control and Prevention; CNS, central nervous system; DMSA, dimercaptosuccinic acid; ECG, electrocardiogram; GI, gastrointestinal; ICU, intensive care unit; IQ, intelligence quotient; LFT, liver function tests; OSHA, Occupational Safety and Health Administration; RBC, red blood cell.

Whole-bowel irrigation may be useful with ingestions of foreign bodies, drug packets, slow-release medications, and heavy metals. Electrolyte/polyethylene glycol solution (e.g., Golytely, Colyte) is given orally or by gastric tube up to a rate of 2 L/h. Cathartic salts (magnesium citrate) and saccharides (sorbitol, mannitol) promote evacuation of the rectum but have not been shown to of benefit in poison decontamination. Dilution of corrosive acids and alkali is accomplished by having the pt drink 5 mL water per kg body weight. Endoscopy or surgical intervention may be required in large foreign-body ingestion, concretions of ingested material (heavy metals, lithium, salicylate, or sustained-release tablets), and when ingested drug packets leak or rupture.

Skin and eyes are decontaminated by washing with copious amounts of water or saline.

ENHANCEMENT OF ELIMINATION Activated charcoal in repeated doses of 1 g/kg q2–4h is useful for ingestions of drugs with enteral circulation such as carbamazepine, dapsone, diazepam, digoxin, glutethimide, meprobamate, methotrexate, phenobarbital, phenytoin, salicylate, theophylline, and valproic acid.

Forced urinary alkalinization enhances the elimination of chlorophenoxyacetic acid herbicides, chlorpropamide, diflunisal, fluoride, methotrexate, phenobarbital, sulfonamides, and salicylates through ionization and inhibition of tubular reabsorption. Sodium bicarbonate, 1–2 ampules per liter of 0.45% NaCl, is given at a rate sufficient to maintain urine pH ≥7.5 and urine output at 3–6 mL/kg per h. Acid diuresis is no longer recommended.

Hemodialysis may be useful in severe poisoning due to barbiturates, bromide, chloral hydrate, ethanol, ethylene glycol, isopropyl alcohol, lithium, heavy metals, methanol, procainamide, and salicylate. Peritoneal dialysis is less effective. Hemoperfusion may be indicated for chloramphenicol, disopyramide, and hypnotic-sedative overdose, but is no longer widely available. Exchange transfusion removes poisons affecting red blood cells (arsine, sodium chlorate causing hemolysis, methemoglobinemia, sulfhemoglobinemia).

The features of specific toxic syndromes and approaches to treatment are summarized in Table 32-3. The features of selected heavy metal toxicity and approaches to treatment are summarized in Table 32-4. Readers are encouraged to contact poison control centers for additional information (*www.aapcc.org/DNN/*).

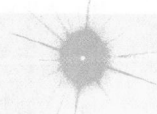

For a more detailed discussion, see Hu H: Heavy Metal Poisoning, Chap. e49 and Mycyk MB: Poisoning and Drug Overdosage, Chap. e50; in HPIM-18.

CHAPTER **33**
Bioterrorism

MICROBIAL BIOTERRORISM

Microbial bioterrorism refers to the use of microbial pathogens as weapons of terror that target civilian populations. A primary goal of bioterrorism is not necessarily to produce mass casualties but to destroy the morale of a society through creating fear and uncertainty. The events of September 11, 2001, followed by the anthrax attacks through the U.S. Postal Service, illustrate the vulnerability of the American public to terrorist attacks, including those that use microbes. The key to combating bioterrorist attacks is a highly functioning system of public health surveillance and education that rapidly identifies and effectively contains the attack.

Agents of microbial bioterrorism may be used in their natural form or may be deliberately modified to maximize their deleterious effect. Modifications that increase the deleterious effect of a biologic agent include genetic alteration of microbes to produce antimicrobial resistance, creation of fine-particle aerosols, chemical treatment to stabilize and prolong infectivity, and alteration of the host range through changes in surface protein receptors. Certain of these approaches fall under the category of *weaponization*, a term that describes the processing of microbes or toxins in a manner that enhances their deleterious effect after release. The key features that characterize an effective biologic weapon are summarized in Table 33-1.

The U.S. Centers for Disease Control and Prevention (CDC) has classified microbial agents that could potentially be used in bioterrorism

---

TABLE 33-1 KEY FEATURES OF BIOLOGIC AGENTS USED AS BIOWEAPONS

1. High morbidity and mortality
2. Potential for person-to-person spread
3. Low infective dose and highly infectious by aerosol
4. Lack of rapid diagnostic capability
5. Lack of universally available effective vaccine
6. Potential to cause anxiety
7. Availability of pathogen and feasibility of production
8. Environmental stability
9. Database of prior research and development
10. Potential to be "weaponized"

Source: From L Borio et al: JAMA 287:2391, 2002; with permission.

TABLE 33-2 CDC CATEGORY A, B, AND C AGENTS

Category A
Anthrax (*Bacillus anthracis*)
Botulism (*Clostridium botulinum* toxin)
Plague (*Yersinia pestis*)
Smallpox (Variola major)
Tularemia (*Francisella tularensis*)
Viral hemorrhagic fevers
Arenaviruses: Lassa, New World (Machupo, Junin, Guanarito, and Sabia)
Bunyaviridae: Crimean-Congo, Rift Valley
Filoviridae: Ebola, Marburg
Category B
Brucellosis (*Brucella* spp.)
Epsilon toxin of *Clostridium perfringens*
Food safety threats (e.g., *Salmonella* spp., *Escherichia coli* 0157:H7, *Shigella*)
Glanders (*Burkholderia mallei*)
Melioidosis (*B. pseudomallei*)
Psittacosis (*Chlamydia psittaci*)
Q fever (*Coxiella burnetii*)
Ricin toxin from *Ricinus communis* (castor beans)
Staphylococcal enterotoxin B
Typhus fever (*Rickettsia prowazekii*)
Viral encephalitis [alphaviruses (e.g., Venezuelan, eastern, and western equine encephalitis)]
Water safety threats (e.g., *Vibrio cholerae, Cryptosporidium parvum*)
Category C
Emerging infectious diseases threats such as Nipah, hantavirus, SARS coronavirus, and pandemic influenza.

Abbreviations: SARS, severe acute respiratory syndrome.
Source: Centers for Disease Control and Prevention and the National Institute of Allergy and Infectious Diseases.

attacks into three categories: A, B, and C (Table 33-2). Category A agents are the highest-priority pathogens. They pose the greatest risk to national security because they (1) can be easily disseminated or transmitted from person to person, (2) are associated with high case-fatality rates, (3) have potential to cause significant public panic and social disruption, and (4) require special action and public health preparedness.

■ CATEGORY A AGENTS

Anthrax (*Bacillus Anthracis*)

Anthrax as a Bioweapon Anthrax in many ways is the prototypic bioweapon. Although it is only rarely spread by person-to-person contact, it has many of the other features of an ideal biologic weapon listed in Table 33-1. The potential impact of anthrax as a bioweapon is illustrated by the apparent accidental release in 1979 of anthrax spores from a Soviet bioweapons facility in Sverdlosk, Russia. As a result of this atmospheric release of anthrax spores, at least 77 cases of anthrax (of which 66 were fatal) occurred in individuals within an area 4 km downwind of the facility. Deaths were noted in livestock up to 50 km from the facility. The interval between probable exposure and onset of symptoms ranged from 2 to 43 days, with the majority of cases occurring within 2 weeks. In September of 2001 the American public was exposed to anthrax spores delivered through the U.S. Postal Service. There were 22 confirmed cases: 11 cases of inhaled anthrax (5 died) and 11 cases of cutaneous anthrax (no deaths). Cases occurred in individuals who opened contaminated letters as well as in postal workers involved in processing the mail.

Microbiology and Clinical Features (See also Chaps. 138 and 221, HPIM-18)

- Anthrax is caused by infections with *B. anthracis*, a gram-positive, non-motile, spore-forming rod that is found in soil and predominantly causes disease in cattle, goats, and sheep.
- Spores can remain viable for decades in the environment and be difficult to destroy with standard decontamination procedures. These properties make anthrax an ideal bioweapon.
- Naturally occurring human infection generally results from exposure to infected animals or contaminated animal products.

  There are three major clinical forms of anthrax:

1. *Gastrointestinal anthrax* is rare and is unlikely to result from a bioterrorism event.
2. *Cutaneous anthrax* follows introduction of spores through an opening in the skin. The lesion begins as a papule followed by the development of a black eschar. Prior to the availability of antibiotics, about 20% of cutaneous anthrax cases were fatal.
3. *Inhalation anthrax* is the form most likely to result in serious illness and death in a bioterrorism attack. It occurs following inhalation of spores that become deposited in the alveolar spaces. The spores are phagocytosed by alveolar macrophages and are transported to regional lymph nodes where they germinate. Following germination, rapid bacterial growth and toxin production occur. Subsequent hematologic dissemination leads to cardiovascular collapse and death. The earliest symptoms are typically those of a viral-like prodrome with fever, malaise, and abdominal/chest symptoms that rapidly progress to a septic shock picture. Widening of the mediastinum and pleural effusions are typical findings on chest radiography. Once considered 100% fatal, experience from the Sverdlosk and U.S. Postal outbreaks indicate that with prompt initiation of appropriate antibiotic therapy, survival may be >50%. Awareness of the possibility of the diagnosis of anthrax is critical to the prompt initiation of therapy.

| **TREATMENT** | Anthrax (See Table 33-3) |

Anthrax can be successfully treated if the disease is promptly recognized and appropriate antibiotic therapy is initiated.

- Penicillin, ciprofloxacin, and doxycycline are currently licensed for the treatment of anthrax.
- Clindamycin and rifampin have in vitro activity against the organism and may be used as part of the treatment regimen.
- Pts with inhalation anthrax are not contagious and do not require special isolation procedures.

Vaccination and Prevention

- Currently there is a single vaccine licensed for use, produced from a cell-free culture supernatant of an attenuated strain of *B. anthracis* (Stern strain).
- Current recommendation for postexposure prophylaxis is 60 days of antibiotics (see Table 33-1); recent animal studies have suggested that postexposure vaccination may be of some additional benefit.

Plague (*Yersinia Pestis*) (See also Chap. 100)

Plague as a Bioweapon Although plague lacks the environmental stability of anthrax, the highly contagious nature of the infection and the high mortality rate make it a potentially important agent of bioterrorism. As a bioweapon, plague would likely be delivered via an aerosol leading to primary pneumonic plague. In such an attack, person-to-person transmission of plague via respiratory aerosol could lead to large numbers of secondary cases.

Microbiology and Clinical Features See Chap. 100.

| **TREATMENT** | Plague See Table 33-3 and Chap. 100. |

Smallpox (Variola major and V. minor) (See also Chaps. 183 and 221, HPIM-18)

Smallpox as a Bioweapon Smallpox as a disease was globally eradicated by 1980 through a worldwide vaccination program. However, with the cessation of smallpox immunization programs in the United States in 1972 (and worldwide in 1980), close to half the U.S. population is fully susceptible to smallpox today. Given the infectious nature and the 10–30% mortality of smallpox in unimmunized individuals, the deliberate release of virus could have devastating effects on the population. In the absence of effective containment measures, an initial infection of 50–100 persons in a first generation of cases could expand by a factor of 10 to 20 with each succeeding generation. These considerations make smallpox a formidable bioweapon.

Microbiology and Clinical Features The disease smallpox is caused by one of two closely related double-strand DNA viruses, V. major and V. minor. Both viruses are members of the Orthopoxvirus genus of the Poxviridae family. Infection with V. minor is generally less severe, with low mortality rates; thus, V. major is the only one considered as a potential bioweapon.

TABLE 33-3 CLINICAL SYNDROMES, PREVENTION, AND TREATMENT STRATEGIES FOR DISEASES CAUSED BY CATEGORY A AGENTS

Agent	Clinical Syndrome	Incubation Period	Diagnosis	Treatment	Prophylaxis
Bacillus anthracis (anthrax)	Cutaneous lesion	1–12 days	Culture, Gram stain, PCR, Wright stain of peripheral smear	Postexposure	Anthrax vaccine adsorbed
	Papule to eschar			Ciprofloxacin, 500 mg, PO bid × 60 d *or*	Recombinant protective antigen vaccines are under study
	Inhalational disease	1–60 days		Doxycycline, 100 mg PO bid × 60 d *or*	
	Fever, malaise, chest and abdominal discomfort			Amoxicillin, 500 mg PO q8h, likely to be effective if strain penicillin sensitive	
	Pleural effusion, widened mediastinum on chest x-ray			*Active disease:*	
				Ciprofloxacin, 400 mg IV q12h *or* Doxycycline, 100 mg IV q12h *plus*	
				Clindamycin, 900 mg IV q8h and/or rifampin, 300 mg IV q12h; switch to PO when stable × 60 d total	
				Antitoxin strategies:	
				Neutralizing monoclonal and polyclonal antibodies are under study	

(continued)

195

TABLE 33-3 CLINICAL SYNDROMES, PREVENTION, AND TREATMENT STRATEGIES FOR DISEASES CAUSED BY CATEGORY A AGENTS **(CONTINUED)**

Agent	Clinical Syndrome	Incubation Period	Diagnosis	Treatment	Prophylaxis
Yersinia pestis (pneumonic plague)	Fever, cough, dyspnea, hemoptysis Infiltrates and consolidation on chest x-ray	1–6 days	Culture, Gram stain, direct fluorescent antibody, PCR	Gentamicin, 2.0 mg/kg IV loading then 1.7 mg/kg q8h IV *or* Streptomycin, 1.0 g q12h IM or IV Alternatives include doxycycline, 100 mg bid PO or IV; chloramphenicol, 500 mg qid PO or IV	Doxycycline, 100 mg PO bid (ciprofloxacin may also be active)
Variola major (smallpox)	Fever, malaise, headache, backache, emesis Maculopapular to vesicular to pustular skin lesions	7–17 days	Culture, PCR, electron microscopy	Supportive measures; consideration for cidofovir, anti-vaccinia immunoglobulin	Formalin-fixed vaccine (FDA licensed; not available) Vaccinia immunization
Francisella tularensis (tularemia)	Fever, chills, malaise, myalgia, chest discomfort, dyspnea, headache, skin rash, pharyngitis, conjunctivitis Hilar adenopathy on chest x-ray	1–14 days	Gram stain, culture, immunohistochemistry, PCR	Streptomycin, 1 g IM bid *or* Gentamicin, 5 mg/kg per day div q8h IV for 14 days *or* Doxycycline, 100 mg IV bid *or* Chloramphenicol, 15 mg/kg up to 1 gm IV qid *or* Ciprofloxacin, 400 mg IV bid	Doxycycline, 100 mg PO bid × 14 days *or* Ciprofloxacin, 500 mg PO bid × 14 days

Agent	Symptoms	Incubation	Diagnosis	Treatment	Prophylaxis
Viral hemorrhagic fevers	Fever, myalgia, rash, encephalitis, prostration	2–21 days	RT-PCR, serologic testing for antigen or antibody Viral isolation by CDC or U.S. Army Medical Research Institute of Infectious Diseases (USAMRIID)	Supportive measures Ribavirin 30 mg/kg up to 2 g × 1, followed by 16 mg/kg IV up to 1 g q6h for 4 days, followed by 8 mg/kg IV up to 0.5 g q8h × 6 days	No known chemoprophylaxis Consideration for ribavirin in high-risk situations
Botulinum toxin (*Clostridium botulinum*)	Dry mouth, blurred vision, ptosis, weakness, dysarthria, dysphagia, dizziness, respiratory failure, progressive paralysis, dilated pupils	12–72 h	Mouse bioassay, toxin immunoassay	Supportive measures including ventilation, HBAT equine antitoxin from the CDC Emergency Operations Center, 770-488-7100	Administration of antitoxin

Abbreviations: CDC, Centers for Disease Control and Prevention; FDA, U.S. Food and Drug Administration; HBAT, heptavalent botulinum antitoxin; PCR, polymerase chain reaction; RT-PCR, reverse transcriptase PCR.

Infection with V. major typically occurs following contact with an infected person from the time that a maculopapular rash appears through scabbing of the pustular lesions. Infection is thought to occur from inhalation of virus-containing saliva droplets from oropharyngeal lesions. Contaminated clothing or linen can also spread infection. About 12–14 days following initial exposure the pt develops high fever, malaise, vomiting, headache, back pain, and a maculopapular rash that begins on the face and extremities and spreads to the trunk. The skin lesions evolve into vesicles that eventually become pustular with scabs. The oral mucosa also develops macular lesions that progress to ulcers. Smallpox is associated with a 10–30% mortality. Historically, about 5–10% of naturally occurring cases manifest as highly virulent atypical forms, classified as *hemorrhagic* and *malignant*. These are difficult to recognize due to their atypical manifestations. Both forms have similar onset of a severe prostrating illness characterized by high fever, severe headache, and abdominal and back pain. In the hemorrhagic form, cutaneous erythema develops followed by petechiae and hemorrhage into the skin and mucous membranes. In the malignant form, confluent skin lesions develop but never progress to the pustular stage. Both of these forms are often fatal, with death occurring in 5–6 days.

TREATMENT Smallpox

Treatment is supportive. There is no licensed specific antiviral therapy for smallpox; however, certain candidate drugs look promising in preclinical testing in animal models. Smallpox is highly infectious to close contacts; pts who are suspected cases should be handled with strict isolation procedures.

Vaccination and Prevention Smallpox is a preventable disease following immunization with vaccinia. Past and current experience indicates that the smallpox vaccine is associated with a very low incidence of severe complications (see Table 221-4, p. 1775, HPIM-18). The current dilemma facing our society regarding assessment of the risk/benefit of smallpox vaccination is that, while the risks of vaccination are known, the risk of someone deliberately and effectively releasing smallpox into the general population is unknown. Given the rare, but potentially severe complications associated with smallpox vaccination using the currently available vaccine together with the current level of threat, it has been decided by public health authorities that vaccination of the general population is not indicated.

Tularemia (*Francisella Tularensis*) (See also Chap. 100)

Tularemia as a Bioweapon Tularemia has been studied as a biologic agent since the mid-twentieth century. Reportedly, both the United States and the former Soviet Union had active programs investigating this organism as a possible bioweapon. It has been suggested that the Soviet program extended into the era of molecular biology and that some strains of *F. tularensis* may have been genetically engineered to be resistant to commonly used antibiotics. *F. tularensis* is extremely infectious and can cause significant morbidity and mortality. These facts make it reasonable to consider this organism as a possible bioweapon that could be disseminated by either aerosol or contamination of food or drinking water.

Microbiology and Clinical Features See Chap. 100.

TREATMENT Tularemia See Table 33-3 and Chap. 100.

Viral Hemorrhagic Fevers (See also Chap. 113)

Hemorrhagic Fever Viruses as Bioweapons Several of the hemorrhagic fever viruses have been reported to have been weaponized by the former Soviet Union and the United States. Nonhuman primate studies indicate that infection can be established with very few virions and that infectious aerosol preparations can be produced.

Microbiology and Clinical Features See Chap. 113.

TREATMENT Viral Hemorrhagic Fevers See Table 33-3 and Chap. 113.

Botulinum Toxin (*Clostridium botulinum*) (See also Chap. 101)

Botulinum Toxin as a Bioweapon In a bioterrorism attack, botulinum toxin would likely be dispersed as an aerosol or used to contaminate food. Contamination of the water supply is possible, but the toxin would likely be degraded by chlorine used to purify drinking water. The toxin can also be inactivated by heating food to >85°C for >5 min. The United States, the former Soviet Union, and Iraq have all acknowledged studying botulinum toxin as a potential bioweapon. Unique among the Category A agents for not being a live organism, botulinum toxin is one of the most potent and lethal toxins known to man. It has been estimated that 1 g of toxin is sufficient to kill 1 million people if adequately dispersed.

Microbiology and Clinical Features See Chap. 101.

TREATMENT Botulinum Toxin See Table 33-3 and Chap. 101.

■ CATEGORY B AND C AGENTS (SEE TABLE 33-2)

Category B agents are the next highest priority and include agents that are moderately easy to disseminate, produce moderate morbidity and low mortality, and require enhanced diagnostic capacity.

Category C agents are the third highest priority agents in the biodefense agenda. These agents include emerging pathogens, such as SARS (severe acute respiratory syndrome) coronavirus or a pandemic influenza virus, to which the general population lacks immunity. Category C agents could be engineered for mass dissemination in the future. It is important to note that these categories are empirical, and, depending on future circumstances, the priority ratings for a given microbial agent may change.

■ PREVENTION AND PREPAREDNESS

As indicated above, a diverse array of agents have the potential to be used against a civilian population in a bioterrorism attack. The medical profession must maintain a high index of suspicion that unusual clinical presentations or clustering of rare diseases may not be a chance occurrence, but rather the first sign of a bioterrorism attack. Possible early indicators of a bioterrorism attack could include:

- The occurrence of rare diseases in healthy populations
- The occurrence of unexpectedly large numbers of a rare infection
- The appearance in an urban population of an infectious disease that is usually confined to rural settings

Given the importance of rapid diagnosis and early treatment for many of these diseases, it is important that the medical care team report any suspected cases of bioterrorism immediately to local and state health authorities and/or the CDC (888-246-2675).

CHEMICAL BIOTERRORISM

The use of chemical warfare agents (CWAs) as weapons of terror against civilian populations is a potential threat that must be addressed by public health officials and the medical profession. The use of both nerve agents and sulfur mustard by Iraq against Iranian military and Kurdish civilians and the sarin attacks in 1994–1995 in Japan underscore this threat.

A detailed description of the various CWAs can be found in Chap. 222, HPIM-18, and on the CDC website at *www.bt.cdc.gov/agent/agentlistchem.asp*. In this section only vesicants and nerve agents will be discussed, as these are considered the most likely agents to be used in a terrorist attack.

■ VESICANTS (SULFUR MUSTARD, NITROGEN MUSTARD, LEWISITE)

Sulfur mustard is the prototype for this group of CWAs and was first used on the battlefields of Europe in World War I. This agent constitutes both a vapor and liquid threat to exposed epithelial surfaces. The organs most commonly affected are the skin, eyes, and airways. Exposure to large quantities of sulfur mustard can result in bone marrow toxicity. Sulfur mustard dissolves slowly in aqueous media such as sweat or tears, but once dissolved it forms reactive compounds that react with cellular proteins, membranes, and importantly DNA. Much of the biologic damage from this agent appears to result from DNA alkylation and cross-linking in rapidly dividing cells in the corneal epithelium, skin, bronchial mucosal epithelium, GI epithelium, and bone marrow. Sulfur mustard reacts with tissue within minutes of entering the body.

Clinical Features

The topical effects of sulfur mustard occur in the skin, airways, and eyes. Absorption of the agent may produce effects in the bone marrow and GI tract (direct injury to the GI tract may occur if sulfur mustard is ingested in contaminated food or water).

- *Skin:* erythema is the mildest and earliest manifestation; involved areas of skin then develop vesicles that coalesce to form bullae; high-dose exposure may lead to coagulation necrosis within bullae.

- *Airways*: initial and, with mild exposures, the only airway manifestations are burning of the nares, epistaxis, sinus pain, and pharyngeal pain. With exposure to higher concentrations, damage to the trachea and lower airways may occur, producing laryngitis, cough, and dyspnea. With large exposures, necrosis of the airway mucosa occurs leading to pseudomembrane formation and airway obstruction. Secondary infection may occur due to bacterial invasion of denuded respiratory mucosa.
- *Eyes*: the eyes are the most sensitive organ to injury by sulfur mustard. Exposure to low concentrations may produce only erythema and irritation. Exposure to higher concentrations produces progressively more severe conjunctivitis, photophobia, blepharospasm pain, and corneal damage.
- GI tract manifestations include nausea and vomiting, lasting up to 24 h.
- Bone marrow suppression, with peaks at 7–14 days following exposure, may result in sepsis due to leukopenia.

TREATMENT ▶ Sulfur Mustard

Immediate decontamination is essential to minimize damage. Immediately remove clothing and gently wash skin with soap and water. Eyes should be flushed with copious amounts of water or saline. Subsequent medical care is supportive. Cutaneous vesicles should be left intact. Larger bullae should be debrided and treated with topical antibiotic preparations. Intensive care similar to that given to severe burn pts is required for pts with severe exposure. Oxygen may be required for mild/moderate respiratory exposure. Intubation and mechanical ventilation may be necessary for laryngeal spasm and severe lower airway damage. Pseudomembranes should be removed by suctioning; bronchodilators are of benefit for bronchospasm. The use of granulocyte colony-stimulating factor and/or stem cell transplantation may be effective for severe bone marrow suppression.

■ NERVE AGENTS

The organophosphorus nerve agents are the deadliest of the CWAs and work by inhibiting synaptic acetylcholinesterase, creating an acute cholinergic crisis. The "classic" organophosphorus nerve agents are tabun, sarin, soman, cyclosarin, and VX. All agents are liquid at standard temperature and pressure. With the exception of VX, all these agents are highly volatile, and the spilling of even a small amount of liquid agent represents a serious vapor hazard.

Mechanism

Inhibition of acetylcholinesterase accounts for the major life-threatening effects of these agents. At the cholinergic synapse, the enzyme acetylcholinesterase functions as a "turn off" switch to regulate cholinergic synaptic transmission. Inhibition of this enzyme allows released acetylcholine to accumulate, resulting in end-organ overstimulation and leading to what is clinically referred to as *cholinergic crisis*.

Clinical Features

The clinical manifestations of nerve agent exposure are identical for vapor and liquid exposure routes. Initial manifestations include miosis, blurred vision, headache, and copious oropharyngeal secretions. Once the agent enters the bloodstream (usually via inhalation of vapors) manifestations of cholinergic overload include nausea, vomiting, abdominal cramping, muscle twitching, difficulty breathing, cardiovascular instability, loss of consciousness, seizures, and central apnea. The onset of symptoms following vapor exposure is rapid (seconds to minutes). Liquid exposure to nerve agents results in differences in speed of onset and order of symptoms. Contact of a nerve agent with intact skin produces localized sweating followed by localized muscle fasciculations. Once in the muscle, the agent enters the circulation and causes the symptoms described above.

TREATMENT   Nerve Agents

Since nerve agents have a short circulating half-life, improvement should be rapid if exposure is terminated and supportive care and appropriate antidotes are given. Thus, the treatment of acute nerve agent poisoning involves decontamination, respiratory support, antidotes.

1. *Decontamination*: Procedures are the same as those described above for sulfur mustard.
2. *Respiratory support*: Death from nerve agent exposure is usually due to respiratory failure. Ventilation will be complicated by increased airway resistance and secretions. Atropine should be given before mechanical ventilation is instituted.
3. *Antidotal therapy* (see Table 33-4):
   a. *Atropine*: Generally the preferred anticholinergic agent of choice for treating acute nerve agent poisoning. Atropine rapidly reverses cholinergic overload at muscarinic synapses but has little effect at nicotinic synapses. Thus, atropine can rapidly treat the life-threatening respiratory effects of nerve agents but will probably not help neuromuscular effects. The field loading dose is 2–6 mg IM, with repeat doses given every 5–10 min until breathing and secretions improve. In the mildly affected pt with miosis and no systemic symptoms, atropine or homoatropine eye drops may suffice.
   b. *Oxime therapy*: Oximes are nucleophiles that help restore normal enzyme function by reactivating the cholinesterase whose active site has been occupied and bound by the nerve agent. The oxime available in the United States is 2-pralidoxime chloride (2-PAM Cl). Treatment with 2-PAM may cause blood pressure elevation.
   c. *Anticonvulsant*: Seizures caused by nerve agents do not respond to the usual anticonvulsants such as phenytoin, phenobarbital, carbamazepine, valproate, and lamotrigine. The only class of drugs known to have efficacy in treating nerve agent–induced seizures are the benzodiazepines. Diazepam is the only benzodiazepine approved by the U.S. Food and Drug Administration for the treatment of seizures (although other benzodiazepines have been shown to work well in animal models of nerve agent–induced seizures).

TABLE 33-4 ANTIDOTE RECOMMENDATIONS FOLLOWING EXPOSURE TO NERVE AGENTS

Antidotes

Patient Age	Mild/Moderate Effects[a]	Severe Effects[b]	Other Treatment
Infants (0–2 yrs)	Atropine: 0.05 mg/kg IM, or 0.02 mg/kg IV; and 2-PAM chloride: 15 mg/kg IM or IV slowly	Atropine: 0.1 mg/kg IM, or 0.02 mg/kg IV; and 2-PAM chloride: 25 mg/kg IM, or 15 mg/kg IV slowly	Assisted ventilation after antidotes for severe exposure.
Child (2–10 yrs)	Atropine: 1 mg IM, or 0.02 mg/kg IV; and 2-PAM chloride[c]: 15 mg/kg IM or IV slowly	Atropine: 2 mg IM, or 0.02 mg/kg IV; and 2-PAM chloride[c]: 25 mg/kg IM, or 15 mg/kg IV slowly	Repeat atropine (2 mg IM, or 1 mg IM for infants) at 5- to 10-min intervals until secretions have diminished and breathing is comfortable or airway resistance has returned to near normal.
Adolescent (>10 yrs)	Atropine: 2 mg IM, or 0.02 mg/kg IV; and 2-PAM chloride[c]: 15 mg/kg IM or IV slowly	Atropine: 4 mg IM, or 0.02 mg/kg IV; and 2-PAM chloride[c]: 25 mg/kg IM, or 15 mg/kg IV slowly	Phentolamine for 2-PAM-induced hypertension: (5 mg IV for adults; 1 mg IV for children).
Adult	Atropine: 2–4 mg IM or IV; and 2-PAM chloride: 600 mg IM, or 15 mg/kg IV slowly	Atropine: 6 mg IM; and 2-PAM chloride: 1800 mg IM, or 15 mg/kg IV slowly	Diazepam for convulsions: (0.2–0.5 mg IV for infants <5 years; 1 mg IV for children >5 years; 5 mg IV for adults).
Elderly, frail	Atropine: 1 mg IM; and 2-PAM chloride: 10 mg/kg IM, or 5–10 mg/kg IV slowly	Atropine: 2–4 mg IM; and 2-PAM chloride: 25 mg/kg IM, or 5–10 mg/kg IV slowly	

[a]Mild/moderate effects include localized sweating, muscle fasciculations, nausea, vomiting, weakness, dyspnea.

[b]If calculated dose exceeds the adult IM dose, adjust accordingly.

Source: State of New York, Department of Health.

[c]Severe effects include unconsciousness, convulsions, apnea, flaccid paralysis.

Note: 2-PAM chloride is pralidoxime chloride or protopam chloride.

RADIATION BIOTERRORISM

Nuclear or radiation-related devices represent a third category of weapon that could be used in a terrorism attack. There are two major types of attacks that could occur. The first is the use of radiologic dispersal devices that cause the dispersal of radioactive material without detonation of a nuclear explosion. Such devices could use conventional explosives to disperse radio-nuclides. The second, and less probable, scenario would be the use of actual nuclear weapons by terrorists against a civilian target. In addition to weaponization, detrimental human exposure has also resulted from unintentional breaches in radiation containment. The consequences of radiation sickness remain the same for accidental exposure as they do for deliberate release.

■ TYPES OF RADIATION

Alpha radiation consists of heavy, positively charged particles containing two protons and two neutrons. Due to their large size, alpha particles have limited penetrating power. Cloth and human skin can usually prevent alpha particles from penetrating into the body. If alpha particles are internalized, they can cause significant cellular damage.

Beta radiation consists of electrons and can travel only short distances in tissue. Plastic layers and clothing can stop most beta particles. Higher energy beta particles can cause injury to the basal stratum of skin similar to a thermal burn.

Gamma radiation and *x-rays* are forms of electromagnetic radiation discharged from the atomic nucleus. Sometimes referred to as *penetrating radiation*, both gamma and x-rays easily penetrate matter and are the principle type of radiation to cause whole-body exposure (see below).

Neutron particles are heavy and uncharged; often emitted during a nuclear detonation. Their ability to penetrate tissues is variable, depending upon their energy. They are less likely to be generated in various scenarios of radiation bioterrorism.

The commonly used units of radiation are the *rad* and the *gray*. The rad is the energy deposited within living matter and is equal to 100 ergs/g of tissue. The rad has been replaced by the SI unit of the gray (Gy). 100 rad = 1 Gy.

■ TYPES OF EXPOSURE

Whole-body exposure represents deposition of radiation energy over the entire body. Alpha and beta particles have limited penetration power and do not cause significant whole-body exposure unless they are internalized in large amounts. Whole-body exposure from gamma rays, x-rays, or high-energy neutron particles can penetrate the body, causing damage to multiple tissues and organs.

External contamination results from fallout of radioactive particles landing on the body surface, clothing, and hair. This is the dominant form of contamination likely to occur in a terrorist strike that utilizes a dispersal device. The most likely contaminants would emit alpha and beta radiation. Alpha particles do not penetrate the skin and thus would produce minimal systemic damage. Beta emitters can cause significant cutaneous burns. Gamma emitters not only cause cutaneous burns but can also cause significant internal damage.

Internal contamination will occur when radioactive material is inhaled, is ingested, or is able to enter the body via a disruption in the skin. The respiratory tract is the main portal of entrance for internal contamination, and the lung is the organ at greatest risk. Radioactive material entering the GI tract will be absorbed according to its chemical structure and solubility. Penetration through the skin usually occurs when wounds or burns have disrupted the cutaneous barrier. Absorbed radioactive materials will travel throughout the body. Liver, kidney, adipose tissue, and bone tend to bind and retain radioactive material more than do other tissues.

Localized exposure results from close contact between highly radioactive material and a part of the body, resulting in discrete damage to the skin and deeper structures.

■ ACUTE RADIATION SICKNESS

Radiation interactions with atoms can result in ionization and free radical formation that damages tissue by disrupting chemical bonds and molecular structures in the cell, including DNA. Radiation can lead to cell death; cells that recover may have DNA mutations that pose a higher risk for malignant transformation. Cell sensitivity to radiation damage increases as replication rate increases. Bone marrow and mucosal surfaces in the GI tract have high mitotic activity and thus are significantly more prone to radiation damage than slowly dividing tissues such as bone and muscle. Acute radiation sickness (ARS) can develop following exposure of all or most of the human body to ionizing radiation. The clinical manifestations of ARS reflect the dose and type of radiation as well as the parts of the body that are exposed.

Clinical Features

ARS produces signs and symptoms related to damage of three major organ systems: GI tract, bone marrow, and neurovascular. The type and dose of radiation and the part of the body exposed will determine the dominant clinical picture.

- There are four major stages of ARS:
  1. *Prodrome* occurs between hours to 4 days after exposure and lasts from hours to days. Manifestations include nausea, vomiting, anorexia, and diarrhea.
  2. The *latent stage* follows the prodrome and is associated with minimal or no symptoms. It most commonly lasts up to 2 weeks, but can last as long as 6 weeks.
  3. *Illness* follows the latent stage.
  4. *Death or recovery* is the final stage of ARS.
- The higher the radiation dose, the shorter and more severe the stage.
- At low radiation doses (0.7–4 Gy), bone marrow suppression occurs and constitutes the main illness. The pt may develop bleeding or infection secondary to thrombocytopenia and leukopenia. The bone marrow will generally recover in most pts. Care is supportive (transfusion, antibiotics, colony-stimulating factors).
- With exposure to 6–8 Gy, the clinical picture is more complicated; the bone marrow may not recover and death will ensue. Damage to the GI mucosa producing diarrhea, hemorrhage, sepsis, fluid and electrolyte imbalance may occur and complicate the clinical picture.

- Whole-body exposure to >10 Gy is usually fatal. In addition to severe bone marrow and GI tract damage, a neurovascular syndrome characterized by vascular collapse, seizures, and death may occur (especially at doses >20 Gy).

TREATMENT   Acute Radiation Sickness

Treatment of ARS is largely supportive (Fig. 33-1).

1. Persons contaminated either externally or internally should be decontaminated as soon as possible. Contaminated clothes should be removed; showering or washing the entire skin and hair is very important. A radiation detector should be used to check for residual contamination. Decontamination of medical personnel should occur following emergency treatment and decontamination of the pt.

2. Treatment for the hematopoietic system includes appropriate therapy for neutropenia and infection, transfusion of blood products as needed, and hematopoietic growth factors. The value of bone marrow transplantation in this situation is unknown.

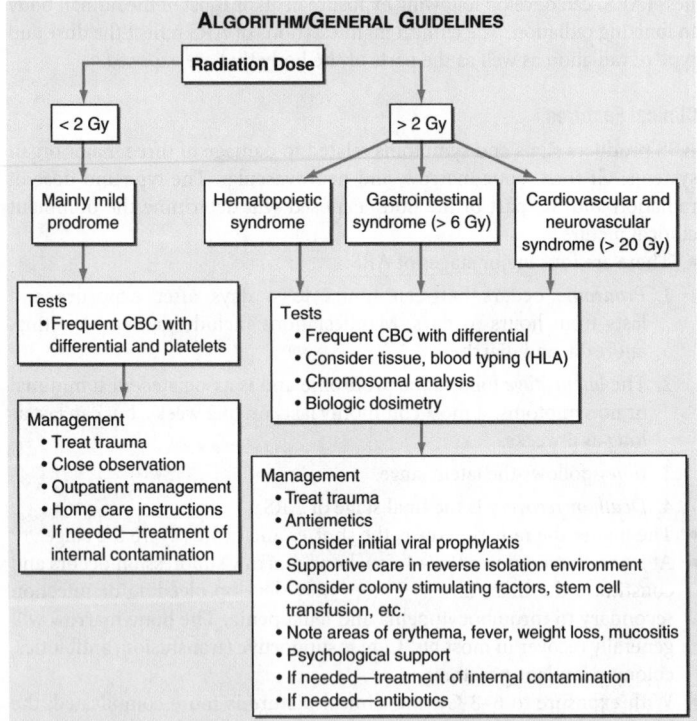

ALGORITHM/GENERAL GUIDELINES

Radiation Dose

< 2 Gy

Mainly mild prodrome

> 2 Gy

Hematopoietic syndrome

Gastrointestinal syndrome (> 6 Gy)

Cardiovascular and neurovascular syndrome (> 20 Gy)

Tests
• Frequent CBC with differential and platelets

Tests
• Frequent CBC with differential
• Consider tissue, blood typing (HLA)
• Chromosomal analysis
• Biologic dosimetry

Management
• Treat trauma
• Close observation
• Outpatient management
• Home care instructions
• If needed—treatment of internal contamination

Management
• Treat trauma
• Antiemetics
• Consider initial viral prophylaxis
• Supportive care in reverse isolation environment
• Consider colony stimulating factors, stem cell transfusion, etc.
• Note areas of erythema, fever, weight loss, mucositis
• Psychological support
• If needed—treatment of internal contamination
• If needed—antibiotics

FIGURE 33-1 General guidelines for treatment of radiation casualties. CBC, complete blood count.

3. Partial or total parenteral nutrition is appropriate supportive therapy for pts with significant injury to the GI mucosa.

4. Treatment of internal radionuclide contamination is aimed at reducing absorption and enhancing elimination of the ingested material (Table 223-2, p. 1794, HPIM-18).

   a. Clearance of the GI tract may be achieved by gastric lavage, emetics, or purgatives, laxatives, ion exchange resins, and aluminum-containing antacids.

   b. Administration of *blocking agents* is aimed at preventing the entrance of radioactive materials into tissues (e.g., potassium iodide, which blocks the uptake of radioactive iodine by the thyroid).

   c. *Diluting agents* decrease the absorption of the radionuclide (e.g., water in the treatment of tritium contamination).

   d. *Mobilizing agents* are most effective when given immediately; however, they may still be effective for up to 2 weeks following exposure. Examples include antithyroid drugs, glucocorticoids, ammonium chloride, diuretics, expectorants, and inhalants. All of these should induce the release of radionuclides from tissues.

   e. *Chelating agents* bind many radioactive materials, after which the complexes are excreted from the body.

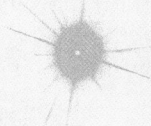

For a more detailed discussion, see Lane HC, Fauci AS: Microbial Bioterrorism, Chap. 221, p. 1768; Hurst CG, Newmark J, Romano JA: Chemical Terrorism, Chap. 222, p. 1779; and Tochner ZA, Glatstein E: Radiation Terrorism, Chap. 223, p. 1788, in HPIM-18.

CHAPTER **34**
Fever, Hyperthermia, and Rash

■ **DEFINITIONS**

- *Temperature:* The hypothalamic thermoregulatory center balances excess heat production from metabolic activity in muscle and liver with heat dissipation from the skin and lungs to maintain a normal body temperature of 36.8° ± 0.4°C (98.2° ± 0.7°F), with diurnal variation (lower in A.M., higher in P.M.).
- *Fever:* an elevation of body temperature (>37.2°C/98.9°F in the morning and >37.7°C/99.9°F in the evening) in conjunction with an increase in the hypothalamic set point
- *Fever of unknown origin* (*FUO*): generally refers to temperatures >38.3°C (>101°F) on several occasions over a defined period, with unrevealing investigations into its cause. FUO can be classified further into several categories:

  - *Classic FUO:* fever lasting >3 weeks where 3 outpt visits, 3 days in the hospital, *or* 1 week of "intelligent and invasive" ambulatory investigation does not elucidate a cause
  - *Nosocomial FUO:* at least 3 days of investigation and 2 days of culture incubation failing to elucidate a cause of fever in a hospitalized pt with no infection on admission
  - *Neutropenic FUO:* at least 3 days of investigation and 2 days of culture incubation failing to elucidate a cause of fever in a pt whose neutrophil count is <500/μL or is expected to fall to that level within 1–2 days
  - *HIV-associated FUO:* fever in an HIV-infected pt, lasting >4 weeks for outpatients or >3 days for hospitalized pts, where appropriate investigation (including 2 days' incubation of cultures) does not reveal a cause

- *Hyperpyrexia:* temperatures >41.5°C (>106.7°F) that can occur with severe infections but more commonly occur with CNS hemorrhages
- *Hyperthermia:* an uncontrolled increase in body temperature that exceeds the body's ability to lose heat *without* a change in the hypothalamic set point. Hyperthermia does not involve pyrogenic molecules.
- *Pyrogen:* any fever-causing substance, including exogenous pyrogens (e.g., microbial toxins, lipopolysaccharide, superantigens) and pyrogenic cytokines (e.g., IL-1, IL-6, TNF)

FEVER

- **Pathogenesis:** The hypothalamic set point increases, causing peripheral vasoconstriction (i.e., heat conservation). The pt feels cold as a result of blood shunting to the internal organs. Mechanisms of heat production (e.g., shivering, increased hepatic thermogenesis) help to raise the body temperature to the new set point. Increases in peripheral prostaglandin E_2 account for the nonspecific myalgias and arthralgias that often accompany fever. When the set point is lowered again by resolution or treatment of fever, processes of heat loss (e.g., peripheral vasodilation and sweating) commence.
- **Etiology** Most fevers are associated with self-limited infections (usually viral) and have causes that are easily identified.

APPROACH TO THE PATIENT   Fever

- *History:* A meticulous history is essential, with particular attention to the chronology of events (e.g., in the case of rash: the site of onset and the direction and rate of spread; see below) and the relation of symptoms to medications, pet exposure, sick contacts, sexual contacts, travel, trauma, and the presence of prosthetic materials.
- *Physical examination:* A thorough physical examination should be performed. A consistent site for taking temperatures should be used. Temperature–pulse dissociations (relative bradycardia) should be noted, if present (sometimes present, for example, with typhoid fever, brucellosis, leptospirosis, factitious fever). Close attention should be paid to any rash, with precise definition of its salient features.
  1. Lesion type (e.g., macule, papule, nodule, vesicle, pustule, purpura, ulcer; see Chap. 65 for details), configuration (e.g., annular or target), arrangement, distribution (e.g., central or peripheral)
  2. Classification of rash
     a. Centrally distributed maculopapular eruptions (e.g., viral exanthems, exanthematous drug-induced eruptions)
     b. Peripheral eruptions (e.g., Rocky Mountain spotted fever, secondary syphilis, bacterial endocarditis)
     c. Confluent desquamative erythemas (e.g., toxic shock syndrome)
     d. Vesiculobullous eruptions (e.g., varicella, primary HSV infection, ecthyma gangrenosum)
     e. Urticaria-like eruptions: in the presence of fever, usually due to urticarial vasculitis caused by serum sickness, connective-tissue disease, infection (hepatitis B virus, enteroviral, or parasitic infection), or malignancy (particularly lymphoma)
     f. Nodular eruptions (e.g., disseminated fungal infection, erythema nodosum, Sweet's syndrome)
     g. Purpuric eruptions (e.g., meningococcemia, viral hemorrhagic fever, disseminated gonococcemia)

h. Eruptions with ulcers or eschars (e.g., rickettsial diseases, tularemia, anthrax)
- *Laboratory tests:* CBC with differential, ESR, and C-reactive protein; other tests as indicated by history and physical exam

TREATMENT   Fever

- The use of antipyretics is not contraindicated in common viral or bacterial infections and can relieve symptoms without slowing resolution of infection. Withholding of antipyretics may be useful, however, in evaluating the effectiveness of a particular antibiotic or in diagnosing conditions with temperature–pulse dissociations or relapsing fevers (e.g., infection with *Plasmodium* or *Borrelia* species).
- Treatment of fever in pts with preexisting impairment of cardiac, pulmonary, or CNS function is recommended to reduce oxygen demand.
- Aspirin, NSAIDs, and glucocorticoids are effective antipyretics. Acetaminophen is preferred because it does not mask signs of inflammation, does not impair platelet function, and is not associated with Reye's syndrome.
- Hyperpyretic pts should be treated with cooling blankets in addition to oral antipyretics.

FEVER OF UNKNOWN ORIGIN

- **Etiology:** The likely etiologies differ with the category of FUO.
  - *Classic FUO*: Etiologies to consider include:
    - Infection—e.g., extrapulmonary tuberculosis; EBV, CMV, or HIV infection; occult abscesses; endocarditis; fungal disease. Infections remain a leading diagnosable cause of FUO, accounting for ~25% of cases in recent studies.
    - Neoplasm—e.g., colon cancer
    - Miscellaneous noninfectious inflammatory diseases—e.g., systemic rheumatologic disease, vasculitis, granulomatous disease. In pts >50 years old, giant-cell arteritis accounts for 15–20% of FUO cases.
    - Miscellaneous diseases—e.g., pulmonary embolism, hereditary fever syndromes, drug fever, factitious fevers
  - *Nosocomial FUO*: More than 50% of cases are due to infection (e.g., infected foreign bodies or catheters, *Clostridium difficile* colitis, sinusitis). Noninfectious causes (e.g., drug fever, pulmonary embolism, acalculous cholecystitis) account for ~25% of cases.
  - *Neutropenic FUO*: More than 50–60% of pts with febrile neutropenia are infected, and 20% are bacteremic. *Candida* and *Aspergillus* infections are common.
  - *HIV-associated FUO*: More than 80% of pts are infected, with the specific infectious etiology dependent on the extent of immunosuppression and the geographic region. Drug fever and lymphoma are also possible etiologies.

APPROACH TO THE
PATIENT ▶ FUO

The workup must consider the pt's country of origin, recent and remote travel, environmental exposures associated with hobbies, and pets. An approach to diagnosis of FUO is illustrated in Fig. 34-1.

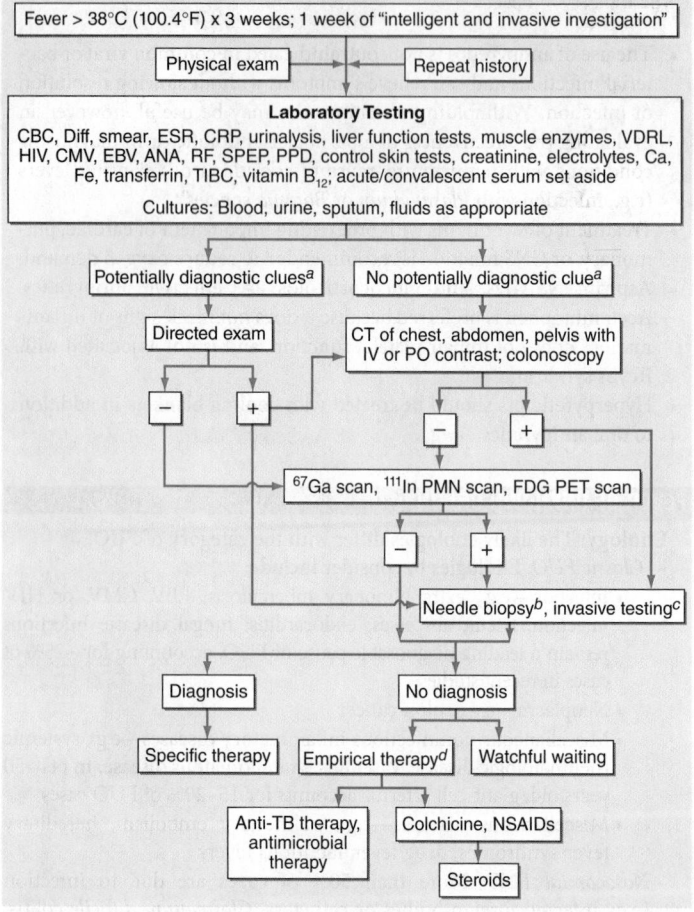

Fever > 38°C (100.4°F) x 3 weeks; 1 week of "intelligent and invasive investigation"

Physical exam ◀──── Repeat history

Laboratory Testing
CBC, Diff, smear, ESR, CRP, urinalysis, liver function tests, muscle enzymes, VDRL, HIV, CMV, EBV, ANA, RF, SPEP, PPD, control skin tests, creatinine, electrolytes, Ca, Fe, transferrin, TIBC, vitamin B_{12}; acute/convalescent serum set aside

Cultures: Blood, urine, sputum, fluids as appropriate

Potentially diagnostic clues[a] — No potentially diagnostic clue[a]

Directed exam — CT of chest, abdomen, pelvis with IV or PO contrast; colonoscopy

− +   − +

^{67}Ga scan, ^{111}In PMN scan, FDG PET scan

− +

Needle biopsy[b], invasive testing[c]

Diagnosis — No diagnosis

Specific therapy Empirical therapy[d] Watchful waiting

Anti-TB therapy, antimicrobial therapy   Colchicine, NSAIDs

Steroids

[a]"Potentially diagnostic clues," as outlined by de Kleijn and colleagues (1997, Part II), may be key findings in the history, localizing signs, or key symptoms. [b]Needle biopsy of liver as well as any other tissue indicated by "potentially diagnostic clues." [c]Invasive testing could involve laparoscopy. [d]Empirical therapy is a last resort, given the good prognosis of most patients with FUO persisting without a diagnosis.

FIGURE 34-1 Approach to the patient with classic FUO. ANA, antinuclear antibody; CBC, complete blood count; CMV, cytomegalovirus; CRP, C-reactive protein; CT, computed tomography; Diff, differential; EBV, Epstein-Barr virus; ESR, erythrocyte sedimentation rate; FDG, fluorodeoxy-glucose F18; NSAIDs, nonsteroidal anti-inflammatory drugs; PET, positron emission tomography; PMN, polymorphonuclear leukocyte; PPD, purified protein derivative; RF, rheumatoid factor; SPEP, serum protein electrophoresis; TB, tuberculosis; TIBC, total iron-binding capacity; VDRL, Venereal Disease Research Laboratory test.

TREATMENT FUO

The emphasis in pts with classic FUO is on continued observation and examination, with the avoidance of "shotgun" empirical therapy.
- Vital-sign instability, neutropenia, and immunosuppressive conditions may prompt earlier empirical anti-infective therapies.
- The use of glucocorticoids and NSAIDs should be avoided unless infection has been largely ruled out and unless inflammatory disease is both probable and debilitating or threatening.

Prognosis: When no underlying source of FUO is identified after prolonged observation (>6 months), the prognosis is generally good.

HYPERTHERMIA

- **Etiology:** Exogenous heat exposure (e.g., heat stroke) and endogenous heat production (e.g., drug-induced hyperthermia, malignant hyperthermia) are two mechanisms by which hyperthermia can result in dangerously high internal temperatures.
  - *Heat stroke*: thermoregulatory failure in association with a warm environment; can be categorized as *exertional* (e.g., due to exercise in high heat or humidity) or *nonexertional* (typically occurring in either very young or elderly individuals during heat waves)
  - *Drug-induced hyperthermia*: caused by drugs such as monoamine oxidase inhibitors (MAOIs), tricyclic antidepressants, amphetamines, and cocaine and other illicit agents
  - *Malignant hyperthermia*: hyperthermic and systemic response (e.g., muscle rigidity, rhabdomyolysis, cardiovascular instability) in pts with a genetic abnormality that causes a rapid increase in intracellular calcium in response to inhalational anesthetics or succinylcholine. This rare condition is often fatal.
  - *Neuroleptic malignant syndrome*: caused by use of neuroleptic agents (e.g., haloperidol) or withdrawal of dopaminergic drugs and characterized by "lead-pipe" muscle rigidity, extrapyramidal side effects, autonomic dysregulation, and hyperthermia
  - *Serotonin syndrome*: caused by selective serotonin reuptake inhibitors (SSRIs), MAOIs, and other serotonergic drugs. Serotonin syndrome can be distinguished clinically from neuroleptic malignant syndrome by the presence of diarrhea, tremor, and myoclonus rather than lead-pipe rigidity.
- **Clinical Features:** high core temperature in association with an appropriate history (heat exposure, certain drug treatments) and dry skin, hallucinations, delirium, pupil dilation, muscle rigidity, and/or elevated levels of creatine phosphokinase
- **Diagnosis:** It can be difficult to distinguish fever from hyperthermia. The clinical history is often most useful (e.g., a history of heat exposure or treatment with drugs that interfere with thermoregulation).
  - *Hyperthermic* pts have hot, dry skin; antipyretic agents do not lower the body temperature.

- *Febrile* pts can have cold skin (as a result of vasoconstriction) or hot, moist skin; antipyretics usually result in some lowering of the body temperature.

TREATMENT Hyperthermia

- Physical cooling by external physical means (e.g., sponging, fans, cooling blankets, ice baths) or internal cooling (e.g., gastric or peritoneal lavage with iced saline). In extreme cases, hemodialysis or cardiopulmonary bypass with cooling of blood may be necessary.
- IV fluids, given the risk of dehydration
- Pharmacologic agents can be used, as appropriate.
  - Malignant hyperthermia, neuroleptic malignant syndrome, and drug-induced hyperthermia should be treated with dantrolene (1–2.5 mg/kg IV q6h for at least 24–48 h); dantrolene may also be helpful in serotonin syndrome and thyrotoxicosis.
  - Neuroleptic malignant syndrome also may be treated with bromocriptine, levodopa, amantadine, or nifedipine or by induction of muscle paralysis with curare and pancuronium.
  - Tricyclic antidepressant overdose may be treated with physostigmine.

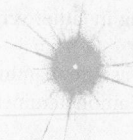

For a more detailed discussion, see Kaye KM, Kaye ET: Atlas of Rashes Associated With Fever, Chap. e7 and Dinarello CA, Porat R: Fever and Hyperthermia, Chap. 16, p. 143; Kaye ET, Kaye KM: Fever and Rash, Chap. 17, p. 148; and Gelfand JA, Callahan MV: Fever of Unknown Origin, Chap. 18, p. 158, in HPIM-18.

CHAPTER **35**
Generalized Fatigue

Fatigue is one of the most common complaints related by pts. It usually refers to nonspecific sense of a low energy level, or the feeling that near exhaustion is reached after relatively little exertion. Fatigue should be distinguished from true neurologic *weakness*, which describes a reduction in the normal power of one or more muscles (Chap. 59). It is not uncommon for pts, especially the elderly, to present with generalized failure to thrive, which may include components of fatigue and weakness, depending on the cause.

■ CLINICAL MANIFESTATIONS

Because the causes of generalized fatigue are numerous, a thorough history, review of systems (ROS), and physical examination are paramount to narrow the focus to likely causes. The history and ROS should focus on the temporal onset of fatigue and its progression. Has it lasted days, weeks, or months? Activities of daily living, exercise, eating habits/appetite, sexual practices, and sleep habits should be reviewed. Features of depression or dementia should be sought. Travel history and possible exposures to infectious agents should be reviewed, along with the medication list. The ROS may elicit important clues as to organ system involvement. The past medical history may elucidate potential precursors to the current presentation, such as previous malignancy or cardiac problems. The physical exam should specifically assess weight and nutritional status, lymphadenopathy, hepatosplenomegaly, abdominal masses, pallor, rash, heart failure, new murmurs, painful joints or trigger points, and evidence of weakness or neurologic abnormalities. A finding of true weakness or paralysis should prompt consideration of neurologic disorders (Chap. 59).

■ DIFFERENTIAL DIAGNOSIS

Determining the cause of fatigue can be one of the most challenging diagnostic problems in medicine because the differential diagnosis is very broad, including infection, malignancy, cardiac disease, endocrine disorders, neurologic disease, depression, or serious abnormalities of virtually any organ system, as well as side effects of many medications (Table 35-1). Symptoms of fever and weight loss will focus attention on infectious causes, whereas symptoms of progressive dyspnea might point toward cardiac, pulmonary, or renal causes. A presentation that includes arthralgia suggests the possibility of a rheumatologic disorder. A previous malignancy, thought to be cured or in remission, may have recurred or metastasized widely. A previous history of valvular heart disease or cardiomyopathy may identify a condition that has decompensated. Treatment for Graves' disease may have resulted in hypothyroidism. Changes in medication should always be pursued, whether discontinued or recently started. Almost any new medication has the potential to cause fatigue. However, a temporal association with a new medication should not eliminate other causes, as many pts may have received new medications in an effort to address their complaints. Medications and their dosages should be carefully assessed, especially in elderly pts, in whom polypharmacy and inappropriate or misunderstood dosing is a frequent cause of fatigue. The time course for presentation is also valuable. Indolent presentations over months to years are more likely to be associated with slowly progressive organ failure or endocrinopathies, whereas a more rapid course over weeks to months suggests infection or malignancy.

■ LABORATORY TESTING

Laboratory testing and imaging should be guided by the history and physical exam. However, a CBC with differential, electrolytes, BUN, creatinine, glucose, calcium, and LFTs are useful in most pts with undifferentiated fatigue, as these tests will rule out many causes and may provide clues to unsuspected disorders. Similarly, a CXR is useful to evaluate many possible disorders rapidly, including heart failure, pulmonary disease, or occult malignancy that may be detected in the lungs or bony structures. Subsequent testing should be based on the initial results and clinical assessment of the likely differential diagnoses. For example, a finding of anemia would dictate the need to assess whether it has features of iron deficiency or hemolysis, thereby narrowing potential causes. Hyponatremia might be caused by SIADH, hypothyroidism, adrenal insufficiency, or medications or by underlying cardiac, pulmonary, liver, or renal dysfunction. An elevated WBC count would raise the possibility of infection or malignancy. Thus, the approach is generally one of gathering information in a serial but cost-effective manner to narrow the differential diagnosis progressively.

TABLE 35-1 POTENTIAL CAUSES OF GENERALIZED FATIGUE

Disease Category	Examples
Infection	HIV, TB, Lyme disease, endocarditis, hepatitis, sinusitis, fungal, Epstein-Barr virus (EBV), malaria (chronic phase)
Inflammatory disease	RA, polymyalgia rheumatica, chronic fatigue syndrome, fibromyalgia, sarcoidosis
Cancer	Lung, GI, breast, prostate, leukemia, lymphoma, metastases
Psychiatric	Depression, alcoholism, chronic anxiety
Metabolic	Hypothyroidism, hyperthyroidism, diabetes mellitus, Addison's disease, hyperparathyroidism, hypogonadism, hypopituitarism (TSH, ACTH, growth hormone deficiency), McArdle's disease
Electrolyte imbalance	Hypercalcemia, hypokalemia, hyponatremia, hypomagnesemia,
Nutrition, vitamin deficiency	Starvation, obesity, iron deficiency, vitamin B_{12}, folic acid deficiency, vitamin C deficiency (scurvy), thiamine deficiency (beriberi)
Neurologic	Multiple sclerosis, myasthenia gravis, dementia
Cardiac	Heart failure, CAD, valvular disease, cardiomyopathy
Pulmonary	COPD, pulmonary hypertension, chronic pulmonary emboli, sarcoidosis
Sleep disturbances	Sleep apnea, insomnia, restless leg syndrome
Gastrointestinal	Celiac disease, Crohn's, ulcerative colitis, chronic hepatitis, cirrhosis
Hematologic	Anemia
Renal	Renal failure
Medication	Sedatives, antihistamines, narcotics, β blockers, and many other medications

| **TREATMENT** | Generalized Fatigue |

Treatment should be based on the diagnosis, if known. Many conditions, such as metabolic, nutritional, or endocrine disorders, can be corrected quickly by appropriate treatment of the underlying causes. Specific treatment can also be initiated for many infections, such as TB, sinusitis, or endocarditis. Pts with chronic conditions such as COPD, heart failure, renal failure, or liver disease may benefit from interventions that enhance organ function or correct associated metabolic problems, and it may be possible to gradually improve physical conditioning. In pts with cancer, fatigue may be caused by chemotherapy or radiation and may resolve with time; treatment of associated anemia, nutritional deficiency, hyponatremia, or hypercalcemia may increase energy levels. Replacement therapy in endocrine deficiencies typically results in improvement. Treatment of depression or sleep disorders, whether a primary cause of fatigue or secondary to a medical disorder, may be beneficial. Withdrawal of medications that potentially contribute to fatigue should be considered, recognizing that other medications may need to be substituted for the underlying condition. In elderly pts, appropriate medication dose adjustments (typically lowering the dose) and restricting the regimen to only essential drugs may improve fatigue.

CHRONIC FATIGUE SYNDROME

Chronic fatigue syndrome (CFS) is characterized by debilitating fatigue and several associated physical, constitutional, and neuropsychological complaints. The majority of pts (~75%) are women, generally 30–45 years old. The CDC has developed diagnostic criteria for CFS based upon symptoms and the exclusion of other illnesses (Table 35-2). The cause is uncertain, although clinical manifestations often follow an infectious illness (Q fever, Lyme disease, mononucleosis or another viral illness). Many studies have attempted, without success, to link CFS to infection with EBV, a retrovirus (including a murine leukemia virus–related retrovirus), or an enterovirus. Physical or psychological stress is also often identified as a precipitating factor. Depression is present in half to two-thirds of pts, and some experts believe that CFS is fundamentally a psychiatric disorder.

CFS remains a diagnosis of exclusion, and no laboratory test can establish the diagnosis or measure its severity. CFS does not appear to progress but typically has a protracted course. The median annual recovery rate is 5% (range, 0–31%) with an improvement rate of 39% (range, 8–63%).

The management of CFS commences with acknowledgement by the physician that the pt's daily functioning is impaired. The pt should be informed of the current understanding of CFS (or lack thereof) and be offered general advice about disease management. NSAIDs alleviate headache, diffuse pain, and feverishness. Antihistamines or decongestants may be helpful for symptoms of rhinitis and sinusitis. Although the pt may be averse to psychiatric diagnoses, features of depression and anxiety may justify treatment. Nonsedating antidepressants improve mood and disordered sleep

TABLE 35-2 CDC CRITERIA FOR DIAGNOSIS OF CHRONIC FATIGUE SYNDROME

A case of chronic fatigue syndrome is defined by the presence of:

1. Clinically evaluated, unexplained, persistent or relapsing fatigue that is of new or definite onset; is not the result of ongoing exertion; is not alleviated by rest; and results in substantial reduction of previous levels of occupational, educational, social, or personal activities; and

2. Four or more of the following symptoms that persist or recur during six or more consecutive months of illness and that do not predate the fatigue:

   • Impaired memory or concentration
   • Sore throat that is frequent or recurring
   • Tender cervical or axillary nodes
   • Muscle pain
   • Multi-joint pain without redness or swelling
   • Headaches of a new pattern or severity
   • Unrefreshing sleep
   • Postexertional malaise lasting ≥ 24 h

Abbreviation: CDC, Centers for Disease Control and Prevention.
Source: www.cdc.gov/cfs/toolkit/

and may attenuate the fatigue. Cognitive behavioral therapy (CBT) and graded exercise therapy (GET) have been found to be effective treatment strategies in some pts.

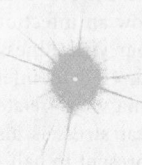

For a more detailed discussion, see Aminoff MJ: Weakness and Paralysis, Chap. 22, p. 181; Czeisler CA, Winkelman JW, Richardson GS: Sleep Disorders, Chap. 27, p. 213; Robertson RG, Jameson LJ: Involuntary Weight Loss, Chap. 80, p. 641; Bleijenberg G, van der Meer JWM: Chronic Fatigue Syndrome, Chap. 389, p. 3519; Reus VI: Mental Disorders, Chap. 391, p. 3529, in HPIM-18.

CHAPTER **36**
Weight Loss

Significant unintentional weight loss in a previously healthy individual is often a harbinger of underlying systemic disease. The routine medical history should always include inquiry about changes in weight. Rapid fluctuations of weight over days suggest loss or gain of fluid, whereas long-term changes usually involve loss of tissue mass. Loss of 5% of body weight over 6–12 months should prompt further evaluation. Gradual weight loss is physiologic in persons over age 80, but this demographic group also has a high risk for malignancy or other serious illness.

■ ETIOLOGY

The principal causes of involuntary weight loss can be assigned to four categories: (1) malignant neoplasms, (2) chronic inflammatory or infectious diseases, (3) metabolic disorders, or (4) psychiatric disorders (Table 36-1). In older persons the most common causes of weight loss are depression,

TABLE 36-1 CAUSES OF WEIGHT LOSS

Cancer	Medications
Endocrine and metabolic causes	Sedatives
Hyperthyroidism	Antibiotics
Diabetes mellitus	Nonsteroidal anti-inflammatory drugs
Pheochromocytoma	
Adrenal insufficiency	Serotonin reuptake inhibitors
Gastrointestinal disorders	Metformin
Malabsorption	Levodopa
Obstruction	ACE inhibitors
Peptic ulcer	Other drugs
Inflammatory bowel disease	Disorders of the mouth and teeth
Pancreatitis	Caries
Pernicious anemia	Dysgeusia
Cardiac disorders	Age-related factors
Chronic ischemia	Physiologic changes
Chronic congestive heart failure	Decreased taste and smell
Respiratory disorders	Functional disabilities
Emphysema	Neurologic causes
Chronic obstructive pulmonary disease	Stroke
	Parkinson's disease
	Neuromuscular disorders
Renal insufficiency	Dementia
Rheumatologic disease	Social causes
Infections	Isolation
HIV	Economic hardship
Tuberculosis	Psychiatric and behavioral causes
Parasitic infection	Depression
Subacute bacterial endocarditis	Anxiety
	Bereavement
	Alcoholism
	Eating disorders
	Increased activity or exercise
	Idiopathic

cancer, and benign gastrointestinal disease. Lung and GI cancers are the most common malignancies in pts presenting with weight loss. In younger individuals, diabetes mellitus, hyperthyroidism, anorexia nervosa, and infection, especially with HIV, should be considered.

■ CLINICAL FEATURES

Before extensive evaluation is undertaken, it is important to confirm that weight loss has occurred (up to 50% of claims of weight loss cannot be substantiated). In the absence of documentation, changes in belt notch size or the fit of clothing may help to determine loss of weight.

The *history* should include questions about fever, pain, shortness of breath or cough, palpitations, and evidence of neurologic disease. A history of GI symptoms should be obtained, including difficulty eating, dysgeusia, dysphagia, anorexia, nausea, and change in bowel habits. Travel history, use of cigarettes, alcohol, and all medications should be reviewed, and pts should be questioned about previous illness or surgery as well as diseases in family members. Risk factors for HIV should be assessed. Signs of depression, evidence of dementia, and social factors, including isolation, loneliness, and financial issues that might affect food intake, should be considered.

Physical examination should begin with weight determination and documentation of vital signs. The skin should be examined for pallor, jaundice, turgor, surgical scars, and stigmata of systemic disease. Evaluation for oral thrush, dental disease, thyroid gland enlargement, and adenopathy and for respiratory, cardiac, or abdominal abnormalities should be performed. All men should have a rectal examination, including the prostate; all women should have a pelvic examination; and both should have testing of the stool for occult blood. Neurologic examination should include mental status assessment and screening for depression.

Initial *laboratory evaluation* is shown in Table 36-2, with appropriate treatment based on the underlying cause of the weight loss. If an etiology of weight loss is not found, careful clinical follow-up, rather than persistent undirected testing, is reasonable. The absence of abnormal laboratory tests is a favorable prognostic sign.

TABLE 36-2 SCREENING TESTS FOR EVALUATION OF INVOLUNTARY WEIGHT LOSS

Initial testing	Additional testing
CBC	HIV test
Electrolytes, calcium, glucose	Upper and/or lower gastrointestinal endoscopy
Renal and liver function tests	
Urinalysis	Abdominal CT scan or MRI
Thyroid-stimulating hormone	Chest CT scan
Chest x-ray	
Recommended cancer screening	

TREATMENT Weight Loss

Treatment of weight loss should be directed at correcting the underlying physical cause or social circumstance. In specific situations, nutritional supplements and medications (megestrol acetate, dronabinol, or growth hormone) may be effective for stimulating appetite or increasing weight.

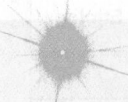

For a more detailed discussion, see Robertson RG, Jameson JL: Involuntary Weight Loss, Chap. 80, p. 641, in HPIM-18.

CHAPTER **37**
Chest Pain

There is little correlation between the severity of chest pain and the seriousness of its cause. The range of disorders that cause chest discomfort is shown in Table 37-1.

TABLE 37-1 DIFFERENTIAL DIAGNOSES OF PATIENTS ADMITTED TO HOSPITAL WITH ACUTE CHEST PAIN RULED NOT MYOCARDIAL INFARCTION

Diagnosis	Percentage
Gastroesophageal disease[a]	42
Gastroesophageal reflux	
Esophageal motility disorders	
Peptic ulcer	
Gallstones	
Ischemic heart disease	31
Chest wall syndromes	28
Pericarditis	4
Pleuritis/pneumonia	2
Pulmonary embolism	2
Lung cancer	1.5
Aortic aneurysm	1
Aortic stenosis	1
Herpes zoster	1

[a]In order of frequency.
Source: Fruergaard P et al: Eur Heart J 17:1028, 1996.

■ POTENTIALLY SERIOUS CAUSES

The differential diagnosis of chest pain is shown in Figs. 37-1 and 37-2. It is useful to characterize the chest pain as (1) new, acute, and ongoing; (2) recurrent, episodic; and (3) persistent, e.g., for days at a time.

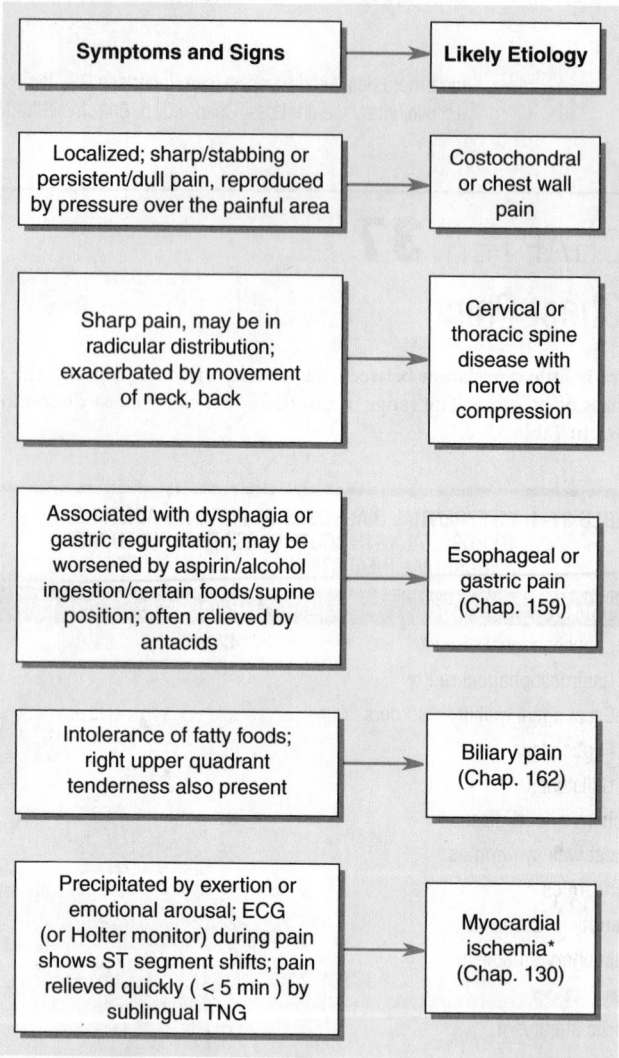

FIGURE 37-1 Differential diagnosis of recurrent chest pain. *If myocardial ischemia suspected, also consider aortic valve disease (Chap. 123) and hypertrophic obstructive cardiomyopathy (Chap. 124) if systolic murmur present.

	Acute myocardial infarction (Chaps. 128 and 129)	Aortic dissection (Chap. 134)	Acute pericarditis (Chap. 125)	Pulmonary embolism (Chap. 142)	Acute pneumothorax (Chap. 144)	Rupture of esophagus
Description of pain	Oppressive, constrictive, or squeezing; may radiate to arm(s), neck, back	"Tearing" or "ripping", may travel from anterior chest to mid-back	Crushing, sharp, pleuritic; relieved by sitting forward	Pleuritic, sharp; possibly accompanied by cough/hemoptysis	Very sharp, pleuritic	Intense substernal and epigastric; accompanied by vomiting ± hematemesis
Background history	Less severe, similar pain on exertion; + coronary risk factors	Hypertension or Marfan syndrome (Chap. 169)	Recent upper respiratory tract infection, or other conditions which predispose to pericarditis (Chap. 125)	Recent surgery or other immobilization	Recent chest trauma, or history of chronic obstructive lung disease	Recent recurrent vomiting/retching
Key Physical findings	Diaphoresis, pallor; S4 common; S3 less common	Weak, asymmetric peripheral pulses; possible diastolic murmur of aortic insufficiency (Chap. 123)	Pericardial friction rub (usually 3 components, best heard by sitting patient forward)	Tachypnea; possible pleural friction rub	Tachypnea; breath sounds & hyperresonance over affected lung field	Subcutaneous emphysema; audible crepitus adjacent to the sternum
Consider						
Confirmatory tests	• Serial ECGs • Serial cardiac markers (esp. troponins,CK)	• CXR – widened mediastinal silhouette • MRI, CT, or transesophageal echogram: intimal flap visualized • Aortic angiogram: definitive diagnosis	• ECG: diffuse ST elevation and PR segment depression • Echogram: pericardial effusion often visualized	• Normal D-dimer makes diagnosis unlikely • CT angiography or lung scan: V/Q mismatch • Pulmonary angiogram: arterial luminal filling defects	• CXR: radiolucency within pleural space; poss. collapse of adjacent lung segment; if tension pneumothorax, mediastinum is shifted to opp. side	• CXR: pneumo-mediastinum • Esophageal endoscopy is diagnostic

FIGURE 37-2 Differential diagnosis of acute chest pain.

Myocardial Ischemia Angina Pectoris

Substernal pressure, squeezing, constriction, with radiation typically to left arm; usually on exertion, especially after meals or with emotional arousal. Characteristically relieved by rest and nitroglycerin.

Acute Myocardial Infarction (Chaps. 128 and 129)

Similar to angina but usually more severe, of longer duration ($\geq$30 min), and not immediately relieved by rest or nitroglycerin. S_3 and S_4 common.

Pulmonary Embolism (Chap. 142)

May be substernal or lateral, pleuritic in nature, and associated with hemoptysis, tachycardia, and hypoxemia.

Aortic Dissection (Chap. 134)

Very severe, in center of chest, a sharp "ripping" quality, radiates to back, not affected by changes in position. May be associated with weak or absent peripheral pulses.

Mediastinal Emphysema

Sharp, intense, localized to substernal region; often associated with audible crepitus.

Acute Pericarditis (Chap. 125)

Usually steady, crushing, substernal; often has pleuritic component aggravated by cough, deep inspiration, supine position, and relieved by sitting upright; one-, two-, or three-component pericardial friction rub often audible.

Pleurisy

Due to inflammation; less commonly tumor and pneumothorax. Usually unilateral, knifelike, superficial, aggravated by cough and respiration.

■ LESS SERIOUS CAUSES

Costochondral Pain

In anterior chest, usually sharply localized, may be brief and darting or a persistent dull ache. Can be reproduced by pressure on costochondral and/or chondrosternal junctions. In Tietze's syndrome (costochondritis), joints are swollen, red, and tender.

Chest Wall Pain

Due to strain of muscles or ligaments from excessive exercise or rib fracture from trauma; accompanied by local tenderness.

Esophageal Pain

Deep thoracic discomfort; may be accompanied by dysphagia and regurgitation.

Emotional Disorders

Prolonged ache or dartlike, brief, flashing pain; associated with fatigue, emotional strain.

■ **OTHER CAUSES**

(1) Cervical disk disease; (2) osteoarthritis of cervical or thoracic spine; (3) abdominal disorders: peptic ulcer, hiatus hernia, pancreatitis, biliary colic; (4) tracheobronchitis, pneumonia; (5) diseases of the breast (inflammation, tumor); (6) intercostal neuritis (herpes zoster).

APPROACH TO THE PATIENT	Chest Pain

A meticulous history of the behavior of pain, what precipitates it and what relieves it, aids diagnosis of recurrent chest pain. Fig. 37-2 presents clues to diagnosis and workup of acute, life-threatening chest pain.

An ECG is key to the initial evaluation to rapidly distinguish pts with acute ST-elevation MI, who typically warrant immediate reperfusion therapies (Chap. 128).

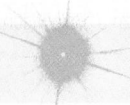

For a more detailed discussion, see Lee TH: Chest Discomfort, Chap. 12, p. 102, in HPIM-18.

CHAPTER **38**
Palpitations

Palpitations represent an intermittent or sustained awareness of the heartbeat, often described by the pt as a thumping, pounding, or fluttering sensation in the chest. The symptom may reflect a cardiac etiology, an extracardiac cause [hyperthyroidism, use of stimulants (e.g., caffeine, cocaine)], or a high catecholamine state (e.g., exercise, anxiety, pheochromocytoma). Contributory cardiac dysrhythmias include atrial or ventricular premature beats or, when sustained and regular, supraventricular or ventricular tachyarrhythmias (Chap. 132). *Irregular* sustained palpitations are often due to atrial fibrillation. Asking the pt to "tap out" the sense of palpitation can help distinguish regular from irregular rhythms.

APPROACH TO THE PATIENT	Palpitations

Palpitations are often benign but may represent an important dysrhythmia if associated with hemodynamic compromise (lightheadedness, syncope, angina, dyspnea) or if found in pts with preexisting CAD, ventricular dysfunction, hypertrophic cardiomyopathy, aortic stenosis, or other valvular disease.

Helpful diagnostic studies include *electrocardiography* (if symptoms present at time of recording), *exercise testing* (if exertion typically precipitates the sense of palpitation or if underlying CAD is suspected), and *echocardiography* (if structural heart disease is suspected). If symptoms are episodic, ambulatory electrocardiographic monitoring can be diagnostic, including use of a Holter monitor (24–48 h of monitoring), event/loop monitor (for 2–4 weeks), or implantable loop monitor (for 1–2 years). Helpful laboratory studies may include testing for hypokalemia, hypomagnesemia, and/or hyperthyroidism.

For pts with benign atrial or ventricular premature beats in the absence of structural heart disease, therapeutic strategies include reduction of ethanol and caffeine intake, reassurance, and consideration of beta-blocker therapy for symptomatic suppression. Treatment of more serious dysrhythmias is presented in Chaps. 131 and 132.

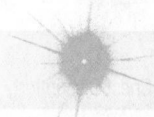

For a more detailed discussion, see Loscalzo J: Palpitations, Chap. 37, p. 295, in HPIM-18.

CHAPTER 39
Dyspnea

▪ DEFINITION

Dyspnea, a subjective experience of uncomfortable breathing, is a symptom that often results from increased work of inhalation and exhalation. Assessment begins by determining the quality and intensity of the discomfort. Dyspnea typically results from cardiopulmonary problems that cause an increased drive to breathe, an increased work of breathing, and/or stimulation of specific receptors in the heart, lungs, or vasculature.

▪ CAUSES

Respiratory System Dyspnea

- *Airway disease:* Asthma and COPD are common causes of dyspnea associated with increased work of breathing. Bronchospasm can cause chest tightness and hyperventilation. Hypoxemia and hypercapnia can result from ventilation-perfusion mismatch.
- *Chest wall disorders:* Chest wall stiffness (e.g., kyphoscoliosis) and neuromuscular weakness (e.g., myasthenia gravis) cause increased work of breathing.
- *Lung parenchymal disorders:* Interstitial lung diseases (Chap. 143) cause reduced lung compliance and increased work of breathing. Ventilation-perfusion mismatch and pulmonary fibrosis may lead to hypoxemia. Stimulation of lung receptors can cause hyperventilation.

Cardiovascular System Dyspnea

- *Left heart disorders:* Elevations of left-ventricular end-diastolic and pulmonary capillary wedge pressures lead to dyspnea related to stimulation of pulmonary receptors and hypoxemia from ventilation-perfusion mismatch.
- *Pulmonary vascular disorders:* Pulmonary emboli, primary pulmonary arterial hypertension, and pulmonary vasculitis stimulate pulmonary receptors via increased pulmonary artery pressures. Hyperventilation and hypoxemia also may contribute to dyspnea.
- *Pericardial diseases:* Constrictive pericarditis and pericardial tamponade cause increased intracardiac and pulmonary arterial pressures, leading to dyspnea.

Dyspnea with Normal Respiratory and Cardiovascular Systems

Anemia can cause dyspnea, especially with exertion. Obesity is associated with dyspnea due to high cardiac output and impaired ventilatory function. Deconditioning may contribute as well.

APPROACH TO THE PATIENT | **Dyspnea (See** Fig. 39-1**)**

History: Obtain description of discomfort, including the impact of position, infections, and environmental exposures. Orthopnea is commonly observed in congestive heart failure (CHF). Nocturnal dyspnea is seen in CHF and asthma. Intermittent dyspnea suggests myocardial ischemia, asthma, or pulmonary embolism.

Physical examination: Assess increased work of breathing indicated by accessory ventilatory muscle use. Determine if chest movement is symmetric. Use percussion (dullness or hyperresonance) and auscultation (decreased or adventitious breath sounds) to assess the lungs. Cardiac exam should note jugular venous distention, heart murmurs, and S3 or S4 gallops. Clubbing can relate to interstitial lung disease or lung cancer. To evaluate exertional dyspnea, reproduce the dyspnea with observation while assessing pulse oximetry.

Radiographic studies: Chest radiograph should be obtained as initial evaluation. Chest CT can be used subsequently to assess lung parenchyma (e.g., emphysema or interstitial lung disease) and pulmonary embolism.

Laboratory studies: ECG should be obtained; echocardiography can assess left ventricular dysfunction, pulmonary hypertension, and valvular disease. Pulmonary function tests to consider include spirometry, lung volumes, and diffusing capacity. Methacholine challenge testing can assess for asthma in subjects with normal spirometry. Cardiopulmonary exercise testing can determine whether pulmonary or cardiac disease limits exercise capacity.

TREATMENT | **Dyspnea**

Ideally, treatment involves correcting the underlying problem that caused dyspnea. Supplemental oxygen is required for significant oxygen desaturation at rest or with exertion. Pulmonary rehabilitation is helpful in COPD.

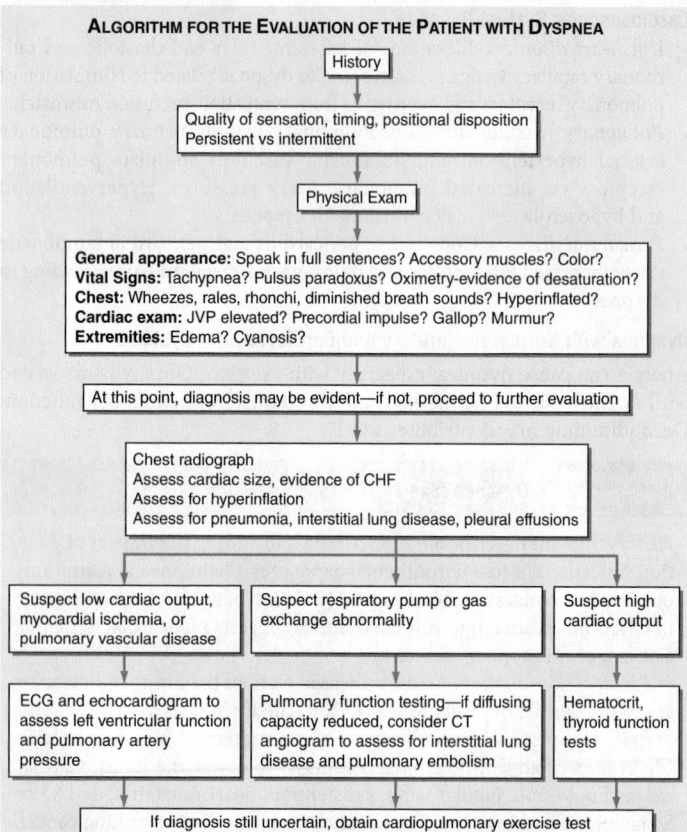

FIGURE 39-1 An algorithm for the evaluation of the pt with dyspnea. JVP, jugular venous pulse; CHF, congestive heart failure; ECG, electrocardiogram. (*Adapted from RM Schwartzstein, D Feller-Kopman, in Primary Cardiology, 2nd ed. E Braunwald, L Goldman (eds): Philadelphia, Saunders, 2003.*)

Pulmonary Edema

Cardiogenic pulmonary edema results from cardiac abnormalities that cause increased pulmonary venous pressure leading to interstitial edema; with greater pressures, alveolar edema and pleural effusions develop. Symptoms include exertional dyspnea and orthopnea. Physical examination can reveal S3 gallop, elevated jugular venous pressure, and peripheral edema. Chest radiographs show prominent vascular markings in the upper lung zones. With increased severity, CXRs demonstrate perihilar alveolar opacities progressing to diffuse parenchymal abnormalities.

Noncardiogenic pulmonary edema results from damage to the pulmonary capillary lining. Hypoxemia relates to intrapulmonary shunt; decreased pulmonary compliance is observed. Clinical impact can range from mild dyspnea to severe respiratory failure. Normal intracardiac pressures are typically observed. Etiologies may be direct injury (e.g., aspiration, smoke inhalation, pneumonia, oxygen toxicity, or chest trauma), indirect injury (e.g., sepsis, pancreatitis, and leukoagglutination reactions), or pulmonary vascular (e.g., high altitude and neurogenic pulmonary edema). Chest radiograph typically shows normal heart size and diffuse alveolar infiltrates; pleural effusions are atypical. Hypoxemia in noncardiogenic pulmonary edema often requires treatment with high concentrations of oxygen.

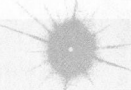

For a more detailed discussion, see Schwartzstein RM: Dyspnea, Chap. 33, p. 277, HPIM-18.

CHAPTER **40**
Cyanosis

Bluish discoloration of the skin and/or mucous membranes is usually due to elevated quantity of reduced hemoglobin [>40 g/L (>4 g/dL)] in the capillary blood vessels. Findings are most apparent in the lips, nail beds, ears, and malar eminences.

■ CENTRAL CYANOSIS

Results from arterial desaturation or presence of an abnormal hemoglobin. Usually evident when arterial saturation is ≤85%, or ≤75% in dark-skinned individuals. Etiologies include:

1. *Impaired pulmonary function:* Poorly ventilated alveoli or impaired oxygen diffusion; most frequent in pneumonia, pulmonary edema, and chronic obstructive pulmonary disease (COPD); in COPD with cyanosis, polycythemia is often present.
2. *Anatomic vascular shunting*: Shunting of desaturated venous blood into the arterial circulation may result from congenital heart disease or pulmonary AV fistula.
3. *Decreased inspired O_2*: Cyanosis may develop in ascents to altitudes >4000 m (>13,000 ft).
4. *Abnormal hemoglobins*: Methemoglobinemia, sulfhemoglobinemia, and mutant hemoglobins with low oxygen affinity (see Chap. 104, HPIM-18).

■ PERIPHERAL CYANOSIS

Occurs with normal arterial O_2 saturation with increased extraction of O_2 from capillary blood caused by decreased localized blood flow. Contributors include vasoconstriction due to cold exposure, decreased cardiac output

TABLE 40-1 CAUSES OF CYANOSIS

Central Cyanosis
Decreased arterial oxygen saturation
Decreased atmospheric pressure—high altitude
Impaired pulmonary function
Alveolar hypoventilation
Uneven relationships between pulmonary ventilation and perfusion (perfusion of hypoventilated alveoli)
Impaired oxygen diffusion
Anatomic shunts
Certain types of congenital heart disease
Pulmonary arteriovenous fistulas
Multiple small intrapulmonary shunts
Hemoglobin with low affinity for oxygen
Hemoglobin abnormalities
Methemoglobinemia—hereditary, acquired
Sulfhemoglobinemia—acquired
Carboxyhemoglobinemia (not true cyanosis)

Peripheral Cyanosis
Reduced cardiac output
Cold exposure
Redistribution of blood flow from extremities
Arterial obstruction
Venous obstruction

(e.g., in shock, Chap. 12), heart failure (Chap. 133), and peripheral vascular disease (Chap. 135) with arterial obstruction or vasospasm (Table 40-1). Local (e.g., thrombophlebitis) or central (e.g., constrictive pericarditis) venous hypertension intensifies cyanosis.

APPROACH TO THE PATIENT   **Cyanosis**

- Inquire about duration (cyanosis since birth suggests congenital heart disease) and exposures (drugs or chemicals that result in abnormal hemoglobins).
- Differentiate central from peripheral cyanosis by examining nailbeds, lips, and mucous membranes. Peripheral cyanosis is most intense in nailbeds and may resolve with gentle warming of extremities.
- Check for clubbing, i.e., selective enlargement of the distal segments of fingers and toes, due to proliferation of connective tissue. Clubbing

may be hereditary, idiopathic, or acquired in association with lung cancer, infective endocarditis, bronchiectasis, or hepatic cirrhosis. Combination of clubbing and cyanosis is frequent in congenital heart disease and occasionally in pulmonary disease (lung abscess, pulmonary AV shunts, but *not* with uncomplicated obstructive lung disease).

- Examine chest for evidence of pulmonary disease, pulmonary edema, or murmurs associated with congenital heart disease.
- If cyanosis is localized to an extremity, evaluate for peripheral vascular obstruction.
- Obtain arterial blood gas to measure systemic O_2 saturation. Repeat while pt inhales 100% O_2; if saturation fails to increase to >95%, intravascular shunting of blood bypassing the lungs is likely (e.g., right-to-left intracardiac shunts).
- Evaluate for abnormal hemoglobins (e.g., hemoglobin electrophoresis, spectroscopy, measurement of methemoglobin level).

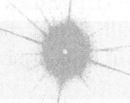

For a more detailed discussion, see Loscalzo J: Hypoxia and Cyanosis, Chap. 35, p. 287, in HPIM-18.

CHAPTER **41**
Cough and Hemoptysis

COUGH

■ ETIOLOGY

Acute cough, which is defined as duration <21 days, is usually related to respiratory infection, aspiration, or inhalation of respiratory irritants. Subacute cough (present for 3–8 weeks) is often related to persistent inflammation from a tracheobronchitis episode. Chronic cough (>8 weeks in duration) can be caused by many pulmonary and cardiac diseases. Chronic bronchitis related to cigarette smoking is a common cause. If the chest radiograph and physical examination are unremarkable, other common causes of chronic cough include cough-variant asthma, gastroesophageal reflux disease (GERD), postnasal drip related to sinus disease, and medications including angiotensin-converting enzyme (ACE) inhibitors. Irritation of tympanic membranes and chronic eosinophilic bronchitis also can cause chronic cough with a normal chest radiograph. Ineffective cough can predispose to serious respiratory infections due to difficulty clearing lower respiratory secretions; abnormal airway secretions (e.g., due to bronchiectasis) or tracheomalacia can contribute. Weakness or pain limiting abdominal and intercostal muscle use also can lead to ineffective cough.

■ **CLINICAL ASSESSMENT**

Key historic issues include triggers for onset of cough, determinants of increased or decreased cough, and sputum production. Symptoms of nasopharyngeal disease should be assessed, including postnasal drip, sneezing, and rhinorrhea. GERD may be suggested by heartburn, hoarseness, and frequent eructation. Cough-variant asthma is suggested by noting the relationship of cough onset to asthmatic triggers. Usage of ACE inhibitors, but not angiotensin receptor blockers, can cause cough long after treatment is initiated.

On physical examination, signs of cardiopulmonary diseases should be assessed, including adventitious lung sounds and digital clubbing. Examination of the nasal passages, posterior pharyngeal wall, auditory canals, and tympanic membranes should be performed.

Laboratory evaluation should include chest radiography. Spirometry with bronchodilator testing can assess for reversible airflow obstruction. With normal spirometry, methacholine challenge testing can be used to assess for asthma. Sputum should be sent for routine bacterial and possibly mycobacterial cultures. Sputum cytology can reveal malignant cells in lung cancer and eosinophils in eosinophilic bronchitis. Esophageal pH probes can be used to assess for GERD. Chest CT should be considered in pts with normal chest radiographs who fail to improve with treatment. Evaluation of hemoptysis is discussed below.

| TREATMENT | Chronic Cough |

In pts with chronic cough and a normal chest x-ray, empiric treatment is directed at the most likely cause based on the history and physical examination. If treatment directed at one empiric cause fails, empiric treatment of an alternative etiology can be considered. Postnasal drip treatment may include antihistamines, nasal corticosteroids, and/ or antibiotics. GERD can be treated with antacids, type 2 histamine blockers, or proton pump inhibitors. Cough-variant asthma is treated with inhaled glucocorticoids and as-needed inhaled beta agonists. Pts on ACE inhibitors should be given a 1-month trial of discontinuing this medication. Chronic eosinophilic bronchitis often improves with inhaled glucocorticoid treatment. Symptomatic treatment of cough can include narcotics such as codeine; however, somnolence, constipation, and addiction can result. Dextromethorphan and benzonatate have fewer side effects but reduced efficacy.

HEMOPTYSIS

■ **ETIOLOGY**

Hemoptysis, expectoration of blood from the respiratory tract, must be differentiated from expectorated blood originating from the nasopharynx and gastrointestinal tract. Acute bronchitis is the most common cause of hemoptysis in the U.S.; tuberculosis is the leading cause worldwide.

Hemoptysis originating from the alveoli is known as diffuse alveolar hemorrhage (DAH). DAH can be caused by inflammatory diseases including Wegener's granulomatosis, systemic lupus erythematosus, and Goodpasture's disease. Within the first 100 days after bone marrow transplant, inflammatory DAH can cause severe hypoxemia. Noninflammatory DAH usually results from inhalational injuries from toxic exposures, such as smoke inhalation or cocaine.

Hemoptysis most commonly originates from small- to medium-sized bronchi. Since the bleeding source is usually bronchial arteries, there is potential for rapid blood loss. Airway hemoptysis is often caused by viral or bacterial bronchitis. Pts with bronchiectasis have increased risk of hemoptysis. Pneumonia can cause hemoptysis, especially if cavitation (e.g., tuberculosis) and/or necrotizing pneumonia (e.g., *Klebsiella pneumoniae* and *Staphylococcus aureus*) develop. Paragonimiasis, a helminthic infection common in pts from Southeast Asia and China, can cause hemoptysis and must be differentiated from tuberculosis. Although only 10% of lung cancer pts have hemoptysis at diagnosis, cancers developing in central airways (e.g., squamous cell carcinoma, small cell carcinoma, and carcinoid tumors) often cause hemoptysis. Cancers that metastasize to the lungs can cause hemoptysis less commonly.

Pulmonary vascular sources of hemoptysis include congestive heart failure, which usually causes pink, frothy sputum. Pulmonary embolism with infarction and pulmonary arteriovenous malformations are additional pulmonary vascular etiologies to consider.

■ CLINICAL ASSESSMENT

The approaches to assess and treat hemoptysis are shown in Fig. 41-1. History should determine whether the bleeding source is likely the respiratory tract or an alternative source (e.g., nasopharynx, upper GI tract). The quantity of expectorated blood should be estimated, as it influences the urgency of evaluation and treatment. Massive hemoptysis, variably defined as 200–600 mL within 24 h, requires emergent care. The presence of purulent or frothy secretions should be assessed. History of previous hemoptysis episodes and cigarette smoking should be ascertained. Fever and chills should be assessed as potential indicators of acute infection. Recent inhalation of illicit drugs and other toxins should be determined.

Physical examination should include assessment of the nares for epistaxis, and evaluation of the heart and lungs. Pedal edema could indicate congestive heart failure if symmetric, and deep-vein thrombosis with pulmonary embolism if asymmetric. Clubbing could indicate lung cancer or bronchiectasis. Assessment of vital signs and oxygen saturation can provide information about hemodynamic stability and respiratory compromise.

Radiographic evaluation with a chest x-ray should be performed. Chest CT may be helpful to assess for bronchiectasis, pneumonia, lung cancer, and pulmonary embolism. Laboratory studies include a complete blood count and coagulation studies; renal function and urinalysis should be assessed, with additional blood tests including ANCA, anti-GBM, and ANA if diffuse alveolar hemorrhage is suspected. Sputum should be sent for Gram's stain and routine culture as well as AFB smear and culture.

Bronchoscopy is often required to complete the evaluation. In massive hemoptysis, rigid bronchoscopy may be necessary.

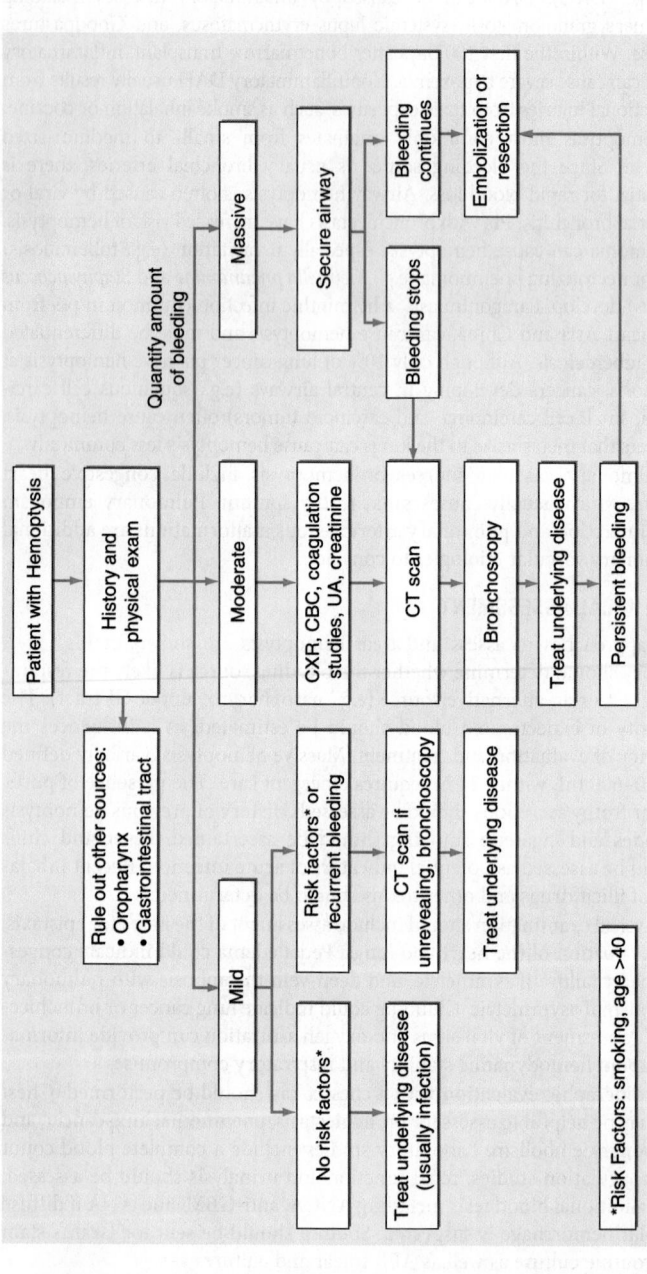

FIGURE 41-1 An algorithm for the evaluation of hemoptysis. CBC, complete blood count; CT, computed tomography; CXR, chest x-ray; UA, urinalysis. (*From Kritek P and Fanta C: HPIM-18.*)

TREATMENT Hemoptysis

As shown in Fig. 41-1, massive hemoptysis may require endotracheal intubation and mechanical ventilation to provide airway stabilization. If the source of bleeding can be identified, isolating the bleeding lung with an endobronchial blocker or double-lumen endotracheal tube is optimal. Pts should be positioned with the bleeding side down. If bleeding persists, bronchial arterial embolization by angiography may be beneficial; however, risk of spinal artery embolization is an important potential adverse event. As a last resort, surgical resection can be considered to stop the bleeding. Cough suppression, typically with narcotics, is desirable.

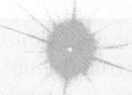

For a more detailed discussion, see Kritek P, Fanta C: Cough and Hemoptysis, Chap. 34, p. 282, in HPIM-18.

CHAPTER **42**
Edema

■ DEFINITION

Soft tissue swelling due to abnormal expansion of interstitial fluid volume. Edema fluid is a plasma transudate that accumulates when movement of fluid from vascular to interstitial space is favored. Since detectable generalized edema in the adult reflects a gain of ≥ 3 L, renal retention of salt and water is necessary for edema to occur. Distribution of edema can be an important guide to cause.

Localized Edema

Limited to a particular organ or vascular bed; easily distinguished from generalized edema. Unilateral extremity edema is usually due to venous or lymphatic obstruction (e.g., deep venous thrombosis, tumor obstruction, primary lymphedema). Stasis edema of a paralyzed lower extremity also may occur. Allergic reactions ("angioedema") and superior vena caval obstruction are causes of localized facial edema. Bilateral lower-extremity edema may have localized causes, e.g., inferior vena caval obstruction, compression due to ascites, abdominal mass. Ascites (fluid in peritoneal cavity) and hydrothorax (in pleural space) also may present as isolated localized edema, due to inflammation or neoplasm.

Generalized Edema

Soft tissue swelling of most or all regions of the body. Bilateral lower-extremity swelling, more pronounced after standing for several hours, and pulmonary edema are usually cardiac in origin. Periorbital edema noted on awakening often results from renal disease and impaired Na excretion.

Ascites and edema of lower extremities and scrotum are frequent in cirrhosis, nephrotic syndrome, or CHF.

In *CHF*, diminished cardiac output and arterial underfilling result in both decreased renal perfusion and increased venous pressure with resultant renal Na retention due to renal vasoconstriction, intrarenal blood flow redistribution, direct Na-retentive effects of norepinephrine and angiotensin II, and secondary hyperaldosteronism.

In *cirrhosis*, arteriovenous shunts and peripheral vasodilation lower renal perfusion, resulting in Na retention. Ascites accumulates when increased intrahepatic vascular resistance produces portal hypertension. As in heart failure, the effects of excess intrarenal and circulating norepinephrine, angiotensin II, and aldosterone lead to renal Na retention and worsening edema. Reduced serum albumin and increased abdominal pressure also promote lower-extremity edema.

In acute or chronic *renal failure*, edema occurs if Na intake exceeds kidneys' ability to excrete Na secondary to marked reductions in glomerular filtration. Severe hypoalbuminemia [<25 g/L (2.5 g/dL)] of any cause (e.g., nephrotic

TABLE 42-1 DRUGS ASSOCIATED WITH EDEMA FORMATION

Nonsteroidal anti-inflammatory drugs

Antihypertensive agents

  Direct arterial/arteriolar vasodilators

    Hydralazine

    Clonidine

    Methyldopa

    Guanethidine

    Minoxidil

  Calcium channel antagonists

  α-Adrenergic antagonists

  Thiazolidinediones

Steroid hormones

  Glucocorticoids

  Anabolic steroids

  Estrogens

  Progestins

Cyclosporine

Growth hormone

Immunotherapies

  Interleukin 2

  OKT3 monoclonal antibody

Source: From GM Chertow, in E Braunwald, L Goldman (eds): *Cardiology for the Primary Care Physician,* 2nd ed. Philadelphia, Saunders, 2003.

syndrome, nutritional deficiency, chronic liver disease) may lower plasma oncotic pressure, promoting fluid transudation into interstitium; lowering of effective blood volume stimulates renal Na retention and causes edema.

Less common causes of generalized edema: *idiopathic edema*, a syndrome of recurrent rapid weight gain and edema in women of reproductive age; *hypothyroidism*, in which myxedema is typically located in the pretibial region; *drugs* (Table 42-1).

TREATMENT Edema

Primary management is to identify and treat the underlying cause of edema (Fig. 42-1).

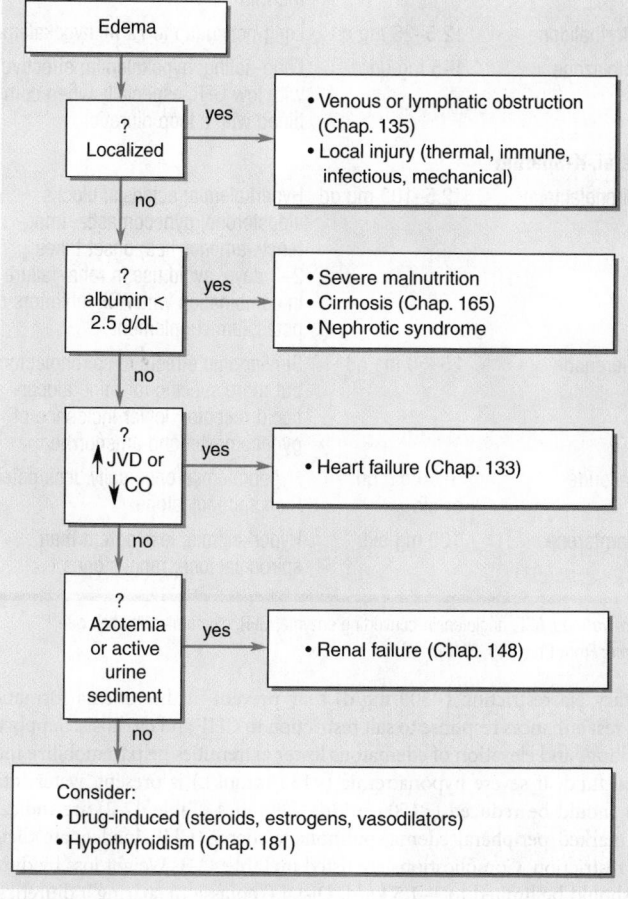

FIGURE 42-1 Diagnostic approach to edema. CO, cardiac output; JVD, jugular venous distention. (*From Chap. 49: HMOM-17.*)

TABLE 42-2 DIURETICS FOR EDEMA

Drug	Usual Dose	Comments
Loop (May be administered PO or IV)		
Furosemide	20–120 mg qd or bid	Short-acting; potent; effective with low GFR
Bumetanide	0.5–2 mg qd or bid	Better oral absorption than furosemide, but shorter duration of action
Torsemide	20–200 mg qd	Better oral absorption than furosemide, longer duration of action
Distal, K-Losing		
Hydrochlorothiazide	12.5–25 mg qd	Causes hypokalemia; need GFR >25 mL/min
Chlorthalidone	12.5–25 mg qd	Long-acting (up to 72 h); hypokalemia
Metolazone	1–5 mg qd	Long-acting; hypokalemia; effective with low GFR, especially when combined with a loop diuretic
Distal, K-Sparing		
Spironolactone	12.5–100 mg qd	Hyperkalemia; acidosis; blocks aldosterone; gynecomastia, impotence, amenorrhea; onset takes 2–3 days; avoid use in renal failure or in combination with ACE inhibitors or potassium supplement
Eplerenone	25–50 mg qd	Similar side effects to spironolactone, but more specific for mineralocorticoid receptor; lower incidence of gynecomastia and amenorrhea
Amiloride	5–10 mg qd or bid	Hyperkalemia; once daily; less potent than spironolactone
Triamterene	100 mg bid	Hyperkalemia; less potent than spironolactone; renal stones

Abbreviations: ACE, angiotensin-converting enzyme; GFR, glomerular filtration rate.
Source: From Chap. 49, HMOM-17.

Dietary Na restriction (<500 mg/d) may prevent further edema formation. Bed rest enhances response to salt restriction in CHF and cirrhosis. Supportive stockings and elevation of edematous lower extremities help to mobilize interstitial fluid. If severe hyponatremia (<132 mmol/L) is present, water intake also should be reduced (<1500 mL/d). Diuretics (Table 42-2) are indicated for marked peripheral edema, pulmonary edema, CHF, inadequate dietary salt restriction. Complications are listed in Table 42-3. Weight loss by diuretics should be limited to 1–1.5 kg/d. Distal ("potassium sparing") diuretics or metolazone may be added to loop diuretics for enhanced effect. Note that intestinal edema may impair absorption of oral diuretics and reduce effectiveness. When desired weight is achieved, diuretic doses should be reduced.

Evaluation

The initial steps in evaluating the pt with jaundice are to determine whether (1) hyperbilirubinemia is conjugated or unconjugated, and (2) other biochemical liver tests are abnormal (Figs. 48-1 and 48-2, Tables 48-2 and 48-3). Essential clinical examination includes history (especially duration of jaundice, pruritus, associated pain, risk factors for parenterally transmitted diseases, medications, ethanol use, travel history, surgery, pregnancy, presence of any accompanying symptoms), physical examination (hepatomegaly, tenderness over liver, palpable gallbladder, splenomegaly, gynecomastia, testicular atrophy, other stigmata of chronic liver disease), blood liver tests (see below), and complete blood count.

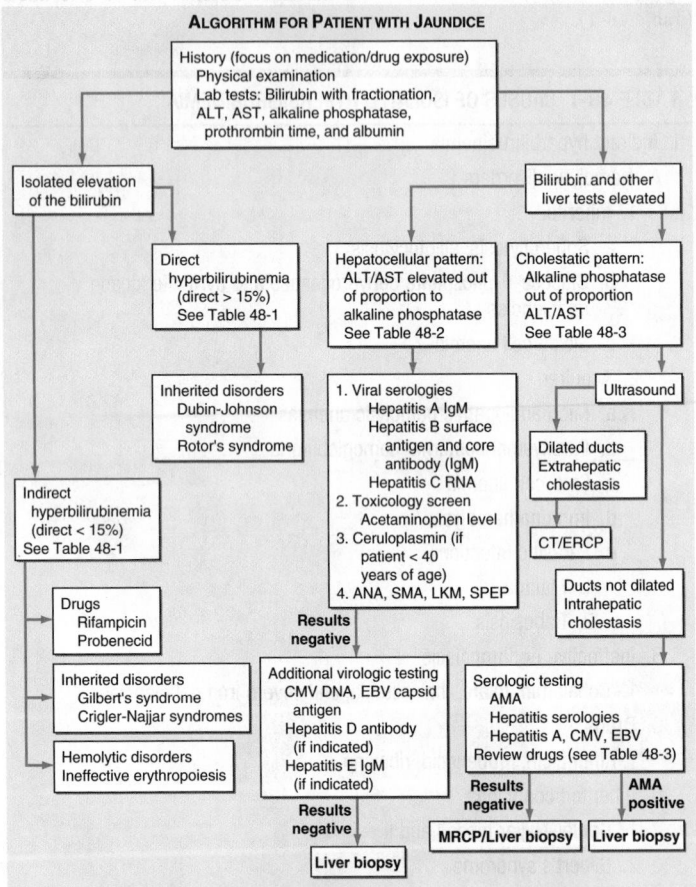

FIGURE 48-1 Evaluation of the pt with jaundice. ALT, alanine aminotransferase; AMA, antimitochondrial antibody; ANA, antinuclear antibody; AST, aspartate aminotransferase; CMV, cytomegalovirus; EBV, Epstein-Barr virus; LKM, liver-kidney microsomal antibody; MRCP, magnetic resonance cholangiopancreatography; SMA, smooth-muscle antibody; SPEP, serum protein electrophoresis.

TABLE 42-3 COMPLICATIONS OF DIURETICS

Common	Uncommon
Volume depletion	Interstitial nephritis (thiazides, furosemide)
Prerenal azotemia	Pancreatitis (thiazides)
Potassium depletion	Loss of hearing (loop diuretics)
Hyponatremia (thiazides)	Anemia, leukopenia, thrombocytopenia (thiazides)
Metabolic alkalosis	
Hypercholesterolemia	
Hyperglycemia (thiazides)	
Hyperkalemia (K-sparing)	
Hypomagnesemia	
Hyperuricemia	
Hypercalcemia (thiazides)	
GI complaints	
Rash (thiazides)	

Source: From Chap. 49, HMOM-17.

In *CHF* (Chap. 133), avoid overdiuresis because it may bring a fall in cardiac output and prerenal azotemia. Avoid diuretic-induced hypokalemia, which predisposes to digitalis toxicity.

In *cirrhosis* and other hepatic causes of edema, spironolactone is the initial diuretic of choice but may produce acidosis and hyperkalemia. Thiazides or small doses of loop diuretics may also be added. However, renal failure may result from volume depletion. Overdiuresis may result in hyponatremia, hypokalemia, and alkalosis, which may worsen hepatic encephalopathy (Chap. 165).

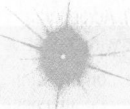

For a more detailed discussion, see Braunwald E, Loscalzo J: Edema, Chap. 36, p. 290, in HPIM-18.

CHAPTER **43**
Abdominal Pain

Numerous causes, ranging from acute, life-threatening emergencies to chronic functional disease and disorders of several organ systems, can generate abdominal pain. Evaluation of acute pain requires rapid assessment of likely causes and early initiation of appropriate therapy. A more detailed and time-consuming approach to diagnosis may be followed in less acute situations. Table 43-1 lists the common causes of abdominal pain.

TABLE 43-1 COMMON ETIOLOGIES OF ABDOMINAL PAIN

Mucosal or muscle inflammation in hollow viscera: Peptic disease (ulcers, erosions, inflammation), hemorrhagic gastritis, gastroesophageal reflux, appendicitis, diverticulitis, cholecystitis, cholangitis, inflammatory bowel diseases (Crohn's, ulcerative colitis), infectious gastroenteritis, mesenteric lymphadenitis, colitis, cystitis, or pyelonephritis

Visceral spasm or distention: Intestinal obstruction (adhesions, tumor, intussusception), appendiceal obstruction with appendicitis, strangulation of hernia, irritable bowel syndrome (muscle hypertrophy and spasm), acute biliary obstruction, pancreatic ductal obstruction (chronic pancreatitis, stone), ureteral obstruction (kidney stone, blood clot), fallopian tubes (tubal pregnancy)

Vascular disorders: Mesenteric thromboembolic disease (arterial or venous), arterial dissection or rupture (e.g., aortic aneurysm), occlusion from external pressure or torsion (e.g., volvulus, hernia, tumor, adhesions, intussusception), hemoglobinopathy (esp. sickle cell disease)

Distention or inflammation of visceral surfaces: Hepatic capsule (hepatitis, hemorrhage, tumor, Budd-Chiari syndrome, Fitz-Hugh-Curtis syndrome), renal capsule (tumor, infection, infarction, venous occlusion), splenic capsule (hemorrhage, abscess, infarction), pancreas (pancreatitis, pseudocyst, abscess, tumor), ovary (hemorrhage into cyst, ectopic pregnancy, abscess)

Peritoneal inflammation: Bacterial infection (perforated viscus, pelvic inflammatory disease, infected ascites), intestinal infarction, chemical irritation, pancreatitis, perforated viscus (esp. stomach and duodenum), reactive inflammation (neighboring abscess, incl. diverticulitis, pleuropulmonary infection or inflammation), serositis (collagen-vascular diseases, familial Mediterranean fever), ovulation (mittelschmerz).

Abdominal wall disorders: Trauma, hernias, muscle inflammation or infection, hematoma (trauma, anticoagulant therapy), traction from mesentery (e.g., adhesions)

Toxins: Lead poisoning, black widow spider bite

Metabolic disorders: Uremia, ketoacidosis (diabetic, alcoholic), Addisonian crisis, porphyria, angioedema (C1 esterase deficiency), narcotic withdrawal

Neurologic disorders: Herpes zoster, tabes dorsalis, causalgia, compression or inflammation of spinal roots, (e.g., arthritis, herniated disk, tumor, abscess), psychogenic

Referred pain: From heart, lungs, esophagus, genitalia (e.g., cardiac ischemia, pneumonia, pneumothorax, pulmonary embolism, esophagitis, esophageal spasm, esophageal rupture)

APPROACH TO THE PATIENT **Abdominal Pain**

History: History is of critical diagnostic importance. Physical exam may be unrevealing or misleading, and laboratory and radiologic exams delayed or unhelpful.

CHARACTERISTIC FEATURES OF ABDOMINAL PAIN

Duration and Pattern: These provide clues to nature and severity, although acute abdominal crisis may occasionally present insidiously or on a background of chronic pain.

Type and location provide a rough guide to nature of disease. *Visceral pain* (due to distention of a hollow viscus) localizes poorly and is often perceived in the midline. Intestinal pain tends to be crampy; when originating proximal to the ileocecal valve, it usually localizes above and around the umbilicus. Pain of colonic origin is perceived in the hypogastrium and lower quadrants. Pain from biliary or ureteral obstruction often causes pts to writhe in discomfort. *Somatic pain* (due to peritoneal inflammation) is usually sharper and more precisely localized to the diseased region (e.g., acute appendicitis; capsular distention of liver, kidney, or spleen), exacerbated by movement, causing pts to remain still. Pattern of radiation may be helpful: right shoulder (hepatobiliary origin), left shoulder (splenic), midback (pancreatic), flank (proximal urinary tract), groin (genital or distal urinary tract).

Factors that precipitate or relieve pain: Ask about its relationship to eating (e.g., upper GI, biliary, pancreatic, ischemic bowel disease), defecation (colorectal), urination (genitourinary or colorectal), respiratory (pleuropulmonary, hepatobiliary), position (pancreatic, gastroesophageal reflux, musculoskeletal), menstrual cycle/ menarche (tuboovarian, endometrial, including endometriosis), exertion (coronary/intestinal ischemia, musculoskeletal), medication or specific foods (motility disorders, food intolerance, gastroesophageal reflux, porphyria, adrenal insufficiency, ketoacidosis, toxins), and stress (motility disorders, nonulcer dyspepsia, irritable bowel syndrome).

Associated symptoms: Look for fevers/chills (infection, inflammatory disease, infarction), weight loss (tumor, inflammatory disease, malabsorption, ischemia), nausea/vomiting (obstruction, infection, inflammatory disease, metabolic disease), dysphagia/odynophagia (esophageal), early satiety (gastric), hematemesis (esophageal, gastric, duodenal), constipation (colorectal, perianal, genitourinary), jaundice (hepatobiliary, hemolytic), diarrhea (inflammatory disease, infection, malabsorption, secretory tumors, ischemia, genitourinary), dysuria/ hematuria/vaginal or penile discharge (genitourinary), hematochezia (colorectal or, rarely, urinary), skin/joint/eye disorders (inflammatory disease, bacterial or viral infection).

Predisposing factors: Inquire about family history (inflammatory disease, tumors, pancreatitis), hypertension and atherosclerotic disease (ischemia), diabetes mellitus (motility disorders, ketoacidosis), connective tissue disease (motility disorders, serositis), depression (motility disorders, tumors), smoking (ischemia), recent smoking cessation (inflammatory disease), ethanol use (motility disorders, hepatobiliary, pancreatic, gastritis, peptic ulcer disease).

lithiasis) vs. still (peritonitis, perforation)], position (a pt leaning forward may have pancreatitis or gastric perforation into the lesser sac), presence of fever or hypothermia, hyperventilation, cyanosis, bowel sounds, direct or rebound abdominal tenderness, pulsating abdominal mass, abdominal bruits, ascites, rectal blood, rectal or pelvic tenderness, and evidence of coagulopathy. Useful laboratory studies include hematocrit (may be normal with acute hemorrhage or misleadingly high with dehydration), WBC with differential count, arterial blood gases, serum electrolytes, BUN, creatinine, glucose, lipase or amylase, and UA. Females of reproductive age should have a pregnancy test. Radiologic studies should include supine and upright abdominal films (left lateral decubitus view if upright unobtainable) to evaluate bowel caliber and presence of free peritoneal air, cross-table lateral film to assess aortic diameter; CT (when available) to detect evidence of bowel perforation, inflammation, solid organ infarction, retroperitoneal bleeding, abscess, or tumor. Abdominal paracentesis (or peritoneal lavage in cases of trauma) can detect evidence of bleeding or peritonitis. Abdominal ultrasound (when available) reveals evidence of abscess, cholecystitis, biliary or ureteral obstruction, or hematoma and is used to determine aortic diameter.

■ DIAGNOSTIC STRATEGIES

The initial decision point is based on whether the pt is hemodynamically stable. If not, one must suspect a vascular catastrophe such as a leaking abdominal aortic aneurysm. Such pts receive limited resuscitation and move immediately to surgical exploration. If the pt is hemodynamically stable, the next decision point is whether the abdomen is rigid. Rigid abdomens are most often due to perforation or obstruction. The diagnosis can generally be made by a chest and plain abdominal radiograph.

If the abdomen is not rigid, the causes may be grouped based on whether the pain is poorly localized or well localized. In the presence of poorly localized pain, one should assess whether an aortic aneurysm is possible. If so, a CT scan can make the diagnosis; if not, early appendicitis, early obstruction, mesenteric ischemia, inflammatory bowel disease, pancreatitis, and metabolic problems are all in the differential diagnosis.

Pain localized to the epigastrium may be of cardiac origin or due to esophageal inflammation or perforation, gastritis, peptic ulcer disease, biliary colic or cholecystitis, or pancreatitis. Pain localized to the right upper quadrant includes those same entities plus pyelonephritis or nephrolithiasis, hepatic abscess, subdiaphragmatic abscess, pulmonary embolus, or pneumonia, or it may be of musculoskeletal origin. Additional considerations with left upper quadrant localization are infarcted or ruptured spleen, splenomegaly, and gastric or peptic ulcer. Right lower quadrant pain may be from appendicitis, Meckel's diverticulum, Crohn's disease, diverticulitis, mesenteric adenitis, rectus sheath hematoma, psoas abscess, ovarian abscess or torsion, ectopic pregnancy, salpingitis, familial fever syndromes, uterolithiasis, or herpes zoster. Left lower quadrant pain may be due to diverticulitis, perforated neoplasm, or other entities previously mentioned.

TREATMENT	Acute, Catastrophic Abdominal Pain

IV fluids, correction of life-threatening acid-base disturbances, and assessment of need for emergent surgery are the first priority; careful follow-up with frequent reexamination (when possible, by the same examiner) is essential. Relieve the pain. The use of narcotic analgesia is controversial. Traditionally, narcotic analgesics were withheld pending establishment of diagnosis and therapeutic plan, since masking of diagnostic signs may delay needed intervention. However, evidence that narcotics actually mask a diagnosis is sparse.

For a more detailed discussion, see Silen W: Abdominal Pain, Chap. 13, p. 108, in HPIM-18.

CHAPTER **44**
Nausea, Vomiting, and Indigestion

NAUSEA AND VOMITING

Nausea refers to the imminent desire to vomit and often precedes or accompanies vomiting. *Vomiting* refers to the forceful expulsion of gastric contents through the mouth. *Retching* refers to labored rhythmic respiratory activity that precedes emesis. *Regurgitation* refers to the gentle expulsion of gastric contents in the absence of nausea and abdominal diaphragmatic muscular contraction. *Rumination* refers to the regurgitation, rechewing, and reswallowing of food from the stomach.

■ PATHOPHYSIOLOGY

Gastric contents are propelled into the esophagus when there is relaxation of the gastric fundus and gastroesophageal sphincter followed by a rapid increase in intraabdominal pressure produced by contraction of the abdominal and diaphragmatic musculature. Increased intrathoracic pressure results in further movement of the material to the mouth. Reflex elevation of the soft palate and closure of the glottis protect the nasopharynx and trachea and complete the act of vomiting. Vomiting is controlled by two brainstem areas, the vomiting center and chemoreceptor trigger zone. Activation of the chemoreceptor trigger zone results in impulses to the vomiting center, which controls the physical act of vomiting.

■ ETIOLOGY

Nausea and vomiting are manifestations of a large number of disorders (Table 44-1).

TABLE 44-1 CAUSES OF NAUSEA AND VOMITING

Intraperitoneal	Extraperitoneal	Medications/Metabolic Disorders
Obstructing disorders	Cardiopulmonary disease	Drugs
Pyloric obstruction	Cardiomyopathy	Cancer chemotherapy
Small bowel obstruction	Myocardial infarction	Antibiotics
Colonic obstruction	Labyrinthine disease	Cardiac antiarrhythmics
Superior mesenteric artery syndrome	Motion sickness	Digoxin
Enteric infections	Labyrinthitis	Oral hypoglycemics
Viral	Malignancy	Oral contraceptives
Bacterial	Intracerebral disorders	Endocrine/metabolic disease
Inflammatory diseases	Malignancy	Pregnancy
Cholecystitis	Hemorrhage	Uremia
Pancreatitis	Abscess	Ketoacidosis
Appendicitis	Hydrocephalus	Thyroid and parathyroid disease
Hepatitis	Psychiatric illness	Adrenal insufficiency
Altered sensorimotor function	Anorexia and bulimia nervosa	Toxins
Gastroparesis	Depression	Liver failure
Intestinal pseudo-obstruction	Postoperative vomiting	Ethanol
Gastroesophageal reflux		
Chronic idiopathic nausea		
Functional vomiting		
Cyclic vomiting syndrome		
Biliary colic		
Abdominal irradiation		

■ EVALUATION

The history, including a careful drug history, and the timing and character of the vomitus can be helpful. For example, vomiting that occurs predominantly in the morning is often seen in pregnancy, uremia, and alcoholic gastritis; feculent emesis implies distal intestinal obstruction or gastrocolic fistula; projectile vomiting suggests increased intracranial pressure; vomiting during or shortly after a meal may be due to psychogenic causes or peptic ulcer disease. Associated symptoms may also be helpful: vertigo and tinnitus in Ménière's disease, relief of abdominal pain with vomiting in peptic ulcer, and early satiety in gastroparesis. Plain radiographs can suggest diagnoses such as intestinal obstruction. The upper GI series assesses motility of the proximal GI tract as well as the mucosa. Other studies may be indicated, such as gastric emptying scans (diabetic gastroparesis) and CT scan of the brain.

■ **COMPLICATIONS**

Rupture of the esophagus (Boerhaave's syndrome), hematemesis from a mucosal tear (Mallory-Weiss syndrome), dehydration, malnutrition, dental caries and erosions, metabolic alkalosis, hypokalemia, and aspiration pneumonitis.

TREATMENT Nausea and Vomiting

Treatment is aimed at correcting the specific cause. The effectiveness of antiemetic medications depends on etiology of symptoms, pt responsiveness, and side effects. Antihistamines such as meclizine and dimenhydrinate are effective for nausea due to inner ear dysfunction. Anticholinergics such as scopolamine are effective for nausea associated with motion sickness. Haloperidol and phenothiazine derivatives such as prochlorperazine are often effective in controlling mild nausea and vomiting, but sedation, hypotension, and parkinsonian symptoms are common side effects. Selective dopamine antagonists such as metoclopramide may be superior to the phenothiazines in treating severe nausea and vomiting and are particularly useful in treatment of gastroparesis. IV metoclopramide may be effective as prophylaxis against nausea when given before chemotherapy. Ondansetron and granisetron, serotonin receptor blockers, and glucocorticoids are used for treating nausea and vomiting associated with cancer chemotherapy. Aprepitant, a neurokinin receptor blocker, is effective at controlling nausea from highly emetic drugs like cisplatin. Erythromycin is effective in some pts with gastroparesis.

INDIGESTION

Indigestion is a nonspecific term that encompasses a variety of upper abdominal complaints including heartburn, regurgitation, and dyspepsia (upper abdominal discomfort or pain). These symptoms are overwhelmingly due to gastroesophageal reflux disease (GERD).

■ **PATHOPHYSIOLOGY**

GERD occurs as a consequence of acid reflux into the esophagus from the stomach, gastric motor dysfunction, or visceral afferent hypersensitivity. A wide variety of situations promote GERD: increased gastric contents (from a large meal, gastric stasis, or acid hypersecretion), physical factors (lying down, bending over), increased pressure on the stomach (tight clothes, obesity, ascites, pregnancy), and loss (usually intermittent) of lower esophageal sphincter tone (diseases such as scleroderma, smoking, anticholinergics, calcium antagonists). Hiatal hernia also promotes acid flow into the esophagus.

◼ NATURAL HISTORY

Heartburn is reported once monthly by 40% of Americans and daily by 7%. Functional dyspepsia is defined as >3 months of dyspepsia without an organic cause. Functional dyspepsia is the cause of symptoms in 60% of pts with dyspeptic symptoms. However, peptic ulcer disease from either *Helicobacter pylori* infection or ingestion of nonsteroidal anti-inflammatory drugs (NSAIDs) is present in 15% of cases.

In most cases, the esophagus is not damaged, but 5% of pts develop esophageal ulcers and some form strictures; 8–20% develop glandular epithelial cell metaplasia, termed *Barrett's esophagus*, which can progress to adenocarcinoma.

Extraesophageal manifestations include asthma, laryngitis, chronic cough, aspiration pneumonitis, chronic bronchitis, sleep apnea, dental caries, halitosis, and hiccups.

◼ EVALUATION

The presence of dysphagia, odynophagia, unexplained weight loss, recurrent vomiting leading to dehydration, occult or gross bleeding, or a palpable mass or adenopathy are "alarm" signals that demand directed radiographic, endoscopic, and surgical evaluation. Pts without alarm features are generally treated empirically. Individuals >45 years can be tested for the presence of *H. pylori*. Pts positive for the infection are treated to eradicate the organism. Pts who fail to respond to *H. pylori* treatment, those >45 years old, and those with alarm factors generally undergo upper GI endoscopy.

| TREATMENT | Indigestion |

Weight reduction; elevation of the head of the bed; and avoidance of large meals, smoking, caffeine, alcohol, chocolate, fatty food, citrus juices, and NSAIDs may prevent GERD. Antacids are widely used. Clinical trials suggest that proton pump inhibitors (omeprazole) are more effective than histamine receptor blockers (ranitidine) in pts with or without esophageal erosions. *H. pylori* eradication regimens are discussed in Chap. 158. Motor stimulants like metoclopramide and erythromycin may be useful in a subset of pts with postprandial distress.

Surgical techniques (Nissen fundoplication, Belsey procedure) work best in young individuals whose symptoms have improved on proton pump inhibitors and who otherwise may require lifelong therapy. They can be used in the rare pts who are refractory to medical management. Clinical trials have not documented the superiority of one over another.

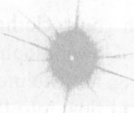

For a more detailed discussion, see Hasler WL: Nausea, Vomiting, and Indigestion, Chap. 39, p. 301, in HPIM-18.

CHAPTER **45**
Dysphagia

DYSPHAGIA

Dysphagia is difficulty moving food or liquid through the mouth, pharynx, and esophagus. The pt senses swallowed material sticking along the path. *Odynophagia* is pain on swallowing. *Globus pharyngeus* is the sensation of a lump lodged in the throat, with swallowing unaffected.

■ PATHOPHYSIOLOGY

Dysphagia is caused by two main mechanisms: mechanical obstruction or motor dysfunction. Mechanical causes of dysphagia can be luminal (e.g., large food bolus, foreign body), intrinsic to the esophagus (e.g., inflammation, webs and rings, strictures, tumors), or extrinsic to the esophagus (e.g., cervical spondylitis, enlarged thyroid or mediastinal mass, vascular compression). The motor function abnormalities that cause dysphagia may be related to defects in initiating the swallowing reflex (e.g., tongue paralysis, lack of saliva, lesions affecting sensory components of cranial nerves X and XI), disorders of the pharyngeal and esophageal striated muscle (e.g., muscle disorders such as polymyositis and dermatomyositis, neurologic lesions such as myasthenia gravis, polio, or amyotrophic lateral sclerosis), and disorders of the esophageal smooth muscle (e.g., achalasia, scleroderma, myotonic dystrophy).

APPROACH TO THE PATIENT | Dysphagia

History can provide a presumptive diagnosis in about 80% of pts. Difficulty only with solids implies mechanical dysphagia. Difficulty with both solids and liquids may occur late in the course of mechanical dysphagia but is an early sign of motor dysphagia. Pts can sometimes pinpoint the site of food sticking. Weight loss out of proportion to the degree of dysphagia may be a sign of underlying malignancy. Hoarseness may be related to involvement of the larynx in the primary disease process (e.g., neuromuscular disorders), neoplastic disruption of the recurrent laryngeal nerve, or laryngitis from gastroesophageal reflux.

Physical exam may reveal signs of skeletal muscle, neurologic, or oropharyngeal diseases. Neck exam can reveal masses impinging on the esophagus. Skin changes might suggest the systemic nature of the underlying disease (e.g., scleroderma).

Dysphagia is nearly always a symptom of organic disease rather than a functional complaint. If oropharyngeal dysphagia is suspected, video-fluoroscopy of swallowing may be diagnostic. Mechanical dysphagia can be evaluated by barium swallow and esophagogastroscopy with endoscopic biopsy. Barium swallow and esophageal motility studies can show the presence of motor dysphagia. An algorithm outlining an approach to the pt with dysphagia is shown in Fig. 45-1.

■ OROPHARYNGEAL DYSPHAGIA

Pt has difficulty initiating the swallow; food sticks at the level of the suprasternal notch; nasopharyngeal regurgitation and aspiration may be present.

Causes include the following: for solids only, carcinoma, aberrant vessel, congenital or acquired web (Plummer-Vinson syndrome in iron deficiency), cervical osteophyte; for solids and liquids, cricopharyngeal bar (e.g., hypertensive or hypotensive upper esophageal sphincter), Zenker's diverticulum (outpouching in the posterior midline at the intersection of the pharynx and the cricopharyngeus muscle), myasthenia gravis, glucocorticoid myopathy, hyperthyroidism, hypothyroidism, myotonic dystrophy, amyotrophic lateral sclerosis, multiple sclerosis, Parkinson's disease, stroke, bulbar palsy, pseudobulbar palsy.

■ ESOPHAGEAL DYSPHAGIA

Food sticks in the mid or lower sternal area; can be associated with regurgitation, aspiration, odynophagia. Causes include the following: for solids only, lower esophageal ring (Schatzki's ring—symptoms are usually intermittent), peptic stricture (heartburn accompanies this), carcinoma, lye stricture; for solids and liquids, diffuse esophageal spasm (occurs with chest pain and is intermittent), scleroderma (progressive and occurs with heartburn), achalasia (progressive and occurs without heartburn).

NONCARDIAC CHEST PAIN

Of pts presenting with chest pain, 30% have an esophageal source rather than angina. History and physical exam often cannot distinguish cardiac from noncardiac pain. Exclude cardiac disease first. Causes include the following: gastroesophageal reflux disease, esophageal motility disorders, peptic ulcer disease, gallstones, psychiatric disease (anxiety, panic attacks, depression).

■ EVALUATION

Consider a trial of antireflux therapy (omeprazole); if no response, 24-h ambulatory luminal pH monitoring; if negative, esophageal manometry may show motor disorder. Trial of imipramine, 50 mg PO qhs, may be worthwhile. Consider psychiatric evaluation in selected cases.

ESOPHAGEAL MOTILITY DISORDERS

Pts may have a spectrum of manometric findings ranging from nonspecific abnormalities to defined clinical entities.

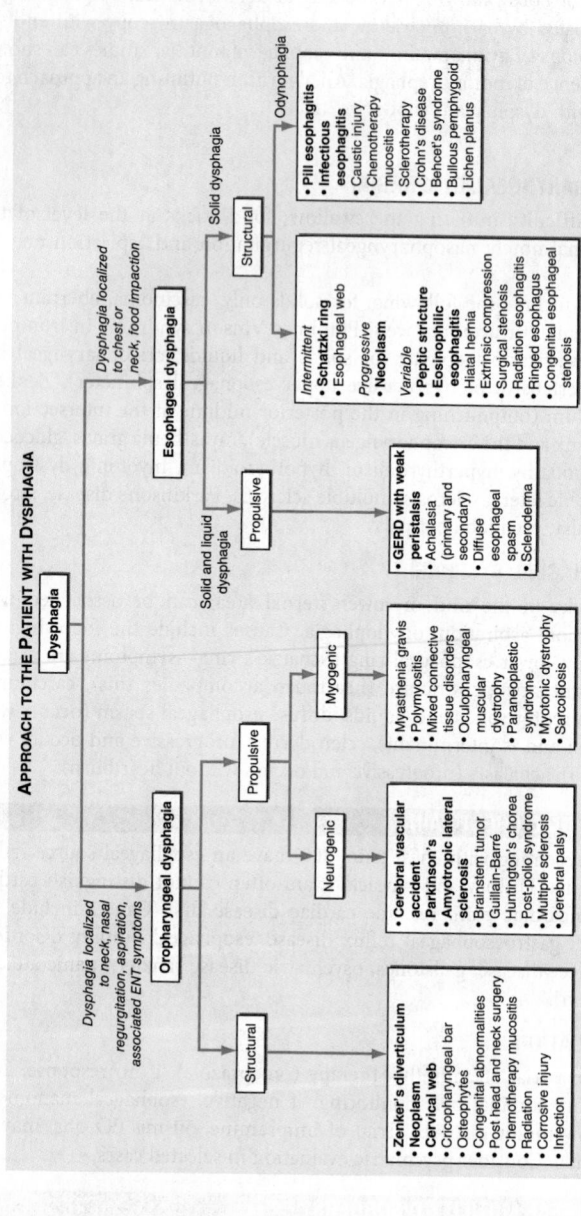

FIGURE 45-1 Approach to the pt with dysphagia. Etiologies in bold print are the most common. ENT, ear, nose, and throat; GERD, gastroesophageal reflux disease.

■ ACHALASIA

Motor obstruction caused by hypertensive lower esophageal sphincter (LES), incomplete relaxation of LES, or loss of peristalsis in smooth-muscle portion of esophagus. Causes include the following: primary (idiopathic) or secondary due to Chagas' disease, lymphoma, carcinoma, chronic idiopathic intestinal pseudoobstruction, ischemia, neurotropic viruses, drugs, toxins, radiation therapy, postvagotomy.

■ EVALUATION

Chest x-ray shows absence of gastric air bubble. Barium swallow shows dilated esophagus with distal beaklike narrowing and air-fluid level. Endoscopy is done to rule out cancer, particularly in persons >50 years. Manometry shows normal or elevated LES pressure, decreased LES relaxation, absent peristalsis.

> **TREATMENT** Achalasia
>
> Pneumatic balloon dilatation is effective in 85%, with 3–5% risk of perforation or bleeding. Injection of botulinum toxin at endoscopy to relax LES is safe and effective, but effects last only ~12 months. Myotomy of LES (Heller procedure) is effective, but 10–30% of pts develop gastroesophageal reflux. Nifedipine, 10–20 mg, or isosorbide dinitrate, 5–10 mg SL ac, may avert need for dilatation or surgery. Sildenafil may also augment swallow-induced relaxation of the LES.

■ SPASTIC DISORDERS

Diffuse esophageal spasm involves multiple spontaneous and swallow-induced contractions of the esophageal body that are of simultaneous onset and long duration and are recurrent. Causes include the following: primary (idiopathic) or secondary due to gastroesophageal reflux disease, emotional stress, diabetes, alcoholism, neuropathy, radiation therapy, ischemia, or collagen vascular disease.

An important variant is nutcracker esophagus: high-amplitude (>180 mmHg) peristaltic contractions; particularly associated with chest pain or dysphagia, but correlation between symptoms and manometry is inconsistent. Condition may resolve over time or evolve into diffuse spasm; associated with increased frequency of depression, anxiety, and somatization.

■ EVALUATION

Barium swallow shows corkscrew esophagus, pseudodiverticula, and diffuse spasm. Manometry shows spasm with multiple simultaneous esophageal contractions of high amplitude and long duration. In nutcracker esophagus, the contractions are peristaltic and of high amplitude. If heart disease has been ruled out, edrophonium, ergonovine, or bethanechol can be used to provoke spasm.

> **TREATMENT**   Spastic Disorders
>
> Anticholinergics are usually of limited value; nitrates (isosorbide dinitrate, 5–10 mg PO ac) and calcium antagonists (nifedipine, 10–20 mg PO ac) are more effective. Those refractory to medical management may benefit from balloon dilatation. Rare pts require surgical intervention: longitudinal myotomy of esophageal circular muscle. Treatment of concomitant depression or other psychological disturbance may help.

■ SCLERODERMA

Atrophy of the esophageal smooth muscle and fibrosis can make the esophagus aperistaltic and lead to an incompetent LES with attendant reflux esophagitis and stricture. Treatment of gastroesophageal reflux disease is discussed in Chap. 44.

ESOPHAGEAL INFLAMMATION

■ VIRAL ESOPHAGITIS

Herpesviruses I and II, varicella-zoster virus, and cytomegalovirus (CMV) can all cause esophagitis; particularly common in immunocompromised pts (e.g., AIDS). Odynophagia, dysphagia, fever, and bleeding are symptoms and signs. Diagnosis is made by endoscopy with biopsy, brush cytology, and culture.

> **TREATMENT**   Viral Esophagitis
>
> Disease is usually self-limited in the immunocompetent person; viscous lidocaine can relieve pain; in prolonged cases and in immunocompromised hosts, herpes and varicella esophagitis are treated with acyclovir, 5–10 mg/kg IV q8h for 10–14 d, then 200–400 mg PO 5 times a day for a week or valacyclovir 1 g PO tid for 7 days. CMV is treated with ganciclovir, 5 mg/kg IV q12h, until healing occurs, which may take weeks. Oral valganciclovir (900 mg bid) is an effective alternative to parenteral treatment. In nonresponders, foscarnet, 90 mg/kg IV q12h for 21 days, may be effective.

■ *CANDIDA* ESOPHAGITIS

In immunocompromised hosts, or those with malignancy, diabetes, hypoparathyroidism, hemoglobinopathy, systemic lupus erythematosus, corrosive esophageal injury, candidal esophageal infection may present with odynophagia, dysphagia, and oral thrush (50%). Diagnosis is made on endoscopy by identifying yellow-white plaques or nodules on friable red mucosa. Characteristic hyphae are seen on KOH stain. In pts with AIDS, the development of symptoms may prompt an empirical therapeutic trial.

> **TREATMENT**   *Candida* Esophagitis
>
> Oral nystatin (100,000 U/mL), 5 mL q6h, or clotrimazole, 10-mg tablet sucked q6h, is effective. In immunocompromised hosts, fluconazole, 200 mg PO on day 1 followed by 100 mg daily for 1–2 weeks, is treatment of

choice; alternatives include itraconazole, 200 mg PO bid, or ketoconazole, 200–400 mg PO daily; long-term maintenance therapy is often required. Poorly responsive pts may respond to higher doses of fluconazole (400 mg/d) or to amphotericin, 10–15 mg IV q6h for a total dose of 300–500 mg.

◼ PILL-RELATED ESOPHAGITIS

Doxycycline, tetracycline, aspirin, nonsteroidal anti-inflammatory drugs, KCl, quinidine, ferrous sulfate, clindamycin, alprenolol, and alendronate can induce local inflammation in the esophagus. Predisposing factors include recumbency after swallowing pills with small sips of water and anatomic factors impinging on the esophagus and slowing transit.

> **TREATMENT**   Pill-Related Esophagitis
>
> Withdraw offending drug, use antacids, and dilate any resulting stricture.

◼ EOSINOPHILIC ESOPHAGITIS

Mucosal inflammation with eosinophils with submucosal fibrosis can be seen especially in pts with food allergies. This diagnosis relies on the presence of symptoms of esophagitis with the appropriate findings on esophageal biopsy. Eotaxin 3, an eosinophil chemokine, has been implicated in its etiology. IL-5 and TARC (thymus and activation-related chemokine) levels may be elevated. Treatment involves a 12-week course of swallowed fluticasone (440 µg bid) using a metered-dose inhaler.

◼ OTHER CAUSES OF ESOPHAGITIS IN AIDS

Mycobacteria, *Cryptosporidium*, *Pneumocystis*, idiopathic esophageal ulcers, and giant ulcers (possible cytopathic effect of HIV) can occur. Ulcers may respond to systemic glucocorticoids.

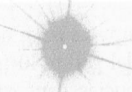

For a more detailed discussion, see Hirano I, Kahrilas PJ: Dysphagia, Chap. 38, p. 297; and Kahrilas PJ, Hirano I: Diseases of the Esophagus, Chap. 292, p. 2427, in HPIM-18.

CHAPTER **46**
Diarrhea, Constipation, and Malabsorption

NORMAL GASTROINTESTINAL FUNCTION
◼ ABSORPTION OF FLUID AND ELECTROLYTES

Fluid delivery to the GI tract is 8–10 L/d, including 2 L/d ingested; most is absorbed in small bowel. Colonic absorption is normally 0.05–2 L/d, with capacity for 6 L/d if required. Intestinal water absorption passively follows active transport of Na⁺, Cl⁻, glucose, and bile salts. Additional transport mechanisms include Cl^-/HCO_3^- exchange, Na^+/H^+ exchange, H^+, K^+, Cl^-, and HCO_3^- secretion, Na^+-glucose cotransport, and active Na^+ transport across the basolateral membrane by Na^+,K^+-ATPase.

■ NUTRIENT ABSORPTION

1. *Proximal small intestine*: iron, calcium, folate, fats (after hydrolysis of triglycerides to fatty acids by pancreatic lipase and colipase), proteins (after hydrolysis by pancreatic and intestinal peptidases), carbohydrates (after hydrolysis by amylases and disaccharidases); triglycerides absorbed as micelles after solubilization by bile salts; amino acids and dipeptides absorbed via specific carriers; sugars absorbed by active transport.
2. *Distal small intestine*: vitamin B_{12}, bile salts, water.
3. *Colon*: water, electrolytes.

■ INTESTINAL MOTILITY

Allows propulsion of intestinal contents from stomach to anus and separation of components to facilitate nutrient absorption. Propulsion is controlled by neural, myogenic, and hormonal mechanisms; mediated by migrating motor complex, an organized wave of neuromuscular activity that originates in the distal stomach during fasting and migrates slowly down the small intestine. Colonic motility is mediated by local peristalsis to propel feces. Defecation is effected by relaxation of internal anal sphincter in response to rectal distention, with voluntary control by contraction of external anal sphincter.

DIARRHEA

■ PHYSIOLOGY

Formally defined as fecal output >200 g/d on low-fiber (western) diet; also frequently used to connote loose or watery stools. Mediated by one or more of the following mechanisms:

■ OSMOTIC DIARRHEA

Nonabsorbed solutes increase intraluminal oncotic pressure, causing outpouring of water; usually ceases with fasting; stool osmolal gap > 40 (see below). Causes include disaccharidase (e.g., lactase) deficiencies, pancreatic insufficiency, bacterial overgrowth, lactulose or sorbitol ingestion, polyvalent laxative abuse, celiac or tropical sprue, and short bowel syndrome. Lactase deficiency can be either primary (more prevalent in blacks and Asians, usually presenting in early adulthood) or secondary (from viral, bacterial, or protozoal gastroenteritis, celiac or tropical sprue, or kwashiorkor).

■ SECRETORY DIARRHEA

Active ion secretion causes obligatory water loss; diarrhea is usually watery, often profuse, unaffected by fasting; stool Na^+ and K^+ are elevated with osmolal gap <40. Causes include viral infections (e.g., rotavirus, Norwalk virus), bacterial infections (e.g., cholera, enterotoxigenic *Escherichia coli*, *Staphylococcus aureus*), protozoa (e.g., *Giardia*, *Isospora*, *Cryptosporidium*), AIDS-associated disorders (including mycobacterial and HIV-induced), medications (e.g., theophylline, colchicine, prostaglandins, diuretics), Zollinger-Ellison syndrome (excess gastrin production), vasoactive intestinal peptide (VIP)-producing tumors, carcinoid tumors (histamine and sero-tonin), medullary thyroid carcinoma (prostaglandins and calcitonin), systemic mastocytosis, basophilic leukemia, distal colonic villous adenomas (direct secretion of potassium-rich fluid), collagenous and microscopic colitis, and choleraic diarrhea (from ileal malabsorption of bile salts).

■ EXUDATIVE DIARRHEA

Inflammation, necrosis, and sloughing of colonic mucosa; may include component of secretory diarrhea due to prostaglandin release by inflammatory cells; stools usually contain polymorphonuclear leukocytes as well as occult or gross blood. Causes include bacterial infections [e.g., *Campylobacter*, *Salmonella*, *Shigella*, *Yersinia*, invasive or enterotoxigenic *E. coli*, *Vibrio parahaemolyticus*, *Clostridium difficile* colitis (frequently antibiotic-induced)], colonic parasites (e.g., *Entamoeba histolytica*), Crohn's disease, ulcerative proctocolitis, idiopathic inflammatory bowel disease, radiation enterocolitis, cancer chemotherapeutic agents, and intestinal ischemia.

■ ALTERED INTESTINAL MOTILITY

Alteration of coordinated control of intestinal propulsion; diarrhea often intermittent or alternating with constipation. Causes include diabetes mellitus, adrenal insufficiency, hyperthyroidism, collagen-vascular diseases, parasitic infestations, gastrin and VIP hypersecretory states, amyloidosis, laxatives (esp. magnesium-containing agents), antibiotics (esp. erythromycin), cholinergic agents, primary neurologic dysfunction (e.g., Parkinson's disease, traumatic neuropathy), fecal impaction, diverticular disease, and irritable bowel syndrome. Blood in intestinal lumen is cathartic, and major upper GI bleeding leads to diarrhea from increased motility.

■ DECREASED ABSORPTIVE SURFACE

Usually arises from surgical manipulation (e.g., extensive bowel resection or rearrangement) that leaves inadequate absorptive surface for fat and carbohydrate digestion and fluid and electrolyte absorption; occurs spontaneously from enteroenteric fistulas (esp. gastrocolic).

■ EVALUATION HISTORY

Diarrhea must be distinguished from fecal incontinence, change in stool caliber, rectal bleeding, and small, frequent, but otherwise normal stools. Careful medication history is essential. Alternating diarrhea and constipation suggests fixed colonic obstruction (e.g., from carcinoma) or irritable bowel syndrome. A sudden, acute course, often with nausea, vomiting, and fever, is typical of viral and bacterial infections, diverticulitis, ischemia, radiation enterocolitis, or drug-induced diarrhea and may be the initial presentation of inflammatory bowel disease. More than 90% of acute diarrheal illnesses are infectious in etiology. A longer (>4 weeks), more insidious course suggests malabsorption, inflammatory bowel disease, metabolic or endocrine disturbance, pancreatic insufficiency, laxative abuse, ischemia, neoplasm (hypersecretory state or partial obstruction), or irritable bowel syndrome. Parasitic and certain forms of bacterial enteritis can also produce chronic symptoms. Particularly foul-smelling or oily stool suggests fat

TABLE 46-1 INFECTIOUS CAUSES OF DIARRHEA IN PATIENTS WITH AIDS

Nonopportunistic Pathogens	Opportunistic Pathogens
Shigella	Protozoa
Salmonella	Cryptosporidium
Campylobacter	Isospora belli
Entamoeba histolytica	Microsporidia
Chlamydia	Blastocystis hominis
Neisseria gonorrhoeae	Viruses
Treponema pallidum and other spirochetes	Cytomegalovirus
Giardia lamblia	Herpes simplex
	Adenovirus
	HIV
	Bacteria
	Mycobacterium avium complex

malabsorption. Fecal impaction may cause apparent diarrhea because only liquids pass partial obstruction. Several infectious causes of diarrhea are associated with an immunocompromised state (Table 46-1).

■ **PHYSICAL EXAMINATION**

Signs of dehydration are often prominent in severe, acute diarrhea. Fever and abdominal tenderness suggest infection or inflammatory disease but are often absent in viral enteritis. Evidence of malnutrition suggests chronic course. Certain signs are frequently associated with specific deficiency states secondary to malabsorption (e.g., cheilosis with riboflavin or iron deficiency, glossitis with B$_{12}$, folate deficiency). Questions to address in pts with chronic diarrhea are shown in Table 46-2.

TABLE 46-2 PHYSICAL EXAMINATION IN PATIENTS WITH CHRONIC DIARRHEA

1. Are there general features to suggest malabsorption or inflammatory bowel disease (IBD) such as anemia, dermatitis herpetiformis, edema, or clubbing?

2. Are there features to suggest underlying autonomic neuropathy or collagen-vascular disease in the pupils, orthostasis, skin, hands, or joints?

3. Is there an abdominal mass or tenderness?

4. Are there any abnormalities of rectal mucosa, rectal defects, or altered anal sphincter functions?

5. Are there any mucocutaneous manifestations of systemic disease such as dermatitis herpetiformis (celiac disease), erythema nodosum (ulcerative colitis), flushing (carcinoid), or oral ulcers for IBD or celiac disease?

■ STOOL EXAMINATION

Culture for bacterial pathogens, examination for leukocytes, measurement of *C. difficile* toxin, and examination for ova and parasites are important components of evaluation of pts with severe, protracted, or bloody diarrhea. Presence of blood (fecal occult blood test) or leukocytes (Wright's stain) suggests inflammation (e.g., ulcerative colitis, Crohn's disease, infection, or ischemia). Gram's stain of stool can be diagnostic of *Staphylococcus*, *Campylobacter*, or *Candida* infection. Steatorrhea (determined with Sudan III stain of stool sample or 72-h quantitative fecal fat analysis) suggests malabsorption or pancreatic insufficiency. Measurement of Na^+ and K^+ levels in fecal water helps to distinguish osmotic from other types of diarrhea; osmotic diarrhea is implied by stool osmolal gap > 40, where stool osmolal gap = $osmol_{serum} [2 \times (Na^+ + K^+)_{stool}]$.

■ LABORATORY STUDIES

Complete blood count may indicate anemia (acute or chronic blood loss or malabsorption of iron, folate, or B_{12}), leukocytosis (inflammation), eosinophilia (parasitic, neoplastic, and inflammatory bowel diseases). Serum levels of calcium, albumin, iron, cholesterol, folate, B_{12}, vitamin D, and carotene; serum iron-binding capacity; and prothrombin time can provide evidence of intestinal malabsorption or maldigestion.

■ OTHER STUDIES

D-Xylose absorption test is a convenient screen for small-bowel absorptive function. Small-bowel biopsy is especially useful for evaluating intestinal malabsorption. Specialized studies include Schilling test (B_{12} malabsorption), lactose H_2 breath test (carbohydrate malabsorption), [^{14}C]xylose and lactulose H_2 breath tests (bacterial overgrowth), glycocholic breath test (ileal malabsorption), triolein breath test (fat malabsorption), and bentiromide and secretin tests (pancreatic insufficiency). Sigmoidoscopy or colonoscopy with biopsy is useful in the diagnosis of colitis (esp. pseudomembranous, ischemic, microscopic); it may not allow distinction between infectious and noninfectious (esp. idiopathic ulcerative) colitis. Barium contrast x-ray studies may suggest malabsorption (thickened bowel folds), inflammatory bowel disease (ileitis or colitis), tuberculosis (ileocecal inflammation), neoplasm, intestinal fistula, or motility disorders.

| TREATMENT | Diarrhea |

An approach to the management of acute diarrheal illnesses is shown in Fig. 46-1. Symptomatic therapy includes vigorous rehydration (IV or with oral glucose-electrolyte solutions), electrolyte replacement, binders of osmotically active substances (e.g., kaolin-pectin), and opiates to decrease bowel motility (e.g., loperamide, diphenoxylate); opiates may be contraindicated in infectious or inflammatory causes of diarrhea. An approach to the management of chronic diarrhea is shown in Fig. 46-2.

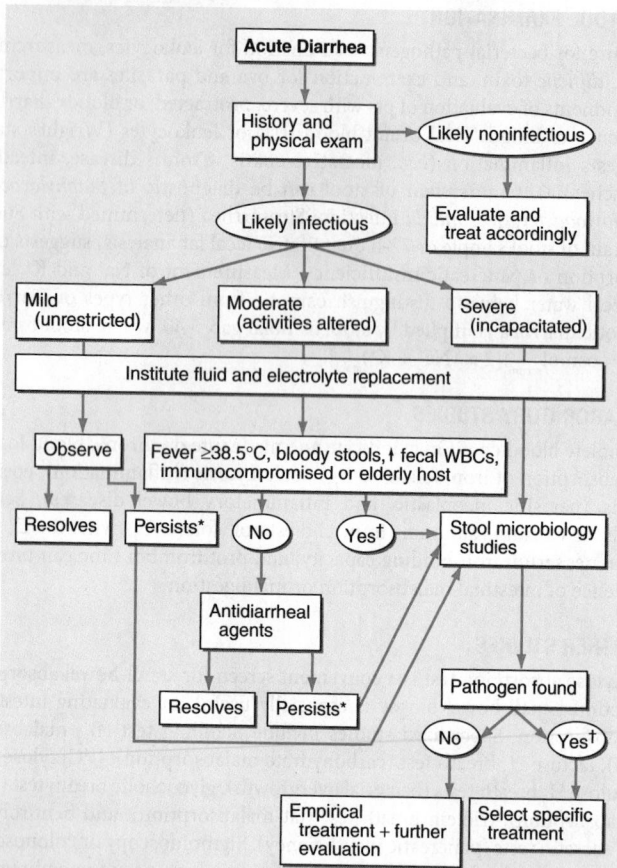

FIGURE 46-1 Algorithm for the management of acute diarrhea. Before evaluation, consider empiric RX with (*) metronidazole and with (†) quinolone.

MALABSORPTION SYNDROMES

Intestinal malabsorption of ingested nutrients may produce osmotic diarrhea, steatorrhea, or specific deficiencies (e.g., iron; folate; B$_{12}$; vitamins A, D, E, and K). Table 46-3 lists common causes of intestinal malabsorption. Protein-losing enteropathy may result from several causes of malabsorption; it is associated with hypoalbuminemia and can be detected by measuring stool α_1-antitrypsin or radiolabeled albumin levels. Therapy is directed at the underlying disease.

CONSTIPATION

Defined as decrease in frequency of stools to <1 per week or difficulty in defecation; may result in abdominal pain, distention, and fecal impaction, with consequent obstruction or, rarely, perforation. Constipation is a frequent and often subjective complaint. Contributory factors may include inactivity, low-fiber diet, and inadequate allotment of time for defecation.

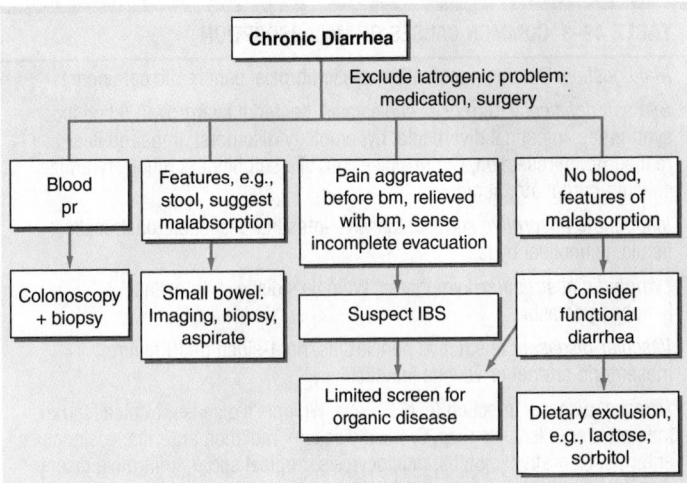

FIGURE 46-2 Algorithm for the management of chronic diarrhea based on accompanying symptoms or features (*A*) or based on a limited screening for organic disease (*B*). pr, per rectum; bm, bowel movement; IBS, irritable bowel syndrome; Hb, hemoglobin; Alb, albumin; MCV, mean corpuscular volume; MCH, mean corpuscular hemoglobin; OSM, osmolality. (*Reprinted from M Camilleri: Clin Gastrol Hepatol. 2:198, 2004.*)

■ SPECIFIC CAUSES

Altered colonic motility due to neurologic dysfunction (diabetes mellitus, spinal cord injury, multiple sclerosis, Chagas' disease, Hirschsprung's disease, chronic idiopathic intestinal pseudoobstruction, idiopathic megacolon), scleroderma, drugs (esp. anticholinergic agents, opiates, aluminum- or

TABLE 46-3 COMMON CAUSES OF MALABSORPTION

Maldigestion: Chronic pancreatitis, cystic fibrosis, pancreatic carcinoma

Bile salt deficiency: Cirrhosis, cholestasis, bacterial overgrowth (blind loop syndromes, intestinal diverticula, hypomotility disorders), impaired ileal reabsorption (resection, Crohn's disease), bile salt binders (cholestyramine, calcium carbonate, neomycin)

Inadequate absorptive surface: Massive intestinal resection, gastrocolic fistula, jejunoileal bypass

Lymphatic obstruction: Lymphoma, Whipple's disease, intestinal lymphangiectasia

Vascular disease: Constrictive pericarditis, right-sided heart failure, mesenteric arterial or venous insufficiency

Mucosal disease: Infection (esp. *Giardia*, Whipple's disease, tropical sprue), inflammatory diseases (esp. Crohn's disease), radiation enteritis, eosinophilic enteritis, ulcerative jejunitis, mastocytosis, tropical sprue, infiltrative disorders (amyloidosis, scleroderma, lymphoma, collagenous sprue, microscopic colitis), biochemical abnormalities (gluten-sensitive enteropathy, disaccharidase deficiency, hypogammaglobulinemia, abetalipoproteinemia, amino acid transport deficiencies), endocrine disorders (diabetes mellitus, hypoparathyroidism, adrenal insufficiency, hyperthyroidism, Zollinger-Ellison syndrome, carcinoid syndrome)

calcium-based antacids, calcium channel blockers, iron supplements, sucralfate), hypothyroidism, Cushing's syndrome, hypokalemia, hypercalcemia, dehydration, mechanical causes (colorectal tumors, diverticulitis, volvulus, hernias, intussusception), and anorectal pain (from fissures, hemorrhoids, abscesses, or proctitis) leading to retention, constipation, and fecal impaction.

TREATMENT   Constipation

A management approach is shown in Fig. 46-3. In absence of identifiable cause, constipation may improve with reassurance, exercise, increased dietary fiber, bulking agents (e.g., psyllium), and increased fluid intake. Specific therapies include removal of bowel obstruction (fecalith, tumor), discontinuance of nonessential hypomotility agents (esp. aluminum- or calcium-containing antacids, opiates), or substitution of magnesium-based antacids for aluminum-based antacids. For symptomatic relief, magnesium-containing agents or other cathartics are occasionally needed. With severe hypo- or dysmotility or in presence of opiates, osmotically active agents (e.g., oral lactulose, intestinal polyethylene glycol–containing lavage solutions) and oral or rectal emollient laxatives (e.g., docusate salts) and mineral oil are most effective.

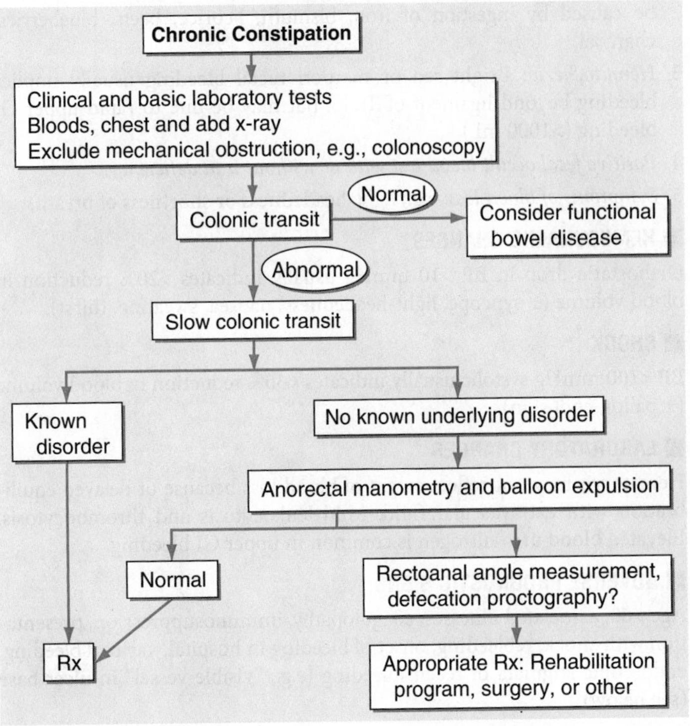

Chronic Constipation

↓

Clinical and basic laboratory tests
Bloods, chest and abd x-ray
Exclude mechanical obstruction, e.g., colonoscopy

↓

Colonic transit —— (Normal) ——→ Consider functional bowel disease

(Abnormal)

↓

Slow colonic transit

↓

Known disorder

No known underlying disorder

↓

Anorectal manometry and balloon expulsion

Normal

Rectoanal angle measurement, defecation proctography?

↓

Rx

Appropriate Rx: Rehabilitation program, surgery, or other

FIGURE 46-3 Algorithm for the management of chronic constipation.

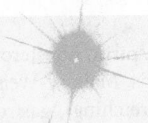

For a more detailed discussion, see Camilleri M, Murray JA: Diarrhea and Constipation, Chap. 40, p. 308; and Binder HJ: Disorders of Absorption, Chap. 294, p. 2460, in HPIM-18.

CHAPTER **47**
Gastrointestinal Bleeding

PRESENTATION

1. *Hematemesis*: Vomiting of blood or altered blood ("coffee grounds") indicates bleeding proximal to ligament of Treitz.

2. *Melena*: Altered (black) blood per rectum (>100 mL blood required for one melenic stool) usually indicates bleeding proximal to ligament of Treitz but may be as distal as ascending colon; pseudomelena may

be caused by ingestion of iron, bismuth, licorice, beets, blueberries, charcoal.

3. *Hematochezia*: Bright red or maroon rectal bleeding usually implies bleeding beyond ligament of Treitz but may be due to rapid upper GI bleeding (>1000 mL).

4. *Positive fecal occult blood test with or without iron deficiency*.

5. *Symptoms of blood loss*: e.g., light-headedness or shortness of breath.

■ HEMODYNAMIC CHANGES

Orthostatic drop in BP >10 mmHg usually indicates >20% reduction in blood volume (± syncope, light-headedness, nausea, sweating, thirst).

■ SHOCK

BP <100 mmHg systolic usually indicates <30% reduction in blood volume (± pallor, cool skin).

■ LABORATORY CHANGES

Hematocrit may not reflect extent of blood loss because of delayed equilibration with extravascular fluid. Mild leukocytosis and thrombocytosis. Elevated blood urea nitrogen is common in upper GI bleeding.

■ ADVERSE PROGNOSTIC SIGNS

Age >60, associated illnesses, coagulopathy, immunosuppression, presentation with shock, rebleeding, onset of bleeding in hospital, variceal bleeding, endoscopic stigmata of recent bleeding [e.g., "visible vessel" in ulcer base (see below)].

UPPER GI BLEEDING

■ CAUSES

Common

Peptic ulcer (accounts for ~50%), gastropathy [alcohol, aspirin, nonsteroidal anti-inflammatory drugs (NSAIDs), stress], esophagitis, Mallory-Weiss tear (mucosal tear at gastroesophageal junction due to retching), gastroesophageal varices.

Less Common

Swallowed blood (nosebleed); esophageal, gastric, or intestinal neoplasm; anticoagulant and fibrinolytic therapy; hypertrophic gastropathy (Ménétrier's disease); aortic aneurysm; aortoenteric fistula (from aortic graft); arteriovenous malformation; telangiectases (Osler-Rendu-Weber syndrome); Dieulafoy lesion (ectatic submucosal vessel); vasculitis; connective tissue disease (pseudoxanthoma elasticum, Ehlers-Danlos syndrome); blood dyscrasias; neurofibroma; amyloidosis; hemobilia (biliary origin).

■ EVALUATION

After hemodynamic resuscitation (see below and Fig. 47-1).

- History and physical examination: Drugs (increased risk of upper and lower GI tract bleeding with aspirin and NSAIDs), prior ulcer, bleeding

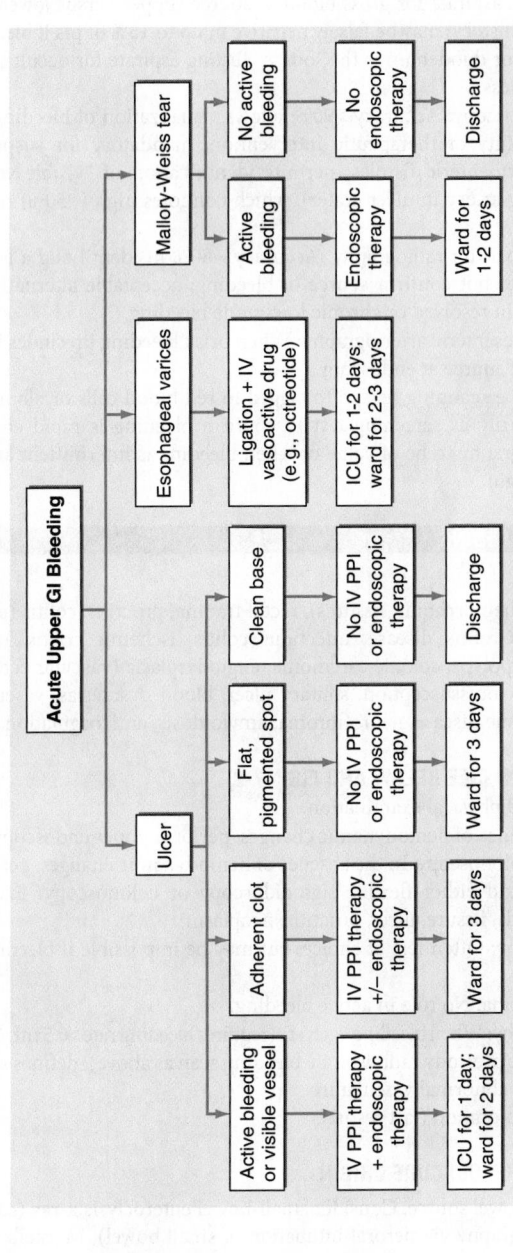

FIGURE 47-1 Suggested algorithm for pts with acute upper GI bleeding. Recommendations on level of care and time of discharge assume pt is stabilized without further bleeding or other concomitant medical problems. ICU, intensive care unit; PPI, proton pump inhibitor.

263

history, family history, features of cirrhosis or vasculitis, etc. Hyperactive bowel sounds favor upper GI source.

- Nasogastric aspirate for gross blood, if source (upper versus lower) not clear from history; may be falsely negative in up to 16% of pts if bleeding has ceased or duodenum is the source. Testing aspirate for occult blood is meaningless.
- Upper endoscopy: Accuracy >90%; allows visualization of bleeding site and possibility of therapeutic intervention; mandatory for suspected varices, aortoenteric fistulas; permits identification of "visible vessel" (protruding artery in ulcer crater), which connotes high (~50%) risk of rebleeding.
- Upper GI barium radiography: Accuracy ~80% in identifying a lesion, though does not confirm source of bleeding; acceptable alternative to endoscopy in resolved or chronic low-grade bleeding.
- Selective mesenteric arteriography: When brisk bleeding precludes identification of source at endoscopy.
- Radioisotope scanning (e.g., ^{99}Tc tagged to red blood cells or albumin); used primarily as screening test to confirm bleeding is rapid enough for arteriography to be of value or when bleeding is intermittent and of unclear origin.

LOWER GI BLEEDING

■ CAUSES

Anal lesions (hemorrhoids, fissures), rectal trauma, proctitis, colitis (ulcerative colitis, Crohn's disease, infectious colitis, ischemic colitis, radiation), colonic polyps, colonic carcinoma, angiodysplasia (vascular ectasia), diverticulosis, intussusception, solitary ulcer, blood dyscrasias, vasculitis, connective tissue disease, neurofibroma, amyloidosis, anticoagulation.

■ EVALUATION (SEE BELOW AND FIG. 47-2)

- History and physical examination.
- In the presence of hemodynamic changes, perform upper endoscopy followed by colonoscopy. In the absence of hemodynamic changes, perform anoscopy and either flexible sigmoidoscopy or colonoscopy: Exclude hemorrhoids, fissure, ulcer, proctitis, neoplasm.
- Colonoscopy: Often test of choice, but may be impossible if bleeding is massive.
- Barium enema: No role in active bleeding.
- Arteriography: When bleeding is severe (requires bleeding rate >0.5 mL/min; may require prestudy radioisotope bleeding scan as above); defines site of bleeding or abnormal vasculature.
- Surgical exploration (last resort).

■ BLEEDING OF OBSCURE ORIGIN

Often small-bowel source. Consider small-bowel enteroclysis x-ray (careful barium radiography via peroral intubation of small bowel), Meckel's scan, enteroscopy (small-bowel endoscopy), or exploratory laparotomy with intraoperative enteroscopy.

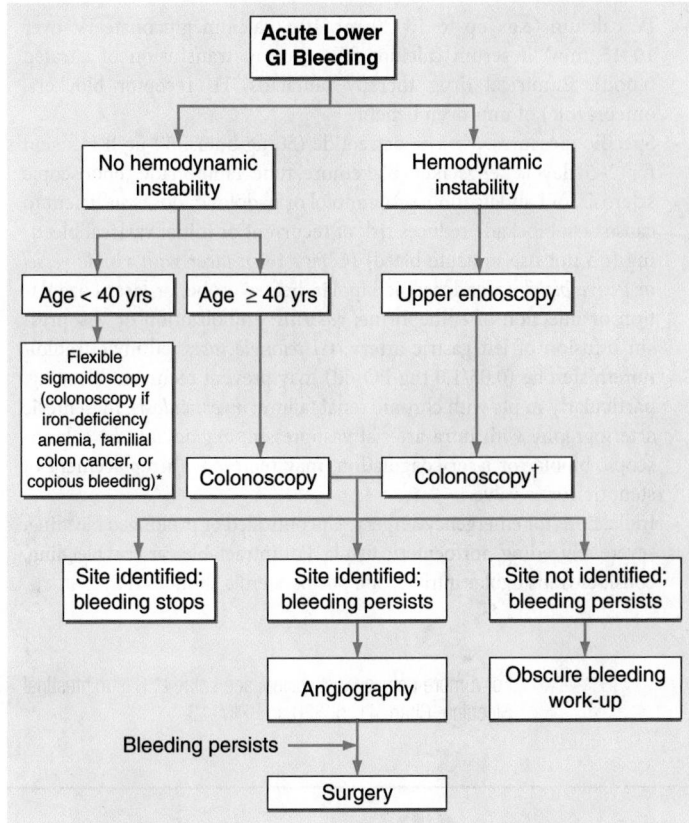

FIGURE 47-2 Suggested algorithm for pts with acute lower gastrointestinal bleeding. *Some suggest colonoscopy for any degree of rectal bleeding in pts <40 years as well. †If massive bleeding does not allow time for colonic lavage, proceed to angiography.

TREATMENT Upper and Lower GI Bleeding

- Venous access with large-bore IV (14–18 gauge); central venous line for major bleed and pts with cardiac disease; monitor vital signs, urine output, Hct (fall may lag). Gastric lavage of unproven benefit but clears stomach before endoscopy. Iced saline may lyse clots; room-temperature tap water may be preferable. Intubation may be required to protect airway.
- Type and cross-match blood (6 units for major bleed).
- Surgical standby when bleeding is massive.
- Support blood pressure with isotonic fluids (normal saline); albumin and fresh-frozen plasma in cirrhotics. Packed red blood cells when available (whole blood if massive bleeding); maintain Hct >25–30. Fresh-frozen plasma and vitamin K (10 mg SC or IV) in cirrhotics with coagulopathy.

- IV calcium (e.g., up to 10–20 mL 10% calcium gluconate IV over 10–15 min) if serum calcium falls (due to transfusion of citrated blood). Empirical drug therapy (antacids, H$_2$ receptor blockers, omeprazole) of unproven benefit.
- Specific measures: *Varices*: octreotide (50-µg bolus, 50-µg/h infusion for 2–5 days), Sengstaken-Blakemore tube tamponade, endoscopic sclerosis, or band ligation; propranolol or nadolol in doses sufficient to cause beta blockade reduces risk of recurrent or initial variceal bleeding (do not use in acute bleed) (Chap. 166); *ulcer with visible vessel or active bleeding*: endoscopic bipolar, heater-probe, or laser coagulation or injection of epinephrine; *gastritis*: embolization or vasopressin infusion of left gastric artery; *GI telangiectases*: ethinylestradiol/norethisterone (0.05/1.0 mg PO qd) may prevent recurrent bleeding, particularly in pts with chronic renal failure; *diverticulosis*: mesenteric arteriography with intra-arterial vasopressin; *angiodysplasia*: colonoscopic bipolar or laser coagulation, may regress with replacement of stenotic aortic valve.
- Indications for emergency surgery: Uncontrolled or prolonged bleeding, severe rebleeding, aortoenteric fistula. For intractable variceal bleeding, consider transjugular intrahepatic portosystemic shunt (TIPS).

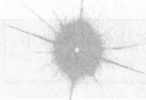

For a more detailed discussion, see Laine L: Gastrointestinal Bleeding, Chap. 41, p. 320, in HPIM-18.

CHAPTER 48
Jaundice and Evaluation of Liver Function

■ JAUNDICE

Definition

Yellow skin pigmentation caused by elevation in serum bilirubin level (also termed *icterus*); often more easily discernible in sclerae. Scleral icterus becomes clinically evident at a serum bilirubin level of ≥51 µmol/L (≥3 mg/dL); yellow skin discoloration also occurs with elevated serum carotene levels but without pigmentation of the sclerae.

Bilirubin Metabolism

Bilirubin is the major breakdown product of hemoglobin released from senescent erythrocytes. Initially, it is bound to albumin, transported into the liver, conjugated to a water-soluble form (glucuronide) by glucuronosyl transferase, excreted into the bile, and converted to urobilinogen in the colon. Urobilinogen is mostly excreted in the stool; a small portion is reabsorbed and excreted by the kidney. Bilirubin can be filtered by the kidney only in its conjugated form (measured as the "direct" fraction); thus, increased *direct* serum bilirubin level is associated with bilirubinuria. Increased bilirubin production and excretion (even without hyperbilirubinemia, as in hemolysis) produce elevated urinary urobilinogen levels.

Etiology

Hyperbilirubinemia occurs as a result of (1) overproduction; (2) impaired uptake, conjugation, or excretion of bilirubin; (3) regurgitation of unconjugated or conjugated bilirubin from damaged hepatocytes or bile ducts (Table 48-1).

TABLE 48-1 CAUSES OF ISOLATED HYPERBILIRUBINEMIA

I. Indirect hyperbilirubinemia

   A. Hemolytic disorders

      1. Inherited

         a. Spherocytosis, elliptocytosis

         b. Glucose-6-phosphate dehydrogenase and pyruvate kinase deficiencies

         c. Sickle cell anemia

      2. Acquired

         a. Microangiopathic hemolytic anemias

         b. Paroxysmal nocturnal hemoglobinuria

         c. Spur cell anemia

         d. Immune hemolysis

         e. Parasitic infections

            1. Malaria

            2. Babesiosis

   B. Ineffective erythropoiesis

      1. Cobalamin, folate, thalassemia, and severe iron deficiencies

   C. Drugs

      1. Rifampicin, probenecid, ribavirin

   D. Inherited conditions

      1. Crigler-Najjar types I and II

      2. Gilbert's syndrome

II. Direct hyperbilirubinemia

   A. Inherited conditions

      1. Dubin-Johnson syndrome

      2. Rotor's syndrome

Physical examination: *Evaluate abdomen* for prior trauma or surgery, current trauma; abdominal distention, fluid, or air; direct, rebound, and referred tenderness; liver and spleen size; masses, bruits, altered bowel sounds, hernias, arterial masses. Rectal examination assesses presence and location of tenderness, masses, blood (gross or occult). Pelvic examination in women is essential. *General examination*: evaluate for evidence of hemodynamic instability, acid-base disturbances, nutritional deficiency, coagulopathy, arterial occlusive disease, stigmata of liver disease, cardiac dysfunction, lymphadenopathy, and skin lesions.

Routine laboratory and radiologic studies: Choices depend on clinical setting (esp. severity of pain, rapidity of onset) and may include complete blood count, serum electrolytes, coagulation parameters, serum glucose, and biochemical tests of liver, kidney, and pancreatic function; chest x-ray to determine the presence of diseases involving heart, lung, mediastinum, and pleura; electrocardiogram is helpful to exclude referred pain from cardiac disease; plain abdominal radiographs to evaluate bowel displacement, intestinal distention, fluid and gas pattern, free peritoneal air, liver size, and abdominal calcifications (e.g., gallstones, renal stones, chronic pancreatitis).

Special studies: These include abdominal ultrasonography (to visualize biliary ducts, gallbladder, liver, pancreas, and kidneys); CT to identify masses, abscesses, evidence of inflammation (bowel wall thickening, mesenteric "stranding," lymphadenopathy), aortic aneurysm; barium contrast radiographs (barium swallow, upper GI series, small-bowel follow-through, barium enema); upper GI endoscopy, sigmoidoscopy, or colonoscopy; cholangiography (endoscopic, percutaneous, or via MRI), angiography (direct or via CT or MRI), and radionuclide scanning. In selected cases, percutaneous biopsy, laparoscopy, and exploratory laparotomy may be required.

ACUTE, CATASTROPHIC ABDOMINAL PAIN

Intense abdominal pain of acute onset or pain associated with syncope, hypotension, or toxic appearance necessitates rapid yet orderly evaluation. Consider obstruction, perforation, or rupture of hollow viscus; dissection or rupture of major blood vessels (esp. aortic aneurysm); ulceration; abdominal sepsis; ketoacidosis; and adrenal crisis.

■ BRIEF HISTORY AND PHYSICAL EXAMINATION

Historic features of importance include age; time of onset of the pain; activity of the pt when the pain began; location and character of the pain; radiation to other sites; presence of nausea, vomiting, or anorexia; temporal changes; changes in bowel habits; and menstrual history. Physical exam should focus on the pt's overall appearance [writhing in pain (ureteral

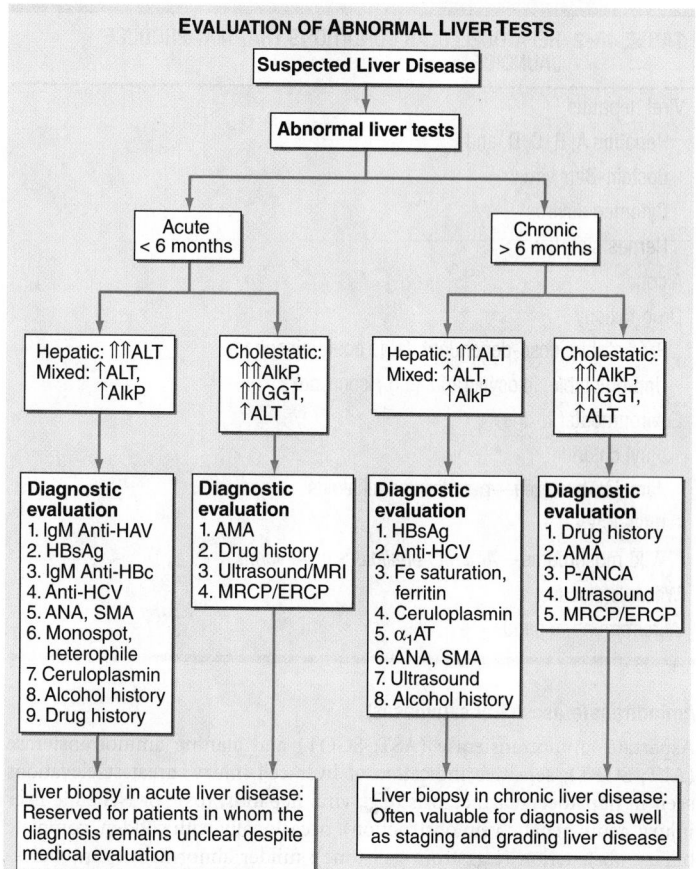

FIGURE 48-2 Algorithm for evaluation of abnormal liver tests.

Gilbert's Syndrome

Impaired conjugation of bilirubin due to reduced bilirubin UDP glucuronosyl transferase activity. Results in mild unconjugated hyperbilirubinemia, almost always <103 μmol/L (<6 mg/dL). Affects 3–7% of the population; males/females 2–7:1.

■ BLOOD TESTS OF LIVER FUNCTION

Used to detect presence of liver disease (Fig. 48-2), discriminate among different types of liver disease (Table 48-4), gauge the extent of known liver damage, and follow response to treatment.

Bilirubin

Provides indication of hepatic uptake, metabolic (conjugation) and excretory functions; conjugated fraction (direct) distinguished from unconjugated by chemical assay (Table 48-1).

TABLE 48-2   HEPATOCELLULAR CONDITIONS THAT MAY PRODUCE JAUNDICE

Viral hepatitis
   Hepatitis A, B, C, D, and E
   Epstein-Barr virus
   Cytomegalovirus
   Herpes simplex
Alcohol
Drug toxicity
   Predictable, dose-dependent, (e.g., acetaminophen)
   Unpredictable, idiosyncratic, (e.g., isoniazid)
Environmental toxins
   Vinyl chloride
   Jamaica bush tea—pyrrolizidine alkaloids
   Kava Kava
   Wild mushrooms—*Amanita phalloides* or *A. verna*
Wilson's disease
Autoimmune hepatitis

Aminotransferases (Transaminases)

Aspartate aminotransferase (AST; SGOT) and alanine aminotransferase (ALT; SGPT); sensitive indicators of liver cell injury; greatest elevations seen in hepatocellular necrosis (e.g., viral hepatitis, toxic or ischemic liver injury, acute hepatic vein obstruction), occasionally with sudden, complete biliary obstruction (e.g., from gallstone); milder abnormalities in cholestatic, cirrhotic, and infiltrative disease; poor correlation between degree of liver cell damage and level of aminotransferases; ALT more specific measure of liver injury, since AST also found in striated muscle and other organs; ethanol-induced liver injury usually produces modest increases with more prominent elevation of AST than ALT.

Alkaline Phosphatase

Sensitive indicator of cholestasis, biliary obstruction (enzyme increases more quickly than serum bilirubin), and liver infiltration; mild elevations in other forms of liver disease; limited specificity because of wide tissue distribution; elevations also seen in normal childhood, pregnancy, and bone diseases; tissue-specific isoenzymes can be distinguished by fractionation or by differences in heat stability (liver enzyme activity stable under conditions that destroy bone enzyme activity).

5′-Nucleotidase (5′-NT)

Pattern of elevation in hepatobiliary disease similar to alkaline phosphatase; has greater specificity for liver disorders; used to determine whether liver

TABLE 48-3 CHOLESTATIC CONDITIONS THAT MAY PRODUCE JAUNDICE

I. Intrahepatic

  A. Viral hepatitis

    1. Fibrosing cholestatic hepatitis—hepatitis B and C

    2. Hepatitis A, Epstein-Barr virus, cytomegalovirus

  B. Alcoholic hepatitis

  C. Drug toxicity

    1. Pure cholestasis—anabolic and contraceptive steroids

    2. Cholestatic hepatitis—chlorpromazine, erythromycin estolate

    3. Chronic cholestasis—chlorpromazine and prochlorperazine

  D. Primary biliary cirrhosis

  E. Primary sclerosing cholangitis

  F. Vanishing bile duct syndrome

    1. Chronic rejection of liver transplants

    2. Sarcoidosis

    3. Drugs

  G. Inherited

    1. Progressive familial intrahepatic cholestasis

    2. Benign recurrent cholestasis

  H. Cholestasis of pregnancy

  I. Total parenteral nutrition

  J. Nonhepatobiliary sepsis

  K. Benign postoperative cholestasis

  L. Paraneoplastic syndrome

  M. Venoocclusive disease

  N. Graft-versus-host disease

  O. Infiltrative disease

    1. TB

    2. Lymphoma

    3. Amyloidosis

II. Extrahepatic

  A. Malignant

    1. Cholangiocarcinoma

    2. Pancreatic cancer

    3. Gallbladder cancer

    4. Ampullary cancer

    5. Malignant involvement of the porta hepatis lymph nodes

(*continued*)

TABLE 48-3 CHOLESTATIC CONDITIONS THAT MAY PRODUCE JAUNDICE (CONTINUED)

B. Benign
  1. Choledocholithiasis
  2. Postoperative biliary structures
  3. Primary sclerosing cholangitis
  4. Chronic pancreatitis
  5. AIDS cholangiopathy
  6. Mirizzi syndrome
  7. Parasitic disease (ascariasis)

---

is source of elevation in serum alkaline phosphatase, esp. in children, pregnant women, pts with possible concomitant bone disease.

γ-Glutamyltranspeptidase (GGT)

Correlates with serum alkaline phosphatase activity. Elevation is less specific for cholestasis than alkaline phosphatase or 5′-NT.

TABLE 48-4 LIVER TEST PATTERNS IN HEPATOBILIARY DISORDERS

Type of Disorder	Bilirubin	Aminotransferases
Hemolysis/Gilbert's syndrome	Normal to 86 µmol/L (5 mg/dL) 85% due to indirect fractions No bilirubinuria	Normal
Acute hepatocellular necrosis (viral and drug hepatitis, hepatotoxins, acute heart failure)	Both fractions may be elevated Peak usually follows aminotransferases Bilirubinuria	Elevated, often >500 IU ALT >AST
Chronic hepatocellular disorders	Both fractions may be elevated Bilirubinuria	Elevated, but usually <300 IU
Alcoholic hepatitis Cirrhosis	Both fractions may be elevated Bilirubinuria	AST:ALT > 2 suggests alcoholic hepatitis or cirrhosis
Intra- and extra-hepatic cholestasis (Obstructive jaundice)	Both fractions may be elevated Bilirubinuria	Normal to moderate elevation Rarely >500 IU
Infiltrative diseases (tumor, granulomata); partial bile duct obstruction	Usually normal	Normal to slight elevation

TABLE 48-4   LIVER TEST PATTERNS IN HEPATOBILIARY DISORDERS (CONTINUED)

Alkaline Phosphatase	Albumin	Prothrombin Time
Normal	Normal	Normal
Normal to <3 times normal elevation	Normal	Usually normal. If >5 × above control and not corrected by parenteral vitamin K, suggests poor prognosis
Normal to <3 times normal elevation	Often decreased	Often prolonged Fails to correct with parenteral vitamin K
Normal to <3 times normal elevation	Often decreased	Often prolonged Fails to correct with parenteral vitamin K
Elevated, often >4 times normal elevation	Normal, unless chronic	Normal If prolonged, will correct with parenteral vitamin K
Elevated, often >4 times normal elevation Fractionate, or confirm liver origin with 5′ nucleotidase or γ glutamyl transpeptidase	Normal	Normal

Coagulation Factors (See also Chap. 70)

Measure of clotting factor activity; prolongation results from clotting factor deficiency or inactivity; all clotting factors except factor VIII are synthesized in the liver, and deficiency can occur rapidly from widespread liver disease as in hepatitis, toxic injury, or cirrhosis; single best acute measure of hepatic synthetic function; helpful in Dx and prognosis of acute liver disease. Clotting factors II, VII, IX, X function only in the presence of the fat-soluble vitamin K; PT prolongation from fat malabsorption distinguished from hepatic disease by rapid and complete response to vitamin K replacement.

Albumin

Decreased serum levels result from decreased hepatic synthesis (chronic liver disease or prolonged malnutrition) or excessive losses in urine or stool; insensitive indicator of acute hepatic dysfunction, since serum half-life is 2–3 weeks; in pts with chronic liver disease, degree of hypoalbuminemia correlates with severity of liver dysfunction.

Globulin

Mild polyclonal hyperglobulinemia often seen in chronic liver diseases; marked elevation frequently seen in *autoimmune* chronic active hepatitis.

Ammonia

Elevated blood levels result from deficiency of hepatic detoxification pathways and portal-systemic shunting, as in fulminant hepatitis, hepatotoxin exposure, and severe portal hypertension (e.g., from cirrhosis); elevation of blood ammonia does not correlate well with hepatic function or the presence or degree of acute encephalopathy.

■ HEPATOBILIARY IMAGING PROCEDURES

Ultrasonography (US)

Rapid, noninvasive examination of abdominal structures; no radiation exposure; relatively low cost, equipment portable; images and interpretation strongly dependent on expertise of examiner; particularly valuable for detecting biliary duct dilatation and gallbladder stones (>95%); much less sensitive for intraductal stones (~60%); most sensitive means of detecting ascites; moderately sensitive for detecting hepatic masses but excellent for discriminating solid from cystic structures; useful in directing percutaneous needle biopsies of suspicious lesions; Doppler US useful to determine patency and flow in portal, hepatic veins and portal-systemic shunts; imaging improved by presence of ascites but severely hindered by bowel gas; endoscopic US less affected by bowel gas and is sensitive for determination of depth of tumor invasion through bowel wall.

CT

Particularly useful for detecting, differentiating, and directing percutaneous needle biopsy of abdominal masses, cysts, and lymphadenopathy; imaging enhanced by intestinal or intravenous contrast dye and unaffected by intestinal gas; somewhat less sensitive than US for detecting stones in gallbladder but more sensitive for choledocholithiasis; may be useful in distinguishing certain forms of diffuse hepatic disease (e.g., fatty infiltration, iron overload).

MRI

Most sensitive detection of hepatic masses and cysts; allows easy differentiation of hemangiomas from other hepatic tumors; most accurate noninvasive means of assessing hepatic and portal vein patency, vascular invasion by tumor; useful for monitoring iron, copper deposition in liver (e.g., in hemochromatosis, Wilson's disease). Magnetic resonance cholangiopancreatography (MRCP) can be useful for visualizing the head of the pancreas and the pancreatic and biliary ducts.

Radionuclide Scanning

Using various radiolabeled compounds, different scanning methods allow sensitive assessment of biliary excretion (HIDA, PIPIDA, DISIDA scans), parenchymal changes (technetium sulfur colloid liver/spleen scan), and selected inflammatory and neoplastic processes (gallium scan); HIDA and related scans particularly useful for assessing biliary patency and excluding acute cholecystitis in situations where US is not diagnostic; CT, MRI, and colloid scans have similar sensitivity for detecting liver tumors and metastases; CT and combination of colloidal liver and lung scans sensitive for detecting right subphrenic (suprahepatic) abscesses.

Cholangiography

Most sensitive means of detecting biliary ductal calculi, biliary tumors, sclerosing cholangitis, choledochal cysts, fistulas, and bile duct leaks; may be performed via endoscopic (transampullary) or percutaneous (transhepatic) route; allows sampling of bile and ductal epithelium for cytologic analysis and culture; allows placement of biliary drainage catheter and stricture dilatation; endoscopic route (ERCP) permits manometric evaluation of sphincter of Oddi, sphincterotomy, and stone extraction.

Angiography

Most accurate means of determining portal pressures and assessing patency and direction of flow in portal and hepatic veins; highly sensitive for detecting small vascular lesions and hepatic tumors (esp. primary hepatocellular carcinoma); "gold standard" for differentiating hemangiomas from solid tumors; most accurate means of studying vascular anatomy in preparation for complicated hepatobiliary surgery (e.g., portal-systemic shunting, biliary reconstruction) and determining resectability of hepatobiliary and pancreatic tumors. Similar anatomic information (but not intravascular pressures) can often be obtained noninvasively by CT- and MR-based techniques.

Percutaneous Liver Biopsy

Most accurate in disorders causing diffuse changes throughout the liver; subject to sampling error in focal infiltrative disorders such as metastasis; should not be the initial procedure in the Dx of cholestasis.

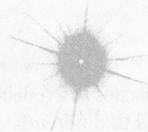

For a more detailed discussion, see Pratt DS, Kaplan MM: Jaundice, Chap. 42, p. 324; Ghany M, Hoofnagle JH: Approach to the Patient With Liver Disease, Chap 301, p. 2520; and Pratt DS, Kaplan MM: Evaluation of Liver Function, Chap. 302, p. 2527, in HPIM-18.

CHAPTER **49**
Ascites

■ DEFINITION

Accumulation of fluid within the peritoneal cavity. Small amounts may be asymptomatic; increasing amounts cause abdominal distention and discomfort, anorexia, nausea, early satiety, heartburn, flank pain, and respiratory distress.

■ DETECTION

Physical Examination

Bulging flanks, fluid wave, shifting dullness, "puddle sign" (dullness over dependent abdomen with pt on hands and knees). May be associated with penile or scrotal edema, umbilical or inguinal herniation, pleural effusion.

Evaluation should include rectal and pelvic examination, assessment of liver and spleen. Palmar erythema and spider angiomata seen in cirrhosis. Periumbilical nodule (*Sister Mary Joseph's nodule*) suggests metastatic disease from a pelvic or GI tumor.

Ultrasonography/CT

Very sensitive; able to distinguish fluid from cystic masses.

■ EVALUATION

Diagnostic paracentesis (50–100 mL) essential. Routine evaluation includes gross inspection, protein, albumin, glucose, cell count and differential, Gram's and acid-fast stains, culture, cytology; in selected cases check amylase, LDH, triglycerides, culture for tuberculosis (TB). Rarely, laparoscopy or even exploratory laparotomy may be required. Ascites due to CHF (e.g., pericardial constriction) may require evaluation by right-sided heart catheterization.

Differential Diagnosis

More than 90% of cases due to cirrhosis, neoplasm, CHF, TB.

Diseases of peritoneum: Infections (bacterial, tuberculous, fungal, parasitic), neoplasms, connective tissue disease, miscellaneous (Whipple's disease, familial Mediterranean fever, endometriosis, starch peritonitis, etc.).

Diseases not involving peritoneum: Cirrhosis, CHF, Budd-Chiari syndrome, hepatic venoocclusive disease, hypoalbuminemia (nephrotic syndrome, protein-losing enteropathy, malnutrition), miscellaneous (myxedema, ovarian diseases, pancreatic disease, chylous ascites).

Pathophysiologic Classification Using Serum-Ascites Albumin Gradient (SAAG)

Difference in albumin concentrations between serum and ascites as a reflection of imbalances in hydrostatic pressures and can be used to differentiate between potential causes of ascites (Fig. 49-1).

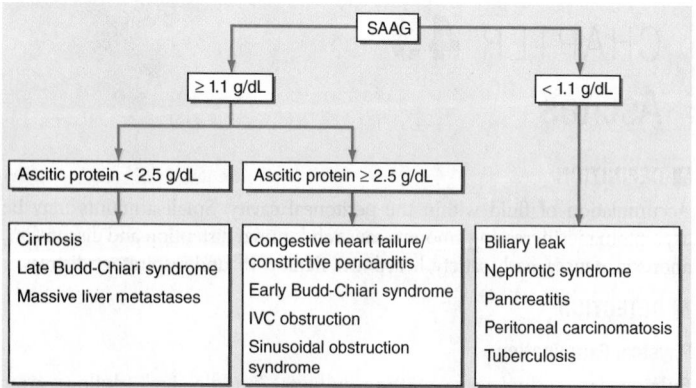

FIGURE 49-1 Algorithm for the diagnosis of ascites according to the serum-ascites albumin gradient (SAAG). IVC, inferior vena cava.

■ **CIRRHOTIC ASCITES**

Pathogenesis

Contributing factors: (1) portal hypertension, (2) hypoalbuminemia, (3) hepatic lymph, (4) renal sodium retention–secondary to hyperaldosteronism, increased sympathetic nervous system activity (renin-angiotensin production). Initiating event may be peripheral arterial vasodilation triggered by endotoxin and cytokines and mediated by nitric oxide.

| TREATMENT | Cirrhotic Ascites |

Maximum mobilization ~700 mL/d (peripheral edema may be mobilized faster).

1. Rigid salt restriction (<2 g Na/d).
2. For moderate ascites, diuretics usually necessary; spironolactone 100–200 mg/d PO (can be increased to 400 mg/d if low-sodium diet is confirmed and fluid not mobilized); furosemide 40–80 mg/d PO or IV may be added if necessary (greater risk of hepatorenal syndrome, encephalopathy), can increase to maximum of 120–160 mg/d until effect achieved or complication occurs.
3. Monitor weight, urinary Na and K, serum electrolytes, and creatinine. If ascites is still present with the above measures this is defined as *refractory ascites*. Treatment modalities include:
   a. Repeated large-volume paracentesis (5 L) with IV infusions of albumin (10 g/L ascites removed).
   b. Consider transjugular intrahepatic portosystemic shunt (TIPS). While TIPS manages the ascites, it has not been found to improve survival and is often associated with encephalopathy.

Prognosis for pts with cirrhotic ascites is poor with <50% survival 2 years after onset of ascites. Consider liver transplantation in appropriate candidates with the onset of ascites (Chap. 165).

■ **COMPLICATIONS**

Spontaneous Bacterial Peritonitis

Suspect in cirrhotic pt with ascites and fever, abdominal pain, worsening ascites, ileus, hypotension, worsening jaundice, or encephalopathy; low ascitic protein concentration (low opsonic activity) is predisposing factor. Diagnosis suggested by ascitic fluid PMN cell count >250/μL; confirmed by positive culture (usually *Escherichia coli* and other gut bacteria; however, gram-positive bacteria including *Streptococcus viridans, Staphylococcus aureus,* and *Enterococcus* spp. also can be found). Initial treatment: Cefotaxime 2 g IV q8h. Risk is increased in pts with variceal bleeding and prophylaxis against spontaneous bacterial peritonitis is recommended when a pt presents with upper GI bleeding.

Hepatorenal Syndrome (HRS)

Functional renal failure without renal pathology; occurs in 10% of pts with advanced cirrhosis or acute liver failure. Thought to result from altered renal hemodynamics. Two types: type 1 HRS–decrease in renal function within 1–2 weeks of presentation; type 2 HRS–associated with a rise in serum creatinine but is associated with a better outcome. Often seen in pts with refractory ascites. Treatment: midodrine along with octreotide and IV albumin. For either type 1 or 2 HRS, prognosis is poor in the absence of liver transplantation.

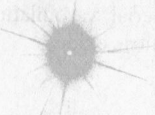

> For a more detailed discussion, see Corey KE, Friedman LS: Abdominal Swelling and Ascites, Chap. 43, p. 330; and Bacon BR: Cirrhosis and Its Complications, Chap. 308, p. 2592, in HPIM-18.

CHAPTER 50
Lymphadenopathy and Splenomegaly

LYMPHADENOPATHY

Exposure to antigen through a break in the skin or mucosa results in antigen being taken up by an antigen-presenting cell and carried via lymphatic channels to the nearest lymph node. Lymph channels course throughout the body except for the brain and the bones. Lymph enters the node through the afferent vessel and leaves through an efferent vessel. As antigen-presenting cells pass through lymph nodes, they present antigen to lymphocytes residing there. Lymphocytes in a node are constantly being replaced by antigen-naïve lymphocytes from the blood. They are retained in the node via special homing receptors. B cells populate the lymphoid follicles in the cortex; T cells populate the paracortical regions. When a B cell encounters an antigen to which its surface immunoglobulin can bind, it stays in the follicle for a few days and forms a germinal center where the immunoglobulin gene is mutated in an effort to make an antibody with higher affinity for the antigen. The B cell then migrates to the medullary region, differentiates into a plasma cell, and secretes immunoglobulin into the efferent lymph.

When a T cell in the node encounters an antigen it recognizes, it proliferates and joins the efferent lymph. The efferent lymph laden with antibodies and T cells specific for the inciting antigen passes through several nodes on its way to the thoracic duct, which drains lymph from most of the body. From the thoracic duct, lymph enters the bloodstream at the left subclavian vein. Lymph from the head and neck and the right arm drains into the right subclavian vein. From the bloodstream, the antibody and T cells localize to the site of infection.

Lymphadenopathy may be caused by infections, immunologic diseases, malignancies, lipid storage diseases, or other disorders of uncertain etiology (e.g., sarcoidosis, Castleman's disease; Table 50-1). The two major mechanisms of lymphadenopathy are *hyperplasia*, in response to immunologic or infectious stimuli, and *infiltration*, by cancer cells or lipid- or glycoprotein-laden macrophages.

TABLE 50-1 DISEASES ASSOCIATED WITH LYMPHADENOPATHY

1. Infectious diseases
   a. Viral—infectious mononucleosis syndromes (EBV, CMV), infectious hepatitis, herpes simplex, herpesvirus 6, varicella-zoster virus, rubella, measles, adenovirus, HIV, epidemic keratoconjunctivitis, vaccinia, herpesvirus 8
   b. Bacterial—streptococci, staphylococci, cat-scratch disease, brucellosis, tularemia, plague, chancroid, melioidosis, glanders, tuberculosis, atypical mycobacterial infection, primary and secondary syphilis, diphtheria, leprosy
   c. Fungal—histoplasmosis, coccidioidomycosis, paracoccidioidomycosis
   d. Chlamydial—lymphogranuloma venereum, trachoma
   e. Parasitic—toxoplasmosis, leishmaniasis, trypanosomiasis, filariasis
   f. Rickettsial—scrub typhus, rickettsialpox, Q fever
2. Immunologic diseases
   a. Rheumatoid arthritis
   b. Juvenile rheumatoid arthritis
   c. Mixed connective tissue disease
   d. Systemic lupus erythematosus
   e. Dermatomyositis
   f. Sjögren's syndrome
   g. Serum sickness
   h. Drug hypersensitivity—diphenylhydantoin, hydralazine, allopurinol, primidone, gold, carbamazepine, etc.
   i. Angioimmunoblastic lymphadenopathy
   j. Primary biliary cirrhosis
   k. Graft-versus-host disease
   l. Silicone-associated
   m. Autoimmune lymphoproliferative syndrome
3. Malignant diseases
   a. Hematologic—Hodgkin's disease, non-Hodgkin's lymphomas, acute or chronic lymphocytic leukemia, hairy cell leukemia, malignant histiocytosis, amyloidosis
   b. Metastatic—from numerous primary sites
4. Lipid storage diseases—Gaucher's, Niemann-Pick, Fabry, Tangier
5. Endocrine diseases—hyperthyroidism
6. Other disorders
   a. Castleman's disease (giant lymph node hyperplasia)
   b. Sarcoidosis
   c. Dermatopathic lymphadenitis
   d. Lymphomatoid granulomatosis

(continued)

| TABLE 50-1 | DISEASES ASSOCIATED WITH LYMPHADENOPATHY (CONTINUED) |

e. Histiocytic necrotizing lymphadenitis (Kikuchi's disease)

f. Sinus histiocytosis with massive lymphadenopathy (Rosai-Dorfman disease)

g. Mucocutaneous lymph node syndrome (Kawasaki's disease)

h. Histiocytosis X

i. Familial Mediterranean fever

j. Severe hypertriglyceridemia

k. Vascular transformation of sinuses

l. Inflammatory pseudotumor of lymph node

m. Congestive heart failure

Abbreviations: CMV, cytomegalovirus; EBV, Epstein-Barr virus.

APPROACH TO THE PATIENT   Lymphadenopathy

HISTORY   Age, occupation, animal exposures, sexual orientation, substance abuse history, medication history, and concomitant symptoms influence diagnostic workup. Adenopathy is more commonly malignant in origin in those over age 40. Farmers have an increased incidence of brucellosis and lymphoma. Male homosexuals may have AIDS-associated adenopathy. Alcohol and tobacco abuse increase risk of malignancy. Phenytoin may induce adenopathy. The concomitant presence of cervical adenopathy with sore throat or with fever, night sweats, and weight loss suggests particular diagnoses (mononucleosis in the former instance, Hodgkin's disease in the latter).

PHYSICAL EXAMINATION   Location of adenopathy, size, node texture, and the presence of tenderness are important in differential diagnosis. Generalized adenopathy (three or more anatomic regions) implies systemic infection or lymphoma. Subclavian or scalene adenopathy is always abnormal and should be biopsied. Nodes >4 cm should be biopsied immediately. Rock-hard nodes fixed to surrounding soft tissue are usually a sign of metastatic carcinoma. Tender nodes are most often benign.

LABORATORY TESTS   Usually lab tests are not required in the setting of localized adenopathy. If generalized adenopathy is noted, an excisional node biopsy should be performed for diagnosis, rather than a panoply of laboratory tests.

TREATMENT   Lymphadenopathy

Pts over age 40, those with scalene or supraclavicular adenopathy, those with lymph nodes >4 cm in diameter, and those with hard nontender nodes should undergo immediate excisional biopsy. In younger pts with smaller nodes that are rubbery in consistency or tender, a period of observation for 7–14 days is reasonable. Empirical antibiotics are not indicated. If the nodes shrink, no further evaluation is necessary. If they enlarge, excisional biopsy is indicated.

SPLENOMEGALY

Just as the lymph nodes are specialized to fight pathogens in the tissues, the spleen is the lymphoid organ specialized to fight bloodborne pathogens. It has no afferent lymphatics. The spleen has specialized areas like the lymph node for making antibodies (follicles) and amplifying antigen-specific T cells (periarteriolar lymphatic sheath, or PALS). In addition, it has a well-developed reticuloendothelial system for removing particles and antibody-coated bacteria. The flow of blood through the spleen permits it to filter pathogens from the blood and to maintain quality control over erythrocytes (RBCs)—those that are old and nondeformable are destroyed, and intracellular inclusions (sometimes including pathogens such as *Babesia* and *Plasmodium*) are culled from the cells in a process called *pitting*. Under certain conditions, the spleen can generate hematopoietic cells in place of the marrow.

The normal spleen is about 12 cm in length and 7 cm in width and is not normally palpable. Dullness from the spleen can be percussed between the ninth and eleventh ribs with the pt lying on the right side. Palpation is best performed with the pt supine with knees flexed. The spleen may be felt as it descends when the pt inspires. Physical diagnosis is not sensitive. CT or ultrasound are superior tests.

Spleen enlargement occurs by three basic mechanisms: (1) hyperplasia or hypertrophy due to an increase in demand for splenic function (e.g., hereditary spherocytosis where demand for removal of defective RBCs is high or immune hyperplasia in response to systemic infection or immune diseases); (2) passive vascular congestion due to portal hypertension; and (3) infiltration with malignant cells, lipid- or glycoprotein-laden macrophages, or amyloid (Table 50-2). Massive enlargement, with spleen palpable >8 cm below the left costal margin, usually signifies a lymphoproliferative or myeloproliferative disorder.

Peripheral blood RBC count, white blood cell count, and platelet count may be normal, decreased, or increased depending on the underlying disorder. Decreases in one or more cell lineages could indicate hypersplenism, increased destruction. In cases with hypersplenism, the spleen is removed and the cytopenia is generally reversed. In the absence of hypersplenism, most causes of splenomegaly are diagnosed on the basis of signs and symptoms and laboratory abnormalities associated with the underlying disorder. Splenectomy is rarely performed for diagnostic purposes.

Individuals who have had splenectomy are at increased risk of sepsis from a variety of organisms including pneumococcus and *Haemophilus influenzae*. Vaccines for these agents should be given before splenectomy is performed. Splenectomy compromises the immune response to these T-independent antigens.

TABLE 50-2 DISEASES ASSOCIATED WITH SPLENOMEGALY GROUPED BY PATHOGENIC MECHANISM

Enlargement Due to Increased Demand for Splenic Function

Reticuloendothelial system hyperplasia (for removal of defective erythrocytes)

　Spherocytosis

　Early sickle cell anemia

　Ovalocytosis

　Thalassemia major

　Hemoglobinopathies

　Paroxysmal nocturnal hemoglobinuria

　Pernicious anemia

Immune hyperplasia

　Response to infection (viral, bacterial, fungal, parasitic)

　　Infectious mononucleosis

　　AIDS

　　Viral hepatitis

　　Cytomegalovirus

　　Subacute bacterial endocarditis

　　Bacterial septicemia

　　Congenital syphilis

　　Splenic abscess

　　Tuberculosis

　　Histoplasmosis

　　Malaria

Leishmaniasis

Trypanosomiasis

Ehrlichiosis

Disordered immunoregulation

　Rheumatoid arthritis (Felty's syndrome)

　Systemic lupus erythematosus

　Collagen vascular diseases

　Serum sickness

　Immune hemolytic anemias

　Immune thrombocytopenias

　Immune neutropenias

　Drug reactions

　Angioimmunoblastic lymphadenopathy

　Sarcoidosis

　Thyrotoxicosis (benign lymphoid hypertrophy)

　Interleukin 2 therapy

Extramedullary hematopoiesis

　Myelofibrosis

　Marrow damage by toxins, radiation, strontium

　Marrow infiltration by tumors, leukemias, Gaucher's disease

Enlargement Due to Abnormal Splenic or Portal Blood Flow

Cirrhosis

Hepatic vein obstruction

Portal vein obstruction, intrahepatic or extrahepatic

Cavernous transformation of the portal vein

Splenic vein obstruction

Splenic artery aneurysm

Hepatic schistosomiasis

Congestive heart failure

Hepatic echinococcosis

Portal hypertension (any cause including the above): "Banti's disease"

TABLE 50-2 DISEASES ASSOCIATED WITH SPLENOMEGALY GROUPED BY PATHOGENIC MECHANISM (CONTINUED)

Infiltration of the Spleen	
Intracellular or extracellular depositions	Hodgkin's disease
Amyloidosis	Myeloproliferative syndromes (e.g., polycythemia vera, essential thrombocytosis)
Gaucher's disease	
Niemann-Pick disease	Angiosarcomas
Tangier disease	Metastatic tumors (melanoma is most common)
Hurler's syndrome and other mucopolysaccharidoses	
	Eosinophilic granuloma
Hyperlipidemias	Histiocytosis X
Benign and malignant cellular infiltrations	Hamartomas
Leukemias (acute, chronic, lymphoid, myeloid, monocytic)	Hemangiomas, fibromas, lymphangiomas
Lymphomas	Splenic cysts
Unknown Etiology	
Idiopathic splenomegaly	Iron-deficiency anemia
Berylliosis	

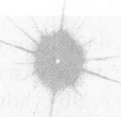

For a more detailed discussion, see Henry PH, Longo DL: Enlargement of Lymph Nodes and Spleen, Chap. 59, p. 465, in HPIM-18.

CHAPTER **51**
Anemia and Polycythemia

ANEMIA

According to World Health Organization criteria, anemia is defined as blood hemoglobin (Hb) concentration <130 g/L (<13 g/dL) or hematocrit (Hct) <39% in adult males; Hb <120 g/L (<12 g/dL) or Hct <37% in adult females.

Signs and symptoms of anemia are varied, depending on the level of anemia and the time course over which it developed. Acute anemia is nearly always due to blood loss or hemolysis. In acute blood loss, hypovolemia dominates the clinical picture; hypotension and decreased organ perfusion are the main issues. Symptoms associated with more chronic onset vary with the age of the pt and the adequacy of blood supply to critical organs. Moderate anemia is associated with fatigue, loss of stamina, breathlessness, and tachycardia. The pt's skin and mucous membranes may appear pale. If the palmar creases are lighter in color than the surrounding skin with the fingers extended, Hb level is often <80 g/L (8 g/dL). In pts with coronary artery disease, anginal episodes may appear or increase in frequency and severity. In pts with carotid artery disease, lightheadedness or dizziness may develop.

A physiologic approach to anemia diagnosis is based on the understanding that a decrease in circulating red blood cells (RBCs) can be related to either inadequate production of RBCs or increased RBC destruction or loss. Within the category of inadequate production, erythropoiesis can be either ineffective, due to an erythrocyte maturation defect (which usually results in RBCs that are too small or too large), or hypoproliferative (which usually results in RBCs of normal size, but too few of them).

Basic evaluations include (1) reticulocyte index (RI), and (2) review of blood smear and RBC indices [chiefly mean corpuscular volume (MCV)] (Fig. 51-1).

The RI is a measure of RBC production. The reticulocyte count is corrected for the Hct level and for early release of marrow reticulocytes into the circulation, which leads to an increase in the lifespan of the circulating reticulocyte beyond the usual 1 day. Thus, RI = (% reticulocytes × pt Hct/45%) × (1/shift correction factor). The shift correction factor varies with the Hct: 1.5 for Hct = 35%, 2 for Hct = 25%, 2.5 for Hct = 15%. RI < 2–2.5% implies inadequate RBC production for the particular level of anemia; RI > 2.5% implies excessive RBC destruction or loss.

If the anemia is associated with a low RI, RBC morphology helps distinguish a maturation disorder from hypoproliferative marrow states. Cytoplasmic maturation defects such as iron deficiency or Hb synthesis problems produce smaller RBCs, MCV < 80; nuclear maturation defects such as B_{12} and folate deficiency and drug effects produce larger RBCs, MCV >100. In hypoproliferative marrow states, RBCs are generally normal in morphology but too few are produced. Bone marrow examination is often helpful in the evaluation of anemia but is done most frequently to diagnose hypoproliferative marrow states.

Other laboratory tests indicated to evaluate particular forms of anemia depend on the initial classification based on the pathophysiology of the defect. These are discussed in more detail in Chap. 68.

POLYCYTHEMIA (ERYTHROCYTOSIS)

Polycythemia is an increase above the normal range of RBCs in the circulation. Concern that the Hb level may be abnormally high should be triggered at a level of 170 g/L (17 g/dL) in men and 150 g/L (15 g/dL) in women. Polycythemia is usually found incidentally at routine blood count. Relative erythrocytosis, due to plasma volume loss (e.g., severe dehydration, burns),

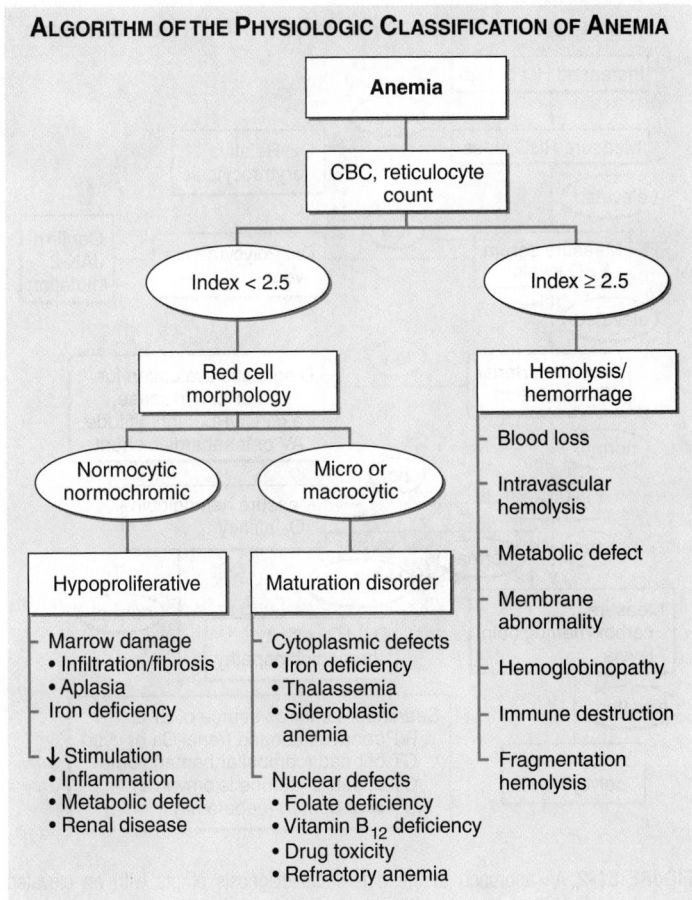

ALGORITHM OF THE PHYSIOLOGIC CLASSIFICATION OF ANEMIA

FIGURE 51-1 The physiologic classification of anemia. CBC, complete blood count.

does not represent a true increase in total RBC mass. Absolute erythrocytosis is a true increase in total RBC mass.

■ CAUSES

Polycythemia vera (a clonal myeloproliferative disorder), erythropoietin-producing neoplasms (e.g., renal cancer, cerebellar hemangioma), chronic hypoxemia (e.g., high altitude, pulmonary disease), carboxyhemoglobin excess (e.g., smokers), high-affinity hemoglobin variants, Cushing's syndrome, androgen excess. Polycythemia vera is distinguished from secondary polycythemia by the presence of splenomegaly, leukocytosis, thrombocytosis, and elevated vitamin B$_{12}$ levels, and by decreased erythropoietin levels. An approach to evaluate polycythemic pts is shown in Fig. 51-2.

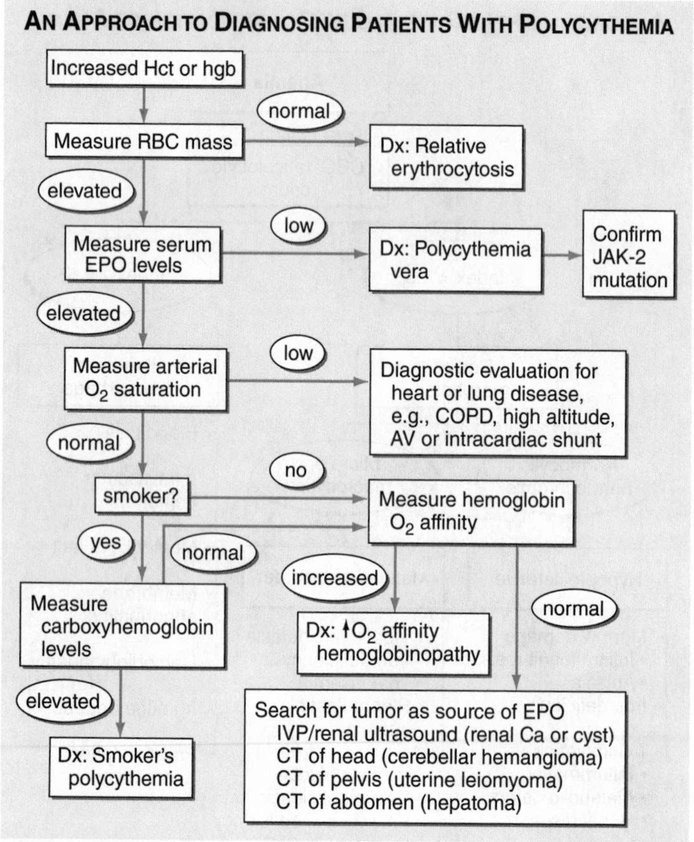

AN APPROACH TO DIAGNOSING PATIENTS WITH POLYCYTHEMIA

Increased Hct or hgb

Measure RBC mass ──(normal)──→ Dx: Relative erythrocytosis

(elevated)

Measure serum EPO levels ──(low)──→ Dx: Polycythemia vera ──→ Confirm JAK-2 mutation

(elevated)

Measure arterial O_2 saturation ──(low)──→ Diagnostic evaluation for heart or lung disease, e.g., COPD, high altitude, AV or intracardiac shunt

(normal)

smoker? ──(no)──→ Measure hemoglobin O_2 affinity

(yes)   (normal)   (increased)   (normal)

Measure carboxyhemoglobin levels

Dx: ↑O_2 affinity hemoglobinopathy

Search for tumor as source of EPO
IVP/renal ultrasound (renal Ca or cyst)
CT of head (cerebellar hemangioma)
CT of pelvis (uterine leiomyoma)
CT of abdomen (hepatoma)

(elevated)

Dx: Smoker's polycythemia

FIGURE 51-2 An approach to the differential diagnosis of pts with an elevated hemoglobin (possible polycythemia). AV, atrioventricular; COPD, chronic obstructive pulmonary disease; EPO, erythropoietin; Hct, hematocrit; IVP, intravenous pyelogram; RBC, red blood cell.

◼ COMPLICATIONS

Hyperviscosity (with diminished O_2 delivery) with risk of ischemic organ injury and thrombosis (venous or arterial) are most common.

TREATMENT	Polycythemia

Phlebotomy recommended for Hct ≥ 55%, regardless of cause, to low-normal range.

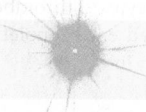

For a more detailed discussion, see Adamson JW, Longo DL: Anemia and Polycythemia, Chap. 57, p. 448, in HPIM-18.

CHAPTER **52**
Azotemia and Urinary Abnormalities

■ ABNORMALITIES OF RENAL FUNCTION, AZOTEMIA

Azotemia is the retention of nitrogenous waste products excreted by the kidney. Increased levels of blood urea nitrogen (BUN) [>10.7 mmol/L (>30 mg/dL)] and creatinine [>133 μmol/L (>1.5 mg/dL)] are ordinarily indicative of impaired renal function. Renal function can be estimated by determining the clearance of creatinine (CL_{cr}) (normal >100 mL/min); this can be directly measured from a 24-h urine collection using the following equation:

$$\text{Creatinine clearance (mL/min)} = (uCr \times uV)/(sCr \times 1440)$$

1. Where uCr is urine creatinine in mg/dL
2. Where sCr is serum creatinine in mg/dL
3. Where uV is 24-h urine volume in mL
4. Where 1440 represents number of minutes in 24 h

The "adequacy" or "completeness" of the collection is estimated by the urinary volume and creatinine content; creatinine is produced from muscle and excreted at a relatively constant rate. For a 20- to 50-year-old man, creatinine excretion should be 18.5–25.0 mg/kg body weight; for a woman of the same age, it should be 16.5–22.4 mg/kg body weight. For example, an 80-kg man should excrete between ~1500 and 2000 mg of creatinine in an "adequate" collection. Creatinine excretion is also influenced by age and muscle mass. Notably, creatinine is an imperfect measure of glomerular filtration rate (GFR), since it is both filtered by glomeruli and secreted by proximal tubular cells; the relative contribution of tubular secretion increases with advancing renal dysfunction, such that creatinine clearance will provide an overestimate of the "true" GFR in pts with chronic kidney disease. Isotopic markers that are filtered and not secreted (e.g., iothalamate) provide more accurate estimates of GFR.

A formula that allows for an estimate of creatinine clearance in men that accounts for age-related decreases in GFR, body weight, and sex has been derived by Cockcroft-Gault:

$$\text{Creatinine clearance (mL/min)}$$
$$= (140 \text{ age}) \times \text{lean body weight (kg)/plasma creatinine (mg/dL)} \times 72$$

This value should be multiplied by 0.85 for women.

GFR may also be estimated using serum creatinine–based equations derived from the Modification of Diet in Renal Disease Study. This "eGFR" is now reported with serum creatinine by most clinical laboratories in the United States and is the basis for the National Kidney Foundation classification of chronic kidney disease (Table 52-1).

TABLE 52-1 THE CLASSIFICATION OF CHRONIC KIDNEY DISEASE (NATIONAL KIDNEY FOUNDATION GUIDELINES)

Kidney Damage Stage	Description	eGFR (mL/min per 1.73 m²)
0	With risk factors for CKD[a]	>90
1	With evidence of kidney damage[b]	>90
2	Mild decrease in GFR	60–89
3	Moderate decrease in GFR	30–59
4	Severe decrease in GFR	15–29
5	Kidney failure	<15

[a]Diabetes, high blood pressure, family history, older age, African ancestry.
[b]Abnormal urinalysis, hematuria, proteinuria, albuminuria.
Abbreviations: CKD, chronic kidney disease; eGFR, estimated glomerular filtration rate; GFR, glomerular filtration rate.

Manifestations of impaired renal function include volume overload, hypertension, electrolyte abnormalities (e.g., hyperkalemia, hypocalcemia, hyperphosphatemia), metabolic acidosis, and hormonal disturbances (e.g., insulin resistance, functional vitamin D deficiency, secondary hyperparathyroidism). When severe, the symptom complex of "uremia" may develop, encompassing one or more of the following symptoms and signs: anorexia, dysgeusia, nausea, vomiting, lethargy, confusion, asterixis, pleuritis, pericarditis, enteritis, pruritus, sleep and taste disturbance, nitrogenous fetor.

An approach to the pt with azotemia is shown in Fig. 52-1.

◼ ABNORMALITIES OF URINE VOLUME

Oliguria

This refers to reduced urine output, usually defined as <400 mL/d. *Oligoanuria* refers to a more marked reduction in urine output, i.e., <100 mL/d. *Anuria* indicates the complete absence of urine output. Oliguria most often occurs in the setting of volume depletion and/or renal hypoperfusion, resulting in "prerenal azotemia" and acute renal failure (Chap. 148). Anuria can be caused by complete bilateral urinary tract obstruction; a vascular catastrophe (dissection or arterial occlusion); renal vein thrombosis; renal cortical necrosis; severe acute tubular necrosis; nonsteroidal anti-inflammatory drugs, angiotensin-converting enzyme (ACE) inhibitors, and/or angiotensin receptor blockers; and hypovolemic, cardiogenic, or septic shock. Oliguria is never normal, since at least 400 mL of maximally concentrated urine must be produced to excrete the obligate daily osmolar load.

Polyuria

Polyuria is defined as a urine output >3 L/d. It is often accompanied by nocturia and urinary frequency and must be differentiated from other more common conditions associated with lower urinary tract pathology and

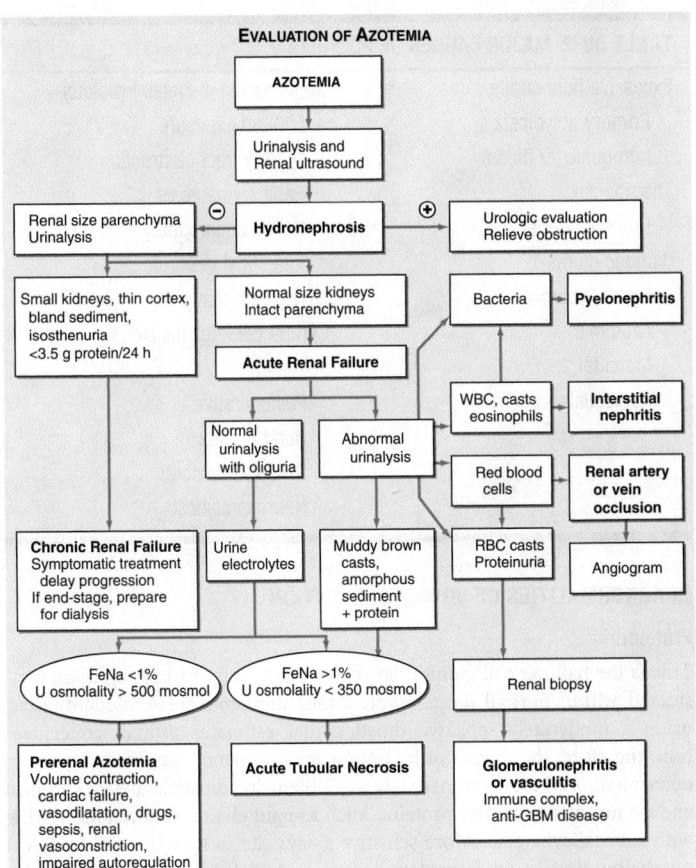

FIGURE 52-1 Approach to the pt with azotemia. FeNa, fractional excretion of sodium; GBM, glomerular basement membrane; RBC, red blood cell; WBC, white blood cell. (*From Lin J and Denker BM: HPIM-18.*)

urinary urgency or frequency (e.g., cystitis, prostatism). It is often accompanied by hypernatremia (Chap. 2). Polyuria (Table 52-2) can occur as a response to a solute load (e.g., hyperglycemia) or to an abnormality in arginine vasopressin [AVP; also known as antidiuretic hormone (ADH)] action. Diabetes insipidus is termed *central* if due to the insufficient hypothalamic production of AVP and *nephrogenic* if the result of renal insensitivity to the action of AVP. Excess fluid intake can lead to polyuria, but primary polydipsia rarely results in changes in plasma osmolality unless urinary diluting capacity is impaired. Tubulointerstitial diseases, lithium therapy, and resolving acute tubular necrosis or urinary tract obstruction can be associated with nephrogenic diabetes insipidus, which is more rarely caused by mutations in the V2 AVP receptor or the AVP-regulated water channel, aquaporin 2.

The approach to the pt with polyuria is shown in Fig. 52-2.

TABLE 52-2 MAJOR CAUSES OF POLYURIA

Excessive fluid intake	Nephrogenic diabetes insipidus
Primary polydipsia	Lithium exposure
Iatrogenic (IV fluids)	Urinary tract obstruction
Therapeutic	Papillary necrosis
Diuretic agents	Reflux nephropathy
Osmotic diuresis	Interstitial nephritis
Hyperglycemia	Hypercalcemia
Azotemia	Central diabetes insipidus
Mannitol	Tumor
Radiocontrast	Postoperative
	Head trauma
	Basilar meningitis
	Neurosarcoidosis

■ ABNORMALITIES OF URINE COMPOSITION

Proteinuria

This is the hallmark of glomerular disease. Levels up to 150 mg/d are considered within normal limits. Typical measurements are semiquantitative, using a moderately sensitive dipstick that estimates protein concentration; therefore, the degree of hydration may influence the dipstick protein determination. Most commercially available urine dipsticks detect albumin and do not detect smaller proteins, such as light chains, that require testing with sulfosalicylic acid. More sensitive assays can in turn be used to detect microalbuminuria, an important screening tool for diabetic nephropathy. A urine albumin to creatinine ratio >30 mg/g defines the presence of micro-albuminuria.

Formal assessment of urinary protein excretion requires a 24-h urine protein collection (see "Abnormalities of Renal Function, Azotemia," above). The ratio of protein to creatinine in a random, "spot" urine can also provide a rough estimate of protein excretion; for example, a protein/creatinine ratio of 3.0 correlates to ~3.0 g of proteinuria per day.

Urinary protein excretion rates between 500 mg/d and 3 g/d are nonspecific and can be seen in a variety of renal diseases (including hypertensive nephrosclerosis, interstitial nephritis, vascular disease, and other primary renal diseases with little or no glomerular involvement). Transient, lesser degrees of proteinuria (500 mg/d to 1.5 g/d) may be seen after vigorous exercise, changes in body position, fever, or congestive heart failure. Protein excretion rates >3 g/d are termed *nephrotic range proteinuria* in that they may be accompanied by hypoalbuminemia, hypercholesterolemia, and edema (the nephrotic syndrome). Nephrotic syndrome can be associated with a variety of extrarenal complications (Chap. 152). Massive degrees of proteinuria (>10 g/d) can be seen with minimal change

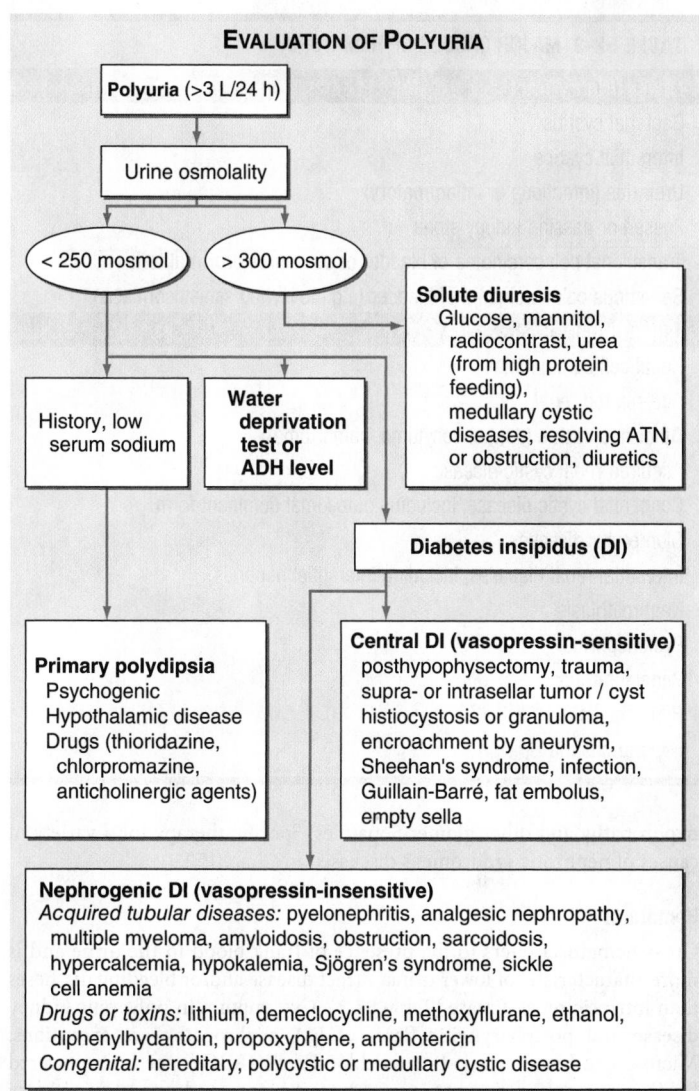

FIGURE 52-2 Approach to the pt with polyuria. ADH, antidiuretic hormone; ATN, acute tubular necrosis. (*From Lin J and Denker BM: HPIM-18.*)

disease, primary focal segmental sclerosis (FSGS), membranous nephropathy, collapsing glomerulopathy (a subtype of primary FSGS), and HIV-associated nephropathy.

Pharmacologic inhibition of ACE or blockade of angiotensin II should be employed to reduce proteinuria; successful reduction of proteinuria decreases the rate of progression to end-stage renal disease in diabetic

TABLE 52-3 MAJOR CAUSES OF HEMATURIA

Lower Urinary Tract
Bacterial cystitis
Interstitial cystitis
Urethritis (infectious or inflammatory)
Passed or passing kidney stone
Transitional cell carcinoma of bladder or structures proximal to it
Squamous cell carcinoma of bladder (e.g., following schistosomiasis)

Upper Urinary Tract
Renal cell carcinoma
Age-related renal cysts
Other neoplasms (e.g., oncocytoma, hamartoma)
Acquired renal cystic disease
Congenital cystic disease, including autosomal dominant form
Glomerular diseases
Interstitial renal diseases, including interstitial nephritis
Nephrolithiasis
Pyelonephritis
Renal infarction
Hypercalciuria
Hyperuricosuria

nephropathy and other glomerulopathies. Specific therapy for a variety of causes of nephrotic syndrome is discussed in Chap. 152.

Hematuria

Gross hematuria refers to the presence of frank blood in the urine and is more characteristic of lower urinary tract disease and/or bleeding diatheses than intrinsic renal disease (Table 52-3). Cyst rupture in polycystic kidney disease and postpharyngitic flares of IgA nephropathy are exceptions. Microscopic hematuria [>1–2 red blood cells (RBCs) per high-powered field] accompanied by proteinuria, hypertension, and an active urinary sediment (the "nephritic syndrome") is most likely related to an inflammatory glomerulonephritis, classically poststreptococcal glomerulonephritis (Chap. 152).

Free hemoglobin and myoglobin are detected by dipstick; a negative urinary sediment with strongly heme-positive dipstick is characteristic of either hemolysis or rhabdomyolysis, which can be differentiated by clinical history and laboratory testing. RBC casts are not a sensitive finding but when seen are highly specific for glomerulonephritis. Specificity of urinalysis can be enhanced by examining urine with a phase contrast microscope capable of detecting dysmorphic red cells ("acanthocytes") associated with glomerular disease.

The approach to the pt with hematuria is shown in Fig. 52-3.

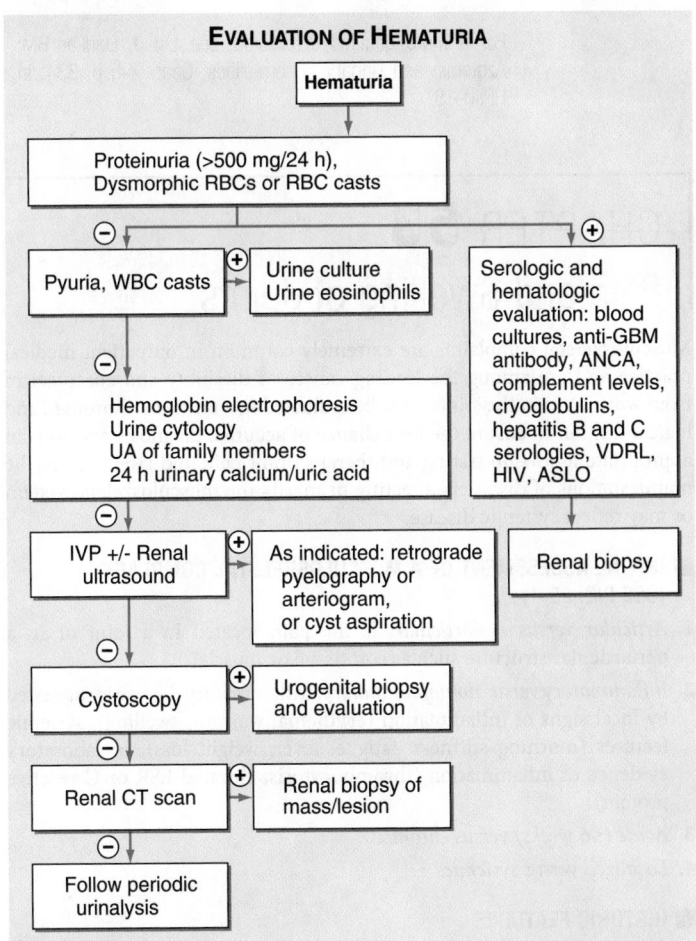

FIGURE 52-3 Approach to the pt with hematuria. ANCA, antineutrophil cytoplasmic antibody; ASLO, antistreptolysin O; CT, computed tomography; GBM, glomerular basement membrane; IVP, intravenous pyelography; RBC, red blood cell; UA, urinalysis; VDRL, Venereal Disease Research Laboratory; WBC, white blood cell. (*From Lin J and Denker BM: HPIM-18.*)

Pyuria

This may accompany hematuria in inflammatory glomerular diseases. Isolated pyuria is most commonly observed in association with an infection of the upper or lower urinary tract. Pyuria may also occur with allergic interstitial nephritis (often with a preponderance of eosinophils), transplant rejection, and noninfectious, nonallergic tubulointerstitial diseases, including atheroembolic renal disease. The finding of "sterile" pyuria (i.e., urinary white blood cells without bacteria) in the appropriate clinical setting should raise suspicion of renal tuberculosis.

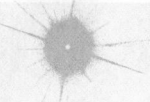

For a more detailed discussion, see Lin J, Denker BM: Azotemia and Urinary Abnormalities, Chap. 44, p. 334, in HPIM-18.

CHAPTER **53**
Pain and Swelling of Joints

Musculoskeletal complaints are extremely common in outpatient medical practice and are among the leading causes of disability and absenteeism from work. Pain in the joints must be evaluated in a uniform, thorough, and logical fashion to ensure the best chance of accurate diagnosis and to plan appropriate follow-up testing and therapy. Joint pain and swelling may be manifestations of disorders affecting primarily the musculoskeletal system or may reflect systemic disease.

▉ INITIAL ASSESSMENT OF A MUSCULOSKELETAL COMPLAINT (SEE FIG. 53-1)

1. *Articular versus nonarticular.* Is the pain located in a joint or in a periarticular structure such as soft tissue or muscle?
2. *Inflammatory versus noninflammatory.* Inflammatory disease is suggested by local signs of inflammation (erythema, warmth, swelling); systemic features (morning stiffness, fatigue, fever, weight loss); or laboratory evidence of inflammation (thrombocytosis, elevated ESR or C-reactive protein).
3. *Acute (≤6 weeks) versus chronic.*
4. *Localized versus systemic.*

▉ HISTORIC FEATURES

- Age, sex, race, and family history
- Symptom onset (abrupt or gradual), evolution (chronic constant, intermittent, migratory, additive), and duration (acute versus chronic)
- Number and distribution of involved structures: monarticular (one joint), oligoarticular (2–3 joints), polyarticular (>3 joints); symmetry
- Other articular features: morning stiffness, effect of movement, features that improve/worsen Sx
- Extraarticular Sx: e.g., fever, rash, weight loss, visual change, dyspnea, diarrhea, dysuria, numbness, weakness
- Recent events: e.g., trauma, drug administration, travel, other illnesses

▉ PHYSICAL EXAMINATION

Complete examination is essential: particular attention to skin, mucous membranes, nails (may reveal characteristic pitting in psoriasis), eyes. Careful and thorough examination of involved and uninvolved joints and periarticular structures; this should proceed in an organized fashion from

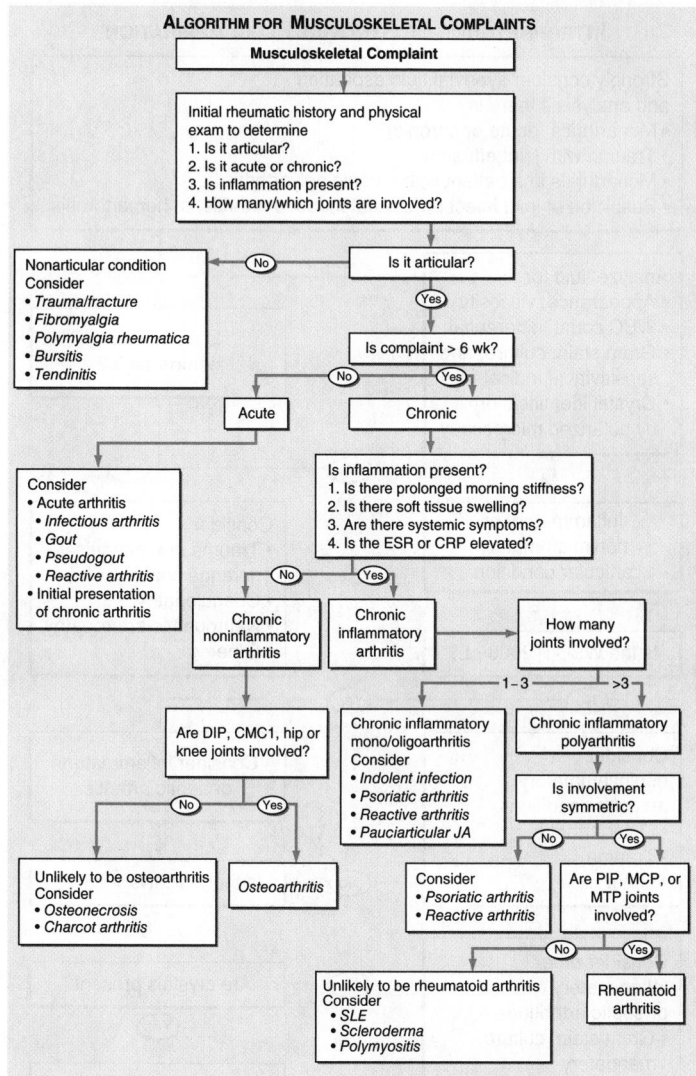

FIGURE 53-1 Algorithm for the diagnosis of musculoskeletal complaints. An approach to formulating a differential diagnosis (shown in italics). CMC, carpometacarpal; CRP, C-reactive protein; DIP, distal interphalangeal; ESR, erythrocyte sedimentation rate; JA, juvenile arthritis; MCP, metacarpophalangeal; MTP, metatarsophalangeal; PIP, proximal interphalangeal; SLE, systemic lupus erythematosus.

head to foot or from extremities inward toward axial skeleton; special attention should be paid to identifying the presence or absence of:

• Warmth and/or erythema
• Swelling

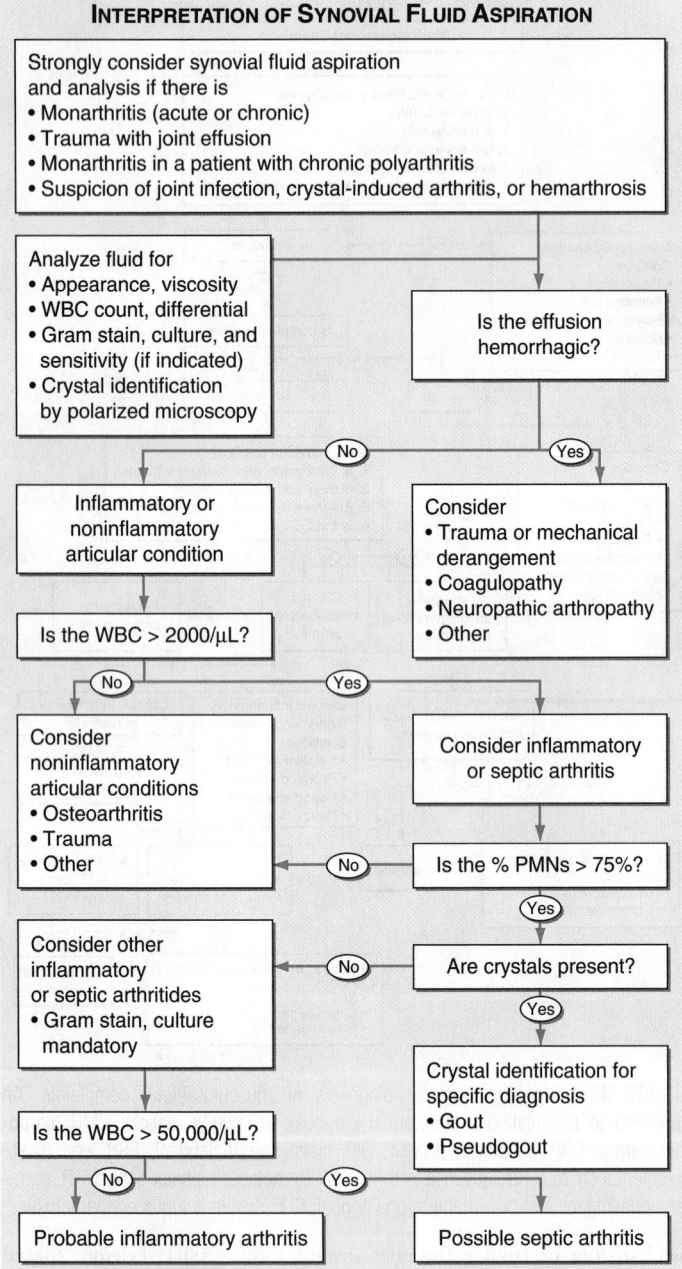

FIGURE 53-2 Algorithmic approach to the use and interpretation of synovial fluid aspiration and analysis. PMNs, polymorphonuclear leukocytes; WBC, white blood cell count.

- Synovial thickening
- Subluxation, dislocation, joint deformity
- Joint instability
- Limitations to active and passive range of motion
- Crepitus
- Periarticular changes
- Muscular changes including weakness, atrophy

■ LABORATORY INVESTIGATIONS

Additional evaluation usually indicated for monarticular, traumatic, inflammatory, or chronic conditions or for conditions accompanied by neurologic changes or systemic manifestations.

- For all evaluations: include CBC, ESR, or C-reactive protein
- Where there are suggestive clinical features, include: rheumatoid factor, ANA, antineutrophilic cytoplasmic antibodies (ANCA), antistreptolysin O titer, Lyme antibodies
- Where systemic disease is present or suspected: renal/hepatic function tests, UA
- Uric acid: useful only when gout diagnosed and therapy contemplated
- CPK, aldolase: consider with muscle pain, weakness
- Synovial fluid aspiration and analysis: always indicated for acute monarthritis or when infectious or crystal-induced arthropathy is suspected. Should be examined for (1) appearance, viscosity; (2) cell count and differential (suspect septic joint if WBC count > 50,000/μL); (3) crystals using polarizing microscope; (4) Gram's stain, cultures (Fig. 53-2).

■ DIAGNOSTIC IMAGING

Conventional radiography using plain x-rays is a valuable tool in the diagnosis and staging of articular disorders (Table 53-1).

Additional imaging procedures, including ultrasound, radionuclide scintigraphy, CT, and MRI, may be helpful in selected clinical settings.

■ SPECIAL CONSIDERATIONS IN THE ELDERLY PATIENT

The evaluation of joint and musculoskeletal disorders in the elderly pt presents a special challenge given the frequently insidious onset and chronicity of disease in this age group, the confounding effect of other medical

TABLE 53-1 APPLICATIONS FOR CONVENTIONAL RADIOGRAPHY IN ARTICULAR DISEASE

Trauma
Suspected chronic joint or bone infection
Progressive joint disability
Monarticular involvement
Baseline assessment of a chronic articular process
When therapeutic alterations are considered (such as for rheumatoid arthritis)

conditions, and the increased variability of many diagnostic tests in the geriatric population. Although virtually all musculoskeletal conditions may afflict the elderly, certain disorders are especially frequent. Special attention should be paid to identifying the potential rheumatic consequences of intercurrent medical conditions and therapies when evaluating the geriatric pt with musculoskeletal complaints.

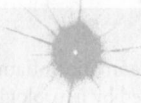

> For a more detailed discussion, see Cush JJ, Lipsky PE: Approach to Articular and Musculoskeletal Disorders, Chap. 331, p. 2818, in HPIM-18.

CHAPTER **54**
Back and Neck Pain

LOW BACK PAIN

The cost of low back pain (LBP) in the United States is ~$100 billion annually. Back symptoms are the most common cause of disability in those <45 years; LBP is the second most common cause of visiting a physician in the United States; ~1% of the United States population is disabled because of back pain.

■ TYPES OF LOW BACK PAIN

- *Local pain*—caused by stretching of pain-sensitive structures that compress or irritate nerve endings; pain (i.e., tears, stretching) located near the affected part of the back.
- *Pain referred to the back*—abdominal or pelvic origin; back pain unaffected by routine movements.
- *Pain of spine origin*—restricted to the back or referred to lower limbs or buttock. Diseases of upper lumbar spine refer pain to upper lumbar region, groin, or anterior thighs. Diseases of lower lumbar spine refer pain to buttocks, posterior thighs, or rarely the calves or feet.
- *Radicular back pain*—radiates from spine to leg in specific nerve root territory. Coughing, sneezing, lifting heavy objects, or straining may elicit pain.
- *Pain associated with muscle spasm*—diverse causes; accompanied by taut paraspinal muscles and abnormal posture.

■ EXAMINATION

Include abdomen, pelvis, and rectum to search for visceral sources of pain. Inspection may reveal scoliosis or muscle spasm. Palpation may elicit pain over a diseased spine segment. Pain from hip may be confused with spine pain; manual internal/external rotation of leg at hip (knee and hip in flexion) reproduces the hip pain.

Straight leg raising (SLR) sign—elicited by passive flexion of leg at the hip with pt in supine position; maneuver stretches L5/S1 nerve roots and sciatic nerve passing posterior to the hip; SLR sign is positive if maneuver reproduces the pain. Crossed SLR sign—positive when SLR on one leg reproduces symptoms in opposite leg or buttocks; nerve/nerve root lesion is on the painful side. Reverse SLR sign—passive extension of leg backwards with pt standing; maneuver stretches L2–L4 nerve roots, lumbosacral plexus, and femoral nerve passing anterior to the hip.

Neurologic exam—search for focal atrophy, weakness, reflex loss, diminished sensation in a dermatomal distribution. Findings with radiculopathy are summarized in Table 54-1.

TABLE 54-1 LUMBOSACRAL RADICULOPATHY—NEUROLOGIC FEATURES

Lumbosacral Nerve Roots	Examination Findings			Pain Distribution
	Reflex	Sensory	Motor	
L2[a]	—	Upper anterior thigh	Psoas (hip flexion)	Anterior thigh
L3[a]	—	Lower anterior thigh	Psoas (hip flexion)	Anterior thigh, knee
		Anterior knee	Quadriceps (knee extension)	
			Thigh adduction	
L4[a]	Quadriceps (knee)	Medial calf	Quadriceps (knee extension)[b]	Knee, medial calf
			Thigh adduction	Anterolateral thigh
			Tibialis anterior (foot dorsiflexion)	
L5[c]	—	Dorsal surface—foot	Peroneii (foot eversion)[b]	Lateral calf, dorsal foot, posterolateral thigh, buttocks
		Lateral calf	Tibialis anterior (foot dorsiflexion)	
			Gluteus medius (hip abduction)	
			Toe dorsiflexors	
S1[c]	Gastrocnemius/ soleus (ankle)	Plantar surface—foot	Gastrocnemius/ soleus (foot plantar flexion)[b]	Bottom foot, posterior calf, posterior thigh, buttocks
		Lateral aspect—foot	Abductor hallucis (toe flexors)[b]	
			Gluteus maximus (hip extension)	

[a]Reverse straight leg–raising sign present—see "Examination of the Back."
[b]These muscles receive the majority of innervation from this root.
[c]Straight leg–raising sign present—see "Examination of the Back."

TABLE 54-2 ACUTE LOW BACK PAIN: RISK FACTORS FOR AN IMPORTANT STRUCTURAL CAUSE

History
Pain worse at rest or at night
Prior history of cancer
History of chronic infection (esp. lung, urinary tract, skin)
History of trauma
Incontinence
Age >70 years
Intravenous drug use
Glucocorticoid use
History of a rapidly progressive neurologic deficit

Examination
Unexplained fever
Unexplained weight loss
Percussion tenderness over the spine
Abdominal, rectal, or pelvic mass
Patrick's sign or heel percussion sign
Straight leg or reverse straight leg–raising signs
Progressive focal neurologic deficit

■ LABORATORY EVALUATION

"Routine" laboratory studies and lumbar spine x-rays are rarely needed for acute LBP (<3 months) but indicated when risk factors for serious underlying disease are present (Table 54-2). MRI and CT-myelography are tests of choice for anatomic definition of spine disease. Electromyography (EMG) and nerve conduction studies useful for functional assessment of peripheral nervous system.

■ ETIOLOGY

Lumbar Disk Disease

Common cause of low back and leg pain; usually at L4-L5 or L5-S1 levels. Dermatomal sensory loss, reduction or loss of deep tendon reflexes, or myotomal pattern of weakness more informative than pain pattern for localization. Usually unilateral; can be bilateral with large central disk herniations compressing multiple nerve roots and causing cauda equina syndrome (Chap. 200).

Indications for lumbar disk surgery:

- Progressive motor weakness on exam or progressive nerve root injury demonstrated on EMG
- Cauda equina syndrome or spinal cord compression usually indicated by abnormal bowel or bladder function

Incapacitating nerve root pain despite conservative treatment for at least 6–8 weeks: Trials indicate surgery leads to more rapid pain relief but no difference at 1–2 years compared with nonsurgical treatment.

Spinal Stenosis

A narrowed spinal canal producing neurogenic claudication, i.e., back, buttock, and/or leg pain induced by walking or standing and relieved by sitting. Symptoms are usually bilateral. Unlike vascular claudication, symptoms are provoked by standing without walking. Unlike lumbar disk disease, symptoms are relieved by sitting. Focal neurologic deficits common; severe neurologic deficits (paralysis, incontinence) rare. Stenosis results from acquired (75%), congenital, or mixed acquired/congenital factors.

- Symptomatic treatment adequate for mild disease
- Surgery indicated when medical therapy does not allow for activities of daily living or if focal neurologic signs are present. Most pts treated surgically experience relief of back and leg pain; 25% develop recurrent stenosis within 7–10 years.

Trauma

Low back strain or *sprain* used to describe minor, self-limited injuries associated with LBP. *Vertebral fractures* from trauma result in anterior wedging or compression of vertebral bodies; burst fractures involving vertebral body and posterior spine elements can occur. Neurologic impairment common with vertebral fractures; early surgical intervention indicated. CT scans used to screen for spine disease in moderate to severe trauma; superior to routine x-rays for bony disease. Most common cause of *nontraumatic fracture* is osteoporosis; others are osteomalacia, hyperparathyroidism, hyperthyroidism, multiple myeloma, or metastatic carcinoma.

Spondylolisthesis

Slippage of anterior spine forward, leaving posterior elements behind; L4-L5 > L5-S1 levels; can produce LBP or radiculopathy/cauda equina syndrome (Chap. 200).

Osteoarthritis (Spondylosis)

Back pain induced by spine movement and associated with stiffness. Increases with age; radiologic findings do not correlate with severity of pain. Osteophytes or combined disc-osteophytes may cause or contribute to central spinal canal stenosis, lateral recess stenosis, or neural foraminal narrowing.

Vertebral Metastases

Back pain most common neurologic symptom in pts with systemic cancer and may be presenting complaint; pain typically not relieved by rest. Metastatic carcinoma, multiple myeloma, and lymphomas frequently involve spine. MRI or CT-myelography demonstrates vertebral body metastasis; disk space is spared.

Vertebral Osteomyelitis

Back pain unrelieved by rest; focal spine tenderness, elevated ESR. Primary source of infection is usually lung, urinary tract, or skin; IV drug abuse a risk factor. Destruction of the vertebral bodies and disk space common. Lumbar spinal epidural abscess presents as back pain and fever; exam may be normal or show radicular findings, spinal cord involvement, or cauda equina syndrome. Extent of abscess best defined by MRI.

Lumbar Adhesive Arachnoiditis

May follow inflammation within subarachnoid space; fibrosis results in clumping of nerve roots, best seen by MRI; treatment is unsatisfactory.

Immune Disorders

Ankylosing spondylitis, rheumatoid arthritis, Reiter's syndrome, psoriatic arthritis, and chronic inflammatory bowel disease. Ankylosing spondylitis—typically male <40 years with nocturnal back pain and morning stiffness, elevated ESR and presence of HLA-B27; pain unrelieved by rest but improves with exercise.

Osteoporosis

Loss of bone substance resulting from hyperparathyroidism, chronic glucocorticoid use, immobilization, other medical disorders, or increasing age (particularly in females). Sole manifestation may be back pain exacerbated by movement. Can also occur in the upper back.

Visceral Diseases (Table 54-3)

Pelvis refers pain to sacral region, lower abdomen to mid-lumbar region, upper abdomen to lower thoracic or upper lumbar region. Local signs are absent; normal movements of the spine are painless. A contained rupture of an abdominal aortic aneurysm may produce isolated back pain.

TABLE 54-3 VISCERAL CAUSES OF LOW BACK PAIN

Stomach (posterior wall)—gallbladder—gallstones
Pancreas—tumor, cyst, pancreatitis
Retroperitoneal—hemorrhage, tumor, pyelonephritis
Vascular—abdominal aortic aneurysm, renal artery and vein thrombosis
Colon—colitis, diverticulitis, neoplasm
Uterosacral ligaments—endometriosis, carcinoma
Uterine malposition
Menstrual pain
Neoplastic infiltration of nerves
Radiation neurosis of tumors/nerves
Prostate—carcinoma, prostatitis
Kidney—renal stones, inflammatory disease, neoplasm, infection

Other

Chronic LBP with no clear cause; psychiatric disorders, substance abuse may be associated.

| TREATMENT | Low Back Pain |

ACUTE LOW BACK PAIN (ALBP)
- Pain of <3 months' duration.
- When leg pain absent, prognosis is excellent; full recovery in 85%.
- Management controversial; few well-controlled clinical trials exist.
- If "risk factors" (Table 54-2) are absent, initial treatment is symptomatic and no diagnostic tests necessary.
- Clinical trials do not show benefit from bed rest >2 days. Possible benefits of early activity—cardiovascular conditioning, disk and cartilage nutrition, bone and muscle strength, increased endorphin levels.
- A short course of lumbar spinal manipulation or physical therapy is a reasonable option.
- Proof lacking to support acupuncture, ultrasound, diathermy, transcutaneous electrical nerve stimulation, biofeedback, magnets, traction, or electrical stimulation.
- Self-application of ice or heat or use of shoe insoles is optional given low cost and risk.
- Spine infections, fractures, tumors, or rapidly progressive neurologic deficits require urgent diagnostic evaluation.
- Drug treatment of ALBP includes NSAIDs and acetaminophen (Chap. 6).
- Muscle relaxants (cyclobenzaprine) may be useful but sedation is a common side effect.
- Opioids are not clearly superior to NSAIDs or acetaminophen for ALBP.
- No evidence to support oral or injected epidural glucocorticoids.

CHRONIC LOW BACK PAIN (CLBP)
- Pain lasting >12 weeks; differential diagnosis includes most conditions described above.
- CLBP causes can be clarified by neuroimaging and EMG/nerve conduction studies; diagnosis of radiculopathy secure when results concordant with findings on neurologic exam. Treatment should not be based on neuroimaging alone: up to one-third of asymptomatic young adults have a herniated lumbar disk by CT or MRI.
- Management is not amenable to a simple algorithmic approach. Treatment based on identification of underlying cause; when specific cause not found, conservative management necessary.
- Drug treatment and comfort measures similar to those described for ALBP.
- Evidence supports the use of exercise therapy; effective in returning some pts to work, diminishing pain, and improving walking distances.
- Cognitive-behavioral therapy may have some use; long-term results unclear.

- Alternative therapies including spinal manipulation, acupuncture, and massage are frequently tried; trials are mixed as to their effectiveness.
- Some pts report short-term pain relief with percutaneous electrical nerve stimulation, but a recent evidence-based guideline failed to show efficacy.
- Epidural glucocorticoids and facet joint injections are not effective in the absence of radiculopathy.
- Surgical intervention for chronic LBP without radiculopathy is controversial, and clinical trials do not support its use.

NECK AND SHOULDER PAIN

Usually arises from diseases of the cervical spine and soft tissues of the neck; typically precipitated by movement and may be accompanied by focal tenderness and limitation of motion.

■ ETIOLOGY

Trauma to the Cervical Spine

Trauma to the cervical spine (fractures, subluxation) places the spine at risk for compression; immediate immobilization of the neck is essential to minimize movement of unstable cervical spine segments.

Whiplash injury is due to trauma (usually automobile accidents) causing cervical musculoligamentous injury due to hyperflexion or hyperextension. This diagnosis is not applied to pts with fractures, disk herniation, head injury, focal neurologic findings, or altered consciousness.

Cervical Disk Disease

Herniation of a lower cervical disk is a common cause of neck, shoulder, arm, or hand pain or tingling. Neck pain (worse with movement), stiffness, and limited range of neck motion are common. With nerve root compression, pain may radiate into a shoulder or arm. Extension and lateral rotation of the neck narrows the intervertebral foramen and may reproduce radicular symptoms (Spurling's sign). In young individuals, acute radiculopathy from a ruptured disk is often traumatic. *Subacute radiculopathy* is less likely to be related to a specific traumatic incident and may involve both disk disease and spondylosis. Clinical features of cervical nerve root lesions are summarized in Table 54-4.

Cervical Spondylosis

Osteoarthritis of the cervical spine may produce neck pain that radiates into the back of the head, shoulders, or arms; can also be source of headaches in the posterior occipital region. A combined radiculopathy and myelopathy may occur. An electrical sensation elicited by neck flexion and radiating down the spine from the neck (Lhermitte's symptom) usually indicates spinal cord involvement. MRI or CT-myelography can define the anatomic abnormalities, and EMG and nerve conduction studies can quantify the severity and localize the levels of nerve root injury.

TABLE 54-4 CERVICAL RADICULOPATHY—NEUROLOGIC FEATURES

| Cervical Nerve Roots | Examination Findings | | | Pain Distribution |
	Reflex	Sensory	Motor	
C5	Biceps	Over lateral deltoid	Supraspinatus[a] (initial arm abduction) Infraspinatus[a] (arm external rotation) Deltoid[a] (arm abduction) Biceps (arm flexion)	Lateral arm, medial scapula
C6	Biceps	Thumb, index fingers Radial hand/forearm	Biceps (arm flexion) Pronator teres (internal forearm rotation)	Lateral forearm, thumb, index finger
C7	Triceps	Middle fingers Dorsum forearm	Triceps[a] (arm extension) Wrist extensors[a] Extensor digitorum[a] (finger extension)	Posterior arm, dorsal forearm, lateral hand
C8	Finger flexors	Little finger Medial hand and forearm	Abductor pollicis brevis (abduction D1) First dorsal interosseous (abduction D2) Abductor digiti minimi (abduction D5)	4th and 5th fingers, medial forearm
T1	Finger flexors	Axilla and medial arm	Abductor pollicis brevis (abduction D1) First dorsal interosseous (abduction D2) Abductor digiti minimi (abduction D5)	Medial arm, axilla

[a]These muscles receive the majority of innervation from this root.

Other Causes of Neck Pain

Includes *rheumatoid arthritis* of the cervical apophyseal joints, ankylosing spondylitis, *herpes zoster* (shingles), *neoplasms* metastatic to the cervical spine, *infections* (osteomyelitis and epidural abscess), and *metabolic bone diseases*. Neck pain may also be referred from the heart with coronary artery ischemia (cervical angina syndrome).

Thoracic Outlet

An anatomic region containing the first rib, the subclavian artery and vein, the brachial plexus, the clavicle, and the lung apex. Injury may result in posture- or movement-induced pain around the shoulder and supraclavicular region. *True neurogenic thoracic outlet syndrome* is uncommon and results from compression of the lower trunk of the brachial plexus by an anomalous band of tissue; treatment consists of surgical division of the band. *Arterial thoracic outlet syndrome* results from compression of the subclavian artery by a cervical rib; treatment is with thrombolysis or anticoagulation, and surgical excision of the cervical rib. *Disputed thoracic outlet syndrome* includes a large number of pts with chronic arm and shoulder pain of unclear cause; surgery is controversial, and treatment is often unsuccessful.

Brachial Plexus and Nerves

Pain from injury to the brachial plexus or peripheral nerves can mimic pain of cervical spine origin. *Neoplastic infiltration* can produce this syndrome, as can *postradiation fibrosis* (pain less often present). *Acute brachial neuritis* consists of acute onset of severe shoulder or scapular pain followed over days by weakness of proximal arm and shoulder girdle muscles innervated by the upper brachial plexus; onset often preceded by an infection or immunization.

Shoulder

If signs of radiculopathy are absent, differential diagnosis includes mechanical shoulder pain (tendinitis, bursitis, rotator cuff tear, dislocation, adhesive capsulitis, and cuff impingement under the acromion) and referred pain [subdiaphragmatic irritation, angina, Pancoast (apical lung) tumor]. Mechanical pain is often worse at night, associated with shoulder tenderness, and aggravated by abduction, internal rotation, or extension of the arm.

TREATMENT   Neck and Shoulder Pain

- Indications for cervical disk surgery are similar to those for lumbar disk; however, with cervical disease, an aggressive approach is indicated if spinal cord injury is threatened.

NECK PAIN WITHOUT RADICULOPATHY

- Spontaneous improvement is expected for most acute neck pain.
- Symptomatic treatment of neck pain includes analgesic medications.
- If not related to trauma, supervised exercise appears to be effective.
- No valid clinical evidence to support cervical fusion or cervical disc arthroplasty.

- No evidence to support radiofrequency neurotomy or cervical facet injections.

NECK PAIN WITH RADICULOPATHY

- Natural history is favorable and many will improve without specific therapy.
- NSAIDs, with or without muscle relaxants are appropriate initial therapy.
- Soft cervical collars are modestly helpful in limiting movements that exacerbate pain.
- *Cervical spondylosis* with bony, compressive cervical radiculopathy is generally treated with surgical decompression to interrupt the progression of neurologic signs.
- Surgical options for *cervical herniated disks* consist of anterior cervical discectomy alone, laminectomy with discectomy, discectomy with fusion, and disk arthroplasty. The cumulative risk of subsequent radiculopathy or myelopathy at cervical segments adjacent to the fusion is ~3% per year.
- Indications for surgery include a progressive radicular motor deficit, pain that limits function and fails to respond to conservative management, or spinal cord compression.

For more detailed discussion, see Engstrom JW, Deyo RA: Back and Neck Pain, Chap. 15, p. 129, in HPIM-18.

CHAPTER **55**
Headache

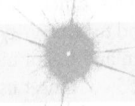

APPROACH TO THE PATIENT | Headache

Headache is among the most common reasons that pts seek medical attention. Headache can be either primary or secondary (Table 55-1). First step—distinguish serious from benign etiologies. Symptoms that raise suspicion for a serious cause are listed in Table 55-2. Intensity of head pain rarely has diagnostic value; most pts who present to emergency ward with worst headache of their lives have migraine. Headache location can suggest involvement of local structures (temporal pain in giant cell arteritis, facial pain in sinusitis). Ruptured aneurysm (instant onset), cluster headache (peak over 3–5 min), and migraine (onset over minutes to hours) differ in time to peak intensity. Provocation by environmental factors suggests a benign cause.

TABLE 55-1 COMMON CAUSES OF HEADACHE

Primary Headache		Secondary Headache	
Type	%	Type	%
Tension-type	69	Systemic infection	63
Migraine	16	Head injury	4
Idiopathic stabbing	2	Vascular disorders	1
Exertional	1	Subarachnoid hemorrhage	<1
Cluster	0.1	Brain tumor	0.1

Source: After J Olesen et al: *The Headaches.* Philadelphia, Lippincott, Williams & Wilkins, 2005.

Complete neurologic exam is important in the evaluation of headache. If exam is abnormal or if serious underlying cause is suspected, an imaging study (CT or MRI) is indicated as a first step. Lumbar puncture (LP) is required when meningitis (stiff neck, fever) or subarachnoid hemorrhage (after negative imaging) is a possibility. The psychological state of the pt should also be evaluated since a relationship exists between pain and depression.

■ MIGRAINE

A benign and recurring syndrome of headache associated with other symptoms of neurologic dysfunction in varying admixtures. Second to tension-type as most common cause of headache; afflicts ~15% of women and 6% of men annually. Diagnostic criteria for migraine are listed in Table 55-3. Onset usually in childhood, adolescence, or early adulthood; however, initial attack may occur at any age. Family history often positive. Women may have increased sensitivity to attacks during menstrual cycle. Classic triad: premonitory visual (scotoma or scintillations), sensory, or motor symptoms; unilateral throbbing headache; and nausea and vomiting. Most pts do not have visual aura or other

TABLE 55-2 HEADACHE SYMPTOMS THAT SUGGEST A SERIOUS UNDERLYING DISORDER

"Worst" headache ever

First severe headache

Subacute worsening over days or weeks

Abnormal neurologic examination

Fever or unexplained systemic signs

Vomiting that precedes headache

Pain induced by bending, lifting, cough

Pain that disturbs sleep or presents immediately upon awakening

Known systemic illness

Onset after age 55

Pain associated with local tenderness, e.g., region of temporal artery

TABLE 55-3 SIMPLIFIED DIAGNOSTIC CRITERIA FOR MIGRAINE

Repeated attacks of headache lasting 4–72 h in pts with a normal physical examination, no other reasonable cause for the headache, and:

At least 2 of the following features:	Plus at least 1 of the following features:
Unilateral pain	Nausea/vomiting
Throbbing pain	Photophobia and phonophobia
Aggravation by movement	
Moderate or severe intensity	

Source: Adapted from the International Headache Society Classification (Headache Classification Committee of the International Headache Society, 2004).

premonitory symptoms and are therefore referred to as having "common migraine." Photo- and phonophobia common. Vertigo may occur. Focal neurologic disturbances without headache or vomiting (migraine equivalents) may also occur. An attack lasting 4–72 h is typical, as is relief after sleep. Attacks may be triggered by glare, bright lights, sounds, hunger, stress, physical exertion, hormonal fluctuations, lack of sleep, alcohol, or other chemical stimulation.

TREATMENT Migraine

- Three approaches to migraine treatment: nonpharmacologic (such as the avoidance of pt-specific triggers; information for pts is available at *www.achenet.org*); drug treatment of acute attacks (Tables 55-4 and 55-5); and prophylaxis (Table 55-6).
- Drug treatment necessary for most migraine pts, but avoidance or management of environmental triggers is sufficient for some.
- General principles of pharmacologic treatment:
  - Response rates vary from 50—70%.
  - Initial drug choice is empirical—influenced by age, coexisting illnesses, and side effect profile.
  - Efficacy of prophylactic treatment may take several months to assess with each drug.
  - When an acute attack requires additional medication 60 min after the first dose, then the initial drug dose should be increased for subsequent attacks.
- Mild to moderate acute migraine attacks often respond to over-the-counter (OTC) NSAIDs when taken early in the attack.
- Triptans are widely used also but many have recurrence of pain after initial relief.
- There is less frequent headache recurrence when using ergots, but more frequent side effects.
- For prophylaxis, tricyclic antidepressants are a good first choice for young people with difficulty falling asleep; verapamil is often a first choice for prophylaxis in the elderly.

TABLE 55-4 TREATMENT OF ACUTE MIGRAINE

Drug	Trade Name	Dosage
Simple Analgesics		
Acetaminophen, aspirin, caffeine	Excedrin Migraine	Two tablets or caplets q6h (max 8 per day)
NSAIDs		
Naproxen	Aleve, Anaprox, generic	220–550 mg PO bid
Ibuprofen	Advil, Motrin, generic	400 mg PO q3–4h
Tolfenamic acid	Clotam Rapid	200 mg PO. May repeat ×1 after 1–2 h
5-HT$_1$ Agonists		
Oral		
Ergotamine	Ergomar	One 2-mg sublingual tablet at onset and q½h (max 3 per day, 5 per week)
Ergotamine 1 mg, caffeine 100 mg	Ercaf, Wigraine	One or two tablets at onset, then one tablet q½h (max 6 per day, 10 per week)
Naratriptan	Amerge	2.5-mg tablet at onset; may repeat once after 4 h
Rizatriptan	Maxalt	5- or 10-mg tablet at onset; may repeat after 2 h (max 30 mg/d)
	Maxalt-MLT	
Sumatriptan	Imitrex	50- or 100-mg tablet at onset; may repeat after 2 h (max 200 mg/d)
Frovatriptan	Frova	2.5-mg tablet at onset, may repeat after 2 h (max 5 mg/d)
Almotriptan	Axert	12.5-mg tablet at onset, may repeat after 2 h (max 25 mg/d)
Eletriptan	Relpax	40 or 80 mg
Zolmitriptan	Zomig	2.5-mg tablet at onset; may repeat after 2 h (max 10 mg/d)
	Zomig Rapimelt	
Nasal		
Dihydroergotamine	Migranal Nasal Spray	Prior to nasal spray, the pump must be primed 4 times; 1 spray (0.5 mg) is administered, followed in 15 min by a second spray
Sumatriptan	Imitrex Nasal Spray	5- or 20-mg intranasal spray as 4 sprays of 5 mg or a single 20-mg spray (may repeat once after 2 h, not to exceed a dose of 40 mg/d)
Zolmitriptan	Zomig	5-mg intranasal spray as one spray (may repeat once after 2 h, not to exceed a dose of 10 mg/d)

TABLE 55-4 TREATMENT OF ACUTE MIGRAINE (CONTINUED)

Drug	Trade Name	Dosage
Parenteral		
Dihydroergotamine	DHE-45	1 mg IV, IM, or SC at onset and q1h (max 3 mg/d, 6 mg per week)
Sumatriptan	Imitrex Injection	6 mg SC at onset (may repeat once after 1 h for max of 2 doses in 24 h)
Dopamine Antagonists		
Oral		
Metoclopramide	Reglan,[a] generic[a]	5–10 mg/d
Prochlorperazine	Compazine,[a] generic[a]	1–25 mg/d
Parenteral		
Chlorpromazine	Generic[a]	0.1 mg/kg IV at 2 mg/min; max 35 mg/d
Metoclopramide	Reglan,[a] generic	10 mg IV
Prochlorperazine	Compazine,[a] generic[a]	10 mg IV
Other		
Oral		
Acetaminophen, 325 mg, *plus* dichloralphenazone, 100 mg, *plus* isometheptene, 65 mg	Midrin, Duradrin, generic	Two capsules at onset followed by 1 capsule q1h (max 5 capsules)
Nasal		
Butorphanol	Stadol[a]	1 mg (1 spray in 1 nostril), may repeat if necessary in 1–2 h
Parenteral		
Narcotics	Generic[a]	Multiple preparations and dosages; see Table 6-2

[a]Not all drugs are specifically indicated by the FDA for migraine. Local regulations and guidelines should be consulted.

Note: Antiemetics (e.g., domperidone 10 mg or ondansetron 4 or 8 mg) or prokinetics (e.g., metoclopramide 10 mg) are sometimes useful adjuncts.

Abbreviations: NSAIDs, nonsteroidal anti-inflammatory drugs; 5-HT, 5-hydroxytryptamine.

TABLE 55-5 CLINICAL STRATIFICATION OF ACUTE SPECIFIC MIGRAINE TREATMENTS

Clinical Situation	Treatment Options
Failed NSAIDS/analgesics	**First tier**
	Sumatriptan 50 mg or 100 mg PO
	Almotriptan 12.5 mg PO
	Rizatriptan 10 mg PO
	Eletriptan 40 mg PO
	Zolmitriptan 2.5 mg PO
	Slower effect/better tolerability
	Naratriptan 2.5 mg PO
	Frovatriptan 2.5 mg PO
	Infrequent headache
	Ergotamine 1–2 mg PO
	Dihydroergotamine nasal spray 2 mg
Early nausea or difficulties taking tablets	Zolmitriptan 5 mg nasal spray
	Sumatriptan 20 mg nasal spray
	Rizatriptan 10 mg MLT wafer
Headache recurrence	Ergotamine 2 mg (most effective PR/usually with caffeine)
	Naratriptan 2.5 mg PO
	Almotriptan 12.5 mg PO
	Eletriptan 40 mg
Tolerating acute treatments poorly	Naratriptan 2.5 mg
	Almotriptan 12.5 mg
Early vomiting	Zolmitriptan 5 mg nasal spray
	Sumatriptan 25 mg PR
	Sumatriptan 6 mg SC
Menses-related headache	**Prevention**
	Ergotamine PO at night
	Estrogen patches
	Treatment
	Triptans
	Dihydroergotamine nasal spray
Very rapidly developing symptoms	Zolmitriptan 5 mg nasal spray
	Sumatriptan 6 mg SC
	Dihydroergotamine 1 mg IM

TABLE 55-6 PREVENTIVE TREATMENTS IN MIGRAINE[a]

Drug	Dose	Selected Side Effects
Pizotifen[b]	0.5–2 mg qd	Weight gain
		Drowsiness
Beta blocker		
Propranolol	40–120 mg bid	Reduced energy
		Tiredness
		Postural symptoms
		Contraindicated in asthma
Tricyclics		
Amitriptyline	10–75 mg at night	Drowsiness
Dothiepin	25–75 mg at night	
Nortriptyline[c]	25–75 mg at night	
Anticonvulsants		
Topiramate	25–200 mg/d	Paresthesias
		Cognitive symptoms
		Weight loss
		Glaucoma
		Caution with nephrolithiasis
Valproate	400–600 mg bid	Drowsiness
		Weight gain
		Tremor
		Hair loss
		Fetal abnormalities
		Hematologic or liver abnormalities
Gabapentin	900–3600 mg qd	Dizziness
		Sedation
Serotonergic drugs		
Methysergide	1–4 mg qd	Drowsiness
		Leg cramps
		Hair loss
		Retroperitoneal fibrosis (1-month drug holiday is required every 6 months)
Flunarizine[b]	5–15 mg qd	Drowsiness
		Weight gain
		Depression
		Parkinsonism

(continued)

TABLE 55-6 PREVENTIVE TREATMENTS IN MIGRAINE[a] (CONTINUED)

Drug	Dose	Selected Side Effects
No convincing evidence from controlled trials		
Verapamil		
Controlled trials demonstrate *no effect*		
Nimodipine		
Clonidine		
SSRIs: fluoxetine		

[a]Commonly used preventives are listed with typical doses and common side effects. Not all listed medicines are approved by the FDA; local regulations and guidelines should be consulted.
[b]Not available in the United States.
[c]Some pts may only need a total dose of 10 mg, although generally 1–1.5 mg/kg body weight is required.

Tension-Type Headache

Common in all age groups. Pain is described as bilateral tight, bandlike discomfort. May persist for hours or days; usually builds slowly.

- Pain can be managed generally with simple analgesics such as acetaminophen, aspirin, or NSAIDs.
- Often related to stress; responds to behavioral approaches including relaxation.
- Amitriptyline may be helpful for chronic (>15 days per month) tension-type headache prophylaxis.

Cluster Headache

Rare form of primary headache; population frequency 0.1%. Characterized by episodes of recurrent, deep, unilateral, retroorbital searing pain. Unilateral lacrimation and nasal and conjunctival congestion may be present. Visual complaints, nausea, or vomiting are rare. Unlike migraine, pts with cluster tend to move about during attacks. A core feature is periodicity. Typically, daily bouts of one to two attacks of relatively short-duration unilateral pain for 8–10 weeks a year; usually followed by a pain-free interval that averages a little less than a year. Alcohol provokes attacks in 70%.

- Prophylaxis with verapamil (40–80 mg twice daily to start), lithium (400–800 mg/d), prednisone (60 mg/d for 7 days followed by a taper over 21 days), or ergotamine (1–2 mg suppository 1–2 h before expected attack).
- High-flow oxygen (10–12 L/min for 15–20 min) or sumatriptan (6 mg SC or 20-mg nasal spray) is useful for the acute attack.
- Deep-brain stimulation of the posterior hypothalamic gray matter is successful for refractory cases as is the less-invasive approach of occipital nerve stimulation.

Post-Concussion Headache

Common following motor vehicle collisions, other head trauma; severe injury or loss of consciousness often not present. Symptoms of headache, dizziness, vertigo, impaired memory, poor concentration, irritability; typically remits after several weeks to months. Neurologic examination and neuroimaging studies normal. Not a functional disorder; cause unknown and treatment usually not satisfactory.

Lumbar Puncture Headache

Typical onset within 48 h after LP; follows 10–30% of LPs. Positional: onset when pt sits or stands, relief by lying flat. Most cases remit spontaneously in ≤1 week. Oral or IV caffeine (500 mg IV over 2 hours) successful in 85%; epidural blood patch effective immediately in refractory cases.

Cough Headache

Transient severe head pain with coughing, bending, lifting, sneezing, or stooping; lasts for several minutes; men > women. Usually benign, but posterior fossa mass lesion in some pts; therefore consider brain MRI.

Indomethacin-Responsive Headaches

A diverse set of disorders that respond often exquisitely to indomethacin includes:
- *Paroxysmal hemicrania*: Frequent unilateral, severe, short-lasting episodes of headache that are often retroorbital and associated with autonomic phenomena such as lacrimation and nasal congestion.
- *Hemicrania continua*: Moderate and continuous unilateral pain associated with fluctuations of severe pain that may be associated with autonomic features.
- *Primary stabbing headache*: Stabbing pain confined to the head or rarely the face lasting from 1 to many seconds or minutes.
- *Primary cough headache*
- *Primary exertional headache*: Has features similar to cough headache and migraine; usually precipitated by any form of exercise.

■ FACIAL PAIN

Most common cause of facial pain is dental; triggered by hot, cold, or sweet foods. Exposure to cold repeatedly induces dental pain. Trigeminal neuralgia consists of paroxysmal, electric shock–like episodes of pain in the distribution of trigeminal nerve; occipital neuralgia presents as lancinating occipital pain. These disorders are discussed in Chap. 199.

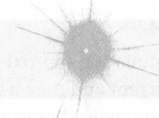

For a more detailed discussion, see Goadsby PJ, Raskin NH: Headache, Chap. 14, p. 112, in HPIM-18.

CHAPTER **56**
Syncope

Syncope is a transient, self-limited loss of consciousness and postural tone due to reduced cerebral blood flow. It may occur suddenly, without warning, or may be preceded by presyncopal symptoms such as lightheadedness or faintness, weakness, fatigue, nausea, dimming vision, ringing in ears, or sweating. The syncopal pt appears pale and has a faint, rapid, or irregular pulse. Breathing may be almost imperceptible; transient myoclonic or clonic movements may occur. Recovery of consciousness is prompt if pt is maintained in a horizontal position and cerebral perfusion is restored.

APPROACH TO THE PATIENT	Syncope

The cause may be apparent only at the time of the event, leaving few, if any, clues when the pt is seen by the physician. Other disorders must be distinguished from syncope, including seizures, vertebrobasilar ischemia, hypoxemia, and hypoglycemia (see below). First consider serious underlying etiologies; among these are massive internal hemorrhage, myocardial infarction (can be painless), and cardiac arrhythmias. In elderly pts, a sudden faint without obvious cause should raise the question of complete heart block or a tachyarrhythmia. Loss of consciousness in particular situations, such as during venipuncture or micturition, suggests a benign abnormality of vascular tone. The position of the pt at the time of the syncopal episode is important; syncope in the supine position is unlikely to be vasovagal and suggests arrhythmia or seizure. Medications must be considered, including nonprescription drugs or health store supplements, with particular attention to recent changes. Symptoms of impotence, bowel and bladder difficulties, disturbed sweating, or an abnormal neurologic exam suggest a primary neurogenic cause. An algorithmic approach is presented in Fig. 56-1.

◼ ETIOLOGY

Syncope is usually due to a neurally mediated disorder, orthostatic hypotension, or an underlying cardiac condition (Table 56-1). Not infrequently the cause is multifactorial.

Neurocardiogenic (Vasovagal and Vasodepressor) Syncope

The common faint, experienced by normal persons, accounts for approximately half of all episodes of syncope. It is frequently recurrent and may be provoked by hot or crowded environment, alcohol, fatigue, pain, hunger, prolonged standing, or stressful situations.

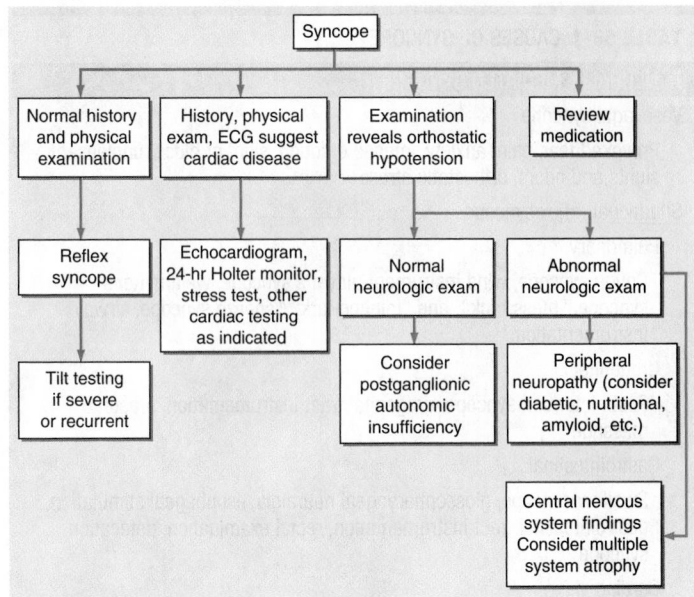

FIGURE 56-1 Approach to the pt with syncope.

Postural (Orthostatic) Hypotension

Sudden rising from a recumbent position or standing quietly are precipitating circumstances. Cause of syncope in 30% of elderly; polypharmacy with antihypertensive or antidepressant drugs often a contributor; physical deconditioning may also play a role. Also occurs with autonomic nervous system disorders, either peripheral (diabetes, nutritional, or amyloid polyneuropathy) or central (multiple system atrophy, Parkinson's disease). Some cases are idiopathic.

▇ DIFFERENTIAL DIAGNOSIS

Seizures

The differential diagnosis is often between syncope and a generalized seizure. Syncope is more likely if the event was provoked by acute pain or anxiety or occurred immediately after arising from a lying or sitting position; seizures are typically not related to posture. Pts with syncope often describe a stereotyped transition from consciousness to unconsciousness that develops over a few seconds. Seizures occur either very abruptly without a transition or are preceded by premonitory symptoms such as an epigastric rising sensation, perception of odd odors, or racing thoughts. Pallor is seen during syncope; cyanosis is usually seen during a seizure. The duration of unconsciousness is usually very brief (i.e., seconds) in syncope and more prolonged (i.e., >5 min) in a seizure. Injury from falling and incontinence are common in seizure, rare in syncope. Whereas tonic-clonic movements are the hallmark of a generalized seizure, myoclonic and other movements also occur in 90% of syncopal episodes and eyewitnesses will often have a difficult time distinguishing between the two etiologies.

TABLE 56-1 CAUSES OF SYNCOPE

A. NEURALLY MEDIATED SYNCOPE

Vasovagal syncope

Provoked fear, pain, anxiety, intense emotion, sight of blood, unpleasant sights and odors, orthostatic stress

Situational reflex syncope

Pulmonary

Cough syncope, wind instrument player's syncope, weightlifter's syncope, "mess trick"[a] and "fainting lark,"[b] sneeze syncope, airway instrumentation

Urogenital

Postmicturition syncope, urogenital tract instrumentation, prostatic massage

Gastrointestinal

Swallow syncope, glossopharyngeal neuralgia, esophageal stimulation, gastrointestinal tract instrumentation, rectal examination, defecation syncope

Cardiac

Swallow syncope, glossopharyngeal neuralgia, esophageal stimulation, gastrointestinal tract instrumentation, rectal examination, defecation syncope

Carotid sinus

Carotid sinus sensitivity, carotid sinus massage

Ocular

Ocular pressure, ocular examination, ocular surgery

B. ORTHOSTATIC HYPOTENSION

Primary autonomic failure due to idiopathic central and peripheral neurodegenerative diseases—the "synucleinopathies"

Lewy body diseases

Parkinson's disease

Lewy body dementia

Pure autonomic failure

Multiple system atrophy (Shy-Drager syndrome)

Secondary autonomic failure due to autonomic peripheral neuropathies

Diabetes

Hereditary amyloidosis (familial amyloid polyneuropathy)

Primary amyloidosis (AL amyloidosis; immunoglobulin light chain associated)

Hereditary sensory and autonomic neuropathies (HSAN) (especially type III—familial dysautonomia)

Idiopathic immune-mediated autonomic neuropathy

TABLE 56-1 CAUSES OF SYNCOPE (CONTINUED)

B. ORTHOSTATIC HYPOTENSION

    Autoimmune autonomic ganglionopathy

    Sjögren's syndrome

    Paraneoplastic autonomic neuropathy

    HIV neuropathy

Postprandial hypotension

Iatrogenic (drug-induced)

Volume depletion

C. CARDIAC SYNCOPE

Arrhythmias

    Sinus node dysfunction

    Atrioventricular dysfunction

    Supraventricular tachycardias

    Ventricular tachycardias

    Inherited channelopathies

Cardiac structural disease

    Valvular disease

    Myocardial ischemia

    Obstructive and other cardiomyopathies

    Atrial myxoma

    Pericardial effusions and tamponade

[a]Hyperventilation for 1 minute, followed by sudden chest compression.
[b]Hyperventilation (20 breaths) in a squatting position, rapid rise to standing, then Valsalva.

Hypoglycemia

Severe hypoglycemia is usually due to a serious disease. Hunger is a premonitory feature that is not typical in syncope. The glucose level at the time of a spell is diagnostic.

Cataplexy

Abrupt partial or complete loss of muscular tone triggered by strong emotions; occurs in 60–75% of narcolepsy pts. Unlike syncope, consciousness is maintained throughout the attacks. No premonitory symptoms.

Psychiatric Disorders

Apparent loss of consciousness can be present in generalized anxiety, panic disorders, major depression, and somatization disorder. Frequently resembles presyncope, although the symptoms are not accompanied by prodromal symptoms and are not relieved by recumbency. Attacks can often be reproduced by hyperventilation and have associated symptoms of panic attacks such as a feeling of impending doom, air hunger, palpitations, and tingling of the fingers and perioral region. Such pts are rarely injured despite numerous falls. There are no clinically significant hemodynamic changes.

TREATMENT Syncope

Therapy is determined by the underlying cause.
- Pts with neurally mediated syncope should be instructed to avoid situations or stimuli that provoke attacks.
- Drug therapy may be necessary for resistant neurally medicated syncope. β-adrenergic antagonists (metoprolol 25–50 mg twice daily; atenolol 25–50 mg/d; or nadolol 10–20 mg twice daily; all starting doses) are the most widely used agents; serotonin reuptake inhibitors (paroxetine 20–40 mg/d, or sertraline 25–50 mg/d) and bupropion SR (150 mg/d) are also effective.
- Pts with orthostatic hypotension should first be treated with removal of vasoactive medications. Then consider nonpharmacologic (pt education regarding moves from supine to upright, increasing fluids and salt in diet) and finally pharmacologic methods such as the mineralo-corticoid fludrocortisone acetate and vasoconstricting agents such as midodrine and pseudoephedrine.

Management of refractory orthostatic hypotension is discussed in Chap. 198.

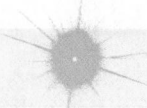

For a more detailed discussion, see Freeman R: Syncope, Chap. 20, p. 171, in HPIM-18.

CHAPTER **57**
Dizziness and Vertigo

APPROACH TO THE PATIENT Dizziness or Vertigo

The term *dizziness* is used by pts to describe a variety of head sensations or gait unsteadiness. With a careful history, distinguishing between *faintness* (presyncope; Chap. 56) and *vertigo* (an illusory or hallucinatory sense of movement of the body or the environment, most often a feeling of spinning) is usually possible.

When the meaning of *dizziness* is uncertain, provocative tests to reproduce the symptoms may be helpful. Valsalva maneuver, hyperventilation, or postural changes leading to orthostasis may reproduce faintness. Rapid rotation in a swivel chair is a simple provocative test to reproduce vertigo.

Benign positional vertigo is identified by the Dix-Hallpike maneuver to elicit vertigo and the characteristic nystagmus; the pt begins in a sitting position with head turned 45 degrees; holding the back of the head, examiner gently lowers pt to supine position with head extended backward 20 degrees and observes for nystagmus; after 30 s the pt is raised to sitting position and after 1 min rest the maneuver is repeated on other side.

If a central cause for the vertigo is suspected (e.g., signs of peripheral vertigo are absent or other neurologic abnormalities are present), then prompt evaluation for central pathology is required. The initial test is usually an MRI scan of the posterior fossa. Distinguishing between central and peripheral etiologies can be accomplished with vestibular function tests, including videonystagmography and simple bedside exams including the *head impulse test* (rapid, small amplitude head rotations while pt instructed to fixate on the examiner's face; if peripheral, a catch-up saccade is seen at the end of the rotation) and *dynamic visual acuity* (measure acuity at rest and with head rotated back and forth by examiner; a drop in acuity of more than one line on a near card or Snellen chart indicates vestibular dysfunction).

■ FAINTNESS

Faintness is usually described as light-headedness followed by visual blurring and postural swaying along with a feeling of warmth, diaphoresis, and nausea. It is a symptom of insufficient blood, oxygen, or, rarely, glucose supply to the brain. It can occur prior to a syncopal event of any etiology (Chap. 56) and with hyperventilation or hypoglycemia. Lightheadedness can rarely occur during an aura before a seizure. Chronic lightheadedness is a common somatic complaint with depression.

■ VERTIGO

Usually due to a disturbance in the vestibular system; abnormalities in the visual or somatosensory systems may also contribute to vertigo. Frequently accompanied by nausea, postural unsteadiness, and gait ataxia; may be provoked or worsened by head movement.

Physiologic vertigo results from unfamiliar head movement (seasickness) or a mismatch between visual-proprioceptive-vestibular system inputs (height vertigo, visual vertigo during motion picture chase scenes). True vertigo almost never occurs as a presyncopal symptom.

Pathologic vertigo may be caused by a peripheral (labyrinth or eighth nerve) or central CNS lesion. Distinguishing between these causes is the essential first step in diagnosis (Table 57-1) as central lesions require urgent imaging, usually with MRI.

Peripheral Vertigo

Usually severe, accompanied by nausea and emesis. Tinnitus, a feeling of ear fullness, or hearing loss may occur. A characteristic jerk nystagmus is almost always present. The nystagmus does not change direction with a change in direction of gaze; it is usually horizontal with a torsional component and has its fast phase away from the side of the lesion. It is inhibited by visual fixation. The pt senses spinning motion away from the lesion and

TABLE 57-1 FEATURES OF PERIPHERAL AND CENTRAL VERTIGO

Sign or Symptom	Peripheral (Labyrinth or Vestibular Nerve)	Central (Brainstem or Cerebellum)
Direction of associated nystagmus	Unidirectional; fast phase opposite lesion[a]	Bidirectional (direction-changing) or unidirectional
Purely horizontal nystagmus without torsional component	Uncommon	May be present
Purely vertical or purely torsional nystagmus	Never present[b]	May be present
Visual fixation	Inhibits nystagmus	No inhibition
Tinnitus and/or deafness	Often present	Usually absent
Associated central nervous system abnormalities	None	Extremely common (e.g., diplopia, hiccups, cranial neuropathies, dysarthria)
Common causes	Benign paroxysmal positional vertigo, infection (labyrinthitis), vestibular neuritis, Ménière's disease, labyrinthine ischemia, trauma, toxin	Vascular, demyelinating, neoplasm

[a]In Ménière's disease, the direction of the fast phase is variable.
[b]Combined vertical-torsional nystagmus suggests benign paroxysmal positional vertigo.

tends to have difficulty walking, with falls towards the side of the lesion, particularly in the darkness or with eyes closed. No other neurologic abnormalities are present.

Acute prolonged vertigo may be caused by infection, trauma, or ischemia. Often no specific etiology is found, and the nonspecific term *acute labyrinthitis* (or *vestibular neuritis*) is used to describe the event. *Acute bilateral labyrinthine dysfunction* is usually due to drugs (aminoglycoside antibiotics), alcohol, or a neurodegenerative disorder. *Recurrent labyrinthine dysfunction* with signs and symptoms of cochlear disease is usually due to *Ménière's disease* (recurrent vertigo accompanied by tinnitus and deafness). Positional vertigo is usually precipitated by a recumbent head position. *Benign paroxysmal positional vertigo* (BPPV) of the posterior semicircular canal is particularly common; the pattern of nystagmus is distinctive. BPPV may follow trauma but is usually idiopathic; it generally abates spontaneously after weeks or months. *Vestibular schwannomas* of the eighth cranial nerve (acoustic neuroma) usually present as hearing loss and tinnitus, sometimes accompanied by facial weakness and sensory loss due to involvement of cranial nerves VII and V. *Psychogenic vertigo* should be suspected in pts with chronic incapacitating vertigo who also have agoraphobia, panic attacks, a normal neurologic exam, and no nystagmus.

TABLE 57-2 TREATMENT OF VERTIGO

Agent[a]	Dose[b]
Antihistamines	
Meclizine	25–50 mg 3 times daily
Dimenhydrinate	50 mg 1–2 times daily
Promethazine	25 mg 2–3 times daily (can also be given rectally and IM)
Benzodiazepines	
Diazepam	2.5 mg 1–3 times daily
Clonazepam	0.25 mg 1–3 times daily
Anticholinergic	
Scopolamine transdermal[c]	Patch
Physical therapy	
Repositioning maneuvers[d]	
Vestibular rehabilitation	
Other	
Diuretics and/or low-sodium (1 g/d) diet[e]	
Antimigraine drugs[f]	
Methylprednisolone[g]	100 mg daily days 1–3; 80 mg daily days 4–6; 60 mg daily days 7–9; 40 mg daily days 10–12; 20 mg daily days 13–15; 10 mg daily days 16–18, 20, 22
Selective serotonin reuptake inhibitors[h]	

[a]All listed drugs are approved by the U.S. Food and Drug Administration, but most are not approved for the treatment of vertigo.
[b]Usual oral (unless otherwise stated) starting dose in adults; a higher maintenance dose can be reached by a gradual increase.
[c]For motion sickness only.
[d]For benign paroxysmal positional vertigo.
[e]For Ménière's disease.
[f]For vestibular migraine.
[g]For acute vestibular neuritis (started within three days of onset).
[h]For psychosomatic vertigo.

Central Vertigo

Identified by associated brainstem or cerebellar signs such as dysarthria, diplopia, dysphagia, hiccups, other cranial nerve abnormalities, weakness, or limb ataxia; depending on the cause, headache may be present. The nystagmus can take almost any form (i.e., vertical or multidirectional) but is often purely horizontal without a torsional component and changes direction with different directions of gaze. Central nystagmus is not inhibited by fixation. Central vertigo may be chronic, mild, and is usually not accompanied by tinnitus or hearing loss. It may be due to vascular, demyelinating, or neoplastic disease. Vertigo may be a manifestation of migraine or, rarely, of temporal lobe epilepsy.

TREATMENT	Vertigo

- Treatment of acute vertigo consists of vestibular suppressant drugs for short-term relief (Table 57-2). They may hinder central compensation, prolonging the duration of symptoms, and therefore should be used sparingly.
- Vestibular rehabilitation promotes central adaptation processes and may habituate motion sensitivity and other symptoms of psychosomatic dizziness.
- BPPV may respond dramatically to repositioning exercises such as the Epley procedure designed to empty particulate debris from the posterior semicircular canal (*www.youtube.com/watch?v=pa6t-Bpg494*).
- For vestibular neuritis, antiviral medications are of no proven benefit unless herpes zoster oticus is present. Some data suggest that glucocorticoids improve the likelihood of recovery in vestibular neuritis.
- Ménière's disease may respond to a low-salt diet (1 g/d) or to a diuretic. Otolaryngology referral is recommended.
- Recurrent episodes of migraine-associated vertigo should be treated with antimigraine therapy (Chap. 55).

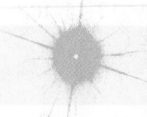

For a more detailed discussion, see Walker MF, Daroff RB: Dizziness, and Vertigo, Chap. 21, p. 178, in HPIM-18.

CHAPTER **58**
Acute Visual Loss and Double Vision

APPROACH TO THE PATIENT	Acute Visual Loss or Double Vision

Accurate measurement of visual acuity in each eye (with glasses) is of primary importance. Additional assessments include testing of pupils, eye movements, ocular alignment, and visual fields. Slit-lamp examination can exclude corneal infection, trauma, glaucoma, uveitis, and cataract. Ophthalmoscopic exam to inspect the optic disc and retina often requires pupillary dilation using 1% tropicamide and 2.5% phenylephrine; risk of provoking an attack of narrow-angle glaucoma is remote.

Visual field mapping by finger confrontation localizes lesions in the visual pathway (Fig. 58-1); formal testing using a perimeter may be necessary. The goal is to determine whether the lesion is anterior to, at, or posterior to the optic chiasm. A scotoma confined to one eye is caused by an anterior lesion affecting the optic nerve or globe; swinging flashlight test may reveal an afferent pupil defect. History and ocular exam are usually sufficient for diagnosis. If a bitemporal hemianopia is present, lesion is located at optic chiasm (e.g., pituitary adenoma, meningioma).

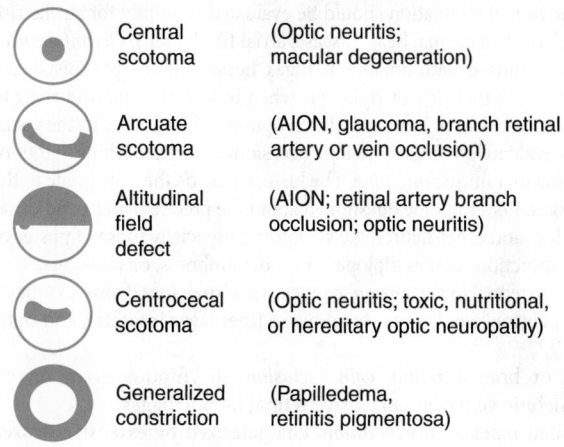

OPTIC NERVE OR RETINA

	Central scotoma	(Optic neuritis; macular degeneration)
	Arcuate scotoma	(AION, glaucoma, branch retinal artery or vein occlusion)
	Altitudinal field defect	(AION; retinal artery branch occlusion; optic neuritis)
	Centrocecal scotoma	(Optic neuritis; toxic, nutritional, or hereditary optic neuropathy)
	Generalized constriction	(Papilledema, retinitis pigmentosa)

OPTIC CHIASM

Left   Right

Bitemporal hemianopia — (Optic chiasm compression by pituitary tumor, meningioma)

RETRO-CHIASMAL PATHWAY

Right homonymous hemianopia — (Lesion of left optic tract, lateral geniculate body, optic radiations, or visual cortex)

Superior right quadrantopia ("Pie in the Sky") — (Lesion of left optic radiations in temporal lobe)

Macular sparing — (Bilateral visual cortex lesions)

FIGURE 58-1 Deficits in visual fields caused by lesions affecting visual pathways.

Homonymous visual field loss signals a retrochiasmal lesion affecting the optic tract, lateral geniculate body, optic radiations, or visual cortex (e.g., stroke, tumor, abscess). Neuroimaging is recommended for any pt with a bitemporal or homonymous hemianopia.

■ TRANSIENT OR SUDDEN VISUAL LOSS

Amaurosis fugax (*transient monocular blindness*; a TIA of the retina) usually occurs from a retinal embolus often arising from severe ipsilateral carotid stenosis. Prolonged occlusion of the central retinal artery results in classic fundus appearance of a milky, infarcted retina with cherry red fovea. Any pt with compromise of the retinal circulation should be evaluated promptly for stroke risk factors (e.g., carotid atheroma, heart disease, atrial fibrillation). *Occipital cortex lesions* can be confused with amaurosis fugax because many pts mistakenly ascribe symptoms to their left or right eye, when in fact they are occurring in the left or right hemifield of both eyes. Interruption of blood flow to the visual cortex causes sudden graying of vision, occasionally with flashing lights or other symptoms that mimic *migraine*. The history may be the only guide to the correct diagnosis. Pts should be questioned about the precise pattern and duration of visual loss and other neurologic symptoms, especially those of posterior circulation dysfunction such as diplopia, vertigo, numbness, or weakness.

Malignant systemic hypertension can cause visual loss from exudates, hemorrhages, cotton-wool spots (focal nerve fiber layer infarcts), and optic disc edema.

In central or branch *retinal vein occlusion*, the fundus exam reveals engorged, phlebitic veins with extensive retinal hemorrhages.

In age-related *macular degeneration*, characterized by extensive drusen and scarring of the pigment epithelium, leakage of blood or fluid from subretinal neovascular membranes can produce sudden central visual loss.

Flashing lights and floaters may indicate a fresh *vitreous detachment*. Separation of the vitreous from the retina is a frequent involutional event in the elderly. It is not harmful unless it creates sufficient traction to produce a *retinal detachment*. *Vitreous hemorrhage* may occur in diabetic pts from retinal neovascularization.

Papilledema refers to optic disc edema from raised intracranial pressure. Transient visual obscurations are common, but visual acuity is not affected unless the papilledema is severe, long-standing, or accompanied by macular exudates or hemorrhage. Enlarged blind spots and peripheral constriction are typical. Neuroimaging should be obtained to exclude an intracranial mass. If negative, an LP is required to confirm elevation of the intracranial pressure. *Pseudotumor cerebri* (idiopathic intracranial hypertension) is a diagnosis of exclusion. Most pts are young, female, and obese; some are found to have occult cerebral venous sinus thrombosis. Treatment is with acetazolamide, repeated LPs, and weight loss; some pts require lumboperitoneal shunting to prevent blindness.

Optic neuritis is a common cause of monocular optic disc swelling and visual loss. If site of inflammation is retrobulbar, fundus will appear normal on initial exam. The typical pt is female, age 15–45, with pain provoked by eye movements. Glucocorticoids, typically IV methylprednisolone (1 g daily for 3 days) followed by oral prednisone (1 mg/kg daily for 11 days), may hasten recovery in severely affected pts but make no difference in final acuity (measured 6 months after the attack). If an MR scan shows multiple demyelinating lesions, treatment for multiple sclerosis (Chap. 202) should be considered. Optic neuritis involving both eyes simultaneously or sequentially suggests neuromyelitis optica.

Anterior ischemic optic neuropathy (AION) is an infarction of the optic nerve head due to inadequate perfusion via the posterior ciliary arteries. Pts have sudden visual loss, often noted on awakening, and painless swelling of the optic disc. It is important to differentiate between nonarteritic (idiopathic) AION and arteritic AION. There is no treatment for nonarteritic AION. In contrast, arteritic AION is caused by *giant cell (temporal) arteritis* and requires immediate glucocorticoid therapy to prevent blindness; temporal artery biopsy establishes the diagnosis. The ESR and C-reactive protein should be checked in any elderly pt with acute optic disc swelling or symptoms suggestive of polymyalgia rheumatica (associated with arteritic AION).

■ DOUBLE VISION (DIPLOPIA)

First step: clarify whether diplopia persists in either eye after covering the opposite eye; if it does the diagnosis is monocular diplopia usually caused by disease intrinsic to the eye with no dire implications for the pt.

If pt has diplopia while being examined, motility testing will usually reveal an abnormality in ocular excursions. However, if the degree of angular separation between the double images is small, the limitation of eye movements may be subtle and difficult to detect. In this situation, the cover test is useful. While the pt is fixating upon a distant target, one eye is covered while observing the other eye for a movement of redress as it takes up fixation. If none is seen, the procedure is repeated with the other eye. With genuine diplopia, this test should reveal ocular malalignment, especially if the head is turned or tilted in the position that gives rise to the worst symptoms.

Common causes of diplopia are summarized in Table 58-1. The physical findings in isolated ocular motor nerve palsies are:

- CN III: Ptosis and deviation of the eye down and outwards, causing vertical and horizontal diplopia. A dilated pupil suggests direct compression of the third nerve; if present, the possibility of an aneurysm of the posterior communicating artery must be considered urgently.
- CN IV: Vertical diplopia with cyclotorsion; the affected eye is slightly elevated, and limitation of depression is seen when the eye is held in adduction. The pt may assume a head tilt to the opposite side (e.g., left head tilt in right fourth nerve paresis).
- CN VI: Horizontal diplopia with crossed eyes; the affected eye cannot abduct.

Isolated ocular motor nerve palsies often occur in pts with hypertension or diabetes. They usually resolve spontaneously over several months.

The development of multiple ocular motor nerve palsies, or diffuse ophthalmoplegia, raises the possibility of myasthenia gravis. In this disease, the pupils are always normal. Systemic weakness may be absent. Multiple ocular motor nerve palsies should be investigated with neuroimaging focusing on the cavernous sinus, superior orbital fissure, and orbital apex where all three nerves are in close proximity. Diplopia that cannot be explained by a single

TABLE 58-1 COMMON CAUSES OF DIPLOPIA

Brainstem stroke (skew deviation, nuclear or fascicular palsy)
Microvascular infarction (III, IV, VI nerve palsy)
Tumor (brainstem, cavernous sinus, superior orbital fissure, orbit)
Multiple sclerosis (internuclear ophthalmoplegia, ocular motor nerve palsy)
Aneurysm (III nerve)
Raised intracranial pressure (VI nerve)
Postviral inflammation
Meningitis (bacterial, fungal, granulomatosis, neoplastic)
Carotid-cavernous fistula or thrombosis
Herpes zoster
Tolosa-Hunt syndrome
Wernicke-Korsakoff syndrome
Botulism
Myasthenia gravis
Guillain-Barré or Fisher syndrome
Graves' disease
Orbital pseudotumor
Orbital myositis
Trauma
Orbital cellulitis

ocular motor nerve palsy may also be caused by carcinomatous or fungal meningitis, Graves' disease, Guillain-Barré syndrome (especially the Miller Fisher variant), or Tolosa-Hunt syndrome.

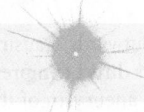

For a more detailed discussion, see Horton JC: Disorders of the Eye, Chap. 28, p. 224, in HPIM-18.

CHAPTER **59**
Weakness and Paralysis

APPROACH TO THE PATIENT | Weakness or Paralysis

Weakness is a reduction of power in one or more muscles. *Paralysis* indicates weakness that is so severe that the muscle cannot be contracted at all, whereas *paresis* refers to weakness that is mild or moderate. The prefix *hemi-* refers to one half of the body, *para-* to both legs, and *quadri-* to all four limbs. The suffix *-plegia* signifies severe weakness or paralysis.

TABLE 59-1 SIGNS THAT DISTINGUISH THE ORIGIN OF WEAKNESS

Sign	Upper Motor Neuron	Lower Motor Neuron	Myopathic
Atrophy	None	Severe	Mild
Fasciculations	None	Common	None
Tone	Spastic	Decreased	Normal/decreased
Distribution of weakness	Pyramidal/regional	Distal/segmental	Proximal
Tendon reflexes	Hyperactive	Hypoactive/absent	Normal/hypoactive
Babinski sign	Present	Absent	Absent

TABLE 59-2 COMMON CAUSES OF WEAKNESS

Upper Motor Neuron

Cortex: ischemia; hemorrhage; intrinsic mass lesion (primary or metastatic cancer, abscess); extrinsic mass lesion (subdural hematoma); degenerative (amyotrophic lateral sclerosis)

Subcortical white matter/internal capsule: ischemia; hemorrhage; intrinsic mass lesion (primary or metastatic cancer, abscess); immunologic (multiple sclerosis); infectious (progressive multifocal leukoencephalopathy)

Brainstem: ischemia; immunologic (multiple sclerosis)

Spinal cord: extrinsic compression (cervical spondylosis, metastatic cancer, epidural abscess); immunologic (multiple sclerosis, transverse myelitis); infectious (AIDS-associated myelopathy, HTLV-I–associated myelopathy, tabes dorsalis); nutritional deficiency (subacute combined degeneration)

Motor Unit

Spinal motor neuron: degenerative (amyotrophic lateral sclerosis); infectious (poliomyelitis)

Spinal root: compressive (degenerative disc disease); immunologic (Guillain-Barré syndrome); infectious (AIDS-associated polyradiculopathy, Lyme disease)

Peripheral nerve: metabolic (diabetes mellitus, uremia, porphyria); toxic (ethanol, heavy metals, many drugs, diphtheria); nutritional (B_{12} deficiency); inflammatory (polyarteritis nodosa); hereditary (Charcot-Marie-Tooth); immunologic (paraneoplastic, paraproteinemia); infectious (AIDS-associated polyneuropathies and mononeuritis multiplex); compressive (entrapment)

Neuromuscular junction: immunologic (myasthenia gravis); toxic (botulism, aminoglycosides)

Muscle: inflammatory (polymyositis, inclusion body myositis); degenerative (muscular dystrophy); toxic (glucocorticoids, ethanol, AZT); infectious (trichinosis); metabolic (hypothyroid, periodic paralyses); congenital (central core disease)

TABLE 59-3 CLINICAL DIFFERENTIATION OF WEAKNESS ARISING FROM DIFFERENT AREAS OF THE NERVOUS SYSTEM

Location of Lesion	Pattern of Weakness	Associated Signs
Upper motor neuron		
Cerebral cortex	Hemiparesis (face and arm predominantly, or leg predominantly)	Hemisensory loss, seizures, homonymous hemianopia or quadrantanopia, aphasia, apraxias, gaze preference
Internal capsule	Hemiparesis (face, arm, leg may be equally affected)	Hemisensory deficit; homonymous hemianopia or quadrantanopia
Brainstem	Hemiparesis (arm and leg; face may not be involved at all)	Vertigo, nausea and vomiting, ataxia and dysarthria, eye movement abnormalities, cranial nerve dysfunction, altered level of consciousness, Horner's syndrome
Spinal cord	Quadriparesis if mid-cervical or above	Sensory level; bowel and bladder dysfunction
	Paraparesis if low cervical or thoracic	
	Hemiparesis below level of lesion (Brown-Séquard)	Contralateral pain/temperature loss below level of lesion
Motor unit		
Spinal motor neuron	Diffuse weakness, may involve control of speech and swallowing	Muscle fasciculations and atrophy; no sensory loss
Spinal root	Radicular pattern of weakness	Dermatomal sensory loss; radicular pain common with compressive lesions
Peripheral nerve		
Polyneuropathy	Distal weakness, usually feet more than hands; usually symmetric	Distal sensory loss, usually feet more than hands
Mononeuropathy	Weakness in distribution of single nerve	Sensory loss in distribution of single nerve
Neuromuscular junction	Fatigable weakness, usually with ocular involvement producing diplopia and ptosis	No sensory loss; no reflex changes
Muscle	Proximal weakness	No sensory loss; diminished reflexes only when severe; may have muscle tenderness

Increased *fatigability* or limitation in function due to pain or articular stiffness is often confused with weakness by pts. Increased time is sometimes required for full power to be exerted, and this *bradykinesia* may be misinterpreted as weakness. Severe proprioceptive sensory loss may also lead to complaints of weakness because adequate feedback information about the direction and power of movements is lacking. Finally, *apraxia*, a disorder of planning and initiating a skilled or learned movement, is sometimes mistaken for weakness.

The history should focus on the tempo of development of weakness, presence of sensory and other neurologic symptoms, medication history, predisposing medical conditions, and family history.

Weakness or paralysis is typically accompanied by other neurologic abnormalities that help to indicate the site of the responsible lesion (Table 59-1). It is important to distinguish weakness arising from disorders of upper motor neurons (i.e., motor neurons in the cerebral cortex and their axons that descend through the subcortical white matter, internal capsule, brainstem, and spinal cord) from disorders of the motor unit (i.e., lower motor neurons in the ventral horn of the spinal cord and their axons in the spinal roots and peripheral nerves, neuromuscular junction, and skeletal muscle).

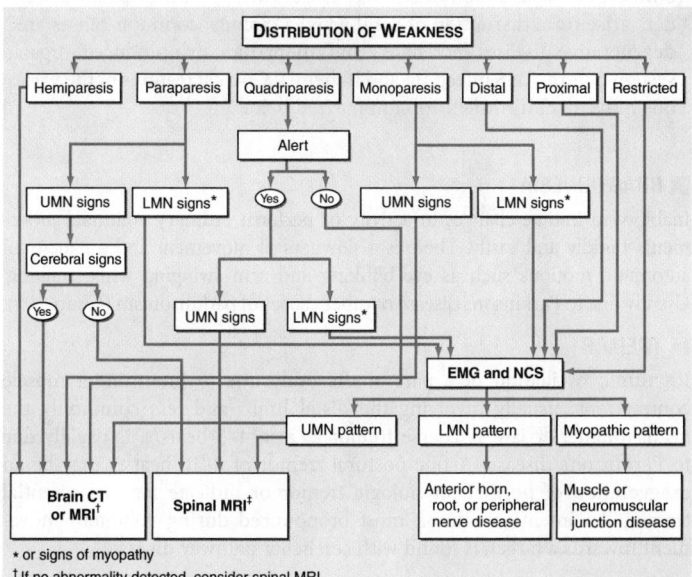

* or signs of myopathy
† If no abnormality detected, consider spinal MRI.
‡ If no abnormality detected, consider myelogram or brain MRI.

FIGURE 59-1 An algorithm for the initial workup of a pt with weakness. CT, computed tomography; EMG, electromyography; LMN, lower motor neuron; MRI, magnetic resonance imaging; NCS, nerve conduction studies; UMN, upper motor neuron.

Table 59-2 lists common causes of weakness by the primary site of pathology. Table 59-3 summarizes patterns with lesions of different parts of the nervous system.

An algorithm for the initial workup of weakness is shown in Fig. 59-1.

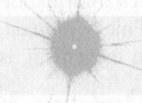

For a more detailed discussion, see Aminoff MJ: Weakness and Paralysis, Chap. 22, p. 181, in HPIM-18.

CHAPTER **60**
Tremor and Movement Disorders

APPROACH TO THE PATIENT | **Movement Disorders**

Divided into akinetic rigid forms, with muscle rigidity and slowness of movement, and hyperkinetic forms, with involuntary movements. In both types, preservation of strength is the rule. Most movement disorders arise from disruption of basal ganglia circuits; common causes are degenerative diseases (hereditary and idiopathic), drug-induced, organ system failure, CNS infection, and ischemia. Clinical features of the various movement disorders are summarized below.

■ BRADYKINESIA

Inability to initiate changes in activity or perform ordinary volitional movements rapidly and easily. There is a slowness of movement and a paucity of automatic motions such as eye blinking and arm swinging while walking. Usually due to Parkinson's disease or other causes of parkinsonism (Chap. 195).

■ TREMOR

Rhythmic oscillation of a part of the body due to intermittent muscle contractions, usually involving the distal limbs and less commonly the head, tongue, or jaw. A coarse tremor at rest, 4–5 beats/s, is usually due to Parkinson's disease. A fine postural tremor of 8–10 beats/s may be an exaggeration of normal physiologic tremor or indicate familial essential tremor. An intention tremor, most pronounced during voluntary movement towards a target, is found with cerebellar pathway disease.

■ ESSENTIAL TREMOR (ET)

This is the most common movement disorder. The tremor of ET must be distinguished from early Parkinson's disease (Table 60-1). The pathophysiology of ET is unknown. Approximately 50% of cases have a positive family history with autosomal dominant inheritance; *LINGO1* was recently

TABLE 60-1 ADVANCED EXAMINATION PEARLS: DIFFERENTIATING ESSENTIAL TREMOR FROM PARKINSONIAN TREMOR

	Essential Tremor	Parkinsonian Tremor
Speed	5–10 Hz	4–6 Hz
Symmetry	Bilateral	Usually asymmetric
Most common component	Postural	Rest
Other parkinsonian symptoms	Absent	Present
Helped with alcohol	Usually	Rarely
Family history	Present often	Usually absent

identified in some early onset familial cases. Many pts with ET have mild symptoms and require no treatment.

- When activities of daily living such as eating and writing are impaired, therapy with propranolol (20–80 mg/d) or primidone (12.5–750 mg/d) leads to benefit in 50% of pts.
- Surgical therapies targeting the thalamus may be effective in refractory cases.

■ DYSTONIA

Consists of sustained or repetitive involuntary muscle contractions, frequently causing twisting movements and abnormal posture. Dystonias may be generalized or focal.

Focal dystonias are common and include blepharospasm of the eyelids; spasmodic dysphonia involving the vocal cords; oromandibular dystonia of the face, lips, tongue, and jaw; cervical dystonia of the neck musculature (torticollis); and limb dystonias that are often task-specific such as writer's cramp, playing a musical instrument (musician's cramp), or putting in golf (yips).

Idiopathic torsional dystonia is a predominantly childhood-onset form of generalized dystonia with an autosomal dominant pattern of inheritance that mainly affects Ashkenazi Jewish families; most are linked to a mutation in the *DYT1* gene on chromosome 9. Other generalized dystonias occur as a consequence of drugs such as antiemetics, neuroleptics, and treatments for Parkinson's disease.

- Therapy for focal dystonias usually involves botulinum toxin injections into the affected musculature.
- All forms of dystonia may respond to anticholinergic medications (e.g., trihexyphenidyl 20–120 mg/d), baclofen, or tetrabenazine.
- Surgical therapies, including deep brain stimulation (DBS), may be effective in refractory cases.

■ CHOREOATHETOSIS

A combination of chorea (rapid, graceful, dance-like movements) and athetosis (slow, distal, writhing movements). The two usually exist together, though one may be more prominent. Choreic movements are the predominant involuntary movements in rheumatic (Sydenham's) chorea and Huntington's disease. Systemic lupus erythematosus is the most common systemic disorder that causes chorea, but it can also be seen in pts with hyperthyroidism, various autoimmune disorders, infections including HIV, metabolic alterations, and in association with a wide variety of medications. Hemiballismus is a violent form of chorea that comprises wild, flinging movements on one side of the body; the most common cause is a lesion (often infarct or hemorrhage) of the subthalamic nucleus. Athetosis is prominent in some forms of cerebral palsy. Chronic neuroleptic use may lead to tardive dyskinesia, in which choreoathetotic movements are usually restricted to the buccal, lingual, and mandibular areas.

■ HUNTINGTON'S DISEASE (HD)

This is a progressive, fatal, autosomal dominant disorder characterized by motor, behavioral, and cognitive dysfunction. Onset is typically between the ages of 25 and 45 years. Rapid, nonpatterned, semipurposeful, involuntary choreiform movements are the hallmark feature; dysarthria, gait disturbance, and oculomotor abnormalities also occur. In late stages, chorea becomes less prominent, and the picture is dominated by dystonia, rigidity, bradykinesia, myoclonus, and spasticity. HD pts eventually develop behavioral and cognitive disturbances that can be a major source of disability. HD is inherited as an autosomal dominant disorder and is caused by an expansion in the number of polyglutamine (CAG) repeats in the coding sequence of the *HTT* gene on chromosome 4 encoding the protein huntingtin.

- Treatment involves a multidisciplinary approach with medical, neuropsychiatric, social, and genetic counseling for pts and their families.
- Dopamine-blocking agents may control the chorea; tetrabenazine may cause secondary parkinsonism
- Depression and anxiety should be treated with appropriate antidepressant and antianxiety drugs
- Psychosis can be treated with atypical neuroleptic agents.
- No disease-modifying agents currently exist.

■ TICS

Brief, rapid, recurrent, and seemingly purposeless stereotyped muscle contractions. Gilles de la Tourette syndrome (TS) is a neurobehavioral, multiple tic disorder that may involve motor tics (especially twitches of the face, neck, and shoulders) and vocal tics (grunts, words, coprolalia, echolalia). Pts may experience an irresistible urge to express tics but characteristically can voluntarily suppress them for short periods of time. Onset is usually between 2 and 15 years of age, and tics often lessen or even disappear in adulthood.

- Drug treatment is only indicated when tics are disabling and interfere with quality of life.
- Therapy is generally initiated with clonidine, starting at low dose, or guanfacine (0.5–2 mg/d). If these agents are not effective, neuroleptics may be used.

■ MYOCLONUS

Rapid (<100 ms), brief, shocklike, jerky, movements that are usually multifocal. Like asterixis, often indicates a diffuse encephalopathy. Following cardiac arrest, diffuse cerebral hypoxia may produce multifocal myoclonus.

Spinal cord injury can also cause myoclonus. Myoclonus occurs in normal individuals when waking up or falling asleep.

- Treatment of myoclonus, indicated only when function is impaired, consists of treating the underlying condition or removing an offending agent.
- Drug therapies include valproic acid (800–3000 mg/d), piracetam (8–20 g/d), clonazepam (2–15 mg/d), or primidone (500–1000 mg/d). Levetiracetam may be particularly effective.

■ ASTERIXIS

Brief, arrhythmic interruptions of sustained voluntary muscle contraction, usually observed as a brief lapse of posture of wrists in dorsiflexion with arms outstretched; "negative myoclonus." This "liver flap" may be seen in any encephalopathy related to drug intoxication, organ system failure, or CNS infection.

Therapy is correction of the underlying disorder.

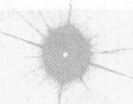

> For a more detailed discussion, see Olanow CW, Schapira AHV: Parkinson's Disease and Other Movement Disorders, Chap. 372, p. 3317, in HPIM-18.

CHAPTER **61**
Aphasia

Aphasias are disturbances in the comprehension or production of spoken or written language. Clinical examination should assess spontaneous speech (fluency), comprehension, repetition, naming, reading, and writing. A classification scheme is presented in Table 61-1. In nearly all right-handed individuals and many left-handed pts, language localization is in the left hemisphere.

■ CLINICAL FEATURES

Wernicke's Aphasia

Although speech sounds grammatical, melodic, and effortless (fluent), it is virtually incomprehensible due to errors in word usage, structure, and tense and the presence of paraphasic errors and neologisms ("jargon"). Comprehension of written and spoken material is severely impaired, as are reading, writing, and repetition. The pt usually seems unaware of the deficit. Associated symptoms can include parietal lobe sensory deficits and homonymous hemianopia. Motor disturbances are rare.

Lesion is located in posterior perisylvian region. Most common cause is embolism to the inferior division of dominant middle cerebral artery (MCA); less commonly intracerebral hemorrhage, severe head trauma, or tumor is responsible.

TABLE 61-1 CLINICAL FEATURES OF APHASIAS AND RELATED CONDITIONS

	Comprehension	Repetition of Spoken Language	Naming	Fluency
Wernicke's	Impaired	Impaired	Impaired	Preserved or increased
Broca's	Preserved (except grammar)	Impaired	Impaired	Decreased
Global	Impaired	Impaired	Impaired	Decreased
Conduction	Preserved	Impaired	Impaired	Preserved
Nonfluent (motor) transcortical	Preserved	Preserved	Impaired	Impaired
Fluent (sensory) transcortical	Impaired	Preserved	Impaired	Preserved
Isolation	Impaired	Echolalia	Impaired	No purposeful speech
Anomic	Preserved	Preserved	Impaired	Preserved except for word-finding pauses
Pure word deafness	Impaired only for spoken language	Impaired	Preserved	Preserved
Pure alexia	Impaired only for reading	Preserved	Preserved	Preserved

Broca's Aphasia

Speech output is sparse (nonfluent), slow, labored, interrupted by many word-finding pauses, and usually dysarthric; output may be reduced to a grunt or single word. Naming and repetition also impaired. Most pts have severe writing impairment. Comprehension of written and spoken language is relatively preserved. The pt is often aware of and visibly frustrated by deficit. With large lesions, a dense hemiparesis may occur, and eyes may deviate toward side of lesion. More commonly, lesser degrees of contralateral face and arm weakness are present. Sensory loss is rarely found, and visual fields are intact.

Lesion involves dominant inferior frontal gyrus (Broca's area), although cortical and subcortical areas along superior sylvian fissure and insula are often involved. Commonly caused by vascular lesions involving the superior division of the MCA; less commonly due to tumor, intracerebral hemorrhage, or abscess.

Global Aphasia

All aspects of speech and language are impaired. Pt cannot read, write, or repeat and has poor auditory comprehension. Speech output is minimal and nonfluent. Hemiplegia, hemisensory loss, and homonymous hemianopia are usually present. Syndrome represents the combined dysfunction of Wernicke's and Broca's areas, usually resulting from proximal occlusion of MCA supplying dominant hemisphere (less commonly hemorrhage, trauma, or tumor).

Conduction Aphasia

Speech output is fluent but paraphasic, comprehension of spoken language is intact, and repetition is severely impaired, as are naming and writing. Lesion spares, but functionally disconnects, Wernicke's and Broca's areas. Most cases are embolic, involving supramarginal gyrus of dominant parietal lobe, dominant superior temporal lobe, or arcuate fasciculus.

■ LABORATORY EVALUATION

CT scan or MRI usually identifies the location and nature of the causative lesion.

| TREATMENT | Aphasia |

- Speech therapy may be helpful in treatment of certain types of aphasia.
- When the lesion is caused by a stroke, recovery of language function generally peaks within 2–6 months, after which time further progress is limited.

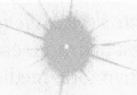

For a more detailed discussion, see Mesulam M-M: Aphasia, Memory Loss, and Other Focal Cerebral Disorders, Chap. 26, p. 202 in HPIM-18.

CHAPTER **62**
Sleep Disorders

Disorders of sleep are among the most common problems seen by clinicians. More than one-half of adults experience at least intermittent sleep disturbances, and 50–70 million Americans suffer from a chronic sleep disturbance.

| APPROACH TO THE PATIENT | Sleep Disorders |

Pts may complain of (1) difficulty in initiating and maintaining sleep (insomnia); (2) excessive daytime sleepiness, fatigue, or tiredness; (3) behavioral phenomena occurring during sleep [sleepwalking, rapid eye movement (REM) behavioral disorder, periodic leg movements of sleep, etc.]; or (4) circadian rhythm disorders associated with jet lag, shift work, and delayed sleep phase syndrome. A careful history of sleep habits and reports from the sleep partner (e.g., heavy snoring, falling asleep while driving) are a cornerstone of diagnosis. Pts with excessive sleepiness should be advised to avoid all driving until effective therapy has been achieved. Completion of a day-by-day sleep-work-drug log for at least 2 weeks is often helpful. Work and sleep times (including daytime naps and nocturnal awakenings) as well as drug and alcohol use, including caffeine and hypnotics, should be noted each day. Objective sleep laboratory recording is necessary to evaluate specific disorders such as sleep apnea and narcolepsy.

■ INSOMNIA

Insomnia, or the complaint of inadequate sleep, may be subdivided into difficulty falling asleep (*sleep onset insomnia*), frequent or sustained awakenings (*sleep maintenance insomnia*), early morning awakenings (*sleep offset insomnia*), or persistent sleepiness/fatigue despite sleep of adequate duration (*nonrestorative sleep*). An insomnia complaint lasting one to several nights is termed *transient insomnia* and is typically due to situational stress or a change in sleep schedule or environment (e.g., jet lag). *Short-term insomnia* lasts from a few days up to 3 weeks; it is often associated with more protracted stress such as recovery from surgery or short-term illness. *Long-term (chronic) insomnia* lasts for months or years and, in contrast to short-term insomnia, requires a thorough evaluation for underlying causes. Chronic insomnia is often a waxing and waning disorder, with spontaneous or stress-induced exacerbations.

All insomnias can be exacerbated and perpetuated by behaviors that are not conducive to initiating or maintaining sleep. *Inadequate sleep hygiene* is characterized by a behavior pattern prior to sleep, and/or a bedroom environment, that is not conducive to sleep. In preference to hypnotic medications, the pt should attempt to avoid stressful activities before bed, reserve the bedroom environment for sleeping, and maintain regular rising times.

Adjustment Insomnia (Acute Insomnia)

Acute insomnia can occur after a change in the sleeping environment (e.g., in an unfamiliar hotel or hospital bed) or before or after a significant life event or anxiety-provoking situation. Treatment is symptomatic, with intermittent use of hypnotics and resolution of the underlying stress.

Psychophysiologic Insomnia

These pts are preoccupied with a perceived inability to sleep adequately at night. Rigorous attention should be paid to sleep hygiene and correction of counterproductive, arousing behaviors before bedtime. Behavioral therapies are the treatment of choice.

Drugs and Medications

Caffeine is probably the most common pharmacologic cause of insomnia. Alcohol and nicotine can also interfere with sleep, despite the fact that many pts use these agents to relax and promote sleep. A number of prescribed medications, including antidepressants, sympathomimetics, and glucocorticoids, can produce insomnia. In addition, severe rebound insomnia can result from the acute withdrawal of hypnotics, especially following use of high doses of benzodiazepines with a short half-life. For this reason, doses of hypnotics should be low to moderate and prolonged drug tapering is encouraged.

Movement Disorders

Pts with *restless legs syndrome* (RLS) complain of creeping dysesthesias deep within the calves or feet associated with an irresistible urge to move the affected limbs; symptoms are typically worse at night. Iron deficiency and renal failure can cause secondary RLS. One-third of pts have multiple affected family members. Treatment is with dopaminergic drugs (pramipexole 0.25–0.5 mg daily at 8 P.M. or ropinirole 0.5–4.0 mg daily at 8 P.M.). *Periodic limb movements of sleep* (PLMS) consists of stereotyped extensions of the great toe and dorsiflexion of the foot recurring every 20–40 s during non-REM sleep. Treatment options include dopaminergic medications or benzodiazepines.

Other Neurologic Disorders

A variety of neurologic disorders produce sleep disruption through both indirect, nonspecific mechanisms (e.g., neck or back pain) or by impairment of central neural structures involved in the generation and control of sleep itself. Common disorders to consider include *dementia* from any cause, *epilepsy*, *Parkinson's disease*, and *migraine*.

Psychiatric Disorders

Approximately 80% of pts with mental disorders complain of impaired sleep. The underlying diagnosis may be depression, mania, an anxiety disorder, or schizophrenia.

Medical Disorders

In *asthma*, daily variation in airway resistance results in marked increases in asthmatic symptoms at night, especially during sleep. Treatment of asthma with theophylline-based compounds, adrenergic agonists, or glucocorticoids can independently disrupt sleep. Inhaled glucocorticoids that do not disrupt sleep may provide a useful alternative to oral drugs. *Cardiac ischemia* is also associated with sleep disruption; the ischemia itself may result from increases in sympathetic tone as a result of sleep apnea. Pts may present with complaints of nightmares or vivid dreams. *Paroxysmal nocturnal dyspnea* can also occur from cardiac ischemia that causes pulmonary congestion exacerbated by the recumbent posture. *Chronic obstructive pulmonary disease, cystic fibrosis, hyperthyroidism, menopause, gastroesophageal reflux, chronic renal failure*, and *liver failure* are other causes.

TREATMENT ▸ Insomnia

INSOMNIA WITHOUT IDENTIFIABLE CAUSE Primary insomnia is a diagnosis of exclusion.

- Treatment directed toward behavior therapies for anxiety and negative conditioning; pharmacotherapy and/or psychotherapy for mood/anxiety disorders; an emphasis on good sleep hygiene; and intermittent hypnotics for exacerbations of insomnia.

- Cognitive therapy emphasizes understanding the nature of normal sleep, the circadian rhythm, the use of light therapy, and visual imagery to block unwanted thought intrusions.
- Behavioral modification involves bedtime restriction, set schedules, and careful sleep environment practices.
- Judicious use of benzodiazepine receptor agonists with short half-lives can be effective; options include zaleplon (5–20 mg), zolpidem (5–10 mg), triazolam (0.125–0.25 mg), eszopiclone (1–3 mg). Limit use to 2–4 weeks maximum for acute insomnia or intermittent use for chronic.

■ DISORDERS OF EXCESSIVE DAYTIME SLEEPINESS

Differentiation of sleepiness from subjective complaints of fatigue may be difficult. Quantification of daytime sleepiness can be performed in a sleep laboratory using a multiple sleep latency test (MSLT), the repeated daytime measurement of sleep latency under standardized conditions. Common causes are summarized in Table 62-1.

Sleep Apnea Syndromes

Respiratory dysfunction during sleep is a common cause of excessive daytime sleepiness and/or disturbed nocturnal sleep, affecting an estimated 2–5 million individuals in the United States. Episodes may be due to occlusion of the airway (*obstructive sleep apnea*), absence of respiratory effort (*central sleep apnea*), or a combination of these factors (*mixed sleep apnea*). Obstruction is exacerbated by obesity, supine posture, sedatives (especially alcohol), nasal obstruction, and hypothyroidism. Sleep apnea is particularly prevalent in overweight men and in the elderly and is undiagnosed in 80–90% of affected individuals. Treatment consists of correction of the above factors, positive airway pressure devices, oral appliances, and sometimes surgery (Chap. 146).

Narcolepsy

A disorder of excessive daytime sleepiness and intrusion of REM-related sleep phenomena into wakefulness (cataplexy, hypnagogic hallucinations, and sleep paralysis). *Cataplexy*, the abrupt loss of muscle tone in arms, legs, or face, is precipitated by emotional stimuli such as laughter or sadness. Symptoms of narcolepsy (Table 62-2) typically begin in the second decade, although the onset ranges from ages 5–50. The prevalence is 1 in 4000. Narcolepsy has a genetic basis; almost all narcoleptics with cataplexy are positive for HLA DQB1*0602. Hypothalamic neurons containing the neuropeptide hypocretin (orexin) regulate the sleep/wake cycle and loss of these cells, possibly due to autoimmunity, has been implicated in narcolepsy. Diagnosis is made with sleep studies confirming a short daytime sleep latency and a rapid transition to REM sleep.

| TREATMENT | Narcolepsy |

- Somnolence is treated with modafinil (200–400 mg/d given as a single dose).
- Older stimulants such as methylphenidate (10 mg bid to 20 mg qid) or dextroamphetamine (10 mg bid) are alternatives, particularly in refractory pts.

TABLE 62-1 EVALUATION OF THE PATIENT WITH THE COMPLAINT OF EXCESSIVE DAYTIME SOMNOLENCE

Findings on History and Physical Examination	Diagnostic Evaluation	Diagnosis	Therapy
Obesity, snoring, hypertension	Polysomnography with respiratory monitoring	Obstructive sleep apnea	Continuous positive airway pressure; ENT surgery (e.g., uvulopalatopharyngoplasty); dental appliance; pharmacologic therapy (e.g., protriptyline); weight loss
Cataplexy, hypnogogic hallucinations, sleep paralysis, family history	Polysomnography with multiple sleep latency testing	Narcolepsy-cataplexy syndrome	Stimulants (e.g., modafinil, methylphenidate); REM-suppressant antidepressants (e.g., protriptyline); genetic counseling
Restless legs, disturbed sleep, predisposing medical condition (e.g., iron deficiency or renal failure)	Assessment for predisposing medical conditions	Restless legs syndrome	Treatment of predisposing condition, if possible; dopamine agonists (e.g., pramipexole, ropinirole)
Disturbed sleep, predisposing medical conditions (e.g., asthma), and/or predisposing medical therapies (e.g., theophylline)	Sleep-wake diary recording	Insomnias (see text)	Treatment of predisposing condition and/or change in therapy, if possible; behavioral therapy; short-acting benzodiazepine receptor agonist (e.g., zolpidem)

Abbreviations: EMG, electromyogram; ENT, ears, nose, throat; REM, rapid eye movement.

TABLE 62-2 PREVALENCE OF SYMPTOMS IN NARCOLEPSY

Symptom	Prevalence, %
Excessive daytime somnolence	100
Disturbed sleep	87
Cataplexy	76
Hypnagogic hallucinations	68
Sleep paralysis	64
Memory problems	50

Source: Modified from TA Roth, L Merlotti in SA Burton et al (eds). *Narcolepsy 3rd International Symposium: Selected Symposium Proceedings,* Chicago, Matrix Communications, 1989.

- Cataplexy, hypnagogic hallucinations, and sleep paralysis respond to the tricyclic antidepressants protriptyline (10–40 mg/d) and clomipramine (25–50 mg/d) and to the selective serotonin uptake inhibitor fluoxetine (10–20 mg/d). Alternatively, γ-hydroxybutyrate (GHB) given at bedtime, and 4 h later, is effective in reducing daytime cataplectic episodes.
- Adequate nocturnal sleep time and the use of short naps are other useful preventative measures.

■ CIRCADIAN RHYTHM SLEEP DISORDERS

Insomnia or hypersomnia may occur in disorders of sleep timing rather than sleep generation. Such conditions may be (1) organic—due to a defect in the hypothalamic circadian pacemaker or its input from entraining stimuli, or (2) environmental—due to a disruption of exposure to entraining stimuli (light/dark cycle). Examples of the latter include jet-lag disorder and shift work. Shift work sleepiness can be treated with modafinil (200 mg, taken 30–60 min before the start of each night shift) as well as properly timed exposure to bright light. Safety programs should promote education about sleep and increase awareness of the hazards associated with night work.

Delayed sleep phase syndrome is characterized by late sleep onset and awakening with otherwise normal sleep architecture. Bright-light phototherapy in the morning hours or melatonin therapy during the evening hours may be effective.

Advanced sleep phase syndrome moves sleep onset to the early evening hours with early morning awakening. These pts may benefit from bright-light phototherapy during the evening hours. Some autosomal dominant cases result from mutations in a gene (*PER2*) involved in regulation of the circadian clock.

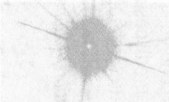

For a more detailed discussion, see Czeisler CA, Winkleman JW, Richardson GS: Sleep Disorders, Chap. 27, p. 213, in HPIM-18.

CHAPTER 63

Common Disorders of Vision and Hearing

DISORDERS OF THE EYE

APPROACH TO THE PATIENT | **Eye Disorders**

The history and examination permit accurate diagnosis of most eye disorders without need for laboratory or imaging studies. The essential ocular exam includes assessment of the visual acuity, pupil reactions, eye movements, eye alignment, visual fields, and intraocular pressure. The lids, conjunctiva, cornea, anterior chamber, iris, and lens are examined with a slit lamp. The fundus is viewed with an ophthalmoscope.

Acute visual loss or double vision in a pt with quiet, uninflamed eyes often signifies a serious ocular or neurologic disorder and should be managed emergently (Chap. 58). Paradoxically, the occurrence of a red eye, even if painful, has less dire implications as long as visual acuity is spared.

■ SPECIFIC DISORDERS

Red or Painful Eye

Common causes are listed in Table 63-1.

Minor Trauma This may result in corneal abrasion, subconjunctival hemorrhage, or foreign body. The integrity of the corneal epithelium is assessed by placing a drop of fluorescein in the eye and looking with a slit lamp (using cobalt-blue light) or a blue penlight. The conjunctival fornices should be searched carefully for foreign bodies by pulling the lower lid down and everting the upper lid.

TREATMENT | **Minor Trauma**

- Chemical splashes and foreign bodies are treated by copious saline irrigation.
- Foreign body can be removed with a moistened cotton-tipped applicator after a drop of topical anesthetic
- Corneal abrasions may require application of a topical antibiotic, a mydriatic agent (1% cyclopentolate), and an eye patch.

343

TABLE 63-1 CAUSES OF A RED OR PAINFUL EYE

Blunt or penetrating trauma

Chemical exposure

Corneal abrasion

Foreign body

Contact lens (overuse or infection)

Corneal exposure (5th, 7th nerve palsy, ectropion)

Subconjunctival hemorrhage

Blepharitis

Conjunctivitis (infectious or allergic)

Corneal ulcer

Herpes keratitis

Herpes zoster ophthalmicus

Keratoconjunctivitis sicca (dry eye)

Dacryocystitis

Episcleritis

Scleritis

Anterior uveitis (iritis or iridocyclitis)

Endophthalmitis

Acute angle-closure glaucoma

Medicamentosus

Pinguecula

Pterygium

Proptosis (retrobulbar mass, orbital cellulitis, Graves' ophthalmopathy, orbital pseudotumor, carotid-cavernous fistula)

Infection Infection of the eyelids and conjunctiva (blepharoconjunctivitis) produces redness and irritation but should not cause visual loss or pain. Adenovirus is the most common viral cause of "pink eye." It produces a thin, watery discharge, whereas bacterial infection causes a more mucopurulent exudate. On slit-lamp exam one should confirm that the cornea is not affected, by observing that it remains clear and lustrous. Corneal infection (keratitis) is a more serious condition than blepharoconjunctivitis because it can cause scarring, perforation, and permanent visual loss. Worldwide, the two leading causes of blindness from keratitis are trachoma from chlamydial infection and vitamin A deficiency from malnutrition; in the United States, contact lenses play a major role. A dendritic pattern of corneal fluorescein staining is pathognomonic of herpes simplex keratitis but is seen in only a minority of cases.

| **TREATMENT** | Infection |

- Strict handwashing and broad-spectrum topical antibiotics for blepharoconjunctivitis (sulfacetamide 10%, polymyxin-bacitracin-neomycin, or trimethoprim-polymyxin).
- Keratitis requires empirical antibiotics (usually topical and subconjunctival) pending culture results from corneal scrapings.
- Herpes keratitis is treated with topical antiviral agents, cycloplegics, and oral acyclovir.

Inflammation Eye inflammation, without infection, can produce episcleritis, scleritis, or uveitis (iritis or iridocyclitis). Most cases are idiopathic, but some occur in conjunction with autoimmune disease. There is no discharge. A ciliary flush results from injection of deep conjunctival and episcleral vessels near the corneal limbus. The diagnosis of uveitis hinges on the slit-lamp observation of inflammatory cells floating in the aqueous humor of the anterior chamber or deposited on the corneal endothelium (keratic precipitates).

| **TREATMENT** | Inflammation |

- Mydriatic agents (to reduce pain and prevent the formation of synechiae), NSAIDs, and topical glucocorticoids. (*Note:* prolonged treatment with ocular glucocorticoids can cause cataract and glaucoma.)

Acute Angle-Closure Glaucoma This is a rare but frequently misdiagnosed cause of a red, painful eye. Because the anterior chamber is shallow, aqueous outflow via the anterior chamber angle becomes blocked by the peripheral iris. Intraocular pressure rises abruptly, causing ocular pain, injection, corneal edema, obscurations, headache, nausea, and blurred vision. The key diagnostic step is measurement of the intraocular pressure during an attack.

| **TREATMENT** | Acute Angle-Closure Glaucoma |

- The acute attack is broken by constricting the pupil with a drop of pilocarpine and by lowering the intraocular pressure with acetazolamide (PO or IV), topical beta blockers, prostaglandin analogues, and α_2-adrenergic agonists.
- If these measures fail, laser therapy can be used to create a hole in the peripheral iris to relieve papillary block.

Chronic Visual Loss

Most common causes are listed in Table 63-2.

Cataract A cloudy lens sufficient to reduce vision, due principally to aging. The formation of cataract occurs more rapidly in pts with a history of ocular

TABLE 63-2 CAUSES OF CHRONIC, PROGRESSIVE VISUAL LOSS

Cataract
Glaucoma
Macular degeneration
Diabetic retinopathy
Optic nerve or optic chiasm tumor
Intraocular tumor
Retinitis pigmentosa
Epiretinal membrane
Macular hole

trauma, uveitis, or diabetes mellitus. Radiation and glucocorticoid treatment can induce a cataract as a side effect. It is treated by surgical extraction and replacement with an artificial intraocular lens.

Glaucoma An insidious optic neuropathy that leads to slowly progressive visual loss, usually associated with elevated intraocular pressure. Angle closure accounts for only a few cases; most pts have open angles and no identifiable cause for their pressure elevation. The diagnosis is made by documenting arcuate (nerve fiber bundle) scotomas on visual field exam, observing "cupping" of the optic disc (Fig. 63-1), and measuring intraocular pressure.

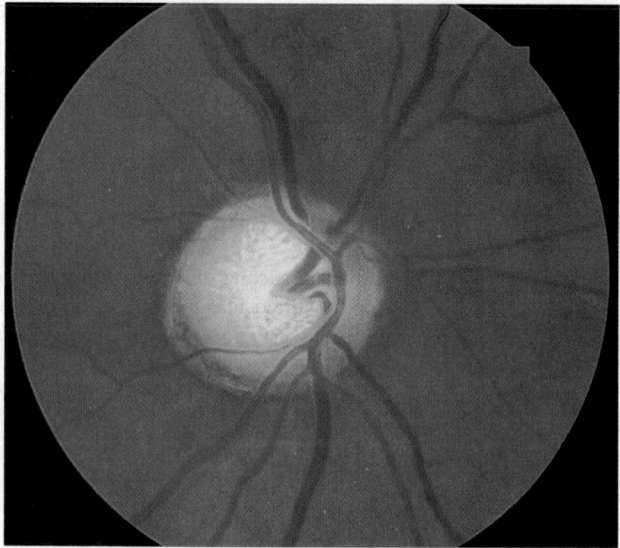

FIGURE 63-1 Glaucoma results in "cupping" as the neural rim is destroyed and the central cup becomes enlarged and excavated. The cup-to-disc ratio is about 0.7/1.0 in this pt.

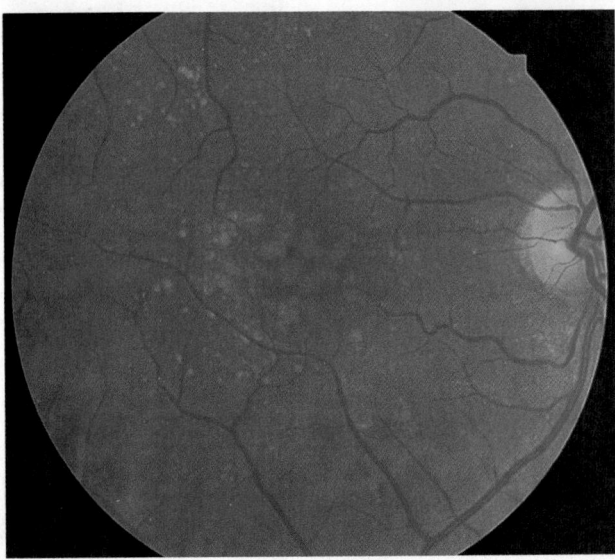

FIGURE 63-2 Age-related macular degeneration begins with the accumulation of drusen within the macula. They appear as scattered yellow subretinal deposits.

TREATMENT Glaucoma

- Topical adrenergic agonists, cholinergic agonists, beta blockers, prostaglandin analogues, and oral carbonic anhydrase inhibitors (to lower intraocular pressure) are used for treatment.
- Laser treatment of the trabecular meshwork in the anterior chamber angle improves aqueous outflow from the eye.
- If medical and laser treatments fail, a surgical filter (trabeculectomy) or valve must be placed.

Macular Degeneration This occurs in both a "dry" and "wet" form. In the dry form, clumps of extracellular material, called *drusen*, are deposited beneath the retinal pigment epithelium (Fig. 63-2). As they accumulate, vision is slowly lost. In the wet form, neovascular proliferation occurs beneath the retinal pigment epithelium. Bleeding from these neovascular vessels can cause sudden, central visual loss in the elderly, although usually blurring of vision is more gradual. Macular exam shows drusen and subretinal hemorrhage.

TREATMENT Macular Degeneration

- Treatment with vitamins C and E, beta carotene, and zinc may retard dry macular degeneration.

- Wet macular degeneration can be treated with vascular endothelial growth factor antagonists directly injected into the vitreous cavity on a monthly basis.

Diabetic Retinopathy A leading cause of blindness in the United States. Appears in most pts years after onset of diabetes. Background diabetic retinopathy consists of intraretinal hemorrhage, exudates, nerve fiber layer infarcts (cotton-wool spots), and macular edema. Proliferative diabetic retinopathy is characterized by ingrowth of neovascular vessels on the retinal surface, causing blindness from vitreous hemorrhage, retinal detachment, and glaucoma (Fig. 63-3).

TREATMENT	Diabetic Retinopathy

- All diabetics should be examined regularly by an ophthalmologist for surveillance of diabetic retinopathy.
- Neovascularization is treated by panretinal laser photocoagulation to prevent complications.

Tumors Tumors of the optic nerve or chiasm are comparatively rare, but often escape detection because they produce insidious visual loss and few physical findings, except for optic disc pallor. Pituitary tumor is the most common lesion. It causes bitemporal or monocular visual loss. Melanoma is the most common primary tumor of the eye itself.

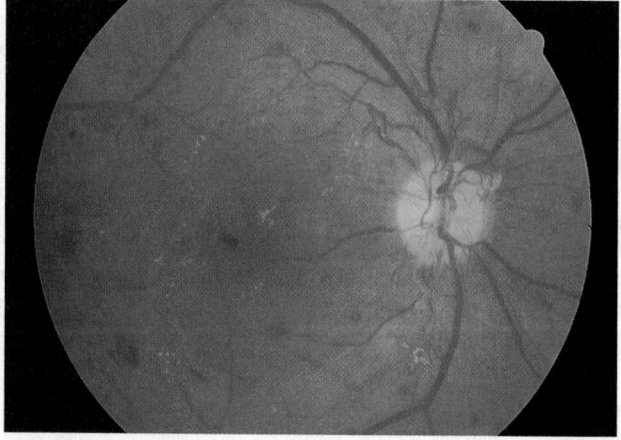

FIGURE 63-3 Diabetic retinopathy results in scattered hemorrhages, yellow exudates, and neovascularization. This pt has neovascular vessels proliferating from the optic disc, requiring urgent pan retinal laser photocoagulation.

TREATMENT	Tumors

- Large pituitary tumors producing chiasm compression are removed transsphenoidally.
- In some cases, small tumors can be observed or controlled pharmacologically (e.g., bromocriptine for prolactinoma).

HEARING DISORDERS

Nearly 10% of the adult population has some hearing loss; up to one-third of individuals over the age of 65 have hearing loss of sufficient magnitude to require a hearing aid. Hearing loss can result from disorders of the auricle, external auditory canal, middle ear, inner ear, or central auditory pathways. *In general, lesions in the auricle, external auditory canal, or middle ear cause conductive hearing losses, while lesions in the inner ear or eighth nerve cause sensorineural hearing losses.*

APPROACH TO THE PATIENT	Hearing Impairment

The goal is to determine (1) the nature of the hearing impairment (sensorineural vs. conductive vs. mixed), (2) the severity of the impairment, (3) the anatomy of the impairment, and (4) the etiology. Ascertain onset (sudden vs. insidious), progression (rapid vs. slow), and whether symptoms are unilateral or bilateral. Ask about tinnitus, vertigo, imbalance, aural fullness, otorrhea, headache, and facial or other cranial nerve symptoms. Prior head trauma, exposure to ototoxins, occupational or recreational noise exposure, or family history of hearing impairment also important.

Exam should include the auricle, external ear canal, and tympanic membrane. The external ear canal of the elderly is often dry and fragile; it is preferable to clean cerumen with wall-mounted suction and cerumen loops and to avoid irrigation. Inspect the nose, nasopharynx, cranial nerves, and upper respiratory tract. Unilateral serous effusion should prompt a fiberoptic exam of the nasopharynx to exclude neoplasm.

The Weber and Rinne tests differentiate conductive from sensorineural hearing losses. *Rinne test*: the tines of a vibrating tuning fork (512 Hz) are held near the opening of the external auditory canal, and then the stem is placed on the mastoid process. Normally, and with sensorineural hearing loss, air conduction is louder than bone conduction; however, with conductive hearing loss, bone conduction is louder. *Weber test*: the stem of a vibrating tuning fork is placed on the forehead in the midline. With a unilateral conductive hearing loss, the tone is perceived in the affected ear; with a unilateral sensorineural hearing loss, the tone is perceived in the unaffected ear.

■ LABORATORY EVALUATION

Audiologic Assessment *Pure tone audiometry* assesses hearing acuity for pure tones. Speech recognition requires greater synchronous neural firing than necessary for appreciation of pure tones; clarity of hearing is tested in *speech audiometry.* *Tympanometry* measures impedance of middle ear to sound; useful in diagnosis of middle-ear effusions. *Otoacoustic emissions* (OAE), measured with microphones inserted in external auditory canal, indicate that outer hair cells of the organ of Corti are intact; useful to assess auditory thresholds and distinguish sensory from neural hearing loss. *Electrocochleography* measures earliest evoked potentials generated in cochlea and auditory nerve; useful in diagnosis of Ménière's disease. *Brainstem auditory evoked responses* (BAER) localize site of sensorineural hearing loss.

Imaging Studies CT of temporal bone with fine 0.3–0.6 mm cuts can define the caliber of the external auditory canal, integrity of the ossicular chain, presence of middle ear or mastoid disease, inner-ear malformations, and bone erosion (chronic otitis media and cholesteatoma). MRI superior to CT for imaging of retrocochlear structures including cerebellopontine angle (vestibular schwannoma) and brainstem.

■ CAUSES OF HEARING LOSS (FIG. 63-4)

Conductive Hearing Loss

May result from obstruction of the external auditory canal by cerumen, debris, and foreign bodies; swelling of the lining of the canal; atresia of the ear canal; neoplasms of the canal; perforations of the tympanic membrane; disruption of the ossicular chain, as occurs with necrosis of the long process of the incus in trauma or infection; otosclerosis; and fluid, scarring, or neoplasms in the middle ear. Hearing loss with otorrhea most likely due to otitis media or cholesteatoma.

Cholesteatoma, i.e., stratified squamous epithelium in the middle ear or mastoid, is a benign, slowly growing lesion that destroys bone and normal ear tissue. A chronically draining ear that fails to respond to appropriate antibiotic therapy suggests cholesteatoma; surgery is required.

Conductive hearing loss with a normal ear canal and intact tympanic membrane suggests ossicular pathology. Fixation of the stapes from *otosclerosis* is a common cause of low-frequency conductive hearing loss; onset is between the late teens to the forties. In women, the hearing loss is often first noticeable during pregnancy. A hearing aid or a surgical stapedectomy can provide auditory rehabilitation.

Eustachian tube dysfunction is common and may predispose to acute otitis media (AOM) or serous otitis media (SOM). Trauma, AOM, or chronic otitis media are the usual factors responsible for tympanic membrane perforation. While small perforations often heal spontaneously, larger defects usually require surgical tympanoplasty (>90% effective). Otoscopy is usually sufficient to diagnose AOM, SOM, chronic otitis media, cerumen impaction, tympanic membrane perforation, and eustachian tube dysfunction.

Sensorineural Hearing Loss

Damage to hair cells of the organ of Corti may be caused by intense noise, viral infections, ototoxic drugs (e.g., salicylates, quinine and its analogues, aminoglycoside antibiotics, diuretics such as furosemide and ethacrynic

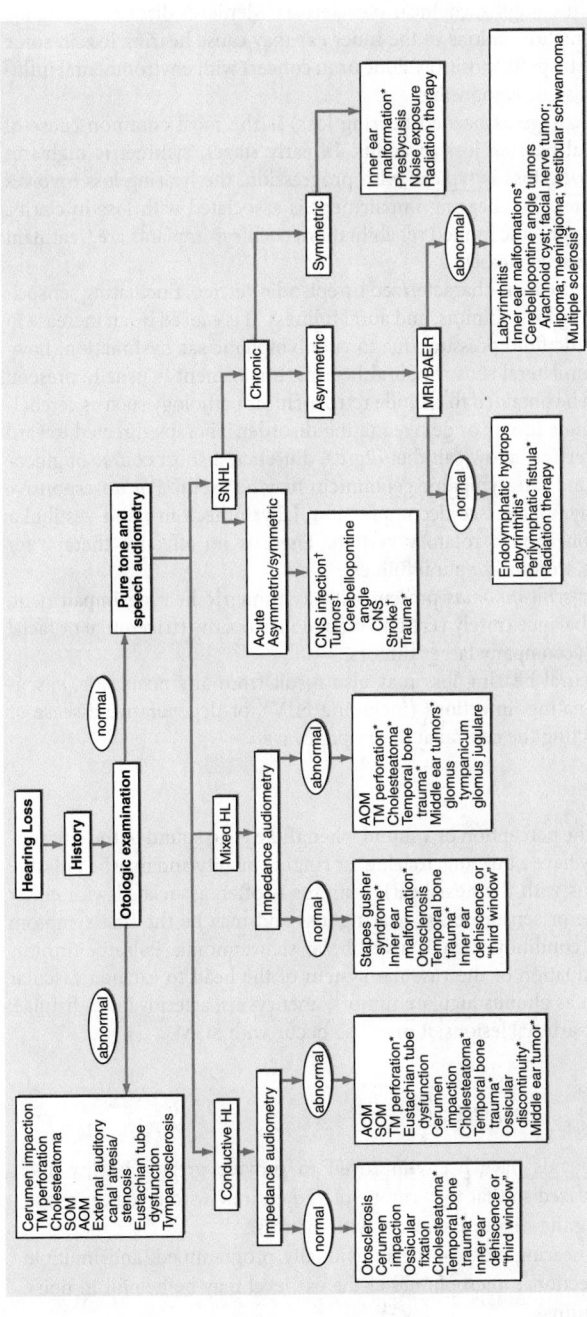

FIGURE 63-4 An algorithm for the approach to hearing loss. AOM, acute otitis media; HL, hearing loss; SNHL, sensorineural hearing loss; SOM, serous otitis media; TM, tympanic membrane; *, CT scan of temporal bone; †, MRI scan.

acid, and chemotherapeutic agents such as cisplatin), fractures of the temporal bone, meningitis, cochlear otosclerosis, Ménière's disease, and aging. Congenital malformations of the inner ear may cause hearing loss in some adults. Genetic predisposition alone or in concert with environmental influences may also be responsible.

Presbycusis (age-associated hearing loss) is the most common cause of sensorineural hearing loss in adults. In early stages, symmetric high frequency hearing loss is typical; with progression, the hearing loss involves all frequencies. The hearing impairment is associated with loss in clarity. Hearing aids provide limited rehabilitation; cochlear implants are treatment of choice for severe cases.

Ménière's disease is characterized by episodic vertigo, fluctuating sensorineural hearing loss, tinnitus, and aural fullness. It is caused by an increase in endolymphatic fluid pressure due to endolymphatic sac dysfunction. Low-frequency, unilateral sensorineural hearing impairment is usually present. MRI should be obtained to exclude retrocochlear pathology such as cerebellopontine angle tumor or demyelinating disorder. Therapy directed toward control of vertigo; a low-salt diet (2g/d), diuretics, a short course of glucocorticoids, and intratympanic gentamicin may be useful. For unresponsive cases, endolymphatic sac decompression, labyrinthectomy, and vestibular nerve section abolish rotatory vertigo. There is no effective therapy for hearing loss, tinnitus, or aural fullness.

Vestibular schwannomas present with asymmetric hearing impairment, tinnitus, imbalance (rarely vertigo); cranial neuropathy (trigeminal or facial nerve) may accompany larger tumors.

Sensorineural hearing loss may also result from any neoplastic, vascular, demyelinating, infectious (including HIV), or degenerative disease or trauma affecting the central auditory pathways.

Tinnitus

Defined as the perception of a sound when there is no sound in the environment. It may have a buzzing, roaring, or ringing quality and may be pulsatile (synchronous with the heartbeat). Tinnitus is often associated with either a conductive or sensorineural hearing loss and may be the first symptom of a serious condition such as a vestibular schwannoma. Pulsatile tinnitus requires evaluation of the vascular system of the head to exclude vascular tumors such as glomus jugulare tumors, aneurysms, arteriovenous fistulae, and stenotic arterial lesions; it may also occur with SOM.

TREATMENT   Hearing Loss

- Hearing aids have been improved to provide greater fidelity and miniaturized so that they can be placed entirely within the ear canal, reducing the stigma associated with their use.
- Digital hearing aids can be individually programmed, and multiple and directional microphones at the ear level may be helpful in noisy surroundings.

- If the hearing aid provides inadequate rehabilitation, cochlear implants can be effective.
- Treatment of tinnitus is problematic. Relief of the tinnitus may be obtained by masking it with background music. Hearing aids are also helpful in tinnitus suppression, as are tinnitus maskers, devices that present a sound to the affected ear that is more pleasant to listen to than the tinnitus. Antidepressants have also shown some benefit.
- Hard-of-hearing individuals often benefit from a reduction in unnecessary noise to enhance the signal-to-noise ratio. Speech comprehension is aided by lip-reading; the face of the speaker should be well illuminated and easily seen.

■ PREVENTION

Conductive hearing losses may be prevented by prompt antibiotic therapy for AOM and by ventilation of the middle ear with tympanostomy tubes in middle-ear effusions lasting ≥12 weeks. Loss of vestibular function and deafness due to aminoglycoside antibiotics can largely be prevented by monitoring of serum peak and trough levels.

Ten million Americans have noise-induced hearing loss, and 20 million are exposed to hazardous noise in their employment. Noise-induced hearing loss can be prevented by avoidance of exposure to loud noise or by regular use of ear plugs or fluid-filled muffs to attenuate intense sound.

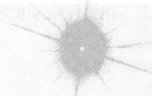

For a more detailed discussion, see Horton JC: Disorders of the Eye, Chap. 28, p. 224; and Lalwani AK: Disorders of Hearing, Chap. 30, p. 248, in HPIM-18.

CHAPTER **64**
Sinusitis, Pharyngitis, Otitis, and Other Upper Respiratory Tract Infections

- Upper respiratory tract infections (URIs) are among the leading causes of lost time from work or school.
- Distinguishing pts with primary viral URI from those with primary bacterial URI is difficult since the signs and symptoms are the same.
- URIs are often treated with antibiotics even though bacteria cause only 25% of cases. Inappropriate prescribing of antibiotics for URIs is a

leading cause of antibiotic resistance in common community-acquired pathogens such as *Streptococcus pneumoniae*.

NONSPECIFIC URIs

- **Definition:** Nonspecific URIs (the "common cold") have no prominent localizing features.
- **Etiology:** A wide variety of viruses (e.g., rhinoviruses, coronaviruses, parainfluenza viruses, influenza viruses, adenoviruses) can cause non-specific URIs.
- **Clinical manifestations:** an acute, mild, self-limited catarrhal syndrome, typically characterized by rhinorrhea, nasal congestion, cough, and sore throat
  - Hoarseness, malaise, sneezing, and fever are more variable.
  - The median duration of symptoms is ~1 week (range, 2–10 days).
- **Treatment:** Symptom-based treatment (e.g., with decongestants, NSAIDs, dextromethorphan, throat lozenges) is typically all that is required.
  - Because secondary bacterial URI complicates only 0.5–2% of colds, antibiotics are not indicated.
  - Purulent nasal and throat secretions are poor predictors of bacterial infection.

SINUS INFECTIONS

- Rhinosinusitis is an inflammatory condition most commonly involving the maxillary sinus; next, in order of frequency, are the ethmoid, frontal, and sphenoid sinuses.
- Sinusitis accounts for millions of visits to primary care physicians each year and is the fifth most common diagnosis for which antibiotics are prescribed.

◼ ACUTE SINUSITIS

- **Definition:** sinusitis of <4 weeks' duration
- **Etiology:** Infectious and noninfectious causes lead to sinus ostial obstruction and retention of mucus.
  - Infectious causes include viruses (e.g., rhinovirus, parainfluenza virus, influenza virus) and bacteria [e.g., *S. pneumoniae*, nontypable *Haemophilus influenzae*, and (in children) *Moraxella catarrhalis*].
    - In immunocompromised pts, fungi (e.g., *Rhizopus*, *Mucor*, and occasionally *Aspergillus*) can be involved.
    - Nosocomial cases are often polymicrobial and involve *Staphylococcus aureus* and gram-negative bacilli.
  - Noninfectious causes include allergic rhinitis, barotrauma, and exposure to chemical irritants.
- **Clinical manifestations:** Common manifestations include nasal drainage, congestion, facial pain or pressure, and headache.
  - Tooth pain and halitosis can be associated with bacterial sinusitis.
  - Pain localizes to the involved sinus and is often worse when the pt bends over or is supine.

- Advanced frontal sinusitis can present as "Pott's puffy tumor": swelling and pitting edema over the frontal bone from a communicating subperiosteal abscess.
- Life-threatening complications include meningitis, epidural abscess, and brain abscess.
- **Diagnosis:** It is difficult to distinguish viral from bacterial sinusitis clinically, although viral cases greatly outnumber bacterial cases.
  - Only 40–50% of pts with symptoms of >10 days' duration, purulent nasal drainage, nasal obstruction, and facial pain have bacterial sinusitis.
  - If fungal sinusitis is a consideration, biopsies of involved areas should be performed.
  - Except in nosocomial cases, sinus CT or radiography is not recommended for acute sinusitis. Nosocomial sinusitis should be confirmed by sinus CT, with sinus aspirates sent for culture and susceptibility testing (ideally before antimicrobial therapy is initiated).

TREATMENT ⟩ Acute Sinusitis

- Most pts improve without antibiotic therapy.
- For pts with mild to moderate symptoms, treatment should focus on symptom relief and facilitation of sinus drainage (e.g., oral and topical decongestants, nasal saline lavage).
- Pts without improvement after 10 days or with severe disease at presentation should be given antibiotics.
  - See Table 64-1 for recommended regimens for adults.
  - Up to 10% of pts do not respond to initial antimicrobial therapy; consultation with an otolaryngologist about possible sinus aspiration and/or lavage should be considered in these cases.
- Surgery should be considered for pts with severe disease, intracranial complications, or invasive fungal sinusitis.

■ CHRONIC SINUSITIS

- **Definition:** sinusitis of >12 weeks' duration
- **Etiology:** commonly associated with bacterial or fungal infection
- **Chronic bacterial sinusitis:** Impaired mucociliary clearance leads to repeated infections as opposed to one persistent infection.
  - Pts have constant nasal congestion and sinus pressure, with periods of increased severity.
  - Sinus CT can define the extent of disease, detect an underlying anatomic defect or obstructing process, and assess response to treatment.
  - Endoscopy-derived tissue samples for histology and culture should be obtained to guide treatment.
  - Repeated courses of antibiotics are required, often for 3–4 weeks at a time. Adjunctive measures include intranasal administration of glucocorticoids, sinus irrigation, and surgical evaluation.

TABLE 64-1 GUIDELINES FOR THE DIAGNOSIS AND TREATMENT OF SELECTED UPPER RESPIRATORY TRACT INFECTIONS IN ADULTS[a]

Syndrome, Diagnostic Criteria	Treatment Recommendations
Acute sinusitis[b]	*Initial therapy*
Moderate symptoms (e.g., nasal purulence/congestion or cough) for >10 d *or*	Amoxicillin, 500 mg PO tid or 875 mg PO bid
	Penicillin allergy
	TMP-SMX, 1 DS tablet PO bid for 10–14 d
Severe symptoms of any duration, including unilateral/focal facial swelling or tooth pain	*Exposure to antibiotics within 30 d or >30% prevalence of penicillin-resistant S. pneumoniae*
	Amoxicillin/clavulanate (extended-release), 2000 mg PO bid; *or*
	Antipneumococcal fluoroquinolone (e.g., levofloxacin, 500 mg PO qd)
	Recent treatment failure
	Amoxicillin/clavulanate (extended-release), 2000 mg PO bid; *or*
	Amoxicillin, 1500 mg bid, *plus* clindamycin, 300 mg PO qid; *or*
	Antipneumococcal fluoroquinolone (e.g., levofloxacin, 500 mg PO qd)
Acute otitis media[c]	*Initial therapy*
Mild to moderate severity	Observation alone (antibiotic therapy deferred for 48–72 h and management limited to symptom relief)
Mild to moderate severity after observation period	Amoxicillin, 2 g PO qd in divided doses (bid or tid); *or*
	Cefdinir, 600 mg PO qd in 1 dose or divided doses (bid); *or*
	Cefuroxime, 500 mg PO bid; *or*
	Azithromycin, 500 mg PO on day 1 followed by 250 mg PO qd for 4 d
	Antibiotic exposure within 30 d[c] or recent treatment failure[c,d]
	Amoxicillin, 875 mg PO bid, *plus* clavulanate, 125 mg PO bid; *or*
	Ceftriaxone, 1 g IV/IM qd for 3 d; *or*
	Clindamycin, 300 mg PO tid
Severe disease	*Initial therapy*
Middle-ear effusion *and* acute onset of signs and symptoms	Amoxicillin, 875 mg PO bid, *plus* clavulanate, 125 mg PO bid; *or*
	Ceftriaxone, 1 g IV/IM qd for 3 d

TABLE 64-1 GUIDELINES FOR THE DIAGNOSIS AND TREATMENT OF SELECTED UPPER RESPIRATORY TRACT INFECTIONS IN ADULTS[a] (CONTINUED)

of middle-ear inflammation, including temperature ≥39.0°C (102°F) *or* moderate to severe otalgia	*Antibiotic exposure within 30 d[c] or recent treatment failure[c,d]* Ceftriaxone, 1 g IV/IM qd for 3 d; *or* Clindamycin, 300 mg PO tid; *or* Consider tympanocentesis with culture

Acute pharyngitis[b]
 	
  Clinical suspicion of streptococcal pharyngitis (e.g., fever, tonsillar swelling, exudate, enlarged/tender anterior cervical lymph nodes, absence of cough or coryza)[e] *with:*
 	
  History of rheumatic fever *or*
 	
  Documented household exposure *or*
 	
  Positive rapid strep screen
	Initial therapy
	
	Penicillin VK, 500 mg PO tid; *or*
	
	Amoxicillin, 500 mg PO bid; *or*
	
	Erythromycin, 250 mg PO qid; *or*
	
	Benzathine penicillin G, single dose of 1.2 million units IM

[a]For detailed information on diagnosis and treatment in children, see Tables 31-1, 31-2, and 31-3 in HPIM-18.
[b]Unless otherwise specified, the duration of therapy is generally 10 d, with appropriate follow-up.
[c]The duration of therapy is 5–7 d (10 d for pts with severe disease).
[d]Failure to improve and/or clinical worsening after 48–72 h of observation or treatment.
[e]Some organizations support treating adults who have these symptoms and signs without administering a rapid streptococcal antigen test.
Abbreviations: DS, double-strength; TMP-SMX, trimethoprim-sulfamethoxazole.
Sources: Rosenfeld RM et al: Otolaryngol Head Neck Surg 137(3 Suppl):S1, 2007; American Academy of Pediatrics Subcommittee on Management of Sinusitis and Committee on Quality Improvement: Pediatrics 108:798, 2001; American Academy of Pediatrics Subcommittee on Management of Acute Otitis Media: Pediatrics 113:1451, 2004; RJ Cooper et al: Ann Intern Med 134:509, 2001; and B Schwartz et al: Pediatrics 101:171, 1998.

- **Chronic fungal sinusitis:** a noninvasive disease in immunocompetent hosts, typically due to *Aspergillus* species and dematiaceous molds. Recurrence is common.
  - Mild, indolent disease is usually cured with endoscopic surgery and without antifungal agents.
  - Unilateral disease with a mycetoma (fungus ball) in the sinus is treated with surgery and—if bony erosion has occurred—antifungal agents.

- Allergic fungal sinusitis, seen in pts with nasal polyps and asthma, presents as pansinusitis and thick, eosinophil-laden mucus with the consistency of peanut butter.

INFECTIONS OF THE EAR AND MASTOID

■ EXTERNAL EAR INFECTIONS

In the absence of local or regional adenopathy, consider noninfectious causes of inflammation, among which trauma, insect bites, and environmental exposures are more commonly implicated than are autoimmune diseases (e.g., lupus) or vasculitides [e.g., granulomatosis with polyangiitis (Wegener's)].

- *Auricular cellulitis*: Tenderness, erythema, swelling, and warmth of the external ear, particularly the lobule, follow minor trauma. Treat with warm compresses and antibiotics active against *S. aureus* and streptococci (e.g., dicloxacillin).
- *Perichondritis*: Infection of the perichondrium of the auricular cartilage follows minor trauma (e.g., ear piercing). The infection may closely resemble auricular cellulitis, although the lobule is less often involved in perichondritis.
  - Treatment requires systemic antibiotics active against the most common etiologic agents, *Pseudomonas aeruginosa* and *S. aureus*, and typically consists of an antipseudomonal penicillin or a penicillinase-resistant penicillin (e.g., nafcillin) plus an antipseudomonal quinolone (e.g., ciprofloxacin). Surgical drainage may be needed; resolution can take weeks.
  - If perichondritis fails to respond to adequate therapy, consider noninfectious inflammatory etiologies (e.g., relapsing polychondritis).
- *Otitis externa*: a collection of diseases involving primarily the auditory meatus and resulting from a combination of heat and retained moisture, with desquamation and maceration of the epithelium of the outer ear canal. All forms are predominantly bacterial in origin; *P. aeruginosa* and *S. aureus* are the most common pathogens.
  - *Acute localized otitis externa*: furunculosis in the outer third of the ear canal, usually due to *S. aureus*. Treatment consists of an oral antistaphylococcal penicillin (e.g., dicloxacillin), with surgical drainage in cases of abscess formation.
  - *Acute diffuse otitis externa* (swimmer's ear): infection in macerated, irritated canals that is typically due to *P. aeruginosa* and is characterized by severe pain, erythema, and swelling of the canal and white clumpy discharge from the ear. Treatment includes cleansing of the canal to remove debris and use of topical antibiotics (e.g., preparations with neomycin and polymyxin), with or without glucocorticoids to reduce inflammation.
  - *Chronic otitis externa*: erythematous, scaling, pruritic, nonpainful dermatitis that usually arises from persistent drainage from a chronic middle-ear infection, other causes of repeated irritation, or rare chronic infections such as tuberculosis or leprosy. Treatment consists of identifying and eliminating the offending process; successful resolution is frequently difficult.

– *Malignant or necrotizing otitis externa*: a slowly progressive infection characterized by purulent otorrhea, an erythematous swollen ear and external canal, and severe otalgia out of proportion to exam findings, with granulation tissue present in the posteroinferior wall of the canal, near the junction of bone and cartilage

- This potentially life-threatening disease, which occurs primarily in elderly diabetic or immunocompromised pts, can involve the base of the skull, meninges, cranial nerves, and brain.
- *P. aeruginosa* is the most common etiologic agent, but other gram-negative bacilli, *S. aureus*, *Staphylococcus epidermidis*, and *Aspergillus* have been reported.
- A biopsy specimen of the granulation tissue (or of deeper tissues) should be obtained for culture.
- Treatment involves systemic antibiotics for 6–8 weeks and consists of antipseudomonal agents (e.g., piperacillin, ceftazidime) with an aminoglycoside or a fluoroquinolone; antibiotic drops active against *Pseudomonas*, combined with glucocorticoids, are used as adjunctive therapies.
- Recurs in up to 20% of cases. Aggressive glycemic control in diabetic pts helps with treatment and prevention of recurrence.

▓ MIDDLE-EAR INFECTIONS

Eustachian tube dysfunction, often in association with URIs, causes inflammation with a sterile transudate. Viral or bacterial superinfection often occurs.

- *Acute otitis media:* typically follows a viral URI, which can directly cause viral otitis media or predispose to bacterial otitis media
  - **Etiology:** *S. pneumoniae* is isolated in up to 35% of cases; nontypable *H. influenzae* and *M. catarrhalis* are other common causes of bacterial otitis media. Concern is increasing about community-acquired methicillin-resistant *S. aureus* (MRSA) as an emerging etiologic agent. Viruses (e.g., RSV, influenza virus, rhinovirus, enterovirus) have been recovered either alone or with bacteria in up to 40% of cases.
  - **Clinical manifestations:** The tympanic membrane is immobile, erythematous, bulging, or retracted and can perforate spontaneously.
    - Other findings may include otalgia, otorrhea, decreased hearing, fever, and irritability.
    - In isolation, erythema of the tympanic membrane is nonspecific as it is common in association with inflammation of the upper respiratory mucosa.
  - **Treatment:** Most cases of mild to moderate disease resolve within 1 week without specific treatment. Relief of symptoms with analgesic agents and NSAIDs typically suffices.
    - Indications for antibiotic therapy and treatment regimens are listed in Table 64-1.
    - Antibiotic prophylaxis and surgical interventions offer little benefit in recurrent acute otitis media.
- *Serous otitis media:* Also known as otitis media with effusion, this condition can persist for weeks (e.g., acute effusions) or months (e.g., after

an episode of acute otitis media) without signs of infection and is associated with significant hearing loss in the affected ear.

- The majority of cases resolve spontaneously within 3 months without antibiotic therapy.
- Antibiotic therapy or myringotomy with tympanostomy tubes is reserved for pts with bilateral effusions that have persisted for at least 3 months and are associated with bilateral hearing loss.

- *Chronic otitis media*: persistent or recurrent purulent otorrhea with tympanic membrane perforation, usually associated with conductive hearing loss
  - Inactive disease, characterized by a central perforation of the tympanic membrane, is treated with repeated courses of topical antibiotic drops during periods of drainage.
  - Active disease involves formation of a cholesteatoma that may enlarge and ultimately lead to erosion of bone, meningitis, and brain abscess; surgical treatment is required.

- *Mastoiditis*: accumulation of purulent exudate in the mastoid air cells that erodes surrounding bones and causes abscess-like cavities
  - Pts have pain, erythema, and mastoid process swelling causing displacement of the pinna along with the signs and symptoms of otitis media.
  - Rare complications include subperiosteal abscess, deep neck abscess, and septic thrombosis of the lateral sinus.
  - Broad-spectrum empirical IV antibiotic regimens targeting *S. pneumoniae*, *H. influenzae*, and *M. catarrhalis* can be narrowed once culture results are available; mastoidectomy is reserved for complicated cases or pts in whom medical management fails.

INFECTIONS OF THE PHARYNX AND ORAL CAVITY

- Sore throat is the most common presenting symptom and one of the most common reasons for ambulatory care visits by adults and children.

ACUTE PHARYNGITIS

- **Etiology:** Respiratory viruses are the most common identifiable cause, although ~30% of cases have no etiology identified.
  - Viruses: Rhinoviruses and coronaviruses cause ~20% and ~5% of cases, respectively; influenza virus, parainfluenza virus, HSV, coxsackievirus, EBV, and HIV are other important viral causes.
  - Bacteria: Group A *Streptococcus* (GAS) accounts for 5–15% of adult cases. *Fusobacterium necrophorum* is increasingly identified as a cause of pharyngitis in adolescents and is isolated nearly as often as GAS. Other bacterial causes include streptococci of groups C and G, *Neisseria gonorrhoeae*, *Corynebacterium diphtheriae*, and anaerobic bacteria.

- **Clinical manifestations:** Specific signs and symptoms sometimes suggest that one etiology is more likely than another.
  - Respiratory viruses: Symptoms usually are not severe and are associated with coryza without fever, tender cervical lymphadenopathy, or pharyngeal exudates.
  - Influenza virus and adenovirus: evidenced by severe exudative pharyngitis with fever

- HSV: presents as pharyngeal inflammation and exudates with vesicles and ulcers on the palate
- Coxsackievirus (herpangina): characterized by small vesicles on the soft palate and uvula that form shallow white ulcers
- EBV and CMV: present as exudative pharyngitis in association with other signs of infectious mononucleosis
- HIV: associated with fever, acute pharyngitis, myalgias, malaise, and sometimes a maculopapular rash
- Streptococci: Presentation ranges from mild disease to profound pharyngeal pain, fever, chills, abdominal pain, and a hyperemic pharyngeal membrane with tonsillar hypertrophy and exudates; coryzal symptoms are absent.
- Other bacteria: often present as exudative pharyngitis without other specific findings
- **Diagnosis:** The primary goal of diagnostic testing is to identify cases of GAS pharyngitis.
  - Rapid antigen-detection tests for GAS offer good specificity (>90%) but variable sensitivity (65–90%); throat cultures are not routinely recommended for adults in the setting of negative rapid testing.
  - Other bacterial causes may be missed on routine testing if specific cultures are not requested.
  - If HIV is being considered, testing for HIV RNA should be performed.
- **Treatment:** Antibiotic therapy for GAS infection is outlined in Table 64-1 and is recommended to prevent the development of rheumatic fever.
  - Symptom-based treatment of viral pharyngitis is generally sufficient.
  - Specific antiviral therapy may be helpful in selected cases of influenza and HSV infection.

■ ORAL INFECTIONS

Oral-labial herpesvirus infections and oropharyngeal candidiasis are discussed in Chaps. 108 and 115, respectively.

INFECTIONS OF THE LARYNX AND EPIGLOTTIS

- *Laryngitis*: Acute laryngitis is a common syndrome caused by nearly all the major respiratory viruses and by some bacteria (e.g., GAS, *C. diphtheriae*, and *M. catarrhalis*). Chronic cases of infectious laryngitis are much less common in developed countries than in low-income countries and are caused by *Mycobacterium tuberculosis*, endemic fungi (e.g., *Histoplasma, Blastomyces, Coccidioides*), and *Cryptococcus*.
  - Pts are hoarse, exhibit reduced vocal pitch or aphonia, and have coryzal symptoms.
  - Treatment of acute laryngitis consists of humidification, voice rest, and—if GAS is cultured—antibiotic administration. Treatment of chronic laryngitis depends on the pathogen, whose identification usually requires biopsy with culture.
- *Epiglottitis*: acute, rapidly progressive cellulitis of the epiglottis and adjacent structures that can result in complete—and sometimes fatal—airway obstruction

- Epiglottitis is caused by GAS, *S. pneumoniae*, *Haemophilus parainfluenzae*, and *S. aureus*; pediatric cases due to *H. influenzae* type b are now rare because of vaccination.
- Symptoms include fever, severe sore throat, and systemic toxicity, and pts often drool while sitting forward. Examination may reveal respiratory distress, inspiratory stridor, and chest wall retractions.
- Direct visualization in the exam room (i.e., with a tongue blade) should not be performed, given the risk of complete airway obstruction. Direct fiberoptic laryngoscopy in a controlled environment (e.g., an operating room) may be performed for diagnosis, procurement of specimens for culture, and placement of an endotracheal tube.
- Treatment focuses on protection of the airway. After blood and epiglottis samples are obtained for cultures, IV antibiotics active against *H. influenzae* (e.g., ampicillin/sulbactam or a second- or third-generation cephalosporin) should be given for 7–10 days.

INFECTIONS OF DEEP NECK STRUCTURES

These infections, which include Ludwig's angina, Lemierre's syndrome, and retropharyngeal abscess, are discussed in Chap. 101.

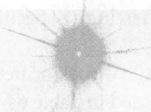

For a more detailed discussion, see Rubin MA et al: Pharyngitis, Sinusitis, Otitis, and Other Upper Respiratory Tract Infections, Chap. 31, p. 255, in HPIM-18.

CHAPTER **65**
General Examination of the Skin

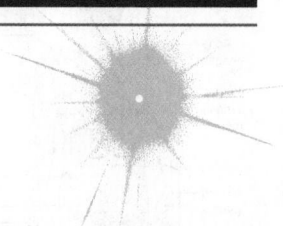

As dermatologic evaluation relies heavily on the objective cutaneous appearance, physical examination is often performed prior to taking a complete history in pts presenting with a skin problem. A differential diagnosis can usually be generated on the basis of a thorough examination with precise descriptions of the skin lesion(s) and narrowed with pertinent facts from the history. Laboratory or diagnostic procedures are then used, when appropriate, to clarify the diagnosis.

PHYSICAL EXAMINATION

Examination of skin should take place in a well-illuminated room with pt completely disrobed. Helpful ancillary equipment includes a hand lens and a pocket flashlight to provide peripheral illumination of lesions. An ideal examination includes evaluation of the skin, hair, nails and mucous membranes. The examination often begins with an assessment of the entire skin viewed at a distance, which is then narrowed down to focus on the individual lesions.

■ DISTRIBUTION

As illustrated in Fig. 65-1, the distribution of skin lesions can provide valuable clues to the identification of the disorder: generalized (systemic diseases); sun-exposed (SLE, photoallergic, phototoxic, polymorphous light eruption, porphyria cutanea tarda); dermatomal (herpes zoster); extensor surfaces (elbows and knees in psoriasis); flexural surfaces (antecubital and popliteal fossae in atopic dermatitis).

■ ARRANGEMENT AND SHAPE

Can describe individual or multiple lesions: *Linear* (contact dermatitis such as poison ivy); *annular*—"ring-shaped" lesion (erythema chronicum migrans, erythema annulare centrificum, tinea corporis); *iris* or *target lesion*—two or three concentric circles of differing hue (erythema multiforme); *nummular*—"coin-shaped" (nummular eczema); *morbilliform*—"measles-like" with small confluent papules coalescing into unusual shapes (measles, drug eruption); *herpetiform*—grouped vesicles, papules, or erosions (herpes simplex).

■ PRIMARY LESIONS

Cutaneous changes caused directly by disease process (Table 65-1).

■ SECONDARY LESIONS

Changes in area of primary pathology often due to secondary events, e.g., scratching, secondary infection, bleeding (Table 65-2).

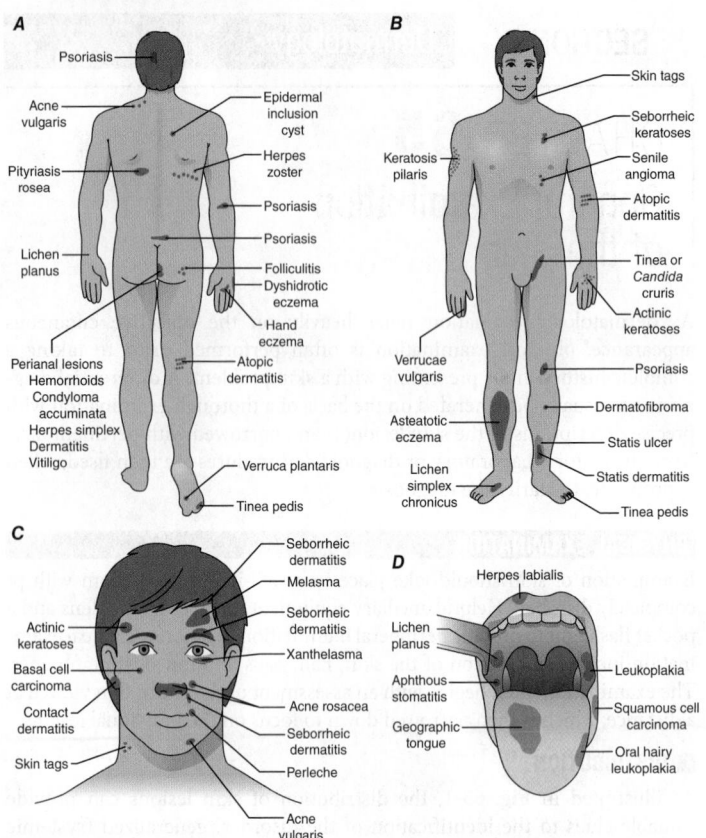

FIGURE 65-1 The distribution of some common dermatologic diseases and lesions.

■ OTHER DESCRIPTIVE TERMS

Color, e.g., violaceous, erythematous; physical characteristics, e.g., warm, tender; sharpness of edge, surface contour—flat-topped, pedunculated (on a stalk), verrucous (wartlike), umbilicated (containing a central depression).

HISTORY

A complete history should be obtained, with special attention being paid to the following points:

1. Evolution of the lesion—site of onset, manner in which eruption progressed or spread, duration, periods of resolution or improvement in chronic eruptions

2. Symptoms associated with the eruption—itching, burning, pain, numbness; what has relieved symptoms; time of day when symptoms are most severe

3. Current or recent medications—both prescription and over-the-counter

4. Associated systemic symptoms (e.g., malaise, fatigue, arthralgias)

5. Ongoing or previous illnesses

TABLE 65-1 DESCRIPTION OF PRIMARY SKIN LESIONS

Macule: A flat, colored lesion, <2 cm in diameter, not raised above the surface of the surrounding skin. A "freckle," or ephelid, is a prototype pigmented macule.

Patch: A large (>2 cm) flat lesion with a color different from the surrounding skin. This differs from a macule only in size.

Papule: A small, solid lesion, <0.5 cm in diameter, raised above the surface of the surrounding skin and hence palpable (e.g., a closed comedone, or whitehead, in acne).

Nodule: A larger (0.5–5.0 cm), firm lesion raised above the surface of the surrounding skin. This differs from a papule only in size (e.g., a dermal nevomelanocytic nevus).

Tumor: A solid, raised growth >5 cm in diameter.

Plaque: A large (>1 cm), flat-topped, raised lesion; edges may either be distinct (e.g., in psoriasis) or gradually blend with surrounding skin (e.g., in eczematous dermatitis).

Vesicle: A small, fluid-filled lesion, <0.5 cm in diameter, raised above the plane of surrounding skin. Fluid is often visible, and the lesions are translucent [e.g., vesicles in allergic contact dermatitis caused by *Toxicodendron* (poison ivy)].

Pustule: A vesicle filled with leukocytes. ***Note:*** The presence of pustules does not necessarily signify the existence of an infection.

Bulla: A fluid-filled, raised, often translucent lesion >0.5 cm in diameter.

Wheal: A raised, erythematous, edematous papule or plaque, usually representing short-lived vasodilatation and vasopermeability.

Telangiectasia: A dilated, superficial blood vessel.

6. History of allergies
7. Presence of photosensitivity
8. Review of systems
9. Family history
10. Social, sexual, or travel history

ADDITIONAL DIAGNOSTIC PROCEDURES

■ SKIN BIOPSY

Minor surgical procedure. Choice of site very important.

■ POTASSIUM HYDROXIDE PREPARATION

Useful for detection of dermatophyte or yeast. Scale is collected from advancing edge of a scaling lesion by gently scraping with side of a microscope slide or a scalpel blade. Nail lesions are best sampled by trimming back nail and scraping subungual debris. A drop of 10–20% potassium hydroxide is added to slide, and coverslip is applied. The slide may be gently heated and examined under microscope. This technique can be utilized to identify hyphae in dermatophyte infections, pseudohyphae and budding yeast in *Candida* infections, and "spaghetti and meatballs" yeast forms in tinea versicolor.

TABLE 65-2 DESCRIPTION OF SECONDARY SKIN LESIONS

Lichenification: A distinctive thickening of the skin that is characterized by accentuated skin-fold markings.

Scale: Excessive accumulation of stratum corneum.

Crust: Dried exudate of body fluids that may be either yellow (i.e., serous crust) or red (i.e., hemorrhagic crust).

Erosion: Loss of epidermis without an associated loss of dermis.

Ulcer: Loss of epidermis and at least a portion of the underlying dermis.

Excoriation: Linear, angular erosions that may be covered by crust and are caused by scratching.

Atrophy: An acquired loss of substance. In the skin, this may appear as a depression with intact epidermis (i.e., loss of dermal or subcutaneous tissue) or as sites of shiny, delicate, wrinkled lesions (i.e., epidermal atrophy).

Scar: A change in the skin secondary to trauma or inflammation. Sites may be erythematous, hypopigmented, or hyperpigmented depending on their age or character. Sites on hair-bearing areas may be characterized by destruction of hair follicles.

■ TZANCK PREPARATION

Useful for determining presence of herpes viruses (herpes simplex virus or herpes zoster virus). Optimal lesion to sample is an early vesicle. Lesion is gently unroofed with no. 15 scalpel blade, and base of vesicle is gently scraped with belly of blade (keep blade perpendicular to skin surface to prevent laceration). Scrapings are transferred to slide and stained with Wright's or Giemsa stain. A positive preparation has multinucleated giant cells. Culture or immunofluorescence testing must be performed to identify the specific virus.

■ DIASCOPY

Assesses whether a lesion blanches with pressure. Done by pressing a magnifying lens or microscope slide on lesion and observing changes in vascularity. For example, hemangiomas will usually blanch; purpuric lesions will not.

■ WOOD'S LIGHT EXAMINATION

Useful for detecting bacterial or fungal infection or accentuating features of some skin lesions.

■ PATCH TESTS

To document cutaneous sensitivity to specific antigen.

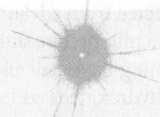

For a more detailed discussion, see Lawley TJ, Yancey KB: Approach to the Patient With a Skin Disorder, Chap. 51, p. 389, in HPIM-18.

CHAPTER **66**
Common Skin Conditions

PAPULOSQUAMOUS DISORDERS

Disorders exhibiting papules and scale.

■ PSORIASIS

A chronic, recurrent disorder. Classic lesion is a well-marginated, erythematous plaque with silvery-white surface scale. Distribution includes extensor surfaces (i.e., knees, elbows, and buttocks); may also involve palms and scalp (particularly anterior scalp margin). Associated findings include psoriatic arthritis (Chap. 172) and nail changes (onycholysis, pitting or thickening of nail plate with accumulation of subungual debris).

TREATMENT   Psoriasis

Maintain cutaneous hydration; topical glucocorticoids; topical vitamin D analogue (calcipotriol) and retinoid (tazarotene); UV light (PUVA when UV used in combination with psoralens); for severe disease methotrexate or cyclosporine; acitretin can also be used but is teratogenic. Alefacept (dimeric fusion protein: LFA-3/Fc human IgG1), or ustekinumab (human monoclonal antibody that blocks IL-12 and IL-23) can be considered for chronic, moderate to severe plaque psoriasis. Etanercept (dimeric fusion protein: TNF receptor/Fc human IgG1), infliximab, and adalimumab (monoclonal antibodies directed against TNF) are approved for psoriatic arthritis and psoriasis.

■ PITYRIASIS ROSEA

A self-limited condition lasting 3–8 weeks. Initially, there is a single 2- to 6-cm annular salmon-colored patch (herald patch) with a peripheral rim of scale, followed in days to weeks by a generalized eruption involving the trunk and proximal extremities. Individual lesions are similar to but smaller than the herald patch and are arranged in symmetric fashion with long axis of each individual lesion along skin lines of cleavage. Appearance may be similar to that of secondary syphilis.

TREATMENT   Pityriasis Rosea

Disorder is self-limited, so treatment is directed at symptoms; oral antihistamines for pruritus; topical glucocorticoids; UV-B phototherapy in some cases.

■ LICHEN PLANUS

Disorder of unknown cause; can follow administration of certain drugs and in chronic graft-versus-host disease; lesions are pruritic, polygonal, flat-topped, and violaceous. Course is variable, but most pts have spontaneous remissions 6–24 months after onset of disease.

TREATMENT   Lichen Planus

Topical glucocorticoids.

ECZEMATOUS DISORDERS

■ ECZEMA

Eczema, or dermatitis, is a reaction pattern that presents with variable clinical and histologic findings; it is the final common expression for a number of disorders.

■ ATOPIC DERMATITIS

One aspect of atopic triad of hayfever, asthma, and eczema. Usually an intermittent, chronic, severely pruritic, eczematous dermatitis with scaly erythematous patches, vesiculation, crusting, and fissuring. Lesions are most commonly on flexures, with prominent involvement of antecubital and popliteal fossae; generalized erythroderma in severe cases.

TREATMENT   Eczema and Atopic Dermatitis

Avoidance of irritants; cutaneous hydration; topical glucocorticoids; treatment of infected lesions [often with *Staphylococcus aureus* (SA)—consider community-acquired methicillin-resistant strains (CA-MRSA)]. Systemic glucocorticoids only for severe exacerbations unresponsive to topical conservative therapy.

■ ALLERGIC CONTACT DERMATITIS

A delayed hypersensitivity reaction that occurs after cutaneous exposure to an antigenic substance. Lesions occur at site of contact and are vesicular, weeping, crusting; linear arrangement of vesicles is common. Most frequent allergens are resin from plants of the genus *Toxicodendron* (poison ivy, oak, sumac), nickel, rubber, and cosmetics.

TREATMENT   Allergic Contact Dermatitis

Avoidance of sensitizing agent; topical glucocorticoids; consideration of systemic glucocorticoids over 2–3 weeks for widespread disease.

■ IRRITANT CONTACT DERMATITIS

Inflammation of the skin due to direct injury by an exogenous agent. The most common area of involvement is the hands, where dermatitis is initiated or aggravated by chronic exposure to water and detergents. Features may include skin dryness, cracking, erythema, edema.

| **TREATMENT** | Irritant Contact Dermatitis |

Avoidance of irritants; barriers (use of protective gloves); topical gluco-corticoids; treatment of secondary bacterial or dermatophyte infection.

■ SEBORRHEIC DERMATITIS

A chronic noninfectious process characterized by erythematous patches with greasy yellowish scale. Lesions are generally on scalp, eyebrows, naso-labial folds, axillae, central chest, and posterior auricular area.

| **TREATMENT** | Seborrheic Dermatitis |

Nonfluorinated topical glucocorticoids; shampoos containing coal tar, salicylic acid, or selenium sulfide.

INFECTIONS

■ IMPETIGO

A superficial infection of skin secondary to either *S. aureus* or group A β-hemolytic streptococci. The primary lesion is a superficial pustule that ruptures and forms a "honey-colored" crust. Tense bullae are associated with *S. aureus* infections (bullous impetigo). Lesions may occur anywhere but commonly involve the face. Impetigo and *furunculosis* (painful ery-thematous nodule, or boil) have gained prominence because of increasing incidence of CA-MRSA.

| **TREATMENT** | Impetigo |

Gentle debridement of adherent crusts with soaks and topical antibiotics; appropriate oral antibiotics depending on organism (Chap. 86).

■ ERYSIPELAS

Superficial cellulitis, most commonly on face, characterized by a bright red, sharply demarcated, intensely painful, warm plaque. Because of superficial location of infection and associated edema, surface of plaque may exhibit a *peau d'orange* (orange peel) appearance. Most commonly due to infection with group A β-hemolytic streptococci, occurring at sites of trauma or other breaks in skin.

| **TREATMENT** | Erysipelas |

Appropriate antibiotics depending on organism (Chap. 86).

■ HERPES SIMPLEX (SEE ALSO CHAP. 108)

Recurrent eruption characterized by grouped vesicles on an erythematous base that progress to erosions; often secondarily infected with staphylococci or streptococci. Infections frequently involve mucocutaneous surfaces around the oral cavity, genitals, or anus. Can also cause severe visceral disease including esophagitis, pneumonitis, encephalitis, and disseminated herpes simplex virus infection. Tzanck preparation of an unroofed early vesicle reveals multinucleated giant cells.

TREATMENT   Herpes Simplex

Will differ based on disease manifestations and level of immune competence (Chap. 108); appropriate antibiotics for secondary infections, depending on organism.

■ HERPES ZOSTER (SEE ALSO CHAP. 108)

Eruption of grouped vesicles on an erythematous base usually limited to a single dermatome ("shingles"); disseminated lesions can also occur, especially in immunocompromised pts. Tzanck preparation reveals multinucleated giant cells; indistinguishable from herpes simplex except by culture. Postherpetic neuralgia, lasting months to years, may occur, especially in the elderly.

TREATMENT   Herpes Zoster

Will differ based on disease manifestations and level of immune competence (Chap. 108).

■ DERMATOPHYTE INFECTION

Skin fungus, may involve any area of body; due to infection of stratum corneum, nail plate, or hair. Appearance may vary from mild scaliness to florid inflammatory dermatitis. Common sites of infection include the foot (tinea pedis), nails (tinea unguium), groin (tinea cruris), or scalp (tinea capitis). Classic lesion of tinea corporis ("ringworm") is an erythematous papulosquamous patch, often with central clearing and scale along peripheral advancing border. Hyphae are often seen on KOH preparation, although tinea capitis and tinea corporis may require culture or biopsy.

TREATMENT   Dermatophyte Infection

Depends on affected site and type of infection. Topical imidazoles, triazoles, and allylamines may be effective. Haloprogin, undecylenic acid, ciclopirox olamine, and tolnaftate are also effective, but nystatin is not active against dermatophytes. Griseofulvin, 500 mg/d, if systemic therapy required. Itraconazole or terbinafine may be effective for nail infections.

■ CANDIDIASIS

Fungal infection caused by a related group of yeasts. Manifestations may be localized to the skin or rarely systemic and life-threatening. Predisposing factors include diabetes mellitus, cellular immune deficiencies, and HIV (Chap. 114). Frequent sites include the oral cavity, chronically wet macerated areas, around nails, intertriginous areas. Diagnosed by clinical pattern and demonstration of yeast on KOH preparation or culture.

> **TREATMENT**   Candidiasis
>
> (See also Chap. 115) Removal of predisposing factors; topical nystatin or azoles; systemic therapy reserved for immunosuppressed pts, unresponsive chronic or recurrent disease; vulvovaginal candidiasis may respond to a single dose of fluconazole, 150 mg.

■ WARTS

Cutaneous neoplasms caused by human papilloma viruses (HPVs). Typically dome-shaped lesions with irregular filamentous surface. Propensity for the face, arms, and legs; often spread by shaving. HPVs are also associated with genital or perianal lesions and play a role in the development of cancer of the uterine cervix and external genitalia in females (Chap. 92).

> **TREATMENT**   Warts
>
> Cryotherapy with liquid nitrogen, keratinolytic agents (salicylic acid). For genital warts, application of podophyllin solution is effective but can be associated with marked local reactions; topical imiquimod also has been used.

ACNE

■ ACNE VULGARIS

Usually a self-limited disorder of teenagers and young adults. Comedones (small cysts formed in hair follicles) are clinical hallmark; often accompanied by inflammatory lesions of papules, pustules, or nodules. May scar in severe cases.

> **TREATMENT**   Acne Vulgaris
>
> Careful cleaning and removal of oils; oral tetracycline or erythromycin; topical antibacterials (e.g., benzoyl peroxide), topical retinoic acid. Systemic isotretinoin only for unresponsive severe nodulocystic acne (risk of severe adverse events including teratogenicity and possible association with depression).

■ ACNE ROSACEA

Inflammatory disorder affecting predominantly the central face, rarely affecting pts <30 years of age. Tendency toward exaggerated flushing, with eventual superimposition of papules, pustules, and telangiectases. May lead to rhinophyma and ocular problems.

> **TREATMENT**   Acne Rosacea
>
> Oral tetracycline, 250–1000 mg/d; topical metronidazole and topical nonfluorinated glucocorticoids may be useful.

VASCULAR DISORDERS

ERYTHEMA NODOSUM

Septal panniculitis characterized by erythematous, warm, tender subcutaneous nodular lesions typically over anterior tibia. Lesions are usually flush with skin surface but are indurated and have appearance of an erythematous/violaceous bruise. Lesions usually resolve spontaneously in 3–6 weeks without scarring. Commonly seen in sarcoidosis, administration of certain drugs (esp. sulfonamides, oral contraceptives, and estrogens), and a wide range of infections including streptococcal and tubercular; may be idiopathic.

> **TREATMENT**   Erythema Nodosum
>
> Identification and treatment/removal of underlying cause. NSAIDs for severe or recurrent lesions; systemic glucocorticoids are effective but dangerous if underlying infection is not appreciated.

ERYTHEMA MULTIFORME

A reaction pattern of skin consisting of a variety of lesions but most commonly erythematous papules and bullae. "Target" or "iris" lesion is characteristic and consists of concentric circles of erythema and normal flesh-colored skin, often with a central vesicle or bulla.

Distribution of lesions classically acral, esp. palms and soles. Three most common causes are drug reaction (particularly penicillins and sulfonamides) or concurrent herpetic or *Mycoplasma* infection. Can rarely affect mucosal surfaces and internal organs (erythema multiforme major or Stevens-Johnson syndrome).

> **TREATMENT**   Erythema Multiforme
>
> Provocative agent should be sought and eliminated if drug-related. In mild cases limited to skin, only symptomatic treatment is needed (antihistamines, NSAID). For Stevens-Johnson, systemic glucocorticoids have been used but are controversial; prevention of secondary infection and maintenance of nutrition and fluid/electrolyte balance are critical.

URTICARIA

A common disorder, either acute or chronic, characterized by evanescent (individual lesions lasting <24 h), pruritic, edematous, pink to erythematous plaques with a whitish halo around margin of individual lesions. Lesions range in size from papules to giant coalescent lesions (10–20 cm in diameter). Often due to drugs, systemic infection, or foods (esp. shellfish). Food additives such as tartrazine dye (FD&C yellow no. 5), benzoate, or salicylates have also been implicated. If individual lesions last >24 h, consider diagnosis of urticarial vasculitis.

TREATMENT	Urticaria

See Chap. 167.

■ VASCULITIS

Palpable purpura (nonblanching, elevated lesions) is the cutaneous hallmark of vasculitis. Other lesions include petechiae (esp. early lesions), necrosis with ulceration, bullae, and urticarial lesions (urticarial vasculitis). Lesions usually most prominent on lower extremities. Associations include infections, collagen-vascular disease, primary systemic vasculitides, malignancy, hepatitis B and C, drugs (esp. thiazides), and inflammatory bowel disease. May occur as an idiopathic, predominantly cutaneous vasculitis.

TREATMENT	Vasculitis

Will differ based on cause. Pursue identification and treatment/elimination of an exogenous cause or underlying disease. If part of a systemic vasculitis, treat based on major organ-threatening features (Chap. 170). Immunosuppressive therapy should be avoided in idiopathic, predominantly cutaneous vasculitis as disease frequently does not respond and rarely causes irreversible organ system dysfunction.

CUTANEOUS DRUG REACTIONS

Cutaneous reactions are among the most frequent medication toxicities. These can have a wide range of severity and manifestations including urticaria, photosensitivity, erythema multiforme, fixed drug reactions, erythema nodosum, vasculitis, lichenoid reactions, bullous drug reactions, Stevens-Johnson syndrome, and toxic epidermal necrolysis (TEN). Diagnosis is usually made by appearance and careful medication history.

TREATMENT	Cutaneous Drug Reactions

Withdrawal of the medication. Treatment based on nature and severity of cutaneous pathology.

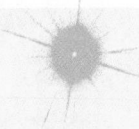

For a more detailed discussion, see Lawley LP, McCall CO, Lawley TJ: Eczema, Psoriasis, Cutaneous Infections, Acne, and Other Common Skin Disorders, Chap. 52, p. 395; Shinkai K, Stern RS, Wintroub BU: Cutaneous Drug Reactions, Chap. 55, p. 432; and Bolognia JL, Braverman IM: Skin Manifestations of Internal Disease, Chap. 53, p. 405, in HPIM-18.

CHAPTER **67**
Examination of Blood Smears and Bone Marrow

BLOOD SMEARS

■ ERYTHROCYTE (RBC) MORPHOLOGY

- Normal: 7.5-μm diameter. Roughly the size of the nucleus of a small lymphocyte.
- *Reticulocytes* (Wright's stain)—large, grayish-blue, admixed with pink (polychromasia).
- *Anisocytosis*—variation in RBC size; large cells imply delay in erythroid precursor DNA synthesis caused by folate or B_{12} deficiency or drug effect; small cells imply a defect in hemoglobin synthesis caused by iron deficiency or abnormal hemoglobin genes.
- *Poikilocytosis*—abnormal RBC shapes; the following are examples:
  1. *Acanthocytes* (spur cells)—irregularly spiculated; abetalipoproteinemia, severe liver disease, rarely anorexia nervosa.
  2. *Echinocytes* (burr cells)—regularly shaped, uniformly distributed spiny projections; uremia, RBC volume loss.
  3. *Elliptocytes*—elliptical; hereditary elliptocytosis.
  4. *Schistocytes* (schizocytes)—fragmented cells of varying sizes and shapes; microangiopathic or macroangiopathic hemolytic anemia.
  5. *Sickled cells*—elongated, crescentic; sickle cell anemias.
  6. *Spherocytes*—small hyperchromic cells lacking normal central pallor; hereditary spherocytosis, extravascular hemolysis as in autoimmune hemolytic anemia, G6PD deficiency.
  7. *Target cells*—central and outer rim staining with intervening ring of pallor; liver disease, thalassemia, hemoglobin C and sickle C diseases.
  8. *Teardrop cells*—myelofibrosis, other infiltrative processes of marrow (e.g., carcinoma).
  9. *Rouleaux formation*—alignment of RBCs in stacks; may be artifactual or due to paraproteinemia (e.g., multiple myeloma, macroglobulinemia).

■ RBC INCLUSIONS

- *Howell-Jolly bodies*—1-μm-diameter basophilic cytoplasmic inclusion that represents a residual nuclear fragment, usually single; asplenic pts.
- *Basophilic stippling*—multiple, punctate basophilic cytoplasmic inclusions composed of precipitated mitochondria and ribosomes; lead poisoning, thalassemia, myelofibrosis.

- *Pappenheimer (iron) bodies*—iron-containing granules usually composed of mitochondria and ribosomes resemble basophilic stippling but also stain with Prussian blue; lead poisoning, other sideroblastic anemias.
- *Heinz bodies*—spherical inclusions of precipitated hemoglobin seen only with supravital stains, such as crystal violet; G6PD deficiency (after oxidant stress such as infection, certain drugs), unstable hemoglobin variants.
- *Parasites*—characteristic intracytoplasmic inclusions; malaria, babesiosis.

▉ LEUKOCYTE INCLUSIONS AND NUCLEAR CONTOUR ABNORMALITIES

- *Toxic granulations*—dark cytoplasmic granules; bacterial infection.
- *Döhle bodies*—1- to 2-μm blue, oval cytoplasmic inclusions; bacterial infection, Chédiak-Higashi anomaly.
- *Auer rods*—eosinophilic, rodlike cytoplasmic inclusions; acute myeloid leukemia (some cases).
- *Hypersegmentation*—neutrophil nuclei contain more than the usual 2–4 lobes; usually >5% have ≥5 lobes or a single cell with 7 lobes is adequate to make the diagnosis; folate or B_{12} deficiency, drug effects.
- *Hyposegmentation*—neutrophil nuclei contain fewer lobes than normal, either one or two: Pelger-Hüet anomaly, pseudo-Pelger-Hüet or acquired Pelger-Hüet anomaly in acute leukemia.

▉ PLATELET ABNORMALITIES

- *Platelet clumping*—an in vitro artifact—is often readily detectable on smear; can lead to falsely low platelet count by automated cell counters.
- *Giant platelets*—can be a sign of a very young platelet or increased platelet production or abnormal karyocyte maturation; if the platelets are >5-6 μm in diameter, they may not be counted as platelets by electronic counters.

BONE MARROW

Aspiration assesses cell morphology. *Biopsy* assesses overall marrow architecture, including degree of cellularity. Biopsy should precede aspiration to avoid aspiration artifact (mainly hemorrhage) in the specimen.

▉ INDICATIONS

Aspiration

Hypoproliferative or unexplained anemia, leukopenia, or thrombocytopenia, suspected leukemia or myeloma or marrow defect, evaluation of iron stores, workup of some cases of fever of unknown origin.

Special Tests

Histochemical staining (leukemias), cytogenetic studies (leukemias, lymphomas), microbiology (bacterial, mycobacterial, fungal cultures), Prussian blue (iron) stain (assessment of iron stores, diagnosis of sideroblastic anemias).

Biopsy

Performed in addition to aspiration for pancytopenia (aplastic anemia), metastatic tumor, granulomatous infection (e.g., mycobacteria, brucellosis, histoplasmosis), myelofibrosis, lipid storage disease (e.g., Gaucher's, Niemann-Pick), any case with "dry tap" on aspiration; evaluation of marrow cellularity. When biopsy and aspirate are both planned, the biopsy should be performed first because of the risk of bleeding artifact from biopsy of an aspiration site.

Special Tests

Histochemical staining (e.g., acid phosphatase for metastatic prostate carcinoma), immunoperoxidase staining (e.g., immunoglobulin or cell surface marker detection in multiple myeloma, leukemia, or lymphoma; lysozyme detection in monocytic leukemia), reticulin staining (increased in myelofibrosis), microbiologic staining (e.g., acid-fast staining for mycobacteria).

■ INTERPRETATION

Cellularity

Defined as percentage of space occupied by hematopoietic cells. The space that is not hematopoietic tissue is usually fat. Cellularity decreases with age after age 65 years from about 50% to 25–30% with a corresponding increase in fat.

Erythroid:Granulocytic (E:G) Ratio

Normally about 1:2, the E:G ratio is decreased in acute and chronic infection, leukemoid reactions (e.g., chronic inflammation, metastatic tumor), acute and chronic myeloid leukemia, myelodysplastic disorders ("preleukemia"), and pure red cell aplasia; increased in agranulocytosis, anemias with erythroid hyperplasia (megaloblastic, iron-deficiency, thalassemia, hemorrhage, hemolysis, sideroblastic), and erythrocytosis (excessive RBC production); normal in aplastic anemia (though marrow hypocellular), myelofibrosis (marrow hypocellular), multiple myeloma, lymphoma, anemia of chronic disease. Some centers use the term M:E (myeloid to erythroid) ratio; normal value is 2:1 and increases with diseases that promote myeloid activity or inhibit erythroid activity and decreases with diseases that inhibit myeloid activity or promote erythroid activity.

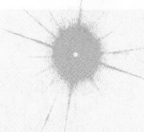

For a more detailed discussion, see Adamson JW, Longo DL: Anemia and Polycythemia, Chap. 57, p. 448; Holland SM, Gallin JI: Disorders of Granulocytes and Monocytes, Chap. 60, p. 472; Longo DL: Atlas of Hematology and Analysis of Peripheral Blood Smears, Chap. e17 in HPIM-18.

CHAPTER **68**
Red Blood Cell Disorders

Anemia is a common clinical problem in medicine. A physiologic approach (outlined in Chap. 51) provides the most efficient path to diagnosis and management. Anemias arise either because red blood cell (RBC) production is inadequate or because RBC lifespan (normally 120 days) is shortened through loss from the circulation or destruction.

HYPOPROLIFERATIVE ANEMIAS

These are the most common anemias. Usually the RBC morphology is normal and the reticulocyte index (RI) is low. Marrow damage, early iron deficiency, and decreased erythropoietin production or action may produce anemia of this type.

Marrow damage may be caused by infiltration of the marrow with tumor or fibrosis that crowds out normal erythroid precursors or by the absence of erythroid precursors (aplastic anemia) as a consequence of exposure to drugs, radiation, chemicals, viruses (e.g., hepatitis), autoimmune mechanisms, or genetic factors, either hereditary (e.g., Fanconi's anemia) or acquired (e.g., paroxysmal nocturnal hemoglobinuria). Most cases of aplasia are idiopathic. The tumor or fibrosis that infiltrates the marrow may originate in the marrow (as in leukemia or myelofibrosis) or be secondary to processes originating outside the marrow (as in metastatic cancer or myelophthisis).

Early iron-deficiency anemia (or iron-deficient erythropoiesis) is associated with a decrease in serum ferritin levels (<15 µg/L), moderately elevated

	Normal	Negative iron balance	Iron-deficient erythropoiesis	Iron-deficiency anemia
Iron stores				
Erythron iron				
Marrow iron stores	1-3+	0-1+	0	0
Serum ferritin (µg/L)	50-200	<20	<15	<15
TIBC (µg/dL)	300-360	>360	>380	>400
SI (µg/dL)	50-150	NL	<50	<30
Saturation (%)	30-50	NL	<20	<10
Marrow sideroblasts (%)	40-60	NL	<10	<10
RBC protoporphyrin (µg/dL)	30-50	NL	>100	>200
RBC morphology	NL	NL	NL	Microcytic/ hypochromic

FIGURE 68-1 Measurements of marrow iron stores, serum ferritin, and total iron-binding capacity (TIBC) are sensitive to early iron-store depletion. Iron-deficient erythropoiesis is recognized from additional abnormalities in the serum iron (SI), percent transferrin saturation, the pattern of marrow sideroblasts, and the red cell protoporphyrin level. Pts with iron-deficiency anemia demonstrate all the same abnormalities plus hypochromic microcytic anemia. (*From RS Hillman, CA Finch: Red Cell Manual, 7th. ed, Philadelphia, Davis, 1996, with permission.*)

TABLE 68-1 DIAGNOSIS OF HYPOPROLIFERATIVE ANEMIAS

Tests	Iron Deficiency	Inflammation	Renal Disease	Hypometabolic States
Anemia	Mild to severe	Mild	Mild to severe	Mild
MCV (fL)	60–90	80–90	90	90
Morphology	Normo-microcytic	Normocytic	Normocytic	Normocytic
SI	<30	<50	Normal	Normal
TIBC	>360	<300	Normal	Normal
Saturation (%)	<10	10–20	Normal	Normal
Serum ferritin (μg/L)	<15	30–200	115–150	Normal
Iron stores	0	2–4+	1–4+	Normal

Abbreviations: MCV, mean corpuscular volume; SI, serum iron; TIBC, total iron-binding capacity.

total iron-binding capacity (TIBC) (>380 μg/dL), serum iron (SI) level <50 μg/dL, and an iron saturation of <30% but >10% (Fig. 68-1). RBC morphology is generally normal until iron deficiency is severe (see below).

Decreased stimulation of erythropoiesis can be a consequence of inadequate erythropoietin production [e.g., renal disease destroying the renal tubular cells that produce it or hypometabolic states (endocrine deficiency or protein starvation) in which insufficient erythropoietin is produced] or of inadequate erythropoietin action. The anemia of chronic disease is a common entity. It is multifactorial in pathogenesis: inhibition of erythropoietin production, inhibition of iron reutilization (which blocks the response to erythropoietin), and inhibition of erythroid colony proliferation by inflammatory cytokines (e.g., tumor necrosis factor, interferon γ). Hepcidin, a small iron-binding molecule produced by the liver during an acute-phase inflammatory response, may bind iron and prevent its reutilization in hemoglobin synthesis. The laboratory tests shown in Table 68-1 may assist in the differential diagnosis of hypoproliferative anemias. Measurement of hepcidin in the urine is not yet practical or widely available.

MATURATION DISORDERS

These result from either defective hemoglobin synthesis, leading to cytoplasmic maturation defects and small relatively empty red cells, or abnormally slow DNA replication, leading to nuclear maturation defects and large full red cells. Defects in hemoglobin synthesis usually result from insufficient iron supply (iron deficiency) or decreased globin production (thalassemia) or are idiopathic (sideroblastic anemia). Defects in DNA synthesis are usually due to nutritional problems (vitamin B_{12} and folate deficiency), toxic (methotrexate or other cancer chemotherapeutic agent) exposure, or intrinsic marrow maturation defects (refractory anemia, myelodysplasia).

TABLE 68-2 DIAGNOSIS OF MICROCYTIC ANEMIA

Tests	Iron Deficiency	Inflammation	Thalassemia	Sideroblastic Anemia
Smear	Micro/hypo	Normal micro/hypo	Micro/hypo with targeting	Variable
SI	<30	<50	Normal to high	Normal to high
TIBC	>360	<300	Normal	Normal
Percent saturation	<10	10–20	30–80	30–80
Ferritin (µg/L)	<15	30–200	50–300	50–300
Hemoglobin pattern on electrophoresis	Normal	Normal	Abnormal with β thalassemia; can be normal with α thalassemia	Normal

Abbreviations: SI, serum iron; TIBC, total iron-binding capacity.

Laboratory tests useful in the differential diagnosis of the microcytic anemias are shown in Table 68-2. Mean corpuscular volume (MCV) is generally 60–80 fL. Increased lactate dehydrogenase (LDH) and indirect bilirubin levels suggest an increase in RBC destruction and favor a cause other than iron deficiency. Iron status is best assessed by measuring SI, TIBC, and ferritin levels. Macrocytic MCVs are >94 fL. Folate status is best assessed by measuring red blood cell folate levels. Vitamin B_{12} status is best assessed by measuring serum B_{12}, homocysteine, and methylmalonic acid levels. Homocysteine and methylmalonic acid levels are elevated in the setting of B_{12} deficiency.

ANEMIA DUE TO RBC DESTRUCTION OR ACUTE BLOOD LOSS

■ BLOOD LOSS

Trauma, GI hemorrhage (may be occult) are common causes; less common are genitourinary sources (menorrhagia, gross hematuria), internal bleeding such as intraperitoneal from spleen or organ rupture, retroperitoneal, iliopsoas hemorrhage (e.g., in hip fractures). Acute bleeding is associated with manifestations of hypovolemia, reticulocytosis, macrocytosis; chronic bleeding is associated with iron deficiency, hypochromia, microcytosis.

■ HEMOLYSIS

Causes are listed in Table 68-3.

1. *Intracellular RBC abnormalities*—most are inherited enzyme defects [glucose-6-phosphate dehydrogenase (G6PD) deficiency > pyruvate kinase deficiency], hemoglobinopathies, sickle cell anemia and variants, thalassemia, unstable hemoglobin variants.

2. *G6PD deficiency*—leads to episodes of hemolysis precipitated by ingestion of drugs that induce oxidant stress on RBCs. These include

TABLE 68-3 CLASSIFICATION OF HEMOLYTIC ANEMIAS[a]

	Intracorpuscular Defects	Extracorpuscular Factors
Hereditary	Hemoglobinopathies	Familial (atypical) hemolytic uremic syndrome
	Enzymopathies	
	Membrane-cytoskeletal defects	
Acquired	Paroxysmal nocturnal hemoglobinuria (PNH)	Mechanical destruction (microangiopathic)
		Toxic agents
		Drugs
		Infectious
		Autoimmune

[a]Hereditary causes correlate with intracorpuscular defects because these defects are due to inherited mutations. The one exception is PNH because the defect is due to an acquired somatic mutation. Similarly, acquired causes correlate with extracorpuscular factors because mostly these factors are exogenous. The one exception is familial hemolytic uremic syndrome (HUS; often referred to as atypical HUS) because here an inherited abnormality allows complement activation to be excessive, with bouts of production of membrane attack complex capable of destroying normal red cells.

antimalarials (chloroquine), sulfonamides, analgesics (phenacetin), and other miscellaneous drugs (Table 68-4).

3. *Sickle cell anemia*—characterized by a single-amino-acid change in β globin (valine for glutamic acid in the 6th residue) that produces a molecule of decreased solubility, especially in the absence of O_2. Although anemia and chronic hemolysis are present, the major disease manifestations relate to vasoocclusion from misshapen sickled RBCs. Infarcts in lung, bone, spleen, retina, brain, and other organs lead to symptoms and dysfunction (Fig. 68-2).

4. *Membrane abnormalities* (rare)—spur cell anemia (cirrhosis, anorexia nervosa), paroxysmal nocturnal hemoglobinuria, hereditary spherocytosis (increased RBC osmotic fragility, spherocytes), hereditary elliptocytosis (causes mild hemolytic anemia).

5. *Immunohemolytic anemia* (positive Coombs' test, spherocytes). Two types: (a) *warm antibody* (usually IgG)—idiopathic, lymphoma, chronic lymphocytic leukemia, systemic lupus erythematosus, drugs (e.g., methyldopa, penicillins, quinine, quinidine, isoniazid, sulfonamides); and (b) *cold antibody*—cold agglutinin disease (IgM) due to *Mycoplasma* infection, infectious mononucleosis, lymphoma, idiopathic; paroxysmal cold hemoglobinuria (IgG) due to syphilis, viral infections.

6. *Mechanical trauma* (macro- and microangiopathic hemolytic anemias; schistocytes)—prosthetic heart valves, vasculitis, malignant hypertension, eclampsia, renal graft rejection, giant hemangioma, scleroderma, thrombotic thrombocytopenic purpura, hemolytic-uremic syndrome, disseminated intravascular coagulation, march hemoglobinuria (e.g., marathon runners, bongo drummers).

TABLE 68-4 DRUGS THAT CARRY RISK OF CLINICAL HEMOLYSIS IN PERSONS WITH G6PD DEFICIENCY

	Definite Risk	Possible Risk	Doubtful Risk
Antimalarials	Primaquine Dapsone/chlorpro-guanil[a]	Chloroquine	Quinine
Sulphonamides/sulphones	Sulfamethoxazole Others Dapsone	Sulfasalazine Sulfadimidine	Sulfisoxazole Sulfadiazine
Antibacterial/antibiotics	Cotrimoxazole Nalidixic acid Nitrofurantoin Niridazole	Ciprofloxacin Norfloxacin	Chloramphenicol p-Aminosalicylic acid
Antipyretic/analgesics	Acetanilide Phenazopyridine	Acetylsalicylic acid high dose (>3 g/d)	Acetylsalicylic acid (<3 g/d) Acetaminophen Phenacetin
Other	Naphthalene Methylene blue	Vitamin K analogues Ascorbic acid >1 g Rasburicase	Doxorubicin Probenecid

[a]Marketed as Lapdap from 2003 to 2008.

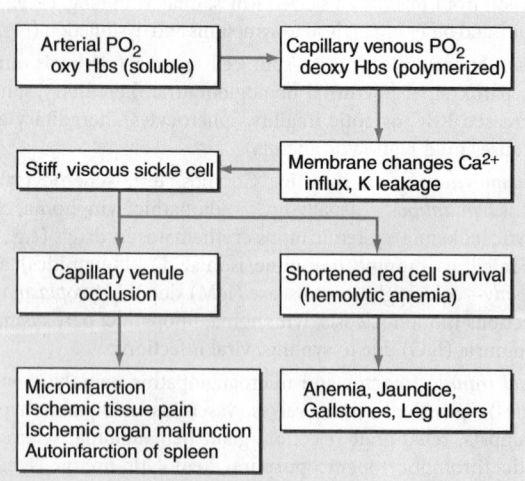

FIGURE 68-2 Pathophysiology of sickle cell crisis.

7. *Direct toxic effect*—infections (e.g., malaria, *Clostridium perfringens* toxin, toxoplasmosis).

8. *Hypersplenism* (pancytopenia may be present).

■ **LABORATORY ABNORMALITIES**

Elevated reticulocyte index, polychromasia and nucleated RBCs on smear; also spherocytes, elliptocytes, schistocytes, or target, spur, or sickle cells may be present depending on disorder; elevated unconjugated serum bilirubin and LDH, elevated plasma hemoglobin, low or absent haptoglobin; urine hemosiderin present in intravascular but not extravascular hemolysis, Coombs' test (immunohemolytic anemias), osmotic fragility test (hereditary spherocytosis), hemoglobin electrophoresis (sickle cell anemia, thalassemia), G6PD assay (best performed after resolution of hemolytic episode to prevent false-negative result).

| **TREATMENT** | Anemia |

GENERAL APPROACHES The acuteness and severity of the anemia determine whether transfusion therapy with packed RBCs is indicated. Rapid occurrence of severe anemia (e.g., after acute GI hemorrhage resulting in Hct <25%, following volume repletion) or development of angina or other symptoms is an indication for transfusion. Hct should increase 3–4% [Hb by 10 g/L (1 g/dL)] with each unit of packed RBCs, assuming no ongoing losses. Chronic anemia (e.g., vitamin B_{12} deficiency), even when severe, may not require transfusion therapy if the pt is compensated and specific therapy (e.g., vitamin B_{12}) is instituted.

SPECIFIC DISORDERS

1. *Iron deficiency*: find and treat cause of blood loss, oral iron (e.g., $FeSO_4$ 300 mg tid).

2. *Folate deficiency*: common in malnourished, alcoholics; less common now than before folate food supplementation; folic acid 1 mg PO qd (5 mg qd for pts with malabsorption).

3. *Vitamin B_{12} deficiency*: can be managed either with parenteral vitamin B_{12} 100 µg IM qd for 7 d, then 100–1000 µg IM per month or with 2 mg oral crystalline vitamin B_{12} per day. An inhaled formulation is also available.

4. *Anemia of chronic disease*: treat underlying disease; in uremia use recombinant human erythropoietin, 50–150 U/kg three times a week; role of erythropoietin in other forms of anemia of chronic disease is less clear; response more likely if serum erythropoietin levels are low. Target Hb 9–10 g/dL.

5. *Sickle cell anemia*: hydroxyurea 10–30 mg/kg per day PO increases level of HbF and prevents sickling, treat infections early, supplemental folic acid; painful crises treated with oxygen, analgesics (opioids), hydration, and hypertransfusion; consider allogeneic bone marrow transplantation in pts with increasing frequency of crises.

6. *Thalassemia*: transfusion to maintain Hb >90 g/L (>9 g/dL), folic acid, prevention of Fe overload with deferoxamine (parenteral) or

deferasirox (oral) chelation; consider splenectomy and allogeneic bone marrow transplantation.

7. *Aplastic anemia*: antithymocyte globulin and cyclosporine leads to improvement in 70%, bone marrow transplantation in young pts with a matched donor.

8. *Autoimmune hemolysis*: glucocorticoids, sometimes immunosuppressive agents, danazol, plasmapheresis, rituximab.

9. *G6PD deficiency*: avoid agents known to precipitate hemolysis.

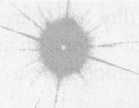

For a more detailed discussion, see Adamson JW, Chap. 103; Benz EJ, Chap. 104; Hoffbrand AV, Chap. 105; Luzzato L, Chap. 106; Young NS, Chap. 107; pp. 844–897, in HPIM-18.

CHAPTER 69
Leukocytosis and Leukopenia

LEUKOCYTOSIS

APPROACH TO THE PATIENT   Leukocytosis

Review smear (? abnormal cells present) and obtain differential count. The normal values for concentration of blood leukocytes are shown in Table 69-1.

■ NEUTROPHILIA

Absolute neutrophil count (polys and bands) >10,000/μL. The pathophysiology of neutrophilia involves increased production, increased marrow mobilization, or decreased margination (adherence to vessel walls).

TABLE 69-1 NORMAL VALUES FOR LEUKOCYTE CONCENTRATION IN BLOOD

Cell Type	Mean, cells/μL	95% Confidence Intervals, cells/μL	Total WBC, %
Neutrophil	3650	1830–7250	30–60%
Lymphocyte	2500	1500–4000	20–50%
Monocyte	430	200–950	2–10%
Eosinophil	150	0–700	0.3–5%
Basophil	30	0–150	0.6–1.8%

Causes

(1) *Exercise, stress*; (2) *infections*—esp. bacterial; smear shows increased numbers of immature neutrophils ("left shift"), toxic granulations, Döhle bodies; (3) *burns*; (4) *tissue necrosis* (e.g., myocardial, pulmonary, renal infarction); (5) *chronic inflammatory disorders* (e.g., gout, vasculitis); (6) *drugs* (e.g., glucocorticoids, epinephrine, lithium); (7) *cytokines* [e.g., granulocyte colony-stimulating factor (G-CSF), granulocyte-macrophage colony-stimulating factor (GM-CSF)]; (8) *myeloproliferative disorders* (Chap. 72); (9) *metabolic* (e.g., ketoacidosis, uremia); (10) *other*—malignant neoplasms, acute hemorrhage or hemolysis, after splenectomy.

■ LEUKEMOID REACTION

Extreme elevation of leukocyte count (>50,000/μL) composed of mature and/or immature neutrophils.

Causes

(1) *Infection* (severe, chronic, e.g., tuberculosis), esp. in children; (2) *hemolysis* (severe); (3) *malignant neoplasms* (esp. carcinoma of the breast, lung, kidney); (4) *cytokines* (e.g., G-CSF, GM-CSF). May be distinguished from chronic myeloid leukemia (CML) by measurement of the leukocyte alkaline phosphatase (LAP) level: elevated in leukemoid reactions, depressed in CML.

■ LEUKOERYTHROBLASTIC REACTION

Similar to leukemoid reaction with addition of nucleated red blood cells (RBCs) and schistocytes on blood smear.

Causes

(1) *Myelophthisis*—invasion of the bone marrow by tumor, fibrosis, granulomatous processes; smear shows "teardrop" RBCs; (2) *myelofibrosis*—same pathophysiology as myelophthisis, but the fibrosis is a primary marrow disorder; (3) *hemorrhage* or *hemolysis* (rarely, in severe cases).

■ LYMPHOCYTOSIS

Absolute lymphocyte count >5000/μL.

Causes

(1) *Infection*—infectious mononucleosis, hepatitis, cytomegalovirus, rubella, pertussis, tuberculosis, brucellosis, syphilis; (2) *endocrine disorders*—thyrotoxicosis, adrenal insufficiency; (3) *neoplasms*—chronic lymphocytic leukemia (CLL), most common cause of lymphocyte count >10,000/μL.

■ MONOCYTOSIS

Absolute monocyte count >800/μL.

Causes

(1) *Infection*—subacute bacterial endocarditis, tuberculosis, brucellosis, rickettsial diseases (e.g., Rocky Mountain spotted fever), malaria, leishmaniasis; (2) *granulomatous diseases*—sarcoidosis, Crohn's disease; (3) *collagen vascular diseases*—rheumatoid arthritis, systemic lupus erythematosus (SLE), polyarteritis nodosa, polymyositis, temporal arteritis; (4) *hematologic diseases*—leukemias, lymphoma, myeloproliferative and myelodysplastic syndromes, hemolytic anemia, chronic idiopathic neutropenia; (5) *malignant neoplasms*.

■ EOSINOPHILIA

Absolute eosinophil count >500/μL.

Causes

(1) *Drugs*, (2) *parasitic infections*, (3) *allergic diseases*, (4) *collagen vascular diseases*, (5) *malignant neoplasms*, (6) *hypereosinophilic syndromes*.

■ BASOPHILIA

Absolute basophil count >100/μL.

Causes

(1) *Allergic diseases*, (2) *myeloproliferative disorders* (esp. CML), (3) *chronic inflammatory disorders* (rarely).

LEUKOPENIA

Total leukocyte count <4300/μL.

■ NEUTROPENIA

Absolute neutrophil count <2000/μL (increased risk of bacterial infection with count <1000/μL). The pathophysiology of neutropenia involves decreased production or increased peripheral destruction.

Causes

(1) *Drugs*—cancer chemotherapeutic agents are most common cause, also phenytoin, carbamazepine, indomethacin, chloramphenicol, penicillins, sulfonamides, cephalosporins, propylthiouracil, phenothiazines, captopril, methyldopa, procainamide, chlorpropamide, thiazides, cimetidine, allopurinol, colchicine, ethanol, penicillamine, and immunosuppressive agents; (2) *infections*—viral (e.g., influenza, hepatitis, infectious mononucleosis, HIV), bacterial (e.g., typhoid fever, miliary tuberculosis, fulminant sepsis), malaria; (3) *nutritional*—B_{12}, folate deficiencies; (4) *benign*—benign ethnic neutropenia (BEN) seen in up to 25% of blacks, no associated risk of infection; (5) *hematologic diseases*—cyclic neutropenia (q21d, with recurrent infections common), leukemia, myelodysplasia (preleukemia), aplastic anemia, bone marrow infiltration (uncommon cause), Chédiak-Higashi syndrome; (6) *hypersplenism*—e.g., Felty's syndrome, congestive splenomegaly, Gaucher's disease; (7) *autoimmune diseases*—idiopathic, SLE, lymphoma (may see positive antineutrophil antibodies).

TREATMENT ▶ **The Febrile, Neutropenic Patient**

(See Chap. 26) In addition to usual sources of infection, consider paranasal sinuses, oral cavity (including teeth and gums), anorectal region; empirical therapy with broad-spectrum antibiotics (e.g., ceftazidime) is indicated after blood and other appropriate cultures are obtained. Prolonged febrile neutropenia (>7 days) leads to increased risk of dis seminated fungal infections; requires addition of antifungal chemotherapy (e.g., amphotericin B). The duration of chemotherapy-induced neutropenia may be shortened by a few days by treatment with the cytokines GM-CSF or G-CSF.

■ **LYMPHOPENIA**

Absolute lymphocyte count <1000/μL.

Causes

(1) *Acute stressful illness*—e.g., myocardial infarction, pneumonia, sepsis; (2) *glucocorticoid therapy*; (3) *lymphoma* (esp. Hodgkin's disease); (4) *immunodeficiency syndromes*—ataxia telangiectasia and Wiskott-Aldrich and DiGeorge syndromes; (5) *immunosuppressive therapy*—e.g., antilymphocyte globulin, cyclophosphamide; (6) *large-field radiation therapy* (esp. for lymphoma); (7) *intestinal lymphangiectasia* (increased lymphocyte loss); (8) *chronic illness*—e.g., congestive heart failure, uremia, SLE, disseminated malignancies; (9) *bone marrow failure/replacement*—e.g., aplastic anemia, miliary tuberculosis.

■ **MONOCYTOPENIA**

Absolute monocyte count <100/μL.

Causes

(1) *Acute stressful illness*, (2) *glucocorticoid therapy*, (3) *aplastic anemia*, (4) *leukemia* (certain types, e.g., hairy cell leukemia), (5) *chemotherapeutic and immunosuppressive agents*.

■ **EOSINOPENIA**

Absolute eosinophil count <50/μL.

Causes

(1) *Acute stressful illness*, (2) *glucocorticoid therapy*.

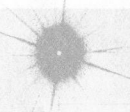 For a more detailed discussion, see Holland SM, Gallin JI: Disorders of Granulocytes and Monocytes, Chap. 60, p. 472; in HPIM-18.

CHAPTER **70**
Bleeding and Thrombotic Disorders

BLEEDING DISORDERS

Bleeding may result from abnormalities of (1) platelets, (2) blood vessel walls, or (3) coagulation. Platelet disorders characteristically produce petechial and purpuric skin lesions and bleeding from mucosal surfaces. Defective coagulation results in ecchymoses, hematomas, and mucosal and, in some disorders, recurrent joint bleeding (hemarthroses).

■ PLATELET DISORDERS

Thrombocytopenia

Normal platelet count is 150,000–350,000/μL. Thrombocytopenia is defined as a platelet count <100,000/μL. Bleeding time, a measurement of platelet function, is abnormally increased if platelet count <100,000/μL; injury or surgery may provoke excess bleeding. Spontaneous bleeding is unusual unless count <20,000/μL; platelet count <10,000/μL is often associated with serious hemorrhage. Bone marrow examination shows increased number of megakaryocytes in disorders associated with accelerated platelet destruction; decreased number in disorders of platelet production. Evaluation of thrombocytopenia is shown in Fig. 70-1.

Causes

(1) Production defects such as marrow injury (e.g., drugs, irradiation), marrow failure (e.g., aplastic anemia), marrow invasion (e.g., carcinoma, leukemia, fibrosis); (2) sequestration due to splenomegaly; (3) accelerated destruction—causes include:

- *Drugs* such as chemotherapeutic agents, thiazides, ethanol, estrogens, sulfonamides, quinidine, quinine, methyldopa.
- *Heparin-induced thrombocytopenia* is seen in 5% of pts receiving >5 days of therapy and is due to in vivo platelet aggregation often from anti–platelet

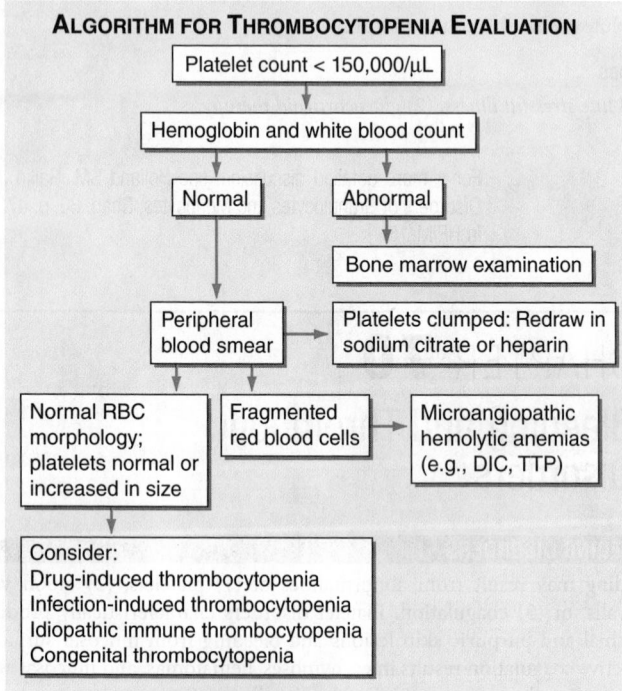

FIGURE 70-1 Algorithm for evaluating the thrombocytopenic pt.

factor 4 antibodies. Arterial and occasionally venous thromboses may result. Despite the low platelets, HIT is a hypercoagulable state.

- *Autoimmune destruction* by an antibody mechanism; may be idiopathic or associated with systemic lupus erythematosus (SLE), lymphoma, HIV.
- *Idiopathic thrombocytopenic purpura* (ITP) has two forms: an acute, self-limited disorder of childhood requiring no specific therapy, and a chronic disorder of adults (esp. women 20–40 years). Chronic ITP may be due to autoantibodies to glycoprotein IIb-IIIa or glycoprotein Ib-IX complexes.
- *Disseminated intravascular coagulation* (DIC)—platelet consumption with coagulation factor depletion [prolonged prothrombin time (PT), partial thromboplastin time (PTT)] and stimulation of fibrinolysis [generation of fibrin split products (FSPs)]. Blood smear shows microangiopathic hemolysis (schistocytes). Causes include infection (esp. meningococcal, pneumococcal, gram-negative bacteremias), extensive burns, trauma, or thrombosis; giant hemangioma, retained dead fetus, heat stroke, mismatched blood transfusion, metastatic carcinoma, acute promyelocytic leukemia.
- *Thrombotic thrombocytopenic purpura* (TTP)—rare disorder characterized by microangiopathic hemolytic anemia, fever, thrombocytopenia, renal dysfunction (and/or hematuria), and neurologic dysfunction caused by failure to cleave von Willebrand factor (vWF) normally.
- *Hemorrhage with extensive transfusion.*

Pseudothrombocytopenia

Platelet clumping secondary to collection of blood in EDTA (0.3% of pts). Examination of blood smear establishes diagnosis.

Thrombocytosis

Platelet count >350,000/μL. Either primary (essential thrombocytosis; Chap. 72) or secondary (reactive); latter secondary to severe hemorrhage, iron deficiency, surgery, after splenectomy (transient), malignant neoplasms (esp. Hodgkin's disease, polycythemia vera), chronic inflammatory diseases (e.g., inflammatory bowel disease), recovery from acute infection, vitamin B_{12} deficiency, drugs (e.g., vincristine, epinephrine). Rebound thrombocytosis may occur after marrow recovery from cytotoxic agents, alcohol, vitamin B_{12} replenishment. Primary thrombocytosis may be complicated by bleeding and/or thrombosis; secondary rarely causes hemostatic problems.

Disorders of Platelet Function

Suggested by the finding of prolonged bleeding time with normal platelet count. Defect is in platelet adhesion, aggregation, or granule release. Causes include (1) drugs—aspirin, other nonsteroidal anti-inflammatory drugs, dipyridamole, clopidogrel or prasugrel, heparin, penicillins, esp. carbenicillin, ticarcillin; (2) uremia; (3) cirrhosis; (4) dysproteinemias; (5) myeloproliferative and myelodysplastic disorders; (6) von Willebrand disease (vWD; see below); (7) cardiopulmonary bypass.

■ HEMOSTATIC DISORDERS DUE TO BLOOD VESSEL WALL DEFECTS

Causes include (1) aging; (2) drugs—e.g., glucocorticoids (chronic therapy), penicillins, sulfonamides; (3) vitamin C deficiency; (4) TTP; (5) hemolytic uremic syndrome; (6) Henoch-Schönlein purpura; (7) paraproteinemias; (8) hereditary hemorrhagic telangiectasia (Osler-Weber-Rendu disease).

■ DISORDERS OF BLOOD COAGULATION

Congenital Disorders

1. *Hemophilia A*—incidence 1:5000; sex-linked recessive deficiency of factor VIII (low plasma factor VIII coagulant activity, but normal amount of factor VIII–related antigen—vWF). Laboratory features: elevated PTT, normal PT.

2. *Hemophilia B* (Christmas disease)—incidence 1:30,000, sex-linked recessive, due to factor IX deficiency. Clinical and laboratory features similar to hemophilia A.

3. *von Willebrand disease*—most common inherited coagulation disorder (1:800–1000), usually autosomal dominant; primary defect is reduced synthesis or chemically abnormal factor VIII–related antigen produced by platelets and endothelium, resulting in abnormal platelet function.

Acquired Disorders

1. *Vitamin K deficiency*—impairs production of factors II (prothrombin), VII, IX, and X; vitamin K is a cofactor in the carboxylation of glutamate residues on prothrombin complex proteins; major source of vitamin K is dietary (esp. green vegetables), with minor production by gut bacteria. Laboratory features: elevated PT and PTT.

2. *Liver disease*—results in deficiencies of all clotting factors except VIII. Laboratory features: elevated PT, normal or elevated PTT.

3. *Other disorders*—DIC, fibrinogen deficiency (liver disease, L-asparaginase therapy, rattlesnake bites), other factor deficiencies, circulating anticoagulants (lymphoma, SLE, idiopathic), massive transfusion (dilutional coagulopathy).

TREATMENT   **Bleeding Disorders**

THROMBOCYTOPENIA CAUSED BY DRUGS Discontinue use of possible offending agents; expect recovery in 7–10 days. Platelet transfusions may be needed if platelet count <10,000/μL.

HEPARIN-INDUCED THROMBOCYTOPENIA Discontinue heparin promptly. A direct thrombin inhibitor such as lepirudin (0.4-mg/kg bolus, 0.15-mg/kg per hour infusion; PTT target 1.5–2.5 × baseline) or argatroban (2-μg/kg per min infusion; PTT target 1.5–3 × baseline) should be used for treatment of thromboses. Do not use low-molecular-weight heparin (LMWH), as antibodies often cross-react.

CHRONIC ITP Prednisone, initially 1–2 mg/kg per day, then slow taper to keep the platelet count >60,000/μL. IV immunoglobulin (2 g/kg in divided doses over 2–5 days) to block phagocytic destruction may be useful. Rituximab is effective in pts refractory to glucocorticoids. Eltrombopag (50 mg PO qd) boosts platelet production and allows delay or avoidance of splenectomy. Splenectomy, danazol (androgen), or other agents (e.g., vincristine, cyclophosphamide, fludarabine) are indicated for refractory pts or those requiring >5–10 mg prednisone daily.

DIC Control of underlying disease most important; platelets, fresh-frozen plasma (FFP) to correct clotting parameters. Heparin may be beneficial in pts with acute promyelocytic leukemia.

TTP Plasmapheresis and FFP infusions (plasma exchange), possibly IV IgG; recovery in two-thirds of cases. Plasmapheresis removes inhibitors of the vWF cleavage enzyme (ADAMTS13), and FFP replaces the enzyme.

DISORDERS OF PLATELET FUNCTION Remove or reverse underlying cause. Dialysis and/or cryoprecipitate infusions (10 bags/24 h) may be helpful for platelet dysfunction associated with uremia.

HEMOSTATIC DISORDERS Withdraw offending drugs, replace vitamin C, plasmapheresis, and plasma infusion for TTP.

HEMOPHILIA A Factor VIII replacement for bleeding or before surgical procedure; degree and duration of replacement depends on severity of bleeding. Give factor VIII (e.g., Recombinate) to obtain a 15% (for mild bleeding) to 50% (for severe bleeding) factor VIII level. The duration should range from a single dose of factor VIII to therapy bid for up to 2 weeks. Dose is calculated as follows:

Factor VIII dose = (Target level – baseline level) × weight (kg) × 0.5 unit/kg

Up to 30% of pts may develop anti–factor VIII antibodies; activated factor VII or factor eight inhibitor bypass agent (FEIBA) may stop or prevent bleeding in these pts.

HEMOPHILIA B Recombinant factor IX (e.g., Benefix), FFP or factor IX concentrates (e.g., Proplex, Konyne). Because of the longer half-life, once-daily treatment is sufficient. Dose is calculated as follows:

Factor IX dose = (Target level – baseline level) × weight (kg) × 1 unit/kg

VON WILLEBRAND DISEASE Desmopressin (1-deamino-8-D-arginine vasopressin) increases release of vWF from endothelial stores in type 1 vWD. It is given IV (0.3 µg/kg) or by nasal spray (2 squirts of 1.5-mg/mL fluid in each nostril). For types 2A, 2M, and 3, cryopre-cipitate (plasma product rich in factor VIII) or factor VIII concentrate (Humate-P, Koate HS) is used: up to 10 bags bid for 48–72 h, depending on the severity of bleeding.

VITAMIN K DEFICIENCY Vitamin K, 10 mg SC or slow IV.

LIVER DISEASE Fresh-frozen plasma.

THROMBOTIC DISORDERS

■ HYPERCOAGULABLE STATE

Consider in pts with recurrent episodes of venous thrombosis [i.e., deep-vein thrombosis (DVT), pulmonary embolism (PE)]. Causes include (1) venous stasis (e.g., pregnancy, immobilization); (2) vasculitis; (3) cancer and myeloproliferative disorders; (4) oral contraceptives; (5) lupus anti-coagulant—antibody to platelet phospholipid, stimulates coagulation;

(6) heparin-induced thrombocytopenia; (7) deficiencies of endogenous anticoagulant factors—antithrombin III, protein C, protein S; (8) factor V Leiden—mutation in factor V (Arg → Glu at position 506) confers resistance to inactivation by protein C, accounts for 25% of cases of recurrent thrombosis; (9) prothrombin gene mutation—Glu → Arg at position 20210 results in increased prothrombin levels; accounts for about 6% of thromboses; (10) other—paroxysmal nocturnal hemoglobinuria, dysfibrinogenemias (abnormal fibrinogen).

The approach to the diagnosis of the pt with DVT and/or PE is discussed in Chap. 142.

TREATMENT　Thrombotic Disorders

Correct underlying disorder whenever possible; long-term warfarin therapy is otherwise indicated.

ANTICOAGULANT AGENTS

1. *Heparin* (Table 70-1)—enhances activity of antithrombin III; parenteral agent of choice. LMWH is the preparation of choice (enoxaparin or dalteparin). It can be administered SC, monitoring of the PTT is unnecessary, and it is less likely to induce antibodies and thrombocytopenia. The usual dose is 100 U/kg SC bid. Unfractionated heparin should be given only if LMWH is unavailable. In adults, the dose of unfractionated heparin is 25,000–40,000 U continuous IV infusion over 24 h following initial IV bolus of 5000 U; monitor by following PTT; should be maintained between 1.5 and 2 times upper normal limit. Prophylactic anticoagulation to lower risk of venous thrombosis recommended in some pts (e.g., postoperative, immobilized) (Table 70-1). Prophylactic doses of unfractionated heparin are 5000 U SC bid or tid. Major complication of unfractionated heparin therapy is hemorrhage—manage by discontinuing heparin; for severe bleeding, administer protamine (1 mg/100 U heparin); results in rapid neutralization.

2. *Warfarin* (Coumadin)—vitamin K antagonist, decreases levels of factors II, VII, IX, X, and anticoagulant proteins C and S. Administered over 2–3 days; initial load of 5–10 mg PO qd followed by titration of daily dose to keep PT 1.5–2 times control PT or 2–3 times if the International Normalized Ratio (INR) method is used. Complications include hemorrhage, warfarin-induced skin necrosis (rare, occurs in persons deficient in protein C), teratogenic effects. Warfarin effect reversed by administration of vitamin K; FFP infused if urgent reversal necessary. Numerous drugs potentiate or antagonize warfarin effect. Potentiating agents include chlorpromazine, chloral hydrate, sulfonamides, chloramphenicol, other broad-spectrum antibiotics, allopurinol, cimetidine, tricyclic antidepressants, disulfiram, laxatives, high-dose salicylates, thyroxine, clofibrate. Some pts who are sensitive to warfarin effects have genetic defects metabolizing the drug. Antagonizing agents include vitamin K, barbiturates, rifampin, cholestyramine, oral contraceptives, thiazides.

TABLE 70-1 ANTICOAGULANT THERAPY WITH LOW-MOLECULAR-WEIGHT AND UNFRACTIONATED HEPARIN

Clinical Indication	Heparin Dose and Schedule	Target PTT[a]	LMWH Dose and Schedule[b]
Venous thrombosis pulmonary embolism			
Treatment	5000 U IV bolus; 1000–1500 U/h	2–2.5	100 U/kg SC bid
Prophylaxis	5000 U SC q8–12h	<1.5	100 U/kg SC bid
Acute myocardial infarction			
With thrombolytic therapy	5000 U IV bolus; 1000 U/h	1.5–2.5	100 U/kg SC bid
With mural thrombus	8000 U SC q8h + warfarin	1.5–2.0	100 U/kg SC bid
Unstable angina	5000 U IV bolus; 1000 U/h	1.5–2.5	100 U/kg SC bid
Prophylaxis			
General surgery	5000 U SC bid	<1.5	100 U/kg SC before and bid
Orthopedic surgery	10,000 U SC bid	1.5	100 U/kg SC before and bid
Medical pts with CHF, MI	10,000 U SC bid	1.5	100 U/kg SC bid

[a]Times normal control; assumes PTT has been standardized to heparin levels so that 1.5–2.5 × normal equals 0.2–0.4 U/mL; if PTT is normal (27–35 s), start with 5000 U bolus 1300 U/h infusion monitoring PTT; if PTT at recheck is <50 s, rebolus with 5000 U and increase infusion by 100 U/h; if PTT at recheck is 50–60 s, increase infusion rate by 100 U/h; if PTT at recheck is 60–85 s, no change; if PTT at recheck is 85–100 s, decrease infusion rate 100 U/h; if PTT at recheck is 100–120 s, stop infusion for 30 min and decrease rate 100 U/h at restart; if PTT at recheck is >120 s, stop infusion for 60 min and decrease rate 200 U/h at restart.
[b]LMWH does not affect PTT, and PTT is not used to adjust dosage.
Abbreviations: CHF, congestive heart failure; LMWH, low-molecular-weight heparin; MI, myocardial infarction; PTT, partial thromboplastin time.

3. *Fondaparinux*—a pentapeptide that directly inhibits factor Xa. It is given at a dose of 2.5 mg SC daily for prophylaxis and 7.5 mg SC daily for treatment of thrombosis and does not require monitoring. Unlike the heparins, it does not bind to platelet factor 4 and does not elicit the antibodies that produce heparin-induced thrombocytopenia. *Apixaban* and *rivaroxaban* are oral factor Xa inhibitors. Apixaban (5 mg PO bid) as effective as warfarin in DVT and more effective in stroke prevention in atrial fibrillation (AF).

4. *Argatroban and lepirudin*—direct thrombin inhibitors. These agents are being compared to LMWH and are commonly used in pts with heparin-induced thrombocytopenia. Both are monitored with the activated PTT. *Dabigatran* (150 mg PO bid) is an oral thrombin inhibitor and is non-inferior to warfarin in both DVT and stroke prevention in AF.

In-hospital anticoagulation is usually initiated with heparin for 4–10 days, with subsequent maintenance on warfarin after an overlap of 3 days. Duration of therapy depends on underlying condition; calf DVT with clear precipitating cause, 3 months; proximal or idiopathic DVT or PE, 6–12 months; recurrent idiopathic DVT, 12 months minimum; embolic disease with ongoing risk factor, long-term, indefinite. The new oral Xa and thrombin inhibitors are easier to use than warfarin but much more expensive.

FIBRINOLYTIC AGENTS Tissue plasminogen activators mediate clot lysis by activating plasmin, which degrades fibrin. Currently available versions include streptokinase, urokinase, anistreplase (acylated plasminogen streptokinase activator complex), and three modestly distinct forms of recombinant tissue plasminogen activator (tPA): alteplase, tenecteplase, and reteplase. Indications include treatment of DVT, with lower incidence of postphlebitic syndrome (chronic venous stasis, skin ulceration) than with heparin therapy; massive PE, arterial embolic occlusion of an extremity, treatment of acute myocardial infarction (MI), unstable angina pectoris. Dosages for fibrinolytic agents: (1) tPA—for acute MI and massive PE (adult >65 kg), 10-mg IV bolus over 1–2 min, then 50 mg IV over 1 h and 40 mg IV over next 2 h (total dose = 100 mg). tPA is slightly more effective but more expensive than streptokinase for treatment of acute MI. (2) Streptokinase—for acute MI, 1.5 million IU IV over 60 min; or 20,000 IU as a bolus intracoronary (IC) infusion, followed by 2000 IU/min for 60 min IC. For PE or arterial or deep-vein thrombosis, 250,000 IU over 30 min, then 100,000 IU/h for 24 h (PE) or 72 h (arterial or deep-vein thrombosis). (3) Urokinase—for PE, 4400 IU/kg IV over 10 min, then 4400 (IU/kg)/h IV for 12 h.

Fibrinolytic therapy is usually followed by a period of anticoagulant therapy with heparin. Fibrinolytic agents are contraindicated in pts with (1) active internal bleeding; (2) recent (<2–3 months) cerebrovascular accident; (3) intracranial neoplasm, aneurysm, or recent head trauma.

ANTIPLATELET AGENTS Aspirin inhibits platelet function by blocking the ability of cyclooxygenase (COX-1) to synthesize thromboxane A2. The thienopyridines (ticlopidine and clopidogrel) inhibit ADP-induced platelet aggregation by blocking its receptor ($P2Y_{12}$). Dipyridamole acts by inhibiting phosphodiesterase, which permits cAMP levels to increase and block activation. Glycoprotein IIb/IIIa (GPIIb/IIIa) antagonists block the integrin receptors on the platelet and prevent platelet aggregation. Three such agents are now in use: abciximab, an Fab antibody fragment that binds to the activated form of GPIIb/IIIa; eptifibatide, a cyclic heptapeptide that includes the KGD tripeptide motif that the GPIIb/IIIa receptor recognizes; and tirofiban, a tyrosine derivative that mimics the KGD motif.

Aspirin (160–325 mg/d) plus clopidogrel (400-mg loading dose then 75 mg/d) may be beneficial in lowering incidence of arterial thrombotic events (stroke, MI) in high-risk pts. Antiplatelet agents are useful in preventing strokes, complications from percutaneous coronary interventions, and progression of unstable angina.

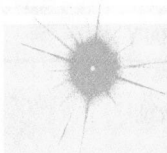

For a more detailed discussion, see Konkle BA: Bleeding and Thrombosis, Chap. 58, p. 457; Konkle BA: Disorders of Platelets and Vessel Wall, Chap. 115, p. 965; Arruda VR, High KA: Coagulation Disorders, Chap. 116, p. 973; Freedman JE, Loscalzo J: Arterial and Venous Thrombosis, Chap. 117, p. 983; and Weitz JI: Antiplatelet, Anticoagulant, and Fibrinolytic Drugs, Chap. 118, p. 988, in HPIM-18.

CHAPTER **71**
Cancer Chemotherapy

■ BIOLOGY OF TUMOR GROWTH

Two essential features of cancer cells are uncontrolled growth and the ability to metastasize. The malignant phenotype of a cell is the end result of a series of genetic changes that remove safeguards restricting cell growth and induce new features that enable the cell to metastasize, including surface receptors for binding to basement membranes, enzymes to poke holes in anatomic barriers, cytokines to facilitate mobility, and angiogenic factors to develop a new vascular lifeline for nutrients and oxygen. These genetic changes usually involve increased or abnormal expression or activity of certain genes known as *proto-oncogenes* (often growth factors or their receptors, enzymes in growth pathways, or transcription factors), deletion or inactivation of tumor-suppressor genes, and defects in DNA repair enzymes. These genetic changes may occur by point mutation, gene amplification, gene rearrangement, or epigenetic changes such as altered gene methylation.

Once cells are malignant, their growth kinetics are similar to those of normal cells but lack regulation. For unclear reasons, tumor growth kinetics follow a Gompertzian curve: as the tumor mass increases, the fraction of dividing cells declines. Thus, by the time a cancer is large enough to be detected clinically, its growth fraction is often small. Unfortunately, tumor growth usually does not stop altogether before the tumor reaches a lethal tumor burden. Cancer cells proceed through the same cell-cycle stages as normal cycling cells: G_1 (period of preparation for DNA synthesis), S (DNA synthesis), G_2 (tetraploid phase preceding mitosis in which integrity of DNA replication is assessed), and M (mitosis). Some noncycling cells may remain in a G_0, or resting, phase for long periods. Certain chemotherapeutic agents are specific for cells in certain phases of the cell cycle.

■ DEVELOPMENT OF DRUG RESISTANCE

Drug resistance can be divided into de novo resistance or acquired resistance. De novo resistance refers to the tendency of many of the most common solid tumors to be unresponsive to chemotherapeutic agents. In acquired resistance, tumors initially responsive to chemotherapy develop

TABLE 71-1 CURABILITY OF CANCERS WITH CHEMOTHERAPY

A. Advanced Cancers with Possible Cure

Acute lymphoid and acute myeloid leukemia (pediatric/adult)

Hodgkin's disease (pediatric/adult)

Lymphomas—certain types (pediatric/adult)

Germ cell neoplasms

    Embryonal carcinoma

    Teratocarcinoma

    Seminoma or dysgerminoma

    Choriocarcinoma

Gestational trophoblastic neoplasia

Pediatric neoplasms

    Wilms' tumor

    Embryonal rhabdomyosarcoma

    Ewing's sarcoma

    Peripheral neuroepithelioma

    Neuroblastoma

Small cell lung carcinoma

Ovarian carcinoma

B. Advanced Cancers Possibly Cured by Chemotherapy and Radiation

Squamous carcinoma (head and neck)

Squamous carcinoma (anus)

Breast carcinoma

Carcinoma of the uterine cervix

Non-small cell lung carcinoma (stage III)

Small cell lung carcinoma

C. Cancers Possibly Cured with Chemotherapy as Adjuvant to Surgery

Breast carcinoma

Colorectal carcinoma[a]

Osteogenic sarcoma

Soft tissue sarcoma

D. Cancers Possibly Cured with "High-Dose" Chemotherapy with Stem Cell Support

Relapsed leukemias, lymphoid and myeloid

Relapsed lymphomas, Hodgkin's and non-Hodgkin's

Chronic myeloid leukemia

Multiple myeloma

E. Cancers Responsive to Chemotherapy with Useful Palliation But Not Cure

Bladder carcinoma

TABLE 71-1 CURABILITY OF CANCERS WITH CHEMOTHERAPY (CONTINUED)

Chronic myeloid leukemia

Hairy cell leukemia

Chronic lymphocytic leukemia

Lymphoma—certain types

Multiple myeloma

Gastric carcinoma

Cervix carcinoma

Endometrial carcinoma

Soft tissue sarcoma

Head and neck cancer

Adrenocortical carcinoma

Islet-cell neoplasms

Breast carcinoma

Colorectal carcinoma

Renal carcinoma

F. Tumor Poorly Responsive in Advanced Stages to Chemotherapy

Pancreatic carcinoma

Biliary-tract neoplasms

Thyroid carcinoma

Carcinoma of the vulva

Non-small cell lung carcinoma

Prostate carcinoma

Melanoma

Hepatocellular carcinoma

Salivary gland cancer

*a*Rectum also receives radiation therapy.

resistance during treatment, usually because resistant clones appear within tumor cell populations (Table 71-1).

Resistance can be specific to single drugs because of (1) defective transport of the drug, (2) decreased activating enzymes, (3) increased drug inactivation, (4) increases in target enzyme levels, or (5) alterations in target molecules. Multiple drug resistance occurs in cells overexpressing the P glycoprotein, a membrane glycoprotein responsible for enhanced efflux of drugs from cells, but there are other mechanisms as well.

■ CATEGORIES OF CHEMOTHERAPEUTIC AGENTS AND MAJOR TOXICITIES

A partial list of toxicities is shown in Table 71-2; some toxicities may apply only to certain members of a group of drugs.

TABLE 71-2 TOXICITIES OF CANCER TREATMENTS

Agent	Toxicities
Alkylating agents	
(add alkyl groups to N-7 or O-6 of guanine)	
Busulfan	Nausea, vomiting, myelosuppression, sterility, alopecia, acute leukemia (rare), hemorrhagic cystitis, pulmonary fibrosis
Chlorambucil	
Cyclophosphamide	
Ifosfamide	
Dacarbazine	
Mechlorethamine	
Nitrosoureas	
Melphalan	
Bendamustine	
Antimetabolites	
(inhibit DNA or RNA synthesis)	
5-Fluorouracil	Nausea, vomiting, myelosuppression, oral ulceration, hepatic toxicity, alopecia, neurologic symptoms
Capecitabine	
Fludarabine	
Cladribine	
Cytarabine	
Methotrexate	
Pemetrexed	
Hydroxyurea	
Pentostatin	
Azathioprine	
Thioguanine	
Tubulin poisons	
(block tubule polymerization or depolymerization)	
Vincristine	Nausea, vomiting, myelosuppression, vesicant effect, ileus, hypersensitivity reaction, peripheral neuropathy, SIADH
Vinblastine	
Vinorelbine	
Paclitaxel	
Docetaxel	
Cabazitaxel	
Nab-paclitaxel	
Estramustine	
Ixabepilone	

TABLE 71-2 TOXICITIES OF CANCER TREATMENTS (CONTINUED)

Agent	Toxicities
Topoisomerase inhibitors	
(interfere with DNA unwinding/repair)	
Doxorubicin	Nausea, vomiting, myelosuppression, vesicant effect, cardiac failure, acute leukemia (rare)
Daunorubicin	
Idarubicin	
Epirubicin	
Etoposide	
Irinotecan	
Topotecan	
Mitoxantrone	
Platinum compounds	
(form DNA adducts, disrupt repair)	
Cisplatin	Nausea, vomiting, myelosuppression, renal toxicity, neurotoxicity
Carboplatin	
Oxaliplatin	
Antibiotics	
(diverse mechanisms)	
Bleomycin	Nausea, vomiting, myelosuppression, cardiac toxicity, lung fibrosis, hypocalcemia, hypersensitivity reaction
Dactinomycin	
Mithramycin	
Mitomycin	
Histone deacetylase inhibitors	
Vorinostat	
Romidepsin	
Hormone and nuclear receptor targeting agents	
Tamoxifen	Nausea, vomiting, hot flashes, gynecomastia, impotence
Raloxifene	
Anastrozole	
Letrozole	
Exemestane	
Tretinoin	
Bexarotene	
Flutamide	
Leuprolide	
Diethylstilbestrol	
Medroxyprogesterone	

(continued)

TABLE 71-2 TOXICITIES OF CANCER TREATMENTS (CONTINUED)

Agent	Toxicities
Biologic agents	
Interferon	Nausea, vomiting, fever, chills, vascular leak, respiratory distress, skin rashes, edema
Interleukin 2	
Rituximab	
Trastuzumab	
Cetuximab	
Panitumomab	
Bevacizumab	
Brentuximab vedotin	
Gemtuzumab ozogamicin	
Denileukin diftitox	
Bortezomib	
Imatinib	
Dasatinib	
Nilotinib	
Gefitinib	
Erlotinib	
Sorafenib	
Sunitinib	
Everolimus	
Temsirolimus	
Radiation therapy	
External beam (teletherapy)	Nausea, vomiting, myelosuppression, tissue damage, late second cancers, heart disease, sterility
Internal implants (brachytherapy)	
Ibritumomab tiuxetan	
Iodine-135 Tositumomab	
Samarium-153 EDTMP	
Strontium-89	

Abbreviation: SIADH, syndrome of inappropriate antidiuretic hormone secretion.

■ COMPLICATIONS OF THERAPY

While the effects of cancer chemotherapeutic agents may be exerted primarily on the malignant cell population, virtually all currently employed regimens have profound effects on normal tissues as well. Every side effect of treatment must be balanced against potential benefits expected, and pts must always be fully apprised of the toxicities they may encounter. While the duration of certain adverse effects may be short-lived, others, such as sterility and the risk of secondary malignancy, have long-term implications; consideration of these effects is important in the use of regimens as adjuvant therapy. The combined toxicity of regimens involving radiotherapy and chemotherapy is greater than that seen with each modality alone. Teratogenesis is a special concern in treating women of childbearing years with radiation or chemotherapy. The most serious late toxicities are sterility (common; from alkylating agents), secondary acute leukemia (rare; from alkylating agents and topoisomerase inhibitors), secondary solid tumors (0.5–1%/year risk for at least 25 years after treatment; from radiation therapy), premature atherosclerosis (3-fold increased risk of fatal myocardial infarction; from radiation therapy that includes the heart), heart failure (rare; from anthracyclines, trastuzumab), and pulmonary fibrosis (rare; from bleomycin).

■ MANAGEMENT OF ACUTE TOXICITIES

Nausea and Vomiting

Mildly to moderately emetogenic agents—prochlorperazine, 5–10 mg PO or 25 mg PR before chemotherapy; effects are enhanced by also administering dexamethasone, 10–20 mg IV. Highly emetogenic agents (such as cisplatin, mechlorethamine, dacarbazine, streptozocin)—ondansetron, 8 mg PO q6h the day before chemotherapy and IV at time of chemotherapy, plus dexamethasone, 20 mg IV at time of chemotherapy. Aprepitant (125 mg PO day 1, 80 mg PO days 2, 3 with or without dexamethasone 8 mg), a substance P/neurokinin 1 receptor blocker, decreases the risk of acute and delayed vomiting from cisplatin.

Neutropenia

Colony-stimulating factors are often used where they have been shown to have little or no benefit. Specific indications for the use of granulocyte colony-stimulating factor or granulocyte-macrophage colony-stimulating factor are provided in Table 71-3.

Anemia

Quality of life is improved by maintaining Hb levels >90 g/L (9 g/dL). This is routinely done with packed red blood cell transfusions. Erythropoietin has the capacity to protect hypoxic cells from dying; its use has resulted in poorer tumor control and is generally discouraged.

Thrombocytopenia

Rarely, treatment may induce a decline in platelet counts. Platelet transfusions are generally triggered at a platelet count of 10,000/μL in pts with solid tumors and at a platelet count of 20,000/μL in pts with acute leukemia. Newer oral thrombopoietin mimetics (e.g., eltrombopag) are promising but have not been widely tested in the setting of cancer chemotherapy.

TABLE 71-3 INDICATIONS FOR THE CLINICAL USE OF G-CSF OR GM-CSF

Preventive uses

With the first cycle of chemotherapy (so-called primary CSF administration)

    Not needed on a routine basis

    Use if the probability of febrile neutropenia is ≥20%

    Use if pt has preexisting neutropenia or active infection

    Age >65 years treated for lymphoma with curative intent or other tumor treated by similar regimens

    Poor performance status

    Extensive prior chemotherapy

    Dose-dense regimens in a clinical trial or with strong evidence of benefit

With subsequent cycles if febrile neutropenia has previously occurred (so-called secondary CSF administration)

    Not needed after short-duration neutropenia without fever

    Use if pt had febrile neutropenia in previous cycle

    Use if prolonged neutropenia (even without fever) delays therapy

Therapeutic uses

Afebrile neutropenic pts

    No evidence of benefit

Febrile neutropenic pts

    No evidence of benefit

    May feel compelled to use in the face of clinical deterioration from sepsis, pneumonia, or fungal infection, but benefit unclear

In bone marrow or peripheral blood stem cell transplantation

    Use to mobilize stem cells from marrow

    Use to hasten myeloid recovery

In acute myeloid leukemia

    G-CSF of minor or no benefit

    GM-CSF of no benefit and may be harmful

In myelodysplastic syndromes

    Not routinely beneficial

    Use intermittently in subset with neutropenia and recurrent infection

What dose and schedule should be used?

G-CSF: 5 mg/kg per day subcutaneously

GM-CSF: 250 mg/m² per day subcutaneously

Peg-filgrastim: one dose of 6 mg 24 h after chemotherapy

When should therapy begin and end?

When indicated, start 24–72 h after chemotherapy

TABLE 71-3 INDICATIONS FOR THE CLINICAL USE OF G-CSF OR GM-CSF (CONTINUED)

Continue until absolute neutrophil count is 10,000/μL

Do not use concurrently with chemotherapy or radiation therapy

Abbreviations: G-CSF, granulocyte colony-stimulating factor; GM-CSF, granulocyte-macrophage colony-stimulating factor.
Source: From the American Society of Clinical Oncology.

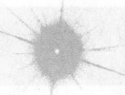

For a more detailed discussion, see Sausville EA, Longo DL: Principles of Cancer Treatment, Chap. 85, p. 689, in HPIM-18.

CHAPTER 72
Myeloid Leukemias, Myelodysplasia, and Myeloproliferative Syndromes

ACUTE MYELOID LEUKEMIA (AML)

AML is a clonal malignancy of myeloid bone marrow precursors in which poorly differentiated cells accumulate in the bone marrow and circulation.

Signs and symptoms occur because of the absence of mature cells normally produced by the bone marrow, including granulocytes (susceptibility to infection) and platelets (susceptibility to bleeding). In addition, if large numbers of immature malignant myeloblasts circulate, they may invade organs and rarely produce dysfunction. There are distinct morphologic subtypes (Table 72-1) that have largely overlapping clinical features. Of note is the propensity of pts with acute promyelocytic leukemia (APL) (FAB M3) to develop bleeding and disseminated intravascular coagulation, especially during induction chemotherapy, because of the release of procoagulants from their cytoplasmic granules.

Incidence and Etiology

In the United States about 13,780 cases have occurred in 2012. AML accounts for about 80% of acute leukemias in adults. Etiology is unknown for the vast majority. Three environmental exposures increase the risk: chronic benzene exposure, radiation exposure, and prior treatment with alkylating agents (especially in addition to radiation therapy) and topoisomerase II inhibitors (e.g., doxorubicin and etoposide). Chronic myeloid leukemia (CML), myelodysplasia, and myeloproliferative syndromes may all evolve into AML. Certain genetic abnormalities are associated with particular morphologic variants: t(15;17) with APL, inv(16) with eosinophilic leukemia; others occur in a number of types. Chromosome 11q23 abnormalities are often

TABLE 72-1 AML CLASSIFICATION SYSTEMS

World Health Organization Classification[a]
AML with recurrent genetic abnormalities
AML with t(8;21)(q22;q22);*RUNX1-RUNX1T1*[b]
AML with inv(16)(p13.1;1q22) or t(16;16)(p13.1;q22);*CBFB-MYH11*[b]
Acute promyelocytic leukemia with t(15;17)(q22;q12); *PML-RARA*[b]
AML with t(9;11)(p22;q23); *MLLT3-MLL*
AML with t(6;9)(p23;q34); *DEK-NUP214*
AML with inv(3)(q21q26.2) or t(3;3)(q21;q26.2); *RPN1-EVI1*
AML (megakaryoblastic) with t(1;22)(p13;q13); *RBM15-MKL1*
Provisional entity: AML with mutated NPM1
Provisional entity: AML with mutated CEBPA
AML with myelodysplasia-related changes
Therapy-related myeloid neoplasms
AML not otherwise specified
AML with minimal differentiation
AML without maturation
AML with maturation
Acute myelomonocytic leukemia
Acute monoblastic and monocytic leukemia
Acute erythroid leukemia
Acute megakaryoblastic leukemia
Acute basophilic leukemia
Acute panmyelosis with myelofibrosis
Myeloid sarcoma
Myeloid proliferations related to Down syndrome
Transient abnormal myelopoiesis
Myeloid leukemia associated with Down syndrome
Blastic plasmacytoid dendritic cell neoplasm
Acute leukemia of ambiguous lineage
Acute undifferentiated leukemia
Mixed phenotype acute leukemia with t(9;22)(q34;q11,20); *BCR-ABL11*
Mixed phenotype acute leukemia with t(v;11q23); *MLL* rearranged
Mixed phenotype acute leukemia, B/myeloid, NOS
Mixed phenotype acute leukemia, T/myeloid, NOS
Provisional entity: Natural killer (NK)-cell lymphoblastic leukemia/lymphoma
French-American-British (FAB) Classification[c]
MO: Minimally differentiated leukemia
MI: Myeloblastic leukemia without maturation

TABLE 72-1 AML CLASSIFICATION SYSTEMS (CONTINUED)

French-American-British (FAB) Classification[c]
M2: Myeloblastic leukemia with maturation
M3: Hypergranular promyelocytic leukemia
M4: Myelomonocytic leukemia
M4Eo: Variant: Increase in abnormal marrow eosinophils
M5: Monocytic leukemia
M6: Erythroleukemia (DiGuglielmo's disease)
M7: Megakaryoblastic leukemia

[a]From SH Swerdlow et al (eds): *World Health Organization Classification of Tumours of Haematopoietic and Lymphoid Tissues.* Lyon, IARC Press, 2008.
[b]Diagnosis is AML regardless of blast count.
[c]From JM Bennett et al: Ann Intern Med 103:620, 1985.
Abbreviation: AML, acute myeloid leukemia.

seen in leukemias developing after exposure to topoisomerase II inhibitors. Chromosome 5 or 7 deletions are seen in leukemias following radiation plus chemotherapy. The particular genetic abnormality has a strong influence on treatment outcome. Expression of MDR1 (multidrug resistance efflux pump) is common in older pts and adversely affects prognosis.

Clinical and Laboratory Features

Initial symptoms of acute leukemia have usually been present for <3 months; a preleukemic syndrome may be present in some 25% of pts with AML. Signs of anemia, pallor, fatigue, weakness, palpitations, and dyspnea on exertion are most common. White blood cell count (WBC) may be low, normal, or markedly elevated; circulating blast cells may or may not be present; with WBC >100 × 10⁹ blasts per liter, leukostasis in lungs and brain may occur. Minor pyogenic infections of the skin are common. Thrombocytopenia leads to spontaneous bleeding, epistaxis, petechiae, conjunctival hemorrhage, gingival bleeding, and bruising, especially with platelet count <20,000/μL. Anorexia and weight loss are common; fever may be present.

Bacterial and fungal infection are common; risk is heightened with total neutrophil count <5000/μL, and breakdown of mucosal and cutaneous barriers aggravates susceptibility; infections may be clinically occult in presence of severe leukopenia, and prompt recognition requires a high degree of clinical suspicion.

Hepatosplenomegaly occurs in about one-third of pts; leukemic meningitis may present with headache, nausea, seizures, papilledema, cranial nerve palsies.

Metabolic abnormalities may include hyponatremia, hypokalemia, elevated serum lactate dehydrogenase (LDH), hyperuricemia, and (rarely) lactic acidosis. With very high blast cell count in the blood, spurious hyperkalemia and hypoglycemia may occur (potassium released from and glucose consumed by tumor cells after the blood was drawn).

TREATMENT   Acute Myeloid Leukemia

Leukemic cell mass at time of presentation may be 10^{11}–10^{12} cells; when total leukemic cell numbers fall below ~10^9, they are no longer detectable in blood or bone marrow and pt appears to be in complete remission (CR). Thus aggressive therapy must continue past the point when initial cell bulk is reduced if leukemia is to be eradicated. Typical phases of chemotherapy include remission induction and postremission therapy, with treatment lasting about 1 year. Figure 72-1 outlines a treatment algorithm.

Supportive care with transfusions of red cells and platelets [from cytomegalovirus (CMV)-seronegative donors, if pt is a candidate for bone marrow transplantation] is very important, as are aggressive prevention, diagnosis, and treatment of infections. Colony-stimulating factors offer little or no benefit; some recommend their use in older pts and those with active infections. Febrile neutropenia should be treated with broad-spectrum antibiotics (e.g., ceftazidime 1 g q8h); if febrile neutropenia persists beyond 7 days, amphotericin B should be added.

About 60–80% of pts will achieve initial remission when treated with cytarabine 100–200 $(mg/m^2)/d$ by continuous infusion for 7 days, and daunorubicin [45 $(mg/m^2)/d]$ or idarubicin [12–13 $(mg/m^2)/d]$ for 3 days. Addition of etoposide may improve CR duration. Half of treated pts enter CR with the first cycle of therapy, and another 25% require two cycles. About 10–30% of pts achieve 5-year disease-free survival and probable cure. Pts achieving a CR who have low risk of relapse [cells contain t(8;21) or inv(16)] receive 3–4 cycles of cytarabine. Those at high risk of relapse may be considered for allogeneic bone marrow transplantation.

Response to treatment after relapse is short, and prognosis for pts who have relapsed is poor. In APL, addition of *trans*-retinoic acid (tretinoin) to chemotherapy induces differentiation of the leukemic cells and may improve outcome. Arsenic trioxide also induces differentiation in APL cells.

Bone marrow transplantation from identical twin or human leukocyte antigen (HLA)-identical sibling is effective treatment for AML. Typical protocol uses high-dose chemotherapy ± total-body irradiation to ablate host marrow, followed by infusion of marrow from donor. Risks are substantial (unless marrow is from identical twin). Complications include graft-versus-host disease, interstitial pneumonitis, opportunistic infections (especially CMV). Comparison between transplantation and high-dose cytarabine as postremission therapy has not produced a clear advantage for either approach. Up to 30% of otherwise end-stage pts with refractory leukemia achieve probable cure from transplantation; results are better when transplant is performed during remission. Results are best for children and young adults.

CHRONIC MYELOID LEUKEMIA (CML)

CML is a clonal malignancy usually characterized by splenomegaly and production of increased numbers of granulocytes; course is initially indolent but eventuates in leukemic phase (blast crisis) that has a poorer prognosis

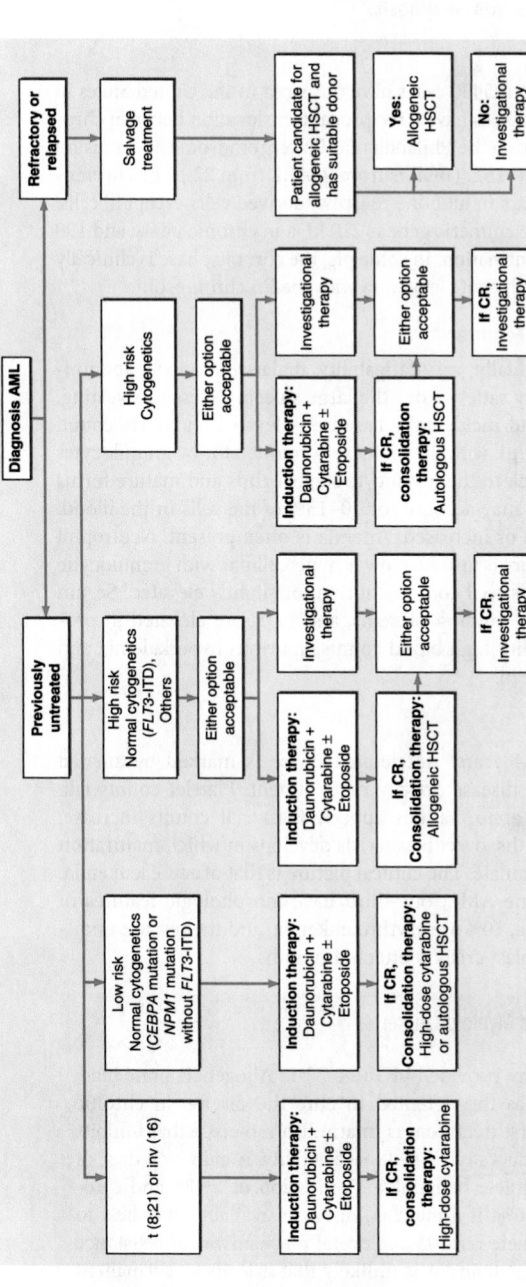

FIGURE 72-1 Flow chart for the therapy of newly diagnosed acute myeloid leukemia. For all forms of AML except acute promyelocytic leukemia (APL), standard therapy includes a 7-day continuous infusion of cytarabine (100–200 mg/m² per day) and a 3-day course of daunorubicin (60–90 mg/m² per day) with or without 3 days of etoposide (only with daunorubicin 60 mg/m² per day) or novel therapies based on their predicted risk of relapse (i.e., risk-stratified therapy). Idarubicin (12–13 mg/m² per day) could be used in place of daunorubicin (not shown). Patients who achieve complete remission undergo postremission consolidation therapy, including sequential courses of high-dose cytarabine, autologous hematopoietic stem cell transplant (HSCT), allogeneic HSCT, or novel therapies, based on their predicted risk of relapse (i.e., risk-stratified therapy). Patients with APL (see text for treatment) usually receive tretinoin together with anthracycline-based chemotherapy for remission induction and then arsenic trioxide followed by consolidation with anthracycline-based chemotherapy and possibly maintenance with tretinoin. The role of cytarabine in APL induction and consolidation is controversial.

407

than de novo AML; rate of progression to blast crisis is variable; overall survival averages 4 years from diagnosis.

Incidence and Etiology

In the United States, about 5430 cases have occurred in the United States in 2012. More than 90% of cases have a reciprocal translocation between chromosomes 9 and 22, creating the Philadelphia (Ph) chromosome and a fusion gene product called *BCR-ABL*. (BCR is from 9, ABL from 22.) The chromosome abnormality appears in all bone marrow–derived cells except T cells. The protein made by the chimeric gene is 210 kDa in chronic phase and 190 kDa in acute blast transformation. In some pts, the chronic phase is clinically silent and pts present with acute leukemia with the Ph chromosome.

Clinical and Laboratory Features

Symptoms develop gradually; easy fatigability, malaise, anorexia, abdominal discomfort and early satiety from the large spleen, excessive sweating. Occasional pts are found incidentally based on elevated leukocyte count. WBC is usually >25,000/μL with the increase accounted for by granulocytes and their precursors back to the myelocyte stage; bands and mature forms predominate. Basophils may account for 10–15% of the cells in the blood. Platelet count is normal or increased. Anemia is often present. Neutrophil alkaline phosphatase score is low. Marrow is hypercellular with granulocytic hyperplasia. Marrow blast cell count is normal or slightly elevated. Serum levels of vitamin B_{12}, B_{12}-binding proteins, and LDH are elevated in proportion to the WBC. With high blood counts, spurious hyperkalemia and hypoglycemia may be seen.

Natural History

Chronic phase lasts 2–4 years. Accelerated phase is marked by anemia disproportionate to the disease activity or treatment. Platelet counts fall. Additional cytogenetic abnormalities appear. Blast cell counts increase. Usually within 6–8 months, overt blast crisis develops in which maturation ceases and blasts predominate. The clinical picture is that of acute leukemia. Half of the cases become AML, one-third have morphologic features of acute lymphoid leukemia, 10% are erythroleukemia, and the rest are undifferentiated. Survival in blast crisis is often <4 months.

TREATMENT | **Chronic Myeloid Leukemia**

Criteria for response are provided in Table 72-2. Allogeneic bone marrow transplantation has the potential to cure the disease in chronic phase. However, the first treatment is imatinib, a molecule that inhibits the chimeric gene product's tyrosine kinase activity. A daily oral dose of 400 mg produces complete hematologic remission of >90% and cytogenetic remission in 76%. If a matched donor is available, it is best to transplant pts in complete remission. Several mechanisms of resistance to imatinib have emerged, and it is unlikely that it leads to permanent remissions when used alone; however, follow-up is not sufficient to draw firm conclusions.

TABLE 72-2 RESPONSE CRITERIA IN CHRONIC MYELOID LEUKEMIA

Hematologic	
Complete response[a]	White blood cell count <10,000/μL, normal morphology
	Normal hemoglobin and platelet counts
Incomplete response	White blood cell count ≥10,000/μL
Cytogenetic	Percentage of bone marrow metaphases with t(9;22)
Complete response	0
Partial response	≤35
Minor response	36–85[b]
No response	85–100
Molecular	Presence of *BCR/ABL* transcript by RT-PCR
Complete response	None
Incomplete response	Any

[a]Complete hematologic response requires the disappearance of splenomegaly.
[b]Up to 15% normal metaphases are occasionally seen at diagnosis (when 30 metaphases are analyzed).
Abbreviation: RT-PCR, reverse transcriptase polymerase chain reaction.

Pts who no longer respond to imatinib may respond to other tyrosine kinase inhibitors such as dasatinib (100 mg PO qd) or nilotinib (400 mg PO bid). The T315I mutation in the *BCR/ABL* gene conveys resistance to all three kinase inhibitors. Allopurinol, 300 mg/d, prevents urate nephropathy. The only curative therapy for the disease is HLA-matched allogeneic bone marrow transplantation. The optimal timing of transplantation is unclear, but transplantation in chronic phase is more effective than transplantation in accelerated phase or blast crisis. Transplantation appears most effective in pts treated within a year of diagnosis. Long-term disease-free survival may be obtained in 50–60% of transplanted pts. Infusion of donor lymphocytes can restore remission in relapsing pts. In pts without a matched donor, autologous transplantation may be helpful using peripheral blood stem cells. Treatment of pts in blast crisis with imatinib can obtain responses, but their durability has not been established.

MYELODYSPLASTIC SYNDROMES (MDS)

These are clonal abnormalities of marrow cells characterized by varying degrees of cytopenias affecting one or more cell lines. The World Health Organization (WHO) classification of myelodysplastic syndromes is shown in Table 72-3. Other terms that have been used to describe one or more of the entities include *preleukemia* and *oligoblastic leukemia*.

TABLE 72-3 WORLD HEALTH ORGANIZATION (WHO) CLASSIFICATION OF MYELODYSPLASTIC SYNDROMES/NEOPLASMS

Name	WHO Estimated Proportion of Patients with MDS	Peripheral Blood: Key Features	Bone Marrow: Key Features
Refractory cytopenias with unilineage dysplasia (RCUD):			
Refractory anemia (RA)	10–20%	Anemia <1% of blasts	Unilineage erythroid dysplasia (in ≥10% of cells) <5% blasts
Refractory neutropenia (RN)	<1%	Neutropenia <1% blasts	Unilineage granulocytic dysplasia <5% blasts
Refractory thrombocytopenia (RT)	<1%	Thrombocytopenia <1% blasts	Unilineage megakaryocytic dysplasia <5% blasts
Refractory anemia with ring sideroblasts (RARS)	3–11%	Anemia No blasts	Unilineage erythroid dysplasia ≥15% of erythroid precursors are ring sideroblasts <5% blasts
Refractory cytopenias with multilineage dysplasia (RCMD)	30%	Cytopenia(s) <1% blasts No Auer rods	Multilineage dysplasia ± ring sideroblasts <5% blasts No Auer rods
Refractory anemia with excess blasts, type 1 (RAEB-1)	40%	Cytopenia(s) <5% blasts No Auer rods	Unilineage or multilineage dysplasia
Refractory anemia with excess blasts, type 2 (RAEB-2)		Cytopenia(s) 5–19% blasts ± Auer rods	Unilineage or multilineage dysplasia 10–19% blasts ± Auer rods

	Peripheral Blood		Bone Marrow
MDS associated with isolated Del(5q) (Del(5q))	Anemia Normal or high platelet count <1% blasts	Uncommon	Isolated 5q31 chromosome deletion Anemia; hypolobated megakaryocytes <5% blasts
Childhood MDS, including refractory cytopenia of childhood (*provisional*) (RCC)	Pancytopenia	<1 %	<5% marrow blasts for RCC Marrow usually hypocellular
MDS, unclassifiable (MDS-U)	Cytopenia ≤1% blasts	?	Does not fit other categories Dysplasia <5% blasts If no dysplasia, MDS-associated karyotype

Note: If peripheral blood blasts are 2–4%, the diagnosis is RAEB-1 even if marrow blasts are <5%. If Auer rods are present, the WHO considers the diagnosis RAEB-2 if the blast proportion is <20% (even if <10%), AML if at least 20% blasts. For all subtypes, peripheral blood monocytes are <1 × 10⁹/L. Bicytopenia may be observed in RCUD subtypes, but pancytopenia with unilineage marrow dysplasia should be classified as MDS-U. Therapy-related MDS (t-MDS), whether due to alkylating agents, topoisomerase II (t-MDS/t-AML) in the WHO classification of AML and precursor lesions. The listing in this table excludes MDS/myeloproliferative neoplasm overlap categories, such as chronic myelomonocytic leukemia, juvenile myelomonocytic leukemia, and the provisional entity RARS with thrombocytosis.
Abbreviation: MDS, myelodysplastic syndrome.

Incidence and Etiology

About 3000 cases occur each year, mainly in persons >50 years old (median age, 68). As in AML, exposure to benzene, radiation, and chemotherapeutic agents may lead to MDS. Chromosome abnormalities occur in up to 80% of cases, including deletion of part or all of chromosomes 5, 7, and 9 (20 or 21 less commonly) and addition of part or all of chromosome 8.

Clinical and Laboratory Features

Symptoms depend on the affected lineages. 85% of pts are anemic, 50% have neutropenia, and about one-third have thrombocytopenia. The pathologic features of MDS are a cellular marrow with varying degrees of cytologic atypia including delayed nuclear maturation, abnormal cytoplasmic maturation, accumulation of ringed sideroblasts (iron-laden mitochondria surrounding the nucleus), uni- or bilobed megakaryocytes, micromegakaryocytes, and increased myeloblasts. Table 72-3 lists features used to identify distinct entities. Prognosis is defined by marrow blast %, karyotype, and lineages affected. The International Prognostic Scoring System is shown in Table 72-4.

TREATMENT   Myelodysplastic Syndromes

Allogeneic bone marrow transplantation is the only curative therapy and may cure 60% of those so treated. However, the majority of pts with MDS are too old to receive transplantation. 5-Azacytidine (75 mg/m² daily × 7, q 4 weeks) can delay transformation to AML by 8–10 months. Decitabine (15 mg/m² by continuous IV infusion, q8h daily × 3, q 6 weeks) may induce responses lasting a median of 1 year in 20% of pts. Lenalidomide (10 mg/d), a thalidomide analogue with fewer central nervous system effects, causes a substantial fraction of pts with the 5q– syndrome to become transfusion-independent. Pts with low erythropoietin levels may respond to erythropoietin, and a minority of pts with neutropenia respond to granulocyte colony-stimulating factor. Supportive care is the cornerstone of treatment.

MYELOPROLIFERATIVE SYNDROMES

The three major myeloproliferative syndromes are polycythemia vera, idiopathic myelofibrosis, and essential thrombocytosis. All are clonal disorders of hematopoietic stem cells and all are associated with a mutation in the *JAK2* kinase (V617F) that results in activation of the kinase. The mutation is seen in 90% of pts with polycythemia vera and ~45% of pts with idiopathic myelofibrosis and essential thrombocytosis.

■ POLYCYTHEMIA VERA

The most common myeloproliferative syndrome, this is characterized by an increase in red blood cell (RBC) mass, massive splenomegaly, and clinical manifestations related to increased blood viscosity, including neurologic symptoms (vertigo, tinnitus, headache, visual disturbances) and thromboses (myocardial infarction, stroke, peripheral vascular disease; uncommonly,

TABLE 72-4 INTERNATIONAL PROGNOSTIC SCORING SYSTEM (IPSS)

Prognostic Variable	Score Value				
	0	0.5	1	1.5	2
Bone marrow blasts (%)	<5%	5–10%		11–20%	21–30%
Karyotype[a]	Good	Intermediate	Poor		
Cytopenia[b] (lineages affected)	0 or 1	2 or 3			

Risk Group Scores	Score
Low	0
Intermediate-1	0.5–1
Intermediate-2	1.5–2
High	≥2.5

[a]Good, normal, -Y, del(5q), del (20q); poor, complex (≥3 abnormalities) or chromosome 7 abnormalities; intermediate, all other abnormalities.
[b]Cytopenias defined as Hb <100 g/L, platelet count <100,000/μL, absolute neutrophil count <1500/μL.

mesenteric and hepatic). It must be distinguished from other causes of increased RBC mass (Chap. 51). This is most readily done by assaying serum erythropoietin levels. Polycythemia vera is associated with very low erythropoietin levels; in other causes of erythrocytosis, erythropoietin levels are high. Pts are effectively managed with phlebotomy. Some pts require splenectomy to control symptoms, and those with severe pruritus may benefit from psoralens and UV light. 20% develop myelofibrosis, <5% acute leukemia.

◼ IDIOPATHIC MYELOFIBROSIS

This rare entity is characterized by marrow fibrosis, myeloid metaplasia with extramedullary hematopoiesis, and splenomegaly. Evaluation of a blood smear reveals teardrop-shaped RBC, nucleated RBC, and some early granulocytic forms, including promyelocytes. However, many entities may lead to marrow fibrosis and extramedullary hematopoiesis, and the diagnosis of primary idiopathic myelofibrosis is made only when the many other potential causes are ruled out. The following diseases are in the differential diagnosis: CML, polycythemia vera, Hodgkin's disease, cancer metastatic to the marrow (especially from breast and prostate), infection (particularly granulomatous infections), and hairy cell leukemia. Supportive therapy is generally used; novel inhibitors of *JAK2* have shown activity in reducing splenomegaly; however, no study has yet shown a particular drug therapy to improve survival.

◼ ESSENTIAL THROMBOCYTOSIS

This is usually noted incidentally upon routine platelet count done in an asymptomatic person. Like myelofibrosis, many conditions can produce elevated platelet counts; thus, the diagnosis is one of exclusion. Platelet count must be >500,000/μL, and known causes of thrombocytosis must be ruled out including CML, iron deficiency, splenectomy, malignancy, infection, hemorrhage, polycythemia vera, myelodysplasia, and recovery from vitamin B_{12} deficiency. Although usually asymptomatic, pts should be treated if they develop migraine headache, transient ischemic attack, or other bleeding or thrombotic disease manifestations. Interferon α is effective therapy, as are anagrelide and hydroxyurea. Treatment should not be given just because the absolute platelet count is high in the absence of other symptoms.

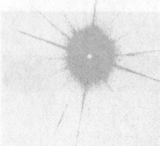

For a more detailed discussion, see Young NS: Aplastic Anemia, Myelodysplasia, and Related Bone Marrow Failure Syndromes, Chap. 107, p. 887; Spivak JL: Polycythemia Vera and Other Myeloproliferative Diseases, Chap. 108, p. 898; and Wetzler M et al: Acute and Chronic Myeloid Leukemia, Chap. 109, p. 905, in HPIM-18.

CHAPTER **73**
Lymphoid Malignancies

■ DEFINITION

Neoplasms of lymphocytes usually represent malignant counterparts of cells at discrete stages of normal lymphocyte differentiation. When bone marrow and peripheral blood involvement dominate the clinical picture, the disease is classified as a *lymphoid leukemia*. When lymph nodes and/or other extranodal sites of disease are the dominant site(s) of involvement, the tumor is called a *lymphoma*. The distinction between lymphoma and leukemia is sometimes blurred; for example, small lymphocytic lymphoma and chronic lymphoid leukemia are tumors of the same cell type and are distinguished arbitrarily on the basis of the absolute number of peripheral blood lymphocytes ($>5 \times 10^9$/L defines leukemia).

■ CLASSIFICATION

Historically, lymphoid tumors have had separate pathologic classifications based on the clinical syndrome—lymphomas according to the Rappaport, Kiel, or Working Formulation systems; acute leukemias according to the French-American-British (FAB) system; Hodgkin's disease according to the Rye classification. Myelomas have generally not been subclassified by pathologic features of the neoplastic cells. The World Health Organization (WHO) has proposed a unifying classification system that brings together all lymphoid neoplasms into a single framework. Although the new system bases the definitions of disease entities on histology, genetic abnormalities, immunophenotype, and clinical features, its organization is based on cell of origin (B cell vs. T cell) and maturation stage (precursor vs. mature) of the tumor, features that are of limited value to the clinician. Table 73-1 lists the disease entities according to a more clinically useful schema based on the clinical manifestations and natural history of the diseases.

TABLE 73-1 CLINICAL SCHEMA OF LYMPHOID NEOPLASMS

Chronic lymphoid leukemias/lymphomas

Chronic lymphocytic leukemia/small lymphocytic lymphoma (99% B cell, 1% T cell)

Prolymphocytic leukemia (90% B cell, 10% T cell)

Large granular lymphocyte leukemia [80% natural killer (NK) cell, 20% T cell]

Hairy cell leukemia (99–100% B cell)

Indolent lymphoma

Follicular center cell lymphoma, grades I and II (100% B cell)

Lymphoplasmacytic lymphoma/Waldenström's macroglobulinemia (100% B cell)

Marginal zone lymphoma (100% B cell)

Extranodal [mucosa-associated lymphatic tissue (MALT) lymphoma]

Nodal (monocytoid B cell lymphoma)

Splenic marginal zone lymphoma

Cutaneous T cell lymphoma (mycosis fungoides) (100% T cell)

Aggressive lymphoma

Diffuse large cell lymphoma (85% B cell, 15% T cell), includes immunoblastic

Follicular center cell lymphoma, grade III (100% B cell)

Mantle cell lymphoma (100% B cell)

Primary mediastinal (thymic) large B cell lymphoma (100% B cell)

Burkitt-like lymphoma (100% B cell)

Peripheral T cell lymphoma (100% T cell)

Angioimmunoblastic lymphoma (100% T cell)

Angiocentric lymphoma (80% T cell, 20% NK cell)

Intestinal T cell lymphoma (100% T cell)

Anaplastic large cell lymphoma (70% T cell, 30% null cell)

Acute lymphoid leukemias/lymphomas

Precursor lymphoblastic leukemia/lymphoma (80% T cell, 20% B cell)

Burkitt's leukemia/lymphoma (100% B cell)

Adult T cell leukemia/lymphoma (100% T cell)

Plasma cell disorders (100% B cell)

Monoclonal gammopathy of uncertain significance

Solitary plasmacytoma

Extramedullary plasmacytoma

Multiple myeloma

Plasma cell leukemia

Hodgkin's disease (cell of origin mainly B cell)

Lymphocyte predominant

Nodular sclerosis

Mixed cellularity

Lymphocyte depleted

■ **INCIDENCE**

Lymphoid tumors are increasing in incidence. Nearly 116,000 cases have been diagnosed in 2012 in the United States (Fig. 73-1).

■ **ETIOLOGY**

The cause(s) for the vast majority of lymphoid neoplasms is unknown. The malignant cells are monoclonal and often contain numerous genetic abnormalities. Some genetic alterations are characteristic of particular histologic entities: t(8;14) in Burkitt's lymphoma, t(14;18) in follicular lymphoma, t(11;14) in mantle cell lymphoma, t(2;5) in anaplastic large cell lymphoma, translocations or mutations involving *bcl*-6 on 3q27 in diffuse large cell lymphoma, and others. In most cases, translocations involve insertion of a distant chromosome segment into the antigen receptor genes (either immunoglobulin or T cell receptor) during the rearrangement of the gene segments that form the receptors.

Three viruses—Epstein-Barr virus (EBV), human herpesvirus 8 (HHV-8) (both herpes family viruses), and human T-lymphotropic virus type I (HTLV-I, a retrovirus)—may cause some lymphoid tumors. EBV has been strongly associated with African Burkitt's lymphoma and the lymphomas that complicate immunodeficiencies (disease-related or iatrogenic). EBV has an uncertain relationship to mixed cellularity Hodgkin's disease and angiocentric lymphoma. HHV-8 causes a rare entity, body cavity lymphoma, mainly in pts with AIDS. HTLV-I is associated with adult T cell leukemia/lymphoma. Both the virus and the disease are endemic to southwestern Japan and the Caribbean.

Gastric *Helicobacter pylori* infection is associated with gastric mucosa-associated lymphoid tissue (MALT) lymphoma and perhaps gastric large cell lymphoma. Eradication of the infection produces durable remissions in about half of pts with gastric MALT lymphoma. MALT lymphomas of other sites are associated with either infection (ocular adnexae, *Chlamydia psittaci*; small intestine, *Campylobacter jejuni*; skin, *Borrelia*) or autoimmunity (salivary gland, Sjögren's syndrome; thyroid gland, Hashimoto's thyroiditis).

Inherited or acquired immunodeficiencies and autoimmune disorders predispose individuals to lymphoma. Lymphoma is 17 times more common in HIV-infected than in HIV-noninfected people. Lymphoma occurs with increased incidence in farmers and meat workers; Hodgkin's disease is increased in wood workers.

■ **DIAGNOSIS AND STAGING**

Excisional biopsy is the standard diagnostic procedure; adequate tissue must be obtained. Tissue undergoes three kinds of studies: (1) light microscopy to discern the pattern of growth and the morphologic features of the malignant cells, (2) flow cytometry for assessment of immunophenotype, and (3) genetic studies (cytogenetics, DNA extraction). Needle aspirates of nodal or extranodal masses are not adequate diagnostic procedures. Leukemia diagnosis and lymphoma staging include generous bilateral iliac crest bone marrow biopsies. Differential diagnosis of adenopathy is reviewed in Chap. 50.

Staging varies with the diagnosis. In acute leukemia, peripheral blood blast counts are most significant in assessing prognosis. In chronic

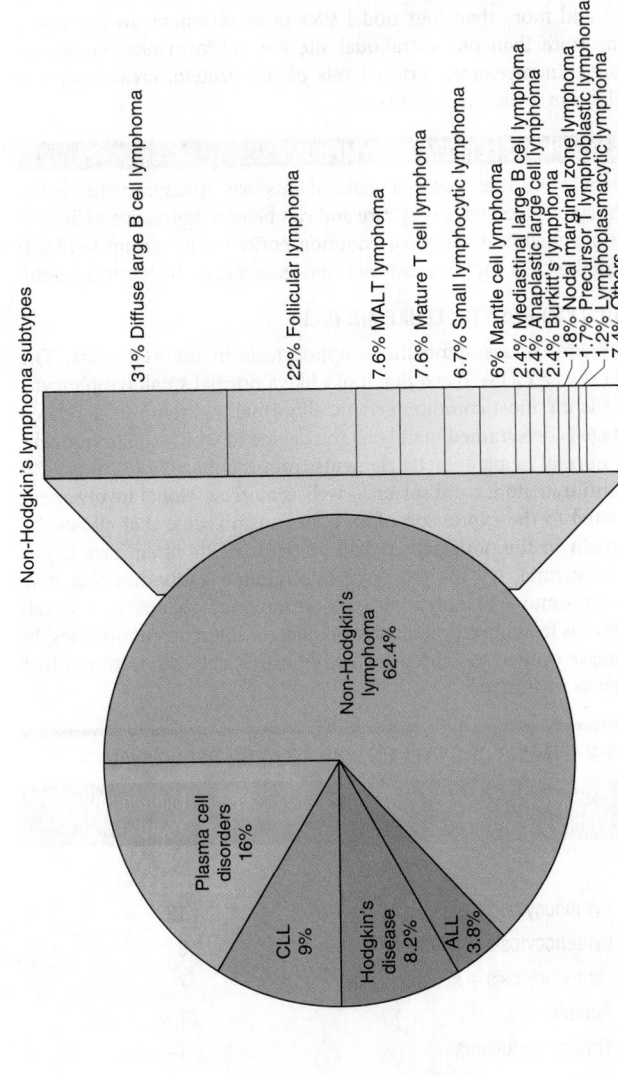

FIGURE 73-1 Relative frequency of lymphoid malignancies. ALL, acute lymphoid leukemia; CLL, chronic lymphoid leukemia; MALT, mucosa-associated lymphoid tissue.

leukemia, peripheral blood red blood cell (RBC) and platelet counts are most significant in assessing prognosis. Non-Hodgkin's lymphomas have five clinical prognostic factors; indolent and aggressive lymphomas share three of these, advanced stage, high lactate dehydrogenase (LDH) levels, and age >60. In follicular lymphoma, the last two factors are Hb <120 g/L (<12 g/dL) and more than four nodal sites of involvement. In aggressive lymphoma, more than one extranodal site and performance status predict outcome. In myeloma, serum levels of paraprotein, creatinine, and β_2-microglobulin levels predict survival.

CHRONIC LYMPHOID LEUKEMIAS/LYMPHOMAS

Most of these entities have a natural history measured in years. (Prolymphocytic leukemia is very rare and can be very aggressive.) Chronic lymphocytic leukemia is the most common entity in this group (~15,000 cases/year in the U.S.) and the most common leukemia in the Western world.

CHRONIC LYMPHOCYTIC LEUKEMIA (CLL)

Usually presents as asymptomatic lymphocytosis in pts >60 years. The malignant cell is a CD5+ B cell that looks like a normal small lymphocyte. Trisomy 12 is the most common genetic abnormality. Prognosis is related to stage; stage is determined mainly by the degree to which the tumor cells crowd out normal hematopoietic elements from the marrow (Table 73-2). Cells may infiltrate nodes and spleen as well as marrow. Nodal involvement may be related to the expression of an adhesion molecule that allows the cells to remain in the node rather than recirculate. Pts often have hypogammaglobulinemia. Up to 20% have autoimmune antibodies that may produce autoimmune hemolytic anemia, thrombocytopenia, or red cell aplasia. Death is from infection, marrow failure, or intercurrent illnesses. In 5%, the disease evolves to aggressive lymphoma (Richter's syndrome) that is refractory to treatment.

TABLE 73-2 STAGING OF B CELL CLL AND RELATION TO SURVIVAL

Stage	Clinical Features	Median Survival, Years
RAI		
0	Lymphocytosis	12
I	Lymphocytosis + adenopathy	9
II	Lymphocytosis + splenomegaly	7
III	Anemia	1–2
IV	Thrombocytopenia	1–2
BINET		
A	No anemia/thrombocytopenia, <3 involved sites	>10
B	No anemia/thrombocytopenia, >3 involved sites	5
C	Anemia and/or thrombocytopenia	2

Subsets of CLL may exist based on whether the immunoglobulin expressed by the tumor cell contains mutations (more indolent course, good prognosis) or retains the germ-line sequence (more aggressive course, poor response to therapy). Methods to distinguish the two subsets clinically are not well defined; CD38+ tumors may have poorer prognosis. The expression of ZAP-70, an intracellular tyrosine kinase normally present in T cells and aberrantly expressed in about 45% of CLL cases, may be a better way to define prognostic subsets. ZAP-70-positive cases usually need treatment within about 3–4 years from diagnosis; ZAP-70-negative cases usually don't require treatment for 8–11 years.

TREATMENT ▶ Chronic Lymphocytic Leukemia

Supportive care is generally given until anemia or thrombocytopenia develop. At that time, tests are indicated to assess the cause of the anemia or thrombocytopenia. Decreased RBC and/or platelet counts related to peripheral destruction may be treated with splenectomy or glucocorticoids without cytotoxic therapy in many cases. If marrow replacement is the mechanism, cytotoxic therapy is indicated. Fludarabine, 25 (mg/m²)/d IV × 5 days every 4 weeks, induces responses in about 75% of pts, complete responses in half. Rituximab (375–500 mg/m² day 1), fludarabine (25 mg/m² days 2–4 on cycle 1 and 1–3 in subsequent cycles), plus cyclophosphamide (250 mg/m² with fludarabine) induces complete responses in nearly 70% of pts but the regimen is associated with significant myelotoxicity. Glucocorticoids increase the risk of infection without adding a substantial antitumor benefit. Monthly IV immunoglobulin (IVIg) significantly reduces risk of serious infection but is expensive and usually reserved for pts who have had a serious infection. Alkylating agents are also active against the tumor. Therapeutic intent is palliative in most pts. Young pts may be candidates for high-dose therapy and autologous or allogeneic hematopoietic cell transplantation; long-term disease-free survival has been noted. Mini-transplant, in which the preparative regimen is immunosuppressive but not myeloablative, may be less toxic and as active or more active in disease treatment than high-dose therapy. Monoclonal antibodies alemtuzumab (anti-CD52) and rituximab (anti-CD20) also are active as single agents.

See Chaps. 110 and e21 in HPIM-18 for discussion of the rarer entities.

INDOLENT LYMPHOMAS

These entities have a natural history measured in years. Median survival is about 10 years. Follicular lymphoma is the most common indolent lymphoma, accounting for about one-third of all lymphoid malignancies.

■ **FOLLICULAR LYMPHOMA**

Usually presents with painless peripheral lymphadenopathy, often involving several nodal regions. "B symptoms" (fever, sweats, weight loss) occur in 10%, less common than with Hodgkin's disease. In about 25%, nodes wax and wane before the pt seeks medical attention. Median age is 55 years. Disease is widespread at diagnosis in 85%. Liver and bone marrow are commonly involved extranodal sites.

The tumor has a follicular or nodular growth pattern reflecting the follicular center origin of the malignant cell. The t(14;18) is present in 85% of cases, resulting in the overexpression of bcl-2, a protein involved in prevention of programmed cell death. The normal follicular center B cell is undergoing active mutation of the immunoglobulin variable regions in an effort to generate antibody of higher affinity for the selecting antigen. Follicular lymphoma cells also have a high rate of mutation that leads to the accumulation of genetic damage. Over time, follicular lymphomas acquire sufficient genetic damage (e.g., mutated p53) to accelerate their growth and evolve into diffuse large B cell lymphomas that are often refractory to treatment. The majority of pts dying from follicular lymphoma have undergone histologic transformation. This transformation occurs at a rate of about 7% per year and is an attribute of the disease, not the treatment.

TREATMENT   Follicular Lymphoma

Only 15% of pts have localized disease, but the majority of these pts are curable with radiation therapy. Although many forms of treatment induce tumor regression in advanced-stage pts, it is not clear that treatment of any kind alters the natural history of disease. No therapy, single-agent alkylators, nucleoside analogues (fludarabine, cladribine), combination chemotherapy, radiation therapy, and biologic agents [interferon (IFN) α, monoclonal antibodies such as rituximab (anti-CD20)] are all considered appropriate. More than 90% of pts are responsive to treatment; complete responses are seen in about 50–75% of pts treated aggressively. The median duration of remission of pts treated with cyclophosphamide, doxorubicin, vincristine, and prednisone (CHOP) + rituximab exceeds 6 years. Younger pts are being treated experimentally with high-dose therapy and autologous hematopoietic stem cells or mini-transplant. It is not yet clear whether this is curative. Radioimmunotherapy with isotopes guided by anti-CD20 antibody (ibritumomab tiuxetan, In-111; tositumomab, I-131) may produce durable responses. Combination chemotherapy with or without IFN maintenance may prolong survival and delay or prevent histologic progression, especially in pts with poor prognostic features. Remissions appear to last longer with chemotherapy plus rituximab; some data suggest that the longer remissions are leading to improved survival.

See Chaps. 110 and e21 in HPIM-18 for discussion of the other indolent lymphomas.

AGGRESSIVE LYMPHOMAS

A large number of pathologic entities share an aggressive natural history; median survival untreated is 6 months, and nearly all untreated pts are dead within 1 year. Pts may present with asymptomatic adenopathy or symptoms referable to involvement of practically any nodal or extranodal site: mediastinal involvement may produce superior vena cava syndrome or pericardial tamponade; retroperitoneal nodes may obstruct ureters; abdominal masses may produce pain, ascites, or GI obstruction or perforation; central nervous system (CNS) involvement may produce confusion, cranial nerve signs, headache, seizures, and/or spinal cord compression; bone involvement may produce pain or pathologic fracture. About 45% of pts have B symptoms.

Diffuse large B cell lymphoma is the most common histologic diagnosis among the aggressive lymphomas, accounting for 35–45% of all lymphomas. Aggressive lymphomas together account for ~60% of all lymphoid tumors. About 85% of aggressive lymphomas are of mature B cell origin; 15% are derived from peripheral (postthymic) T cells.

APPROACH TO THE PATIENT   Aggressive Lymphoma

Early diagnostic biopsy is critical. Pt workup is directed by symptoms and known patterns of disease. Pts with Waldeyer's ring involvement should undergo careful evaluation of the GI tract. Pts with bone or bone marrow involvement should have a lumbar puncture to evaluate meningeal CNS involvement.

TREATMENT   Aggressive Lymphomas

Localized aggressive lymphomas are usually treated with four cycles of CHOP combination chemotherapy ± involved-field radiation therapy. About 85% of these pts are cured. CHOP + rituximab appears to be even more effective than CHOP + radiation therapy. The specific therapy used for pts with more advanced disease is controversial. Six cycles of CHOP + rituximab is the treatment of choice for advanced-stage disease. Outcome is influenced by tumor bulk (usually measured by LDH levels, stage, and number of extranodal sites) and physiologic reserve (usually measured by age and Karnofsky status) (Table 73-3). CHOP + rituximab cures about two-thirds of pts. The use of a sequential high-dose chemotherapy regimen in pts with high-intermediate- and high-risk disease has yielded long-term survival in about 75% of pts in some institutions. Other studies fail to confirm a role for high-dose therapy.

About 30–45% of pts not cured with initial standard combination chemotherapy may be salvaged with high-dose therapy and autologous hematopoietic stem cell transplantation.

Specialized approaches are required for lymphomas involving certain sites (e.g., CNS, stomach) or under certain complicating clinical circumstances (e.g., concurrent illness, AIDS). Lymphomas occurring in iatrogenically immunosuppressed pts may regress when immunosuppressive medication is withheld. Lymphomas occurring post–allogeneic marrow transplant may regress with infusions of donor leukocytes.

Pts with rapidly growing bulky aggressive lymphoma may experience tumor lysis syndrome when treated (Chap. 27); prophylactic measures (hydration, urine alkalinization, allopurinol, rasburicase) may be lifesaving.

TABLE 73-3 INTERNATIONAL PROGNOSTIC INDEX FOR NHL

Five clinical risk factors:

  Age ≥60 years

  Serum lactate dehydrogenase levels elevated

  Performance status ≥2 (ECOG) or ≤70 (Karnofsky)

  Ann Arbor stage III or IV

  >1 site of extranodal involvement

Pts are assigned a number for each risk factor they have

Pts are grouped differently based on the type of lymphoma

For diffuse large B cell lymphoma:

0, 1 factor = low risk:	35% of cases; 5-year survival, 73%
2 factors = low-intermediate risk:	27% of cases; 5-year survival, 51%
3 factors = high-intermediate risk:	22% of cases; 5-year survival, 43%
4, 5 factors = high risk:	16% of cases; 5-year survival, 26%

For diffuse large B cell lymphoma treated with R-CHOP:

0 factor = very good:	10% of cases; 5-year survival, 94%
1, 2 factors = good:	45% of cases; 5-year survival, 79%
3, 4, 5 factors = poor:	45% of cases; 5-year survival, 55%

Abbreviations: ECOG, Eastern Cooperative Oncology Group; R-CHOP, rituximab, cyclophosphamide, doxorubicin, vincristine, prednisone.

ACUTE LYMPHOID LEUKEMIAS/LYMPHOMAS

■ ACUTE LYMPHOBLASTIC LEUKEMIA AND LYMPHOBLASTIC LYMPHOMA

These are more common in children than adults (~6000 total cases/year). The majority of cases have tumor cells that appear to be of thymic origin, and pts may have mediastinal masses. Pts usually present with recent onset of signs of marrow failure (pallor, fatigue, bleeding, fever, infection). Hepatosplenomegaly and adenopathy are common. Males may have testicular enlargement reflecting leukemic involvement. Meningeal involvement may be present at diagnosis or develop later. Elevated LDH, hyponatremia, and hypokalemia may be present, in addition to anemia, thrombocytopenia, and high peripheral blood blast counts. The leukemic cells are more often FAB type L2 in adults than in children, where L1 predominates. Leukemia diagnosis requires at least 20% lymphoblasts in the marrow. Prognosis is adversely affected by high presenting white count, age >35 years, and the presence of t(9;22), t(1;19), and t(4;11) translocations. HOX11 expression identifies a more favorable subset of T cell acute lymphoblastic leukemia.

> **TREATMENT** Acute Lymphoblastic Leukemia and Lymphoblastic Lymphoma

Successful treatment requires intensive induction phase, CNS prophylaxis, and maintenance chemotherapy that extends for about 2 years.

Vincristine, L-asparaginase, cytarabine, daunorubicin, and prednisone are particularly effective agents. Intrathecal or high-dose systemic methotrexate is effective CNS prophylaxis. Long-term survival of 60–65% of pts may be achieved. The role and timing of bone marrow transplantation in primary therapy is debated, but up to 30% of relapsed pts may be cured with salvage transplantation.

■ BURKITT'S LYMPHOMA/LEUKEMIA

This is also more common in children. It is associated with translocations involving the c-*myc* gene on chromosome 8 rearranging with immunoglobulin heavy or light chain genes. Pts often have disseminated disease with large abdominal masses, hepatomegaly, and adenopathy. If a leukemic picture predominates, it is classified as FAB L3.

TREATMENT   Burkitt's Lymphoma/Leukemia

Resection of large abdominal masses improves treatment outcome. Aggressive leukemia regimens that include vincristine, cyclophosphamide, 6-mercaptopurine, doxorubicin, and prednisone are active. CODOX-M and the BFM regimen are the most effective regimens. Cure may be achieved in 50–60%. The need for maintenance therapy is unclear. Prophylaxis against tumor lysis syndrome is important (Chap. 27).

■ ADULT T CELL LEUKEMIA/LYMPHOMA (ATL)

This is very rare; only a small fraction (~2%) of persons infected with HTLV-I go on to develop the disease. Some HTLV-I-infected pts develop spastic paraplegia from spinal cord involvement without developing cancer. The characteristic clinical syndrome of ATL includes high white count without severe anemia or thrombocytopenia, skin infiltration, hepatomegaly, pulmonary infiltrates, meningeal involvement, and opportunistic infections. The tumor cells are CD4+ T cells with cloven hoof- or flower-shaped nuclei. Hypercalcemia occurs in nearly all pts and is related to cytokines produced by the tumor cells.

TREATMENT   Adult T Cell Leukemia/Lymphoma

Aggressive therapy is associated with serious toxicity related to the underlying immunodeficiency. Glucocorticoids relieve hypercalcemia. The tumor is responsive to therapy, but responses are generally short-lived. Zidovudine and IFN may be palliative in some pts.

PLASMA CELL DISORDERS

The hallmark of plasma cell disorders is the production of immunoglobulin molecules or fragments from abnormal plasma cells. The intact immunoglobulin molecule, or the heavy chain or light chain produced by the abnormal plasma cell clone, is detectable in the serum and/or urine and is called the M (for monoclonal) component. The amount of the M component in any given pt reflects the tumor burden in that pt. In some, the presence of a clonal light chain in the urine (Bence Jones protein) is the only tumor product that is detectable. M components may be seen in pts with other lymphoid tumors, nonlymphoid cancers, and noncancerous conditions such as cirrhosis, sarcoidosis, parasitic infestations, and autoimmune diseases.

■ MULTIPLE MYELOMA

A malignant proliferation of plasma cells in the bone marrow (notably not in lymph nodes). Nearly 22,000 new cases are diagnosed each year. Disease manifestations result from tumor expansion, local and remote actions of tumor products, and the host response to the tumor. About 70% of pts have bone pain, usually involving the back and ribs, precipitated by movement. Bone lesions are multiple, lytic, and rarely accompanied by an osteoblastic response. Thus, bone scans are less useful than radiographs. The production of osteoclast-activating cytokines by tumor cells leads to substantial calcium mobilization, hypercalcemia and symptoms related to it. Decreased synthesis and increased catabolism of normal immunoglobulins leads to hypogammaglobulinemia, and a poorly defined tumor product inhibits granulocyte migration. These changes create a susceptibility to bacterial infections, especially the pneumococcus, *Klebsiella pneumoniae*, and *Staphylococcus aureus* affecting the lung and *Escherichia coli* and other gram-negative pathogens affecting the urinary tract. Infections affect at least 75% of pts at some time in their course. Renal failure may affect 25% of pts; its pathogenesis is multifactorial—hypercalcemia, infection, toxic effects of light chains, urate nephropathy, dehydration. Neurologic symptoms may result from hyperviscosity, cryoglobulins, and rarely amyloid deposition in nerves. Anemia occurs in 80% related to myelophthisis and inhibition of erythropoiesis by tumor products. Clotting abnormalities may produce bleeding.

Diagnosis

Marrow plasmacytosis >10%, lytic bone lesions, and a serum and/or urine M component are the classic triad. Monoclonal gammopathy of uncertain significance (MGUS) is much more common than myeloma, affecting about 6% of people over age 70; in general, MGUS is associated with a level of M component <20 g/L, low serum β_2-microglobulin, <10% marrow plasma cells, and no bone lesions. Lifetime risk of progression of MGUS to myeloma is about 25%.

Staging

Disease stage influences survival (Table 73-4).

TREATMENT	Multiple Myeloma

About 10% of pts have very slowly progressive disease and do not require treatment until the paraprotein levels rise above 50 g/L or progressive bone disease occurs. Pts with solitary plasmacytoma and extramedullary plasmacytoma are usually cured with localized radiation therapy. Supportive care includes early treatment of infections; control of

TABLE 73-4 MYELOMA STAGING SYSTEMS

Durie-Salmon Staging System		
Stage	**Criteria**	**Estimated tumor burden, × 10^12 cells/m^2**

I	All of the following:
	1. Hemoglobin >100 g/L (>10 g/dL)
	2. Serum calcium <3 mmol/L (<12 mg/dL)
	3. Normal bone x-ray or solitary lesion
	4. Low M-component production
	  a. IgG level <50 g/L (<5 g/dL)
	  b. IgA level <30 g/L (<3 g/dL)
	  c. Urine light chain <4 g/24 h
		<0.6 (low)

II	Fitting neither I nor III	0.6–1.20 (intermediate)

III	One or more of the following:
	1. Hemoglobin <85 g/L (<8.5 g/dL)
	2. Serum calcium >3 mmol/L (>12 mg/dL)
	3. Advanced lytic bone lesions
	4. High M-component production
	  a. IgG level >70 g/L (>7 g/dL)
	  b. IgA level >50 g/L (>5 g/dL)
	  c. Urine light chains >12 g/24 h
		>1.20 (high)

Level	Stage	Median Survival, Months
Subclassification based on serum creatinine levels		
A <177 μmol/L (<2 mg/dL)	IA	61
B >177 μmol/L (>2 mg/dL)	IIA, B	55
	IIIA	30
	IIIB	15
International Staging System		
β_2M <3.5, alb ≥3.5	I (28%)	62
β_2M <3.5, alb <3.5 or β_2M = 3.5–5.5	II (39%)	44
β_2M >5.5	III (33%)	29

Note: β_2M, serum β_2-microglobulin in mg/L; alb, serum albumin in g/dL; (#), % pts presenting at each stage.

hypercalcemia with glucocorticoids, hydration, and natriuresis; chronic administration of bisphosphonates to antagonize skeletal destruction; and prophylaxis against urate nephropathy and dehydration. Therapy aimed at the tumor is usually palliative. Initial therapy is usually one of several approaches, based on whether the pt is a candidate for high-dose therapy and autologous stem cell transplant. Transplant-eligible (avoid alkylating agents): thalidomide, 400 mg/d PO or 200 mg qhs, plus dexamethasone, 40 mg/d on days 1–4 each month, with or without bortezomib or chemotherapy such as liposomal doxorubicin. Transplant-ineligible: melphalan, 8 mg/m^2 orally for 4–7 days every 4–6 weeks, plus prednisone. About 60% of pts have significant symptomatic improvement plus a 75% decline in the M component. Bortezomib also appears to improve response rates to melphalan. Experimental approaches using sequential high-dose pulses of melphalan plus two successive autologous stem cell transplants have produced complete responses in about 50% of pts <65 years. Long-term follow-up is required to see whether survival is enhanced. Palliatively treated pts generally follow a chronic course for 2–5 years, followed by an acceleration characterized by organ infiltration with myeloma cells and marrow failure. More aggressive treatment may produce median survival of 6 years. New approaches to salvage treatment include bortezomib, 1.3 mg/m^2 on days 1, 4, 8, and 11 every 3 weeks, often used with dexamethasone, vincristine, and/or liposomal doxorubicin. Lenalidomide is also active and increasingly used as maintenance therapy.

■ HODGKIN'S DISEASE

About 9000 new cases are diagnosed each year. Hodgkin's disease (HD) is a tumor of Reed-Sternberg cells, aneuploid cells that usually express CD30 and CD15 but may also express other B or T cell markers. Most tumors are derived from B cells in that immunoglobulin genes are rearranged but not expressed. Most of the cells in an enlarged node are normal lymphoid, plasma cells, monocytes, and eosinophils. The etiology is unknown, but the incidence in both identical twins is 99-fold increased over the expected concordance, suggesting a genetic susceptibility. Distribution of histologic subtypes is 75% nodular sclerosis, 20% mixed cellularity, with lymphocyte predominant and lymphocyte depleted representing about 5%.

Clinical Manifestations

Usually presents with asymptomatic lymph node enlargement or with adenopathy associated with fever, night sweats, weight loss, and sometimes pruritus. Mediastinal adenopathy (common in nodular sclerosing HD) may produce cough. Spread of disease tends to be to contiguous lymph node groups. Superior vena cava obstruction or spinal cord compression may be presenting manifestation. Involvement of bone marrow and liver is rare.

Differential Diagnosis

- Infection—mononucleosis, viral syndromes, *Toxoplasma*, *Histoplasma*, primary tuberculosis

- Other malignancies—especially head and neck cancers
- Sarcoidosis—mediastinal and hilar adenopathy

Immunologic and Hematologic Abnormalities

- Defects in cell-mediated immunity (remains even after successful treatment of lymphoma); cutaneous anergy; diminished antibody production to capsular antigens of *Haemophilus* and pneumococcus
- Anemia; elevated erythrocyte sedimentation rate; leukemoid reaction; eosinophilia; lymphocytopenia; fibrosis and granulomas in marrow

Staging

The Ann Arbor staging classification is shown in Table 73-5. Disease is staged by performing physical exam, chest x-ray, thoracoabdominal CT, bone marrow biopsy; ultrasound examinations, lymphangiogram. Staging laparotomy should be used, especially to evaluate the spleen, if pt has early-stage disease on clinical grounds and radiation therapy is being contemplated. Pathologic staging is unnecessary if the pt is treated with chemotherapy.

TABLE 73-5 THE ANN ARBOR STAGING SYSTEM FOR HODGKIN'S DISEASE

Stage	Definition
I	Involvement of a single lymph node region or lymphoid structure (e.g., spleen, thymus, Waldeyer's ring)
II	Involvement of two or more lymph node regions on the same side of the diaphragm (the mediastinum is a single site; hilar lymph nodes should be considered "lateralized" and, when involved on both sides, constitute stage II disease)
III	Involvement of lymph node regions or lymphoid structures on both sides of the diaphragm
III$_1$	Subdiaphragmatic involvement limited to spleen, splenic hilar nodes, celiac nodes, or portal nodes
III$_2$	Subdiaphragmatic involvement includes paraaortic, iliac, or mesenteric nodes plus structures in III$_1$
IV	Involvement of extranodal site(s) beyond that designated as "E"
	More than one extranodal deposit at any location
	Any involvement of liver or bone marrow
A	No symptoms
B	Unexplained weight loss of >10% of the body weight during the 6 months before staging investigation
	Unexplained, persistent, or recurrent fever with temperatures >38°C during the previous month
	Recurrent drenching night sweats during the previous month
E	Localized, solitary involvement of extralymphatic tissue, excluding liver and bone marrow

---

TREATMENT Hodgkin's Disease

About 85% of pts are curable. Therapy should be performed by experienced clinicians in centers with appropriate facilities. Most pts are clinically staged and treated with chemotherapy alone or combined-modality therapy. Those with localized disease may be treated with radiation therapy alone. Those with stage II disease often receive either two or four cycles of ABVD plus involved-field radiation therapy or Stanford V, a combined-modality program using lower doses of chemotherapy. Those with stage III or IV disease receive six cycles of combination chemotherapy, usually ABVD. Pts with any stage disease accompanied by a large mediastinal mass (greater than one-third the greatest chest diameter) should receive combined-modality therapy with MOPP/ABVD or MOPP-ABV hybrid followed by mantle field radiation therapy. (Radiation plus ABVD is too toxic to the lung.) A persistently positive midtreatment positron emission tomography scan may be an index of risk of relapse and need for additional therapy. About one-half of pts (or more) not cured by their initial chemotherapy regimen may be rescued by high-dose therapy and autologous stem cell transplant. Brentuximab vedotin, an anti-CD30 drug conjugate, has activity in patients relapsing after transplant.

With long-term follow-up, it has become clear that more pts are dying of late fatal toxicities related to radiation therapy (myocardial infarction, stroke, second cancers) than from HD. It may be possible to avoid radiation exposure by using combination chemotherapy alone in early-stage disease as well as in advanced-stage disease.

For a more detailed discussion, see Longo DL: Malignancies of Lymphoid Cells, Chap. 110, p. 919; Munshi NC et al: Plasma Cell Disorders, Chap. 111, p. 936; and Chap. e21 in HPIM-18.

CHAPTER **74**
Skin Cancer

■ MALIGNANT MELANOMA

Most dangerous cutaneous malignancy; high metastatic potential; poor prognosis with metastatic spread.

Incidence

Melanoma has been diagnosed in 76,250 people in the United States in 2011 and caused 9180 deaths.

Predisposing Factors (Table 74-1)

Fair complexion, sun exposure, family history of melanoma, dysplastic nevus syndrome (autosomal dominant disorder with multiple nevi of distinctive

TABLE 74-1 FACTORS ASSOCIATED WITH INCREASED RISK OF MELANOMA

Total body nevi (higher number = higher risk)
Family or personal history
Dysplastic nevi
Light skin/hair/eye color
Poor tanning ability
Freckling
UV exposure/sunburns/tanning booths
CDKN2A mutation
MC1R variants

appearance and cutaneous melanoma, may be associated with 9p deletion), and presence of a giant congenital nevus. Blacks have a low incidence.

Prevention

Sun avoidance lowers risk. Sunscreens are not proven effective.

Types

1. *Superficial spreading melanoma*: Most common; begins with initial radial growth phase before invasion.
2. *Lentigo maligna melanoma*: Very long radial growth phase before invasion, lentigo maligna (Hutchinson's melanotic freckle) is precursor lesion, most common in elderly and in sun-exposed areas (esp. face).
3. *Acral lentiginous*: Most common form in darkly pigmented pts; occurs on palms and soles, mucosal surfaces, in nail beds and mucocutaneous junctions; similar to lentigo maligna melanoma but with more aggressive biologic behavior.
4. *Nodular*: Generally poor prognosis because of invasive growth from onset.

Biology

About half of melanomas carry an activating somatic mutation in the *BRAF* gene, often a valine to glutamate substitution at amino acid 600 (V600E). *N-ras* is mutated in about 20% and rare pts have activating mutations in *c-kit*. These mutations have been targeted by therapeutic agents that appear to have antitumor activity.

Clinical Appearance

Generally pigmented (rarely amelanotic); color of lesions varies, but red, white, and/or blue are common, in addition to brown and/or black. Suspicion should be raised by a pigmented skin lesion that is >6 mm in diameter, asymmetric, has an irregular surface or border, or has variation in color.

Prognosis

Best with thin lesions without evidence of metastatic spread; with increasing thickness or evidence of spread, prognosis worsens. Stage I and II (primary tumor without spread) have 85% 5-year survival. Stage III (palpable regional nodes with tumor) has a 50% 5-year survival when only one node is involved and 15–20% when four or more are involved. Stage IV (disseminated disease) has <5% 5-year survival.

TREATMENT　Malignant Melanoma

Early recognition and local excision for localized disease is best; 1- to 2-cm margins are as effective as 4- to 5-cm margins and do not usually require skin grafting. Elective lymph node dissection offers no advantage in overall survival compared with deferral of surgery until clinical recurrence. Pts with stage II disease may have improved disease-free survival with adjuvant interferon-α 3 million units three times weekly for 12–18 months. In one study, pts with stage III disease had improved survival with adjuvant IFN, 20 million units IV daily × 5 for 4 weeks, then 10 million units SC three times weekly for 11 months. This result was not confirmed in a second study. Metastatic disease may be treated with chemotherapy or immunotherapy. Vemurafenib 960 mg PO bid induces responses in about 50% of pts with *BRAF* mutations. Median survival is about 16 months. The anti-CTLA4 antibody ipilimumab prolongs survival by about 4 months. Dacarbazine (250 mg/m² IV daily × 5 q3w) plus tamoxifen (20 mg/m² PO daily) may induce partial responses in one-quarter of pts. IFN and interleukin 2 (IL-2) at maximum tolerated doses induce partial responses in 15% of pts. Rare long remissions occur with IL-2. Temozolomide is an oral agent related to dacarbazine that has some activity. It can enter the central nervous system (CNS) and is being evaluated with radiation therapy for CNS metastases. No therapy for metastatic disease is curative. Vaccines and adoptive cellular therapies are being tested.

■ BASAL CELL CARCINOMA (BCC)

Most common form of skin cancer; most frequently on sun-exposed skin, esp. face.

Predisposing Factors

Fair complexion, chronic UV exposure, exposure to inorganic arsenic (i.e., Fowler's solution or insecticides such as Paris green), or exposure to ionizing radiation.

Prevention

Avoidance of sun exposure and use of sunscreens lower risk.

Types

Five general types: noduloulcerative (most common), superficial (mimics eczema), pigmented (may be mistaken for melanoma), morpheaform (plaquelike lesion with telangiectasia—with keratotic is most aggressive), keratotic (basosquamous carcinoma).

Clinical Appearance

Classically a pearly, translucent, smooth papule with rolled edges and surface telangiectasia.

TREATMENT Basal Cell Carcinoma

Local removal with electrodesiccation and curettage, excision, cryosurgery, or radiation therapy; metastases are rare but may spread locally. Exceedingly unusual for BCC to cause death. Locally advanced or metastatic disease may respond to vismodegib, an inhibitor of the hedgehog pathway often activated in this disease.

■ SQUAMOUS CELL CARCINOMA (SCC)

Less common than basal cell but more likely to metastasize.

Predisposing Factors

Fair complexion, chronic UV exposure, previous burn or other scar (i.e., scar carcinoma), exposure to inorganic arsenic or ionizing radiation. Actinic keratosis is a premalignant lesion.

Types

Most commonly occurs as an ulcerated nodule or a superficial erosion on the skin. Variants include:

1. *Bowen's disease*: Erythematous patch or plaque, often with scale; noninvasive; involvement limited to epidermis and epidermal appendages (i.e., SCC in situ).

2. *Scar carcinoma*: Suggested by sudden change in previously stable scar, esp. if ulceration or nodules appear.

3. *Verrucous carcinoma*: Most commonly on plantar aspect of foot; low-grade malignancy but may be mistaken for a common wart.

Clinical Appearance

Hyperkeratotic papule or nodule or erosion; nodule may be ulcerated.

TREATMENT Squamous Cell Carcinoma

Local excision and Mohs micrographic surgery are most common; radiation therapy in selected cases. Metastatic disease may be treated with radiation therapy or with combination biologic therapy; 13-*cis*-retinoic acid 1 mg/d PO plus IFN 3 million units/d SC.

Prognosis

Favorable if secondary to UV exposure; less favorable if in sun-protected areas or associated with ionizing radiation.

■ SKIN CANCER PREVENTION

Most skin cancer is related to sun exposure. Encourage pts to avoid the sun and use sunscreen.

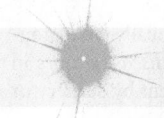

For a more detailed discussion, see Urba WJ et al: Cancer of the Skin, Chap. 87, p. 723, in HPIM-18.

CHAPTER **75**
Head and Neck Cancer

Epithelial cancers may arise from the mucosal surfaces of the head and neck including the sinuses, oral cavity, nasopharynx, oropharynx, hypopharynx, and larynx. These tumors are usually squamous cell cancers. Thyroid cancer is discussed in Chap. 181.

■ INCIDENCE AND EPIDEMIOLOGY

About 52,000 cases are diagnosed each year and 12,000 people die from the disease. Oral cavity, oropharynx, and larynx are the most frequent sites of primary lesions in the United States; nasopharyngeal primaries are more common in the Far East and Mediterranean countries. Alcohol and tobacco (including smokeless) abuse are risk factors. Human papillomavirus (usually types 16 and 18) is associated with some of these cancers.

■ PATHOLOGY

Nasopharyngeal cancer in the Far East has a distinct histology, nonkeratinizing undifferentiated carcinoma with infiltrating lymphocytes called *lymphoepithelioma*, and a distinct etiology, Epstein-Barr virus. Squamous cell head and neck cancer may develop from premalignant lesions (erythroplakia, leukoplakia), and the histologic grade affects prognosis. Pts who have survived head and neck cancer commonly develop a second cancer of the head and neck, lung, or esophagus, presumably reflecting the exposure of the upper aerodigestive mucosa to similar carcinogenic stimuli.

■ GENETIC ALTERATIONS

Chromosomal deletions and mutations have been found in chromosomes 3p, 9p, 17p, and 13q; mutations in p53 have been reported. Cyclin D1 may be overexpressed. Epidermal growth factor receptor is commonly overexpressed.

■ CLINICAL PRESENTATION

Most occur in persons >50 years. Symptoms vary with the primary site. Nasopharynx lesions do not usually cause symptoms until late in the course and then cause unilateral serous otitis media or nasal obstruction or epistaxis. Oral cavity cancers present as nonhealing ulcers, sometimes painful. Oropharyngeal lesions also present late with sore throat or otalgia. Hoarseness may be an early sign of laryngeal cancer. Rare pts present with painless, rock-hard cervical or supraclavicular lymph node enlargement. Staging is based on size of primary tumor and involvement of lymph nodes. Distant metastases occur in <10% of pts.

TREATMENT   Head and Neck Cancer

Three categories of disease are common: localized, locally or regionally advanced, and recurrent or metastatic. *Localized disease* occurs in about one-third of pts and is treated with curative intent by surgery or

radiation therapy. Radiation therapy is preferred for localized larynx cancer to preserve organ function; surgery is used more commonly for oral cavity lesions. Overall 5-year survival is 60–90%, and most recurrences occur within 2 years. *Locally advanced disease* is the most common presentation (>50%). Combined-modality therapy using induction chemotherapy, then surgery followed by concomitant chemotherapy and radiation therapy, is most effective. The use of three cycles of cisplatin (75 mg/m² IV day 1) and docetaxel (75 mg/m² IV day 1) plus 5-fluorouracil (5FU) [750 (mg/m²)/d by 96- to 120-h continuous infusion] before or during radiation therapy is more effective than surgery plus radiation therapy, although mucositis is also more severe; 5-year survival is 34–50%. Cetuximab plus radiation therapy may be more effective than radiation therapy alone. Head and neck cancer pts are frequently malnourished and often have intercurrent illness. Pts with *recurrent* or *metastatic disease* (about 10% of pts) are treated palliatively with cisplatin plus 5FU or paclitaxel (200–250 mg/m² with granulocyte colony-stimulating factor support) or with single-agent chemotherapy (a taxane, methotrexate, cisplatin, or carboplatin). Response rates are usually 30–50% and median survival about 3 months.

■ PREVENTION

The most important intervention is to get the pts to stop smoking. Long-term survival is significantly better in those who stop smoking. Chemopreventive therapy with *cis*-retinoic acid [3 months of 1.5 (mg/kg)/d followed by 9 months of 0.5 (mg/kg)/d PO] may cause regression of leukoplakia but has no consistent effect on development of cancer.

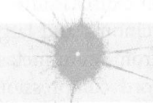

For a more detailed discussion, see Vokes EE: Head and Neck Cancer, Chap. 88, p. 733, in HPIM-18.

CHAPTER **76**
Lung Cancer

■ INCIDENCE

Lung cancer has been diagnosed in about 116,470 men and 109,690 women in the United States in 2012, and 86% of pts die within 5 years. Lung cancer, the leading cause of cancer death, accounts for 28% of all cancer deaths in men and 26% in women. Peak incidence occurs between ages 55 and 65 years. Incidence is decreasing in men and increasing in women.

■ HISTOLOGIC CLASSIFICATION

Four major types account for 88% of primary lung cancers: epidermoid (squamous), 29%; adenocarcinoma (including bronchioloalveolar), 35%;

large cell, 9%; and small cell (or oat cell), 18%. Histology (small cell versus non-small cell types) is a major determinant of treatment approach. Small cell is usually widely disseminated at presentation, while non-small cell may be localized. Epidermoid and small cell typically present as central masses, while adenocarcinomas and large cell usually present as peripheral nodules or masses. Epidermoid and large cell cavitate in 20–30% of pts.

◼ ETIOLOGY

The major cause of lung cancer is tobacco use, particularly cigarette smoking. Lung cancer cells may have ≥10 acquired genetic lesions, most commonly point mutations in *ras* oncogenes; amplification, rearrangement, or transcriptional activation of *myc* family oncogenes; overexpression of *bcl*-2, *Her2/neu*, and telomerase; and deletions involving chromosomes 1p, 1q, 3p12-13, 3p14 (FHIT gene region), 3p21, 3p24-25, 3q, 5q, 9p (p16 and p15 cyclin-dependent kinase inhibitors), 11p13, 11p15, 13q14 (*rb* gene), 16q, and 17p13 (*p53* gene). Loss of 3p and 9p are the earliest events, detectable even in hyperplastic bronchial epithelium; *p53* abnormalities and *ras* point mutations are usually found only in invasive cancers. A small but significant subset of pts with adenocarcinoma have activating mutations in the gene for the EGF receptor, or activating fusion events involving the *alk* or *ros* gene.

◼ CLINICAL MANIFESTATIONS

Only 5–15% are detected while asymptomatic. Central endobronchial tumors cause cough, hemoptysis, wheeze, stridor, dyspnea, pneumonitis. Peripheral lesions cause pain, cough, dyspnea, symptoms of lung abscess resulting from cavitation. Metastatic spread of primary lung cancer may cause tracheal obstruction, dysphagia, hoarseness, Horner's syndrome. Other problems of regional spread include superior vena cava syndrome, pleural effusion, respiratory failure. Extrathoracic metastatic disease affects 50% of pts with epidermoid cancer, 80% with adenocarcinoma and large cell, and >95% with small cell. Clinical problems result from brain metastases, pathologic fractures, liver invasion, and spinal cord compression. Paraneoplastic syndromes may be a presenting finding of lung cancer or first sign of recurrence (Chap. 83). Systemic symptoms occur in 30% and include weight loss, anorexia, fever. Endocrine syndromes occur in 12% and include hypercalcemia (epidermoid), syndrome of inappropriate antidiuretic hormone secretion (small cell), gynecomastia (large cell). Skeletal connective tissue syndromes include clubbing in 30% (most often non-small cell) and hypertrophic pulmonary osteoarthropathy in 1–10% (most often adenocarcinomas), with clubbing, pain, and swelling.

◼ STAGING (SEE TABLE 76-1)

Two parts to staging are (1) determination of location (anatomic staging) and (2) assessment of pt's ability to withstand antitumor treatment (physiologic staging). Non-small cell tumors are staged by the TNM/International Staging System (ISS). The T (tumor), N (regional node involvement), and M (presence or absence of distant metastasis) factors are taken together to define different stage groups. Small cell tumors are staged by two-stage system: limited stage disease—confined to one hemithorax and regional lymph nodes; extensive disease—involvement beyond this. General staging procedures include careful ear, nose, and throat examination; chest x-ray

TABLE 76-1 TUMOR, NODE, METASTASIS INTERNATIONAL STAGING SYSTEM FOR LUNG CANCER

Comparison of Survival by Stage in TNM Sixth and Seventh Editions

Stage	TNM Sixth Edition	TNM Seventh Edition	5-Year Survival, %*
IA	T1N0M0	T1a-T1bN0M0	73
IB	T2N0M0	T2aN0M0	58
IIA	T1N1M0	T1a-T2aN1M0 *or*	46
		T2bN0M0	
IIB	T2N1M0 *or*	T2bN1M0 *or*	36
	T3N0M0	T3N0M0	
IIIA	T3N1M0 *or*	T1a-T3N2M0 *or*	24
	T1-3N2M0	T3N1M0 *or*	
		T4N0-1M0	
IIIB	Any T N3M0	T4N2M0 *or*	9
	T4 Any N M0	T1a-T4N3M0	
IV	Any T Any N M1	Any T Any N M1a *or* M1b	13

	Sixth Edition	Seventh Edition

Tumor (T)

	Sixth Edition	Seventh Edition
T1	Tumor ≤3 cm diameter without invasion more proximal than lobar bronchus	Tumor ≤3 cm diameter, surrounded by lung or visceral pleura, without invasion more proximal than lobar bronchus
T1a		Tumor ≤2 cm in diameter
T1b		Tumor >2 cm but ≤3 cm in diameter
T2	Tumor >3 cm diameter *or* tumor of any size with any of the following:	Tumor >3 cm but ≤7 cm with any of the following:
	Visceral pleural invasion	Involves main bronchus, ≥2 cm distal to carina
	Atelectasis of less than entire lung	Invades visceral pleura
	Proximal extent at least 2 cm from carina	Associated with atelectasis or obstructive pneumonitis extending to hilar region but not involving the entire lung
T2a		Tumor >3 cm but ≤5 cm in diameter
T2b		Tumor >5 cm but ≤7 cm in diameter

(continued)

TABLE 76-1 TUMOR, NODE, METASTASIS INTERNATIONAL STAGING SYSTEM FOR LUNG CANCER (CONTINUED)

	Sixth Edition	Seventh Edition
Tumor (T)		
T3	Tumor of any size that invades any of the following: chest wall, diaphragm, mediastinal pleura, parietal pericardium	Tumor >7 cm or directly invades any of the following: chest wall (including superior sulcus tumors), phrenic nerve, mediastinal pleura, parietal pericardium
	Tumor <2 cm distal to carina	Tumor <2 cm distal to carina but without involvement of carina
		Tumor with associated atelectasis or obstructive pneumonitis of entire lung
		Separate tumor nodule(s) in same lobe
T4	Tumor of any size that invades any of the following: mediastinum, heart or great vessels, trachea, esophagus, vertebral body, carina	Tumor of any size that invades any of the following: mediastinum, heart or great vessels, trachea, recurrent laryngeal nerve, esophagus, vertebral body, carina
	Tumor with malignant pleural or pericardial effusion	Separate tumor nodule(s) in a different ipsilateral lobe
	Separate tumor nodules in same lobe	
Nodes (N)		
N0	No regional lymph node metastasis	No regional lymph node metastasis
N1	Metastasis in ipsilateral peribronchial and/or hilar lymph node(s)	Metastasis in ipsilateral peribronchial and/or hilar lymph node(s) and intrapulmonary node(s), including involvement by direct extensions
N2	Metastasis in ipsilateral mediastinal and/or subcarinal lymph node(s)	Metastasis in ipsilateral mediastinal and/or subcarinal lymph node(s)
N3	Metastasis in contralateral mediastinal, contralateral hilar, ipsilateral or contralateral scalene or supraclavicular lymph node(s)	Metastasis in contralateral mediastinal, hilar, ipsilateral or contralateral scalene or supraclavicular lymph node(s)

TABLE 76-1 TUMOR, NODE, METASTASIS INTERNATIONAL STAGING SYSTEM FOR LUNG CANCER (CONTINUED)

	Sixth Edition	Seventh Edition
Metastasis (M)		
M0	No distant metastasis	No distant metastasis
M1	Distant metastasis (includes tumor nodules in different lobe from primary)	Distant metastasis
M1a		Separate tumor nodules in a contralateral lobe
		Tumor with pleural nodules or malignant pleural or pericardial effusion
M1b		Distant metastasis

*Survival according to the seventh edition.
Source: Bottom portion of table reproduced with permission from P Goldstraw et al: J Thorac Oncol 2:706, 2007.

(CXR); chest and abdominal CT scanning; and positron emission tomography scan. CT scans may suggest mediastinal lymph node involvement and pleural extension in non-small cell lung cancer, but definitive evaluation of mediastinal spread requires histologic examination. Routine radionuclide scans are not obtained in asymptomatic pts. If a mass lesion is on CXR and no obvious contraindications to curative surgical approach are noted, the mediastinum should be investigated. Major contraindications to curative surgery include extrathoracic metastases, superior vena cava syndrome, vocal cord and phrenic nerve paralysis, malignant pleural effusions, metastases to contralateral lung, and histologic diagnosis of small cell cancer.

TREATMENT Lung Cancer (See Table 76-2)

1. Surgery in pts with localized disease and non-small cell cancer; however, majority initially thought to have curative resection ultimately succumb to metastatic disease. Adjuvant chemotherapy [cisplatin, four cycles at 100 mg/m2 plus a second active agent (etoposide, vinblastine, vinorelbine, vindesine, a taxane)] in pts with total resection of stage IIA and IIB disease may modestly extend survival.
2. Solitary pulmonary nodule: factors suggesting resection include cigarette smoking, age ≥35, relatively large (>2 cm) lesion, lack of calcification, chest symptoms, and growth of lesion compared with old CXR. See Fig. 76-1.
3. For unresectable stage II non-small cell lung cancer, combined thoracic radiation therapy and cisplatin-based chemotherapy reduces mortality by about 25% at 1 year.

TABLE 76-2 SUMMARY OF TREATMENT APPROACH TO PATIENTS WITH LUNG CANCER

Non-Small Cell Lung Cancer

Stages IA, IB, IIA, IIB, and some IIIA:

> Surgical resection for stages IA, IB, IIA, and IIB

> Surgical resection with complete-mediastinal lymph node dissection and consideration of neoadjuvant CRx for stage IIIA disease with "minimal N2 involvement" (discovered at thoracotomy or mediastinoscopy)

> Consider postoperative RT for pts found to have N2 disease

> Stage IB: discussion of risk/benefits of adjuvant CRx; not routinely given

> Stage II: Adjuvant CRx

Curative potential RT for "nonoperable" pts

Stage IIIA with selected types of stage T3 tumors:

> Tumors with chest wall invasion (T3): en bloc resection of tumor with involved chest wall and consideration of postoperative RT

> Superior sulcus (Pancoast's) (T3) tumors: preoperative RT (30–45 Gy) and CRx followed by en bloc resection of involved lung and chest wall with postoperative RT

> Proximal airway involvement (<2 cm from carina) without mediastinal nodes: sleeve resection if possible preserving distal normal lung or pneumonectomy

Stages IIIA "advanced, bulky, clinically evident N2 disease" (discovered preoperatively) and IIIB disease that can be included in a tolerable RT port:

> Curative potential concurrent RT + CRx if performance status and general medical condition are reasonable; otherwise, sequential CRx followed by RT, or RT alone

Stage IIIB disease with carinal invasion (T4) but without N2 involvement:

> Consider pneumonectomy with tracheal sleeve resection with direct reanastomosis to contralateral mainstem bronchus

Stage IV and more advanced IIIB disease:

> RT to symptomatic local sites

> CRx for ambulatory pts; consider CRx and bevacizumab for selected pts

> Chest tube drainage of large malignant pleural effusions

> Consider resection of primary tumor and metastasis for isolated brain or adrenal metastases

Small Cell Lung Cancer

Limited stage (good performance status): combination CRx + concurrent chest RT

Extensive stage (good performance status): combination CRx

Complete tumor responders (all stages): consider prophylactic cranial RT

Poor-performance-status pts (all stages):

**TABLE 76-2 SUMMARY OF TREATMENT APPROACH TO PATIENTS WITH
LUNG CANCER (CONTINUED)**

Small Cell Lung Cancer
Modified-dose combination CRx
Palliative RT
Bronchioloalveolar or Adenocarcinoma with EGF Receptor Mutations or ALK rearrangements
Gefitinib or erlotinib, inhibitors of EGF receptor kinase activity
Crizotinib, an alk inhibitor
All Patients
RT for brain metastases, spinal cord compression, weight-bearing lytic bony lesions, symptomatic local lesions (nerve paralyses, obstructed airway, hemoptysis, intrathoracic large venous obstruction, in non-small cell lung cancer and in small cell cancer not responding to CRx)
Appropriate diagnosis and treatment of other medical problems and supportive care during CRx
Encouragement to stop smoking
Entrance into clinical trial, if eligible

Abbreviations: CRx, chemotherapy; EGF, epidermal growth factor; RT, radiotherapy.

4. For unresectable non-small cell cancer, metastatic disease, or refusal of surgery: consider for radiation therapy; addition of cisplatin/taxane-based chemotherapy may reduce death risk by 13% at 2 years and improve quality of life. Pemetrexed has activity in pts with progressive disease.

5. Small cell cancer: combination chemotherapy is standard mode of therapy; response after 6–12 weeks predicts median- and long-term survival.

6. Addition of radiation therapy to chemotherapy in limited-stage small cell lung cancer can increase 5-year survival from about 11% to 20%.

7. Prophylactic cranial irradiation improves survival of limited-stage small cell lung cancer by another 5%.

8. Laser obliteration of tumor through bronchoscopy in presence of bronchial obstruction.

9. Radiation therapy for brain metastases, spinal cord compression, symptomatic masses, bone lesions.

10. Encourage cessation of smoking.

11. Pts with adenocarcinoma carcinoma (3% of all pts with lung cancer): 7% of these have activating mutations in the epidermal growth factor (EGF) receptor. These pts often respond to gefitinib or erlotinib, EGF receptor inhibitors. About 5% of these have activating rearrangements of the *alk* gene and may respond to crizotinib.

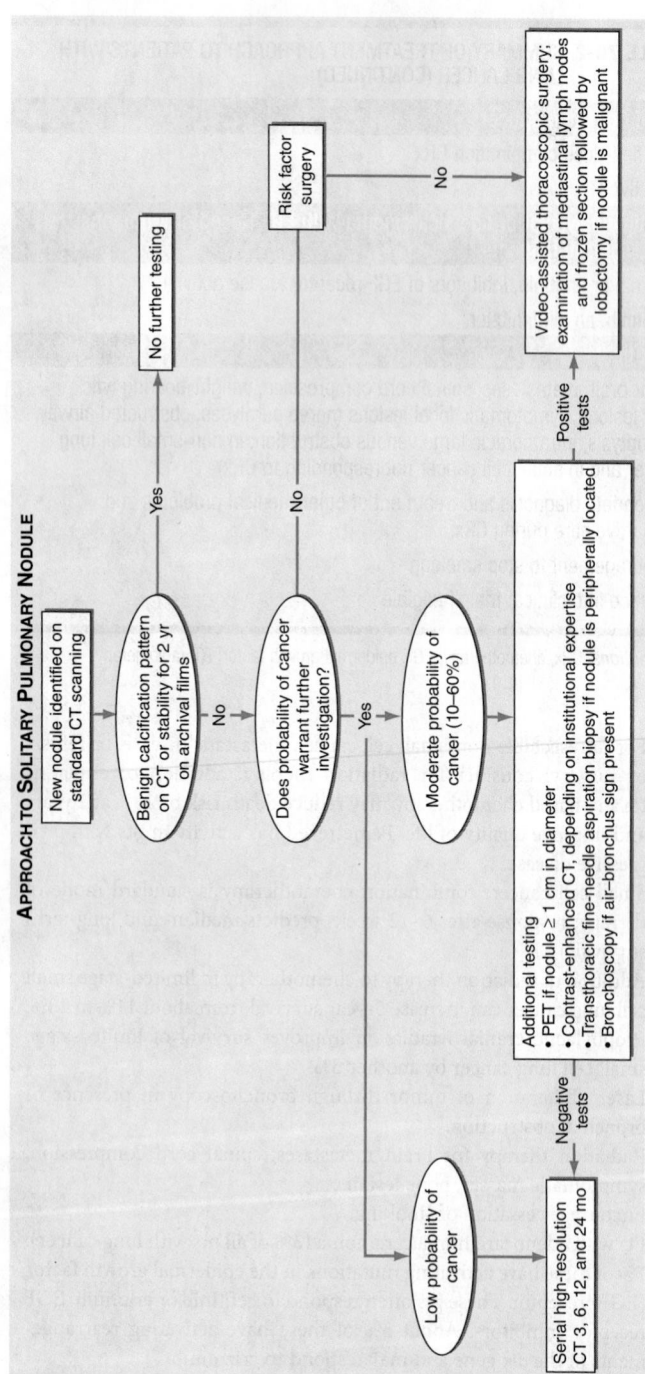

FIGURE 76-1 Approach to solitary pulmonary nodule.

■ PROGNOSIS

At time of diagnosis, only 20% of pts have localized disease. Overall 5-year survival is 30% for males and 50% for females with localized disease and 5% for pts with advanced disease.

■ SCREENING

The National Cancer Institute study of lung cancer screening of high risk pts (age 55 to 74 years with 30+ pack-year smoking history) with low-dose helical CT scan reduced lung cancer mortality by 20% but had only a small effect on overall mortality.

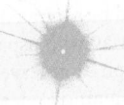

> For a more detailed discussion, see Horn L, Pao W, Johnson DH: Neoplasms of the Lung, Chap. 89, p. 737, in HPIM-18.

CHAPTER **77**
Breast Cancer

■ INCIDENCE AND EPIDEMIOLOGY

The most common tumor in women; 229,060 women in the United States have been diagnosed in 2012 and 40,000 died with breast cancer. Men also get breast cancer; F:M is 150:1. Breast cancer is hormone-dependent. Women with late menarche, early menopause, and first full-term pregnancy by age 18 have a significantly reduced risk. The average American woman has about a 1 in 9 lifetime risk of developing breast cancer. Dietary fat is a controversial risk factor. Oral contraceptives have little, if any, effect on risk and lower the risk of endometrial and ovarian cancer. Voluntary interruption of pregnancy does not increase risk. Estrogen replacement therapy may slightly increase the risk, but the beneficial effects of estrogen on quality of life, bone mineral density, and decreased risk of colorectal cancer appear to be somewhat outnumbered by increases in cardiovascular and thrombotic disease. Women who received therapeutic radiation before age 30 are at increased risk. Breast cancer risk is increased when a sister and mother also had the disease.

■ GENETICS

Perhaps 8–10% of breast cancer is familial. *BRCA-1* mutations account for about 5%. *BRCA-1* maps to chromosome 17q21 and appears to be involved in transcription-coupled DNA repair. Ashkenazi Jewish women have a 1% chance of having a common mutation (deletion of adenine and guanine at position 185). The *BRCA-1* syndrome includes an increased risk of ovarian cancer in women and prostate cancer in men. *BRCA-2* on chromosome 11 may account for 2–3% of breast cancer. Mutations are associated with an increased risk of breast cancer in men and women. Germ-line mutations in p53 (Li-Fraumeni syndrome) are very rare, but breast cancer, sarcomas, and other malignancies occur in such families. Germ-line mutations in *hCHK2* and *PTEN* may account for some familial breast cancer. Sporadic breast cancers show many genetic alterations, including overexpression of *HER2/neu* in 25% of cases, p53 mutations in 40%, and loss of heterozygosity at other loci.

■ DIAGNOSIS

Breast cancer is usually diagnosed by biopsy of a nodule detected by mammogram or by palpation. Women should be strongly encouraged to examine their breasts monthly. In premenopausal women, questionable or nonsuspicious (small) masses should be reexamined in 2–4 weeks (Fig. 77-1). A mass in a premenopausal woman that persists throughout her cycle and any mass in a postmenopausal woman should be aspirated. If the mass is a cyst filled with non-bloody fluid that goes away with aspiration, the pt is returned to routine screening. If the cyst aspiration leaves a residual mass or reveals bloody fluid, the pt should have a mammogram and excisional biopsy. If the mass is solid, the pt should undergo a mammogram and excisional biopsy. Screening mammograms performed every other year beginning at age 50 have been shown to save lives. The controversy regarding screening mammograms beginning at age 40 relates to the following

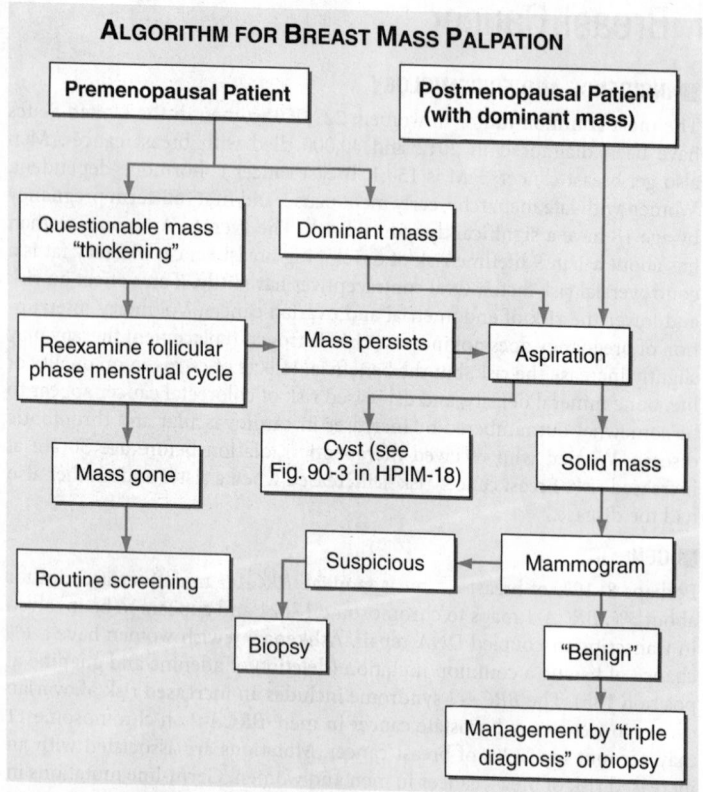

ALGORITHM FOR BREAST MASS PALPATION

FIGURE 77-1 Approach to a palpable breast mass.

facts: (1) the disease is much less common in the 40-to 49-year age group, and screening is generally less successful for less common problems; (2) workup of mammographic abnormalities in the 40- to 49-year age group less commonly diagnoses cancer; and (3) about 50% of women who are screened annually during their forties have an abnormality at some point that requires a diagnostic procedure (usually a biopsy), yet very few evaluations reveal cancer. However, many believe in the value of screening mammography beginning at age 40. After 13–15 years of follow-up, women who start screening at age 40 have a small survival benefit. Women with familial breast cancer more often have false-negative mammograms. MRI is a better screening tool in these women.

■ STAGING

Therapy and prognosis are dictated by stage of disease (Table 77-1). Unless the breast mass is large or fixed to the chest wall, staging of the ipsilateral axilla is performed at the time of lumpectomy (see below). Within pts of a given stage, individual characteristics of the tumor may influence prognosis: expression of estrogen receptor improves prognosis, while overexpression of *HER2/neu*, mutations in p53, high growth fraction, and aneuploidy worsen the prognosis. Breast cancer can spread almost anywhere but commonly goes to bone, lungs, liver, soft tissue, and brain.

TREATMENT	Breast Cancer

Five-year survival rate by stage is shown in Table 77-2. Treatment varies with stage of disease.

Ductal carcinoma in situ is noninvasive tumor present in the breast ducts. Treatment of choice is wide excision with breast radiation therapy. In one study, adjuvant tamoxifen further reduced the risk of recurrence.

Invasive breast cancer can be classified as operable, locally advanced, and metastatic. In operable breast cancer, outcome of primary therapy is the same with modified radical mastectomy or lumpectomy followed by breast radiation therapy. Axillary dissection may be replaced with sentinel node biopsy to evaluate node involvement. The sentinel node is identified by injecting a dye in the tumor site at surgery; the first node in which dye appears is the sentinel node. Women with tumors <1 cm and negative axillary nodes require no additional therapy beyond their primary lumpectomy and breast radiation. Adjuvant combination chemotherapy for 6 months appears to benefit premenopausal women with positive lymph nodes, pre- and postmenopausal women with negative lymph nodes but with large tumors or poor prognostic features, and postmenopausal women with positive lymph nodes whose tumors do not express estrogen receptors. Estrogen receptor–positive tumors >1 cm with or without involvement of lymph nodes are treated with aromatase inhibitors. Women who began treatment with tamoxifen before aromatase inhibitors were approved should switch to an aromatase inhibitor after 5 years of tamoxifen and continue for another 5 years.

Adjuvant chemotherapy is added to hormonal therapy in estrogen receptor–positive, node-positive women and is used without hormonal

TABLE 77-1 STAGING OF BREAST CANCER

Primary Tumor (T)	
T0	No evidence of primary tumor
TIS	Carcinoma in situ
T1	Tumor ≤2 cm
T1a	Tumor >0.1 cm but ≤0.5 cm
T1b	Tumor >0.5 but ≤1 cm
T1c	Tumor >1 cm but ≤2 cm
T2	Tumor >2 cm but ≤5 cm
T3	Tumor >5 cm
T4	Extension to chest wall, inflammation, satellite lesions, ulcerations

Regional Lymph Nodes (N)	
PN0(i–)	No regional lymph node metastasis histologically, negative IHC
PN0(i+)	No regional lymph node metastasis histologically, positive IHC, no IHC cluster greater than 0.2 mm
PN0(mol–)	No regional lymph node metastasis histologically, negative molecular findings (RT-PCR)
PN0(mol+)	No regional lymph node metastasis histologically, positive molecular findings (RT-PCR)
PN1	Metastasis in one to three axillary lymph nodes, or in internal mammary nodes with microscopic disease detected by sentinel lymph node dissection but not clinically apparent
PN1mi	Micrometastasis (>0.2 mm, none >2 mm)
PN1a	Metastasis in one to three axillary lymph nodes
PN1b	Metastasis in internal mammary nodes with microscopic disease detected by sentinel lymph node dissection but not *clinically apparent*[a]
PN1c	Metastasis in one to three axillary lymph nodes and in internal mammary lymph nodes with microscopic disease detected by sentinel lymph node dissection but not clinically apparent.[a] (If associated with greater than three positive axillary lymph nodes, the internal mammary nodes are classified as pN3b to reflect increased tumor burden.)
pN2	Metastasis in four to nine axillary lymph nodes, or in clinically apparent internal mammary lymph nodes in the *absence* of axillary lymph node metastasis
pN3	Metastasis in 10 or more axillary lymph nodes, or in infra-clavicular lymph nodes, or in clinically apparent[a] ipsilateral internal mammary lymph nodes in the *presence* of 1 or more positive axillary lymph nodes; or in more than 3 axillary lymph nodes with clinically negative microscopic metastasis in internal mammary lymph nodes; or in ipsilateral subcarinal lymph nodes

TABLE 77-1 STAGING OF BREAST CANCER (CONTINUED)

Distant Metastasis (M)		
M0	No distant metastasis	
M1	Distant metastasis (includes spread to ipsilateral supraclavicular nodes)	

Stage Grouping		
Stage 0	TIS	N0	M0
Stage I	T1	N0	M0
Stage IIA	T0	N1	M0
	T1	N1	M0
	T2	N0	M0
Stage IIB	T2	N1	M0
	T3	N0	M0
Stage IIIA	T0	N2	M0
	T1	N2	M0
	T2	N2	M0
	T3	N1, N2	M0
Stage IIIB	T4	Any N	M0
	Any T	N3	M0
Stage IIIC	Any T	N3	M0
Stage IV	Any T	Any N	M1

[a]Clinically apparent is defined as detected by imaging studies (excluding lymphoscintigraphy) or by clinical examination.

Abbreviations: IHC, immunohistochemistry; RT-PCR, reverse transcriptase/polymerase chain reaction.

Source: Used with permission of the American Joint Committee on Cancer (AJCC), Chicago, Illinois. The original source for this material is the *AJCC Cancer Staging Manual*, 7th ed. New York, Springer, 2010; *www.springeronline.com*.

therapy in estrogen receptor–negative node-positive women, whether they are pre- or postmenopausal. Various regimens have been used. The most effective regimen appears to be four cycles of doxorubicin, 60 mg/m^2, plus cyclophosphamide, 600 mg/m^2, IV on day 1 of each 3-week cycle followed by four cycles of paclitaxel, 175 mg/m^2, by 3-h infusion on day 1 of each 3-week cycle. In women with HER2+ tumors, trastuzumab augments the ability of chemotherapy to prevent recurrence. The activity of other combinations is being explored. In premenopausal women, ovarian ablation [e.g., with the luteinizing hormone–releasing hormone (LHRH) inhibitor goserelin] may be as effective as adjuvant chemotherapy.

Tamoxifen adjuvant therapy (20 mg/d for 5 years) or an aromatase inhibitor (anastrozole, letrozole, exemestane) is used for postmenopausal women with tumors expressing estrogen receptors whose nodes are

TABLE 77-2 5-YEAR SURVIVAL RATE FOR BREAST CANCER BY STAGE

Stage	5-Year Survival (Percentage of Patients)
0	99
I	92
IIA	82
IIB	65
IIIA	47
IIIB	44
IV	14

Source: Modified from data of the National Cancer Institute—Surveillance, Epidemiology, and End Results (SEER).

positive or whose nodes are negative but with large tumors or poor prognostic features. Breast cancer will recur in about half of pts with localized disease. High-dose adjuvant therapy with marrow support does not appear to benefit even women with high risk of recurrence.

Pts with locally advanced breast cancer benefit from neoadjuvant combination chemotherapy (e.g., CAF: cyclophosphamide 500 mg/m^2, doxorubicin 50 mg/m^2, and 5-fluorouracil 500 mg/m^2 all given IV on days 1 and 8 of a monthly cycle for 6 cycles) followed by surgery plus breast radiation therapy.

Treatment for metastatic disease depends on estrogen receptor status and treatment philosophy. No therapy is known to cure pts with metastatic disease. Randomized trials do not show that the use of high-dose therapy with hematopoietic stem cell support improves survival. Median survival is about 16 months with conventional treatment: aromatase inhibitors for estrogen receptor–positive tumors and combination chemotherapy for receptor-negative tumors. Pts whose tumors express *HER2/neu* have higher response rates by adding trastuzumab (anti-*HER2/neu*) to chemotherapy. Some advocate sequential use of active single agents in the setting of metastatic disease. Active agents in anthracycline- and taxane-resistant disease include capecitabine, vinorelbine, gemcitabine, irinotecan, and platinum agents. Pts progressing on adjuvant tamoxifen may benefit from an aromatase inhibitor such as letrozole or anastrozole. Half of pts who respond to one endocrine therapy will respond to another. Bisphosphonates reduce skeletal complications and may promote antitumor effects of other therapy. Radiation therapy is useful for palliation of symptoms.

◾ PREVENTION

Women with breast cancer have a 0.5% per year risk of developing a second breast cancer. Women at increased risk of breast cancer can reduce their risk by 49% by taking tamoxifen for 5 years. Aromatase inhibitors are probably at least as effective as tamoxifen and are under study. Women with *BRCA-1* mutations can reduce the risk by 90% with simple mastectomy.

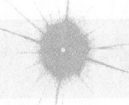

For a more detailed discussion, see Lippman ME: Breast Cancer, Chap. 90, p. 754, in HPIM-18.

CHAPTER **78**
Tumors of the Gastrointestinal Tract

ESOPHAGEAL CARCINOMA

In 2012 in the United States, 17,460 cases and 15,070 deaths; less frequent in women than men. Highest incidence in focal regions of China, Iran, Afghanistan, Siberia, Mongolia. In the United States, blacks more frequently affected than whites; usually presents sixth decade or later; 5-year survival <5% because most pts present with advanced disease.

Pathology

60% squamous cell carcinoma, most commonly in upper two-thirds; <40% adenocarcinoma, usually in distal third, arising in region of columnar metaplasia (Barrett's esophagus), glandular tissue, or as direct extension of proximal gastric adenocarcinoma; lymphoma and melanoma rare. 10% of all esophageal cancers occur in the upper third, 35% in the middle third, and 55% in the lower third.

Risk Factors

Major risk factors for squamous cell carcinoma: ethanol abuse, smoking (combination is synergistic); other risks: lye ingestion and esophageal stricture, radiation exposure, head and neck cancer, achalasia, smoked opiates, Plummer-Vinson syndrome, tylosis, chronic ingestion of extremely hot tea, deficiency of vitamin A, zinc, molybdenum. Barrett's esophagus is a risk for adenocarcinoma.

Clinical Features

Progressive dysphagia (first with solids, then liquids), rapid weight loss common, chest pain (from mediastinal spread), odynophagia, pulmonary aspiration (obstruction, tracheoesophageal fistula), hoarseness (laryngeal nerve palsy), hypercalcemia (parathyroid hormone–related peptide hypersecretion by squamous carcinomas); bleeding infrequent, occasionally severe; examination often unremarkable.

Diagnosis

Double-contrast barium swallow useful as initial test in dysphagia; flexible esophagogastroscopy most sensitive and specific test; pathologic confirmation by combining endoscopic biopsy and cytologic examination of mucosal brushings (neither alone sufficiently sensitive); CT and endoscopic ultrasonography valuable to assess local and nodal spread.

> **TREATMENT** Esophageal Carcinoma
>
> Surgical resection feasible in only 40% of pts; associated with high complication rate (fistula, abscess, aspiration). *Squamous cell carcinoma*: Surgical resection after chemotherapy [5-fluorouracil (5FU), cisplatin] plus radiation therapy prolongs survival and may provide improved cure rate. *Adenocarcinoma*: Curative resection rarely possible; <20% of pts with resectable tumors survive 5 years. Palliative measures include laser ablation, mechanical dilatation, radiotherapy, and a luminal prosthesis to bypass the tumor. Gastrostomy or jejunostomy are frequently required for nutritional support. Preoperative chemotherapy with concurrent radiation therapy is somewhat more effective but more toxic therapy.

GASTRIC CARCINOMA

Highest incidence in Japan, China, Chile, Ireland; incidence decreasing worldwide, eightfold in the United States over past 60 years; in 2012, 21,320 new cases and 10,540 deaths. Male:female = 2:1; peak incidence sixth and seventh decades; overall 5-year survival <15%.

Risk Factors

Increased incidence in lower socioeconomic groups; environmental component is suggested by studies of migrants and their offspring. Several dietary factors correlated with increased incidence: nitrates, smoked foods, heavily salted foods; genetic component suggested by increased incidence in first-degree relatives of affected pts; other risk factors: atrophic gastritis, *Helicobacter pylori* infection, Billroth II gastrectomy, gastrojejunostomy, adenomatous gastric polyps, pernicious anemia, hyperplastic gastric polyps (latter two associated with atrophic gastritis), Ménétrier's disease, slight increased risk with blood group A.

Pathology

Adenocarcinoma in 85%; usually focal (polypoid, ulcerative), two-thirds arising in antrum or lesser curvature, frequently ulcerative ("intestinal type"); less commonly diffuse infiltrative (linitis plastica) or superficial spreading (diffuse lesions more prevalent in younger pts; exhibit less geographic variation; have extremely poor prognosis); spreads primarily to local nodes, liver, peritoneum; systemic spread uncommon; lymphoma accounts for 15% (most frequent extranodal site in immunocompetent pts), either low-grade tumor of mucosa-associated lymphoid tissue (MALT) or aggressive diffuse large B cell lymphoma; leiomyosarcoma or gastrointestinal stromal tumor (GIST) is rare.

Clinical Features

Most commonly presents with progressive upper abdominal discomfort, frequently with weight loss, anorexia, nausea; acute or chronic GI bleeding (mucosal ulceration) common; dysphagia (location in cardia); vomiting (pyloric and widespread disease); early satiety; examination often unrevealing early in course; later, abdominal tenderness, pallor, and cachexia most common signs; palpable mass uncommon; metastatic spread may be manifest by hepatomegaly, ascites, left supraclavicular or scalene adenopathy, periumbilical, ovarian, or prerectal mass (Blumer's shelf), low-grade fever, skin abnormalities (nodules, dermatomyositis, acanthosis nigricans, or multiple seborrheic keratoses). Laboratory findings: iron-deficiency anemia in two-thirds of pts; fecal occult blood in 80%; rarely associated with pancytopenia and microangiopathic hemolytic anemia (from marrow infiltration), leukemoid reaction, migratory thrombophlebitis, or acanthosis nigricans.

Diagnosis

Double-contrast barium swallow useful; gastroscopy most sensitive and specific test; pathologic confirmation by biopsy and cytologic examination of mucosal brushings; superficial biopsies less sensitive for lymphomas (frequently submucosal); important to differentiate benign from malignant gastric ulcers with multiple biopsies and follow-up examinations to demonstrate ulcer healing.

| **TREATMENT** | Gastric Carcinoma |

Adenocarcinoma: Gastrectomy offers only chance of cure (only possible in less than one-third); the rare tumors limited to mucosa are resectable for cure in 80%; deeper invasion, nodal metastases decrease 5-year survival to 20% of pts with resectable tumors in absence of obvious metastatic spread (Table 78-1); CT and endoscopic ultrasonography may aid in determining tumor resectability. Subtotal gastrectomy has similar efficacy to total gastrectomy for distal stomach lesions, but with less morbidity; no clear benefit for resection of spleen and a portion of the pancreas, or for radical lymph node removal. Adjuvant chemotherapy (5FU/leucovorin) plus radiation therapy following primary surgery leads to a 7-month increase in median survival. Neoadjuvant chemotherapy with epirubicin, cisplatin, and 5FU may downstage tumors and increase the efficacy of surgery. Palliative therapy for pain, obstruction, and bleeding includes surgery, endoscopic dilatation, radiation therapy, chemotherapy.

Lymphoma: Low-grade MALT lymphoma is caused by *H. pylori* infection, and eradication of the infection causes complete remissions in 50% of pts; rest are responsive to combination chemotherapy including cyclophosphamide, doxorubicin, vincristine, prednisone (CHOP) plus rituximab. Diffuse large B cell lymphoma may be treated with either CHOP plus rituximab or subtotal gastrectomy followed by chemotherapy; 50–60% 5-year survival.

Leiomyosarcoma: Surgical resection curative in most pts. Tumors expressing the *c-kit* tyrosine kinase (CD117)—GIST—respond to imatinib mesylate in a substantial fraction of cases.

TABLE 78-1 STAGING SYSTEM FOR GASTRIC CARCINOMA

Stage	TNM	Features	Data from ACS	
			No. of Cases, %	5-Year Survival, %
0	T_{is}N0M0	Node negative; limited to mucosa	1	90
IA	T1N0M0	Node negative; invasion of lamina propria or submucosa	7	59
IB	T2N0M0 T1N1M0	Node negative; invasion of muscularis propria	10	44
II	T1N2M0 T2N1M0	Node positive; invasion beyond mucosa but within wall	17	29
		or		
	T3N0M0	Node negative; extension through wall		
IIIA	T2N2M0 T3N1-2M0	Node positive; invasion of muscularis propria or through wall	21	15
IIIB	T4N0-1M0	Node negative; adherence to surrounding tissue	14	9
IIIC	T4N2-3M0	>3 nodes positive; invasion of serosa or adjacent structures		
	T3N3M0	7 or more positive nodes; penetrates wall without invading serosa or adjacent structures		
IV	T4N2M0	Node positive; adherence to surrounding tissue	30	3
		or		
	T1-4N0-2-M1	Distant metastases		

Abbreviations: ACS, American Cancer Society; TNM, tumor, node, metastasis.

BENIGN GASTRIC TUMORS

Much less common than malignant gastric tumors; hyperplastic polyps most common, with adenomas, hamartomas, and leiomyomas rare; 30% of adenomas and occasional hyperplastic polyps are associated with gastric malignancy; polyposis syndromes include Peutz-Jeghers and familial polyposis (hamartomas and adenomas), Gardner's (adenomas), and Cronkhite-Canada (cystic polyps). See "Colonic Polyps," below.

Clinical Features

Usually asymptomatic; occasionally present with bleeding or vague epigastric discomfort.

| TREATMENT | Benign Gastric Tumors |

Endoscopic or surgical excision.

SMALL-BOWEL TUMORS

Clinical Features

Uncommon tumors (~5% of all GI neoplasms); usually present with bleeding, abdominal pain, weight loss, fever, or intestinal obstruction (intermittent or fixed); increased incidence of lymphomas in pts with gluten-sensitive enteropathy, Crohn's disease involving small bowel, AIDS, prior organ transplantation, autoimmune disorders.

Pathology

Usually benign; most common are adenomas (usually duodenal), leiomyomas (intramural), and lipomas (usually ileal); 50% of malignant tumors are adenocarcinoma, usually in duodenum (at or near ampulla of Vater) or proximal jejunum, commonly coexisting with benign adenomas; primary intestinal lymphomas (non-Hodgkin's) account for 25% and occur as focal mass (Western type), which is usually a T cell lymphoma associated with prior celiac disease, or diffuse infiltration (Mediterranean type), which is usually immunoproliferative small-intestinal disease (IPSID; α-heavy chain disease), a B-cell MALT lymphoma associated with *Campylobacter jejuni* infection, which can present as intestinal malabsorption; carcinoid tumors (usually asymptomatic) occasionally produce bleeding or intussusception (see below).

Diagnosis

Endoscopy and biopsy most useful for tumors of duodenum and proximal jejunum; otherwise barium x-ray examination best diagnostic test; direct small-bowel instillation of contrast (enteroclysis) occasionally reveals tumors not seen with routine small-bowel radiography; angiography (to detect plexus of tumor vessels) or laparotomy often required for diagnosis; CT useful to evaluate extent of tumor (esp. lymphomas).

| TREATMENT | Small-Bowel Tumors |

Surgical excision; adjuvant chemotherapy appears helpful for focal lymphoma; IPSID appears to be curable with combination chemotherapy used in aggressive lymphoma plus oral antibiotics (e.g., tetracycline); no proven role for chemotherapy or radiation therapy for other small-bowel tumors.

COLONIC POLYPS

■ TUBULAR ADENOMAS

Present in ~30% of adults; pedunculated or sessile; usually asymptomatic; ~5% cause occult blood in stool; may cause obstruction; overall risk of malignant degeneration correlates with size (<2% if <1.5 cm diam; >10% if >2.5 cm diam) and is higher in sessile polyps; 65% found in rectosigmoid colon; diagnosis by barium enema, sigmoidoscopy, or colonoscopy. *Treatment*: Full colonoscopy to detect synchronous lesions (present in 30%); endoscopic resection (surgery if polyp large or inaccessible by colonoscopy); follow-up surveillance by colonoscopy every 2–3 years.

■ VILLOUS ADENOMAS

Generally larger than tubular adenomas at diagnosis; often sessile; high risk of malignancy (up to 30% when >2 cm); more prevalent in left colon; occasionally associated with potassium-rich secretory diarrhea. *Treatment*: As for tubular adenomas.

■ HYPERPLASTIC POLYPS

Asymptomatic; usually incidental finding at colonoscopy; rarely >5 mm; no malignant potential. No treatment required.

■ HEREDITARY POLYPOSIS SYNDROMES

See Table 78-2.

1. *Familial polyposis coli* (FPC): Diffuse pancolonic adenomatous polyposis (up to several thousand polyps); autosomal dominant inheritance associated with deletion in adenomatous polyposis coli (APC) gene on chromosome 5; colon carcinoma from malignant degeneration of polyp in 100% by age 40. *Treatment*: Prophylactic total colectomy or subtotal colectomy with ileoproctostomy before age 30; subtotal resection avoids ileostomy but necessitates frequent proctoscopic surveillance; periodic colonoscopic or annual radiologic screening of siblings and offspring of pts with FPC until age 35; sulindac and other nonsteroidal anti-inflammatory drugs (NSAIDs) cause regression of polyps and inhibit their development.

2. *Gardner's syndrome*: Variant of FPC with associated soft tissue tumors (epidermoid cysts, osteomas, lipomas, fibromas, desmoids); higher incidence of gastroduodenal polyps, ampullary adenocarcinoma. *Treatment*: As for FPC; surveillance for small-bowel disease with fecal occult blood testing after colectomy.

3. *Turcot's syndrome*: Rare variant of FPC with associated malignant brain tumors. *Treatment*: As for FPC.

4. *Nonpolyposis syndrome*: Familial syndrome with up to 50% risk of colon carcinoma; peak incidence in fifth decade; associated with multiple primary cancers (esp. endometrial); autosomal dominant; due to defective DNA mismatch repair.

5. *Juvenile polyposis*: Multiple benign colonic and small-bowel hamartomas; intestinal bleeding common. Other symptoms: abdominal pain, diarrhea; occasional intussusception. Rarely recur after excision; low risk of

TABLE 78-2 HEREDITABLE (AUTOSOMAL DOMINANT)

Gastrointestinal Polyposis Syndromes

Syndrome	Distribution of Polyps	Histologic Type	Malignant Potential	Associated Lesions
Familial adenomatous polyposis	Large intestine	Adenoma	Common	None
Gardner's syndrome	Large and small intestines	Adenoma	Common	Osteomas, fibromas, lipomas, epidermoid cysts, ampullary cancers, congenital hypertrophy of retinal pigment epithelium
Turcot's syndrome	Large intestine	Adenoma	Common	Brain tumors
Nonpolyposis syndrome (Lynch syndrome)	Large intestine (often proximal)	Adenoma	Common	Endometrial and ovarian tumors
Peutz-Jeghers syndrome	Small and large intestines, stomach	Hamartoma	Rare	Mucocutaneous pigmentation; tumors of the ovary, breast, pancreas, endometrium
Juvenile polyposis	Large and small intestines, stomach	Hamartoma, rarely progressing to adenoma	Rare	Various congenital abnormalities

colon cancer from malignant degeneration of interspersed adenomatous polyps. Prophylactic colectomy controversial.

6. *Peutz-Jeghers syndrome*: Numerous hamartomatous polyps of entire GI tract, though denser in small bowel than colon; GI bleeding common; somewhat increased risk for the development of cancer at GI and non-GI sites. Prophylactic surgery not recommended.

COLORECTAL CANCER

Second most common internal cancer in humans; accounts for 10% of cancer-related deaths in United States; incidence increases dramatically above age 50, nearly equal in men and women. In 2012, 143,460 new cases, 51,690 deaths.

Etiology and Risk Factors

Most colon cancers arise from adenomatous polyps. Genetic steps from polyp to dysplasia to carcinoma in situ to invasive cancer have been defined, including point mutation in K-*ras* proto-oncogene, hypomethylation of DNA leading to enhanced gene expression, allelic loss at the *APC* gene (a tumor suppressor), allelic loss at the *DCC* (deleted in colon cancer) gene on chromosome 18, and loss and mutation of p53 on chromosome 17. Hereditary nonpolyposis colon cancer arises from mutations in the DNA mismatch repair genes, *hMSH2* gene on chromosome 2 and *hMLH1* gene on chromosome 3. Mutations lead to colon and other cancers. Diagnosis requires three or more relatives with colon cancer, one of whom is a first-degree relative; one or more cases diagnosed before age 50; and involvement of at least two generations. Environmental factors also play a role; increased prevalence in developed countries, urban areas, advantaged socioeconomic groups; increased risk in pts with hypercholesterolemia, coronary artery disease; correlation of risk with low-fiber, high-animal-fat diets, although direct effect of diet remains unproven; decreased risk with long-term dietary calcium supplementation and, possibly, daily aspirin ingestion. Risk increased in first-degree relatives of pts; families with increased prevalence of cancer; and pts with history of breast or gynecologic cancer, familial polyposis syndromes, >10-year history of ulcerative colitis or Crohn's colitis, >15-year history of ureterosigmoidostomy. Tumors in pts with strong family history of malignancy are frequently located in right colon and commonly present before age 50; high prevalence in pts with *Streptococcus bovis* bacteremia.

Pathology

Nearly always adenocarcinoma; 75% located distal to the splenic flexure (except in association with polyposis or hereditary cancer syndromes); may be polypoid, sessile, fungating, or constricting; subtype and degree of differentiation do not correlate with course. Degree of invasiveness at surgery (Dukes' classification) is single best predictor of prognosis (Fig. 78-1). Rectosigmoid tumors may spread to lungs early because of systemic paravertebral venous drainage of this area. Other predictors of poor prognosis: preoperative serum carcinoembryonic antigen (CEA) >5 ng/mL (>5 μg/L), poorly differentiated histology, bowel perforation, venous invasion, adherence to adjacent organs, aneuploidy, specific deletions in chromosomes 5, 17, 18, and mutation of *ras* proto-oncogene. 15% have defects in DNA repair.

Clinical Features

Left-sided colon cancers present most commonly with rectal bleeding, altered bowel habits (narrowing, constipation, intermittent diarrhea, tenesmus), and abdominal or back pain; cecal and ascending colon cancers more frequently present with symptoms of anemia, occult blood in stool, or weight loss; other complications: perforation, fistula, volvulus, inguinal hernia; laboratory findings: anemia in 50% of right-sided lesions.

Diagnosis

Early diagnosis aided by screening asymptomatic persons with fecal occult blood testing (see below); >50% of all colon cancers are within reach of a 60-cm flexible sigmoidoscope; air-contrast barium enema will diagnose ~85% of colon cancers not within reach of sigmoidoscope; colonoscopy

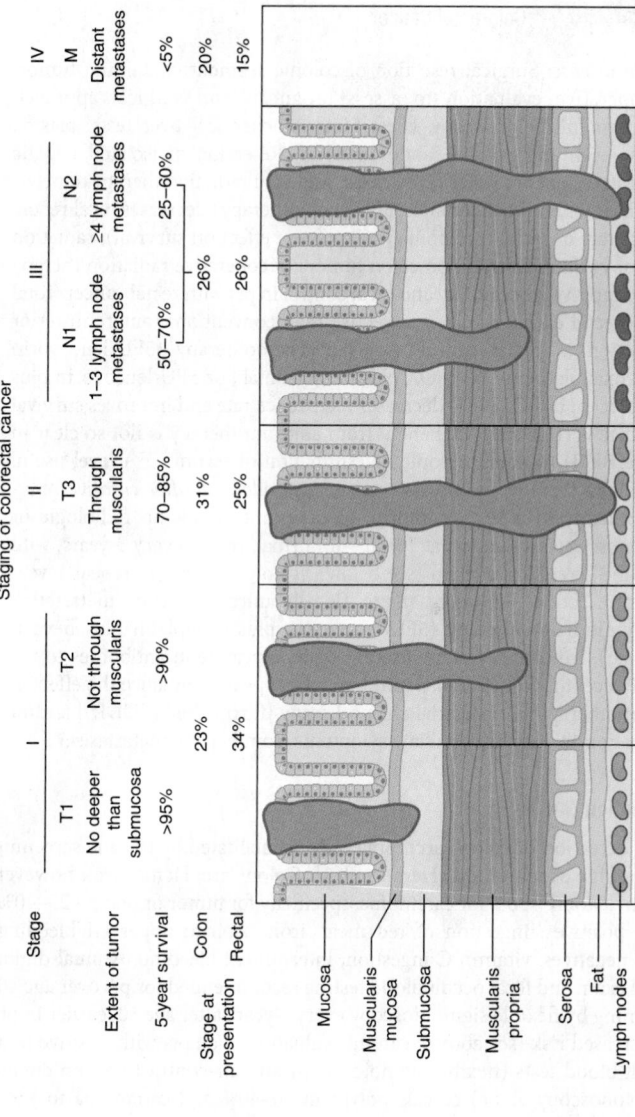

Staging of colorectal cancer

Stage	I		II	III		IV
	T1	T2	T3	N1	N2	M
Extent of tumor	No deeper than submucosa	Not through muscularis	Through muscularis	1–3 lymph node metastases	≥4 lymph node metastases	Distant metastases
5-year survival	>95%	>90%	70–85%	50–70%	25–60%	<5%
Stage at presentation Colon	23%		31%	26%		20%
Rectal	34%		25%	26%		15%

Mucosa
Muscularis mucosa
Submucosa
Muscularis propria
Serosa
Fat
Lymph nodes

FIGURE 78-1 Staging and prognosis for pts with colorectal cancer.

most sensitive and specific, permits tumor biopsy and removal of synchro-nous polyps (thus preventing neoplastic conversion), but is more expensive. Radiographic or virtual colonoscopy has not been shown to be a better diagnostic method than colonoscopy.

TREATMENT Colorectal Cancer

Local disease: Surgical resection of colonic segment containing tumor; preoperative evaluation to assess prognosis and surgical approach includes full colonoscopy, chest films, biochemical liver tests, plasma CEA level, and possible abdominal CT. Resection of isolated hepatic metastases possible in selected cases. Adjuvant radiation therapy to pelvis (with or without concomitant 5FU chemotherapy) decreases local recur-rence rate of rectal carcinoma (no apparent effect on survival); radiation therapy without benefit on colon tumors; preoperative radiation therapy may improve resectability and local control in pts with rectal cancer. Total mesorectal excision is more effective than conventional anteroposterior resection in rectal cancer. Adjuvant chemotherapy (5FU/leucovorin plus oxaliplatin, or FOLFOX plus bevacizumab, or 5FU/leucovorin plus irinotecan, or FOLFIRI) decreases recurrence rate and improves survival of stage C (III); survival benefit from adjuvant therapy is not so clear in stage B (II) tumors; periodic determination of serum CEA level useful to follow therapy and assess recurrence. *Follow-up after curative resec-tion*: Yearly liver tests, complete blood count, follow-up radiologic or colonoscopic evaluation at 1 year—if normal, repeat every 3 years, with routine screening interim (see below); if polyps detected, repeat 1 year after resection. *Advanced tumor* (locally unresectable or metastatic): Systemic chemotherapy (5FU/leucovorin plus oxaliplatin plus bevaci-zumab), irinotecan usually used in second treatment; antibodies to the EGF receptor (cetuximab, panitumumab) appear to enhance the effect of chemotherapy; intraarterial chemotherapy [floxuridine (FUDR)] and/or radiation therapy may palliate symptoms from hepatic metastases.

Prevention

Early detection of colon carcinoma may be facilitated by routine screening of stool for occult blood (Hemoccult II, ColonCare, Hemosure); however, sensitivity only ~50% for carcinoma; specificity for tumor or polyp ~25–40%. False positives: ingestion of red meat, iron, aspirin; upper GI bleeding. False negatives: vitamin C ingestion, intermittent bleeding. Annual digital rectal exam and fecal occult blood testing recommended for pts over age 40, screening by flexible sigmoidoscopy every 3 years after age 50, earlier in pts at increased risk (see above); careful evaluation of all pts with positive fecal occult blood tests (flexible sigmoidoscopy and air-contrast barium enema or colonoscopy alone) reveals polyps in 20–40% and carcinoma in ~5%; screening of asymptomatic persons allows earlier detection of colon cancer (i.e., earlier Dukes' stage) and achieves greater resectability rate; decreased overall mortality from colon carcinoma seen only after 13 years of follow-up. More intensive evaluation of first-degree relatives of pts with colon carcinoma frequently includes screening air-contrast barium enema or colonoscopy after age 40. NSAIDs and cyclooxygenase 2 inhibitors appear to prevent polyp development and induce regression in high-risk groups, but have not been recommended for average-risk pts at this time.

■ ANAL CANCER

Accounts for 1–2% of large-bowel cancer, 6230 cases and 780 deaths in 2012; associated with chronic irritation, e.g., from condyloma acuminata, perianal fissures/fistulas, chronic hemorrhoids, leukoplakia, trauma from anal intercourse. Women are more commonly affected than men. Homosexual men are at increased risk. Human papillomavirus is etiologic. Presents with bleeding, pain, and perianal mass. Radiation therapy plus chemotherapy (5FU and mitomycin) leads to complete response in 80% when the primary lesion is <3 cm. Abdominoperineal resection with permanent colostomy is reserved for those with large lesions or whose disease recurs after chemoradiotherapy.

BENIGN LIVER TUMORS

Hepatocellular adenomas occur most commonly in women in the third or fourth decades who take birth control pills. Most are found incidentally but may cause pain; intratumoral hemorrhage may cause circulatory collapse. 10% may become malignant. Women with these adenomas should stop taking birth control pills. Large tumors near the liver surface may be resected. Focal nodular hyperplasia is also more common in women but seems not to be caused by birth control pills. Lesions are vascular on angiography and have septae and are usually asymptomatic.

HEPATOCELLULAR CARCINOMA

About 28,720 cases in the United States in 2012, but worldwide this may be the most common tumor; 20,550 deaths in 2012 in US. Male:female = 4:1; tumor usually develops in cirrhotic liver in persons in fifth or sixth decade. High incidence in Asia and Africa is related to etiologic relationship between this cancer and hepatitis B and C infections. Aflatoxin exposure contributes to etiology and leaves a molecular signature, a mutation in codon 249 of the gene for p53.

Modes of Presentation

A pt with known liver disease develops an abnormality on ultrasound or rising α fetoprotein (AFP) or des-gamma-carboxy prothrombin (DCP) due to absence of vitamin K; abnormal liver function tests; cachexia, abdominal pain, fever.

Physical Findings

Jaundice, asthenia, itching, tremors, disorientation, hepatomegaly, splenomegaly, ascites, peripheral edema.

TREATMENT   Hepatocellular Carcinoma

Surgical resection or liver transplantation is therapeutic option but rarely successful. Radiofrequency ablation can cause regression of small tumors. Sorafenib may produce partial responses lasting a few months.

Screening and Prevention

Screening populations at risk has given conflicting results. Hepatitis B vaccine prevents the disease. Interferon α (IFN-α) may prevent liver cancer in persons with chronic active hepatitis C disease and possibly in those with hepatitis B. Ribavirin ± IFN-α is most effective treatment of chronic hepatitis C. Teleprevir, a protease inhibitor, is also active.

PANCREATIC CANCER

In 2012 in the United States, about 43,920 new cases and 27,390 deaths. The incidence is decreasing somewhat, but nearly all diagnosed cases are fatal. The tumors are ductal adenocarcinomas and are not usually detected until the disease has spread. About 70% of tumors are in the pancreatic head, 20% in the body, and 10% in the tail. Mutations in K-*ras* have been found in 85% of tumors, and the p16 cyclin-dependent kinase inhibitor on chromosome 9 may also be implicated. Long-standing diabetes, chronic pancreatitis, and smoking increase the risk; coffee-drinking, alcoholism, and cholelithiasis do not. Pts present with pain and weight loss, the pain often relieved by bending forward. Jaundice commonly complicates tumors of the head, due to biliary obstruction. Curative surgical resections are feasible in about 10%. Adjuvant chemotherapy (5FU) may benefit some pts after resection. Gemcitabine plus erlotinib or capecitabine may palliate symptoms in pts with advanced disease.

ENDOCRINE TUMORS OF THE GI TRACT AND PANCREAS

■ CARCINOID TUMOR

Carcinoid tumor accounts for 75% of GI endocrine tumors; incidence is about 15 cases per million population. 90% originate in Kulchitsky cells of the GI tract, most commonly the appendix, ileum, and rectum. Carcinoid tumors of the small bowel and bronchus have a more malignant course than tumors of other sites. About 5% of pts with carcinoid tumors develop symptoms of the carcinoid syndrome, the classic triad being cutaneous flushing, diarrhea, and valvular heart disease. For tumors of GI tract origin, symptoms imply metastases to liver.

Diagnosis can be made by detecting the site of tumor or documenting production of >15 mg/d of the serotonin metabolite 5-hydroxyindoleacetic acid (5-HIAA) in the urine. Octreotide scintigraphy identifies sites of primary and metastatic tumor in about two-thirds of cases.

TREATMENT Carcinoid Tumor

Surgical resection where feasible. Symptoms may be controlled with histamine blockers and octreotide, 150–1500 mg/d in three doses. Hepatic artery embolization and chemotherapy (5FU plus streptozocin or doxorubicin) have been used for metastatic disease. IFN-α at 3–10 million units SC three times a week may relieve symptoms. Prognosis ranges from 95% 5-year survival for localized disease to 20% 5-year survival for those with liver metastases. Median survival of pts with carcinoid syndrome is 2.5 years from the first episode of flushing.

■ PANCREATIC ISLET-CELL TUMORS

Gastrinoma, insulinoma, VIPoma, glucagonoma, and somatostatinoma account for the vast majority of pancreatic islet-cell tumors; their characteristics are shown in Table 78-3. The tumors are named for the dominant hormone they produce. They are generally slow-growing and produce symptoms related to hormone production. *Gastrinomas* and *peptic ulcer disease* constitute the Zollinger-Ellison syndrome. Gastrinomas are rare (4 cases per 10 million population), and in 25–50%, the tumor is a component of a multiple endocrine neoplasia type 1 (MEN 1) syndrome (Chap. 186).

Insulinoma may present with Whipple's triad: fasting hypoglycemia, symptoms of hypoglycemia, and relief after IV glucose. Normal or elevated serum insulin levels in the presence of fasting hypoglycemia are diagnostic. Insulinomas may also be associated with MEN 1.

Verner and Morrison described a syndrome of watery diarrhea, hypokalemia, achlorhydria, and renal failure associated with pancreatic islet tumors that produce vasoactive intestinal polypeptide (VIP). *VIPomas* are rare (1 case per 10 million) but often grow to a large size before producing symptoms.

TABLE 78-3 GASTROINTESTINAL ENDOCRINE TUMOR SYNDROMES

Syndrome	Cell Type	Clinical Features	Percentage Malignant	Major Products
Carcinoid syndrome	Enterochromaffin, enterochromaffin-like	Flushing, diarrhea, wheezing, hypotension	~100	Serotonin, histamine, miscellaneous peptides
Zollinger-Ellison, gastrinoma	Non-β islet cell, duodenal G cell	Peptic ulcers, diarrhea	~70	Gastrin
Insulinoma	Islet β cell	Hypoglycemia	~10	Insulin
VIPoma (Verner-Morrison, WDHA)	Islet D_1 cell	Diarrhea, hypokalemia, hypochlorhydria	~60	Vasoactive intestinal peptide
Glucagonoma	Islet A cell	Mild diabetes mellitus, erythema necrolytica migrans, glossitis	>75	Glucagon
Somatostatinoma	Islet D cell	Diabetes mellitus, diarrhea, steatorrhea, gallstones	~70	Somatostatin

Abbreviation: WDHA, watery diarrhea, hypokalemia, achlorhydria.

Glucagonoma is associated with diabetes mellitus and necrolytic migratory erythema, a characteristic red, raised, scaly rash usually located on the face, abdomen, perineum, and distal extremities. Glucagon levels >1000 ng/L not suppressed by glucose are diagnostic.

The classic triad of *somatostatinoma* is diabetes mellitus, steatorrhea, and cholelithiasis.

Provocative tests may facilitate diagnosis of functional endocrine tumors: tolbutamide enhances somatostatin secretion by somatostatinomas; pentagastrin enhances calcitonin secretion from medullary thyroid (C cell) tumors; secretin enhances gastrin secretion from gastrinomas. If imaging techniques fail to detect tumor masses, angiography or selective venous sampling for hormone determination may reveal the site of tumor. Metastases to nodes and liver should be sought by CT or MRI.

TREATMENT Pancreatic Islet-Cell Tumors

Tumor is surgically removed, if possible. Everolimus 10 mg PO qd or sunitinib 37.5 mg PO qd may produce meaningful delay (~12 months) in progressive disease and prolong survival in pts with metastatic disease. Octreotide inhibits hormone secretion in the majority of cases. IFN-α may reduce symptoms. Streptozotocin plus doxorubicin combination chemotherapy may produce responses in 60–90% of cases. Embolization or chemoembolization of hepatic metastases may be palliative.

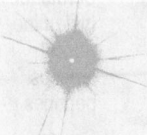
For a more detailed discussion, see Mayer RJ: Gastrointestinal Tract Cancer, Chap. 91, p. 764; Carr BI: Tumors of the Liver and Biliary Tree, Chap. 92, p. 777; Chong I, Cunningham D: Pancreatic Cancer, Chap. 93, p. 786; and Jensen RT: Endocrine Tumors of the Gastrointestinal Tract and Pancreas, Chap. 350, p. 3056, in HPIM-18.

CHAPTER **79**
Genitourinary Tract Cancer

BLADDER CANCER

■ INCIDENCE AND EPIDEMIOLOGY

Annual incidence in the United States is about 73,510 cases with 14,880 deaths. Median age is 65 years. Smoking accounts for 50% of the risk. Exposure to polycyclic aromatic hydrocarbons increases the risk, especially in slow acetylators. Risk is increased in chimney sweeps, dry cleaners, and those involved in aluminum manufacturing. Chronic cyclophosphamide exposure increases risk ninefold. *Schistosoma haematobium* infection also increases risk, especially of squamous histology.

■ ETIOLOGY

Lesions involving chromosome 9q are an early event. Deletions in 17p (p53), 18q (the DCC locus), 13q (RB), 3p, and 5q are characteristic of invasive lesions. Overexpression of epidermal growth factor receptors and *HER2/neu* receptors is common.

■ PATHOLOGY

Over 90% of tumors are derived from transitional epithelium; 3% are squamous, 2% are adenocarcinomas, and <1% are neuroendocrine small cell tumors. Field effects are seen that place all sites lined by transitional epithelium at risk, including the renal pelvis, ureter, bladder, and proximal two-thirds of the urethra; 90% of tumors are in the bladder, 8% in the renal pelvis, and 2% in the ureter or urethra. Histologic grade influences survival. Lesion recurrence is influenced by size, number, and growth pattern of the primary tumor.

■ CLINICAL PRESENTATION

Hematuria is the initial sign in 80–90%; however, cystitis is a more common cause of hematuria (22% of all hematuria) than is bladder cancer (15%). Pts are initially staged and treated by endoscopy. Superficial tumors are removed at endoscopy; muscle invasion requires more extensive surgery.

TREATMENT Bladder Cancer

Management is based on extent of disease: superficial, invasive, or metastatic. Frequency of presentation is 75% superficial, 20% invasive, and 5% metastatic. Superficial lesions are resected at endoscopy. Although complete resection is possible in 80%, 30–80% of cases recur; grade and stage progression occur in 30%. Intravesical instillation of bacille Calmette-Guérin (BCG) reduces the risk of recurrence by 40–45%. Recurrence is monitored every 3 months.

The standard management of muscle-invasive disease is radical cystectomy. 5-year survival is 70% for those without invasion of perivesicular fat or lymph nodes, 50% for those with invasion of fat but not lymph nodes, 35% for those with one node involved, and 10% for those with six or more involved nodes. Pts who cannot withstand radical surgery may have 30–35% 5-year survival with 5000- to 7000-cGy external beam radiation therapy. Bladder sparing may be possible in up to 45% of pts with two cycles of chemotherapy with CMV (methotrexate, 30 mg/m² days 1 and 8, vinblastine, 4 mg/m² days 1 and 8, cisplatin, 100 mg/m² day 2, q21d) followed by 4000-cGy radiation therapy given concurrently with cisplatin.

Metastatic disease is treated with combination chemotherapy. Useful regimens include CMV (see above), M-VAC (methotrexate, 30 mg/m² days 1, 15, 22; vinblastine, 3 mg/m² days 2, 15, 22; doxorubicin, 30 mg/m² day 2; cisplatin, 70 mg/m² day 2; q28d) or cisplatin (70 mg/m² day 2) plus gemcitabine (1000 mg/m² days 1, 8, 15 of a 28-day cycle) or carboplatin plus paclitaxel. About 70% of pts respond to treatment, and 20% have a complete response; 10–15% have long-term disease-free survival.

RENAL CANCER

■ INCIDENCE AND EPIDEMIOLOGY

Annual incidence in the United States is about 65,000 cases with 13,500 deaths. Cigarette smoking accounts for 20–30% of cases. Risk is increased in acquired renal cystic disease. There are two familial forms: a rare autosomal dominant syndrome and von Hippel–Lindau disease. About 35% of pts with von Hippel–Lindau disease develop renal cancer. Incidence is also increased in those with tuberous sclerosis and polycystic kidney disease.

■ ETIOLOGY

Most cases are sporadic; however, the most frequent chromosomal abnormality (occurs in 60%) is deletion or rearrangement of 3p21-26. The von Hippel–Lindau gene has been mapped to that region and appears to have ubiquitin ligase activities that influence regulation of speed of transcription and turnover of damaged proteins. It is unclear how lesions in the gene lead to cancer.

■ PATHOLOGY

Five variants are recognized: clear cell tumors (75%), chromophilic tumors (15%), chromophobic tumors (5%), oncocytic tumors (3%), and collecting duct tumors (2%). Clear cell tumors arise from cells of the proximal convoluted tubules. Chromophilic tumors tend to be bilateral and multifocal and often show trisomy 7 and/or trisomy 17. Chromophobic and eosinophilic tumors less frequently have chromosomal aberrations and follow a more indolent course.

■ CLINICAL PRESENTATION

The classic triad of hematuria, flank pain, and flank mass is seen in only 10–20% of pts; hematuria (40%), flank pain (40%), palpable mass (33%), and weight loss (33%) are the most common individual symptoms. Paraneoplastic syndromes of erythrocytosis (3%), hypercalcemia (5%), and nonmetastatic hepatic dysfunction (Stauffer's syndrome) (15%) may also occur. Workup should include IV pyelography, renal ultrasonography, CT of abdomen and pelvis, chest x-ray (CXR), urinalysis, and urine cytology. Stage I is disease restricted to the kidney, stage II is disease contained within Gerota's fascia, stage III is locally invasive disease involving nodes and/or inferior vena cava, stage IV is invasion of adjacent organs or metastatic sites. Prognosis is related to stage: 66% 5-year survival for I, 64% for II, 42% for III, and 11% for IV.

> **TREATMENT**   Renal Cancer
>
> Radical nephrectomy is standard for stage I, II, and most stage III pts. Surgery may also be indicated in the setting of metastatic disease for intractable local symptoms (bleeding, pain). Response rates of 40–48% have been noted with three different single agents, sunitinib (50 mg/d 4 weeks out of 6), sorafenib (400 mg bid), and temsirolimus (25 mg IV weekly). Sunitinib and sorafenib are thought to be antiangiogenic through inhibition of kinases in tumor cells. Temsirolimus is an inhibitor of mTOR. About 10–15% of pts with advanced-stage disease may benefit from interleukin 2 and/or interferon α (IFN-α). Addition of bevacizumab to IFN-α improves the response rate. Some remissions are durable. Chemotherapy is of little or no benefit.

TESTICULAR CANCER

■ INCIDENCE AND EPIDEMIOLOGY

Annual incidence is about 8590 cases with 360 deaths. Peak age incidence is 20–40. Occurs 4–5 times more frequently in white than black men. Cryptorchid testes are at increased risk. Early orchiopexy may protect against testis cancer. Risk is also increased in testicular feminization syndromes, and Klinefelter syndrome is associated with mediastinal germ cell tumor.

■ ETIOLOGY

The cause is unknown. Disease is associated with a characteristic cytogenetic defect, isochromosome 12p.

■ PATHOLOGY

Two main subtypes are noted: seminoma and nonseminoma. Each accounts for ~50% of cases. Seminoma has a more indolent natural history and is highly sensitive to radiation therapy. Four subtypes of nonseminoma are defined: embryonal carcinoma, teratoma, choriocarcinoma, and endodermal sinus (yolk sac) tumor.

■ CLINICAL PRESENTATION

Painless testicular mass is the classic initial sign. In the presence of pain, differential diagnosis includes epididymitis or orchitis; a brief trial of antibiotics may be undertaken. Staging evaluation includes measurement of serum tumor markers α fetoprotein (AFP) and β-human chorionic gonadotropin (hCG), CXR, and CT scan of abdomen and pelvis. Lymph nodes are staged at resection of the primary tumor through an inguinal approach. Stage I disease is limited to the testis, epididymis, or spermatic cord; stage II involves retroperitoneal nodes; and stage III is disease outside the retroperitoneum. Among seminoma pts, 70% are stage I, 20% are stage II, and 10% are stage III. Among nonseminoma germ cell tumor pts, 33% are found in each stage. hCG may be elevated in either seminoma or nonseminoma, but AFP is elevated only in nonseminoma. 95% of pts are cured if treated appropriately. Primary nonseminoma in the mediastinum is associated with acute leukemia or other hematologic disorders and has a poorer prognosis than testicular primaries (~33%).

TREATMENT   Testicular Cancer (Table 79-1)

For stages I and II seminoma, inguinal orchiectomy followed by retroperitoneal radiation therapy to 2500–3000 cGy is effective. For stages I and II nonseminoma germ cell tumors, inguinal orchiectomy followed by retroperitoneal lymph node dissection is effective. For pts of either histology with bulky nodes or stage III disease, chemotherapy is given. Cisplatin (20 mg/m² days 1–5), etoposide (100 mg/m² days 1–5), and bleomycin (30 U days 2, 9, 16) given every 21 days for four cycles is the standard therapy. If tumor markers return to zero, residual masses are resected. Most are necrotic debris or teratomas. Salvage therapy rescues about 25% of those not cured with primary therapy.

TABLE 79-1 GERM CELL TUMOR STAGING AND TREATMENT

Stage	Extent of Disease	Treatment Seminoma	Nonseminoma
IA	Testis only, no vascular/lymphatic invasion (T1)	Radiation therapy	RPLND or observation
IB	Testis only, with vascular/lymphatic invasion (T2), or extension through tunica albuginea (T2), or involvement of spermatic cord (T3) or scrotum (T4)	Radiation therapy	RPLND or chemotherapy
IIA	Nodes <2 cm	Radiation therapy	RPLND ± adjuvant chemotherapy or chemotherapy followed by RPLND
IIB	Nodes 2–5 cm	Radiation therapy or chemotherapy	Chemotherapy, often followed by RPLND
IIC	Nodes >5 cm	Chemotherapy	Chemotherapy, often followed by RPLND
III	Distant metastases	Chemotherapy	Chemotherapy, often followed by surgery (biopsy or resection)

Abbreviation: RPLND, retroperitoneal lymph node dissection.

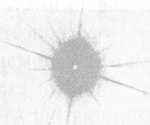

For a more detailed discussion, see Scher HI, Motzer RJ: Bladder and Renal Cell Carcinomas, Chap. 94, p. 790; and Motzer RJ, Bosl GJ: Testicular Cancer, Chap. 96, p. 806, in HPIM-18.

CHAPTER **80**
Gynecologic Cancer

OVARIAN CANCER

■ INCIDENCE AND EPIDEMIOLOGY

Annually in the United States, about 22,000 new cases are found and 15,500 women die of ovarian cancer. Incidence begins to rise in the fifth decade, peaking in the eighth decade. Risk is increased in nulliparous women and reduced by pregnancy (risk decreased about 10% per pregnancy) and oral contraceptives. About 5% of cases are familial.

■ GENETICS

Mutations in *BRCA-1* predispose women to both breast and ovarian cancer. Cytogenetic analysis of epithelial ovarian cancers that are not familial often reveals complex karyotypic abnormalities, including structural lesions on chromosomes 1 and 11 and loss of heterozygosity for loci on chromosomes 3q, 6q, 11q, 13q, and 17. C-*myc*, H-*ras*, K-*ras*, and *HER2/neu* are often mutated or overexpressed. Unlike in colon cancer, a stepwise pathway to ovarian carcinoma is not apparent. Ovarian cancers may also occur in the setting of Lynch syndrome, inherited nonpolyposis colorectal cancer, due to mutations in the genes that repair DNA mismatches. The subset of women with endometrioid histology often have a mutation in ARID1A, a DNA repair complex component.

■ SCREENING

No benefit has been seen from screening women of average risk. Hereditary ovarian cancer accounts for 10% of all cases. Women with *BRCA-1* or *-2* mutations should consider prophylactic bilateral salpingo-oophorectomy by age 40.

■ CLINICAL PRESENTATION

Most pts present with abdominal pain, bloating, urinary symptoms, and weight gain indicative of disease spread beyond the true pelvis. Localized ovarian cancer is usually asymptomatic and detected on routine pelvic examination as a palpable nontender adnexal mass. Most ovarian masses detected incidentally in ovulating women are ovarian cysts that resolve over one to three menstrual cycles. Adnexal masses in postmenopausal women are more often pathologic and should be surgically removed. CA-125 serum levels are ≥35 U/mL in 80–85% of women with ovarian cancer, but other conditions may also cause elevations.

■ PATHOLOGY

Half of ovarian tumors are benign, one-third are malignant, and the rest are tumors of low malignant potential. These borderline lesions have cytologic features of malignancy but do not invade. Malignant epithelial tumors may be of five different types: serous (50%), mucinous (25%), endometrioid (15%), clear cell (5%), and Brenner tumors (1%, derived from urothelial or transitional epithelium). The remaining 4% of ovarian tumors are stromal or germ cell tumors, which are managed like testicular cancer in men (Chap. 79). Histologic grade is an important prognostic factor for the epithelial varieties.

■ STAGING

Extent of disease is ascertained by a surgical procedure that permits visual and manual inspection of all peritoneal surfaces and the diaphragm. Total abdominal hysterectomy, bilateral salpingo-oophorectomy, partial omentectomy, pelvic and paraaortic lymph node sampling, and peritoneal washings should be performed. The staging system and its influence on survival are shown in Table 80-1. About 23% of pts are stage I, 13% are stage II, 47% are stage III, and 16% are stage IV.

TABLE 80-1 STAGING AND SURVIVAL IN GYNECOLOGIC MALIGNANCIES

Stage	Ovarian	5-Year Survival, %	Endometrial	5-Year Survival, %	Cervical	5-Year Survival, %
0	—		—		Carcinoma in situ	100
I	Confined to ovary	90–95	Confined to corpus	89	Confined to uterus	85
II	Confined to pelvis	70–80	Involves corpus and cervix	73	Invades beyond uterus but not pelvic wall	65
III	Intraabdominal spread	25–50	Extends outside the uterus but not outside the true pelvis	52	Extends to pelvic wall and/ or lower third of vagina, or hydronephrosis	35
IV	Spread outside abdomen	1–5	Extends outside the true pelvis or involves the bladder or rectum	17	Invades mucosa of bladder or rectum or extends beyond the true pelvis	7

TREATMENT Ovarian Cancer

Pts with stage I disease, no residual tumor after surgery, and well- or moderately differentiated tumors need no further treatment after surgery and have a 5-year survival of >95%. For stage II pts totally resected and stage I pts with poor histologic grade, adjuvant therapy with single-agent cisplatin or cisplatin plus paclitaxel produces 5-year survival of 80%. Advanced-stage pts should receive paclitaxel, 175 mg/m^2 by 3-h infusion, followed by carboplatin dosed to an area under the curve (AUC) of 7.5 every 3 or 4 weeks. Carboplatin dose is calculated by the Calvert formula: dose = target AUC × (glomerular filtration rate + 25). The complete response rate is about 55%, and median survival is 38 months.

ENDOMETRIAL CANCER

■ INCIDENCE AND EPIDEMIOLOGY

The most common gynecologic cancer—47,000 cases are diagnosed in the United States and 8010 pts die annually. It is primarily a disease of postmenopausal women. Obesity, altered menstrual cycles, infertility, late menopause, and postmenopausal bleeding are commonly encountered in women with endometrial cancer. Women taking tamoxifen to prevent breast cancer recurrence and those taking estrogen replacement therapy are at a modestly increased risk. Peak incidence is in the sixth and seventh decades.

■ CLINICAL PRESENTATION

Abnormal vaginal discharge (90%), abnormal vaginal bleeding (80%), and leukorrhea (10%) are the most common symptoms.

■ PATHOLOGY

Endometrial cancers are adenocarcinomas in 75–80% of cases. The remaining cases include mucinous carcinoma; papillary serous carcinoma; and secretory, ciliate, and clear cell varieties. Prognosis depends on stage, histologic grade, and degree of myometrial invasion.

■ STAGING

Total abdominal hysterectomy and bilateral salpingo-oophorectomy constitute both the staging procedure and the treatment of choice. The staging scheme and its influence on prognosis are shown in Table 80-1. About 75% of pts are stage I, 13% are stage II, 9% are stage III, and 3% are stage IV.

TREATMENT Endometrial Cancer

In women with poor histologic grade, deep myometrial invasion, or extensive involvement of the lower uterine segment or cervix, intracavitary or external-beam radiation therapy is given. If cervical invasion is deep, preoperative radiation therapy may improve the resectability of the tumor. Stage III disease is managed with surgery and radiation therapy. Stage IV disease is usually treated palliatively. Progestational agents such as hydroxy-progesterone or megestrol and the antiestrogen tamoxifen may produce responses in 20% of pts. Doxorubicin, 60 mg/m^2 IV day 1, and cisplatin, 50 mg/m^2 IV day 1, every 3 weeks for 8 cycles produces a 45% response rate.

CERVICAL CANCER

■ INCIDENCE AND EPIDEMIOLOGY

In the United States about 12,120 cases of invasive cervical cancer are diagnosed each year and 50,000 cases of carcinoma in situ are detected by Pap smear. Cervical cancer kills 4220 women a year, 85% of whom never had a Pap smear. It is a major cause of disease in underdeveloped countries and is more common in lower socioeconomic groups, in women with early sexual activity and/or multiple sexual partners, and in smokers. Human papilloma virus (HPV) types 16 and 18 are the major types associated with cervical cancer. The virus attacks the G$_1$ checkpoint of the cell cycle; its E7 protein binds and inactivates Rb protein, and E6 induces the degradation of p53.

■ SCREENING

Women should begin screening when they begin sexual activity or at age 20. After two consecutive negative annual Pap smears, the test should be repeated every 3 years. Abnormal smears dictate the need for a cervical biopsy, usually under colposcopy, with the cervix painted with 3% acetic acid, which shows abnormal areas as white patches. If there is evidence of carcinoma in situ, a cone biopsy is performed, which is therapeutic.

■ PREVENTION

Women and children age 9–26 should consider vaccination with Gardasil to prevent infection with two serotypes of virus (16 and 18) that cause 70% of the cervical cancer in the United States.

■ CLINICAL PRESENTATION

Pts present with abnormal bleeding or postcoital spotting or menometror-rhagia or intermenstrual bleeding. Vaginal discharge, low back pain, and urinary symptoms also may be present.

■ STAGING

Staging is clinical and consists of a pelvic exam under anesthesia with cystoscopy and proctoscopy. Chest x-ray, IV pyelography, and abdominal CT are used to search for metastases. The staging system and its influence on prognosis are shown in Table 80-1. At presentation, 47% of pts are stage I, 28% are stage II, 21% are stage III, and 4% are stage IV.

TREATMENT Cervical Cancer

Carcinoma in situ is cured with cone biopsy. Stage I disease may be treated with radical hysterectomy or radiation therapy. Stages II–IV disease are usually treated with radiation therapy, often with both brachytherapy and teletherapy, or combined-modality therapy. Pelvic exenteration is used uncommonly to control the disease, especially in the setting of centrally recurrent or persistent disease. Women with locally advanced (stage IIB to IVA) disease usually receive concurrent chemotherapy and radiation therapy. The chemotherapy acts as a radiosensitizer. Hydroxyurea, 5-fluorouracil (5FU), and cisplatin have all shown promising results given concurrently with radiation therapy. Cisplatin, 75 mg/m^2 IV over 4 h on day 1, and 5FU, 4 g given by 96-h infusion on days 1–5 of radiation therapy, is a common regimen. Relapse rates are reduced 30–50% by such therapy. Advanced-stage disease is treated palliatively with single agents (cisplatin, irinotecan, ifosfamide).

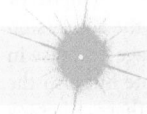

For a more detailed discussion, see Seiden MV: Gynecologic Malignancies, Chap. 97, p. 810, in HPIM-18.

CHAPTER **81**
Prostate Hyperplasia and Carcinoma

PROSTATE HYPERPLASIA

Enlargement of the prostate is nearly universal in aging men. Hyperplasia usually begins by age 45 years, occurs in the area of the prostate gland surrounding the urethra, and produces urinary outflow obstruction. Symptoms develop on average by age 65 in whites and 60 in blacks. Symptoms develop late because hypertrophy of the bladder detrusor compensates for ureteral compression. As obstruction progresses, urinary stream caliber and force diminish, hesitancy in stream initiation develops, and postvoid dribbling occurs. Dysuria and urgency are signs of bladder irritation (perhaps due to inflammation or tumor) and are usually not seen in prostate hyperplasia. As the postvoid residual increases, nocturia and overflow incontinence may develop. Common medications such as tranquilizing drugs and decongestants, infections, or alcohol may precipitate urinary retention. Because of the prevalence of hyperplasia, the relationship to neoplasia is unclear.

On digital rectal exam (DRE), a hyperplastic prostate is smooth, firm, and rubbery in consistency; the median groove may be lost. Prostate-specific antigen (PSA) levels may be elevated but are ≤10 ng/mL unless cancer is also present (see below). Cancer may also be present at lower levels of PSA.

TREATMENT Prostate Hyperplasia

Asymptomatic pts do not require treatment, and those with complications of urethral obstruction such as inability to urinate, renal failure, recurrent urinary tract infection, hematuria, or bladder stones clearly require surgical extirpation of the prostate, usually by transurethral resection (TURP). However, the approach to the remaining pts should be based on the degree of incapacity or discomfort from the disease and the likely side effects of any intervention. If the pt has only mild symptoms, watchful waiting is not harmful and permits an assessment of the rate of symptom progression. If therapy is desired by the pt, two medical approaches may be helpful: terazosin, an α_1-adrenergic blocker (1 mg at bedtime, titrated to symptoms up to 20 mg/d), relaxes the smooth muscle of the bladder neck and increases urine flow; finasteride (5 mg/d) or dutasteride (2.5 mg/d), inhibitors of 5α-reductase, block the conversion of testosterone to dihydrotestosterone and cause an average decrease in prostate size of ~24%. TURP has the greatest success rate but also the greatest risk of complications. Transurethral microwave thermotherapy (TUMT) may be comparably effective to TURP. Direct comparison has not been made between medical and surgical management.

PROSTATE CARCINOMA

Prostate cancer has been diagnosed in 241,740 men in 2012 in the United States—an incidence comparable to that of breast cancer. About 28,170 men have died of prostate cancer in 2012. The early diagnosis of cancers in mildly symptomatic men found on screening to have elevated serum levels of PSA has complicated management. Like most other cancers, incidence is age-related. The disease is more common in blacks than whites. Symptoms are generally similar to and indistinguishable from those of prostate hyperplasia, but those with cancer more often have dysuria and back or hip pain. On histology, 95% are adenocarcinomas. Biologic behavior is affected by histologic grade (Gleason score).

In contrast to hyperplasia, prostate cancer generally originates in the periphery of the gland and may be detectable on DRE as one or more nodules on the posterior surface of the gland, hard in consistency and irregular in shape. An approach to diagnosis is shown in Fig. 81-1. Those with a negative DRE and PSA ≤4 ng/mL may be followed annually. Those with an abnormal DRE or a PSA >10 ng/mL should undergo transrectal ultrasound (TRUS)-guided biopsy. Those with normal DRE and PSA of 4.1–10 ng/mL may be handled differently in different centers. Some would perform TRUS and biopsy any abnormality or follow if no abnormality were found. Some would repeat the PSA in a year and biopsy if the increase over that period were >0.75 ng/mL. Other methods of using PSA to distinguish early cancer from hyperplasia include quantitating bound and free PSA and relating the PSA to the size of the prostate (PSA density). Perhaps one-third of persons with prostate cancer do not have PSA elevations.

Lymphatic spread is assessed surgically; it is present in only 10% of those with Gleason grade 5 or lower and in 70% of those with grade 9 or 10. PSA

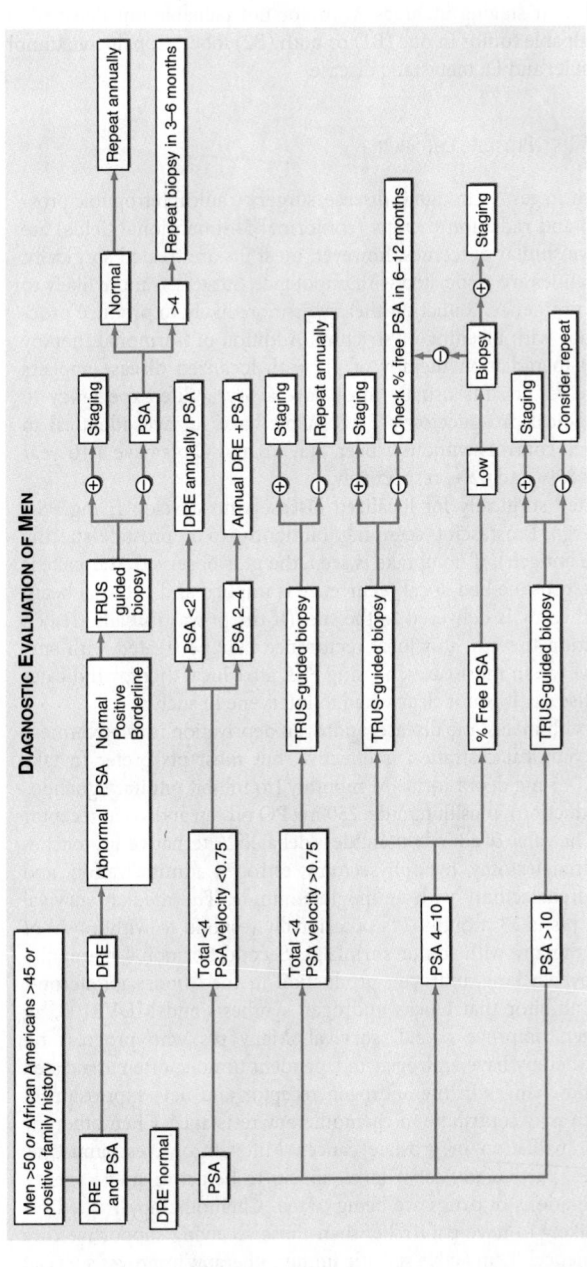

FIGURE 81-1 The use of the annual digital rectal examination (DRE) and measurement of prostate-specific antigen (PSA) as guides for deciding which men should have transrectal ultrasound (TRUS)-guided prostate biopsy. There are at least three schools of thought about what to do if the DRE is negative and the PSA is equivocal (4.1 to 10 ng/mL).

471

level also correlates with spread; only 10% of those with PSA <10 ng/mL have lymphatic spread. Bone is the most common site of distant metastasis. Whitmore-Jewett staging includes A: tumor not palpable but detected at TURP; B: palpable tumor in one (B1) or both (B2) lobes; C: palpable tumor outside capsule; and D: metastatic disease.

TREATMENT   Prostate Carcinoma

For pts with stages A through C disease, surgery (radical retropubic prostatectomy) and radiation therapy (conformal 3-dimensional fields) are said to have similar outcomes; however, most pts are treated surgically. Both modalities are associated with impotence. Surgery is more likely to lead to incontinence. Radiation therapy is more likely to produce proctitis, perhaps with bleeding or stricture. Addition of hormonal therapy (goserelin) to radiation therapy of pts with localized disease appears to improve results. Pts usually must have a 5-year life expectancy to undergo radical prostatectomy. Stage A pts have survival identical to age-matched controls without cancer. Stage B and C pts have a 10-year survival of 82% and 42%, respectively.

Pts treated surgically for localized disease who develop rising PSA may undergo Prostascint scanning (antibody to a prostate-specific membrane antigen). If no uptake is seen, the pt is observed. If uptake is seen in the prostate bed, local recurrence is implied and external beam radiation therapy is delivered to the site. (If the pt was initially treated with radiation therapy, this local recurrence may be treated with surgery.) However, in most cases, a rising PSA after local therapy indicates systemic disease. It is not clear when to intervene in such pts.

For pts with metastatic disease, androgen deprivation is the treatment of choice. Surgical castration is effective, but most pts prefer to take leuprolide, 7.5 mg depot form IM monthly (to inhibit pituitary gonadotropin production), plus flutamide, 250 mg PO tid (an androgen receptor blocker). The value of added flutamide is debated. Alternative approaches include adrenalectomy, hypophysectomy, estrogen administration, and medical adrenalectomy with aminoglutethimide. The median survival of stage D pts is 33 months. Pts occasionally respond to withdrawal of hormonal therapy with tumor shrinkage. Second hormonal manipulations act by blocking androgen production in the tumor; abiraterone, a CYP17 inhibitor that blocks androgen synthesis and MDV3100, an antiandrogen, improve overall survival. Many pts who progress on hormonal therapy have androgen-independent tumors, often associated with genetic changes in the androgen receptor and new expression of bcl-2, which may contribute to chemotherapy resistance. Chemotherapy is used for palliation in prostate cancer. Mitoxantrone, estramustine, and taxanes, particularly cabazitaxel, appear to be active single agents, and combinations of drugs are being tested. Chemotherapy-treated pts are more likely to have pain relief than those receiving supportive care alone. Sipuleucel-T, an active specific immunotherapy, improves survival by about 4 months in hormone-refractory disease without producing any measureable change in the tumor. Bone pain from metastases may be palliated with strontium-89 or samarium-153. Bisphosphonates decrease the incidence of skeletal events.

■ PROSTATE CANCER PREVENTION

Finasteride and dutasteride have been shown to reduce the incidence of prostate cancer by 25%, but no effect on overall survival has been seen with limited follow-up. In addition, the cancers that do occur appear to be shifted to higher Gleason grades, although follow-up is limited to assess the natural history.

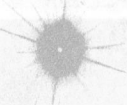

> For a more detailed discussion, see Scher HI: Benign and Malignant Diseases of the Prostate, Chap. 95, p. 796, in HPIM-18.

CHAPTER **82**
Cancer of Unknown Primary Site

Cancer of unknown primary site (CUPS) is defined as follows: biopsy-proven malignancy; primary site unapparent after history, physical exam, chest x-ray, abdominal and pelvic CT, complete blood count, chemistry survey, mammography (women), β-human chorionic gonadotropin (hCG) levels (men), α-fetoprotein (AFP) levels (men), and prostate-specific antigen (PSA) levels (men); and histologic evaluation not consistent with a primary tumor at the biopsy site. CUPS incidence is declining, probably because of better pathology diagnostic criteria; it accounts for about 3% of all cancers today, down from 10–15% 15 years ago. Most pts are over age 60. The tumors are often aneuploid. Cell lines derived from such tumors frequently have abnormalities in chromosome 1.

Clinical Presentation

Pts may present with fatigue, weight loss, pain, bleeding, abdominal swelling, subcutaneous masses, and lymphadenopathy. Once metastatic malignancy is confirmed, diagnostic efforts should be confined to evaluating the presence of potentially curable tumors, such as lymphoma, Hodgkin's disease, germ cell tumor, ovarian cancer, head and neck cancer, and primitive neuroectodermal tumor, or tumors for which therapy may be of significant palliative value such as breast cancer or prostate cancer. In general, efforts to evaluate the presence of these tumor types depend more on the pathologist than on expensive clinical diagnostic testing. Localizing symptoms, a history of carcinogen exposure, or a history of fulguration of skin lesion

TABLE 82-1 POSSIBLE PATHOLOGIC EVALUATION OF BIOPSY SPECIMENS FROM PATIENTS WITH METASTATIC CANCER OF UNKNOWN PRIMARY SITE

Evaluation/Findings	Suggested Primary Site or Neoplasm
Histology (hematoxylin and eosin staining)	
Psammoma bodies, papillary configuration	Ovary, thyroid
Signet ring cells	Stomach
Immunohistology	
Leukocyte common antigen (LCA, CD45)	Lymphoid neoplasm
Leu-M1	Hodgkin's disease
Epithelial membrane antigen	Carcinoma
Cytokeratin	Carcinoma
CEA	Carcinoma
HMB45	Melanoma
Desmin	Sarcoma
Thyroglobulin	Thyroid carcinoma
Calcitonin	Medullary carcinoma of the thyroid
Myoglobin	Rhabdomyosarcoma
PSA/prostatic acid phosphatase	Prostate
AFP	Liver, stomach, germ cell
Placental alkaline phosphatase	Germ cell
β-human chorionic gonadotropin	Germ cell
B, T cell markers	Lymphoid neoplasm
S-100 protein	Neuroendocrine tumor, melanoma
Gross cystic fluid protein	Breast, sweat gland
Estrogen and progesterone receptors	Breast
Factor VIII	Kaposi's sarcoma, angiosarcoma
Thyroid transcription factor 1 (TTF-1)	Lung adenocarcinoma, thyroid
Calretinin, mesothelin	Mesothelioma
URO-III, thrombomodulin	Bladder
Flow Cytometry	
B, T cell markers	Lymphoid neoplasm
Ultrastructure	
Actin-myosin filaments	Rhabdomyosarcoma
Secretory granules	Neuroendocrine tumors
Desmosomes	Carcinoma
Premelanosomes	Melanoma

TABLE 82-1 POSSIBLE PATHOLOGIC EVALUATION OF BIOPSY SPECIMENS FROM PATIENTS WITH METASTATIC CANCER OF UNKNOWN PRIMARY SITE (CONTINUED)

Cytogenetics	
Isochromosome 12p; 12q(−)	Germ cell
t(11;22)	Ewing's sarcoma, primitive neuroectodermal tumor
t(8;14)[a]	Lymphoid neoplasm
3p(−)	Small cell lung carcinoma; renal cell carcinoma, mesothelioma
t(X;18)	Synovial sarcoma
t(12;16)	Myxoid liposarcoma
t(12;22)	Clear cell sarcoma (melanoma of soft parts)
t(2;13)	Alveolar rhabdomyosarcoma
1p(−)	Neuroblastoma
Receptor Analysis	
Estrogen/progesterone receptor	Breast
Molecular Biologic Studies	
Immunoglobulin, *bcl*-2, T cell receptor gene rearrangement	Lymphoid neoplasm

[a]Or any other rearrangement involving an antigen-receptor gene.
Abbreviations: AFP, α-fetoprotein; CEA, carcinoembryonic antigen; PSA, prostate-specific antigen.

may direct some clinical testing; however, the careful light microscopic, ultrastructural, immunologic, karyotypic, and molecular biologic examination of adequate volumes of tumor tissue is the most important feature of the diagnostic workup in the absence of suspicious findings on history and physical exam (Table 82-1).

Histology

About 60% of CUPS tumors are adenocarcinomas, 5% are squamous cell carcinomas, and 30% are poorly differentiated neoplasms not further classified on light microscopy. Expression of cytokeratin subtypes may narrow the range of possible diagnoses (Fig. 82-1).

Prognosis

Pts with squamous cell carcinoma have a median survival of 9 months; those with adenocarcinoma or unclassifiable tumors have a median survival of 4–6 months. Pts in whom a primary site is identified usually have a better prognosis. Limited sites of involvement and neuroendocrine histology are favorable prognostic factors. Pts without a primary diagnosis should be treated palliatively with radiation therapy to symptomatic lesions. All-purpose chemotherapy regimens rarely produce responses but always

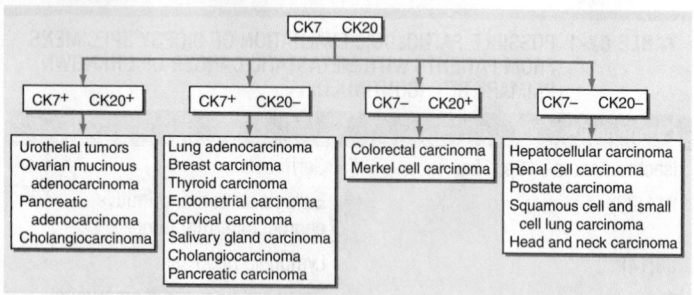

FIGURE 82-1 Approach to cytokeratin (CK7 and CK20) markers used in CUP.

produce toxicity. Certain clinical features may permit individualized therapy.

SYNDROME OF UNRECOGNIZED EXTRAGONADAL GERM CELL CANCER

In pts <50 years with tumor involving midline structures, lung parenchyma, or lymph nodes and evidence of rapid tumor growth, germ cell tumor is a possible diagnosis. Serum tumor markers may or may not be elevated. Cisplatin, etoposide, and bleomycin (Chap. 79) chemotherapy may induce complete responses in ≥25%, and ~15% may be cured. A trial of such therapy should probably also be undertaken in pts whose tumors have abnormalities in chromosome 12.

PERITONEAL CARCINOMATOSIS IN WOMEN

Women who present with pelvic mass or pain and an adenocarcinoma diffusely throughout the peritoneal cavity, but without a clear site of origin, have primary peritoneal papillary serous carcinoma. The presence of psammoma bodies in the tumor or elevated CA-125 levels may favor ovarian origin. Such pts should undergo debulking surgery followed by paclitaxel plus cisplatin or carboplatin combination chemotherapy (Chap. 80). About 20% of pts will respond, and 10% will survive at least 2 years.

CARCINOMA IN AN AXILLARY LYMPH NODE IN WOMEN

Such women should receive adjuvant breast cancer therapy appropriate for their menopausal status even in the absence of a breast mass on physical examination or mammography and undetermined or negative estrogen and progesterone receptors on the tumor (Chap. 77). Unless the ipsilateral breast is radiated, up to 50% of these pts will later develop a breast mass. Although this is a rare clinical situation, long-term survival similar to women with stage II breast cancer is possible.

OSTEOBLASTIC BONE METASTASES IN MEN

The probability of prostate cancer is high; a trial of empirical hormonal therapy (leuprolide and flutamide) is warranted (Chap. 81).

CERVICAL LYMPH NODE METASTASES

Even if panendoscopy fails to reveal a head and neck primary, treatment of such pts with cisplatin and 5-fluorouracil chemotherapy may produce a response; some responses are long-lived (Chap. 75).

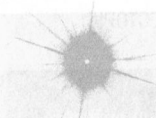

For a more detailed discussion, see Varadhachary GR, Abbruzzese JL: Carcinoma of Unknown Primary, Chap. 99, p. 821, in HPIM-18.

CHAPTER **83**
Paraneoplastic Endocrine Syndromes

Both benign and malignant tumors of nonendocrine tissue can secrete a variety of hormones, principally peptide hormones, and many tumors produce more than one hormone (Table 83-1). At the clinical level, ectopic hormone production is important for two reasons.

First, endocrine syndromes that result may either be the presenting manifestations of the neoplasm or occur late in the course. The endocrine manifestations in some instances are of greater significance than the tumor itself, as in pts with benign or slowly growing malignancies that secrete corticotropin-releasing hormone and cause fulminant Cushing's syndrome. The frequency with which ectopic hormone production is recognized varies with the criteria used for diagnosis. The most common syndromes of clinical import are those of adrenocorticotropic hormone (ACTH) hypersecretion, hypercalcemia, and hypoglycemia. Indeed, ectopic ACTH secretion is responsible for 15–20% of pts with Cushing's syndrome, and ~50% of pts with persistent hypercalcemia have a malignancy rather than hyperparathyroidism. Because of the rapidity of development of hormone secretion in some rapidly growing tumors, diagnosis may require a high index of suspicion, and hormone levels may be elevated out of proportion to the manifestations.

Second, ectopic hormones serve as valuable peripheral markers for neoplasia. Because of the broad spectrum of ectopic hormone secretion, screening measurements of plasma hormone levels for diagnostic purposes are not cost-effective. However, in pts with malignancies that are known to secrete hormones, serial measurements of circulating hormone levels can serve as markers for completeness of tumor excision and for effectiveness of radiation therapy or chemotherapy. Likewise, tumor recurrence may be heralded by reappearance of elevated plasma hormone levels before mass effects of the tumor are evident. However, some tumors at recurrence do not secrete hormones, so hormone measurements cannot be relied on as the sole evidence of tumor activity.

TREATMENT   Paraneoplastic Endocrine Syndromes

Therapy of ectopic hormone-secreting tumors should be directed when possible toward removal of the tumor. When the tumor cannot be removed or is incurable, specific therapy can be directed toward inhibiting

TABLE 83-1   PARANEOPLASTIC SYNDROMES CAUSED BY ECTOPIC HORMONE PRODUCTION

Paraneoplastic Syndrome	Ectopic Hormone	Typical Tumor Types[a]
Common		
Hypercalcemia of malignancy	Parathyroid hormone–related protein (PTHrP)	Squamous cell (head and neck, lung, skin), breast, genitourinary, gastrointestinal
	1,25 dihydroxyvitamin D	Lymphomas
	Parathyroid hormone (PTH) (rare)	Lung, ovary
	Prostaglandin E2 (PGE2) (rare)	Renal, lung
Syndrome of inappropriate antidiuretic hormone secretion (SIADH)	Vasopressin	Lung (squamous, small cell), gastrointestinal, genitourinary, ovary
Cushing's syndrome	Adrenocorticotropic hormone (ACTH)	Lung (small cell, bronchial carcinoid, adenocarcinoma, squamous), thymus, pancreatic islet, medullary thyroid carcinoma
	Corticotropin-releasing hormone (CRH) (rare)	Pancreatic islet, carcinoid, lung, prostate
	Ectopic expression of gastric inhibitory peptide (GIP), luteinizing hormone (LH)/human chorionic gonadotropin (hCG), other G protein–coupled receptors (rare)	Macronodular adrenal hyperplasia
Less common		
Non-islet cell hypoglycemia	Insulin-like growth factor (IGF-II)	Mesenchymal tumors, sarcomas, adrenal, hepatic, gastrointestinal, kidney, prostate
	Insulin (rare)	Cervix (small cell carcinoma)
Male feminization	hCG[b]	Testis (embryonal, seminomas), germinomas, choriocarcinoma, lung, hepatic, pancreatic islet

TABLE 83-1 PARANEOPLASTIC SYNDROMES CAUSED BY ECTOPIC HORMONE PRODUCTION (CONTINUED)

Paraneoplastic Syndrome	Ectopic Hormone	Typical Tumor Types[a]
Less common		
Diarrhea or intestinal hypermotility	Calcitonin[c]	Lung, colon, breast, medullary thyroid carcinoma
	Vasoactive intestinal peptide (VIP)	Pancreas, pheochromocytoma, esophagus
Rare		
Oncogenic osteomalacia	Phosphatonin [fibroblast growth factor 23 (FGF23)]	Hemangiopericytomas, osteoblastomas, fibromas, sarcomas, giant cell tumors, prostate, lung
Acromegaly	Growth hormone–releasing hormone (GHRH)	Pancreatic islet, bronchial and other carcinoids
	Growth hormone (GH)	Lung, pancreatic islet
Hyperthyroidism	Thyroid-stimulating hormone (TSH)	Hydatidiform mole, embryonal tumors, struma ovarii
Hypertension	Renin	Juxtaglomerular tumors, kidney, lung, pancreas, ovary

[a]Only the most common tumor types are listed. For most ectopic hormone syndromes, an extensive list of tumors has been reported to produce one or more hormones.
[b]hCG is produced eutopically by trophoblastic tumors. Certain tumors produce disproportionate amounts of the hCG α or hCG β subunit. High levels of hCG rarely cause hyperthyroidism because of weak binding to the TSH receptor.
[c]Calcitonin is produced eutopically by medullary thyroid carcinoma and is used as a tumor marker.

hormone secretion (octreotide for ectopic acromegaly or mitotane to inhibit adrenal steroidogenesis in the ectopic ACTH syndrome) or blocking the action of the hormone at the tissue level (demeclocycline for inappropriate vasopressin secretion).

■ HYPERCALCEMIA

The most common paraneoplastic syndrome, hypercalcemia of malignancy accounts for 40% of all hypercalcemia. Of cancer pts with hypercalcemia, 80% have humoral hypercalcemia mediated by parathyroid hormone–related peptide; 20% have local osteolytic hypercalcemia mediated by cytokines such as interleukin 1 and tumor necrosis factor. Many tumor types may produce hypercalcemia (Table 83-1). Pts may have malaise, fatigue, confusion, anorexia, bone pain, polyuria, weakness, constipation, nausea, and vomiting. At high calcium levels, confusion, lethargy, coma, and death may ensue. Median survival of hypercalcemic cancer pts is 1–3 months. Treatment with saline hydration, furosemide diuresis, and pamidronate (60–90 mg IV) or zoledronate (4–8 mg IV) controls calcium levels within 2 days and suppresses calcium release for several weeks. Oral bisphosphonates can be used for chronic treatment. In the setting of hematologic malignancies, hypercalcemia may respond to glucocorticoids.

■ HYPONATREMIA

Most commonly discovered in asymptomatic individuals as a result of serum electrolyte measurements, hyponatremia is usually due to tumor secretion of arginine vasopressin, a condition called *syndrome of inappropriate antidiuretic hormone secretion* (SIADH). Atrial natriuretic hormone also may produce hyponatremia. SIADH occurs most commonly in small cell lung cancer (15%) and head and neck cancer (3%). A number of drugs may produce the syndrome. Symptoms of fatigue, poor attention span, nausea, weakness, anorexia, and headache may be controlled by restricting fluid intake to 500 mL/d or blocking the effects of the hormone with 600–1200 mg demeclocycline a day. With severe hyponatremia (<115 meq/L) or in the setting of mental status changes, normal saline infusion plus furosemide may be required; rate of correction should be <1 meq/L per hour to prevent complications.

■ ECTOPIC ACTH SYNDROME

When pro-opiomelanocortin mRNA in the tumor is processed into ACTH, excessive secretion of glucocorticoids and mineralocorticoids may ensue. Pts develop Cushing's syndrome with hypokalemic alkalosis, weakness, hypertension, and hyperglycemia. About half the cases occur in small cell lung cancer. ACTH production adversely affects prognosis. Ketoconazole (400–1200 mg/d) or metyrapone (1–4 g/d) may be used to inhibit adrenal steroid synthesis.

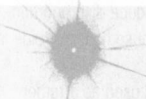

For a more detailed discussion, see Jameson JL, Longo, DL: Paraneoplastic Syndromes: Endocrinologic/Hematologic, Chap. 100, p. 826, in HPIM-18.

CHAPTER **84**
Neurologic Paraneoplastic Syndromes

Paraneoplastic neurologic disorders (PNDs) are cancer-related syndromes that can affect any part of the nervous system; caused by mechanisms other than metastasis or by complications of cancer such as coagulopathy, stroke, metabolic and nutritional conditions, infections, and side effects of cancer therapy. In 60% of pts the neurologic symptoms precede cancer diagnosis.

TABLE 84-1 PARANEOPLASTIC SYNDROMES OF THE NERVOUS SYSTEM

Classic Syndromes: Usually Occur With Cancer Association	Nonclassic Syndromes: May Occur With and Without Cancer Association
Encephalomyelitis	Brainstem encephalitis
Limbic encephalitis	Stiff-person syndrome
Cerebellar degeneration (adults)	Necrotizing myelopathy
Opsoclonus-myoclonus	Motor neuron disease
Subacute sensory neuronopathy	Guillain-Barré syndrome
Gastrointestinal paresis or pseudo-obstruction	Subacute and chronic mixed sensory-motor neuropathies
Dermatomyositis (adults)	Neuropathy associated with plasma cell dyscrasias and lymphoma
Lambert-Eaton myasthenic syndrome	Vasculitis of nerve
Cancer or melanoma associated retinopathy	Pure autonomic neuropathy
	Acute necrotizing myopathy
	Polymyositis
	Vasculitis of muscle
	Optic neuropathy
	BDUMP

Abbreviation: BDUMP, bilateral diffuse uveal melanocytic proliferation.

PNDs occur in 0.5–1% of all cancer pts, but they occur in 2–3% of pts with neuroblastoma or small cell lung cancer (SCLC), and in 30–50% of pts with thymoma or sclerotic myeloma.

■ **CLINICAL FEATURES**

Recognition of a distinctive paraneoplastic syndrome (Table 84-1); should prompt a search for cancer, as prompt treatment of tumor may improve the course of PNDs; many of these disorders also occur without cancer. Diagnosis is based on the clinical pattern, exclusion of other cancer-related disorders, confirmatory serum or CSF antibodies, or electrodiagnostic testing. Most PNDs are mediated by immune responses triggered by neuronal proteins expressed by tumors. PNDs associated with immune responses against intracellular antigens often respond poorly to treatment (Table 84-2), whereas those associated with antibodies to antigens on the neuronal cell surface of the CNS or at neuromuscular synapses are more responsive to immunotherapy (Table 84-3). For any type of PND, if antineuronal antibodies are negative, the diagnosis rests on the demonstration of cancer and the exclusion of other cancer-related or independent disorders. Combined whole-body CT and PET scans often uncover tumors undetected by other tests.

TABLE 84-2 ANTIBODIES TO INTRACELLULAR ANTIGENS, SYNDROMES, AND ASSOCIATED CANCERS

Antibody	Associated Neurologic Syndrome(s)	Tumors
Anti-Hu	Encephalomyelitis, subacute sensory neuronopathy	SCLC
Anti-Yo	Cerebellar degeneration	Ovary, breast
Anti-Ri	Cerebellar degeneration, opsoclonus	Breast, gynecologic, SCLC
Anti-Tr	Cerebellar degeneration	Hodgkin lymphoma
Anti-CV$_2$/CRMP5	Encephalomyelitis, chorea, optic neuritis, uveitis, peripheral neuropathy	SCLC, thymoma, other
Anti-Ma proteins	Limbic, hypothalamic, brainstem encephalitis	Testicular (Ma2), other (Ma)
Anti-amphiphysin	Stiff-person syndrome, encephalomyelitis	Breast, SCLC
Recoverin, bipolar cell antibodies, others[a]	Cancer-associated retinopathy (CAR)	SCLC (CAR), melanoma (MAR)
	Melanoma-associated retinopathy (MAR)	
Anti-GAD	Stiff-person, cerebellar syndromes	Infrequent tumor association (thymoma)

[a]A variety of target antigens have been identified.
Abbreviations: CRMP, collapsing response-mediator protein; SCLC, small cell lung cancer.

PNDs of the Central Nervous System and Dorsal Root Ganglia

MRI and CSF studies are important to rule out neurologic complications due to the direct spread of cancer. In most PNDs the MRI findings are nonspecific. CSF findings typically consist of mild to moderate pleocytosis (<200 mononuclear cells, predominantly lymphocytes), an increase in the protein concentration, intrathecal synthesis of IgG, and a variable presence of oligoclonal bands.

- *Limbic encephalitis* is characterized by confusion, depression, agitation, anxiety, severe short-term memory deficits, partial complex seizures, and dementia; MRI usually shows unilateral or bilateral medial temporal lobe abnormalities.
- *Paraneoplastic cerebellar degeneration* begins as dizziness, oscillopsia, blurry or double vision, nausea, and vomiting; a few days or weeks later, dysarthria, gait and limb ataxia, and variable dysphagia can appear.
- *Opsoclonus-myoclonus syndrome* consists of involuntary, chaotic eye movements in all directions of gaze plus myoclonus; it is frequently associated with ataxia.

TABLE 84-3 ANTIBODIES TO CELL SURFACE OR SYNAPTIC ANTIGENS, SYNDROMES, AND ASSOCIATED TUMORS

Antibody	Neurologic Syndrome	Tumor Type When Associated
Anti-AChR (muscle)[a]	Myasthenia gravis	Thymoma
Anti-AChR (neuronal)[a]	Autonomic neuropathy	SCLC
Anti-VGKC–related proteins[b] (LGI1, Caspr2)	Neuromyotonia, limbic encephalitis	Thymoma, SCLC
Anti-VGCC[c]	LEMS, cerebellar degeneration	SCLC
Anti-NMDAR[d]	Anti-NMDAR encephalitis	Teratoma
Anti-AMPAR[d]	Limbic encephalitis with relapses	SCLC, thymoma, breast
Anti-GABA$_B$R[d]	Limbic encephalitis, seizures	SCLC, neuroendocrine
Glycine receptor[d]	Encephalomyelitis with rigidity, stiff-person syndrome	Lung cancer

[a]A direct pathogenic role of these antibodies has been demonstrated.
[b]Anti-VGKC-related proteins are pathogenic for some types of neuromyotonia.
[c]Anti-VGCC antibodies are pathogenic for LEMS.
[d]These antibodies are strongly suspected to be pathogenic.
Abbreviations: AChR, acetylcholine receptor; AMPAR, α-amino-3-hydroxy-5-methylisoxazole-4-propionic acid receptor; GABA$_B$R, Gamma-amino-butyric acid B receptor; GAD, glutamic acid decarboxylase; LEMS, Lambert-Eaton myasthenic syndrome; NMDAR, N-methyl-d-aspartate receptor; SCLC, small cell lung cancer; VGCC, voltage-gated calcium channel; VGKC, voltage-gated potassium channel.

- *Acute necrotizing myelopathy.* Reports of paraneoplastic spinal cord syndromes have decreased in recent years; it is unclear if this is due to improved oncologic interventions or better detection of nonparaneoplastic etiologies.
- *Paraneoplastic retinopathies* involve cone and rod dysfunction characterized by photosensitivity, progressive loss of vision and color perception, central or ring scotomas, night blindness, and attenuation of photopic and scotopic responses in the electroretinogram (ERG).
- *Dorsal root ganglionopathy* (sensory neuronopathy) is characterized by sensory deficits that may be symmetric or asymmetric, painful dysesthesias, radicular pain, and decreased or absent reflexes; all modalities of sensation can be involved.

PNDs of Nerve and Muscle

These disorders may develop anytime during the course of the neoplastic disease. Serum and urine immunofixation studies should be considered in pts with peripheral neuropathy of unknown cause; detection of a monoclonal gammopathy suggests the need for additional studies to uncover a B cell or plasma cell malignancy. In paraneoplastic neuropathies, diagnostically useful antineuronal antibodies are limited to anti-CV_2/CRMP5 and anti-Hu.

Myasthenia gravis is discussed in Chap. 206, and dermatomyositis in Chap. 207.

TREATMENT   Paraneoplastic Neurologic Disorders

- Treatment of PNDs focuses mainly on recognition and control of the underlying malignancy; a stabilization or improvement of symptoms has been reported in some pts with successful tumor control.
- Variable responses have been described following treatment with glucocorticoids and other immunosuppressive agents as well as IVIg and plasma exchange.
- Those PNDs caused by antibodies to cell surface or synaptic antigens have a much more favorable response to therapy.

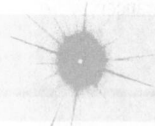

For a more detailed discussion, see Dalmau J, Rosenfeld MR: Paraneoplastic Neurologic Syndromes, Chap. 101, p. 833, in HPIM-18.

CHAPTER **85**

Diagnosis of Infectious
Diseases

The laboratory diagnosis of infection requires the demonstration—either
direct or indirect—of viral, bacterial, fungal, or parasitic agents in tissues,
fluids, or excreta of the host. The traditional detection methods of microscopy and phenotypic characterization are time-consuming and are increasingly being replaced by nucleic acid probe assays.

■ MICROSCOPY

- Wet mounts: the simplest method for microscopic evaluation and useful
  for certain large and/or motile organisms. For example, combining wet
  mounts with dark-field illumination permits detection of spirochetes in
  genital lesions or of *Borrelia* and *Leptospira* in blood.
  - Fungal elements may be identified in skin scrapings with 10% KOH
    wet mount preparations.
  - Some wet mounts use staining to enhance detection and morphologic
    identification—e.g., india ink for visualization of encapsulated crypto-
    cocci in CSF and lactophenol cotton blue for morphologic identifica-
    tion of fungal elements.
- Stains: Staining techniques permit organisms to be seen more clearly.
  - *Gram's stain*: differentiates between organisms with thick peptido-
    glycan cell walls (gram-positive) and those with thin peptidoglycan
    cell walls and outer membranes that can be dissolved with alcohol or
    acetone (gram-negative).
    - This stain is particularly useful for examining sputum samples for
      PMNs and bacteria. The presence of >10 epithelial cells per low-
      power field and multiple bacterial types suggests contamination
      with oral flora.
    - In normally sterile fluids (e.g., CSF, pleural and joint fluid), the
      detection of bacteria suggests an infectious etiology (Fig. 85-1) and
      correlates with the presence of $>10^4$ bacteria/mL.
    - Sensitivity is increased by centrifugation of the sample.
  - *Acid-fast stains*: identify organisms that retain carbol fuchsin dye after
    acid/organic solvation (e.g., *Mycobacterium* spp.). Modification of
    this procedure permits detection of weakly acid-fast organisms (e.g.,
    Nocardia).
  - *Immunofluorescent stains*: utilize antibodies—either labeled directly
    with a fluorescent compound or detected indirectly by a secondary
    immunofluorescent antibody—to detect viral antigens (e.g., CMV,

Gram-Negative Organisms

	GRx only	Oxidase +	Oxidase −	Fastidious	Anaerobic	Curved
Rod		*Pseudomonas* *Aeromonas* *Pasteurella* Others	Enterobacteriaceae Others	*Haemophilus* *Legionella* *Bordetella* *Brucella* *Francisella* Others	*Bacteroides* *Prevotella* *Fusobacterium* Others	*Vibrio* *Campylobacter*
Coccus	*Neisseria* *Branhamella*				*Veillonella* *Acidaminococcus* *Megasphaera*	

Gram-Positive Organisms

	Branching	Spores	Acid-Fast	Catalase +	Catalase −
Rod	*Nocardia* *Actinomyces* *Bifidobacterium*	*Clostridium* *Bacillus*	*Mycobacterium*	*Corynebacterium* *Listeria* Others	*Lactobacillus* Others
Coccus				*Staphylococcus* *Micrococcus* Others	*Streptococcus*

FIGURE 85-1 Interpretation of Gram's stain.

HSV, and respiratory viruses) within cultured cells and difficult-to-grow bacteria (e.g., *Legionella pneumophila*).

■ MACROSCOPIC ANTIGEN DETECTION

- Latex agglutination assays and EIAs are rapid and inexpensive tests that identify bacteria, viruses, or extracellular bacterial toxins by means of their protein or polysaccharide antigens.
- The assays may be performed either directly on clinical specimens or after growth of the organisms in the laboratory.

■ CULTURE

- The success of efforts to culture a specific pathogen often depends on use of appropriate collection and transport procedures in conjunction with a laboratory-processing algorithm suitable for the specimen. Instructions for collection and transport are listed in Table 85-1.
- Bacterial isolation relies on the use of artificial media that support bacterial growth in vitro. Once bacteria are isolated, different methods are used to characterize specific isolates (e.g., phenotyping based on enzymatic and metabolic functions, gas-liquid chromatography, nucleic acid tests).
- Viruses are grown on a monolayer of cultured cells sensitive to infection with the suspected virus. After incubation, cells are examined for cytopathic effects or immunofluorescent studies are performed to detect viral antigens.

■ SEROLOGY

- Measurement of serum antibody provides an indirect marker for past or current infection with a specific pathogen.
- Quantitative assays detect increases in antibody titers, most often with paired serum samples obtained at illness onset and 10–14 days later (i.e., acute- and convalescent-phase samples). A 4-fold increase is regarded as evidence for acute infection.
- Serology can also be used to document protective levels of antibody, particularly in diseases for which vaccines are available (e.g., rubella, VZV infections).

■ NUCLEIC ACID PROBES

- Techniques for the detection and quantitation of specific DNA and RNA base sequences in clinical specimens have become powerful tools for the diagnosis of infection and are useful in four settings:

  1. To detect and/or quantify specific pathogens in clinical specimens (e.g., *Neisseria gonorrhoeae*, HIV)

  2. To identify organisms that are difficult to grow or identify by conventional methods (e.g., *Tropheryma whipplei*, *Legionella*)

  3. To determine whether two or more isolates belong to the same clone or strain

  4. To predict sensitivity (typically of viruses) to chemotherapeutic agents (e.g., HIV, *Mycobacterium tuberculosis*)

- The sensitivity and specificity of probe assays for direct detection are comparable to those of more traditional assays, including EIA and culture.

TABLE 85-1 INSTRUCTIONS FOR COLLECTION AND TRANSPORT OF SPECIMENS FOR CULTURE

Note: It is absolutely essential that the microbiology laboratory be informed of the site of origin of the sample to be cultured and the infections that are suspected. This information determines the selection of culture media and the length of culture time.

Type of Culture (Synonyms)	Specimen	Minimal Volume	Container	Other Considerations
Blood				
Blood, routine (blood culture for aerobes, anaerobes, and yeasts)	Whole blood	10 mL in each of 2 bottles for adults and children; 5 mL, if possible, in aerobic bottles for infants; less for neonates	See below.[a]	See below.[b]
Blood for fungi/ *Mycobacterium* spp.	Whole blood	10 mL in each of 2 bottles, as for routine blood cultures, or in Isolator tube requested from laboratory	Same as for routine blood culture	Specify "hold for extended incubation," since fungal agents may require 4 weeks to grow.
Blood, Isolator (lysis centrifugation)	Whole blood	10 mL	Isolator tubes	Use mainly for isolation of fungi, *Mycobacterium*, and other fastidious aerobes and for elimination of antibiotics from cultured blood in which organisms are concentrated by centrifugation.
Respiratory tract				
Nose	Swab from nares	1 swab	Sterile culturette or similar transport system containing holding medium	Swabs made of calcium alginate may be used.

Throat	Swab of posterior pharynx, ulcerations, or areas of suspected purulence	1 swab	See below.[c]
Sputum	Fresh sputum (not saliva)	2 mL	Commercially available sputum collection system or similar sterile container with screw cap	*Cause for rejection:* Care must be taken to ensure that the specimen is sputum and not saliva. Examination of Gram's stain, with number of epithelial cells and polymorphonuclear leukocytes (PMNs) noted, can be an important part of the evaluation process. Induced sputum specimens should not be rejected.
Bronchial aspirates	Transtracheal aspirate, bronchoscopy specimen, or bronchial aspirate	1 mL of aspirate or brush in transport medium	Sterile aspirate or bronchoscopy tube, bronchoscopy brush in a separate sterile container	Special precautions may be required, depending on diagnostic considerations (e.g., *Pneumocystis*).
Stool				
Stool for routine culture; stool for *Salmonella, Shigella,* and *Campylobacter*	Rectal swab or (preferably) fresh, randomly collected stool	1 g of stool or 2 rectal swabs	Plastic-coated cardboard cup or plastic cup with tight-fitting lid. Other leakproof containers are also acceptable.	If *Vibrio* spp. are suspected, the laboratory must be notified, and appropriate collection/transport methods should be used.
Stool for *Yersinia, Escherichia coli* 0157	Fresh, randomly collected stool	1 g	Plastic-coated cardboard cup or plastic cup with tight-fitting lid	*Limitations:* Procedure requires enrichment techniques.
Stool for *Aeromonas* and *Plesiomonas*	Fresh, randomly collected stool	1 g	Plastic-coated cardboard cup or plastic cup with tight-fitting lid	*Limitations:* Stool should not be cultured for these organisms unless also cultured for other enteric pathogens.

(continued)

TABLE 85-1 INSTRUCTIONS FOR COLLECTION AND TRANSPORT OF SPECIMENS FOR CULTURE (CONTINUED)

Type of Culture (Synonyms)	Specimen	Minimal Volume	Container	Other Considerations
Urogenital tract				
Urine	Clean-voided urine specimen or urine collected by catheter	0.5 mL	Sterile, leak-proof container with screw cap or special urine transfer tube	See below.[d]
Urogenital secretions	Vaginal or urethral secretions, cervical swabs, uterine fluid, prostatic fluid, etc.	1 swab or 0.5 mL of fluid	Vaginal and rectal swabs transported in Amies transport medium or similar holding medium for group B Streptococcus; direct inoculation preferred for Neisseria gonorrhoeae	Vaginal swab samples for "routine culture" should be discouraged whenever possible unless a particular pathogen is suspected. For detection of multiple organisms (e.g., group B Streptococcus, Trichomonas, Chlamydia, or Candida spp.), 1 swab per test should be obtained.
Body fluids, aspirates, and tissues				
Cerebrospinal fluid (lumbar puncture)	Spinal fluid	1 mL for routine cultures; ≥5 mL for Mycobacterium	Sterile tube with tight-fitting cap	Do not refrigerate; transfer to laboratory as soon as possible.
Body fluids	Aseptically aspirated body fluids	1 mL for routine cultures	Sterile tube with tight-fitting cap. Specimen may be left in syringe used for collection if the syringe is capped before transport.	For some body fluids (e.g., peritoneal lavage samples), increased volumes are helpful for isolation of small numbers of bacteria.

Biopsy and aspirated materials	Tissue removed at surgery, bone, anticoagulated bone marrow, biopsy samples, or other specimens from normally sterile areas	Sterile "culturette"-type swab or similar transport system containing holding medium. Sterile bottle or jar should be used for tissue specimens.	Accurate identification of specimen and source is critical. Enough tissue should be collected for both microbiologic and histopathologic evaluations.
Wounds	Purulent material or abscess contents obtained from wound or abscess without contamination by normal microflora	2 swabs or 0.5 mL of aspirated pus	Culturette swab or similar transport system or sterile tube with tight-fitting screw cap. For simultaneous anaerobic cultures, send specimen in anaerobic transport device or closed syringe.	*Collection:* When possible, abscess contents or other fluids should be collected in a syringe (rather than with a swab) to provide an adequate sample volume and an anaerobic environment.

Special recommendations

Fungi	Specimen types listed above may be used. When urine or sputum is cultured for fungi, a first morning specimen usually is preferred.	1 mL or as specified above for individual listing of specimens. Large volumes may be useful for urinary fungi.	Sterile, leakproof container with tight-fitting cap	*Collection:* Specimen should be transported to microbiology laboratory within 1 h of collection. Contamination with normal flora from skin, rectum, vaginal tract, or other body surfaces should be avoided.
Mycobacterium (acid-fast bacilli)	Sputum, tissue, urine, body fluids	10 mL of fluid or small piece of tissue. Swabs should not be used.	Sterile container with tight-fitting cap	Detection of *Mycobacterium* spp. is improved by use of concentration techniques. Smears and cultures of pleural, peritoneal, and pericardial fluids often have low yields. Multiple cultures from the same pt are encouraged. Culturing in liquid media shortens time to detection.

(continued)

TABLE 85-1 INSTRUCTIONS FOR COLLECTION AND TRANSPORT OF SPECIMENS FOR CULTURE (CONTINUED)

Type of Culture (Synonyms)	Specimen	Minimal Volume	Container	Other Considerations
Special recommendations (continued)				
Legionella	Pleural fluid, lung biopsy, bronchoalveolar lavage fluid, bronchial/transbronchial biopsy. Rapid transport to laboratory is critical.	1 mL of fluid; any size tissue sample, although a 0.5-g sample should be obtained when possible	—	—
Anaerobic organisms	Aspirated specimens from abscesses or body fluids	1 mL of aspirated fluid, 1 g of tissue, or 2 swabs	An appropriate anaerobic transport device is required.[e]	Specimens cultured for obligate anaerobes should be cultured for facultative bacteria as well. Fluid or tissue is preferred to swabs.
Viruses[f]	Respiratory secretions, wash aspirates from respiratory tract, nasal swabs, blood samples (including buffy coats), vaginal and rectal swabs, swab specimens from suspicious skin lesions, stool samples (in some cases)	1 mL of fluid, 1 swab, or 1 g of stool in each appropriate transport medium	Fluid or stool samples in sterile containers or swab samples in viral culturette devices (kept on ice but not frozen) are generally suitable. Plasma samples and buffy coats in sterile collection tubes should be kept at 4–8°C. If specimens are to be shipped or kept for a long time, freezing at −80°C is usually adequate.	Most samples for culture are transported in holding medium containing antibiotics to prevent bacterial overgrowth and viral inactivation. Many specimens should be kept cool but not frozen, provided they are transported promptly to the laboratory. Procedures and transport media vary with the agent to be cultured and the duration of transport.

[a]For samples from adults, two bottles (smaller for pediatric samples) should be used: one with dextrose phosphate, tryptic soy, or another appropriate broth and the other with thioglycollate or another broth containing reducing agents appropriate for isolation of obligate anaerobes. For children, from whom only limited volumes of blood can be obtained, only an aerobic culture should be done unless there is specific concern about anaerobic sepsis (e.g., with abdominal infections). For special situations (e.g., suspected fungal infection, culture-negative endocarditis, or mycobacteremia), different blood collection systems may be used (Isolator systems; see table).

[b]Collection: An appropriate disinfecting technique should be used on both the bottle septum and the pt. Do not allow air bubbles to get into anaerobic broth bottles. Special considerations: There is no more important clinical microbiology test than the detection of bloodborne pathogens. The rapid identification of bacterial and fungal agents is a major determinant of pts' survival. Bacteria may be present in blood either continuously (as in endocarditis, overwhelming sepsis, and the early stages of salmonellosis and brucellosis) or intermittently (as in most other bacterial infections, in which bacteria are shed into the blood on a sporadic basis). Most blood culture systems employ two separate bottles containing broth medium: one that is vented in the laboratory for the growth of facultative and aerobic organisms and one that is maintained under anaerobic conditions. In cases of suspected continuous bacteremia/fungemia, two or three samples should be drawn before the start of therapy, with additional sets obtained if fastidious organisms are thought to be involved. For intermittent bacteremia, two or three samples should be obtained at least 1 h apart during the first 24 h.

[c]Normal microflora includes α-hemolytic streptococci, saprophytic *Neisseria* spp., diphtheroids, and *Staphylococcus* spp. Aerobic culture of the throat ("routine") includes screening for and identification of β-hemolytic *Streptococcus* spp. and other potentially pathogenic organisms. Although considered components of the normal microflora, organisms such as *Staphylococcus aureus*, *Haemophilus influenzae*, and *Streptococcus pneumoniae* will be identified by most laboratories, if requested. When *Neisseria gonorrhoeae* or *Corynebacterium diphtheriae* is suspected, a special culture request is recommended.

[d](1) Clean-voided specimens, midvoid specimens, and Foley or indwelling catheter specimens that yield 50,000 organisms/mL and from which no more than three species are isolated should have organisms identified. Neither indwelling catheter tips nor urine from the bag of a catheterized pt should be cultured. (2) Straight-catheterized, bladder-tap, and similar urine specimens should undergo a complete workup (identification and susceptibility testing) for all potentially pathogenic organisms regardless of colony count. (3) Certain clinical problems (e.g., acute dysuria in women) may warrant identification and susceptibility testing of isolates present at concentrations of <50,000 organisms/mL.

[e]Aspirated specimens in capped syringes or other transport devices designed to limit oxygen exposure are suitable for the cultivation of obligate anaerobes. A variety of commercially available transport devices may be used. Contamination of specimens with normal microflora from the skin, rectum, vaginal vault, or another body site should be avoided. Collection containers for aerobic culture (such as dry swabs) and inappropriate specimens (such as refrigerated samples; expectorated sputum; stool; gastric aspirates; and vaginal, throat, nose, and rectal swabs) should be rejected as unsuitable.

[f]Laboratories generally use diverse methods to detect viral agents, and the specific requirements for each specimen should be checked before a sample is sent.

493

- Amplification strategies (e.g., PCR) enhance the sensitivity of RNA or DNA assays, but false-positive findings can result from even low levels of contamination.

■ SUSCEPTIBILITY TESTING

- Susceptibility testing allows the clinician to choose the optimal antimicrobial agents and to identify potential infection-control problems (e.g., the level of methicillin-resistant *Staphylococcus aureus* in a hospital).
- Qualitative measures (e.g., disk/agar diffusion and breakpoint) and quantitative measures [e.g., broth dilution, epsilometer (E-test)] are available.
- Antifungal susceptibility testing is becoming more commonplace; however, testing of some species (e.g., *Aspergillus*) remains technically difficult and is performed primarily in reference labs.

■ CONSIDERATIONS FOR DIAGNOSIS OF PARASITIC INFECTIONS

The cornerstone for the diagnosis of parasitic diseases, as for that of many other infections, is the elicitation of a thorough history of the illness and of epidemiologic factors such as travel, recreational activities, and occupation. Table 85-2 summarizes the diagnosis of some common parasitic infections.

■ INTESTINAL PARASITES

- Most helminths and protozoa can be detected by examination of fecal samples; contamination with urine or water should be avoided.
- Fecal samples should be collected before the ingestion of contrast agents and before treatment with antidiarrheal agents or antacids; these substances alter fecal consistency and interfere with microscopic detection of parasites.
- The collection of three samples on alternate days is recommended because of the cyclic shedding of most parasites in the feces; examination of a single sample can be up to 50% less sensitive.
- Analysis of fecal samples entails macroscopic examination for adult worms or tapeworm segments and microscopic examination that includes direct wet mounts, concentration techniques, and application of permanent stains.
- Alternative diagnostic methods such as sampling of duodenal contents (e.g., for *Giardia lamblia*, *Cryptosporidium*, and *Strongyloides* larvae) and the "cellophane tape" method (e.g., for pinworm ova or *Taenia saginata*) may be required.

■ BLOOD AND TISSUE PARASITES

- Diagnosis of tissue-invasive parasites requires an understanding of the pathophysiology of the parasite in question (e.g., examination of urine sediment to detect *Schistosoma haematobium*).
- The laboratory procedures for detection of parasites in other body fluids are similar to those used for examination of feces.
- The parasites most commonly detected in Giemsa-stained blood smears are plasmodia, microfilariae, and African trypanosomes; however, wet mounts may be more sensitive for microfilariae and African trypanosomes, given their motility.
- The timing of blood collection is crucial—e.g., to diagnose *Wuchereria bancrofti* infection, blood must be drawn near midnight, when the nocturnal microfilariae are active.

TABLE 85-2 DIAGNOSIS OF SOME COMMON PARASITIC INFECTIONS

Parasite	Geographic Distribution	Parasite Stage	Body Fluid or Tissue	Diagnosis		
				Serologic Tests	Other	
Blood flukes						
Schistosoma mansoni	Africa, Central and South America, West Indies	Ova, adults	Feces	EIA, WB	Rectal snips, liver biopsy	
S. haematobium	Africa	Ova, adults	Urine	WB	Liver, urine, or bladder biopsy	
S. japonicum	Far East	Ova, adults	Feces	WB	Liver biopsy	
Intestinal roundworms						
Strongyloides stercoralis (strongyloidiasis)	Moist tropics and subtropics	Larvae	Feces, sputum, duodenal fluid	EIA	Dissemination in immunodeficiency	
Intestinal protozoans						
Entamoeba histolytica (amebiasis)	Worldwide, especially tropics	Troph, cyst	Feces, liver	EIA, antigen detection	Ultrasound, liver CT, PCR	
Giardia lamblia (giardiasis)	Worldwide	Troph, cyst	Feces	Antigen detection	String test, DFA, PCR	
Isospora belli	Worldwide	Oocyst	Feces	—	Acid-fast[a]	
Cryptosporidium	Worldwide	Oocyst	Feces	Antigen detection	Acid-fast,[a] DFA, biopsy, PCR	
Blood and tissue protozoans						
Plasmodium species (malaria)	Subtropics and tropics	Asexual	Blood	Limited use	PCR	
Babesia microti (babesiosis)	U.S., especially New England	Asexual	Blood	IIF	Animal species in asplenia, PCR	
Toxoplasma gondii (toxoplasmosis)	Worldwide	Cyst, troph	CNS, eye, muscles, other	EIA, IIF	PCR	

[a]Acid-fastness is best demonstrated by auramine fluorescence or modified acid-fast stain.
Abbreviations: DFA, direct fluorescent antibody; IIF, indirect immunofluorescence; troph, trophozoite; WB, western blot.
Source: Adapted from Reed SL, Davis CE: Chap. e25, HPIM-18.

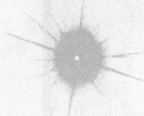

For a more detailed discussion, see McAdam AJ, Onderdonk AB: Laboratory Diagnosis of Infectious Diseases, Chap. e22; and Reed SL, Davis CE: Laboratory Diagnosis of Parasitic Diseases, Chap. e25, in HPIM-18.

CHAPTER **86**
Antibacterial Therapy

Antibacterial agents are among the most commonly prescribed drugs worldwide and can be lifesaving when used appropriately. However, their indiscriminate use (estimated at ~50% of all antibiotic use) drives up the cost of health care, leads to a plethora of side effects and drug interactions, and fosters the emergence of bacterial resistance, rendering previously valuable drugs useless.

MECHANISMS OF DRUG ACTION

Antibacterial agents act on unique targets not found in mammalian cells. *Bactericidal* drugs kill bacteria within their spectrum of activity; *bacteriostatic* drugs inhibit bacterial growth. Table 86-1 summarizes the mechanisms of action of commonly used antibacterial drugs.

- *Inhibition of cell-wall synthesis*: Drugs that inhibit cell-wall synthesis are almost always bactericidal. The cell wall is broken down by bacterial autolysins (cell wall–remodeling enzymes) during normal growth, and this class of antibacterial agents prevents the synthesis of a repaired cell wall. Examples include β-lactam antibiotics (e.g., penicillins, cephalosporins, carbapenems), glycopeptides (vancomycin, teicoplanin), and lipoglycopeptides (telavancin).
- *Inhibition of protein synthesis*: Typically, inhibition takes place through interaction with bacterial ribosomes, which differ in composition from mammalian ribosomes. Except for aminoglycosides, these drugs are bacteriostatic. Examples include aminoglycosides (e.g., gentamicin, tobramycin, streptomycin), macrolides (erythromycin, clarithromycin, azithromycin), ketolides (telithromycin), lincosamides (clindamycin), streptogramins [quinupristin/dalfopristin (Synercid)], chloramphenicol, oxazolidinone (linezolid), tetracyclines (tetracycline, doxycycline, minocycline), and glycylcyclines (tigecycline).
- *Inhibition of bacterial metabolism*: Antimetabolites interfere with bacterial folic acid production, thereby preventing synthesis of thymidine, all purines, and several amino acids. These drugs are generally bacteriostatic, although in some cases they may be bactericidal. Examples include sulfonamides and trimethoprim.
- *Inhibition of nucleic acid synthesis or activity*: Several antibacterial agents have disparate effects on nucleic acids. Examples include fluoroquinolones (ciprofloxacin, levofloxacin, moxifloxacin), rifampin, nitrofurantoin, and metronidazole.

TABLE 86-1 MECHANISMS OF ACTION OF AND RESISTANCE TO MAJOR CLASSES OF ANTIBACTERIAL AGENTS

Antibacterial Agent[a]	Major Cellular Target	Mechanism of Action	Major Mechanisms of Resistance
β-Lactams (penicillins, cephalosporins, carbapenems)	Cell wall	Inhibit cell-wall cross-linking	1. Drug inactivation (β-lactamase) 2. Insensitivity of target (altered penicillin-binding proteins) 3. Decreased permeability (altered gram-negative outer-membrane porins) 4. Active efflux
Vancomycin	Cell wall	Interferes with addition of new cell-wall subunits (muramyl pentapeptides)	Alteration of target (substitution of terminal amino acid of peptidoglycan subunit)
Bacitracin	Cell wall	Prevents addition of cell-wall subunits by inhibiting recycling of membrane lipid carrier	Not defined
Macrolides (erythromycin)	Protein synthesis	Bind to 50S ribosomal subunit	1. Alteration of target (ribosomal methylation and mutation of 23S rRNA) 2. Active efflux
Lincosamides (clindamycin)	Protein synthesis	Bind to 50S ribosomal subunit Block peptide chain elongation	1. Alteration of target (ribosomal methylation) 2. Active efflux
Chloramphenicol	Protein synthesis	Binds to 50S ribosomal subunit Blocks aminoacyl tRNA attachment	1. Drug inactivation (chloramphenicol acetyltransferase) 2. Active efflux
Tetracycline	Protein synthesis	Binds reversibly to 30S ribosomal subunit Blocks binding of aminoacyl tRNA	1. Decreased intracellular drug accumulation (active efflux) 2. Insensitivity of target

(*continued*)

TABLE 86-1 MECHANISMS OF ACTION OF AND RESISTANCE TO MAJOR CLASSES OF ANTIBACTERIAL AGENTS (CONTINUED)

Antibacterial Agent[a]	Major Cellular Target	Mechanism of Action	Major Mechanisms of Resistance
Aminoglycosides (gentamicin)	Protein synthesis	Bind irreversibly to 30S ribosomal subunit Inhibit translocation of peptidyl-tRNA	1. Drug inactivation (aminoglycoside-modifying enzyme) 2. Decreased permeability through gram-negative outer membrane 3. Active efflux 4. Ribosomal methylation
Mupirocin	Protein synthesis	Inhibits isoleucine tRNA synthetase	Mutation of gene for target protein or acquisition of new gene for drug-insensitive target
Streptogramins [quinupristin/dalfopristin (Synercid)]	Protein synthesis	Bind to 50S ribosomal subunit Block peptide chain elongation	1. Alteration of target (ribosomal methylation: dalfopristin) 2. Active efflux (quinupristin) 3. Drug inactivation (quinupristin and dalfopristin)
Linezolid	Protein synthesis	Binds to 50S ribosomal subunit Inhibits initiation of protein synthesis	Alteration of target (mutation of 23S rRNA)
Sulfonamides and trimethoprim	Cell metabolism	Competitively inhibit enzymes involved in two steps of folic acid biosynthesis	Production of insensitive targets [dihydropteroate synthetase (sulfonamides) and dihydrofolate reductase (trimethoprim)] that bypass metabolic block
Rifampin	Nucleic acid synthesis	Inhibits DNA-dependent RNA polymerase	Insensitivity of target (mutation of polymerase gene)

TABLE 86-1 MECHANISMS OF ACTION OF AND RESISTANCE TO MAJOR CLASSES OF ANTIBACTERIAL AGENTS (CONTINUED)

Antibacterial Agent[a]	Major Cellular Target	Mechanism of Action	Major Mechanisms of Resistance
Metronidazole	Nucleic acid synthesis	Intracellularly generates short-lived reactive intermediates that damage DNA by electron transfer system	Not defined
Quinolones (ciprofloxacin)	DNA synthesis	Inhibit activity of DNA gyrase (A subunit) and topoisomerase IV	1. Insensitivity of target (mutation of gyrase genes) 2. Decreased intracellular drug accumulation (active efflux)
Novobiocin	DNA synthesis	Inhibits activity of DNA gyrase (B subunit)	Not defined
Polymyxins (polymyxin B)	Cell membrane	Disrupt membrane permeability by charge alteration	Not defined
Gramicidin	Cell membrane	Forms pores	Not defined
Daptomycin	Cell membrane	Forms channels that disrupt membrane potential	Alteration of membrane charge

[a]Compounds in parentheses are major representatives for the class.

- *Alteration of cell-membrane permeability*: Agents of this class interact with bacterial membranes and are generally bactericidal. Examples include polymyxins (polymyxin B, colistin) and daptomycin.

MECHANISMS OF ANTIBACTERIAL RESISTANCE

- Bacteria can either be intrinsically resistant to an agent (e.g., obligate anaerobic bacteria are resistant to aminoglycosides) or acquire resistance through mutation of resident genes or acquisition of new genes.
- The major mechanisms of resistance used by bacteria are drug inactivation, alteration or overproduction of the antibacterial target, acquisition of a new gene encoding a drug-insensitive target, decreased permeability

to the agent, failure to convert an inactive prodrug to its active derivative, and active efflux of the agent.

- Table 86-1 summarizes specific mechanisms of bacterial resistance to commonly used antibacterial agents.

PHARMACOKINETICS OF ANTIBIOTICS

The *pharmacokinetic profile* refers to drug concentrations in serum and tissue versus time and reflects the processes of absorption, distribution, metabolism, and elimination.

- *Absorption*: systemic bioavailability after PO, IM, or IV administration
  - The IM and IV routes offer 100% bioavailability.
  - Bioavailability after PO administration ranges from 10% (e.g., penicillin G) to nearly 100% (e.g., amoxicillin, clindamycin, metronidazole, fluoroquinolones).
- *Distribution*: The concentration of an antibiotic must exceed the pathogen's minimal inhibitory concentration (MIC) at the site of infection to be effective.
- *Metabolism and elimination*: Antibacterial agents are disposed of by hepatic elimination (metabolism or biliary elimination), renal excretion of the unchanged or metabolized form, or a combination of the two. Understanding the mode of elimination is important in adjusting dosage if elimination is impaired.

PRINCIPLES OF ANTIBACTERIAL CHEMOTHERAPY

- When possible, obtain specimens to identify the etiologic agent (by microscopic examination and culture) before treatment.
- Standard in vitro susceptibility testing assesses only bacteriostasis and is essential to devising a chemotherapeutic regimen. Use local susceptibility patterns to help direct empirical treatment.
- The *pharmacokinetic-pharmacodynamic (PK-PD) profile* of an antibiotic refers to the quantitative relationships among (1) the time course of antibiotic concentrations in serum and tissue, (2) the MIC, and (3) the microbial response (inhibition of growth or rate of killing). Profiles can be categorized as either concentration or time dependent.
  - *Concentration-dependent antibiotics (e.g., fluoroquinolones, aminoglycosides)*: Increasing the ratio of the maximal serum concentration to the MIC (or the ratio of the area under the plasma concentration vs. time curve to the MIC) leads to a more rapid rate of bacterial death. Administration of larger doses (within the confines of toxicity) with longer dosing intervals is the practical application of these relationships.
  - *Time-dependent antibiotics (e.g., β-lactam antibiotics)*: The reduction in bacterial density is proportional to the amount of time that drug concentrations exceed the MIC. While the optimal dosing strategy is continuous infusion, more convenient dosing intervals can be used, with maintenance of the serum drug concentration above the MIC for 30–50% of the dosing interval.
- Once etiology and susceptibility are known, the therapeutic regimen should be changed to one that has the narrowest effective spectrum

TABLE 86-2　MOST CLINICALLY RELEVANT ADVERSE REACTIONS TO COMMON ANTIBACTERIAL DRUGS

Drug	Adverse Event	Comments
β-Lactams	Allergies in ~1–4% of treatment courses	Cephalosporins cause allergy in 2–4% of penicillin-allergic pts. Aztreonam is safe in β-lactam-allergic pts.
	Nonallergic skin reactions	Ampicillin "rash" is common among pts with EBV infection.
	Diarrhea, including *Clostridium difficile* colitis	—
Vancomycin	Anaphylactoid reaction ("red man syndrome")	Give as a 1- to 2-h infusion.
	Nephrotoxicity, ototoxicity, allergy, neutropenia	Thought to be rare, but apparently increasing as larger dosages are used
Telavancin	Taste disturbance, foamy urine, gastrointestinal distress	New drug; full spectrum of adverse reactions unclear
Aminoglycosides	Nephrotoxicity (generally reversible)	Greatest with prolonged therapy in the elderly or with preexisting renal insufficiency. Monitor serum creatinine level every 2–3 days.
	Ototoxicity (often irreversible)	Risk factors similar to those for nephrotoxicity; both vestibular and hearing toxicities
Macrolides/ketolides	Gastrointestinal distress	Most common with erythromycin
	Ototoxicity	High-dose IV erythromycin
	Cardiac toxicity	QTc prolongation and torsades de pointes, especially when inhibitors of erythromycin metabolism are given simultaneously
	Hepatic toxicity (telithromycin)	Warning added to prescribing information (July 2006)
	Respiratory failure in pts with myasthenia gravis (telithromycin)	Warning added to prescribing information (July 2006)
Clindamycin	Diarrhea, including *C. difficile* colitis	—
Sulfonamides	Allergic reactions	Rashes (more common among HIV-infected pts); serious dermal reactions, including erythema multiforme, Stevens-Johnson syndrome, toxic epidermal necrolysis

(continued)

TABLE 86-2   MOST CLINICALLY RELEVANT ADVERSE REACTIONS TO COMMON ANTIBACTERIAL DRUGS (CONTINUED)

Drug	Adverse Event	Comments
	Hematologic reactions	Uncommon; include agranulocytosis and granulocytopenia (more common in HIV-infected pts), hemolytic and megaloblastic anemia, thrombocytopenia
	Renal insufficiency	Crystalluria with sulfadiazine therapy
Fluoroquinolones	Diarrhea, including *C. difficile* colitis	—
	Contraindicated for general use in pts <18 years old and pregnant women	Appear safe in treatment of pulmonary infections in children with cystic fibrosis
	CNS adverse effects (e.g., insomnia)	—
	Miscellaneous: allergies, tendon rupture, dysglycemias, QTc prolongation	Rare, although warnings for tendon rupture have been added to prescribing information
Rifampin	Hepatotoxicity	Rare
	Orange discoloration of urine and body fluids	Common
	Miscellaneous: flu-like symptoms, hemolysis, renal insufficiency	Uncommon; usually related to intermittent administration
Metronidazole	Metallic taste	Common
Tetracyclines/ glycylcyclines	Gastrointestinal distress	Up to 20% with tigecycline
	Esophageal ulceration	Doxycycline (take in A.M. with fluids)
Linezolid	Myelosuppression	Follows long-term treatment
	Ocular and peripheral neuritis	Follows long-term treatment
Daptomycin	Distal muscle pain or weakness	Weekly creatine phosphokinase measurements, especially in pts also receiving statins

and—all else being equal—is least costly. The status of the host (e.g., pregnancy, immunosuppression, hepatic and renal function, other required medications), the site of infection (e.g., CNS infection or endocarditis), and the adverse reaction profile (including contraindications) need to be considered in choosing an appropriate antibacterial agent.

TABLE 86-3 INTERACTIONS OF ANTIBACTERIAL AGENTS WITH OTHER DRUGS

Antibiotic	Interacts with	Potential Consequence (Clinical Significance[a])
Erythromycin/ clarithromycin/ telithromycin	Theophylline	Theophylline toxicity (1)
	Carbamazepine	CNS depression (1)
	Digoxin	Digoxin toxicity (2)
	Triazolam/midazolam	CNS depression (2)
	Ergotamine	Ergotism (1)
	Warfarin	Bleeding (2)
	Cyclosporine/tacrolimus	Nephrotoxicity (1)
	Cisapride	Cardiac arrhythmias (1)
	Statins[b]	Rhabdomyolysis (2)
	Valproate	Valproate toxicity (2)
	Vincristine/vinblastine	Excess neurotoxicity (2)
Quinupristin/ dalfopristin	Similar to erythromycin[c]	—
Fluoroquinolones	Theophylline	Theophylline toxicity (2)[d]
	Antacids/sucralfate/ iron	Subtherapeutic antibiotic levels (1)
Tetracycline	Antacids/sucralfate/ iron	Subtherapeutic antibiotic levels (1)
Trimethoprim- sulfamethoxazole	Phenytoin	Phenytoin toxicity (2)
	Oral hypoglycemics	Hypoglycemia (2)
	Warfarin	Bleeding (1)
	Digoxin	Digoxin toxicity (2)
Metronidazole	Ethanol	Disulfiram-like reactions (2)
	Fluorouracil	Bone marrow suppression (1)
	Warfarin	Bleeding (2)
Rifampin	Warfarin	Clot formation (1)
	Oral contraceptives	Pregnancy (1)
	Cyclosporine/tacrolimus	Rejection (1)
	HIV-1 protease inhibitors	Increased viral load, resistance (1)
	Nonnucleoside reverse- transcriptase inhibitors	Increased viral load, resistance (1)
	Glucocorticoids	Loss of steroid effect (1)

(continued)

TABLE 86-3 INTERACTIONS OF ANTIBACTERIAL AGENTS WITH OTHER DRUGS (CONTINUED)

Antibiotic	Interacts with	Potential Consequence (Clinical Significance[a])
	Methadone	Narcotic withdrawal symptoms (1)
	Digoxin	Subtherapeutic digoxin levels (1)
	Itraconazole	Subtherapeutic itraconazole levels (1)
	Phenytoin	Loss of seizure control (1)
	Statins	Hypercholesterolemia (1)
	Diltiazem	Subtherapeutic diltiazem levels (1)
	Verapamil	Subtherapeutic verapamil levels (1)

[a]1 = well-documented interaction with clinically important consequences; 2 = interaction of uncertain frequency but potential clinical importance.
[b]Lovastatin and simvastatin are most affected; pravastatin and atorvastatin are less likely to have clinically important effects.
[c]The macrolide antibiotics and quinupristin/dalfopristin inhibit the same human metabolic enzyme (CYP3A4), and similar interactions are anticipated.
[d]Ciprofloxacin only. Levofloxacin and moxifloxacin do not inhibit theophylline metabolism.
Note: New interactions are commonly reported after marketing. Consult the most recent prescribing information for updates.

- Although combination chemotherapy usually is not indicated, it is used occasionally to prevent emergence of resistance (e.g., addition of rifampin for staphylococci), for synergistic or additive activity (e.g., β-lactam/aminoglycoside combinations against enterococci), and for therapy directed against multiple potential pathogens (e.g., intraabdominal or brain abscess). Some combination therapies (e.g., penicillin plus tetracycline against pneumococci) have antagonistic effects; i.e., the combination is *worse* than either drug alone.

CHOICE OF ANTIBACTERIAL AGENTS

For current and practical information regarding antimicrobial drugs and treatment regimens for specific indications, consult relevant chapters in HPIM-18. In addition, online references such as the Johns Hopkins antibiotic guide (*www.Hopkins-abxguide.org*) are available. Evidence-based practice guidelines for many infections are available from the Infectious Diseases Society of America (*www.idsociety.org*).

ADVERSE REACTIONS

Adverse reactions are classified as either dose-related (e.g., aminoglycoside-induced nephrotoxicity) or unpredictable. Unpredictable reactions are idiosyncratic or allergic. Table 86-2 summarizes the most clinically relevant adverse reactions to common antibacterial drugs.

DRUG INTERACTIONS

Antimicrobial agents are a common cause of drug–drug interactions, often because of effects on the hepatic P450 system, which is responsible for metabolizing many drugs. Table 86-3 lists the most common and best-documented interactions of antimicrobial agents with other drugs and characterizes the clinical relevance of these interactions. This information is presented only to heighten awareness of potential interactions; to ensure that no drug–drug interactions occur, appropriate sources should be consulted before any antibiotic is prescribed.

> For a more detailed discussion, see Archer GL, Polk RE: Treatment and Prophylaxis of Bacterial Infections, Chap. 133, p. 1133, in HPIM-18. For a discussion of antifungal therapy, see Chaps. 115 and 116 in this manual; for antimycobacterial therapy, see Chap. 103; for antiviral therapy, see Chaps. 108 through 114; and for antiparasitic therapy, see Chaps. 117 and 118.

CHAPTER 87
Health Care–Associated Infections

Hospital-acquired or *nosocomial* infections (defined as those not present or incubating at the time of admission to the hospital) and other health care–associated infections affect an estimated 1.7 million pts, cost $28–33 billion, and contribute to 99,000 deaths in U.S. hospitals each year. Although efforts to lower infection risks have been challenged by the growing numbers of immunocompromised pts, antibiotic-resistant bacteria, fungal and viral superinfections, and invasive procedures and devices, the "zero-tolerance" viewpoint of consumer advocates holds that nearly all health care–associated infections should be avoidable. Accordingly, federal legislation now exists to prevent U.S. hospitals from upgrading Medicare charges to pay for hospital costs resulting from at least 10 specific nosocomial events.

■ PREVENTION OF HOSPITAL-ACQUIRED INFECTIONS

Nosocomial pathogens have reservoirs, are transmitted by largely predictable routes, and require susceptible hosts—features that allow the implementation of monitoring and prevention strategies.

- *Surveillance*: review of microbiology laboratory results, surveys of nursing wards, and use of other mechanisms to keep track of infections acquired after hospital admission. Most hospitals aim surveillance at infections associated with high-level morbidity or great expense. Results of surveillance are expressed as rates and should include a denominator indicating the number of pts exposed to a specific risk (e.g., pts using a mechanical ventilator) or the number of intervention days (e.g., 1000 pt-days on a ventilator).

- *Prevention and control measures:* Hand hygiene is the single most important measure to prevent cross-infection.

  - Health care workers' rates of adherence to hand-hygiene recommendations are abysmally low at <50%.

  - Other measures include identifying and eradicating reservoirs of infection and minimizing use of invasive procedures and catheters.

- *Isolation techniques:* Isolation of infectious pts is a standard component of infection control programs.

  - *Standard precautions:* include hand hygiene and use of gloves when there is a potential for contact with blood, other body fluids, nonintact skin, or mucous membranes during the care of all pts. In certain cases, masks, eye protection, and gowns are used as well.

  - *Transmission-based guidelines:* Airborne, droplet, or contact precautions—for which personnel don (at a minimum) N95 respirators, surgical face masks, or gowns and gloves, respectively—are used to prevent transmission of disease from pts with contagious clinical syndromes. More than one precaution can be used for diseases that have more than one mode of transmission (e.g., contact and airborne isolation for varicella).

■ NOSOCOMIAL AND DEVICE-RELATED INFECTIONS

Nosocomial infections are due to the combined effect of the pt's own flora and the presence of invasive devices in 25–50% of cases. Intensive education, "bundling" of evidence-based interventions, and use of checklists to facilitate adherence can reduce infection rates. Table 87-1 summarizes effective interventions to reduce the incidence of the more common nosocomial infections.

- **Urinary Tract Infections** Approximately 34% of nosocomial infections are UTIs, contributing ~15% to prolongation of hospital stay with an attributable cost of ~$1300.

  - Most nosocomial UTIs are associated with prior instrumentation or indwelling bladder catheterization. The 3–10% risk of infection for each day a catheter remains in place is due to the ascent of bacteria from the periurethral area or via intraluminal contamination of the catheter.

  - In men, condom catheters may lessen the risk of UTI.

  - The most common pathogens are *Escherichia coli*, nosocomial gram-negative bacilli, enterococci, and (particularly for pts in the ICU) *Candida*.

  - For suspected infection in the setting of chronic catheterization, the catheter should be replaced and a freshly voided urine specimen obtained for culture to confirm actual infection as opposed to simple colonization of the catheter.

TABLE 87-1   EXAMPLES OF "BUNDLED INTERVENTIONS" TO PREVENT COMMON HEALTH CARE–ASSOCIATED INFECTIONS AND OTHER ADVERSE EVENTS

Prevention of Central Venous Catheter Infections

Educate personnel about catheter insertion and care.

Use chlorhexidine to prepare the insertion site.

Use maximal barrier precautions during catheter insertion.

Consolidate insertion supplies (e.g., in an insertion kit or cart).

Use a checklist to enhance adherence to the bundle.

Empower nurses to halt insertion if asepsis is breached.

Cleanse pts daily with chlorhexidine.

Ask daily: Is the catheter needed? Remove catheter if not needed or used.

Prevention of Ventilator-Associated Pneumonia and Complications

Elevate head of bed to 30–45 degrees.

Decontaminate oropharynx regularly with chlorhexidine.

Give "sedation vacation," and assess readiness to extubate daily.

Use peptic ulcer disease prophylaxis.

Use deep-vein thrombosis prophylaxis (unless contraindicated).

Prevention of Surgical-Site Infections

Administer prophylactic antibiotics within 1 h before surgery; discontinue within 24 h.

Limit hair removal to the time immediately before surgery; use clippers or do not remove hair at all.

Prepare surgical site with chlorhexidine-alcohol.

Maintain normal perioperative glucose levels (cardiac surgery pts).[a]

Maintain perioperative normothermia (colorectal surgery pts).[a]

Prevention of Urinary Tract Infections

Place bladder catheters only when absolutely needed (e.g., to relieve obstruction), not solely for the provider's convenience.

Use aseptic technique for catheter insertion and urinary tract instrumentation.

Minimize manipulation or opening of drainage systems.

[a]These components of care are supported by clinical trials and experimental evidence in the specified populations; they may prove valuable for other surgical pts as well.
Source: Adapted from information presented at the following website: www.cdc.gov/HAI/InfectionTypes.html

- As with all nosocomial infections, it is useful to repeat the culture to confirm the persistence of infection at the time therapy is initiated.
- **Pneumonia** Accounting for ~13% of nosocomial infections, pneumonia increases the duration of hospital stay by 10 days, accounts for ~$23,000 in extra costs, and is associated with more deaths than are infections at any other body site.

- Bacterial nosocomial pneumonia is caused by aspiration of endogenous or hospital-acquired oropharyngeal flora.
- Risk factors include events that increase colonization with potential pathogens, such as prior antibiotic use, contaminated ventilator equipment, or decreased gastric acidity; events that increase risk of aspiration, such as nasogastric or endotracheal intubation or decreased level of consciousness; and conditions that compromise host defense mechanisms in the lung, such as chronic obstructive pulmonary disease, extremes of age, or upper abdominal surgery.
- Etiologic organisms include community-acquired pathogens (e.g., *Streptococcus pneumoniae*, *Haemophilus influenzae*) early during hospitalization and *Staphylococcus aureus*, *Pseudomonas aeruginosa*, *Klebsiella pneumoniae*, *Enterobacter* species, and *Acinetobacter* species later in the hospital stay.
- Diagnosis can be difficult, as clinical criteria (e.g., fever, leukocytosis, purulent secretions, and new or changing pulmonary infiltrates on chest x-ray) have high sensitivity but low specificity.
  - An etiology should be sought by studies of lower respiratory tract samples protected from upper-tract contamination; quantitative cultures have diagnostic sensitivities in the range of 80%.
  - Febrile pts with nasogastric or nasotracheal tubes should also have sinusitis or otitis media ruled out.
- **Surgical Wound Infections** Making up ~17% of nosocomial infections, surgical wound infections increase the length of hospital stay by 7–10 days and increase costs by $3000–$29,000.
  - These infections often become evident after pts have left the hospital; thus it is difficult to assess the true incidence.
  - Risk factors include the pt's underlying conditions (e.g., diabetes mellitus or obesity) and age, inappropriate timing of antibiotic prophylaxis, the presence of drains, prolonged preoperative hospital stays, shaving of the operative site the day before surgery (rather than just before the procedure), long duration of surgery, and infection at remote sites.
  - These infections are typically caused by the pt's endogenous or hospital-acquired flora. *S. aureus*, coagulase-negative staphylococci, and enteric and anaerobic bacteria are the most common pathogens.
    - *S. aureus*, coagulase-negative staphylococci, and enteric and anaerobic bacteria are the most common pathogens.
    - Group A streptococcal and clostridial infections should be considered in rapidly progressing postoperative infections (manifesting within 24–48 h of a procedure).
  - Clinical assessment of the surgical site may reveal obvious cellulitis or abscess formation; diagnosis of deeper infections requires a high index of suspicion and radiographic imaging.
  - Treatment of postoperative wound infections requires source control (drainage or surgical excision of infected or necrotic material) and antibiotic therapy aimed at the most likely or laboratory-confirmed pathogens.

- **Intravascular Device Infections** Intravascular device–related infections cause ~14% of nosocomial infections, increase the duration of hospital stay by 12 days, add $3700–$29,000 to hospital costs, and have an attributable mortality rate of 12–25%.
  - Catheterization of the femoral vessels is associated with a higher risk of infection in adults.
    - These infections are largely due to the skin flora at the site of catheter insertion, with pathogens migrating extraluminally to the catheter tip.
    - Contamination of the infusate is rare.
    - Coagulase-negative staphylococci, *S. aureus* (≥50% methicillin-resistant isolates), enterococci, nosocomial gram-negative bacilli, and *Candida* are the pathogens most frequently associated with these bacteremias.
  - Infection is suspected on the basis of the catheter site's appearance and/or the presence of fever or bacteremia without another source. The diagnosis is confirmed by isolation of the same bacteria from peripheral-blood cultures and from semiquantitative or quantitative cultures of samples from the vascular catheter tip.
  - In addition to the initiation of appropriate antibiotic treatment, other considerations include the level of risk for endocarditis (relatively high in pts with *S. aureus* bacteremia) and the decision regarding catheter removal, which is often necessary to cure infection.
    - If salvage of the catheter is attempted, the "antibiotic lock" technique (allowing a concentrated antibiotic solution to dwell in the catheter lumen along with systemic antibiotic administration) should be used.
    - If the catheter is changed over a guidewire and cultures of the removed catheter tip are positive, the catheter should be moved to a new site.

■ EPIDEMIC AND EMERGING PROBLEMS

Although outbreaks and emerging pathogens often receive a great deal of press, they account for <5% of nosocomial infections.

- *Influenza*: The main components of infection control—vaccination of the general public and health care workers, early use of antiviral agents for control of outbreaks, and adherence to surveillance and droplet precautions for symptomatic pts—have been effective in controlling influenza, including the 2009 H1N1 pandemic.
- *Nosocomial diarrhea*: Rates of health care–associated diarrhea have been increasing in recent years.
  - Rates of infection with *Clostridium difficile*—particularly the more virulent BI/NAP1/027 strain—are increasing, especially among older pts. Important infection-control components include judicious antibiotic use; heightened suspicion in cases with atypical presentations; and early diagnosis, treatment, and implementation of contact precautions.
  - Outbreaks of norovirus infection should be suspected in bacterial culture-negative diarrheal syndromes in which nausea and vomiting are prominent aspects. Contact precautions may need to be augmented

by environmental cleaning and active exclusion of ill staff and visitors, who often represent index cases.

- *Chickenpox*: Routine vaccination of children and VZV-susceptible employees has made nosocomial spread less common.

  – If VZV exposure occurs, postexposure prophylaxis with varicella-zoster immune globulin (VZIg) is considered for immunocompromised or pregnant contacts.

  – Varicella vaccine or preemptive administration of acyclovir is an alternative for other susceptible persons.

  – Susceptible employees are furloughed for 8–21 days (or for 28 days if VZIg has been given).

- *Tuberculosis*: Prompt recognition and isolation of cases, use of negative-pressure private rooms with 100% exhaust and at least 6–12 air changes per hour, use of approved N95 respirators, and follow-up skin testing of susceptible, exposed personnel are required.

- *Group A streptococcal infections*: A single nosocomial case, usually involving surgical wounds and the presence of an asymptomatic carrier in the operating room, should trigger an investigation. Health care workers linked to nosocomial transmission of group A streptococci should not be permitted to return to pt care settings until eradication of carriage via antimicrobial therapy has been documented.

- *Fungal infections*: Hospital renovations and disturbance of dusty surfaces can cause fungal spores to become airborne. Routine surveillance of neutropenic pts for infections with filamentous fungi (e.g., *Aspergillus*, *Fusarium*) helps determine whether there are extensive environmental risks.

- *Legionellosis*: If nosocomial cases are detected, environmental samples (e.g., tap water) should be cultured; eradication measures should be pursued if typing of clinical and environmental isolates reveals a correlation.

- *Antibiotic-resistant bacterial infection*: Close laboratory surveillance, strict infection-control practices, and aggressive antibiotic-control policies are the cornerstones of resistance-control efforts.

  – Molecular typing can help distinguish an outbreak of a single isolate (which necessitates an emphasis on hand hygiene and an evaluation of common-source exposures) from a polyclonal outbreak (which necessitates re-emphasis on antibiotic prudence and device bundles).

  – Organisms that raise concerns include methicillin-resistant *S. aureus*, gram-negative organisms that produce carbapenemases and/or extended-spectrum β-lactamases, pan-resistant strains of *Acinetobacter*, and vancomycin-resistant enterococci.

- *Bioterrorism preparedness*: Education, effective systems of internal and external communication, and risk assessment capabilities are key features.

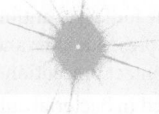

For a more detailed discussion, see Weinstein RA: Health Care–Associated Infections, Chap. 131, p. 1112, in HPIM-18.

CHAPTER **88**
Infections in the Immunocompromised Host

The immunocompromised pt is at increased risk for infection with both common and opportunistic pathogens.

INFECTIONS IN CANCER PTS

Table 88-1 lists the normal barriers to infection whose disruption may permit infections in immunocompromised pts, with particular relevance for the noted cancers. Infection-associated mortality rates among cancer pts have decreased as a result of an evolving approach entailing early use of empirical broad-spectrum antibiotics; empirical antifungal therapy in neutropenic pts who, after 4–7 days of antibiotic treatment, remain febrile without positive cultures; and use of antibiotics for afebrile neutropenic pts as broad-spectrum prophylaxis against infections.

■ SYSTEM-SPECIFIC SYNDROMES

- **Skin infections** Skin lesions of various types are common in pts with cancer and may be the first sign of bacterial or fungal sepsis, particularly in neutropenic pts (those with <500 functional neutrophils/μL).
    - *Cellulitis:* most often caused by group A *Streptococcus* and *Staphylococcus aureus.* Unusual organisms (e.g., *Escherichia coli, Pseudomonas,* fungi) may be involved in neutropenic pts.
    - *Macules or papules:* due to bacteria (e.g., *Pseudomonas aeruginosa* causing ecthyma gangrenosum) or fungi (e.g., *Candida*)
    - *Sweet's syndrome or febrile neutrophilic dermatosis:* Most often seen in neutropenic leukemic pts, it presents as red or bluish-red papules or nodules that form sharply bordered plaques; high fever; and an elevated ESR. The skin lesions are most common on the face, neck, and arms.
    - *Erythema multiforme with mucous membrane involvement:* Often due to HSV infection, it is distinct from Stevens-Johnson syndrome, which is associated with drugs and has a more widespread distribution; both conditions are common in pts with cancer.
    - *Drug rashes:* Rashes associated with drugs, particularly cytokines used in cancer therapy, complicate the differential diagnosis of rashes in pts with cancer.
- **Catheter-related infections** Exit-site infections, often with erythema around the insertion site, are most common.
    - Infections caused by coagulase-negative staphylococci can often be treated medically without catheter removal.
    - Infections caused by other organisms, including *S. aureus, P. aeruginosa, Candida, Stenotrophomonas,* or *Bacillus,* usually require catheter removal.

TABLE 88-1 DISRUPTION OF NORMAL BARRIERS THAT MAY PREDISPOSE TO INFECTIONS IN PATIENTS WITH CANCER

Type of Defense	Specific Lesion	Cells Involved	Organisms	Cancer Association	Disease
Physical barrier	Breaks in skin	Skin epithelial cells	Staphylococci, streptococci	Head and neck, squamous cell carcinoma	Cellulitis, extensive skin infection
Emptying of fluid collections	Occlusion of orifices: ureters, bile duct, colon	Luminal epithelial cells	Gram-negative bacilli	Renal, ovarian, biliary tree, and many metastatic cancers	Rapid, overwhelming bacteremia; urinary tract infection
Lymphatic function	Node dissection	Lymph nodes	Staphylococci, streptococci	Breast cancer surgery	Cellulitis
Splenic clearance of microorganisms	Splenectomy	Splenic reticuloendothelial cells	*Streptococcus pneumoniae, Haemophilus influenzae, Neisseria meningitidis, Babesia, Capnocytophaga canimorsus*	Hodgkin's disease, leukemia, idiopathic thrombocytopenic purpura	Rapid, overwhelming sepsis
Phagocytosis	Lack of granulocytes	Granulocytes (neutrophils)	Staphylococci, streptococci, enteric organisms, fungi	Hairy cell, acute myelocytic, and acute lymphocytic leukemias	Bacteremia
Humoral immunity	Lack of antibody	B cells	*S. pneumoniae, H. influenzae, N. meningitidis*	Chronic lymphocytic leukemia, multiple myeloma	Infections with encapsulated organisms, sinusitis, pneumonia
Cellular immunity	Lack of T cells	T cells and macrophages	*Mycobacterium tuberculosis, Listeria,* herpesviruses, fungi, intracellular parasites	Hodgkin's disease, leukemia, T cell lymphoma	Infections with intracellular bacteria, fungi, parasites

– If a red streak develops over the SC part of a "tunneled" catheter, the device must be removed to prevent extensive cellulitis and tissue necrosis.

- **Upper GI infections** Breakdown of mucosal surfaces due to chemotherapy and infection are common.
  – Oral mucositis is associated with viridans streptococci and HSV.
  – Oral candidal infections (thrush) are common.
  – Esophagitis can be caused by *Candida albicans* and HSV.
- **Lower GI infections** Transmigration of bowel flora across the intestinal epithelium can lead to severe conditions.
  – *Chronic disseminated candidiasis:* results from seeding of organs (e.g., liver, spleen, kidneys) during neutropenia in pts with hematologic malignancy and generally presents symptomatically when neutropenia resolves. Pts have persistent fever unresponsive to antibiotics, abdominal pain, and increased alkaline phosphatase levels. Although biopsies may reveal granulomas, yeasts, or pseudohyphae, the diagnosis is often made on the basis of radiographic studies (CT, MRI). Treatment should be directed to the causative agent; *C. albicans* is usually responsible, but *C. tropicalis* or other *Candida* species are sometimes involved.
  – *Typhlitis (necrotizing colitis):* more common among children than among adults and among pts with acute myelocytic leukemia or acute lymphocytic leukemia than among pts with other forms of cancer. Pts have fever, RLQ tenderness, and diarrhea that is often bloody. The diagnosis is confirmed by documentation of a thickened cecal wall via imaging. Treatment should include antibiotics directed against bowel flora and surgery (in the case of perforation).
- **CNS infections** The susceptibility of pts to specific infections depends on whether they have prolonged neutropenia, defects in cellular immunity (e.g., high-dose glucocorticoid therapy, cytotoxic chemotherapy), or defects in humoral immunity [e.g., pts with chronic lymphocytic leukemia, s/p splenectomy, or s/p bone marrow transplantation (BMT)].
  – *Meningitis:* Consider *Cryptococcus* or *Listeria*, particularly for pts with defects in cellular immunity. Pts with defects in humoral immunity are also at risk for infection with encapsulated bacteria such as *Streptococcus pneumoniae*, *Haemophilus influenzae*, and *Neisseria meningitidis*.
  – *Encephalitis:* Pts with defects in cellular immunity are particularly prone to infection with VZV, JC virus (progressive multifocal leukoencephalopathy), CMV, *Listeria*, HSV, and human herpesvirus type 6.
  – *Brain masses:* most often present as headache with or without fever or neurologic abnormalities. Pts with prolonged neutropenia are at increased risk for a brain abscess due to *Aspergillus*, *Nocardia*, or *Cryptococcus*. Pts with defects in cellular immunity are at increased risk for infection with *Toxoplasma* and EBV (lymphoproliferative disease). A definitive diagnosis may require a biopsy.
- **Pulmonary infections** Pneumonia can be difficult to diagnose in immunocompromised pts, given that many of the conventional findings (e.g., purulent sputum, physical findings suggestive of chest consolidation)

rely on the presence of neutrophils. Radiographic patterns of infiltration can help narrow the differential diagnosis.

– *Localized infiltrate:* Consider bacterial pneumonia (including *Legionella* and mycobacteria), local hemorrhage or embolism, and tumor.

– *Nodular infiltrate:* Consider fungal infection (e.g., *Aspergillus, Mucor*), *Nocardia* infection, and recurrent tumor. In pts with *Aspergillus* infection, hemoptysis may be an ominous sign. A biopsy performed with direct visualization may be required for definitive diagnosis.

– *Diffuse infiltrates:* Consider infection with viruses (particularly CMV), *Chlamydia, Pneumocystis, Toxoplasma,* or mycobacteria. Viruses that cause upper respiratory infections in normal hosts (e.g., influenza, respiratory syncytial) may cause fatal pneumonitis in immunocompromised pts. Noninfectious causes include radiation pneumonitis, CHF, diffuse alveolar hemorrhage (after BMT), and drug-induced lung injury (e.g., bleomycin, alkylating agents).

- **Renal and ureteral infections** These infections are usually associated with obstructing tumor masses.

– *Candida* has a predilection for the kidneys, reaching this site via either hematogenous seeding or retrograde spread from the bladder. Persistent funguria should prompt a search for infection in the kidney (e.g., fungus ball).

– BK virus and adenovirus can cause hemorrhagic cystitis.

APPROACH TO THE PATIENT | Febrile Neutropenia

Approach to Diagnosis and Treatment of Febrile Neutropenic Pts

Figure 88-1 presents an algorithm for the diagnosis and treatment of pts with febrile neutropenia.

- The initial regimen should be refined on the basis of culture data.
- Adding antibiotics to the initial regimen is not appropriate unless there is a clinical or microbiologic reason to do so. The addition of aminoglycosides to β-lactam therapy does not enhance efficacy (but does increase toxicity), even for infections involving *P. aeruginosa.*
- For empirical antifungal treatment, amphotericin B is being supplanted by liposomal formulations of amphotericin B, newer azoles (e.g., voriconazole or posaconazole), and echinocandins (e.g., caspofungin). Echinocandins are useful against infections with azole-resistant *Candida.* Clinical experience related to antiviral therapy is most extensive with acyclovir for HSV and VZV infections. Newer agents (e.g., cidofovir, foscarnet) with a broader spectrum of action have heightened the focus on treatment of viral infections.

– Prophylactic antibiotics (e.g., fluoroquinolones) in pts expected to have prolonged neutropenia or antifungal agents (e.g., fluconazole) in pts with hematopoietic stem cell transplants may prevent infections. *Pneumocystis* prophylaxis is mandatory for pts with acute lymphocytic leukemia and for those receiving glucocorticoid-containing regimens.

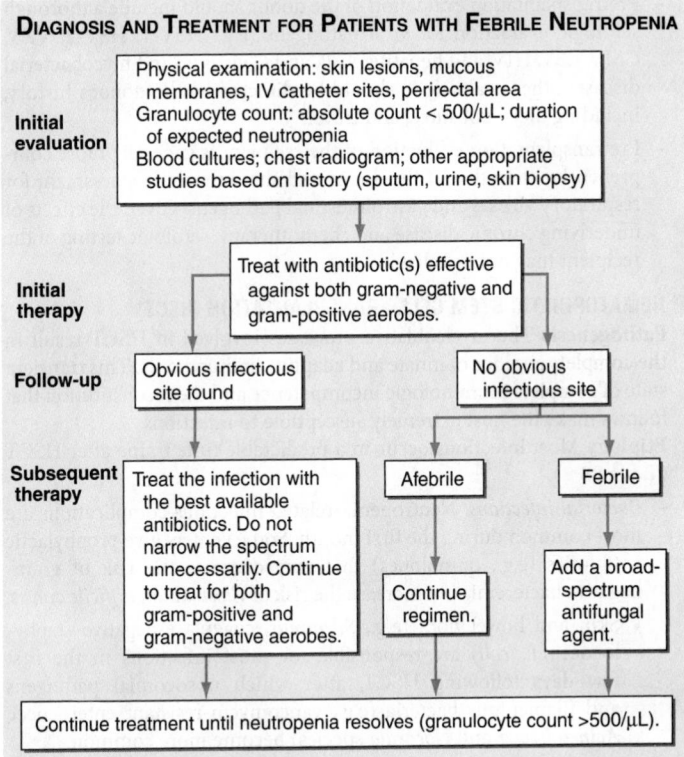

DIAGNOSIS AND TREATMENT FOR PATIENTS WITH FEBRILE NEUTROPENIA

Initial evaluation
Physical examination: skin lesions, mucous membranes, IV catheter sites, perirectal area
Granulocyte count: absolute count < 500/μL; duration of expected neutropenia
Blood cultures; chest radiogram; other appropriate studies based on history (sputum, urine, skin biopsy)

Initial therapy
Treat with antibiotic(s) effective against both gram-negative and gram-positive aerobes.

Follow-up
Obvious infectious site found
No obvious infectious site

Subsequent therapy
Treat the infection with the best available antibiotics. Do not narrow the spectrum unnecessarily. Continue to treat for both gram-positive and gram-negative aerobes.

Afebrile → Continue regimen.

Febrile → Add a broad-spectrum antifungal agent.

Continue treatment until neutropenia resolves (granulocyte count >500/μL).

FIGURE 88-1 Algorithm for the diagnosis and treatment of febrile neutropenic pts. Several general guidelines are useful in the initial treatment of these pts: (1) The agents used should reflect both the epidemiology and the antibiotic resistance pattern of the hospital. (2) A single third-generation cephalosporin constitutes an appropriate initial regimen in many hospitals (if the pattern of resistance justifies its use). (3) Most standard regimens are designed for pts who have not previously received prophylactic antibiotics. The development of fever in a pt receiving antibiotics affects the choice of subsequent therapy (which should target resistant organisms and organisms known to cause infections in pts being treated with the antibiotics already administered). (4) Randomized trials have indicated that it is safe to use oral antibiotic regimens to treat "low-risk" pts who have fever and neutropenia. Outpatients who are expected to remain neutropenic for <10 days and who have no concurrent medical problems (such as hypotension, pulmonary compromise, or abdominal pain) can be classified as low-risk and treated with a broad-spectrum oral regimen.

INFECTIONS IN TRANSPLANT RECIPIENTS

Evaluation of infections in transplant recipients must involve consideration of infectious agents harbored by the donor organ and the recipient's immunosuppressive drug regimen, which increases susceptibility to latent infections (among other infections).

- Pretransplantation evaluation of the donor should include a thorough serologic evaluation for viral pathogens (e.g., HSV-1, HSV-2, VZV, CMV, EBV, HIV, and hepatitis A, B, and C viruses) and mycobacterial disease; other evaluations should be directed by the donor's history, including diet, exposures, and travel.
- Pretransplantation evaluation of the recipient is generally more comprehensive than that of the donor and should include assessment for respiratory viruses and gastrointestinal pathogens. Given the effects of underlying chronic disease and chemotherapy, serologic testing of the recipient may not be reliable.

■ HEMATOPOIETIC STEM CELL TRANSPLANTATION (HSCT)

- **Pathogenesis** The myeloablative processes involved in HSCT result in the complete absence of innate and adaptive immune cells. This transient state of complete immunologic incompetence and the reconstitution that follows make the host extremely susceptible to infections.
- **Etiology** Most infections occur in a predictable time frame after HSCT (Table 88-2).
  - *Bacterial infections*: Neutropenia-related infectious complications are most common during the first month. Some centers give prophylactic antibiotics (e.g., quinolones) that may decrease the risk of gram-negative bacteremia but increase the risk of *Clostridium difficile* colitis.
    - Skin and bowel flora (e.g., *S. aureus*, coagulase-negative staphylococci, *E. coli*) are responsible for most infections in the first few days following HSCT, after which nosocomial pathogens and filamentous bacteria (e.g., vancomycin-resistant enterococci, *Acinetobacter* and *Nocardia* species) become more common.
  - *Fungal infections*: Fungal infections are increasingly common beyond the first week after HSCT, particularly among pts who receive broad-spectrum antibiotics. Infections with *Candida* species are most common, although resistant fungi (e.g., *Aspergillus*, *Fusarium*) are becoming more common because of the increased use of prophylactic fluconazole.
    - Prolonged treatment with glucocorticoids or other immunosuppressive agents increases the risk of infection with *Candida* or *Aspergillus* and of reactivation of endemic fungi even after resolution of neutropenia.
    - Maintenance prophylaxis with trimethoprim-sulfamethoxazole (TMP-SMX; 160/800 mg/d starting 1 month after engraftment and continuing for at least 1 year) is recommended to prevent *Pneumocystis jiroveci* pneumonia.
  - *Parasitic infections*: Prophylaxis with TMP-SMX is also protective against disease caused by *Toxoplasma* as well as against late infections caused by certain bacteria, including *Nocardia*, *Listeria monocytogenes*, *S. pneumoniae*, and *H. influenzae*.
    - Given increasing international travel, parasitic diseases (e.g., caused by *Strongyloides*, *Leishmania*, *Giardia*, *Cryptosporidium*) that are typically restricted to particular environments may be more likely to be reactivated in pts after HSCT.

TABLE 88-2 COMMON INFECTIONS AFTER HSCT

Infection Site	Period after Transplantation		
	Early (<1 Month)	Middle (1–4 Months)	Late (>6 Months)
Disseminated	Aerobic bacteria (gram-negative, gram-positive)	*Nocardia, Candida, Aspergillus,* EBV	Encapsulated bacteria (*Streptococcus pneumoniae, Haemophilus influenzae, Neisseria meningitidis*)
Skin and mucous membranes	HSV	HHV-6	VZV
Lungs	Aerobic bacteria (gram-negative, gram-positive), *Candida, Aspergillus,* other molds, HSV	CMV, seasonal respiratory viruses, *Pneumocystis, Toxoplasma*	*Pneumocystis, S. pneumoniae*
Gastrointestinal tract	*Clostridium difficile*	CMV, adeno-virus	EBV, CMV
Kidney		BK virus, adenovirus	
Brain	HHV-6[a]	HHV-6 *Toxoplasma*	*Toxoplasma,* JC virus (rare)
Bone marrow	HHV-6		

[a] HHV-6, human herpesvirus type 6.

- *Viral infections*: Prophylactic acyclovir or valacyclovir for HSV-seropositive pts reduces rates of mucositis and prevents pneumonia and other HSV manifestations.
  - Zoster generally occurs several months after HSCT and usually is managed readily with acyclovir.
  - Human herpesvirus type 6 delays monocyte and platelet engraftment and may be linked to encephalitis or pneumonitis; the efficacy of antiviral treatment has not been well studied.
  - CMV disease (e.g., interstitial pneumonia, bone marrow suppression, colitis, and graft failure) usually occurs 30–90 days after HSCT. Severe disease is more common among allogeneic transplant recipients and is often associated with graft-versus-host disease, with pneumonia as the foremost cause of death. Preemptive therapy (initiation of antiviral therapy only after CMV is detected in blood) has supplanted prophylactic therapy (treatment of all transplant recipients when either the recipient or the donor is seropositive) because of the toxic side effects associated with ganciclovir.

- EBV lymphoproliferative disease as well as infections caused by respiratory viruses (e.g., respiratory syncytial virus, parainfluenza virus, metapneumovirus, influenza virus, adenovirus) can occur. BK virus (a polyomavirus) has been found in the urine of pts after HSCT and may be associated with hemorrhagic cystitis.

■ SOLID ORGAN TRANSPLANTATION

- **Pathogenesis** After solid organ transplantation, pts do not go through a stage of neutropenia like that seen after HSCT; thus the infections in these two groups of pts differ. However, solid organ transplant recipients are immunosuppressed for longer periods with agents that chronically impair T cell immunity. Moreover, the persistent HLA mismatch between recipient immune cells (e.g., effector T cells) and the donor organ (allograft) places the organ at permanently increased risk of infection.
- **Etiology** As in HSCT, the infection risk depends on the interval since transplantation.
  - *Early infections (<1 month)*: Infections are most commonly caused by extracellular organisms, which originate in surgical wound or anastomotic sites.
  - *Middle-period infections (1–6 months)*: The consequences of suppressing cell-mediated immunity become apparent, and infections result from acquisition—or reactivation—of viruses, mycobacteria, endemic fungi, and parasites.
    - CMV can cause severe systemic disease or infection of transplanted organs; the latter increases the risk of organ rejection, prompting increased immunosuppression that, in turn, increases CMV replication.
    - Diagnosis, treatment, and prophylaxis of CMV infection are the keys to interrupting this cycle.
  - *Late infections (>6 months)*: Infections of this period are similar to those in pts with chronically impaired T cell immunity (e.g., *Listeria*, *Nocardia*, *Rhodococcus*, mycobacteria, various fungi, other intracellular organisms).
    - EBV lymphoproliferative disease occurs most commonly in pts who receive a heart or lung transplant (as well as the most intense immunosuppressive regimens); in these cases, immunosuppression should be decreased or discontinued, if possible, and consideration should be given to treatment with anti–B cell antibodies.
    - Prophylaxis against *Pneumocystis* pneumonia for at least 1 year is generally recommended for all solid organ transplant recipients.
    - The incidence of tuberculosis within the first 12 months after solid organ transplantation is greater than that after HSCT and reflects the prevalence of tuberculosis in the local population.
- **Specific issues** While the above information is generally valid for all organ transplants, there are some organ-specific considerations.
  - *Kidney transplantation*: TMP-SMX prophylaxis for the first 4–6 months decreases the incidence of early and middle-period infections, particularly UTIs related to anatomic alterations resulting from

TABLE 88-3 VACCINATION OF CANCER PATIENTS RECEIVING CHEMOTHERAPY[a]

Vaccine	Use in Indicated Patients		
	Intensive Chemotherapy	Hodgkin's Disease	HSCT
Diphtheria-tetanus[b]	Primary series and boosters as necessary	No special recommendation	3 doses given 6–12 months after transplantation
Poliomyelitis[c]	Complete primary series and boosters	No special recommendation	3 doses given 6–12 months after transplantation
Haemophilus influenzae type b conjugate	Primary series and booster for children	Immunization before treatment and booster 3 months afterward	3 doses given 6–12 months after transplantation
Human papillomavirus	3 doses for girls and women through 26 years of age	3 doses for girls and women through 26 years of age	3 doses for girls and women through 26 years of age
Hepatitis A	As indicated for normal hosts based on occupation and lifestyle	As indicated for normal hosts based on occupation and lifestyle	As indicated for normal hosts based on occupation and lifestyle
Hepatitis B	Same as for normal hosts	As indicated for normal hosts based on occupation and lifestyle	3 doses given 6–12 months after transplantation
23-Valent pneumococcal polysaccharide[d]	Every 5 years	Immunization before treatment and booster 3 months afterward	1 or 2 doses given 6–12 months after transplantation
4-Valent meningococcal[e]	Should be administered to splenectomized pts and pts living in endemic areas, including college students in dormitories	Should be administered to splenectomized pts and pts living in endemic areas, including college students in dormitories	Should be administered to splenectomized pts and pts living in endemic areas, including college students in dormitories
Influenza	Seasonal immunization	Seasonal immunization	Seasonal immunization

(*continued*)

TABLE 88-3 VACCINATION OF CANCER PATIENTS RECEIVING CHEMOTHERAPY[a] (CONTINUED)

	Use in Indicated Patients		
Vaccine	Intensive Chemotherapy	Hodgkin's Disease	HSCT
Measles/mumps/rubella	Contraindicated	Contraindicated during chemotherapy	After 24 months in pts without graft-versus-host disease
Varicella-zoster virus[f]	Contraindicated[g]	Contraindicated	Contraindicated

[a]The latest recommendations by the Advisory Committee on Immunization Practices and the CDC guidelines can be found at *www.cdc.gov/vaccines*.

[b]The Td (tetanus-diphtheria) combination was recommended for adults. Pertussis vaccine was not recommended for people >6 years of age in the past. However, recent data indicate that the Tdap (tetanus–diphtheria–acellular pertussis) product is both safe and efficacious in adults. A single Tdap booster is now recommended for adults.

[c]Live-virus vaccine is contraindicated; inactivated vaccine should be used.

[d]The 13-valent pneumococcal conjugate vaccine is currently recommended for children.

[e]Meningococcal conjugate vaccine (MCV4) is recommended for adults ≤55 years old and meningococcal polysaccharide vaccine (MPSV4) for those ≥56 years old.

[f]Includes both varicella vaccine for children and zoster vaccine for adults.

[g]Contact the manufacturer for more information on use in children with acute lymphocytic leukemia.

surgery. CMV is the predominant pathogen in the middle period; disease is evident in 50% of renal transplant pts presenting with fever 1–4 months after transplantation, prompting many centers to use valacyclovir prophylaxis for high-risk pts. BK viruria and viremia are associated with ureteral strictures, nephropathy, and vasculopathy and require a reduction of immunosuppression to lower rates of graft loss.

– *Heart transplantation*: Mediastinitis, generally caused by typical skin flora and rarely caused by *Mycoplasma hominis*, is an early complication of heart transplantation. The overall incidence of toxoplasmosis (a middle-period infection) is so high in the setting of heart transplantation that serologic screening and some prophylaxis (e.g., TMP-SMX) are always warranted.

– *Lung transplantation*: Pts receiving a lung transplant are predisposed to pneumonia and mediastinitis in the early period. The high incidence of CMV disease (75–100% if either the donor or the recipient is seropositive) indicates the importance of antiviral prophylaxis; late disease may occur once prophylaxis is discontinued, although the pt is generally better able to handle it because of reduced immunosuppression.

– *Liver transplantation*: Bacterial abscesses and peritonitis are common early complications and often result from biliary leaks. Pts receiving a liver transplant have a high incidence of fungal infections correlated with preoperative glucocorticoid use, long-term antimicrobial use, and a high degree of immunosuppression. Recurrent (reactivated) hepatitis B and C infections are problematic; while hepatitis B immunoglobulin administration and prophylaxis with antiviral agents active against hepatitis B virus have been successful in preventing reinfection with hepatitis B virus, reinfection with hepatitis C virus occurs in all pts.

IMMUNIZATIONS IN IMMUNOSUPPRESSED PTS

Recommendations for vaccination of cancer pts receiving chemotherapy, pts with Hodgkin's disease, and hematopoietic stem cell transplant recipients are listed in Table 88-3. In solid organ transplant recipients, the usual vaccines and boosters should be given before immunosuppression. Pts with continued immunosuppression should have pneumococcal vaccination repeated every 5 years and should not receive live vaccines.

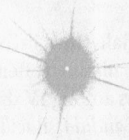

> For a more detailed discussion, see Finberg R: Infections in Patients With Cancer, Chap. 86, p. 712; Madoff LC, Kasper DL: Introduction to Infectious Diseases: Host–Pathogen Interactions, Chap. 119, p. 1007; and Finberg R, Fingeroth J: Infections in Transplant Recipients, Chap. 132, p. 1120, in HPIM-18.

CHAPTER **89**
Infective Endocarditis

Acute endocarditis is a febrile illness that rapidly damages cardiac structures, seeds extracardiac sites hematogenously, and can progress to death within weeks. *Subacute* endocarditis follows an indolent course, rarely causes metastatic infection, and progresses gradually unless complicated by a major embolic event or a ruptured mycotic aneurysm.

- **Epidemiology** In developed countries, the incidence of endocarditis ranges from 2.6 to 7.0 cases per 100,000 population per year, with higher rates among the elderly.
  - Predisposing conditions include congenital heart disease, illicit IV drug use, degenerative valve disease, and intracardiac devices.
  - Chronic rheumatic heart disease is a risk factor in low-income countries.
  - Of endocarditis cases, 16–30% involve prosthetic valves, with the greatest risk during the first 6–12 months after valve replacement.
- **Etiology** Because of their different portals of entry, the causative microorganisms vary among clinical types of endocarditis.
  - In native valve endocarditis (NVE), viridans streptococci, staphylococci, and HACEK organisms [*Haemophilus* spp., *Aggregatibacter* (formerly *Actinobacillus) actinomycetemcomitans, Cardiobacterium hominis, Eikenella corrodens*, and *Kingella kingae*] enter the bloodstream from oral, skin, and upper respiratory tract portals. *Streptococcus*

gallolyticus (formerly *S. bovis*) originates from the gut and is associated with colon polyps or cancer. Enterococci originate from the genitourinary tract.

– Health care–associated NVE, frequently due to *Staphylococcus aureus*, coagulase-negative staphylococci (CoNS), and enterococci, can have a nosocomial onset (55%) or a community onset (45%) in pts who have had extensive contact with the health care system in the preceding 90 days.

– Prosthetic valve endocarditis (PVE) developing within 2 months of surgery is due to intraoperative contamination or a bacteremic postoperative complication and is typically caused by CoNS, *S. aureus*, facultative gram-negative bacilli, diphtheroids, or fungi. Cases beginning >1 year after valve surgery are caused by the same organisms that cause community-acquired NVE. PVE due to CoNS that presents 2–12 months after surgery often represents delayed-onset nosocomial infection.

– Endocarditis occurring among IV drug users, especially that involving the tricuspid valve, is commonly caused by *S. aureus* (often a methicillin-resistant strain). Left-sided valve infections among IV drug users are caused by *Pseudomonas aeruginosa* and *Candida*, *Bacillus*, *Lactobacillus*, and *Corynebacterium* spp. in addition to the usual causes of endocarditis.

– About 5–15% of endocarditis cases are culture negative, and one-third to one-half of these cases are due to prior antibiotic exposure. The remainder of culture-negative cases represent infection by fastidious organisms, such as the nutritionally variant bacteria *Granulicatella* and *Abiotrophia*, HACEK organisms, *Bartonella* spp., *Coxiella burnetii*, *Brucella* spp., and *Tropheryma whipplei*.

• **Pathogenesis** Endothelial injury allows direct infection by more virulent pathogens (e.g., *S. aureus*) or the development of an uninfected platelet-fibrin thrombus [referred to as *nonbacterial thrombotic endocarditis* (NBTE)] that may become infected during transient bacteremia. NBTE arises from cardiac conditions (e.g., mitral regurgitation, aortic stenosis, aortic regurgitation), hypercoagulable states, and the antiphospholipid antibody syndrome. After entering the bloodstream, organisms adhere to the endothelium or sites of NBTE via surface adhesin molecules. The clinical manifestations of endocarditis arise from cytokine production, damage to intracardiac structures, embolization of vegetation fragments, hematogenous infection of sites during bacteremia, and tissue injury due to the deposition of immune complexes.

• **Clinical manifestations** The clinical syndrome is variable and spans a continuum between acute and subacute presentations. The temporal course of disease is dictated in large part by the causative organism: *S. aureus*, β-hemolytic streptococci, pneumococci, and *Staphylococcus lugdunensis* typically present acutely, whereas viridans streptococci, enterococci, CoNS (other than *S. lugdunensis*), and the HACEK group typically present subacutely.

– *Constitutional symptoms*: generally nonspecific, but may include fever, chills, weight loss, myalgias, or arthralgias.

– *Cardiac manifestations*: Heart murmurs, particularly new or worsened regurgitant murmurs, are ultimately heard in 85% of pts with acute NVE.

• CHF develops in 30–40% of pts and is usually due to valvular dysfunction.

• Extension of infection can result in perivalvular abscesses, which in turn may cause intracardiac fistulae. Abscesses may burrow from the aortic root into the ventricular septum and interrupt the conduction system or may burrow through the epicardium and cause pericarditis.

– *Noncardiac manifestations*: Arterial emboli are present in 50% of pts, with hematogenously seeded focal infection most often evident in the skin, spleen, kidneys, bones, and meninges.

• The risk of embolization increases with endocarditis caused by *S. aureus*, vegetations >10 mm in diameter, and infection involving the mitral valve.

• Cerebrovascular emboli presenting as stroke or encephalopathy complicate 15–35% of cases, with one-half of these cases preceding the diagnosis of endocarditis.

– The incidence of stroke decreases dramatically with antibiotic therapy and does not correlate with change in vegetation size.

– Other neurologic complications include aseptic or purulent meningitis, intracranial hemorrhage due to ruptured mycotic aneurysms (focal dilations of arteries at points in the artery wall that have been weakened by infection or where septic emboli have lodged) or hemorrhagic infarcts, seizures, and microabscesses (especially with *S. aureus*).

• Immune complex deposition on the glomerular basement membrane causes glomerulonephritis and renal dysfunction.

• Nonsuppurative peripheral manifestations of subacute endocarditis (e.g., Janeway lesions, Roth's spots) are related to duration of infection and are now rare because of early diagnosis and treatment.

– *Manifestations of specific predisposing conditions*: Underlying conditions may affect the presenting signs and symptoms.

• *IV drug use*: ~50% of endocarditis cases associated with IV drug use are limited to the tricuspid valve and present as fever, faint or no murmur, and prominent pulmonary findings such as cough, pleuritic chest pain, nodular pulmonary infiltrates, or occasional pyopneumothorax. Pts with left-sided cardiac infections present with the typical clinical features of endocarditis.

• *Health care–associated endocarditis*: Manifestations are typical in the absence of a retained intracardiac device. Endocarditis associated with a transvenous pacemaker or an implanted defibrillator may be associated with a generator pocket infection and result in fever, minimal murmur, and pulmonary symptoms due to septic emboli.

• *PVE*: In cases of endocarditis occurring within 60 days of valve surgery, typical symptoms may be masked by comorbidity associated with recent surgery. Paravalvular infection is common in PVE, resulting in partial valve dehiscence, regurgitant murmurs, CHF, or disruption of the conduction system.

- **Diagnosis** A diagnosis of infective endocarditis is established definitively only when vegetations are examined histologically and microbiologically.
  - The Duke criteria (Table 89-1) constitute a highly sensitive and specific diagnostic schema that emphasizes the roles of bacteremia and echocardiographic findings.
    - A clinical diagnosis of definite endocarditis requires fulfillment of 2 major, 1 major plus 3 minor, or 5 minor criteria.
    - A diagnosis of possible endocarditis requires documentation of 1 major plus 1 minor criterion or 3 minor criteria.
  - For antibiotic-naïve pts, three 2-bottle blood culture sets—separated from one another by at least 1 h—should be obtained from different sites within the first 24 h. If blood cultures are negative after 48–72 h, two or three additional cultures should be performed.
  - Serology is helpful in implicating *Brucella, Bartonella, Legionella,* or *C. burnetii* in endocarditis. Examination of the vegetation by histology, culture, direct fluorescent antibody techniques, and/or PCR may be helpful in identifying the causative organism in the absence of a positive blood culture.
  - Echocardiography should be performed to confirm the diagnosis, to verify the size of vegetations, to detect intracardiac complications, and to assess cardiac function.
    - Transthoracic echocardiography (TTE) does not detect vegetations <2 mm in diameter and is not adequate for evaluation of prosthetic valves or detection of intracardiac complications; however, TTE may be used when pts have a low pretest likelihood of endocarditis (<5%).
    - Transesophageal echocardiography (TEE) detects vegetations in >90% of cases of definite endocarditis and is optimal for evaluation of prosthetic valves and detection of abscesses, valve perforation, or intracardiac fistulas.
    - When endocarditis is likely, a negative TEE result does not exclude the diagnosis but warrants repetition of the study in 7–10 days.

TREATMENT Endocarditis

ANTIMICROBIAL THERAPY

- Antimicrobial therapy must be bactericidal and prolonged. See Table 89-2 for organism-specific regimens. Most pts defervesce within 5–7 days.
  - Blood cultures should be repeated until sterile, and results should be rechecked if there is recrudescent fever and at 4–6 weeks after therapy to document cure.
  - If pts are febrile for 7 days despite antibiotic therapy, an evaluation for paravalvular or extracardiac abscesses should be performed.

TABLE 89-1 THE DUKE CRITERIA FOR THE CLINICAL DIAGNOSIS OF INFECTIVE ENDOCARDITIS[a]

Major Criteria

1. Positive blood culture

   Typical microorganism for infective endocarditis from two separate blood cultures

       Viridans streptococci, *Streptococcus gallolyticus*, HACEK group, *Staphylococcus aureus*, *or*

       Community-acquired enterococci in the absence of a primary focus, *or*

   Persistently positive blood culture, defined as recovery of a microorganism consistent with infective endocarditis from:

       Blood cultures drawn >12 h apart; *or*

       All of three or a majority of four or more separate blood cultures, with first and last drawn at least 1 h apart

   Single positive blood culture for *Coxiella burnetii* or phase I IgG antibody titer of >1:800

2. Evidence of endocardial involvement

   Positive echocardiogram[b]

       Oscillating intracardiac mass on valve or supporting structures or in the path of regurgitant jets or in implanted material, in the absence of an alternative anatomic explanation, *or*

       Abscess, *or*

       New partial dehiscence of prosthetic valve, *or*

   New valvular regurgitation (increase or change in preexisting murmur not sufficient)

Minor Criteria

1. Predisposition: predisposing heart condition or injection drug use

2. Fever ≥38.0°C (≥100.4°F)

3. Vascular phenomena: major arterial emboli, septic pulmonary infarcts, mycotic aneurysm, intracranial hemorrhage, conjunctival hemorrhages, Janeway lesions

4. Immunologic phenomena: glomerulonephritis, Osler's nodes, Roth's spots, rheumatoid factor

5. Microbiologic evidence: positive blood culture but not meeting major criterion as noted previously[c] or serologic evidence of active infection with organism consistent with infective endocarditis

[a]See text for details.

[b]Transesophageal echocardiography is recommended for assessing possible prosthetic valve endocarditis or complicated endocarditis.

[c]Excluding single positive cultures for coagulase-negative staphylococci and diphtheroids, which are common culture contaminants, and organisms that do not cause endocarditis frequently, such as gram-negative bacilli.

Abbreviations: HACEK, *Haemophilus* spp., *Aggregatibacter actinomycetemcomitans, Cardiobacterium hominis, Eikenella corrodens, Kingella kingae.*

Source: Adapted from JS Li et al: Clin Infect Dis 30:633, 2000, with permission from the University of Chicago Press.

TABLE 89-2 ANTIBIOTIC TREATMENT FOR INFECTIVE ENDOCARDITIS CAUSED BY COMMON ORGANISMS[a]

Organism	Drug (Dose, Duration)	Comments
Streptococci		
Penicillin-susceptible[b] streptococci, *Streptococcus gallolyticus*	• Penicillin G (2–3 mU IV q4h for 4 weeks)	—
	• Ceftriaxone (2 g/d IV as a single dose for 4 weeks)	Can use ceftriaxone in pts with nonimmediate penicillin allergy
	• Vancomycin[c] (15 mg/kg IV q12h for 4 weeks)	Use vancomycin in pts with severe or immediate β-lactam allergy
	• Penicillin G (2–3 mU IV q4h) or ceftriaxone (2 g IV qd) for 2 weeks *plus* Gentamicin[d] (3 mg/kg qd IV or IM, as a single dose[e] or divided into equal doses q8h for 2 weeks)	Avoid 2-week regimen when risk of aminoglycoside toxicity is increased and in prosthetic valve or complicated endocarditis
Relatively penicillin-resistant[f] streptococci	• Penicillin G (4 mU IV q4h) or ceftriaxone (2 g IV qd) for 4 weeks *plus* Gentamicin[d] (3 mg/kg qd IV or IM, as a single dose[e] or divided into equal doses q8h for 2 weeks)	Penicillin alone at this dose for 6 weeks or with gentamicin during initial 2 weeks is preferred for prosthetic valve endocarditis caused by streptococci with penicillin MICs of ≤0.1 μg/mL
	• Vancomycin[c] as noted above for 4 weeks	—
Moderately penicillin-resistant[g] streptococci, nutritionally variant organisms, or *Gemella morbillorum*	• Penicillin G (4–5 mU IV q4h) or ceftriaxone (2 g IV qd) for 6 weeks *plus* Gentamicin[d] (3 mg/kg qd IV or IM as a single dose[e] or divided into equal doses q8h for 6 weeks)	Preferred for prosthetic valve endocarditis caused by streptococci with penicillin MICs of >0.1 μg/mL
	• Vancomycin[c] as noted above for 4 weeks	—
Enterococci[h]		
	• Penicillin G (4–5 mU IV q4h) *plus* Gentamicin[d] (1 mg/kg IV q8h), both for 4–6 weeks	Can use streptomycin (7.5 mg/kg q12h) in lieu of gentamicin if there is not high-level resistance to streptomycin

TABLE 89-2 ANTIBIOTIC TREATMENT FOR INFECTIVE ENDOCARDITIS CAUSED BY COMMON ORGANISMS[a] (CONTINUED)

Organism	Drug (Dose, Duration)	Comments
Enterococci[h] (continued)		
	• Ampicillin (2 g IV q4h) *plus* Gentamicin[d] (1 mg/kg IV q8h), both for 4–6 weeks	—
	• Vancomycin[c] (15 mg/kg IV q12h) *plus* Gentamicin[d] (1 mg/kg IV q8h), both for 4–6 weeks	Use vancomycin plus gentamicin for penicillin-allergic pts, or desensitize to penicillin
Staphylococci		
Methicillin-susceptible, infecting native valves (no foreign devices)	• Nafcillin or oxacillin (2 g IV q4h for 4–6 weeks)	Can use penicillin (4 mU q4h) if isolate is penicillin-susceptible (does not produce β-lactamase)
	• Cefazolin (2 g IV q8h for 4–6 weeks)	Can use cefazolin regimen for pts with nonimmediate penicillin allergy
	• Vancomycin[c] (15 mg/kg IV q12h for 4–6 weeks)	Use vancomycin for pts with immediate (urticarial) or severe penicillin allergy
Methicillin-resistant, infecting native valves (no foreign devices)	• Vancomycin[c] (15 mg/kg IV q8–12h for 4–6 weeks)	No role for routine use of rifampin
Methicillin-susceptible, infecting prosthetic valves	• Nafcillin or oxacillin (2 g IV q4h for 6–8 weeks) *plus* Gentamicin[d] (1 mg/kg IM or IV q8h for 2 weeks) *plus* Rifampin[i] (300 mg PO q8h for 6–8 weeks)	Use gentamicin during initial 2 weeks; determine susceptibility to gentamicin before initiating rifampin; if pt is highly allergic to penicillin, use regimen for methicillin-resistant staphylococci; if β-lactam allergy is of the minor nonimmediate type, can substitute cefazolin for oxacillin/nafcillin

(continued)

TABLE 89-2 ANTIBIOTIC TREATMENT FOR INFECTIVE ENDOCARDITIS CAUSED BY COMMON ORGANISMS[a] (CONTINUED)

Organism	Drug (Dose, Duration)	Comments
Staphylococci (continued)		
Methicillin-resistant, infecting prosthetic valves	• Vancomycin[c] (15 mg/kg IV q12h for 6–8 weeks) *plus* Gentamicin[d] (1 mg/kg IM or IV q8h for 2 weeks) *plus* Rifampin[i] (300 mg PO q8h for 6–8 weeks)	Use gentamicin during initial 2 weeks; determine gentamicin susceptibility before initiating rifampin
HACEK organisms		
	• Ceftriaxone (2 g/d IV as a single dose for 4 weeks)	Can use another third-generation cephalosporin at comparable dosage
	• Ampicillin/sulbactam (3 g IV q6h for 4 weeks)	—

[a]Doses are for adults with normal renal function. Doses of gentamicin, streptomycin, and vancomycin must be adjusted for reduced renal function. Ideal body weight is used to calculate doses of gentamicin and streptomycin per kilogram (men = 50 kg + 2.3 kg per inch over 5 feet; women = 45.5 kg + 2.3 kg per inch over 5 feet).

[b]MIC, ≤0.1 µg/mL.

[c]Vancomycin dose is based on actual body weight. Adjust for trough level of 10–15 µg/mL for streptococcal and enterococcal infections and 15–20 µg/mL for staphylococcal infections.

[d]Aminoglycosides should not be administered as single daily doses for enterococcal endocarditis and should be introduced as part of the initial treatment. Target peak and trough serum concentrations of divided-dose gentamicin 1 h after a 20- to 30-min infusion or IM injection are ~3.5 µg/mL and ≤1 µg/mL, respectively; target peak and trough serum concentrations of streptomycin (timing as with gentamicin) are 20–35 µg/mL and <10 µg/mL, respectively.

[e]Netilmicin (4 mg/kg qd, as a single dose) can be used in lieu of gentamicin.

[f]MIC, >0.1 µg/mL and <0.5 µg/mL.

[g]MIC, ≥0.5 µg/mL and <8 µg/mL.

[h]Antimicrobial susceptibility must be evaluated.

[i]Rifampin increases warfarin and dicumarol requirements for anticoagulation.

- Pts with acute endocarditis require antibiotic treatment as soon as three sets of blood culture samples are obtained, but pts with subacute disease who are clinically stable should have antibiotics withheld until a diagnosis is made.
- Pts treated with vancomycin or an aminoglycoside should have serum drug levels monitored. Tests to detect renal, hepatic, and/or hematologic toxicity should be performed periodically.

ORGANISM-SPECIFIC THERAPIES
- Endocarditis due to group B, C, or G streptococci should be treated with the regimen recommended for relatively penicillin-resistant streptococci (Table 89-2).

- Enterococci require the synergistic activity of a cell wall–active agent and an aminoglycoside for killing. Enterococci must be tested for high-level resistance to streptomycin and gentamicin. If such resistance is detected, the addition of an aminoglycoside will not produce a synergistic effect; the cell wall–active agent should be given alone for periods of 8–12 weeks, or—for *Enterococcus faecalis*—high-dose ampicillin plus ceftriaxone can be given. If treatment fails or the isolate is resistant to commonly used agents, surgical therapy is advised (see below and Table 89-3). The aminoglycoside can be discontinued in those pts who have responded satisfactorily to therapy if toxicity develops after 2–3 weeks of treatment.
- For staphylococcal endocarditis, the addition of 3–5 days of gentamicin to a β-lactam antibiotic does not improve survival rates and is not recommended.
- Daptomycin [6 mg/kg (or, as some experts prefer, 8–10 mg/kg) IV qd] has been recommended for endocarditis caused by *S. aureus* isolates with a vancomycin MIC of ≥2 µg/mL, although this regimen has not yet been approved by the U.S. Food and Drug Administration. These isolates should be tested to document daptomycin sensitivity.

TABLE 89-3 INDICATIONS FOR CARDIAC SURGICAL INTERVENTION IN PATIENTS WITH ENDOCARDITIS

Surgery required for optimal outcome
Moderate to severe CHF due to valve dysfunction
Partially dehisced unstable prosthetic valve
Persistent bacteremia despite optimal antimicrobial therapy
Lack of effective microbicidal therapy (e.g., fungal or *Brucella* endocarditis)
Staphylococcus aureus PVE with an intracardiac complication
Relapse of PVE after optimal antimicrobial therapy
Surgery to be strongly considered for improved outcome[a]
Perivalvular extension of infection
Poorly responsive *S. aureus* endocarditis involving the aortic or mitral valve
Large (>10-mm diameter) hypermobile vegetations with increased risk of embolism
Persistent unexplained fever (≥10 days) in culture-negative NVE
Poorly responsive or relapsed endocarditis due to highly antibiotic-resistant enterococci or gram-negative bacilli

[a]Surgery must be carefully considered; findings are often combined with other indications to prompt surgery.
Abbreviations: NVE, native valve endocarditis; PVE, prosthetic valve endocarditis.

- Staphylococcal PVE is treated for 6–8 weeks with a multidrug regimen. Rifampin is important because it kills organisms adherent to foreign material. The inclusion of two other agents in addition to rifampin helps prevent the emergence of rifampin resistance in vivo. Susceptibility testing for gentamicin should be performed before rifampin is given; if the strain is resistant, another aminoglycoside, a fluoroquinolone, or another active agent should be substituted.
- Empirical therapy (either before culture results are known or when cultures are negative) depends on epidemiologic clues to etiology (e.g., endocarditis in an IV drug user, health care–associated endocarditis).
  - In the setting of no prior antibiotic therapy and negative blood cultures, *S. aureus*, CoNS, and enterococcal infection are unlikely; empirical therapy in this situation should target nutritionally variant organisms, the HACEK group, and *Bartonella*.
  - If negative cultures are confounded by prior antibiotic therapy, broader empirical therapy is indicated and should cover pathogens inhibited by the prior therapy.

SURGICAL TREATMENT

- Surgery should be considered early in the course of illness in pts with the indications listed in Table 89-3; most of these indications are not absolute, and recommendations are derived from observational studies and expert opinion. Moderate or severe refractory CHF is the major indication for surgical treatment of endocarditis.
- Pts who develop acute aortic regurgitation with preclosure of the mitral valve, a sinus of Valsalva abscess rupture into the right heart, or rupture into the pericardial sac require emergent (same-day) surgery.
- Cardiac surgery should be delayed for 2–3 weeks if possible when the pt has had a nonhemorrhagic embolic stroke and for 4 weeks when the pt has had a hemorrhagic embolic stroke. Ruptured mycotic aneurysms should be treated prior to cardiac surgery.
- The duration of antibiotic therapy after cardiac surgery depends on the indication for surgery.
  - For cases of uncomplicated NVE caused by susceptible organisms with negative valve cultures at surgery, the duration of pre- and postoperative treatment should equal the total duration of recommended therapy, with ~2 weeks of treatment given postoperatively.
  - For endocarditis with paravalvular abscess, partially treated PVE, or culture-positive valves, pts should receive a full course of therapy postoperatively.

- **Outcome** Death and poor outcome are related not to failure of antibiotic therapy but rather to interactions of comorbidities and endocarditis-related end-organ complications.
  - Survival rates are 85–90% for NVE due to viridans streptococci, HACEK organisms, or enterococci as opposed to 55–70% for NVE due to *S. aureus* in pts who are not IV drug users.

TABLE 89-4   HIGH-RISK CARDIAC LESIONS FOR WHICH ENDOCARDITIS PROPHYLAXIS IS ADVISED BEFORE DENTAL PROCEDURES

Prosthetic heart valves
Prior endocarditis
Unrepaired cyanotic congenital heart disease, including palliative shunts or conduits
Completely repaired congenital heart defects during the 6 months after repair
Incompletely repaired congenital heart disease with residual defects adjacent to prosthetic material
Valvulopathy developing after cardiac transplantation

Source: W Wilson et al: Circulation, published online, 9th April, 2007.

- – PVE beginning within 2 months of valve replacement results in mortality rates of 40–50%, whereas rates are only 10–20% in later-onset cases.
- **Prevention** The American Heart Association has reversed earlier recommendations and dramatically restricted recommendations for antibiotic prophylaxis. Prophylaxis is now recommended only for pts at highest risk of severe morbidity and death from endocarditis.
  - – Prophylaxis is recommended only for those dental procedures involving manipulation of gingival tissue or the periapical region of the teeth or perforation of the oral mucosa (including respiratory tract surgery).

TABLE 89-5   ANTIBIOTIC REGIMENS FOR PROPHYLAXIS OF ENDOCARDITIS IN ADULTS WITH HIGH-RISK CARDIAC LESIONS[a,b]

A. Standard oral regimen
1. Amoxicillin: 2 g PO 1 h before procedure
B. Inability to take oral medication
1. Ampicillin: 2 g IV or IM within 1 h before procedure
C. Penicillin allergy
1. Clarithromycin or azithromycin: 500 mg PO 1 h before procedure
2. Cephalexin[c]: 2 g PO 1 h before procedure
3. Clindamycin: 600 mg PO 1 h before procedure
D. Penicillin allergy, inability to take oral medication
1. Cefazolin[c] or ceftriaxone[c]: 1 g IV or IM 30 min before procedure
2. Clindamycin: 600 mg IV or IM 1 h before procedure

[a]Dosing for children: for amoxicillin, ampicillin, cephalexin, or cefadroxil, use 50 mg/kg PO; cefazolin, 25 mg/kg IV; clindamycin, 20 mg/kg PO, 25 mg/kg IV; clarithromycin, 15 mg/kg PO; and vancomycin, 20 mg/kg IV.
[b]For high-risk lesions, see Table 89-4. Prophylaxis is not advised for other lesions.
[c]Do not use cephalosporins in pts with immediate hypersensitivity (urticaria, angioedema, anaphylaxis) to penicillin.
Source: W Wilson et al: Circulation, published online 4/19/2007.

Prophylaxis is not advised for pts undergoing gastrointestinal or genitourinary tract procedures.

– Table 89-4 lists the high-risk cardiac lesions for which prophylaxis is advised, and Table 89-5 lists the recommended antibiotic regimens for this purpose.

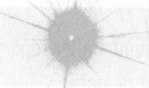

> For a more detailed discussion, see Karchmer AW: Infective Endocarditis, Chap. 124, p. 1052, in HPIM-18.

CHAPTER 90
Intraabdominal Infections

Intraperitoneal infections result when normal anatomic barriers are disrupted. Organisms contained within the bowel or an intraabdominal organ enter the sterile peritoneal cavity, causing peritonitis and—if the infection goes untreated and the pt survives—abscesses.

PERITONITIS

Peritonitis is a life-threatening event that is often accompanied by bacteremia and sepsis. Primary peritonitis has no apparent source, whereas secondary peritonitis is caused by spillage from an intraabdominal viscus; the etiologic organisms and the clinical presentation of these two processes are different.

◼ PRIMARY (SPONTANEOUS) BACTERIAL PERITONITIS

- **Epidemiology** Primary bacterial peritonitis (PBP) is most common among pts with cirrhosis (usually due to alcoholism) and preexisting ascites, but ≤10% of these pts develop PBP. PBP is also described in other settings (e.g., malignancy, hepatitis).
- **Pathogenesis** PBP is due to hematogenous spread of organisms to ascitic fluid in pts in whom a diseased liver and altered portal circulation compromise the liver's filtration function.
- **Microbiology** Enteric gram-negative bacilli such as *Escherichia coli* or gram-positive organisms such as streptococci, enterococci, and pneumococci are the most common etiologic agents.
  - A single organism is typically isolated.
  - If a polymicrobial infection including anaerobes is identified, the diagnosis of PBP should be reconsidered and a source of secondary peritonitis should be sought.
- **Clinical manifestations** Although some pts experience acute-onset abdominal pain or signs of peritoneal irritation, other pts have only nonspecific and nonlocalizing manifestations (e.g., malaise, fatigue, encephalopathy). Fever is common (~80% of pts).

- **Diagnosis** PBP is diagnosed if peritoneal fluid is sampled and contains >250 PMNs/μL.
  - Culture yield is improved if a 10-mL volume of peritoneal fluid is placed directly into blood culture bottles.
  - Blood cultures should be performed because bacteremia is common.

TREATMENT Primary (Spontaneous) Bacterial Peritonitis

- A third-generation cephalosporin (e.g., ceftriaxone, 2 g q24h IV; or cefotaxime, 2 g q8h IV) or piperacillin/tazobactam (3.375 g qid IV) constitutes appropriate empirical treatment.
- The regimen should be narrowed after the etiology is identified.
- Treatment should continue for at least 5 days, but longer courses (up to 2 weeks) may be needed for pts with coexisting bacteremia or for those whose improvement is slow.

- **Prevention** Up to 70% of pts have a recurrence of PBP within 1 year. Prophylaxis with fluoroquinolones (e.g., ciprofloxacin, 750 mg weekly) or trimethoprim-sulfamethoxazole (TMP-SMX; one double-strength tablet daily) reduces this rate to 20% but increases the risk of serious staphylococcal infections over time.

■ SECONDARY PERITONITIS

- **Pathogenesis** Secondary peritonitis develops when bacteria contaminate the peritoneum as a result of spillage from an intraabdominal viscus.
- **Microbiology** Infection almost always involves a mixed flora in which gram-negative bacilli and anaerobes predominate, especially when the contaminating source is colonic. The specific organisms depend on the flora present at the site of the initial process.
- **Clinical manifestations** Initial symptoms may be localized or vague and depend on the primary organ involved. Once infection has spread to the peritoneal cavity, pain increases; pts lie motionless, often with knees drawn up to avoid stretching the nerve fibers of the peritoneal cavity. Coughing or sneezing causes severe, sharp pain. There is marked voluntary and involuntary guarding of anterior abdominal musculature, tenderness (often with rebound), and fever.
- **Diagnosis** Although recovery of organisms from peritoneal fluid is easier in secondary than in primary peritonitis, radiographic studies to find the source of peritoneal contamination or immediate surgical intervention should usually be part of the initial diagnostic evaluation. Abdominal taps are done only to exclude hemoperitoneum in trauma cases.
- **Treatment** Antibiotics aimed at the inciting flora—e.g., penicillin/β-lactamase inhibitor combinations or a combination of a fluoroquinolone or a third-generation cephalosporin plus metronidazole—should be administered early.
  - For critically ill pts in the ICU, imipenem (500 mg q6h IV) or drug combinations such as ampicillin plus metronidazole plus ciprofloxacin should be used.
  - Surgical intervention is often needed.

■ **PERITONITIS IN PTS UNDERGOING CAPD**

- **Pathogenesis** In a phenomenon similar to that seen in intravascular device–related infections, organisms migrate along the catheter, a foreign body that serves as an entry point.
- **Microbiology** CAPD-associated peritonitis usually involves skin organisms, with *Staphylococcus* spp. such as coagulase-negative staphylococci and *Staphylococcus aureus* accounting for ~45% of cases; gram-negative bacilli and fungi (e.g., *Candida*) are occasionally identified.
- **Clinical manifestations** CAPD-associated peritonitis presents similarly to secondary peritonitis, in that diffuse pain and peritoneal signs are common.
- **Diagnosis** Several hundred milliliters of removed dialysis fluid should be centrifuged and sent for culture.
  - Use of blood culture bottles improves the diagnostic yield.
  - The dialysate is usually cloudy and contains >100 WBCs/µL, with >50% neutrophils.
- **Treatment** Empirical therapy should be directed against staphylococcal species and gram-negative bacilli (e.g., cefazolin plus a fluoroquinolone or a third-generation cephalosporin such as ceftazidime). Vancomycin should be used instead of cefazolin if methicillin resistance is prevalent, if the pt has an overt exit-site infection, or if the pt appears toxic.
  - Antibiotics are given by the intraperitoneal route either continuously (e.g., with each exchange) or intermittently (e.g., once daily, with the dose allowed to remain in the peritoneal cavity for 6 h). Severely ill pts should be given the same regimen by the IV route.
  - Catheter removal should be considered if the pt's condition does not improve within 48 h.

INTRAABDOMINAL ABSCESSES

Intraabdominal abscesses are generally diagnosed through radiographic studies, of which abdominal CT is typically most useful.

■ **INTRAPERITONEAL ABSCESSES**

- **Epidemiology** Of intraabdominal abscesses, 74% are intraperitoneal or retroperitoneal, not visceral.
- **Pathogenesis** Most abscesses arise from colonic sources. Abscesses develop in untreated peritonitis as an extension of the disease process and represent host defense activity aimed at containing the infection.
- **Microbiology** *Bacteroides fragilis* accounts for only 0.5% of the normal colonic flora, but is the anaerobe most frequently isolated from intraabdominal abscesses and from blood.
- **Treatment** Antimicrobial therapy is adjunctive to drainage and/or surgical correction of an underlying lesion or process.
  - Diverticular abscesses usually wall off locally, and surgical intervention is not routinely needed.
  - Antimicrobial agents with activity against gram-negative bacilli and anaerobic organisms are indicated (see "Secondary Peritonitis," above).

■ VISCERAL ABSCESSES

Liver Abscess

- **Epidemiology and Microbiology** Liver abscesses account for up to half of visceral intraabdominal abscesses and are caused most commonly by biliary tract disease (due to aerobic gram-negative bacilli or enterococci) and less often by local spread from pelvic and other intraperitoneal sources (due to mixed flora including aerobic and anaerobic species, among which *B. fragilis* is most common) or hematogenous seeding (infection with a single species, usually *S. aureus* or streptococci such as *S. milleri*).
  - Amebic liver abscesses are not uncommon.
  - Amebic serology has yielded positive results in >95% of affected pts.
- **Clinical manifestations** Pts have fever, anorexia, weight loss, nausea, and vomiting, but only ~50% have signs localized to the RUQ, such as pain, tenderness, hepatomegaly, and jaundice. Serum levels of alkaline phosphatase are elevated in ~70% of pts, and leukocytosis is common. One-third to one-half of pts are bacteremic.
- **Treatment** Drainage is the mainstay of treatment, but medical management with long courses of antibiotics can be successful.
  - Empirical therapy is the same as for intraabdominal sepsis and SBP.
  - Percutaneous drainage tends to fail in cases with multiple, sizable abscesses; with viscous abscess contents that plug the pigtail catheter; with associated disease (e.g., of the biliary tract); or with lack of response in 4–7 days.

Splenic Abscess

- **Epidemiology** Splenic abscesses are much less common than liver abscesses and usually develop via hematogenous spread of infection (e.g., due to endocarditis). The diagnosis is often made only after the pt's death; the condition is frequently fatal if left untreated.
- **Microbiology** Splenic abscesses are most often caused by streptococci; *S. aureus* is the next most common cause. Gram-negative bacilli can cause splenic abscess in pts with urinary tract foci, with associated bacteremia, or with infection from another intraabdominal source; salmonellae are fairly commonly isolated, particularly from pts with sickle cell disease.
- **Clinical manifestations** Abdominal pain or splenomegaly occurs in ~50% of cases and pain localized to the LUQ in ~25%. Fever and leukocytosis are common.
- **Treatment** Pts with multiple or complex multilocular abscesses should undergo splenectomy, receive adjunctive antibiotics, and be vaccinated against encapsulated organisms (*Streptococcus pneumoniae*, *Haemophilus influenzae*, and *Neisseria meningitidis*). Percutaneous drainage has been successful for single, small (<3-cm) abscesses and may also be useful for pts at high surgical risk.

Perinephric and Renal Abscesses

- **Epidemiology** Perinephric and renal abscesses are uncommon. More than 75% of these abscesses are due to ascending infection and are preceded by pyelonephritis. The most important risk factor is the presence of renal calculi that produce local obstruction to urinary flow.

- **Microbiology** *E. coli*, *Proteus* spp. (associated with struvite stones), and *Klebsiella* spp. are the most common etiologic agents; *Candida* species are sometimes identified.
- **Clinical manifestations** Clinical signs are nonspecific and include flank pain, abdominal pain, and fever. The diagnosis should be considered if pts with pyelonephritis have persistent fever after 4 or 5 days of treatment, if a urine culture yields a polymicrobial flora in pts with known renal stone disease, or if fever and pyuria occur in conjunction with a sterile urine culture.
- **Treatment** Drainage and the administration of antibiotics active against the organisms recovered are essential. Percutaneous drainage is usually successful for perinephric abscesses.

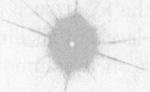

For a more detailed discussion, see Baron MJ, Kasper DL: Intraabdominal Infections and Abscesses, Chap. 127, p. 1077, in HPIM-18.

CHAPTER **91**
Infectious Diarrheas

Acute diarrheal disease, which has an incidence of ~4.6 billion cases worldwide per year, is the second most common infectious cause of death worldwide (after lower respiratory tract infection). The wide range of clinical manifestations is matched by the wide variety of infectious agents involved (Table 91-1). An approach to pts with infectious diarrhea is presented in Fig. 91-1.

NONINFLAMMATORY DIARRHEA

■ TRAVELER'S DIARRHEA
See Chap. 214 for details.

■ BACTERIAL FOOD POISONING
If there is evidence of a common-source outbreak, questions concerning the ingestion of specific foods and the timing of the diarrhea after a meal can provide clues to the bacterial cause of the illness.

- *Staphylococcus aureus*: Enterotoxin is elaborated in food left at room temperature (e.g., at picnics).
  - The incubation period is 1–6 h. Disease lasts <12 h and consists of diarrhea, nausea, vomiting, and abdominal cramping, usually without fever.
  - Most cases are due to contamination from infected human carriers.
- *Bacillus cereus*: Either an *emetic* or a *diarrheal* form of food poisoning can occur.

TABLE 91-1 GASTROINTESTINAL PATHOGENS CAUSING ACUTE DIARRHEA

Mechanism	Location	Illness	Stool Findings	Examples of Pathogens Involved
Noninflammatory (enterotoxin)	Proximal small bowel	Watery diarrhea	No fecal leukocytes; mild or no increase in fecal lactoferrin	*Vibrio cholerae*, enterotoxigenic *Escherichia coli* (LT and/or ST), entero-aggregative *E. coli*, *Clostridium perfringens*, *Bacillus cereus*, *Staphylococcus aureus*, *Aeromonas hydrophila*, *Plesiomonas shigelloides*, rotavirus, norovirus, enteric adenoviruses, *Giardia lamblia*, *Cryptosporidium* spp., *Cyclospora* spp., microsporidia
Inflammatory (invasion or cytotoxin)	Colon or distal small bowel	Dysentery or inflammatory diarrhea	Fecal polymorphonuclear leukocytes; substantial increase in fecal lactoferrin	*Shigella* spp., *Salmonella* spp., *Campylobacter jejuni*, enterohemorrhagic *E. coli*, enteroinvasive *E. coli*, *Yersinia enterocolitica*, *Listeria monocytogenes*, *Vibrio parahaemolyticus*, *Clostridium difficile*, *A. hydrophila*, *P. shigelloides*, *Entamoeba histolytica*, *Klebsiella oxytoca*
Penetrating	Distal small bowel	Enteric fever	Fecal mononuclear leukocytes	*Salmonella typhi*, *Y. enterocolitica*

Abbreviations: LT, heat-labile enterotoxin; ST, heat-stable enterotoxin.
Source: After Steiner TS, Guerrant RL: Principles and syndromes of enteric infection, in *Mandell, Douglas, and Bennett's Principles and Practice of Infectious Diseases*, 7th ed, GL Mandell et al (eds). Philadelphia, Churchill Livingstone, 2010, pp 1335–1351.

- The emetic form presents like *S. aureus* food poisoning, is due to a staphylococcal type of enterotoxin, has an incubation period of 1–6 h, and is associated with contaminated fried rice.
- The diarrheal form has an incubation period of 8–16 h, is caused by an enterotoxin resembling *Escherichia coli* heat-labile toxin (LT), and presents with diarrhea and abdominal cramps without vomiting.

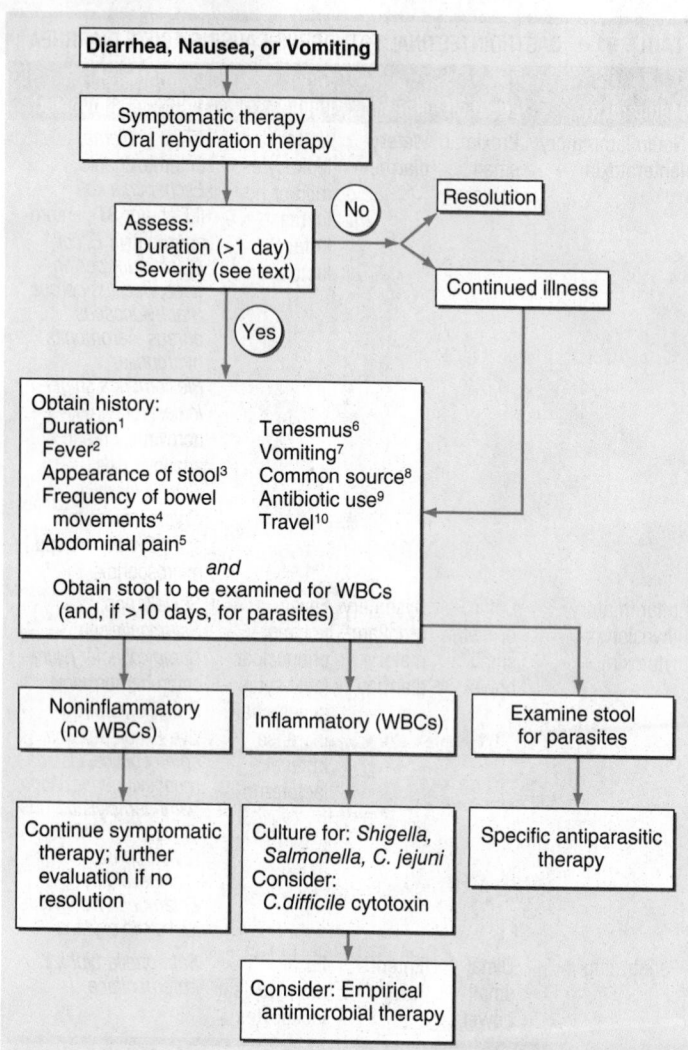

FIGURE 91-1 Clinical algorithm for the approach to pts with community-acquired infectious diarrhea or bacterial food poisoning. Key to superscripts: **1.** Diarrhea lasting >2 weeks is generally defined as chronic; in such cases, many of the causes of acute diarrhea are much less likely, and a new spectrum of causes needs to be considered. **2.** Fever often implies invasive disease, although fever and diarrhea may also result from infection outside the GI tract, as in malaria. **3.** Stools that contain blood or mucus indicate ulceration of the large bowel. Bloody stools without fecal leukocytes should alert the laboratory to the possibility of infection with Shiga toxin–producing entero-hemorrhagic *Escherichia coli*. Bulky white stools suggest a small-intestinal process that is causing malabsorption. Profuse "rice-water" stools suggest cholera or a similar toxigenic process. **4.** Frequent stools over a given period can provide the first warning

- *Clostridium perfringens*: Ingestion of heat-resistant spores in undercooked meat, poultry, or legumes leads to toxin production in the intestinal tract. The incubation period is 8–14 h, after which pts develop ≤24 h of diarrhea and abdominal cramps, without vomiting or fever.

■ CHOLERA

Microbiology

Cholera is caused by *Vibrio cholerae* serogroups O1 (classic and El Tor biotypes) and O139—highly motile, facultatively anaerobic, curved gram-negative rods. The natural habitat of *V. cholerae* is coastal salt water and brackish estuaries. Toxin production causes disease manifestations.

Epidemiology

Currently, >90% of cases reported to the World Health Organization (WHO) are from Africa; however, most cases go unreported or do not have a specific bacterial etiology identified.

- It is estimated that there are >3 million cases annually, with >100,000 deaths.
- Spread takes place by fecal contamination of water and food sources. Infection requires ingestion of a relatively large inoculum (compared with that required for other pathogens) of >10^5 organisms.

Clinical Manifestations

After an incubation period of 24–48 h, pts develop painless watery diarrhea and vomiting that can cause profound, rapidly progressive dehydration and death within hours.

- Volume loss can be >250 mL/kg in the first day.
- Stool has a characteristic "rice-water" appearance: gray cloudy fluid with flecks of mucus; no blood; and a fishy, inoffensive odor.

---

of impending dehydration. **5.** Abdominal pain may be most severe in inflammatory processes like those due to *Shigella*, *Campylobacter*, and necrotizing toxins. Painful abdominal muscle cramps, caused by electrolyte loss, can develop in severe cases of cholera. Bloating is common in giardiasis. An appendicitis-like syndrome should prompt a culture for *Yersinia enterocolitica* with cold enrichment. **6.** Tenesmus (painful rectal spasms with a strong urge to defecate but little passage of stool) may be a feature of cases with proctitis, as in shigellosis or amebiasis. **7.** Vomiting implies an acute infection (e.g., a toxin-mediated illness or food poisoning) but can also be prominent in a variety of systemic illnesses (e.g., malaria) and in intestinal obstruction. **8.** Asking pts whether anyone else they know is sick is a more efficient means of identifying a common source than is constructing a list of recently eaten foods. If a common source seems likely, specific foods can be investigated. See text for a discussion of bacterial food poisoning. **9.** Current antibiotic therapy or a recent history of treatment suggests *Clostridium difficile* diarrhea. Stop antibiotic treatment if possible and consider tests for *C. difficile* toxins. Antibiotic use may increase the risk of other infections, such as salmonellosis. **10.** See Chap. 214 for a discussion of traveler's diarrhea. *[After Steiner TS, Guerrant RL: Principles and syndromes of enteric infection, in Mandell, Douglas, and Bennett's Principles and Practice of Infectious Diseases, 7th ed, GL Mandell et al (eds). Philadelphia, Churchill Livingstone, 2010, pp 1335–1351; RL Guerrant, DA Bobak: N Engl J Med 325:327, 1991; with permission.]*

Diagnosis

Stool cultures on selective medium [e.g., thiosulfate–citrate–bile salts–sucrose (TCBS) agar] can isolate the organism. A point-of-care antigen-detection assay is available for field use.

TREATMENT	Cholera

Rapid fluid replacement is critical, preferably with the WHO's reduced-osmolarity oral rehydration solution (ORS), which contains (per liter of water) Na$^+$, 75 mmol; K$^+$, 20 mmol; Cl$^-$, 65 mmol; citrate, 10 mmol; and glucose, 75 mmol.

- If available, rice-based ORS is considered superior to standard ORS for cholera.
- If ORS is not available, a substitute can be made by adding 0.5 teaspoon of table salt (NaCl; 3.5 g) and 4 tablespoons of table sugar (glucose; 40 g) to 1 L of safe water.
- Severely dehydrated pts should be managed initially with IV hydration (preferably with Ringer's lactate), with the total fluid deficit replaced in the first 3–6 h (half within the first hour).
- A single dose of an effective antibiotic diminishes the duration and volume of stool: doxycycline (300 mg), ciprofloxacin (30 mg/kg, not to exceed 1 g), or azithromycin (1 g).

VIBRIO PARAHAEMOLYTICUS AND NON-01 *V. CHOLERAE*

These infections are linked to ingestion of contaminated seawater or undercooked seafood. After an incubation period of 4 h to 4 days, watery diarrhea, abdominal cramps, nausea, vomiting, and occasionally fever and chills develop. The disease lasts <7 days. Dysentery is a less common presentation. Pts with comorbid disease (e.g., liver disease) sometimes have extraintestinal infections that require antibiotic treatment.

■ NOROVIRUSES AND RELATED HUMAN CALICIVIRUSES

Microbiology and Epidemiology

These single-stranded RNA viruses are common causes of traveler's diarrhea and of viral gastroenteritis in pts of all ages as well as of epidemics worldwide, with a higher prevalence in cold-weather months. In the United States, >90% of outbreaks of nonbacterial gastroenteritis are caused by noroviruses. Very small inocula are required for infection. Thus, although the fecal-oral route is the primary mode of transmission, aerosolization, fomite contact, and person-to-person contact can also result in infection.

Clinical Manifestations

After a 24-h incubation period (range, 12–72 h), pts experience the sudden onset of nausea, vomiting, diarrhea, and/or abdominal cramps with constitutional symptoms (e.g., fever, headache, chills). Stools are loose, watery, and without blood, mucus, or leukocytes. Disease lasts 12–60 h.

Diagnosis

PCR assays and enzyme immunoassays (EIAs) have been developed to detect these viruses in stool and other body fluids, but these techniques are still largely relegated to research and outbreak settings.

> **TREATMENT** Infections with Noroviruses and Related Human Caliciviruses
>
> Only supportive measures are required.

■ ROTAVIRUSES

Microbiology and Epidemiology

Rotavirus is a segmented, double-stranded RNA virus that infects nearly all children worldwide by 3–5 years of age; adults can become infected if exposed.

- Reinfections are progressively less severe.
- Large quantities of virus are shed in the stool during the first week of infection, and transmission takes place both via the fecal-oral route and from person to person.
- Disease incidence peaks in the cooler fall and winter months.

Clinical Manifestations

After an incubation period of 1–3 days, disease onset is abrupt. Vomiting often precedes diarrhea (loose, watery stools without blood or fecal leukocytes), and about one-third of pts have temperatures >39°C. Symptoms resolve within 3–7 days.

Diagnosis

EIAs or viral RNA detection techniques, such as PCR, can identify rotavirus in stool samples.

> **TREATMENT** Rotavirus Infections
>
> Only supportive treatment is needed. Dehydration can be severe, and IV hydration may be needed in pts with frequent vomiting. Avoid antibiotics and antimotility agents.

Prevention

Rotavirus vaccines, two of which are available, are included in the routine vaccination schedule for U.S. infants. Although these vaccines have a lower efficacy (50–70%) in low-resource settings, the WHO recommends their use in all countries worldwide.

■ GIARDIASIS

Microbiology and Epidemiology

Giardia lamblia (also known as *G. intestinalis* or *G. duodenalis*) is a protozoal parasite that inhabits the small intestines of humans and other mammals.

- Cysts are ingested from the environment, excyst in the small intestine, and release flagellated trophozoites that remain in the proximal small intestine. Some trophozoites encyst, with the resulting cysts excreted in feces.

- Transmission occurs via the fecal-oral route, by ingestion of contaminated food and water, or from person to person in settings with poor fecal hygiene (e.g., day-care centers, institutional settings). Infection results from as few as 10 cysts.
- Viable cysts can be eradicated from water by either boiling or filtration. Standard chlorination techniques used to control bacteria do not destroy cysts.
- Young pts, newly exposed pts, and pts with hypogammaglobulinemia are at increased risk—a pattern suggesting a role for humoral immunity in resistance.

Clinical Manifestations

After an incubation period of 5 days to 3 weeks, disease ranges from asymptomatic carriage (most common) to fulminant diarrhea and malabsorption.

- Prominent early symptoms include diarrhea, abdominal pain, bloating, belching, flatus, nausea, and vomiting and usually last >1 week. Fever is rare, as is blood or mucus in stool.
- Chronic giardiasis can be continual or episodic; diarrhea may not be prominent, but increased flatulence, sulfurous belching, and weight loss can occur.
- In some cases, disease can be severe, with malabsorption, growth retardation, dehydration, and/or extraintestinal manifestations (e.g., anterior uveitis, arthritis).

Diagnosis

Giardiasis can be diagnosed by parasite antigen detection in feces and/or identification of cysts (oval, with four nuclei) or trophozoites (pear-shaped, flattened parasites with two nuclei and four pairs of flagella) in stool specimens. Given variability in cyst excretion, multiple samples may need to be examined.

TREATMENT Giardiasis

- Cure rates with metronidazole (250 mg tid for 5 days) are >90%; tinidazole (2 g PO once) may be more effective. Nitazoxanide (500 mg bid for 3 days) is an alternative agent.
- If symptoms persist, continued infection should be documented before re-treatment and possible sources of reinfection sought. Prolonged therapy with metronidazole (750 mg tid for 21 days) has been successful.

■ CRYPTOSPORIDIOSIS

Microbiology and Epidemiology

Cryptosporidial infections are caused by *Cryptosporidium hominis* and *C. parvum*.

- Oocysts are ingested and subsequently excyst, enter intestinal cells, and generate oocysts that are excreted in feces. The 50% infectious dose in immunocompetent individuals is ~132 oocysts.

- Person-to-person transmission of infectious oocysts can occur among close contacts and in day-care settings. Waterborne transmission is common. Oocysts are not killed by routine chlorination.

Clinical Manifestations

After an incubation period of ~1 week, pts may remain asymptomatic or develop watery, nonbloody diarrhea, occasionally with abdominal pain, nausea, anorexia, fever, and/or weight loss lasting 1–2 weeks. In immunocompromised hosts (particularly those with $CD4^+$ T cell counts <100/μL), diarrhea can be profuse and chronic, resulting in severe dehydration, weight loss, and wasting; the biliary tract can be involved.

Diagnosis

On multiple days, fecal samples should be examined for oocysts (4–5 μm in diameter, smaller than most parasites). Modified acid-fast staining, direct immunofluorescent techniques, and EIAs can facilitate diagnosis.

TREATMENT Cryptosporidiosis

- Nitazoxanide (500 mg bid for 3 days) is effective for immunocompetent pts but not for HIV-infected pts; improved immune status due to antiretroviral therapy can alleviate symptoms in the latter pts.
- In addition to antiprotozoal agents, supportive measures include replacement of fluid and electrolytes and use of antidiarrheal agents.

■ CYSTOISOSPORIASIS

Cystoisospora belli (formerly *Isospora belli*) infection is acquired by oocyst ingestion and is most common in tropical and subtropical countries. Acute infection can begin suddenly with fever, abdominal pain, and watery, nonbloody diarrhea and can last for weeks or months. Eosinophilia may occur. Compromised (e.g., HIV-infected) pts may have chronic disease that resembles cryptosporidiosis. Detection of large oocysts (~25 μm) in stool by modified acid-fast staining confirms the diagnosis.

TREATMENT Cystoisosporiasis

- Trimethoprim-sulfamethoxazole (TMP-SMX; 160/800 mg bid for 10 days) is effective therapy for immunocompetent pts.
  - HIV-infected pts should receive prolonged therapy with TMP-SMX (160/800 mg qid for 10 days, followed by 160/800 mg bid, tid, or qid for 3–4 weeks, depending on the clinical response).
  - Pyrimethamine (50–75 mg/d) can be given to pts intolerant of TMP-SMX.
  - Pts with AIDS may need suppressive maintenance therapy (TMP-SMX, 160/800 mg 3 times per week) to prevent relapses.

■ CYCLOSPORIASIS

Cyclospora cayetanensis can be transmitted through water or food (e.g., basil, raspberries). Clinical symptoms include diarrhea, flulike symptoms, flatulence, and burping. Disease can be self-limited or can persist for >1 month. Diagnosis is made by detection of oocysts (spherical, 8–10 μm) in stool; targeted diagnostic studies must be specifically requested.

TREATMENT   Cyclosporiasis

TMP-SMX (160/800 mg bid for 1 week) is effective. Pts with AIDS may need suppressive maintenance therapy to prevent relapses.

INFLAMMATORY DIARRHEA

■ SALMONELLOSIS

Microbiology and Pathogenesis

Salmonellae are facultatively anaerobic gram-negative bacilli that cause infection when 10^3–10^6 organisms are ingested.

- Conditions that reduce gastric acidity or intestinal integrity increase susceptibility to infection.
- Organisms penetrate the small-intestinal mucus layer and traverse the intestinal epithelium through M cells overlying Peyer's patches.
  - *S. typhi* and *S. paratyphi* survive within macrophages, then disseminate throughout the body via lymphatics, and ultimately colonize reticuloendothelial tissues.
  - Nontyphoidal salmonellae most commonly cause gastroenteritis, invading the large- and small-intestinal mucosa and resulting in massive PMN infiltration (as opposed to the mononuclear-cell infiltration seen with typhoid fever).

Epidemiology and Clinical Manifestations

Depending on the specific species, salmonellosis results in typhoid fever or gastroenteritis.

- *Typhoid (enteric) fever:* Typhoid fever is a systemic disease characterized by fever and abdominal pain and caused by dissemination of *S. typhi* or *S. paratyphi*, for which humans are the only hosts.
  - Disease results from ingestion of food or water contaminated by chronic carriers and is rare in developed nations. Worldwide, there are ~22 million cases, with 200,000 deaths annually.
  - After an incubation period of 3–21 days, prolonged fever (>75% of cases), headache (80%), chills (35–45%), anorexia (55%), and abdominal pain (30–40%) are common. Other symptoms may include sweating, cough, malaise, arthralgias, nausea, vomiting, and diarrhea—or, less often, constipation.
  - Physical findings include *rose spots* (faint, salmon-colored, blanching, maculopapular rash), hepatosplenomegaly, epistaxis, and relative bradycardia.
  - Intestinal perforation and/or GI hemorrhage can occur in the third and fourth weeks of illness; neurologic manifestations (e.g., meningitis, Guillain-Barré syndrome) occur in 2–40% of pts.
  - Long-term *Salmonella* carriage (i.e., for >1 year) in urine or stool develops in 1–4% of pts.

- *Nontyphoidal salmonellosis (NTS)*: Most commonly caused by *S. typhimurium* or *S. enteritidis*, NTS typically presents within 6–48 h of exposure as gastroenteritis (nausea, vomiting, nonbloody diarrhea, abdominal cramping, and fever) that lasts 3–7 days.
  - In 2009, there were ~14 million cases of NTS in the United States.
  - Disease is acquired from multiple animal reservoirs. The main mode of transmission is via contaminated food products, such as eggs (*S. enteritidis*), poultry, undercooked meat, dairy products, manufactured or processed foods, and fresh produce. Infection is also acquired during exposure to pets, especially reptiles.
  - Stool cultures remain positive for 4–5 weeks and—in rare cases of chronic carriage—for >1 year.
  - 8% of pts develop bacteremia, usually due to *S. choleraesuis* and *S. dublin*; of these pts, 5–10% develop localized infections (e.g., hepatosplenic abscesses, meningitis, pneumonia, osteomyelitis).
  - Reactive arthritis can follow *Salmonella* gastroenteritis, particularly in persons with the HLA-B27 histocompatibility antigen.

Diagnosis

Positive cultures of blood, stool, or other specimens are required for diagnosis.

TREATMENT Salmonellosis

- *Typhoid fever*: A fluoroquinolone (e.g., ciprofloxacin, 500 mg PO bid) is most effective for susceptible organisms.
  - Pts infected with nalidixic acid–resistant strains (whose susceptibility to ciprofloxacin is reduced) should be treated with ceftriaxone (2–3 g/d IV for 7–14 days), azithromycin (1 g/d PO for 5 days), or high-dose ciprofloxacin (750 mg PO bid or 400 mg IV q8h for 10–14 days).
  - Dexamethasone may be of benefit in severe cases.
- *NTS*: Antibiotic treatment is not recommended in most cases as it does not shorten the duration of symptoms and is associated with increased rates of relapse, a prolonged carrier state, and adverse drug reactions.
  - Antibiotic treatment may be required for infants ≤3 months of age; pts >50 years of age with suspected atherosclerosis; pts with immunosuppression; pts with cardiac, valvular, or endovascular abnormalities; and pts with significant joint disease.
  - Fluoroquinolones or third-generation cephalosporins are given for 2–3 days or until defervescence (if the pt is immunocompetent) or for 1–2 weeks (if the pt is immunocompromised).
  - HIV-infected pts are at high risk for *Salmonella* bacteremia and should receive 4 weeks of oral fluoroquinolone therapy after 1–2 weeks of IV treatment. In cases of relapse, long-term suppression with a fluoroquinolone or TMP-SMX should be considered.
  - Pts with endovascular infections or endocarditis should receive 6 weeks of treatment with a third-generation cephalosporin.

■ **CAMPYLOBACTERIOSIS**

Microbiology

Campylobacters are motile, curved gram-negative rods that are a common bacterial cause of gastroenteritis in the United States. Most cases are caused by *C. jejuni*.

Epidemiology

Campylobacters are common commensals in the GI tract of many food animals and household pets. In the United States, ingestion of contaminated poultry accounts for 30–70% of cases. Transmission to humans occurs via contact with or ingestion of raw or undercooked food products or direct contact with infected animals.

Clinical Manifestations

An incubation period of 2–4 days (range, 1–7 days) is followed by a pro-drome of fever, headache, myalgia, and/or malaise. Within the next 12–48 h, diarrhea (with stools containing blood, mucus, and leukocytes), cramping abdominal pain, and fever develop.

- Most cases are self-limited, but illness persists for >1 week in 10–20% of pts and may be confused with inflammatory bowel disease.
- Species other than *C. jejuni* (e.g., *C. fetus*) can cause a similar illness or prolonged relapsing systemic disease without a primary focus in immu-nocompromised pts.
  - The course may be fulminant, with bacterial seeding of many organs, particularly vascular sites.
  - Fetal death can result from infection in a pregnant pt.
- Three patterns of extraintestinal infection have been noted: (1) transient bacteremia in a normal host with enteritis (benign course, no specific treat-ment needed); (2) sustained bacteremia or focal infection in a normal host; and (3) sustained bacteremia or focal infection in a compromised host.
- Complications include reactive arthritis (particularly in persons with the HLA-B27 phenotype) and Guillain-Barré syndrome (in which campylo-bacters are associated with 20–40% of cases).

Diagnosis

The diagnosis is confirmed by cultures of stool, blood, or other specimens on special media and/or with selective techniques.

TREATMENT Campylobacteriosis

- Fluid and electrolyte replacement is the mainstay of therapy.
- Use of antimotility agents is not recommended, as they are associ-ated with toxic megacolon.
- Antibiotic treatment (erythromycin, 250 mg PO qid for 5–7 days) should be reserved for pts with high fever, bloody or severe diarrhea, persistence for >1 week, and worsening of symptoms. Azithromycin and fluoroquinolones are alternative regimens, although resistance to these drugs is increasing.

■ **SHIGELLOSIS AND INFECTION WITH SHIGA TOXIN–PRODUCING/ENTEROHEMORRHAGIC *E. COLI* (STEC/EHEC)**

Microbiology and Epidemiology

Shigellae are small, gram-negative, nonmotile bacilli that are very closely related to *E. coli*. The four most common *Shigella* serotypes are *S. dysenteriae* type 1, *S. flexneri*, *S. boydii*, and *S. sonnei* (which is more prevalent in the industrialized world). There are no animal reservoirs other than higher primates.

- These bacteria are transmitted from person to person via the fecal-oral route and occasionally via intermediate vectors such as food and water.
- The ability of as few as 100 organisms to cause infection helps explain the high rate of secondary household transmission.
- Shiga toxin and Shiga-like toxins produced by some strains of *E. coli* (including O157:H7) are important factors in disease severity. The toxins target endothelial cells and play a significant role in the microangiopathic complications of *Shigella* and *E. coli* infections, such as hemolytic-uremic syndrome (HUS) and thrombotic thrombocytopenic purpura.
- An analysis of cases occurring in 1966–1997 revealed an incidence of 165 million cases (of which 69% affected children <5 years of age) with 0.5–1.1 million deaths annually; these numbers have likely decreased since then, but multidrug-resistant strains have emerged.

Clinical Manifestations

After an incubation period of 1–4 days, shigellosis evolves through three phases: watery diarrhea, dysentery (bloody mucopurulent stools), and the postinfectious phase.

- Most episodes resolve in 1 week without treatment; with appropriate treatment, recovery takes place within a few days, with no sequelae.
- Complications are largely intestinal (e.g., toxic megacolon, intestinal perforation, rectal prolapse) or metabolic (e.g., hypoglycemia, hyponatremia). Shiga toxin produced by *S. dysenteriae* type 1 is linked to HUS (Coombs-negative hemolytic anemia; thrombocytopenia; and acute renal failure) in developing countries but is rare in industrialized countries, where *E. coli* O157:H7 is a more common cause.

Diagnosis

Shigellosis is diagnosed directly by stool culture. STEC/EHEC infection is diagnosed by screening of stool cultures for *E. coli* strains that do not ferment sorbitol, with subsequent serotyping for O157. Tests to detect Shiga toxins or toxin genes are sensitive, specific, and rapid; this approach detects non-O157 STEC/EHEC and sorbitol-fermenting strains of O157:H7.

TREATMENT **Shigellosis and Infection with STEC/EHEC**

- In the United States, because of the ready transmissibility of *Shigella*, antibiotics are recommended. Fluoroquinolones (e.g., ciprofloxacin, 500 mg bid) are effective, as are ceftriaxone, azithromycin, and pivmecillinam.

- *S. dysenteriae* infection should be treated for 5 days and non-*dysenteriae Shigella* infection for 3 days.
  - Immunocompromised pts should receive 7–10 days of treatment.
- Antibiotic treatment for STEC/EHEC infections should be avoided, since antibiotics may increase the incidence of HUS.
- Rehydration usually is not needed; *Shigella* infection rarely causes significant dehydration. If required, rehydration should be oral, and nutrition should be started as soon as possible. Use of antimotility agents may prolong fever and increase the risk of HUS and toxic megacolon.

■ YERSINIOSIS

Microbiology and Clinical Manifestations

Y. enterocolitica and *Y. pseudotuberculosis* are nonmotile gram-negative rods that cause enteritis or enterocolitis with self-limited diarrhea that lasts an average of 2 weeks as well as mesenteric adenitis (especially common with *Y. pseudotuberculosis*) and terminal ileitis (especially common with *Y. enterocolitica*) that can resemble acute appendicitis. Septicemia can occur in pts with chronic liver disease, malignancy, diabetes mellitus, and other underlying illnesses. Infection has been linked to reactive arthritis in HLA-B27-positive pts.

Diagnosis

Stool culture studies for *Yersinia* must be specifically requested and require the use of special media.

> **TREATMENT**   Yersiniosis
>
> Antibiotics are not indicated for diarrhea caused by yersiniae; supportive measures suffice.

■ AMEBIASIS

Microbiology and Epidemiology

Caused by *Entamoeba histolytica*, amebiasis has a high incidence in developing countries and among travelers, recent immigrants, men who have sex with men, and inmates of institutions in developed nations. Infection follows ingestion of cysts from fecally contaminated water, food, or hands. Motile trophozoites are released from cysts in the small intestine and then cause infection in the large bowel. Trophozoites may be shed in stool (in active dysentery) or encyst. Excreted cysts survive for weeks in a moist environment.

Clinical Manifestations

Most pts harboring *Entamoeba* species are asymptomatic, but some pts develop inflammatory colitis 2–6 weeks after ingestion of amebic cysts.

- Dysentery may develop, with daily passage of 10–12 small stools consisting mostly of blood and mucus. Fewer than 40% of pts have fever.

- Fulminant amebic colitis—characterized by more profuse diarrhea, severe abdominal pain with peritoneal signs, and fever—is more common among young children, pregnant women, and pts taking glucocorticoids.
- Liver abscess is the most common type of extraintestinal infection and can arise months or years after exposure to *E. histolytica*. Pts present with right-upper-quadrant pain, fever, right-sided pleural effusion, and hepatic tenderness and typically do not have active colitis. The abscess can rupture through the diaphragm and metastasize elsewhere (e.g., lung, brain).

Diagnosis

Microscopic examination of three stool samples, often combined with serologic testing, remains the standard diagnostic approach.

- Radiographic demonstration of at least one space-occupying lesion in the liver combined with positive serology confirms the diagnosis of amebic liver abscess. In this setting, serology has a sensitivity of >94% and a specificity of >95%.

TREATMENT Amebiasis

- Tinidazole (2 g/d PO for 3 days) or metronidazole (750 mg PO or IV tid for 5–10 days) is recommended for amebic colitis and amebic liver abscess.
  - >90% of pts respond clinically within 3 days of treatment initiation.
  - Drainage of liver abscesses is rarely needed. Indications for aspiration include the need to rule out pyogenic abscess, a lack of response to treatment after 4 days, an imminent threat of liver-abscess rupture, or the need to prevent left-lobe abscess rupture into the pericardium.
- Pts with either colitis or liver abscesses should also receive a luminal agent to ensure eradication of the infection. Paromomycin (10 mg/kg PO tid for 5–10 days) is the preferred agent; iodoquinol (650 mg PO tid for 20 days) is an alternative.

■ *CLOSTRIDIUM DIFFICILE* INFECTION (CDI)

Microbiology and Epidemiology

C. difficile is an obligately anaerobic, gram-positive, spore-forming bacillus and causes diarrheal illness that is most commonly acquired in the hospital. The disease is acquired almost exclusively in association with antimicrobial treatment; virtually all antibiotics carry a risk of CDI.

- After *C. difficile* colonizes the gut, its spores vegetate, multiply, and secrete toxin A (an enterotoxin) and toxin B (a cytotoxin), causing diarrhea and pseudomembranous colitis. The rate of fecal colonization is often ≥20% among adult pts hospitalized for >1 week; in contrast, the rate is 1–3% among community residents.
- Spores can persist on environmental surfaces in the hospital for months and on the hands of hospital personnel who do not practice adequate hand hygiene.

- Rates and severity of CDI in the United States, Canada, and Europe have increased markedly in the past decade. An epidemic strain accounts for much of the increase and is characterized by production of 16–23 times as much toxin A and toxin B as is documented for control strains, by the presence of a third toxin (binary toxin), and by high-level resistance to fluoroquinolones.

Clinical Manifestations

Most commonly, pts develop diarrhea, with stools that are not grossly bloody and are soft to watery, with a characteristic odor. Pts may have up to 20 bowel movements per day. Fever, abdominal pain, and leukocytosis are common.

- Constipation due to an adynamic ileus can occur. Unexplained leukocytosis (≥15,000 WBCs/μL) in this setting should prompt evaluation for CDI. These pts are at high risk for complications such as toxic megacolon and sepsis.
- *C. difficile* diarrhea recurs after treatment in ~15–30% of cases.

Diagnosis

The diagnosis of CDI is made in a pt with diarrhea (≥3 unformed stools per 24 h for ≥2 days) by detection of the organism, toxin A, or toxin B in stool or identification of pseudomembranes in the colon.

- Most laboratory tests for toxin lack sensitivity, but repeat testing is not recommended.
- Testing of asymptomatic pts (including a test of cure for those who have completed therapy) is not recommended.

TREATMENT   *C. difficile* Infection

- *Primary CDI*: When feasible, discontinuation of ongoing antimicrobial treatment is an effective cure in 15–23% of cases. Prompt initiation of specific therapy is recommended.
  - For mild to moderate disease, metronidazole (500 mg tid for 10 days) is recommended, with extension of therapy if the clinical response is slow.
  - For severe disease (e.g., >15,000 WBCs/μL, serum creatinine levels ≥1.5 times baseline), vancomycin (125 mg qid PO for 10–14 d) is the agent of choice.
- *Recurrent CDI*: The first recurrence should be treated the same as the initial episode.
  - For the second recurrence, an extended, tapered vancomycin regimen (125 mg qid for 10–14 d, then bid for 1 week, then daily for 1 week, then q2–3d for 2–8 weeks) should be used.
  - For multiple recurrences, there is no standard treatment course. Consider repetition of the tapered vancomycin regimen, administration of vancomycin (500 mg qid for 10 days) with *Saccharomyces boulardii* (500 mg bid for 28 d), administration of sequential therapy with vancomycin (125 mg qid for 10–14 d)

followed by rifaximin (400 mg bid for 2 weeks), treatment with nitazoxanide (500 mg bid for 10 d), fecal transplantation, or treatment with IV immunoglobulin (400 mg/kg).

- *Fulminant CDI*: Medical management is complicated by ineffective delivery of oral antibiotics to the intestinal lumen in the setting of ileus. Vancomycin (given via nasogastric tube and by retention enema) combined with IV metronidazole has been used with some success, as has IV tigecycline. Surgical colectomy can be life-saving.

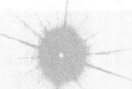

For a more detailed discussion, see LaRocque RC, Ryan ET, Calderwood SB: Acute Infectious Diarrheal Diseases and Bacterial Food Poisoning, Chap. 128, p. 1084; Gerding DN, Johnson S: *Clostridium difficile* Infection, Including Pseudomembranous Colitis, Chap. 129, p. 1091; Russo TA, Johnson JR: Diseases Caused by Gram-Negative Enteric Bacilli, Chap. 149, p. 1246; Pegues DA, Miller SI: Salmonellosis, Chap. 153, p. 1274; Sansonetti P, Bergounioux J: Shigellosis, Chap. 154, p. 1281; Blaser MJ: Infections Due to *Campylobacter* and Related Organisms, Chap. 155, p. 1286; Waldor MK, Ryan ET: Cholera and Other Vibrioses, Chap. 156, p. 1289; Prentice MB: Plague and Other *Yersinia* Infections, Chap. 159, p. 1305; Parashar UD, Glass RI: Viral Gastroenteritis, Chap. 190, p. 1588; Stanley SL Jr: Amebiasis and Infection With Free-Living Amebas, Chap. 209, p. 1683; and Weller PF: Protozoal Intestinal Infections and Trichomoniasis, Chap. 215, p. 1729, in HPIM-18.

CHAPTER **92**
Sexually Transmitted and Reproductive Tract Infections

GENERAL PRINCIPLES

- Worldwide, most adults acquire at least one sexually transmitted infection (STI).
- Three factors determine the initial rate of spread of any STI within a population: rate of sexual exposure of susceptible to infectious people, efficiency of transmission per exposure, and duration of infectivity of those infected.
- STI care and management begin with risk assessment and proceed to clinical assessment, diagnostic testing or screening, syndrome-based treatment to cover the most likely causes, and prevention and control. The "4 C's" of control are contact tracing, ensuring compliance with treatment, and counseling on risk reduction, including condom promotion and provision.

SPECIFIC SYNDROMES

■ URETHRITIS IN MEN

Microbiology and Epidemiology

Most cases are caused by either *Neisseria gonorrhoeae* or *Chlamydia trachomatis*. Other causative organisms include *Mycoplasma genitalium*, *Ureaplasma urealyticum*, *Trichomonas vaginalis*, and herpes simplex virus (HSV). *Chlamydia* causes 30–40% of nongonococcal urethritis (NGU) cases. *M. genitalium* is the probable cause in many *Chlamydia*-negative cases of NGU.

Clinical Manifestations

Urethritis in men produces urethral discharge, dysuria, or both, usually without frequency of urination.

Diagnosis

Pts present with a mucopurulent urethral discharge that can usually be expressed by milking of the urethra; alternatively, a Gram's-stained smear of urethral exudates containing ≥5 PMNs/1000× field confirms the diagnosis.

- Centrifuged sediment of the day's first 20–30 mL of voided urine can be examined instead.
- *N. gonorrhoeae* can be presumptively identified if intracellular gram-negative diplococci are present in Gram's-stained samples.
- Early-morning, first-voided urine should be used in "multiplex" nucleic acid amplification tests (NAATs) for *N. gonorrhoeae* and *C. trachomatis*.

> **TREATMENT**   Urethritis in Men
>
> - Treat urethritis promptly, while test results are pending.
>   - Unless these diseases have been excluded, treat gonorrhea with a single dose of ceftriaxone (250 mg IM), cefpodoxime (400 mg PO), or cefixime (400 mg PO) and treat *Chlamydia* with azithromycin (1 g PO once) or doxycycline (100 mg bid for 7 days); azithromycin may be more effective for *M. genitalium*.
>   - Sexual partners of the index case should receive the same treatment.
> - For recurrent symptoms: With re-exposure, re-treat pt and partner. Without re-exposure, consider infection with *T. vaginalis* (with culture or NAATs of urethral swab and early-morning, first-voided urine) or doxycycline-resistant *M. genitalium* or *Ureaplasma*. Consider treatment with metronidazole, azithromycin (1 g PO once), or both.

■ EPIDIDYMITIS

Microbiology

In sexually active men <35 years old, epididymitis is caused by *C. trachomatis* and, less commonly, by *N. gonorrhoeae*.

- In older men or after urinary tract instrumentation, urinary pathogens are most common.
- In men who practice insertive rectal intercourse, Enterobacteriaceae may be responsible.

Clinical Manifestations

Acute epididymitis—almost always unilateral—produces pain, swelling, and tenderness of the epididymis, with or without symptoms or signs of urethritis. Epididymitis must be differentiated from testicular torsion, tumor, and trauma. If symptoms persist after treatment, a testicular tumor or a chronic granulomatous disease (e.g., tuberculosis) should be considered.

TREATMENT Epididymitis

- Ceftriaxone (250 mg IM once) followed by doxycycline (100 mg PO bid for 10 days) is effective for epididymitis due to *C. trachomatis* and *N. gonorrhoeae*.
- Fluoroquinolones are no longer recommended because of increasing resistance in *N. gonorrhoeae*.

█ URETHRITIS (THE URETHRAL SYNDROME) IN WOMEN

Microbiology and Clinical Manifestations

C. trachomatis, *N. gonorrhoeae*, and occasionally HSV cause symptomatic urethritis—known as *the urethral syndrome* in women—that is characterized by "internal" dysuria (usually without urinary urgency or frequency), pyuria, and an absence of *Escherichia coli* and other uropathogens at counts of ≥10^2/mL in urine.

Diagnosis

Evaluate for infection with *N. gonorrhoeae* or *C. trachomatis* with specific tests (e.g., NAATs on the first 10 mL of voided morning urine).

TREATMENT Urethritis (the Urethral Syndrome) in Women

See "Urethritis in Men," above.

█ VULVOVAGINAL INFECTIONS

Microbiology

A variety of organisms are associated with vulvovaginal infections, including *N. gonorrhoeae* and *C. trachomatis* (particularly when they cause cervicitis), *T. vaginalis*, *Candida albicans*, *Gardnerella vaginalis*, and HSV.

Clinical Manifestations

Vulvovaginal infections encompass a wide array of specific conditions, each of which has different presenting symptoms.

- Unsolicited reporting of abnormal vaginal discharge suggests trichomoniasis or bacterial vaginosis (BV).
  - *Trichomoniasis* is characterized by vulvar irritation and a profuse white or yellow, homogeneous vaginal discharge with a pH that is typically ≥5.
  - *BV* is characterized by vaginal malodor and a slight to moderate increase in white or gray, homogeneous vaginal discharge that uniformly coats the vaginal walls and typically has a pH >4.5.

    – Vaginal trichomoniasis and BV early in pregnancy are associated with premature onset of labor.
- Vulvar conditions such as genital herpes or vulvovaginal candidiasis can cause vulvar pruritus, burning, irritation, or lesions as well as external dysuria (as urine passes over the inflamed vulva or areas of epithelial disruption) or vulvar dyspareunia.

Diagnosis

Evaluation of vulvovaginal symptoms includes a pelvic examination (with a speculum examination) and simple rapid diagnostic tests.
- Examine abnormal vaginal discharge for pH, a fishy odor after mixing with 10% KOH (BV), evidence on microscopy of motile trichomonads and/or clue cells of BV (vaginal epithelial cells coated with coccobacillary organisms) when mixed with saline, or hyphae or pseudohyphae on microscopy when 10% KOH is added (vaginal candidiasis).
- A DNA probe test (the Affirm test) can detect *T. vaginalis*, *C. albicans*, and increased concentrations of *G. vaginalis*.

TREATMENT	Vulvovaginal Infections

- *Vulvovaginal candidiasis*: Miconazole (a single 1200-mg vaginal suppository), clotrimazole (two 100-mg vaginal tablets daily for 3 days), or fluconazole (150 mg PO once) are all effective.
- *Trichomoniasis*: Metronidazole (2 g PO once) or tinidazole is effective. Treatment of sexual partners with the same regimen is the standard of care.
- *BV*: Metronidazole (500 mg PO bid for 7 days) or 2% clindamycin cream (one full applicator vaginally each night for 7 days) is effective, but recurrence is common with both.

■ MUCOPURULENT CERVICITIS

Microbiology

N. gonorrhoeae, *C. trachomatis*, and *M. genitalium* are the primary causative agents. Of note, NAATs for these pathogens, HSV, and *T. vaginalis* have been negative in nearly half of cases.

Clinical Manifestations

Mucopurulent cervicitis represents the "silent partner" of urethritis in men and results from inflammation of the columnar epithelium and subepithelium of the endocervix.

Diagnosis

Yellow mucopurulent discharge from the cervical os, with ≥20 PMNs/1000× field on Gram's stain of cervical mucus, indicates endocervicitis. The presence of intracellular gram-negative diplococci on Gram's stain of cervical mucus is specific but <50% sensitive for gonorrhea; thus NAATs for *N. gonorrhoeae* and *C. trachomatis* are always indicated.

See "Urethritis in Men," above.

■ PELVIC INFLAMMATORY DISEASE (PID)

Microbiology

The agents most often implicated in acute PID—infection that ascends from the cervix or vagina to the endometrium and/or fallopian tubes—include the primary causes of endocervicitis (e.g., *N. gonorrhoeae* and *C. trachomatis*); other organisms (e.g., *M. genitalium*, *Prevotella* spp., peptostreptococci, *E. coli*, *Haemophilus influenzae*, and group B streptococci) account for 25–33% of cases.

Epidemiology

In 2008, there were 104,000 visits to physicians' offices for PID in the United States; there are ~70,000–100,000 hospitalizations related to PID annually.

- Risk factors for PID include cervicitis, BV, a history of salpingitis or recent vaginal douching, menstruation, and recent insertion of an intra-uterine contraceptive device (IUD).
- Oral contraceptive pills decrease risk.

Clinical Manifestations

The presenting symptoms depend on the extent to which the infection has spread.

- *Endometritis*: Pts present with midline abdominal pain and abnormal vaginal bleeding. Lower quadrant, adnexal, or cervical motion or abdominal rebound tenderness is less severe in women with endometritis alone than in women who also have salpingitis.
- *Salpingitis*: Symptoms evolve from mucopurulent cervicitis to endometritis and then to bilateral lower abdominal and pelvic pain caused by salpingitis. Nausea, vomiting, and increased abdominal tenderness may occur if peritonitis develops.
- *Perihepatitis* (Fitz-Hugh–Curtis syndrome): 3–10% of women present with pleuritic upper abdominal pain and tenderness in the right upper quadrant due to perihepatic inflammation. Most cases are due to chlamydial salpingitis.
- *Periappendicitis*: ~5% of pts can have appendiceal serositis without involvement of the intestinal mucosa as a result of gonococcal or chlamydial salpingitis.

Diagnosis

Speculum examination shows evidence of mucopurulent cervicitis in the majority of pts with gonococcal or chlamydial PID; cervical motion tenderness, uterine fundal tenderness, and/or abnormal adnexal tenderness also are usually present. Endocervical swab specimens should be examined by NAATs for *N. gonorrhoeae* and *C. trachomatis*.

TREATMENT Pelvic Inflammatory Disease

- Empirical treatment for PID should be initiated in sexually active young women and in other women who are at risk for PID and who have pelvic or lower abdominal pain with no other explanation as well as cervical motion, uterine, or adnexal tenderness.
- Hospitalization should be considered when (1) the diagnosis is uncertain and surgical emergencies cannot be excluded, (2) the pt is pregnant, (3) pelvic abscess is suspected, (4) severe illness precludes outpatient management, (5) the pt has HIV infection, (6) the pt is unable to follow or tolerate an outpatient regimen, or (7) the pt has failed to respond to outpatient therapy.
- *Outpatient regimen*: Ceftriaxone (250 mg IM once) *plus* doxycycline (100 mg PO bid for 14 days) *plus* metronidazole (500 mg PO bid for 14 days) is effective. Women treated as outpatients should be clinically reevaluated within 72 h.
- *Parenteral regimens*: Parenteral treatment with regimens listed below should be given for ≥48 h after clinical improvement. A 14-day course should be completed with doxycycline (100 mg PO bid); if the clindamycin-containing regimen is used, oral therapy can be given with clindamycin (450 mg PO qid).
  - Cefotetan (2 g IV q12h) or cefoxitin (2 g IV q6h) plus doxycycline (100 mg IV/PO q12h)
  - Clindamycin (900 mg IV q8h) plus gentamicin (loading dose of 2.0 mg/kg IV/IM followed by 1.5 mg/kg q8h)
- Male sex partners should be evaluated and treated empirically for gonorrhea and chlamydial infection.

Prognosis

Late sequelae include infertility (11% after one episode of PID, 23% after two, and 54% after three or more); ectopic pregnancy (sevenfold increase in risk); chronic pelvic pain; and recurrent salpingitis.

◼ ULCERATIVE GENITAL LESIONS

The most common etiologies in the United States are genital herpes, syphilis, and chancroid. See Table 92-1 and sections on individual pathogens below for specific clinical manifestations. Pts with persistent genital ulcers that do not resolve with syndrome-based antimicrobial therapy should have their HIV serologic status assessed if such testing has not previously been performed. Immediate treatment (before all test results are available) is often appropriate to improve response, reduce transmission, and cover pts who might not return for follow-up visits.

◼ PROCTITIS, PROCTOCOLITIS, ENTEROCOLITIS, AND ENTERITIS

Microbiology and Epidemiology

Acquisition of HSV, *N. gonorrhoeae*, or *C. trachomatis* [including lymphogranuloma venereum (LGV) strains of *C. trachomatis*] during receptive

TABLE 92-1 CLINICAL FEATURES OF GENITAL ULCERS

Feature	Syphilis	Herpes	Chancroid	Lymphogranuloma Venereum	Donovanosis
Incubation period	9–90 days	2–7 days	1–14 days	3 days–6 weeks	1–4 weeks (up to 6 months)
Early primary lesions	Papule	Vesicle	Pustule	Papule, pustule, or vesicle	Papule
No. of lesions	Usually one	Multiple	Usually multiple, may coalesce	Usually one; often not detected, despite lymphadenopathy	Variable
Diameter	5–15 mm	1–2 mm	Variable	2–10 mm	Variable
Edges	Sharply demarcated, elevated, round, or oval	Erythematous	Undermined, ragged, irregular	Elevated, round, or oval	Elevated, irregular
Depth	Superficial or deep	Superficial	Excavated	Superficial or deep	Elevated
Base	Smooth, nonpurulent, relatively nonvascular	Serous, erythematous, nonvascular	Purulent, bleeds easily	Variable, nonvascular	Red and velvety, bleeds readily
Induration	Firm	None	Soft	Occasionally firm	Firm
Pain	Uncommon	Frequently tender	Usually very tender	Variable	Uncommon
Lymphadenopathy	Firm, nontender, bilateral	Firm, tender, often bilateral with initial episode	Tender, may suppurate, loculated, usually unilateral	Tender, may suppurate, loculated, usually unilateral	None; pseudobuboes

Source: From RM Ballard, in KK Holmes et al (eds): *Sexually Transmitted Diseases*, 4th ed. New York, McGraw-Hill, 2008.

anorectal intercourse causes most cases of infectious proctitis in women and in men who have sex with men (MSM). Sexually acquired proctocolitis is most often due to *Campylobacter* or *Shigella* species. In MSM without HIV infection, enteritis is often attributable to *Giardia lamblia*.

Clinical Manifestations

Anorectal pain and mucopurulent, bloody rectal discharge suggest proctitis or proctocolitis. Proctitis is more likely to cause tenesmus and constipation, but proctocolitis and enteritis more often cause diarrhea.

- HSV proctitis and LGV proctocolitis can cause severe pain, fever, and systemic manifestations.
- Sacral nerve root radiculopathy, with urinary retention or anal sphincter dysfunction, is associated with primary HSV infection.

Diagnosis

Pts should undergo anoscopy to examine the rectal mucosa and exudates and to obtain specimens for diagnosis.

TREATMENT Proctitis, Proctocolitis, Enterocolitis, Enteritis

- Pending test results, pts should receive empirical treatment for gonorrhea and chlamydial infection with ceftriaxone (125 mg IM once) followed by doxycycline (100 mg bid for 7 days); therapy for syphilis or herpes should be given as indicated.

INDIVIDUAL PATHOGENS

■ GONORRHEA

Microbiology

N. gonorrhoeae, the causative agent of gonorrhea, is a gram-negative, nonmotile, non-spore-forming organism that grows singly and in pairs (i.e., as diplococci).

Epidemiology

The ~299,000 cases reported in the United States in 2008 probably represent only half the true number of cases because of underreporting, self-treatment, and nonspecific treatment without a laboratory diagnosis.

- 40% of reported cases in the U.S. occur in 15- to 19-year-old women and 20- to 24-year-old men.
- Gonorrhea is transmitted from males to females more efficiently than in the opposite direction, with 40–60% of women acquiring gonorrhea during a single unprotected sexual encounter with an infected man. Roughly two-thirds of all infected men are asymptomatic.
- Drug-resistant strains are widespread. Penicillin, ampicillin, and tetracycline are no longer reliable therapeutic agents, and fluoroquinolones are no longer routinely recommended.

Clinical Manifestations

Except in disseminated disease, the sites of infection typically reflect areas involved in sexual contact.

- *Urethritis* and *cervicitis* have an incubation period of 2–7 days and ~10 days, respectively. See above for details.
- *Anorectal gonorrhea* can cause acute proctitis in women (due to the spread of cervical exudate to the rectum) and MSM.
- *Pharyngeal gonorrhea* is usually mild or asymptomatic and results from oral-genital sexual exposure (typically fellatio). Pharyngeal infection almost always coexists with genital infection, resolves spontaneously, and is rarely transmitted to sexual contacts.
- *Ocular gonorrhea* is typically caused by autoinoculation and presents with a markedly swollen eyelid, hyperemia, chemosis, and profuse purulent discharge.
- *Gonorrhea in pregnancy* can have serious consequences for both the mother and the infant.
  - Salpingitis and PID are associated with fetal loss.
  - Third-trimester disease can cause prolonged rupture of membranes, premature delivery, chorioamnionitis, funisitis, and neonatal sepsis.
  - *Ophthalmia neonatorum*, the most common form of gonorrhea among neonates, is preventable by prophylactic ophthalmic ointments (e.g., containing erythromycin or tetracycline), but treatment requires systemic antibiotics.
- *Gonococcal arthritis* results from dissemination of organisms due to gonococcal bacteremia. Pts present during a bacteremic phase (relatively uncommon) or with suppurative arthritis involving one or two joints (most commonly the knees, wrists, ankles, and elbows), with tenosynovitis and skin lesions. Menstruation and complement deficiencies of the membrane attack complex (C5–C9) are risk factors for disseminated disease.

Diagnosis

NAATs, culture, and microscopic examination (for intracellular diplococci) of urogenital samples are used to diagnose gonorrhea. A single culture of endocervical discharge has a sensitivity of 80–90%.

| **TREATMENT** | Gonorrhea |

See Table 92-2.

■ INFECTIONS WITH *CHLAMYDIA TRACHOMATIS*

Microbiology

C. trachomatis organisms are obligate intracellular bacteria that are divided into two biovars: trachoma and LGV. The trachoma biovar causes ocular trachoma and urogenital infections; the LGV biovar causes lymphogranuloma venereum.

Epidemiology

The WHO estimates that >89 million cases of *C. trachomatis* infection occur annually worldwide. The estimated 2–3 million cases per year that occur in the U.S. make *C. trachomatis* infection the most commonly reported infectious disease in this country.

TABLE 92-2 RECOMMENDED TREATMENT FOR GONOCOCCAL INFECTIONS: 2010 GUIDELINES OF THE CENTERS FOR DISEASE CONTROL AND PREVENTION

Diagnosis	Treatment of Choice[a]
Uncomplicated gonococcal infection of the cervix, urethra, pharynx[b], or rectum	
First-line regimens	Ceftriaxone (250 mg IM, single dose)
	or
	Cefixime (400 mg PO, single dose)
	plus
	Treatment for *Chlamydia* if chlamydial infection is not ruled out:
	Azithromycin (1 g PO, single dose)
	or
	Doxycycline (100 mg PO bid for 7 days)
Alternative regimens	Ceftizoxime (500 mg IM, single dose)
	or
	Cefotaxime (500 mg IM, single dose)
	or
	Spectinomycin (2 g IM, single dose)[c,d]
	or
	Cefotetan (1 g IM, single dose) plus probenecid (1 g PO, single dose)[c]
	or
	Cefoxitin (2 g IM, single dose) plus probenecid (1 g PO, single dose)[c]
Epididymitis	See text and Chap. 130, HPIM-18
Pelvic inflammatory disease	See text and Chap. 130, HPIM-18
Gonococcal conjunctivitis in an adult	Ceftriaxone (1 g IM, single dose)[e]
Ophthalmia neonatorum[f]	Ceftriaxone (25–50 mg/kg IV, single dose, not to exceed 125 mg)
Disseminated gonococcal infection[g]	
Initial therapy[h]	
Pt tolerant of β-lactam drugs	Ceftriaxone (1 g IM or IV q24h; recommended)
	or
	Cefotaxime (1 g IV q8h)
	or
	Ceftizoxime (1 g IV q8h)

TABLE 92-2 RECOMMENDED TREATMENT FOR GONOCOCCAL INFECTIONS: 2010 GUIDELINES OF THE CENTERS FOR DISEASE CONTROL AND PREVENTION (CONTINUED)

Diagnosis	Treatment of Choice[a]
Pts allergic to β-lactam drugs	Spectinomycin (2 g IM q12h)[d]
Continuation therapy	Cefixime (400 mg PO bid)
Meningitis or endocarditis	Ceftriaxone (1–2 g IV q12h)[i]

[a]True failure of treatment with a recommended regimen is rare and should prompt an evaluation for reinfection or consideration of an alternative diagnosis.
[b]Ceftriaxone is the only agent recommended for treatment of pharyngeal infection.
[c]Spectinomycin, cefotetan, and cefoxitin, which are alternative agents, currently are unavailable or in short supply in the United States.
[d]Spectinomycin may be ineffective for the treatment of pharyngeal gonorrhea.
[e]Plus lavage of the infected eye with saline solution (once).
[f]Prophylactic regimens are discussed in the text.
[g]Hospitalization is indicated if the diagnosis is uncertain, if the pt has frank arthritis with an effusion, or if the pt cannot be relied on to adhere to treatment.
[h]All initial regimens should be continued for 24–48 h after clinical improvement begins, at which time the switch may be made to one of the continuation regimens to complete a full week of antimicrobial treatment. Treatment for chlamydial infection (as above) should be given if this infection has not been ruled out. Fluoroquinolones may be an option if antimicrobial susceptibility can be documented by culture of the causative organism.
[i]Hospitalization is indicated to exclude suspected meningitis or endocarditis. Treatment should be given in the hospital. The durations are 10–14 days for meningitis and at least 4 weeks for endocarditis.

Clinical Manifestations

80–90% of women and >50% of men with *C. trachomatis* genital infections lack symptoms; other pts have very mild symptoms.

- Urethritis, epididymitis, cervicitis, salpingitis, PID, and proctitis are all discussed above.
- Reactive arthritis (conjunctivitis, urethritis or cervicitis, arthritis, and mucocutaneous lesions) occurs in 1–2% of NGU cases, many of which are due to *C. trachomatis*. More than 80% of pts have the HLA-B27 phenotype.
- LGV is an invasive, systemic STI that—in heterosexual individuals—presents most commonly as painful inguinal lymphadenopathy beginning 2–6 weeks after presumed exposure. Progressive periadenitis results in fluctuant, suppurative nodes with development of multiple draining fistulas. Spontaneous resolution occurs after several months. See Table 92-1 for additional clinical details.

Diagnosis

NAATs of urine or urogenital swabs are the diagnostic tests of choice. Serologic testing may be helpful in the diagnosis of LGV and neonatal pneumonia caused by *C. trachomatis*, but it is not useful in diagnosing uncomplicated urogenital infections.

- See "Specific Syndromes," above.
- LGV should be treated with doxycycline (100 mg PO bid) or erythromycin base (500 mg PO qid) for at least 3 weeks.

■ INFECTIONS DUE TO MYCOPLASMAS

Microbiology and Epidemiology

Mycoplasmas are the smallest free-living organisms known and lack a cell wall. *M. hominis*, *M. genitalium*, *Ureaplasma parvum*, and *U. urealyticum* cause urogenital tract disease. These organisms are commonly present in the vagina of asymptomatic women.

Clinical Manifestations

Ureaplasmas are a common cause of *Chlamydia*-negative NGU. *M. hominis* and *M. genitalium* are associated with PID; *M. hominis* is implicated in 5–10% of cases of postpartum or postabortal fever.

Diagnosis

PCR is most commonly used for detection of urogenital mycoplasmas; culture is possible but can be done primarily at reference laboratories. Serologic testing is not helpful.

TREATMENT   Infections Due to Mycoplasmas

Recommendations for treatment of NGU and PID listed above are appropriate for genital mycoplasmas.

■ SYPHILIS

Microbiology and Epidemiology

Treponema pallidum subspecies *pallidum*—the cause of syphilis—is a thin spiral organism with a cell body surrounded by a trilaminar cytoplasmic membrane. Humans are the only natural host, and the organism cannot be cultured in vitro.

- Cases are acquired by sexual contact with infectious lesions (chancre, mucous patch, skin rash, condyloma latum); nonsexual acquisition through close personal contact, infection in utero, blood transfusion, and organ transplantation is less common.
- There are ~12 million new infections per year worldwide.
  - In the United States, 31,575 cases were reported in 2000.
  - The reported cases of primary and secondary syphilis combined (which better indicate disease activity) increased from <6000 in 2000 to 13,500 in 2008, primarily affecting MSM, many of whom were co-infected with HIV.
- One-third to one-half of sexual contacts of persons with infectious syphilis become infected—a figure that underscores the importance of treating all recently exposed sexual contacts.

Pathogenesis

T. pallidum penetrates intact mucous membranes or microscopic abrasions and, within hours, enters lymphatics and blood to produce systemic infection and metastatic foci. The primary lesion (chancre) appears at the site of inoculation within 4–6 weeks and heals spontaneously. Generalized parenchymal, constitutional, and mucocutaneous manifestations of secondary syphilis appear 6–8 weeks later despite high antibody titers, subsiding in 2–6 weeks. After a latent period, one-third of untreated pts eventually develop tertiary disease (syphilitic gummas, cardiovascular disease, neurologic disease).

Clinical Manifestations

Syphilis progresses through three phases with distinct clinical presentations.

- *Primary syphilis*: A chancre at the site of inoculation (penis, rectum or anal canal, mouth, cervix, labia) is characteristic but often goes unnoticed. See Table 92-1 for clinical details. Regional adenopathy can persist long after the chancre heals.
- *Secondary syphilis*: The protean manifestations of the secondary stage usually include mucocutaneous lesions and generalized nontender lymphadenopathy.
  - Skin lesions can be subtle but are often pale red or pink, nonpruritic macules that are widely distributed over the trunk and extremities, including the palms and soles.
  - In moist intertriginous areas, papules can enlarge and erode to produce broad, highly infectious lesions called *condylomata lata*.
  - Superficial mucosal erosions (*mucous patches*) and constitutional symptoms (e.g., sore throat, fever, malaise) can occur.
  - Less common findings include hepatitis, nephropathy, arthritis, and ocular findings (e.g., optic neuritis, anterior uveitis, iritis).
- *Latent syphilis*: Pts without clinical manifestations but with positive syphilis serology have latent disease. *Early latent* syphilis is limited to the first year after infection, whereas *late latent* syphilis is defined as that of ≥1 year's (or unknown) duration.
- *Tertiary syphilis*: The classic forms of tertiary syphilis include neurosyphilis, cardiovascular syphilis, and gummas.
  - *Neurosyphilis* represents a continuum, with asymptomatic disease occurring early after infection, potentially progressing to general paresis and tabes dorsalis. Symptomatic disease has three main presentations, all of which are now rare (except in pts with advanced HIV infection). *Meningeal* syphilis presents as headache, nausea, vomiting, neck stiffness, cranial nerve involvement, seizures, and changes in mental status within 1 year of infection. *Meningovascular* syphilis presents up to 10 years after infection as a subacute encephalitic prodrome followed by a gradually progressive vascular syndrome. *Parenchymatous* involvement presents at 20 years for general paresis and 25–30 years for tabes dorsalis. A general mnemonic for paresis is *p*ersonality, *a*ffect, *r*eflexes (hyperactive), *e*ye (Argyll Robertson pupils, which react to accommodation but not to light), *s*ensorium (illusions, delusions, hallucinations), *i*ntellect (decrease in recent

memory and orientation, judgment, calculations, insight), and speech. Tabes dorsalis is a demyelination of posterior columns, dorsal roots, and dorsal root ganglia, with ataxic, wide-based gait and footslap; paresthesia; bladder disturbances; impotence; areflexia; and loss of position, deep pain, and temperature sensations.

- *Cardiovascular syphilis* develops in ~10% of untreated pts 10–40 years after infection. Endarteritis obliterans of the vasa vasorum providing the blood supply to large vessels results in aortitis, aortic regurgitation, saccular aneurysm, and coronary ostial stenosis.
- *Gummas* are usually solitary lesions showing granulomatous inflammation with central necrosis. Common sites include the skin and skeletal system; however, any organ (including the brain) may be involved.
- *Congenital syphilis*: Syphilis can be transmitted throughout pregnancy, but fetal disease does not become manifest until after the fourth month of gestation. All pregnant women should be tested for syphilis early in pregnancy.

Diagnosis

Serologic tests—both nontreponemal and treponemal—are the mainstays of diagnosis; changes in antibody titers can also be used to monitor response to therapy.

- Nontreponemal serologic tests that measure IgG and IgM antibodies to a cardiolipin-lecithin-cholesterol antigen complex [e.g., rapid plasma reagin (RPR), Venereal Disease Research Laboratory (VDRL)] are recommended for screening or for quantitation of serum antibody. After therapy for early syphilis, a persistent fall in titer by ≥4-fold is considered an adequate response.
- Treponemal tests, including the agglutination assay (e.g., the Serodia TP-PA test) and the fluorescent treponemal antibody–absorbed (FTA-ABS) test, are used to confirm results from nontreponemal tests. Results remain positive even after successful treatment.
- Lumbar puncture (LP) is recommended for pts with syphilis and neurologic signs or symptoms, an RPR or VDRL titer ≥1:32, or suspected treatment failure and for HIV-infected pts with a CD4+ T cell count <350/μL.
  - CSF exam demonstrates pleocytosis (>5 WBCs/μL) and increased protein levels (>45 mg/dL). A positive CSF VDRL test is specific but not sensitive; an unabsorbed FTA test is sensitive but not specific. A negative unabsorbed FTA test excludes neurosyphilis.
- Pts with syphilis should be evaluated for HIV disease.

TREATMENT Syphilis

- See Table 92-3 for treatment recommendations.
- The Jarisch-Herxheimer reaction is a dramatic reaction to treatment that is most common with initiation of therapy for primary (~50% of pts) or secondary (~90%) syphilis. The reaction is associated with fever, chills, myalgias, tachycardia, headache, tachypnea, and vasodilation. Symptoms subside within 12–24 h without treatment.

TABLE 92-3 RECOMMENDATIONS FOR THE TREATMENT OF SYPHILIS[a]

Stage of Syphilis	Patients without Penicillin Allergy	Patients with Confirmed Penicillin Allergy[b]
Primary, secondary, or early latent	*CSF normal or not examined:* Penicillin G benzathine (single dose of 2.4 mU IM)	*CSF normal or not examined:* Tetracycline HCl (500 mg PO qid) or doxycycline (100 mg PO bid) for 2 weeks
	CSF abnormal: Treat as neurosyphilis	CSF abnormal: Treat as neurosyphilis
Late latent (or latent of uncertain duration), cardiovascular, or benign tertiary	*CSF normal or not examined:* Penicillin G benzathine (2.4 mU IM weekly for 3 weeks)	*CSF normal and pt not infected with HIV:* Tetracycline HCl (500 mg PO qid) or doxycycline (100 mg PO bid) for 4 weeks
		CSF normal and pt infected with HIV: Desensitization and treatment with penicillin if compliance cannot be ensured
	CSF abnormal: Treat as neurosyphilis	CSF abnormal: Treat as neurosyphilis
Neurosyphilis (asymptomatic or symptomatic)	Aqueous crystalline penicillin G (18–24 mU/d IV, given as 3–4 mU q4h or continuous infusion) for 10–14 days *or* Aqueous procaine penicillin G (2.4 mU/d IM) plus oral probenecid (500 mg qid), both for 10–14 days	Desensitization and treatment with penicillin[c]
Syphilis in pregnancy	According to stage	Desensitization and treatment with penicillin

[a]See Table 169-1 in HPIM-18 and text for indications for CSF examination.
[b]Because of documented macrolide resistance in many *T. pallidum* strains in North America, Europe, and China, azithromycin should be used with caution only when treatment with penicillin or doxycycline is not feasible. Azithromycin should not be used for men who have sex with men or for pregnant women.
[c]Limited data suggest that ceftriaxone (2 g/d either IM or IV for 10–14 days) can be used; however, cross-reactivity between penicillin and ceftriaxone is possible.
Abbreviation: mU, million units.
Source: Based on the 2010 Sexually Transmitted Diseases Treatment Guidelines from the Centers for Disease Control and Prevention.

- Response to treatment should be monitored by determination of RPR or VDRL titers at 6 and 12 months in primary and secondary syphilis and at 6, 12, and 24 months in tertiary or latent syphilis.
  - HIV-infected pts should undergo repeat serologic testing at 3, 6, 9, 12, and 24 months, irrespective of the stage of syphilis.
  - Re-treatment should be considered if serologic responses are not adequate (a persistent fall by ≥4-fold) or if clinical signs persist or recur. For these pts, CSF should be examined, with treatment for neurosyphilis if CSF is abnormal and treatment for late latent syphilis if CSF is normal.
  - In treated neurosyphilis, CSF cell counts should be monitored every 6 months until normal. In adequately treated HIV-uninfected pts, an elevated CSF cell count falls to normal in 3–12 months.

■ HERPES SIMPLEX VIRUS INFECTIONS

Microbiology and Epidemiology

HSV is a linear, double-strand DNA virus, with two subtypes (HSV-1 and HSV-2).

- Exposure to HSV at mucosal surfaces or abraded skin sites permits viral entry into cells of the epidermis and dermis, viral replication, entry into neuronal cells, and centrifugal spread throughout the body.
- More than 90% of adults have antibodies to HSV-1 by age 40; 15–20% of the U.S. population has antibodies to HSV-2.
- Unrecognized carriage of HSV-2 and frequent asymptomatic reactivations of virus from the genital tract foster the continued spread of HSV disease.
- Genital lesions caused by HSV-1 have lower recurrence rates in the first year (~55%) than those caused by HSV-2 (~90%).

Clinical Manifestations

See Table 92-1 for clinical details. First episodes of genital herpes due to HSV-1 and HSV-2 present similarly and can be associated with fever, headache, malaise, and myalgias. More than 80% of women with primary genital herpes have cervical or urethral involvement. Local symptoms include pain, dysuria, vaginal and urethral discharge, and tender inguinal lymphadenopathy.

Diagnosis

Isolation of HSV in tissue culture or demonstration of HSV antigens or DNA in scrapings from lesions is the most accurate diagnostic method. PCR is increasingly being used for detection of HSV DNA and is more sensitive than culture at mucosal sites. Staining of scrapings from the base of the lesion with Wright's, Giemsa's (Tzanck preparation), or Papanicolaou's stain to detect giant cells or intranuclear inclusions is well described, but most clinicians are not skilled in these techniques, which furthermore do not differentiate between HSV and VZV.

TREATMENT   HSV Genital Infections

- *First episodes*: Oral acyclovir (400 mg tid), valacyclovir (1 g bid), or famciclovir (250 mg bid) for 7–14 days is effective.
- *Symptomatic recurrent episodes*: Oral acyclovir (800 mg tid for 2 days), valacyclovir (500 mg bid for 3 days), or famciclovir (750 or 1000 mg bid for 1 day, 1500 mg once, or 500 mg stat followed by 250 mg q12h for 3 days) effectively shortens lesion duration.
- *Suppression of recurrent episodes*: Oral acyclovir (400–800 mg bid) or valacyclovir (500 mg qd) is given. Pts with >9 episodes per year should take valacyclovir (1 g qd or 500 mg bid) or famciclovir (250–500 mg bid). Daily valacyclovir appears to be more effective at reducing subclinical shedding than daily famciclovir.

■ CHANCROID (*HAEMOPHILUS DUCREYI* INFECTION)

H. ducreyi is the etiologic agent of chancroid, an STI characterized by genital ulceration and inguinal adenitis. *H. ducreyi* poses a significant health problem in developing countries because of its directly related morbidity and its role in increasing the efficiency of transmission of and degree of susceptibility to HIV infection. See Table 92-1 for clinical details. Culture of *H. ducreyi* from the lesion confirms the diagnosis; PCR is starting to become available.

TREATMENT   Chancroid (*Haemophilus ducreyi* Infection)

- Regimens recommended by the CDC include azithromycin (1 g PO once), ciprofloxacin (500 mg PO bid for 3 days), ceftriaxone (250 mg IM once), and erythromycin base (500 mg tid for 1 week).
- Sexual partners within 10 days preceding the pt's onset of symptoms should be identified and treated, regardless of symptoms.

■ DONOVANOSIS (*KLEBSIELLA GRANULOMATIS* INFECTION)

Microbiology and Epidemiology

Also known as *granuloma inguinale*, donovanosis is caused by *Klebsiella granulomatis*. The infection is endemic in Papua New Guinea, parts of southern Africa, India, French Guyana, Brazil, and aboriginal communities in Australia; few cases are reported in the U.S.

Clinical Manifestations

See Table 92-1 for clinical details. Four types of lesions have been described: (1) the classic ulcerogranulomatous lesion that bleeds readily when touched; (2) a hypertrophic or verrucous ulcer with a raised irregular edge; (3) a necrotic, offensive-smelling ulcer causing tissue destruction; and (4) a sclerotic or cicatricial lesion with fibrous and scar tissue. The genitals are affected in 90% of pts and the inguinal region in 10%.

Diagnosis and Treatment

Diagnosis is often based on identification of typical Donovan bodies (gram-negative intracytoplasmic cysts filled with deeply staining bodies that may have a safety-pin appearance) within large mononuclear cells in smears from lesions or biopsy specimens. PCR is also available. Pts should be treated with azithromycin (1 g on day 1, then 500 mg qd for 7 days or 1 g weekly for 4 weeks); alternative therapy consists of a 14-day course of doxycycline (100 mg bid), trimethoprim-sulfamethoxazole (960 mg bid), erythromycin (500 mg qid), or tetracycline (500 mg qid). If any of the 14-day treatment regimens are chosen, the pts should be monitored until lesions have healed completely.

■ HUMAN PAPILLOMAVIRUS (HPV) INFECTIONS

Microbiology

Papillomaviruses are nonenveloped viruses with a double-strand circular DNA genome. More than 100 HPV types are recognized, and individual types are associated with specific clinical manifestations. For example, HPV types 16, 18, 31, 33, and 45 have been most strongly associated with cervical cancers, and HPV types 6 and 11 cause anogenital warts (*condylomata acuminata*). Most infections, including those with oncogenic types, are self-limited.

Clinical Manifestations

The clinical manifestations of HPV infection depend on the location of lesions and the type of virus. The incubation period is usually 3–4 months but can be as long as 2 years.

- Warts (including plantar warts) appear as flesh-colored to brown and exophytic, with hyperkeratotic papules.
- Anogenital warts are commonly found on the penile shaft (in circumcised men), at the urethral meatus, and in the perianal region (in persons who practice receptive anal intercourse) and may involve the vagina and cervix.

Diagnosis

Most visible warts are diagnosed correctly by history and physical examination alone. Colposcopy is invaluable in assessing vaginal and cervical lesions, and 3–5% acetic acid solution applied to lesions may aid in the diagnosis.

- Papanicolaou smears from cervical or anal scrapings show cytologic evidence of HPV infection.
- Detection of HPV nucleic acids (e.g., PCR, hybrid-capture assay) is the most specific and sensitive method of detection.

> **TREATMENT** Human Papillomavirus Infections
>
> - Many lesions resolve spontaneously. Current treatment is not completely effective, and some agents have significant side effects.
>   - Provider-administered therapy can include cryotherapy, podophyllin resin (10–25%) applied weekly for up to 4 weeks, trichloroacetic acid or bichloroacetic acid (80–90%) applied weekly, surgical excision, intralesionally administered interferon, or laser surgery.
>   - Pt-administered therapy consists of podofilox (0.5% solution or gel applied bid for 3 days; this treatment can be repeated up to 4 times with 4 days between treatment courses) or imiquimod (5% cream applied 3 times/week for up to 16 weeks).

Prevention

A quadrivalent vaccine (Gardasil, Merck) containing HPV types 6, 11, 16, and 18 and a bivalent vaccine (Cervarix, GlaxoSmithKline) containing HPV types 16 and 18 are available. Either vaccine is recommended for administration to girls and young women 9–26 years of age and may be used in males 9–26 years of age.

- HPV types 6 and 11 cause 90% of anogenital warts, and HPV types 16 and 18 cause 70% of cervical cancers.
- Because 30% of cervical cancers are caused by HPV types not included in either vaccine, no changes in clinical cancer-screening programs are currently recommended.

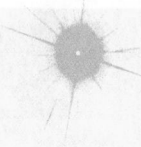

For a more detailed discussion, see Marrazzo JM, Holmes KK: Sexually Transmitted Infections: Overview and Clinical Approach, Chap. 130, p. 1095; Ram S, Rice PA: Gonococcal Infections, Chap. 144, p. 1220; Murphy TF: *Haemophilus* and *Moraxella* Infections, Chap. 145, p. 1228; O'Farrell N: Donovanosis, Chap. 161, p. 1320; Lukehart SA: Syphilis, Chap. 169, p. 1380; Hardy RD: Infections Due to Mycoplasmas, Chap. 175, p. 1417; Gaydos CA, Quinn TC: Chlamydial Infections, Chap. 176, p. 1421; Corey L: Herpes Simplex Virus Infections, Chap. 179, p. 1453; and Reichman RC: Human Papillomavirus Infections, Chap. 185, p. 1481, in HPIM-18.

CHAPTER **93**
Infections of the Skin, Soft Tissues, Joints, and Bones

SKIN AND SOFT TISSUE INFECTIONS

Skin and soft tissue infections are diagnosed principally by a careful history (e.g., temporal progression, travel, animal exposure, bites, trauma, underlying medical conditions) and physical examination (appearance of lesions and distribution). Treatment of common skin infections is summarized in Table 93-1; parenteral treatment is usually given until systemic signs and symptoms have improved. Types of skin lesions include the following:

1. *Vesicles*: due to proliferation of organisms, usually viruses, within the epidermis (e.g., VZV, HSV, coxsackievirus, poxviruses, *Rickettsia akari*)
2. *Bullae*: caused by toxin-producing organisms. Different entities affect different skin levels; for example, staphylococcal scalded-skin syndrome and toxic epidermal necrolysis cause cleavage of the stratum corneum and the stratum germinativum, respectively. Bullae are also seen in necrotizing fasciitis, gas gangrene, and *Vibrio vulnificus* infections.

TABLE 93-1 TREATMENT OF COMMON INFECTIONS OF THE SKIN

Diagnosis/ Condition	Primary Treatment	Alternative Treatment	See Also HPIM-18 Chap(s).
Animal bite (prophylaxis or early infection)[a]	Amoxicillin/ clavulanate, 875/125 mg PO bid	Doxycycline, 100 mg PO bid	e24
Animal bite[a] (established infection)	Ampicillin/ sulbactam, 1.5–3 g IV q6h	Clindamycin, 600– 900 mg IV q8h, *plus* Ciprofloxacin, 400 mg IV q12h, *or* Cefoxitin, 2 g IV q6h	e24
Bacillary angiomatosis	Erythromycin, 500 mg PO qid	Doxycycline, 100 mg PO bid	160
Herpes simplex (primary genital)	Acyclovir, 400 mg PO tid for 10 days	Famciclovir, 250 mg PO tid for 5–10 days, *or* Valacyclovir, 1000 mg PO bid for 10 days	179
Herpes zoster (immunocompetent host >50 years of age)	Acyclovir, 800 mg PO 5 times daily for 7–10 days	Famciclovir, 500 mg PO tid for 7–10 days, *or* Valacyclovir, 1000 mg PO tid for 7 days	180
Cellulitis (staphylococcal or streptococcal[b,c])	Nafcillin or oxacillin, 2 g IV q4–6h	Cefazolin, 1–2 g IV q8h, *or* Ampicillin/ sulbactam, 1.5–3 g IV q6h, *or* Erythromycin, 0.5–1 g IV q6h, *or* Clindamycin, 600– 900 mg IV q8h	135, 136
MRSA skin infection[d]	Vancomycin, 1 g IV q12h	Linezolid, 600 mg IV q12h	135

TABLE 93-1 TREATMENT OF COMMON INFECTIONS OF THE SKIN (CONTINUED)

Diagnosis/ Condition	Primary Treatment	Alternative Treatment	See Also HPIM-18 Chap(s).
Necrotizing fasciitis (group A streptococcal[b])	Clindamycin, 600–900 mg IV q6–8h, *plus* Penicillin G, 4 million units IV q4h	Clindamycin, 600–900 mg IV q6–8h, *plus* Cephalosporin (first- or second-generation)	136
Necrotizing fasciitis (mixed aerobes and anaerobes)	Ampicillin, 2 g IV q4h, *plus* Clindamycin, 600–900 mg IV q6–8h, *plus* Ciprofloxacin, 400 mg IV q6–8h	Vancomycin, 1 g IV q6h, *plus* Metronidazole, 500 mg IV q6h, *plus* Ciprofloxacin, 400 mg IV q6–8h	164
Gas gangrene	Clindamycin, 600–900 mg IV q6–8h, *plus* Penicillin G, 4 million units IV q4–6h	Clindamycin, 600–900 mg IV q6–8h, *plus* Cefoxitin, 2 g IV q6h	142

Note: Parenteral treatment is usually given until systemic signs and symptoms have improved.
[a]*Pasteurella multocida*, a species commonly associated with both dog and cat bites, is resistant to cephalexin, dicloxacillin, clindamycin, and erythromycin. *Eikenella corrodens*, a bacterium commonly associated with human bites, is resistant to clindamycin, penicillinase-resistant penicillins, and metronidazole but is sensitive to trimethoprim-sulfamethoxazole and fluoroquinolones.
[b]The frequency of erythromycin resistance in group A *Streptococcus* is currently ~5% in the United States but has reached 70–100% in some other countries. Most, but not all, erythromycin-resistant group A streptococci are susceptible to clindamycin. Approximately 90–95% of *Staphylococcus aureus* strains are sensitive to clindamycin.
[c]Severe hospital-acquired *S. aureus* infections or community-acquired *S. aureus* infections that are not responding to the β-lactam antibiotics recommended in this table may be caused by methicillin-resistant strains, requiring a switch to vancomycin or linezolid.
[d]Some strains of methicillin-resistant *S. aureus* (MRSA) remain sensitive to tetracycline and trimethoprim-sulfamethoxazole. Daptomycin (4 mg/kg IV q24h) or tigecycline (100-mg loading dose followed by 50 mg IV q12h) are alternative treatments for MRSA.

3. *Crusted lesions*: Impetigo caused by either *Streptococcus pyogenes* (impetigo contagiosa) or *Staphylococcus aureus* (bullous impetigo) usually starts with a bullous phase before development of a golden-brown crust. Crusted lesions are also seen in some systemic fungal infections, dermatophytic infections, and cutaneous mycobacterial infections. It is important to recognize impetigo contagiosa because of its relation to poststreptococcal glomerulonephritis.

4. *Folliculitis*: Localized infection of hair follicles is usually due to *S. aureus*. "Hot-tub folliculitis" is a diffuse condition caused by *Pseudomonas aeruginosa*. Freshwater avian schistosomes cause an allergic reaction after penetrating hair follicles, resulting in "swimmer's itch."

5. *Papular and nodular lesions*: Raised lesions of the skin occur in many different forms and can be caused by *Bartonella* (cat-scratch disease and bacillary angiomatosis), *Treponema pallidum*, human papillomavirus, mycobacteria, and helminths.

6. *Ulcers, with or without eschars*: can be caused by cutaneous anthrax, ulceroglandular tularemia, plague, and mycobacterial infection. Ulcerated lesions on the genitals can be caused by chancroid (painful) or syphilis (painless).

7. *Erysipelas*: abrupt onset of fiery red swelling of the face or extremities, with well-defined indurated margins, intense pain, and rapid progression. *S. pyogenes* is the exclusive cause.

■ CELLULITIS

- **Pathogenesis** Bacteria gain access to the epidermis through breaks in the skin, whether accidental (e.g., cuts, scratches, burns) or iatrogenic (e.g., surgical incisions, IV catheters). The expanding area of erythema may be due to extracellular toxins and/or the host immune response rather than to increasing bacterial numbers.
- **Microbiology** Etiologic causes include commensal flora (e.g., *S. aureus*, *S. pyogenes*) or a wide variety of exogenous flora. With the latter, a thorough history and epidemiologic data may help identify the cause.
  - Examples of exogenous bacteria causing cellulitis include the following: *Pasteurella multocida* after a cat or dog bite; *Capnocytophaga canimorsus* after a dog bite; *Eikenella corrodens* after a human bite; *P. aeruginosa* in association with ecthyma gangrenosum in neutropenic pts, a penetrating injury (stepping on a nail), or hot-tub folliculitis; *Aeromonas hydrophila* after a laceration sustained in fresh water; or *Erysipelothrix rhusiopathiae* after contact with domestic swine and fish.
- **Clinical manifestations** This acute inflammatory condition of the skin is characterized by localized pain, erythema, swelling, and heat.
  - Cellulitis due to *S. aureus* often spreads from a central site of localized infection, such as an abscess or an infected foreign body.
  - *S. pyogenes* can cause a rapidly spreading, diffuse process, often with fever and lymphangitis.
- **Diagnosis** If there is drainage, an open wound, or an obvious portal of entry, Gram's staining and culture may identify the etiology. Aspiration

or biopsy of the leading edge of the cellulitic tissue yields a diagnosis in only 20% of cases.

- **Treatment** See Table 93-1.

■ NECROTIZING FASCIITIS

- **Pathogenesis** Infection, either apparent or inapparent, results from a breach in integrity of the skin or mucous membrane barriers and can be associated with malignancy, a diverticulum, hemorrhoids, or an anal fissure.
  - In the case of infections with no obvious portal of entry, transient bacteremia is thought to seed sites of nonpenetrating trauma (e.g., bruise, muscle strain).
  - Infection spreads to the deep fascia and along fascial planes through venous channels and lymphatics.
- **Microbiology** Necrotizing fasciitis is caused by *S. pyogenes*, mixed aerobic and anaerobic bacteria, or *Clostridium perfringens*; methicillin-resistant *S. aureus* (MRSA) strains that produce the Panton-Valentine leukocidin have also been reported as an occasional cause.
- **Clinical manifestations** The timing of cutaneous manifestations (e.g., violaceous bullae; friable, necrotic skin; induration; brawny edema) depends on whether the infection began superficially (rapid onset) or in deeper structures (slower onset).
  - Early in the disease course, severe pain and unexplained fever may be the only findings.
  - Thrombosis of blood vessels in dermal papillae leads to ischemia of peripheral nerves and anesthesia of the affected area.
  - In later stages, pts appear toxic and often develop shock and multiorgan failure.
- **Diagnosis** Diagnosis is based on clinical presentation. Other findings may include gas detected in deep tissues by imaging studies (particularly with clostridial species but rarely with *S. pyogenes*) and markedly elevated serum creatine phosphokinase levels (in the case of concomitant myositis).
- **Treatment** Emergent surgical exploration to deep fascia and muscle, with removal of necrotic tissue, is essential. Table 93-1 provides recommendations for adjunctive antibiotic therapy.

■ MYOSITIS/MYONECROSIS

- **Clinical manifestations and microbiology** Infections involving the muscle have differing manifestations, depending on the etiology.
  - *Myositis*: can be caused by bacteria (clostridia, streptococci), viruses (influenza virus, dengue virus, coxsackievirus), or parasites (*Trichinella*, *Taenia solium*, *Toxoplasma*). This condition usually manifests with myalgias, but pain can be severe in coxsackievirus, *Trichinella*, and bacterial infections.
  - *Pyomyositis*: a localized muscle infection usually due to *S. aureus*, common in tropical areas, and typically with no known portal of entry.
  - *Myonecrosis*: can be caused by clostridial species (*C. perfringens*, *C. septicum*, *C. histolyticum*, *C. sordellii*) or by mixed aerobic and anaerobic bacteria. Myonecrosis is usually related to trauma; however,

spontaneous gangrene—usually due to *C. septicum*—can occur in pts with neutropenia, GI malignancy, or diverticulosis. Myonecrosis of the uterus, typically due to *C. sordellii*, occurs in women after spontaneous or medically induced abortion and in healthy postpartum women; infection is rapidly and almost uniformly fatal as there are few or no localizing clinical findings.

- **Diagnosis and Treatment** Emergent surgical intervention to visualize deep structures, obtain materials for culture and sensitivity testing, remove necrotic tissue, and reduce compartment pressure is both diagnostic and therapeutic.

  - Empirical antibiotic treatment should target likely etiologies—e.g., vancomycin (1 g IV q12h) for pyomyositis and ampicillin/sulbactam (2–3 g IV q6h) for mixed aerobic-anaerobic infections.

  - For treatment of clostridial myonecrosis (gas gangrene), see Table 93-1.

INFECTIOUS ARTHRITIS

- **Pathogenesis** Joints become infected by hematogenous seeding (the most common route), by spread from a contiguous site of infection, or by direct inoculation (e.g., during trauma or surgery). Acute bacterial infection can rapidly destroy articular cartilage as a result of increased intraarticular pressure and the elicited host immune response.

- **Microbiology** The predominant etiologic agents differ with the pt's age; *S. aureus* is the most common nongonococcal isolate in adults of all ages.

  - In children <5 years old, *S. aureus*, *S. pyogenes*, and *Kingella kingae* predominate.

  - In young adults, *Neisseria gonorrhoeae* is the most common etiology.

  - In adults, *S. aureus* predominates, but gram-negative bacilli, pneumococci, and β-hemolytic streptococci are involved in one-third of cases in older adults.

  - Other causes of septic arthritis include *Borrelia burgdorferi* (Lyme disease), tuberculosis and other mycobacterial infections, fungal infections (e.g., coccidioidomycosis, histoplasmosis), and viral infections (e.g., rubella, mumps, hepatitis B, parvovirus infection).

- **Epidemiology and clinical manifestations** The risk factors and presentation differ depending on whether *N. gonorrhoeae* is the cause.

  - *Nongonococcal bacterial arthritis:* Risk is increased in pts with rheumatoid arthritis, diabetes mellitus, glucocorticoid therapy, hemodialysis, malignancy, and IV drug use.

    - In 90% of pts, one joint is involved—most often the knee, which is followed in frequency by the hip, shoulder, wrist, and elbow; IV drug users often have spinal, sacroiliac, or sternoclavicular joint involvement.

    - Pts have moderate to severe pain, effusion, decreased range of motion, and fever.

  - *Gonococcal arthritis:* Women are 2–3 times more likely than men to develop disseminated gonococcal infection (DGI) and arthritis, particularly during menses and during pregnancy (see Chap. 92).

- DGI presents as fever, chills, rash, and articular symptoms (migratory arthritis). The cutaneous and articular findings result from an immune reaction to circulating gonococci and immune-complex deposition, so that synovial fluid cultures are consistently negative.
  - In true gonococcal arthritis (which always follows DGI), a single joint (hip, knee, ankle, or wrist) is usually involved.
- *Prosthetic joint infections:* complicate 1–4% of joint replacements and are usually acquired intra- or perioperatively.
  - Acute presentations are seen in infections caused by *S. aureus*, pyogenic streptococci, and enteric bacilli.
  - Indolent presentations are seen in infections caused by coagulase-negative staphylococci and diphtheroids.
- *Reactive arthritis:* follows ~1% of cases of nongonococcal urethritis and 2% of enteric infections (e.g., *Yersinia enterocolitica*, *Shigella flexneri*, *Campylobacter jejuni*, *Salmonella* spp.). Only a minority of pts have the other classic findings associated with reactive arthritis, including urethritis, conjunctivitis, uveitis, oral ulcers, and rash.
- **Diagnosis** If there is concern about joint infection, examination of synovial fluid from the affected joint is essential. There is considerable overlap in the cell counts due to different etiologies, but synovial fluid culture and examination for crystals (to rule out gout and pseudogout) can help narrow the diagnosis.
  - *Normal* synovial fluid contains <180 cells (mostly mononuclear)/μL. *Acute bacterial infection* of joints results in synovial fluid cell counts averaging 100,000/μL (range, 25,000–250,000/μL), with >90% PMNs. Synovial fluid in *gonococcal arthritis* contains >50,000 cells/μL, but results of Gram's staining are usually negative, and cultures of synovial fluid are positive in <40% of cases. Other mucosal sites should be cultured to diagnose gonorrhea. Pts with septic arthritis due to *mycobacteria* or *fungi* can have 10,000–30,000 cells/μL in synovial fluid, with 50–70% PMNs. Synovial fluid cell counts in *noninfectious inflammatory arthritides* are typically 30,000–50,000/μL.
  - Gram's staining of synovial fluid should be performed, and injection directly into blood culture bottles can increase the yield of synovial fluid cultures.
  - Blood cultures are positive in 50–70% of cases due to *S. aureus* but are less commonly positive with other organisms.
  - Plain radiographs show soft tissue swelling, joint space widening, and displacement of tissue planes by distended capsule. Narrowing of the joint space and bony erosions suggest advanced disease.

TREATMENT Infectious Arthritis

- Drainage of pus and necrotic debris is needed to cure infection and to prevent destruction of cartilage, postinfectious degenerative arthritis, and joint deformity or instability.

- A third-generation cephalosporin (cefotaxime, 1 g IV q8h; or ceftriaxone, 1–2 g IV q24h) provides adequate empirical coverage for most community-acquired infections in adults when smears demonstrate no organisms. Vancomycin (1 g IV q12h) should be used to cover the possibility of MRSA when there are gram-positive cocci on the smear.
  - In IV drug users and other susceptible pts, treatment for gram-negative organisms such as *P. aeruginosa* should be considered.
  - If a pathogen is identified by culture, treatment should be adjusted according to the specific bacterial organism and its antibiotic susceptibility.
- Treatment for *S. aureus* should be given for 4 weeks, that for enteric gram-negative bacilli for 3–4 weeks, and that for pneumococci or streptococci for 2 weeks. Treatment of gonococcal arthritis should commence with ceftriaxone (1 g/d) until improvement; the 7-day course can be completed with an oral fluoroquinolone (e.g., ciprofloxacin, 500 mg bid). If fluoroquinolone resistance is not prevalent, a fluoroquinolone can be given for the entire course.
- Prosthetic joint infections should be treated with surgery and high-dose IV antibiotics for 4–6 weeks. The prosthesis often has to be removed; to avoid joint removal, antibiotic suppression of infection may be tried. A 3- to 6-month course of ciprofloxacin and rifampin has been successful in *S. aureus* prosthetic joint infections of relatively short duration, although prospective trials confirming the efficacy of this regimen are still needed.

OSTEOMYELITIS

- **Pathogenesis** Osteomyelitis is typically caused either by direct spread from a contiguous focus of infection or by hematogenous spread. Areas of bone or contiguous surrounding tissue that have abnormal viability, blood supply, sensation, or edema are at increased risk for bacterial infection. Bacteria can colonize and persist in these areas, partly because of the decreased immunosurveillance resulting from compromised blood flow and—in the case of some organisms, such as *S. aureus*—elaboration of bacterial adhesins and toxins.
- **Epidemiology** In the U.S., 0.1–1.8% of otherwise healthy adults are affected by acute osteomyelitis; 30–40% of adults with diabetes develop osteomyelitis after a foot puncture. Orthopedic surgery (particularly with implantation of hardware), obesity, diabetes, trauma, bacteremia, poor circulation, and older age are risk factors for osteomyelitis.
- **Microbiology** Table 93-2 lists organisms that cause osteomyelitis.
  - *S. aureus* is the most common cause.
  - The overlapping circulations of the urinary tract and the spine may be a source of vertebral osteomyelitis due to urinary tract pathogens such as *Escherichia coli* and *Klebsiella*.

TABLE 93-2 MICROORGANISMS THAT CAUSE OSTEOMYELITIS

Organism	Comment
Frequently encountered bacteria	
Staphylococcus aureus	Most likely bacterial pathogen
	Aggressive, invasive
	Often metastatic foci with bacteremia
	Should consider surgery early
Staphylococci other than *S. aureus* (coagulase-negative)	Usually associated with foreign material or implants
	Biofilm production
Streptococci	May spread rapidly through soft tissues
Enterobacteriaceae (*Escherichia coli, Klebsiella*, others)	Considerable variation in antibiotic susceptibility
	Increasing antibiotic resistance with overuse
	May become resistant to antibiotics during therapy
Pseudomonas aeruginosa	Increasingly resistant to antibiotics
	Frequent successor to other bacteria when initial therapy fails
	May be related to contamination
Unusual organisms	
Anaerobic bacteria	Usually mixed with aerobic bacteria
	May be synergistic
	Survival dependent on devitalized tissue
Bartonella henselae	Associated with cat scratches and probably with fleas
Brucella spp.	Prominent in developing countries, especially with unpasteurized milk
Fungi	*Candida* the most likely genus
	Considerable variation in susceptibility, depending on species
	Surgery sometimes helpful if infection is invasive
Mycobacterium tuberculosis	May involve any bone
	Vertebral osteomyelitis common in some countries
Mycobacteria other than *M. tuberculosis*	Need special culture media for recovery
Viruses	Some associated viral infections, including varicella and variola

TABLE 93-3 ANTIBIOTICS FOR THE TREATMENT OF OSTEOMYELITIS

Organism	Antimicrobial Agent	Dosing	Comments
Methicillin-susceptible *Staphylococcus aureus*	Oxacillin or nafcillin	2 g IV q6h	May be more active than cephalosporins
			More difficult than cephalosporins to administer for long periods
	Cephalosporins	Cefazolin: 2 g IV q8h	Ceftriaxone advantageous with OPAT
		Ceftriaxone: 1–2 g IV q24h	
	Clindamycin[a]	600–900 mg IV q8h	Not well studied for osteomyelitis
			Oral form possible (300–600 mg q8h)
			Resistance significant and increasing
			Toxicity different from that of β-lactam antibiotics
Methicillin-resistant *S. aureus*	Vancomycin	15 mg/kg IV q12h	Strains with an MIC of ≥2 µg/mL may not respond well.
	Daptomycin[a]	4–6 mg/kg IV q24h	Promising, but concern about adverse effects with prolonged therapy
	Linezolid[a]	600 mg IV or PO q12h	Effectiveness and adverse effects with prolonged therapy unclear
			Bacteriostatic
Streptococci	Penicillin	5 mU IV q6h or 20 mU/d by continuous infusion	Not all streptococci are susceptible.
			Ceftriaxone (1 g/d IV or IM) and ampicillin (12 g/d IV) are alternatives.
Enterococci	Penicillin *plus* Gentamicin	As above 5 mg/kg daily IV	If strain is susceptible
	Vancomycin	As above	If strain is susceptible

TABLE 93-3 ANTIBIOTICS FOR THE TREATMENT OF OSTEOMYELITIS (CONTINUED)

Organism	Antimicrobial Agent	Dosing	Comments
Enterobacteriaceae (*Escherichia coli*, *Klebsiella*, other)	Ceftriaxone or another cephalosporin	As above	If strain is susceptible
	Ciprofloxacin	400 mg IV q8–12h	Oral form possible (500–750 mg q8–12h)
Pseudomonas aeruginosa	Ciprofloxacin	As above	Resistance may develop during therapy; if strain is resistant, drugs to consider include cefepime and ceftazidime.

[a]Not approved for use in osteomyelitis by the U.S. Food and Drug Administration.
Abbreviations: MIC, minimal inhibitory concentration; OPAT, outpatient parenteral antimicrobial therapy.

- **Clinical manifestations** Pts generally have a febrile illness, with localized pain and tenderness. A history of surgery or trauma in the affected region—even in the remote past—should raise suspicion.
- **Diagnosis** Radiographic studies and occasionally invasive sampling of lesions are needed to confirm the diagnosis.
  - X-rays of the affected region may demonstrate bone loss, sequestra, periosteal elevation, or swelling, but many of these findings may become apparent only after the infection has continued for several weeks.
  - CT and especially MRI scans offer increased sensitivity in detecting osteomyelitis.
  - Needle aspiration or biopsy of lesions allows histologic confirmation of disease and may permit identification of the etiologic agent.
- **Treatment** Table 93-3 lists antibiotics for the treatment of osteomyelitis due to common pathogens. Empirical antibiotic therapy should target staphylococci and often includes cefazolin or an antistaphylococcal penicillin (oxacillin or nafcillin).
  - The optimal route and duration of therapy remain controversial, but a 4- to 6-week course of IV therapy is the usual recommended minimum; pediatric studies are providing increasing evidence that shorter courses and oral agents may be adequate.
  - Serial measurement of inflammatory markers (ESR, C-reactive protein) can serve as a surrogate marker of response to treatment in some infections (particularly in cases due to *S. aureus*).

– Given the prolonged treatment necessary, outpatient parenteral antibiotic therapy is increasingly being used and is both safe and effective.

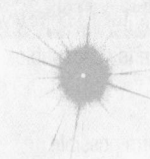

For a more detailed discussion, see Stevens DL: Infections of the Skin, Muscles, and Soft Tissues, Chap. 125, p. 1064; Tice AD: Osteomyelitis, Chap. 126, p. 1071; Wang F: Molluscum Contagiosum, Monkeypox, and Other Poxvirus Infections, Chap. 183, p. 1476; and Madoff LC: Infectious Arthritis, Chap. 334, p. 2842, in HPIM-18.

CHAPTER 94
Pneumococcal Infections

■ MICROBIOLOGY

- *Streptococcus pneumoniae* (the pneumococcus) is a gram-positive coccus that grows in chains, causes α-hemolysis on blood agar, is bile soluble, and is sensitive to optochin.
- Nearly every clinical isolate has a polysaccharide capsule that protects the bacteria from phagocytosis in the absence of type-specific antibody; 92 distinct capsules have been identified.

■ EPIDEMIOLOGY

- In industrialized countries, children serve as the major vectors of pneumococcal transmission: 20–50% of children <5 years old have asymptomatic nasopharyngeal colonization with *S. pneumoniae* (compared with 5–15% of young and middle-aged adults). Colonization rates for all age groups are even higher in low-income countries.
- Rates of pneumococcal disease vary by season (higher in winter), gender (higher for males), and underlying medical condition (e.g., splenic dysfunction; chronic respiratory, heart, liver, and kidney disease; immunosuppression).
- The introduction and widespread use (in industrialized countries) of pneumococcal conjugate vaccines have led to dramatic changes in the epidemiology of invasive pneumococcal disease; rates have fallen by >75% among infants and children in the U.S.

■ PATHOGENESIS

- Nasopharyngeal colonization can persist for many months, resulting in the development of type-specific serum IgG that ultimately leads to pneumococcal clearance from the nasopharynx. Accordingly, pneumococcal disease is usually associated with recent acquisition of a new colonizing serotype.
- Once the nasopharynx has been colonized, the bacteria spread either via the bloodstream to distant sites (e.g., brain, joint, bones) or locally to contiguous areas (e.g., middle ear, lungs).

- Local cytokine production, particularly after intercurrent viral infections, facilitates pneumococcal adherence; bacterial factors such as peptidoglycan and teichoic acid induce inflammation, result in characteristic pathology, and permit bacterial invasion.

◼ CLINICAL MANIFESTATIONS AND DIAGNOSIS

The clinical manifestations of pneumococcal disease depend on the site of infection and the duration of illness.

Pneumonia

Pneumococcal pneumonia—the most common serious pneumococcal syndrome—is difficult to distinguish from pneumonia of other etiologies on the basis of clinical findings.

- Pts often present with fever, abrupt-onset cough and dyspnea, and sputum production.
  - Pts may also have pleuritic chest pain, shaking chills, or myalgias.
  - Among the elderly, presenting symptoms may be less specific, with confusion and malaise but without fever or cough.
- On physical examination, adults may have tachypnea (>30 breaths/min) and tachycardia, crackles on chest auscultation, and dullness to percussion of the chest in areas of consolidation.
  - In some cases, hypotension, bronchial breathing, a pleural rub, or cyanosis may be present.
  - Upper abdominal pain may be present if the diaphragmatic pleura is involved.
- Pneumococcal pneumonia is generally diagnosed by Gram's staining and culture of sputum.
  - While culture results are awaited, chest x-rays—which classically demonstrate lobar or segmental consolidation—may provide some adjunctive evidence, although they may be normal early in the course of illness or with dehydration.
  - Blood cultures are positive for pneumococci in <30% of cases.
  - Leukocytosis (>15,000/μL) is common; leukopenia is documented in <10% of cases and is associated with a fatal outcome.
  - A positive pneumococcal urinary antigen test has a high predictive value among adults, in whom the prevalence of nasopharyngeal colonization is low.
- Empyema occurs in <5% of cases and should be considered when a pleural effusion is accompanied by fever and leukocytosis after 4–5 days of appropriate antibiotic therapy. Pleural fluid with frank pus, bacteria, or a pH of ≤7.1 indicates empyema and requires aggressive drainage.

Meningitis

S. pneumoniae is among the most common causes of meningitis in both adults and children. Pneumococcal meningitis can present as a primary syndrome or as a complication of other pneumococcal conditions (e.g., otitis media, infected skull fracture, bacteremia). Pneumococcal meningitis is indistinguishable from other causes of pyogenic meningitis.

- Pts have fever, headache, neck stiffness, photophobia, and occasionally seizures and confusion.
- On examination, pts have a toxic appearance, altered consciousness, bradycardia, and hypertension (indicative of increased intracranial pressure). Kernig's or Brudzinski's sign or cranial nerve palsies (particularly of the third and sixth cranial nerves) are noted in a small fraction of adult pts.
- Diagnosis of pneumococcal meningitis relies on examination of CSF, which reveals an elevated protein level, elevated WBC count, and reduced glucose concentration; the etiologic agent can be specifically identified by culture, antigen testing, or PCR. A blood culture positive for *S. pneumoniae* in conjunction with clinical manifestations of meningitis is also considered confirmatory.

Other Invasive Syndromes

S. pneumoniae can affect virtually any body site and cause invasive syndromes, including bacteremia, osteomyelitis, septic arthritis, endocarditis, pericarditis, and peritonitis. The essential diagnostic approach is collection of fluid from the site of infection by sterile technique and examination by Gram's staining, culture, and—when relevant—capsular antigen assay or PCR. Hemolytic-uremic syndrome can complicate invasive pneumococcal disease.

Noninvasive Syndromes

Sinusitis and otitis media are the two most common noninvasive syndromes caused by *S. pneumoniae*; the latter is the most common pneumococcal syndrome and most often affects young children. See Chap. 64 for more detail.

TREATMENT Pneumococcal Infections

- Penicillin remains the cornerstone of treatment for pneumococcal disease caused by sensitive isolates, with daily doses ranging from 50,000 U/kg for minor infections to 300,000 U/kg for meningitis. Macrolides and cephalosporins are alternatives for penicillin-allergic pts but otherwise offer no advantage over penicillin.
- Strains resistant to β-lactam drugs are increasing in frequency, and antibiotic recommendations are typically based on the minimal inhibitory concentration against the isolate, particularly in cases of invasive disease.

PNEUMONIA
- *Outpatient treatment:* Amoxicillin (1 g PO q8h) is effective for virtually all cases of pneumococcal pneumonia. Fluoroquinolones (e.g., levofloxacin, 500–750 mg/d; or moxifloxacin, 400 mg/d) are also highly likely to be effective in the U.S., although they are much more expensive than amoxicillin. Clindamycin and azithromycin are effective in 90% and 80% of cases, respectively.
- *Inpatient treatment:* For pts with noncritical illness, β-lactam antibiotics are recommended—e.g., penicillin (3–4 mU IV q4h), ampicillin (1–2 g IV q6h), or ceftriaxone (1 g IV q12–24h). For pts with critical illness, vancomycin may be added, with its use reviewed once susceptibility data are available.

- *Treatment duration:* The optimal duration of treatment is uncertain, but continuation of antibiotics for at least 5 days after the pt becomes afebrile seems prudent.

MENINGITIS

- Because of the increased prevalence of resistant pneumococci, first-line therapy should include vancomycin (1 g IV q12h) plus a third-generation cephalosporin (ceftriaxone, 2 g IV q12h; or cefotaxime, 2 g IV q4h). Rifampin (600 mg/d) can be substituted for the third-generation cephalosporin in pts hypersensitive to β-lactam agents.
- The antibiotic regimen should be adjusted appropriately once susceptibility data are available. If the isolate is resistant to penicillin and cephalosporins, both vancomycin and the cephalosporin should be continued.
- A repeat LP should be considered after 48 h if the organism is not sensitive to penicillin and information on cephalosporin sensitivity is not yet available, if the pt's clinical condition does not improve or deteriorates, or if the pt has received dexamethasone, which may compromise clinical evaluation.
- In adults with community-acquired bacterial meningitis, dexamethasone should be given before or in conjunction with the first dose of antibiotics, as glucocorticoids have been demonstrated to significantly reduce rates of mortality, severe hearing loss, and neurologic sequelae; the data are not clear as to whether this practice is also beneficial in children.

■ PREVENTION

- All persons ≥65 years old and those 2–64 years old who are at increased risk of pneumococcal disease should receive the 23-valent pneumococcal polysaccharide vaccine (PPV23), which contains capsular polysaccharide from the 23 most prevalent serotypes of *S. pneumoniae*.
  - Persons >2 years old with continuing increased risk should be revaccinated every 5 years.
  - Persons whose only indication for vaccination is an age of ≥65 years do not need to be revaccinated.
- The efficacy of PPV23 is controversial; it appears to be effective against invasive pneumococcal disease but less effective or ineffective against nonbacteremic pneumococcal pneumonia.
- The duration of protection conferred by PPV23 is ~5 years.
- The poor response of infants and young children to pneumococcal polysaccharide vaccines prompted the development of pneumococcal conjugate vaccines. In the U.S., the current recommendation is for infants to be routinely vaccinated with the conjugate vaccine PCV13, which contains the 13 serotypes most associated with disease.
  - Pneumococcal conjugate vaccines are highly effective at providing protection against vaccine-serotype invasive pneumococcal disease, pneumonia, otitis media, nasopharyngeal colonization, and all-cause mortality.

– In the U.S., there has been a >90% reduction in vaccine-serotype invasive pneumococcal disease among the whole population, including indirect protection of unvaccinated adults.

> For a more detailed discussion, see Goldblatt D, O'Brien KL: Pneumococcal Infections, Chap. 134, p. 1151, in HPIM-18.

CHAPTER **95**
Staphylococcal Infections

■ MICROBIOLOGY

Staphylococci are gram-positive cocci that form grapelike clusters on Gram's stain; they are catalase positive (unlike streptococci), nonmotile, aerobic, and facultatively anaerobic. *Staphylococcus aureus*, which is distinguished from other staphylococci by its production of coagulase, is the most virulent species.

■ *S. AUREUS* INFECTIONS

Epidemiology

S. aureus is an important cause of community-acquired infections and is the leading cause of nosocomial infections.

- *S. aureus* is a component of the normal human flora, most frequently colonizing the anterior nares but also colonizing the skin (particularly damaged skin), vagina, axilla, perineum, and oropharynx. These sites of colonization are reservoirs for future infection.
- Of healthy persons, 25–50% may be persistently or transiently colonized with *S. aureus*, and the rate is especially high among insulin-dependent diabetic pts, HIV-infected persons, injection drug users, hemodialysis pts, and pts with skin damage.
- Methicillin-resistant *S. aureus* (MRSA) is common in hospitals, and its prevalence is increasing dramatically in community settings among individuals without prior medical exposure.
  - In the United States, strain USA300 (defined by pulsed-field gel electrophoresis) causes most community-acquired MRSA (CA-MRSA) infections and can cause severe disease in immunocompetent pts.
  - Outbreaks of CA-MRSA infection occur among diverse groups, including prisoners, athletes, and drug users.

Pathogenesis

S. aureus is a pyogenic pathogen known for its capacity to induce abscess formation.

- **Invasive Disease** For invasive *S. aureus* infection to occur, some or all of the following steps are necessary:
  - *Colonization/inoculation:* Bacteria colonize tissue surfaces or are inoculated directly into tissue—e.g., as a result of minor abrasions or via IV access catheters.

- *Invasion:* Bacteria replicate at the site of infection and elaborate enzymes that facilitate survival and local spread. CA-MRSA isolates that produce the Panton-Valentine leukocidin toxin have been linked to more serious infections.
- *Evasion of host defense mechanisms:* S. aureus possesses an antiphagocytic polysaccharide microcapsule that facilitates evasion of host defenses and plays a role in abscess formation. Organisms can survive in a quiescent state in various tissues and then cause recrudescent infections when conditions are suitable.
- *Metastatic spread:* S. aureus can survive in PMNs and may use these cells to spread to and seed other tissue sites.
- **Toxin-Mediated Disease** S. aureus produces three types of toxin: cytotoxins, pyrogenic toxin superantigens, and exfoliative toxins.
  - Antitoxin antibodies are protective against toxin-mediated staphylococcal illness.
  - Enterotoxins and toxic shock syndrome toxin 1 (TSST-1) act as "superantigens" or T cell mitogens and cause the release of large amounts of inflammatory mediators, producing multisystem disease that includes fever, rash, and hypotension.

Diagnosis

S. aureus infections are readily diagnosed by Gram's stain and microscopic examination of infected tissue.

- Routine cultures of infected material usually yield positive results, and blood cultures are sometimes positive even when infections are localized to extravascular sites.
- PCR assays have been developed for rapid testing and are increasingly being used.

Clinical Syndromes

Skin and Soft Tissue Infections S. aureus causes a variety of cutaneous infections characterized by pus-containing blisters, many of which can also be caused by group A streptococci and other streptococcal species. Predisposing factors include skin disease (e.g., eczema), skin damage (e.g., minor trauma), injections, and poor personal hygiene.

- Infections can be superficial (e.g., folliculitis, cellulitis, impetigo) or deep and painful (e.g., furuncles, carbuncles, hidradenitis suppurativa).
  - Carbuncles (often located in the lower neck) are more severe and painful than furuncles (boils that extend from hair follicles) and are due to coalesced lesions extending to deeper SC tissue.
  - Mastitis in lactating women can range from superficial cellulitis to abscess.

Musculoskeletal Infections See Chap. 93 for additional details.

- S. aureus is the most common cause of *osteomyelitis* arising from either hematogenous dissemination or contiguous spread from a soft tissue site (e.g., diabetic or vascular ulcers).
  - Hematogenous osteomyelitis in adults is often vertebral and occurs in pts with endocarditis, pts undergoing hemodialysis, injection drug

users, or diabetics. Intense back pain and fever can occur, but infections may also be clinically occult.

- *Epidural abscess* is a serious complication that can present as trouble voiding or walking or as radicular pain in addition to symptoms of osteomyelitis; neurologic compromise can develop in the absence of timely treatment, which often requires surgical intervention.
- Osteomyelitis from contiguous soft tissue infections is suggested by exposure of bone, a draining fistulous tract, failure to heal, or continued drainage.

• *S. aureus* is the most common cause of *septic arthritis* in native joints of both adults and children. *S. aureus* septic arthritis in adults may result from trauma, surgery, or hematogenous dissemination.

- The joints most commonly affected are the knees, shoulders, hips, and phalanges.
- Examination of synovial fluid reveals >50,000 PMNs/μL and gram-positive cocci in clusters on Gram's stain.

• *Pyomyositis*, an infection of skeletal muscles that is seen in tropical climates and in seriously compromised pts (including HIV-infected pts), causes fever, swelling, and pain overlying involved muscle and is usually due to *S. aureus*.

Respiratory Tract Infections

• Newborns and infants can develop serious infections characterized by fever, dyspnea, and respiratory failure; pneumatoceles (shaggy, thin-walled cavities), pneumothorax, and empyema are known complications.

• Community-acquired pneumonia usually follows viral infections (e.g., after influenza) and manifests as fever, bloody sputum production, and midlung-field pneumatoceles or multiple patchy pulmonary infiltrates.

• Nosocomial pneumonia is commonly seen in intubated pts.

- The clinical presentation resembles that of pneumonia of other bacterial etiologies.
- Pts produce an increased volume of purulent sputum and develop fever, new pulmonary infiltrates, and respiratory distress.

Bacteremia and Sepsis The incidence of metastatic seeding during bacteremia has been estimated to be as high as 31%.

• Bones, joints, kidneys, and lungs are most commonly infected.

• Diabetes, HIV infection, and renal insufficiency are often seen in association with *S. aureus* bacteremia and increase the risk of complications.

Infective Endocarditis (See also Chap. 89)

S. aureus is the leading cause of endocarditis worldwide and accounts for 25–35% of cases.

• The incidence is increasing as a result of injection drug use, hemodialysis, intravascular prosthetic devices, and immunosuppression.

• Mortality rates range from 20% to 40% despite the availability of effective antibiotics.

• The four clinical settings in which *S. aureus* endocarditis is encountered are (1) right-sided endocarditis in association with injection drug use,

(2) left-sided native-valve endocarditis, (3) prosthetic-valve endocarditis, and (4) nosocomial endocarditis.

Urinary Tract Infections UTIs due to *S. aureus* are uncommon and suggest hematogenous dissemination.

Prosthetic Device–Related Infections Compared with coagulase-negative staphylococci, *S. aureus* causes more acute disease, with localized and systemic manifestations that tend to be rapidly progressive. Successful treatment usually involves removal of the prosthetic device.

CA-MRSA Infections While the skin and soft tissues are the most common sites of infection associated with CA-MRSA, 5–10% of these infections are invasive and potentially life-threatening (e.g., necrotizing fasciitis, necrotic pneumonia, sepsis, purpura fulminans).

Toxin-Mediated Disease Each class of toxin produced by *S. aureus* results in a characteristic syndrome.

- *Food poisoning*: results from inoculation of toxin-producing *S. aureus* into food by colonized food handlers, with subsequent toxin elaboration in growth-promoting foods (e.g., custard, potato salad, processed meat).
  - The heat-stable toxin is not destroyed even if heating kills the bacteria.
  - Because the disease is caused by preformed toxins, its onset is rapid and explosive, occurring within 1–6 h of ingestion of contaminated food.
  - The chief signs and symptoms are nausea and vomiting, but diarrhea, hypotension, and dehydration may occur. Fever is absent.
  - Symptoms resolve within 8–10 h; treatment is entirely supportive.
- *Toxic shock syndrome (TSS)*: results from elaboration of an enterotoxin (many nonmenstrual TSS cases) or TSST-1 (some nonmenstrual cases and >90% of menstrual cases).
  - Although the specific toxin may differ, the clinical presentation is similar in menstrual and nonmenstrual cases.
  - Diagnosis is based on a constellation of clinical findings. Table 95-1 summarizes the case definition for staphylococcal TSS.
  - Menstrual cases occur 2–3 days after menses begin.
  - Illness occurs only in people who lack antibody to the toxin.
- *Staphylococcal scalded-skin syndrome (SSSS)*: most often affects newborns and children. Fragility of the skin, with tender, thick-walled, fluid-filled bullae, can lead to exfoliation of most of the skin surface. Nikolsky's sign is positive when gentle pressure on bullae causes rupture of lesions and leaves denuded underlying skin.

Prevention

Hand washing and careful attention to appropriate isolation procedures prevent the spread of *S. aureus* infection. Elimination of nasal carriage of *S. aureus* (e.g., with mupirocin) has reduced the incidence of postsurgical infection and the rates of infection among hemodialysis and peritoneal dialysis pts.

TABLE 95-1 CASE DEFINITION OF *S. AUREUS* TOXIC SHOCK SYNDROME

1. Fever: temperature of ≥38.9°C (≥102°F)
2. Hypotension: systolic blood pressure of ≤90 mmHg or orthostatic hypotension (orthostatic drop in diastolic blood pressure by ≥15 mmHg, orthostatic syncope, or orthostatic dizziness)
3. Diffuse macular rash, with desquamation 1–2 weeks after onset (including palms and soles)
4. Multisystem involvement (≥3 of the following)
   a. Hepatic: bilirubin or aminotransferase levels ≥2 times normal
   b. Hematologic: platelet count ≤100,000/μL
   c. Renal: blood urea nitrogen or serum creatinine level ≥2 times the normal upper limit
   d. Mucous membranes: vaginal, oropharyngeal, or conjunctival hyperemia
   e. GI: vomiting or diarrhea at onset of illness
   f. Muscular: severe myalgias or serum creatine phosphokinase level ≥2 times the upper limit
   g. CNS: disorientation or alteration in consciousness without focal neurologic signs and in the absence of fever and hypotension
5. Negative serologic or other tests for measles, leptospirosis, and Rocky Mountain spotted fever as well as negative blood or CSF cultures for organisms other than *S. aureus*

Source: M Wharton et al: Case definitions for public health surveillance. MMWR 39:1, 1990; with permission.

◼ INFECTIONS CAUSED BY COAGULASE-NEGATIVE STAPHYLOCOCCI (CoNS)

Microbiology

CoNS are generally less virulent than *S. aureus* but are important and common causes of prosthetic-device infections.

- Of CoNS species, *S. epidermidis* most often causes disease. This organism is a normal component of the skin, oropharyngeal, and vaginal flora.
- *S. saprophyticus* is a cause of UTIs.
- *S. lugdunensis* and *S. schleiferi* are more virulent than other CoNS species and cause serious infections, possibly because they apparently share more virulence determinants with *S. aureus* than do other CoNS species.

Pathogenesis

CoNS are uniquely adapted to cause prosthetic-device infections because they can elaborate an extracellular polysaccharide (glycocalyx or slime) that forms a biofilm on the device surface, protecting bacteria from host defenses as well as from antibiotic treatment while allowing bacterial survival.

Clinical Syndromes

CoNS cause diverse prosthetic device–related infections. Signs of localized infection are usually subtle, disease progression is slow, and systemic findings are limited. Fever and mild leukocytosis may be documented. Infections not associated with prosthetic devices are infrequent, but up to 5% of native-valve endocarditis cases have been due to CoNS in some series.

Diagnosis

CoNS are readily detected by standard methods, but distinguishing infection from colonization is often problematic because CoNS are common contaminants of cultures of blood and other sites. Only 10–25% of blood cultures positive for CoNS reflect true bacteremia.

TREATMENT Staphylococcal Infections

- Suppurative collections should be surgically drained. The emergence of CA-MRSA has increased the importance of culturing material from all collections to identify the pathogen and determine its antimicrobial susceptibility.
- In most cases of prosthetic-device infection, the device should be removed, although some CoNS infections can be managed medically.
- Antibiotic therapy for *S. aureus* infection is generally prolonged (i.e., 4–8 weeks), particularly if blood cultures remain positive 48–96 h after initiation of therapy, if the infection was acquired in the community, if a removable focus of infection is not removed, or if cutaneous or embolic manifestations of infection occur. For immunocompetent pts in whom shorter therapy is planned, a transesophageal echocardiogram to rule out endocarditis is warranted.
- Antimicrobial therapy for serious staphylococcal infections is summarized in Table 95-2.
  - Penicillinase-resistant β-lactams, such as nafcillin, oxacillin, and cephalosporins, are highly effective against penicillin-resistant strains.
  - The incidence of MRSA is high in hospital settings, and strains intermediately or fully resistant to vancomycin have been described. In general, vancomycin is less reliably bactericidal than the β-lactams and should be used only when absolutely indicated.
  - Among newer antistaphylococcal agents, daptomycin is bactericidal but is not effective in pulmonary infections; quinupristin/dalfopristin is typically bactericidal but is only bacteriostatic against isolates resistant to erythromycin or clindamycin; linezolid is bacteriostatic and offers similar bioavailability after oral or parenteral administration; and telavancin—a derivative of vancomycin—is active against strains with reduced susceptibility to vancomycin (VISA). Tigecycline, a broad-spectrum minocycline analogue, is bacteriostatic against MRSA.
    - Other alternatives include the quinolones, but resistance to these drugs is increasing, especially among MRSA strains.
    - Trimethoprim-sulfamethoxazole (TMP-SMX) and minocycline have been used successfully to treat MRSA infections in cases of vancomycin toxicity or intolerance.
    - Although some drugs have been used in combination (e.g., rifampin, aminoglycosides, fusidic acid), clinical studies have not demonstrated a therapeutic benefit.
- Special considerations for treatment include:
- *Uncomplicated skin and soft tissue infections:* Oral agents are usually adequate.

TABLE 95-2 ANTIMICROBIAL THERAPY FOR STAPHYLOCOCCAL INFECTIONS[a]

Sensitivity/Resistance of Isolate	Drug of Choice	Alternative(s)	Comments
Parenteral therapy for serious infections			
Sensitive to penicillin	Penicillin G (4 mU q4h)	Nafcillin or oxacillin (2 g q4h), cefazolin (2 g q8h), vancomycin (1 g q12h[b])	Fewer than 5% of isolates are sensitive to penicillin.
Sensitive to methicillin	Nafcillin or oxacillin (2 g q4h)	Cefazolin (2 g q8h[c]), vancomycin (15–20 mg/kg q8–12h[b])	Pts with penicillin allergy can be treated with a cephalosporin if the allergy does not involve an anaphylactic or accelerated reaction; desensitization to β-lactams may be indicated in selected cases of serious infection when maximal bactericidal activity is needed (e.g., prosthetic-valve endocarditis[c]). Type A β-lactamase may rapidly hydrolyze cefazolin and reduce its efficacy in endocarditis. Vancomycin is a less effective option.
Resistant to methicillin	Vancomycin (15–20 mg/kg q8–12h[b])	Daptomycin (6 mg/kg q24h[b,c]) for bacteremia, endocarditis, and complicated skin infections; linezolid (600 mg q12h except: 400 mg q12h for uncomplicated skin infections); quinupristin/dalfopristin (7.5 mg/kg q8h)	Sensitivity testing is necessary before an alternative drug is used. Adjunctive drugs (those that should be used only in combination with other antimicrobial agents) include gentamicin (1 mg/kg q8h[b]), rifampin (300 mg PO q8h), and fusidic acid (500 mg q8h; not readily available in the United States). For some serious infections, higher doses of daptomycin have been used. Quinupristin/dalfopristin is bactericidal against methicillin-resistant isolates unless the strain is resistant to erythromycin or clindamycin. The efficacy of adjunctive therapy is not well established in many settings. Both linezolid and quinupristin/dalfopristin have had in vitro activity against most VISA and VRSA strains. See footnote for treatment of prosthetic-valve endocarditis.[d]
Resistant to methicillin with intermediate or complete resistance to vancomycin[e]	Uncertain	Same as for methicillin-resistant strains; check antibiotic susceptibilities	Same as for methicillin-resistant strains; check antibiotic susceptibilities.

Not yet known (i.e., empirical therapy)	Vancomycin (15–20 mg/kg q8–12h[b])	—	Empirical therapy is given when the susceptibility of the isolate is not known. Vancomycin with or without an aminoglycoside is recommended for suspected community- or hospital-acquired *S. aureus* infections because of the increased frequency of methicillin-resistant strains in the community.
Oral therapy for skin and soft tissue infections			
Sensitive to methicillin	Dicloxacillin (500 mg qid), cephalexin (500 mg qid)	Minocycline or doxycycline (100 mg q12h[b]), TMP-SMX (1 or 2 ds tablets bid), clindamycin (300–450 mg/kg tid)	It is important to know the antibiotic susceptibility of isolates in the specific geographic region. All drainage should be cultured.
Resistant to methicillin	Clindamycin (300–450 mg/kg tid), TMP-SMX (1 or 2 ds tablets bid), minocycline or doxycycline (100 mg q12h[b]), linezolid (400–600 mg bid)		It is important to know the antibiotic susceptibility of isolates in the specific geographic region. All drainage should be cultured.

[a]Recommended dosages are for adults with normal renal and hepatic function.

[b]The dosage must be adjusted for pts with reduced creatinine clearance.

[c]Daptomycin cannot be used for pneumonia.

[d]For the treatment of prosthetic-valve endocarditis, the addition of gentamicin (1 mg/kg q8h) and rifampin (300 mg PO q8h) is recommended, with adjustment of the gentamicin dosage if the creatinine clearance rate is reduced.

[e]Vancomycin-resistant *S. aureus* isolates from clinical infections have been reported.

Abbreviations: TMP-SMX, trimethoprim-sulfamethoxazole; ds, double-strength; VISA, vancomycin-intermediate *S. aureus*; VRSA, vancomycin-resistant *S. aureus*.

Source: Modified with permission from FD Lowy: N Engl J Med 339:520, 1998 (© 1998 Massachusetts Medical Society. All rights reserved.) and from DL Stevens et al: Clin Infect Dis 41:1373, 2006, and Med Lett 48:13, 2006.

- *Native-valve endocarditis:* A β-lactam is recommended for MSSA and vancomycin (1 g q12h) for MRSA. Treatment should continue for 4–6 weeks.
- *Prosthetic-valve endocarditis:* Surgery is often needed in addition to antibiotics. A β-lactam drug (or vancomycin if MRSA is involved) with gentamicin and rifampin is indicated.
- *Hematogenous osteomyelitis or septic arthritis:* A 4-week treatment course is adequate for children, but adults require longer courses. Joint infections require repeated aspiration or arthroscopy to prevent damage from inflammatory cells.
- *Chronic osteomyelitis:* Surgical debridement—in addition to antibiotic therapy—is needed in most cases.
- *Prosthetic-joint infections:* Ciprofloxacin and rifampin have been used successfully in combination, particularly when the prosthesis cannot be removed.
- *TSS:* Supportive therapy and removal of tampons or other packing material or debridement of an infected site are most important. The role of antibiotics is less clear, but a clindamycin/semisynthetic penicillin combination is recommended.
  – Clindamycin is recommended because it is a protein synthesis inhibitor and has been shown to decrease toxin synthesis in vitro; its efficacy in vivo is less clear.
  – IV immunoglobulin may be helpful.

For a more detailed discussion, see Lowy FD: Staphylococcal Infections, Chap. 135, p. 1160, in HPIM-18.

CHAPTER **96**

Streptococcal/Enterococcal Infections, Diphtheria, and Other Infections Caused by Corynebacteria and Related Species

STREPTOCOCCAL AND ENTEROCOCCAL INFECTIONS

■ MICROBIOLOGY

Streptococci and enterococci are gram-positive cocci that form chains when grown in liquid media.

- Culture on blood agar reveals three hemolytic patterns:
  – α-Hemolysis results in partial hemolysis that imparts a greenish appearance to agar. This pattern is seen with *S. pneumoniae* and viridans streptococci.

- β-Hemolysis results in complete hemolysis around a colony. This pattern is seen with streptococci of Lancefield groups A, B, C, and G. Lancefield grouping is based on cell-wall carbohydrate antigens.
- γ-Hemolysis describes the absence of hemolytic ability. This pattern is typical of enterococci, nonenterococcal group D streptococci, and anaerobic streptococci.

- Streptococci and enterococci colonize the respiratory, GI, and genitourinary tracts as part of the normal flora. Several of these species are also important causes of human diseases.

GROUP A *STREPTOCOCCUS* (GAS)

Epidemiology and Pathogenesis

GAS (*S. pyogenes*) causes suppurative infections and is associated with postinfectious syndromes such as acute rheumatic fever (ARF) and post-streptococcal glomerulonephritis (PSGN).

- Up to 20% of people may have asymptomatic pharyngeal colonization with GAS.

  - Pharyngitis due to GAS is one of the most common bacterial infections of childhood.

  - GAS accounts for 20–40% of all cases of exudative pharyngitis in children >3 years of age.

- The incidence of all GAS infections is ~10-fold higher in low-income than in high-income countries. Worldwide, GAS contributes to ~500,000 deaths per year.

- The major surface protein (M protein) and the hyaluronic acid polysaccharide capsule protect GAS against phagocytic ingestion and killing.

- GAS makes a large number of extracellular products that may contribute to local and systemic toxicity; these include streptolysins S and O, streptokinase, DNases, and the pyrogenic exotoxins that cause the rash of scarlet fever and contribute to the pathogenesis of toxic shock syndrome (TSS) and necrotizing fasciitis.

- Respiratory droplets provide the usual route of transmission, although other mechanisms have been described.

Clinical Manifestations

Pharyngitis After an incubation period of 1–4 days, pts develop sore throat, fever, chills, malaise, and GI manifestations.

- Examination may reveal an erythematous and swollen pharyngeal mucosa, purulent exudates over the posterior pharynx and tonsillar pillars, and tender anterior cervical adenopathy.
- Viral pharyngitis is the more likely diagnosis when pts have coryza, hoarseness, conjunctivitis, or mucosal ulcers.
- Throat culture is the gold standard for diagnosis.

  - Latex agglutination or enzyme immunoassay is highly specific (>95%) and can be relied on for a rapid, definitive diagnosis.

  - Given a variable sensitivity of 55–90%, a negative rapid-assay result should be confirmed with a throat culture.

TABLE 96-1 TREATMENT OF GROUP A STREPTOCOCCAL INFECTIONS

Infection	Treatment[a]
Pharyngitis	Benzathine penicillin G, 1.2 mU IM; *or* penicillin V, 250 mg PO tid or 500 mg PO bid × 10 days
	(Children <27 kg: Benzathine penicillin G, 600,000 units IM; *or* penicillin V, 250 mg PO bid or tid × 10 days)
Impetigo	Same as pharyngitis
Erysipelas/cellulitis	Severe: Penicillin G, 1–2 mU IV q4h
	Mild to moderate: Procaine penicillin, 1.2 mU IM bid
Necrotizing fasciitis/myositis	Surgical debridement; *plus* penicillin G, 2–4 mU IV q4h; *plus* clindamycin,[b] 600–900 mg q8h
Pneumonia/empyema	Penicillin G, 2–4 mU IV q4h; *plus* drainage of empyema
Streptococcal toxic shock syndrome	Penicillin G, 2–4 mU IV q4h; *plus* clindamycin,[b] 600–900 mg q8h; *plus* IV immunoglobulin,[b] 2 g/kg as a single dose

[a]Penicillin allergy: A first-generation cephalosporin, such as cephalexin or cefadroxil, may be substituted for penicillin in cases of penicillin allergy if the nature of the allergy is not an immediate hypersensitivity reaction (anaphylaxis or urticaria) or another potentially life-threatening manifestation (e.g., severe rash and fever). Alternative agents for oral therapy are erythromycin (10 mg/kg PO qid, up to a maximum of 250 mg per dose) and azithromycin (a 5-day treatment course at a dose of 12 mg/kg once daily, up to a maximum of 500 mg/d). Vancomycin is an alternative for parenteral therapy.
[b]Efficacy unproven, but recommended by several experts.

TREATMENT GAS Pharyngitis

- See Table 96-1 for recommended treatments.
  - The primary goal of treatment is to prevent suppurative complications (e.g., lymphadenitis, abscess, sinusitis, bacteremia, pneumonia) and ARF; therapy does not seem to reduce the duration of symptoms or prevent PSGN.
  - Follow-up cultures after completion of therapy are not routinely recommended.
- Asymptomatic pharyngeal GAS carriage usually is not treated; however, when the pt is a potential source of infection in others (e.g., health care workers), penicillin V (500 mg PO qid for 10 days) with rifampin (600 mg PO bid for the final 4 days) is used.

Scarlet Fever Scarlet fever is the designation for GAS infection—usually pharyngitis—associated with a characteristic rash. It is much less common now than in the past.

- The rash typically appears in the first 2 days of illness over the upper trunk and spreads to the extremities but not to the palms and soles. The skin has a sandpaper feel.
- Other findings include strawberry tongue (enlarged papillae on a coated tongue) and Pastia's lines (accentuation of rash in skin folds).
- Rash improves in 6–9 days, with desquamation on palms and soles.

Skin and Soft Tissue Infections See Chap. 93 for further discussion of clinical manifestations and treatment.

- *Impetigo*: A superficial skin infection, impetigo is most often seen in young children in warmer months or climates and under poor hygienic conditions.
  - Red papular lesions evolve into pustules that ultimately form characteristic honeycomb-like crusts, usually affecting the facial areas around the nose and mouth and the legs. Pts are usually afebrile.
  - GAS impetigo is associated with PSGN.
  - For treatment, see Table 96-1. Given an increasing incidence of impetigo due to *Staphylococcus aureus*, empirical antibiotic therapy should cover GAS and *S. aureus*.
    - Thus dicloxacillin or cephalexin (250 mg PO qid for 10 days) is used.
    - Topical mupirocin ointment is also effective.
- *Cellulitis*: GAS cellulitis develops at anatomic sites where normal lymphatic drainage has been disrupted (e.g., due to surgery or prior cellulitis). When skin integrity is breached, organisms may enter at sites distant from the area of cellulitis.
  - GAS may cause rapidly developing postoperative wound infections with a thin exudate.
  - *Erysipelas* is a form of cellulitis characterized by pain, fever, and acute onset of bright red swelling that is sharply demarcated from normal skin.
    - It usually involves the malar facial area or the lower extremities and is caused almost exclusively by GAS.
    - The skin often has a *peau d'orange* texture, and blebs or bullae may form after 2 or 3 days.
  - For treatment of erysipelas or cellulitis known to be due to GAS, see Table 96-1; empirical treatment should be directed against GAS and *S. aureus*.
- *Necrotizing fasciitis*: See Chap. 93 for details. GAS causes ~60% of cases of necrotizing fasciitis. For treatment, see Table 96-1.

Pneumonia and Empyema GAS is an occasional cause of pneumonia in previously healthy pts.

- Pts have pleuritic chest pain, fever, chills, and dyspnea; ~50% have accompanying pleural effusions that—unlike the sterile parapneumonic effusions of pneumococcal pneumonia—are almost always infected and should be drained quickly to avoid loculation.
- For treatment, see Table 96-1.

TABLE 96-2 PROPOSED CASE DEFINITION FOR STREPTOCOCCAL TOXIC SHOCK SYNDROME[a]

I. Isolation of group A streptococci (*S. pyogenes*)
    A. From a normally sterile site
    B. From a nonsterile site
II. Clinical signs of severity
    A. Hypotension *and*
    B. ≥2 of the following signs:
        1. Renal impairment
        2. Coagulopathy
        3. Liver function impairment
        4. Adult respiratory distress syndrome
        5. Generalized erythematous macular rash that may desquamate
        6. Soft tissue necrosis, including necrotizing fasciitis or myositis; *or* gangrene

[a]An illness fulfilling criteria IA, IIA, and IIB is defined as a *definite* case. An illness fulfilling criteria IB, IIA, and IIB is defined as a *probable* case if no other etiology for the illness is identified.
Source: Modified from Working Group on Severe Streptococcal Infections, JAMA 269:390, 1993.

Bacteremia In most cases of GAS bacteremia, a focus is readily identifiable. Bacteremia occurs occasionally with cellulitis and frequently with necrotizing fasciitis.
- If no focus is immediately evident, a diagnosis of endocarditis, occult abscess, or osteomyelitis should be considered.

Toxic Shock Syndrome Unlike those with TSS due to *S. aureus*, pts with streptococcal TSS generally lack a rash, have bacteremia, and have an associated soft-tissue infection (cellulitis, necrotizing fasciitis, or myositis).
- Table 96-2 presents a proposed case definition for streptococcal TSS.
- The mortality rate for streptococcal TSS is ~30%, with most deaths due to shock and respiratory failure.
- For treatment, see Table 96-1.

Prevention

Although household contacts of individuals with invasive GAS infection are at increased risk of infection, the attack rate is low enough that antibiotic prophylaxis is not routinely recommended.

■ STREPTOCOCCI OF GROUPS C AND G

- Streptococci of groups C and G cause infections similar to those caused by GAS, including cellulitis, bacteremia (particularly in elderly or chronically ill pts), pneumonia, and soft tissue infections.
- Strains that form small colonies (<0.5 mm) on blood agar are generally of the *S. milleri* group (*S. intermedius*, *S. anginosus*); large-colony groups C and G streptococci are now considered a single species (*S. dysgalactiae* subsp. *equisimilis*).

- Treatment is the same as for similar syndromes due to GAS.
  - Although it has not been shown to be superior, the addition of gentamicin (1 mg/kg IV q8h) is recommended by some experts for endocarditis or septic arthritis due to group C or G streptococci because of a poor clinical response to penicillin alone.
  - Joint infections can require repeated aspiration or open drainage for cure.

◼ GROUP B *STREPTOCOCCUS* (GBS)

- GBS is a major cause of meningitis and sepsis in neonates and a common cause of peripartum fever in women.
  - About half of the infants delivered vaginally to mothers colonized with GBS (5–40% of women) become colonized, but only 1–2% develop infection.
  - With maternal colonization, the risk of neonatal GBS infection is high if delivery is preterm or if the mother has an early rupture of membranes (>24 h before delivery), prolonged labor, fever, or chorioamnionitis.
- Widespread prenatal screening for GBS has reduced the incidence of neonatal infection to 0.8 cases per 1000 live births; adults now account for a larger proportion of invasive GBS infections than do newborns.

Neonatal Infections

- *Early-onset infection* occurs within the first week of life (median age, 20 h). The infection is acquired within the maternal genital tract during birth.
  - Neonates typically have respiratory distress, lethargy, and hypotension.
  - Bacteremia is noted in ~100% of cases, pneumonia in one-third to one-half, and meningitis in one-third.
- *Late-onset infection* develops in infants >1 week old and generally ≤3 months of age (mean age, 3–4 weeks). The organism is acquired during delivery or during later contact with a source.
  - Meningitis is the most common manifestation.
  - Infants present with lethargy, fever, irritability, poor feeding, and occasionally seizures.

> **TREATMENT** GBS Infections in Neonates
>
> - Penicillin is the agent of choice for all GBS infections.
>   - Empirical therapy for suspected bacterial sepsis consists of ampicillin and gentamicin while cultures are pending.
>   - Many physicians continue to give gentamicin until the pt improves clinically.

Prevention

Identification of high-risk mothers and prophylactic administration of ampicillin or penicillin during delivery reduce the risk of neonatal infection.

- Maternal screening for anogenital colonization with GBS at 35–37 weeks of pregnancy is currently recommended.

- Women who have previously given birth to an infant with GBS disease, who have a history of GBS bacteriuria during pregnancy, or who have an unknown culture status but risk factors noted above should receive intrapartum prophylaxis (usually 5 mU of penicillin G followed by 2.5 mU q4h until delivery).
  - Cefazolin can be used for pts with a penicillin allergy who are at low risk for anaphylaxis.
  - If the mother is at risk for anaphylaxis and the GBS isolate is known to be susceptible, clindamycin or erythromycin can be used; otherwise, vancomycin is indicated.

Infections in Adults

Most GBS infections in adults are related to pregnancy and parturition. Other GBS infections are seen in the elderly, especially pts with underlying conditions such as diabetes mellitus or cancer.

- Cellulitis and soft tissue infection, urinary tract infection (UTI), pneumonia, endocarditis, and septic arthritis are most common.
- Penicillin (12 mU/d for localized infections and 18–24 mU/d for endocarditis or meningitis, in divided doses) is recommended. Vancomycin is an acceptable alternative for penicillin-allergic pts.
- Relapse or recurrent invasive infection occurs in ~4% of cases.

■ NONENTEROCOCCAL GROUP D STREPTOCOCCI

The main nonenterococcal group D streptococci that cause human infections are *S. gallolyticus, S. pasteurianus, S. infantarius,* and *S. lutetiensis* (previously classified together as *S. bovis*).

- These organisms have been associated with GI malignancies and other bowel lesions, which are found in ≥60% of pts presenting with group D streptococcal endocarditis.
- Unlike enterococcal endocarditis, group D streptococcal endocarditis can be adequately treated with penicillin alone.

■ VIRIDANS STREPTOCOCCI

- Many viridans streptococcal species are part of the normal oral flora, residing in close association with the teeth and gingiva. Minor trauma such as flossing or tooth-brushing can cause transient bacteremia.
- Viridans streptococci have a predilection to cause endocarditis. Moreover, they are often part of a mixed flora in sinus infections and brain and liver abscesses.
- Bacteremia is common in neutropenic pts, who can develop a sepsis syndrome with high fever and shock. Risk factors in these pts include chemotherapy with high-dose cytosine arabinoside, prior treatment with trimethoprim-sulfamethoxazole (TMP-SMX) or a fluoroquinolone, mucositis, or therapy with antacids or histamine antagonists.
- The *S. milleri* group (including *S. intermedius, S. anginosus,* and *S. constellatus*) differs from other viridans streptococci in both hemolytic pattern (i.e., they may be α-, β-, or γ-hemolytic) and clinical syndromes. These organisms commonly cause suppurative infections, especially abscesses of brain and viscera, as well as respiratory tract infections such as pneumonia, empyema, and lung abscess.

- Neutropenic pts should receive vancomycin pending susceptibility testing; other pts may be treated with penicillin.

■ *ABIOTROPHIA* AND *GRANULICATELLA* SPECIES (NUTRITIONALLY VARIANT STREPTOCOCCI)

- The organisms formerly known as nutritionally variant streptococci are now classified as *Abiotrophia defectiva* and three species within the genus *Granulicatella*. These fastidious organisms require media that are enriched (e.g., with vitamin B_6) for growth.
- These organisms are more frequently associated with treatment failure and relapse in cases of endocarditis than are viridans streptococci. Thus gentamicin (1 mg/kg q8h) must be added to the penicillin regimen.

■ ENTEROCOCCAL INFECTIONS

Microbiology

Enterococci are gram-positive cocci that are observed as single cells, diplococci, or short chains.

- Enterococci share many morphologic and phenotypic characteristics with streptococci and thus were previously classified as the latter.
- Enterococci are generally nonhemolytic when cultured on blood agar plates.
- Enterococci are inherently resistant to a variety of commonly used antibiotics. *E. faecium* is the most resistant species, with >80% of U.S. isolates resistant to vancomycin (VRE) and >90% resistant to ampicillin. In contrast, only ~7% of *E. faecalis* isolates are resistant to vancomycin and ~4% to ampicillin.

Epidemiology

Although 18 enterococcal species have been isolated from human infections, *E. faecalis* and *E. faecium* cause the overwhelming majority of enterococcal infections.

- Enterococci are the second most common cause of nosocomial infection (after staphylococci), with roughly equal numbers of cases caused by *E. faecalis* and *E. faecium*.
- Colonization with VRE (as opposed to antibiotic-susceptible strains) predisposes to enterococcal infection. Risk factors for VRE colonization include prolonged hospitalization; long antibiotic courses; hospitalization in long-term-care facilities, surgical units, and/or ICUs; organ transplantation; renal failure; high APACHE scores; and physical proximity to pts colonized with VRE.

Clinical Manifestations

Enterococci cause UTIs, especially in pts who have undergone instrumentation; chronic prostatitis; bacteremia related to intravascular catheters; bacterial endocarditis of both native and prosthetic valves (usually with a subacute presentation); meningitis, particularly in pts who have undergone neurosurgery; soft tissue infections, particularly involving surgical wounds; and neonatal infections. These organisms can also be a component of mixed intraabdominal infections.

| **TREATMENT** | Enterococcal Infections |

- Given low cure rates with β-lactam monotherapy, combination therapy with a β-lactam plus gentamicin or streptomycin is recommended for serious enterococcal infections. High-level resistance to aminoglycosides (i.e., minimal inhibitory concentrations of >500 and >2000 µg/mL for gentamicin and streptomycin, respectively) abolishes the synergism otherwise obtained by adding an aminoglycoside to a cell wall–active agent. This phenotype must be assessed in isolates from serious infections.
- For *E. faecium* isolates resistant to ampicillin:
  - Daptomycin, quinupristin/dalfopristin, or linezolid plus another active agent (doxycycline with rifampin, tigecycline, or a fluoroquinolone) may be used.
  - If daptomycin is used and if high-level resistance is not noted, an aminoglycoside should be added to the regimen.
- If high-level aminoglycoside resistance is present, two other active agents should be used.

CORYNEBACTERIAL AND RELATED INFECTIONS

■ *CORYNEBACTERIUM DIPHTHERIAE*

Microbiology

C. diphtheriae, the causative agent of the nasopharyngeal and skin infection known as diphtheria, is a club-shaped, gram-positive, unencapsulated, nonmotile, nonsporulating rod.

- The bacteria often form clusters of parallel arrays (palisades) in culture, referred to as *Chinese characters*.
- Some strains produce diphtheria toxin, which can cause myocarditis, polyneuropathy, and other systemic toxicities and is associated with the formation of pseudomembranes in the pharynx during respiratory infection.

Epidemiology and Pathogenesis

As a result of routine immunization, fewer than five cases of diphtheria are diagnosed per year in the United States.

- Low-income countries in Africa and Asia continue to have significant outbreaks; globally, there were ~7000 cases of diphtheria in 2008 and ~5000 deaths related to diphtheria in 2004.
- *C. diphtheriae* is transmitted via the aerosol route, primarily during close contact.
- Diphtheria toxin—the primary virulence factor—irreversibly inhibits protein synthesis, thereby causing the death of the cell.

Clinical Manifestations

- *Respiratory diphtheria*: Upper respiratory tract illness due to *C. diphtheriae* typically has a 2- to 5-day incubation period and is diagnosed on the basis of a constellation of sore throat; low-grade fever; and a tonsillar, pharyngeal, or nasal pseudomembrane.

- Unlike that of GAS pharyngitis, the pseudomembrane of diphtheria is tightly adherent; dislodging the membrane usually causes bleeding.
- Massive swelling of the tonsils and "bull-neck" diphtheria resulting from submandibular and paratracheal edema can develop. This illness is further characterized by foul breath, thick speech, and stridorous breathing.
- Respiratory tract obstruction due to swelling and sloughing of the pseudomembrane can be fatal.
- Neurologic manifestations may appear during the first 2 weeks of illness, beginning with dysphagia and nasal dysarthria and progressing to cranial nerve involvement (e.g., weakness of the tongue, facial numbness, blurred vision due to ciliary paralysis).
  • Several weeks later, a generalized sensorimotor polyneuropathy with prominent autonomic dysfunction (including hypotension) may occur.
  • Pts who survive the acute phase gradually improve.
• *Cutaneous diphtheria*: This variable dermatosis is generally characterized by punched-out ulcerative lesions with necrotic sloughing or pseudomembrane formation. Pts typically present to medical care because of nonhealing or enlarging ulcers; the lesions rarely exceed 5 cm in diameter.

Diagnosis

A definitive diagnosis is based on compatible clinical findings and detection of *C. diphtheriae* or toxigenic *C. ulcerans* (by isolation or histologic identification) in local lesions.
• The laboratory should be notified that diphtheria is being considered, and appropriate selective media must be used.
• In the U.S., respiratory diphtheria is a notifiable disease; cutaneous diphtheria is not.

TREATMENT   Diphtheria

• Diphtheria antitoxin is the most important component of treatment and should be given as soon as possible. To obtain antitoxin, contact the Emergency Operations Center at the CDC (770-488-7100). See *www.cdc.gov/vaccines/vpd-vac/diphtheria/dat/dat-main.htm* for further information.
• Antibiotic therapy is administered for 14 days to prevent transmission to contacts. The recommended options are (1) procaine penicillin G (600,000 U IM q12h in adults; 12,500–25,000 U/kg IM q12h in children) until the pt can take oral penicillin V (125–250 mg qid); or (2) erythromycin (500 mg IV q6h in adults; 40–50 mg/kg per day IV in 2–4 divided doses in children) until the pt can take oral erythromycin (500 mg qid).
  - Rifampin and clindamycin are other options for pts who cannot tolerate penicillin or erythromycin.
  - Cultures should document eradication of the organism 1 and 14 days after completion of antibiotic therapy. If the organism is not

eradicated after 2 weeks of therapy, an additional 10-day course followed by repeat cultures is recommended.

- Respiratory isolation and close monitoring of cardiac and respiratory functions should be instituted.

Prognosis

Risk factors for death include a long interval between onset of local disease and antitoxin administration; bull-neck diphtheria; myocarditis with ventricular tachycardia; atrial fibrillation; complete heart block; an age of >60 years or <6 months; alcoholism; extensive pseudomembrane elongation; and laryngeal, tracheal, or bronchial involvement.

Prevention

DTaP (diphtheria and tetanus toxoids and acellular pertussis vaccine adsorbed) is recommended for primary immunization of children up to age 7 years; Tdap (tetanus toxoid, reduced diphtheria toxoid, and acellular pertussis) is recommended as the booster vaccine for children 11–12 years old and as the catch-up vaccine for children 7–10 and 13–18 years old.

- Td (tetanus and diphtheria toxoids) is recommended for routine booster use in adults at 10-year intervals or for tetanus-prone wounds. When >10 years have elapsed since the last Td dose, adults 19–64 years old should receive a single dose of Tdap.
- Close contacts of pts with respiratory diphtheria should have throat specimens cultured for *C. diphtheriae*, should receive a 7- to 10-day course of oral erythromycin or one dose of benzathine penicillin (1.2 mU for persons ≥6 years old; 600,000 U for children <6 years old), and should be vaccinated if immunization status is uncertain.

■ INFECTIONS WITH OTHER CORYNEBACTERIA AND RELATED ORGANISMS

Nondiphtherial *Corynebacterium* species and related organisms are common components of the normal human flora. Although frequently considered contaminants, these bacteria are associated with invasive disease in immunocompromised hosts.

- *C. ulcerans* infection is a zoonosis that causes diphtheria-like illness and requires similar treatment.
- *C. jeikeium* infects pts with cancer or severe immunodeficiency and can cause severe sepsis, endocarditis, device-related infections, pneumonia, and soft tissue infections. Treatment consists of removal of the source of infection and administration of vancomycin.
- *C. urealyticum* is a cause of sepsis and nosocomial UTI, including *alkaline-encrusted cystitis* (a chronic inflammatory bladder infection associated with deposition of ammonium magnesium phosphate on the surface and walls of ulcerating lesions in the bladder). Vancomycin is an effective therapeutic agent.
- *Rhodococcus* species appear as spherical to long, curved, clubbed gram-positive rods that are often acid-fast. The most common presentation—nodular cavitary pneumonia of the upper lobe (similar to tuberculosis

and nocardiosis) in an immunocompromised host—often occurs in conjunction with HIV infection. Vancomycin is the drug of choice, but macrolides, clindamycin, rifampin, and TMP-SMX have also been used to treat these infections.

• *Arcanobacterium haemolyticum* can cause pharyngitis and chronic skin ulcers, often in association with a scarlatiniform rash similar to that caused by GAS. The organism is susceptible to β-lactam agents, macrolides, fluoroquinolones, clindamycin, vancomycin, and doxycycline. Penicillin resistance has been reported.

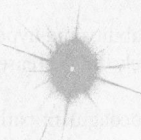

For a more detailed discussion, see Wessels MR: Streptococcal Infections, Chap. 136, p. 1171; Arias CA, Murray BE: Enterococcal Infections, Chap. 137, p. 1180; and Bishai WR, Murphy JR: Diphtheria and Other Infections Caused by Corynebacteria and Related Species, Chap. 138, p. 1188, in HPIM-18.

CHAPTER **97**
Meningococcal and Listerial Infections

MENINGOCOCCAL INFECTIONS

• **Etiology and Microbiology** *Neisseria meningitidis* is a catalase- and oxidase-positive, gram-negative aerobic diplococcus with a polysaccharide capsule that colonizes humans only.
  – Of the 13 identified serogroups, only 5—A, B, C, Y, and W135—account for the majority of cases of invasive disease.
  – Serogroups A and W135 cause recurrent epidemics in sub-Saharan Africa. Serogroup B can cause hyperendemic disease, and serogroups C and Y cause sporadic disease and small outbreaks.
• **Epidemiology** Up to 500,000 cases of meningococcal disease occur worldwide each year, with a mortality rate of ~10%.
  – Most commonly, meningococci asymptomatically colonize the nasopharynx; such asymptomatic nasopharyngeal carriage is detected in >25% of healthy adolescents and adults.
  – Patterns of meningococcal disease include epidemics, outbreaks (e.g., in colleges, refugee camps), hyperendemic disease, and sporadic or endemic cases.
  – Although most countries have predominantly sporadic cases (0.3–5 cases per 100,000 population), epidemics in sub-Saharan Africa can have rates as high as 1000 cases per 100,000 population.
  – Rates of meningococcal disease are highest among infants, with a second peak in adolescents and young adults (15–25 years of age).

- Other risk factors for meningococcal disease include complement deficiency (C5–C9), close contact with carriers, exposure to tobacco smoke, and a recent URI caused by a virus or *Mycoplasma* species.

- **Pathogenesis** Meningococci colonizing the upper respiratory tract invade the bloodstream through the mucosa only rarely, usually within a few days after an invasive strain is acquired.

  - The capsule is an important virulence factor, providing resistance to phagocytosis and helping prevent desiccation during transmission between hosts.

  - Severity of disease is related to the degree of endotoxemia and the magnitude of the inflammatory response.

  - Endothelial injury leads to increased vascular permeability and hypovolemia, resulting in vasoconstriction and ultimately in decreased cardiac output.

  - Intravascular thrombosis caused by activation of procoagulant pathways and down-regulation of anticoagulant pathways results in the characteristic purpura fulminans often seen in meningococcemia.

- **Clinical Manifestations** The most common clinical syndromes are meningitis and meningococcal septicemia, with disease usually developing within 4 days of organism acquisition.

  - A nonblanching rash (petechial or purpuric) develops in >80% of cases; early in the illness, the rash is often absent or may be indistinguishable from viral rashes.

  - Meningococcal meningitis alone (without septicemia) accounts for 30–50% of cases.

    - This meningitis is indistinguishable from other forms of bacterial meningitis unless there is an associated petechial or purpuric rash.

    - Classic signs of meningitis (e.g., headache, neck stiffness, photophobia) are often absent or difficult to discern in infants and young children.

  - Meningococcal septicemia alone accounts for ~20% of cases and initially may present as an influenza-like illness (e.g., fever, headache, myalgias, vomiting, abdominal pain).

    - May progress to shock (e.g., tachycardia, poor peripheral perfusion, oliguria), decreased level of consciousness due to decreased cerebral perfusion, spontaneous hemorrhage (pulmonary, gastric, or cerebral), and ultimately multiorgan failure and death.

    - Poor prognostic factors include an absence of meningismus, hypotension, relatively low temperature (<38°C), leukopenia, and thrombocytopenia.

  - Chronic meningococcemia presents as repeated episodes of petechial rash associated with fever, joint pain, features of arthritis, and splenomegaly that may progress to acute meningococcal septicemia if untreated.

    - Chronic meningococcemia is rarely recognized.

    - This condition is occasionally associated with complement deficiencies or inadequate sulfonamide therapy.

  - Postmeningococcal reactive disease is an immune complex–mediated disease that occurs 4–10 days after onset of meningococcal disease.

- Manifestations can include a maculopapular or vasculitic rash (2% of cases), arthritis (≤8% of cases), iritis (1% of cases), or serositis. These features resolve spontaneously without sequelae.
  - Less common clinical manifestations include pneumonia, pyogenic arthritis, osteomyelitis, purulent pericarditis, endophthalmitis, conjunctivitis, or primary peritonitis.
- **Diagnosis** Although meningococcal infections are often diagnosed on clinical grounds, blood cultures are positive in ~75% of cases and should be performed to confirm the diagnosis and to facilitate public health investigations.
  - In the setting of fever and petechial rash, elevations in the WBC count and inflammatory marker levels suggest meningococcal disease.
  - With antibiotic pretreatment, blood cultures are generally negative; in contrast, PCR analysis of whole-blood samples is effective for several days after initiation of antibiotics and increases the diagnostic yield by >40%.
  - Unless contraindicated on clinical grounds, LP should be performed in cases of suspected meningococcal meningitis.
    - Gram's staining of CSF is ~80% sensitive, and CSF culture is 90% sensitive. Latex agglutination testing of CSF is insensitive and should be avoided.
    - LP should be avoided in pts with meningococcal septicemia, as positioning for the procedure may adversely affect circulatory status.

TREATMENT Meningococcal Infections

- Initial therapy should focus on urgent clinical issues (e.g., hypovolemic shock, increased intracranial pressure, airway patency) and administration of antibiotic therapy.
- Empirical antibiotic therapy for suspected meningococcal disease consists of a third-generation cephalosporin such as ceftriaxone [75–100 mg/kg per day (maximum, 4 g/d) in one or two divided IV doses] or cefotaxime [200 mg/kg per day (maximum, 8 g/d) in four divided IV doses] to provide coverage both for meningococci and for other, potentially penicillin-resistant organisms that may produce an indistinguishable clinical syndrome.
- Meningococcal meningitis and meningococcal septicemia are conventionally treated for 7 days.
  - A single dose of ceftriaxone has been used successfully in resource-poor settings.
  - Treatment for meningococcal disease at other foci (e.g., pneumonia, arthritis) is usually continued until clinical and laboratory evidence of infection has resolved.
- Little evidence supports other adjunctive therapies (e.g., antibody to lipopolysaccharide, recombinant bactericidal/permeability-increasing protein, activated protein C) in relevant pt populations; these therapies are not currently recommended.

- **Prognosis** Despite the availability of antibiotics and other intensive medical interventions, ~10% of pts die.
  - Necrosis of purpuric lesions leads to scarring and potential need for skin grafting in ~10% of cases.
  - Amputations are required in ~2% of cases.
- **Prevention** Polysaccharide-based and conjugate vaccines exist for primary prevention; secondary cases can be prevented with antibiotic prophylaxis.
  - Meningococcal polysaccharide vaccines are currently formulated as bivalent (serogroups A and C) or quadrivalent (serogroups A, C, Y, and W135) and provide adults with immunity of 2–10 years' duration. Because the B polysaccharide is the same as a polysaccharide expressed in fetuses and is therefore recognized as self, serogroup B strains have not been targeted by polysaccharide vaccines.
  - A variety of meningococcal conjugate vaccines have been developed for administration to children. A quadrivalent formulation (serogroups A, C, Y, and W135) is most common in the United States.
  - Close contacts (i.e., household and kissing contacts) of pts with meningococcal disease should receive prophylaxis with ciprofloxacin, ofloxacin, or ceftriaxone to eradicate nasopharyngeal colonization by *N. meningitidis*.
    - Rifampin fails to eradicate carriage in 15–20% of cases, and emerging resistance has been reported.
    - Pts with meningococcal disease who receive treatment with an antibiotic that does not clear colonization (e.g., penicillin) should also be given a prophylactic agent at the end of therapy.

LISTERIAL INFECTIONS

- **Etiology and Microbiology** *Listeria monocytogenes* is a food-borne pathogen that can cause serious infections, particularly in pregnant women and immunocompromised individuals.
  - The organism is a facultatively anaerobic, nonsporulating, gram-positive rod that demonstrates motility when cultured at low temperatures.
  - *Listeria* is commonly found in processed and unprocessed foods such as soft cheeses, delicatessen meats, hot dogs, milk, and cold salads.
  - After ingestion of food that contains a high bacterial burden, virulence factors expressed by *Listeria* allow internalization into cells, intracellular growth, and cell-to-cell spread.
- **Epidemiology**
  - Recent annual incidences in the United States range from 2 to 9 cases per 1 million population.
  - There is no human-to-human transmission (other than vertical transmission from mother to fetus) or waterborne infection.
- **Clinical Manifestations** *Listeria* causes several clinical syndromes, of which meningitis and septicemia are most common.

- *Gastroenteritis:* Can develop within 48 h after ingestion of contaminated foods containing a large bacterial inoculum.
  - Listeriosis should be considered in outbreaks of gastroenteritis when cultures for other likely pathogens are negative.
  - Sporadic cases appear to be uncommon.
- *Bacteremia:* Pts present with fever, chills, myalgias, and arthralgias. Endocarditis is uncommon and is associated with fatality rates of 35–50%.
- *Meningitis: Listeria* causes ~5–10% of cases of community-acquired meningitis in adults in the United States, with case–fatality rates of 15–26%.
  - Listerial meningitis differs from meningitis of other bacterial etiologies in that its presentation is often subacute and the CSF profile usually reveals <1000 WBCs/μL with a less marked neutrophil predominance.
  - Low glucose levels and a positive Gram's stain are seen in ~30–40% of cases.
- *Meningoencephalitis and focal CNS infection: Listeria* can directly invade the brain parenchyma and cause cerebritis or focal abscess.
  - Of CNS infections, ~10% are macroscopic abscesses, which are sometimes misdiagnosed as tumors.
  - Brainstem invasion can cause severe rhombencephalitis, with asymmetric cranial nerve defects, cerebellar signs, and hemiparetic/hemisensory defects.
- *Infection in pregnant women and neonates:* Listeriosis is a serious infection in pregnancy.
  - Pregnant women are usually bacteremic and present with a nonspecific febrile illness that includes myalgias/arthralgias, backache, and headache; CNS involvement is rare. Infected women usually do well after delivery.
  - Infection develops in 70–90% of fetuses from infected women; almost 50% of infected fetuses die. This risk can be reduced with prepartum treatment.
  - Overwhelming listerial fetal infection—*granulomatosis infantiseptica*—is characterized by miliary microabscesses and granulomas, most often in the skin, liver, and spleen.
  - Late-onset neonatal disease develops ~10–30 days after delivery by mothers with asymptomatic infection.
- **Diagnosis** Timely diagnosis requires that the illness be considered in groups at risk: pregnant women, elderly pts, neonates, immunocompromised pts, and pts with chronic underlying medical conditions (e.g., alcoholism, diabetes).
  - Listeriosis is diagnosed when the organism is cultured from a usually sterile site, such as blood, CSF, or amniotic fluid.
  - Listeriae may be confused with "diphtheroids" or pneumococci in gram-stained CSF or may be gram-variable and confused with *Haemophilus* spp.
  - Serologic tests and PCR assays are not clinically useful at present.

TREATMENT **Listerial Infections**

- Ampicillin (2 g IV q4h) is the drug of choice for the treatment of listerial infections; penicillin is also highly active.
  - Most experts recommend gentamicin (1.0–1.7 mg/kg IV q8h) for synergy.
  - For penicillin-allergic pts, trimethoprim-sulfamethoxazole (15–20 mg of TMP/kg IV daily in divided doses q6–8h) should be given. Cephalosporins are not effective.
  - Neonates should receive ampicillin and gentamicin, dosed by weight.
- The duration of therapy depends on the syndrome: 2 weeks for bacteremia, 3 weeks for meningitis, 6–8 weeks for brain abscess/encephalitis, and 4–6 weeks for endocarditis. Early-onset neonatal disease can be severe and requires >2 weeks of treatment.

- **Prognosis** With prompt therapy, many pts recover fully.
  - However, permanent neurologic sequelae are common in pts with brain abscess or rhombencephalitis.
  - Of live-born treated neonates in one series, 60% recovered fully, 24% died, and 13% were left with neurologic or other complications.
- **Prevention** Pregnant women and other persons at risk for listeriosis should avoid soft cheeses and should avoid or thoroughly reheat ready-to-eat and delicatessen foods, even though the absolute risk posed by these foods is relatively low.

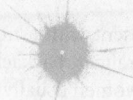

For a more detailed discussion, see Pollard AJ: Meningococcal Infections, Chap. 143, p. 1211; and Hohmann EL, Portnoy DA: *Listeria monocytogenes* Infections, Chap. 139, p. 1194, in HPIM-18.

CHAPTER **98**

Infections Caused by *Haemophilus, Bordetella, Moraxella,* and HACEK Group Organisms

HAEMOPHILUS INFLUENZAE

■ MICROBIOLOGY

H. influenzae is a small, gram-negative, pleomorphic coccobacillus that grows both aerobically and anaerobically.

- Six major serotypes (designated *a* through *f*) have been identified on the basis of antigenically distinct polysaccharide capsules.
- Unencapsulated strains are referred to as nontypable (NTHi).

■ EPIDEMIOLOGY

H. influenzae, an exclusively human pathogen, is spread by airborne droplets or through direct contact with secretions or fomites.

- Type b (Hib) strains are most important clinically, causing systemic invasive disease, primarily in infants and children <6 years of age.
- Widespread use of Hib conjugate vaccine in industrialized countries has dramatically decreased rates of Hib colonization and invasive disease, but the majority of children worldwide remain unimmunized.
- Both typable and nontypable strains can asymptomatically colonize the nasopharynx.

■ PATHOGENESIS

Hib strains cause systemic disease by invasion and systemic spread from the respiratory tract to distant sites (e.g., meninges, bones, joints). In contrast, NTHi strains cause disease by spread from the nasopharynx to contiguous sites (e.g., middle ear, lower respiratory tract).

- The polysaccharide capsule of encapsulated strains is critical for the organism's avoidance of opsonization.
- Levels of maternally derived antibodies to the capsular polysaccharide decline from birth to ~6 months of age and—in the absence of vaccination—remain low until ~2–3 years of age.

■ CLINICAL MANIFESTATIONS

- **Hib infection** The most serious Hib infections are associated with meningitis or epiglottitis.
  - *Meningitis*: primarily affects children <2 years old and presents similarly to meningitis due to other bacterial pathogens.
    - Mortality rates are ~5%.
    - Morbidity rates are high: 6% of pts have sensorineural hearing loss; one-fourth have some significant handicap; and one-half have some neurologic sequelae.
  - *Epiglottitis*: occurs in children 2–7 years old and occasionally in adults. It involves cellulitis of the epiglottis and supraglottic tissues that begins with a sore throat and fever and progresses rapidly to dysphagia, drooling, and airway obstruction.
  - *Other infections*: include cellulitis, pneumonia, osteomyelitis, septic arthritis, and bacteremia without a source.
- **NTHi infection** NTHi is a common cause of lower respiratory tract disease in adults, particularly those with chronic obstructive pulmonary disease (COPD).
  - *COPD exacerbations*: characterized by increased cough, sputum production, and shortness of breath.
  - *Pneumonia*: presents similarly to other bacterial pneumonias, including pneumococcal pneumonia.
  - *Other infections*: NTHi is one of the three most common causes of childhood otitis media and is an important cause of sinusitis (in adults and children) and neonatal bacteremia. It is a less common cause of invasive infections in adults.

■ **DIAGNOSIS**

Recovery of the organism in culture is the most reliable method for diagnosis.

- The presence of gram-negative coccobacilli in gram-stained CSF provides strong evidence for meningitis due to *H. influenzae.*
- Detection of polyribitol ribose phosphate (PRP)—polymers of which form the type b capsule—in CSF allows rapid diagnosis of Hib meningitis before culture results are available.

TREATMENT *H. influenzae* Infections

- Initial therapy for Hib meningitis consists of a third-generation cephalosporin: ceftriaxone (2 g q12h) or cefotaxime (2 g q4–6h) for adults and ceftriaxone (75–100 mg/kg q12h) or cefotaxime (50 mg/kg q6h) for children.
  - Children >2 months of age should receive adjunctive dexamethasone (0.15 mg/kg IV q6h for 2 days) to reduce the incidence of neurologic sequelae.
  - Antibiotic therapy should continue for 7–14 days.
- Antibiotic treatment for invasive infections other than meningitis (e.g., epiglottitis) consists of the same antibiotic but at a dosage different from that given for meningitis—e.g., ceftriaxone (2 g q24h) for adults.
  - Treatment duration depends on the clinical response.
  - A course lasting 1–2 weeks is generally appropriate.
- Most NTHi infections can be treated with oral antibiotics, such as amoxicillin/clavulanate, extended-spectrum cephalosporins, newer macrolides (azithromycin or clarithromycin), and fluoroquinolones (in nonpregnant adults).
  - About 20–35% of NTHi strains produce β-lactamase.
  - The incidence of strains with altered penicillin-binding proteins conferring resistance to ampicillin is increasing in Europe and Japan.

■ **PREVENTION**

Hib vaccine is recommended for all children worldwide; the immunization series should be started at ~2 months of age.

- Secondary attack rates are high among household contacts of pts with Hib disease. All children and adults (except pregnant women) in households with a case of Hib disease and at least one incompletely immunized contact <4 years of age should receive prophylaxis with oral rifampin.
- No vaccines against NTHi disease are currently available.

PERTUSSIS

■ **MICROBIOLOGY AND PATHOGENESIS**

Bordetella pertussis, the etiologic agent of pertussis, is a fastidious gram-negative pleomorphic aerobic bacillus that attaches to ciliated epithelial cells of the nasopharynx, multiplies locally, and produces a wide array of toxins and biologically active products.

- *B. parapertussis* causes a similar, though typically milder, illness.
- The most important toxin in *B. pertussis* is pertussis toxin, which has ADP ribosylating activity. The absence of this toxin in *B. parapertussis* may explain the milder illness.

■ **EPIDEMIOLOGY**

Pertussis is highly communicable. In households, attack rates are 80% among unimmunized contacts and 20% among immunized contacts.

- Pertussis remains an important cause of infant morbidity and death in developing countries, with ~250,000 childhood deaths worldwide in 2004.
- In the United States, although the incidence of pertussis has decreased by >95% because of universal childhood vaccination, 10,454 cases were reported in 2007, with increasing rates among adolescents and adults.
- Persistent cough of >2 weeks' duration in an adult may be due to *B. pertussis* in 12–30% of cases.
- Severe morbidity and mortality are restricted to infants <6 months of age.

■ **CLINICAL MANIFESTATIONS**

After an incubation period of 7–10 days, a prolonged coughing illness begins. Symptoms are usually more severe in infants and young children.

- The initial symptoms (the *catarrhal* phase) are similar to those of the common cold (e.g., coryza, lacrimation, mild cough, low-grade fever, malaise) and last 1–2 weeks.
- The *paroxysmal* phase follows and lasts 2–4 weeks. It is characterized by a hallmark cough that occurs in spasmodic fits of 5–10 coughs each. Vomiting or a "whoop" may follow a coughing fit. Apnea and cyanosis can occur during spasms. Most complications occur during this phase.
- During the subsequent *convalescent* phase, coughing episodes resolve gradually over 1–3 months. For 6–12 months, viral infections may induce a recrudescence of paroxysmal cough.
- Disease manifestations are often atypical in adolescents and adults, with paroxysmal cough and the "whoop" being less common. Post-tussive emesis is the best predictor of pertussis as the cause of prolonged cough in adults.
- Lymphocytosis (an absolute lymphocyte count of >10^5/μL) suggests pertussis in young children, but is not common among affected adolescents and adults.

■ **DIAGNOSIS**

- Cultures of nasopharyngeal secretions—the gold standard for diagnosis—remain positive in untreated cases of pertussis for a mean of 3 weeks after illness onset. Given that the diagnosis often is not considered until the pt is in the paroxysmal phase, there is a small window of opportunity for culture-proven diagnosis.
  - Secretions must be inoculated immediately onto selective media.
  - Results become positive by day 5.
- Compared with culture, PCR of nasopharyngeal specimens is more sensitive and yields positive results longer in both treated and untreated pts.
  - Reporting of pseudo-outbreaks of pertussis based on false-positive PCR results indicates the need for greater standardization.

- Although serology can be useful in pts with symptoms lasting >4 weeks, interpretation of results is complicated by late presentation for medical care and prior immunization.

TREATMENT Pertussis

- Antibiotic therapy does not substantially alter the clinical course unless given early in the catarrhal phase but is effective at eradicating the organism from the nasopharynx.
  - Macrolides (erythromycin, 1–2 g/d for 1–2 weeks; clarithromycin, 250 mg bid for 1 week; or azithromycin, 500-mg load on day 1, then 250 mg/d for 4 days) are the drugs of choice.
  - Trimethoprim-sulfamethoxazole (TMP-SMX; one double-strength tablet PO bid for 2 weeks) is recommended for macrolide-intolerant pts.
- Cough suppressants are ineffective and have no role in management of pertussis.
- Respiratory isolation is required for hospitalized pts until antibiotics have been given for 5 days.

■ PREVENTION
- Chemoprophylaxis with macrolides is recommended for household contacts of pts, especially if there are household members at high risk of severe disease (e.g., children <1 year of age, pregnant women); however, there is no evidence demonstrating that this regimen leads to a decrease in the incidence of clinical disease.
- In addition to the regular childhood immunization schedule, adolescents and adults should receive a one-time booster with an acellular vaccine.

MORAXELLA CATARRHALIS

■ MICROBIOLOGY AND EPIDEMIOLOGY
M. catarrhalis is an unencapsulated gram-negative diplococcus. Part of the normal flora of the upper airways, *M. catarrhalis* colonizes 33–100% of infants; the prevalence of colonization decreases steadily with age.

■ CLINICAL MANIFESTATIONS
- *M. catarrhalis* causes 15–20% of cases of acute otitis media in children. Acute otitis media caused by *M. catarrhalis* or NTHi is clinically milder than cases caused by *S. pneumoniae*, with less fever and a lower frequency of an erythematous, bulging tympanic membrane.
- *M. catarrhalis* accounts for ~20% of cases of acute bacterial sinusitis in children and for a smaller proportion in adults.
- In adults, *M. catarrhalis* is a common cause of exacerbations of chronic obstructive pulmonary disease (COPD), accounting for ~10% of cases.
- *M. catarrhalis* is an infrequent cause of pneumonia. When it occurs, it generally affects elderly pts with underlying cardiopulmonary disease.

■ DIAGNOSIS
Invasive procedures are needed to definitively identify the etiology of otitis media or sinusitis and are generally not performed. Isolation of

M. catarrhalis from sputum samples from pts with COPD is suggestive, but not diagnostic, of *M. catarrhalis* as the cause.

> **TREATMENT**   *M. catarrhalis* **Infections**

- Otitis media in children and exacerbations of COPD in adults are generally managed empirically with antibiotics active against *Streptococcus pneumoniae, Haemophilus influenzae,* and *M. catarrhalis.*
- Most strains of *M. catarrhalis* are susceptible to amoxicillin/clavulanate, extended-spectrum cephalosporins, newer macrolides (e.g., azithromycin, clarithromycin), TMP-SMX, and fluoroquinolones.
- More than 90% of *M. catarrhalis* strains produce a β-lactamase and are resistant to ampicillin.

THE HACEK GROUP
■ MICROBIOLOGY

The HACEK group consists of fastidious, slow-growing, gram-negative bacteria whose growth requires carbon dioxide. Several *Haemophilus* species, *Aggregatibacter* (formerly *Actinobacillus*) *actinomycetemcomitans, Aggregatibacter* (formerly *Haemophilus*) *aphrophilus, Cardiobacterium hominis, Eikenella corrodens,* and *Kingella kingae* make up this group.[1] Normal residents of the oral cavity, HACEK bacteria can cause both local oral infections and severe systemic disease, particularly endocarditis.

■ CLINICAL MANIFESTATIONS
- Up to 3% of cases of infective endocarditis are caused by HACEK organisms; most of these cases are due to *Aggregactibacter* species, *Haemophilus* species, or *C. hominis.*
- Infection typically occurs in pts with underlying valvular disease, often in the setting of a recent dental procedure, nasopharyngeal infection, or tongue piercing or scraping.
- The aortic and mitral valves are most commonly affected.
- Embolization is common, with 28–71% of pts affected.
- Blood cultures can take 30 days to become positive, although most cultures that ultimately yield HACEK bacteria become positive in the first week, especially with newer detection systems such as BACTEC.
- *A. aphrophilus* and *H. parainfluenzae* cause more than half of all cases of HACEK endocarditis. Pts usually present within the first 2 months of illness, and 19–50% of pts develop CHF.
- *A. actinomycetemcomitans* is isolated from soft tissue infections in association with *Actinomyces israelii.* It is associated with severe destructive periodontal disease, which also is frequently evident in pts with endocarditis.
- *C. hominis* most often affects the aortic valve. Long-standing infection usually precedes diagnosis. A second species, *C. valvarum,* has now been described in association with endocarditis.

---

[1] *H. paraphrophilus* is now considered to be encompassed by *A. aphrophilus* as opposed to being a separate species.

TABLE 98-1 TREATMENT OF ENDOCARDITIS AND OTHER SERIOUS INFECTIONS CAUSED BY HACEK GROUP ORGANISMS[a]

Organism	Initial Therapy	Alternative Agents	Comments
Haemophilus or *Aggregatibacter* species	Ceftriaxone (2 g/d)	Ampicillin/ sulbactam (3 g of ampicillin q6h) or fluoroquinolones[b]	Ampicillin ± an amino-glycoside can be used if the organism does not produce β-lactamase.[c]
Cardiobacterium hominis	Ceftriaxone (2 g/d)	Ampicillin/ sulbactam (3 g of ampicillin q6h)	Penicillin (16–18 mU q4h) or ampicillin (2 g q4h) should be used if the organism is susceptible.
Eikenella corrodens	Ampicillin (2 g q4h)	Ceftriaxone (2 g/d) or fluoroquinolones[b]	The organism is typically resistant to clinda-mycin, metronidazole, and aminoglycosides.
Kingella kingae	Ceftriaxone (2 g/d) or ampicillin/ sulbactam (3 g of ampicillin q6h)	Fluoroquinolones[b]	The prevalence of β-lactamase-producing strains is increasing. Efficacy for invasive infections is best demonstrated for first-line treatments.

[a]Susceptibility testing should be performed in all cases to guide therapy.
[b]Fluoroquinolones are not recommended for treatment of children <18 years of age.
[c]European guidelines for endocarditis recommend the addition of gentamicin (3 mg/kg per day in 3 divided doses for 2–4 weeks).

- *E. corrodens* is usually a component of mixed infections and is common in human bite wounds, head and neck soft-tissue infections, endocarditis, and infections in IV drug users.
- *K. kingae* is a common cause of skeletal infections in children <3 years old. Inoculation of clinical specimens (e.g., synovial fluid) into aerobic blood-culture bottles enhances recovery of this organism. Infective endocarditis due to *K. kingae* occurs in older children and adults.

TREATMENT   HACEK Group Infections

- Table 98-1 lists antibiotic regimens used to treat endocarditis and other serious infections caused by HACEK organisms.
- Native-valve endocarditis should be treated for 4 weeks and prosthetic-valve endocarditis for 6 weeks.
- Unlike prosthetic-valve endocarditis caused by other gram-negative organisms, that due to HACEK bacteria can often be cured with antibiotics alone (i.e., without surgery).

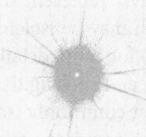

For a more detailed discussion, see Murphy TF: *Haemophilus* and *Moraxella* Infections, Chap. 145, p. 1228; Barlam TF, Kasper DL: Infections Due to the HACEK Group and Miscellaneous Gram-Negative Bacteria, Chap. 146, p. 1233; and Halperin SA: Pertussis and Other *Bordetella* Infections, Chap. 148, p. 1241, in HPIM-18.

CHAPTER **99**
Diseases Caused by Gram-Negative Enteric Bacteria, *Pseudomonas*, and *Legionella*

INFECTIONS CAUSED BY GRAM-NEGATIVE ENTERIC BACTERIA

■ GENERAL CONSIDERATIONS

Gram-negative bacilli (GNB) are normal components of the human colonic flora and/or a number of environmental habitats and can colonize mucosal and skin surfaces, especially in pts in long-term-care facilities and hospital settings. GNB cause a wide variety of infections involving diverse anatomic sites in both healthy and compromised hosts; extraintestinal infections due to *Escherichia coli* and, to a lesser degree, *Klebsiella* and *Proteus* species are most common. Isolation of GNB from any sterile site almost always implies infection, whereas isolation from nonsterile sites requires clinical correlation. Early appropriate antimicrobial therapy improves outcomes. Given worldwide increases in multi-drug-resistant GNB [e.g., due to extended-spectrum β-lactamases (ESBLs) and AmpC β-lactamases], combination empirical antimicrobial therapy pending susceptibility results may be appropriate for critically ill pts.

■ INFECTIONS CAUSED BY EXTRAINTESTINAL PATHOGENIC *E. COLI* (ExPEC)

In contrast to intestinal pathogenic *E. coli*, ExPEC strains are often found in the intestinal flora of healthy individuals but cause disease only when they enter a normally sterile extraintestinal site (e.g., the urinary tract, peritoneal cavity, or lungs). Most ExPEC strains have virulence factor profiles distinct from those of other commensal strains and from those of pathogenic strains that cause intestinal infections.

Clinical Manifestations

The clinical presentation depends in large part on the site of the body infected by ExPEC.

- *Urinary tract infection*: The urinary tract is the site most frequently infected by ExPEC; see Chap. 154 for more details. *E. coli* causes 85–95% of ~6–8 million episodes of acute uncomplicated UTI in premenopausal women.

- *Abdominal and pelvic infection*: The abdomen and pelvis represent the second most common site of infection by ExPEC, which may be isolated in the setting of a polymicrobial infection; see Chap. 90 for more details. Syndromes include peritonitis, intraabdominal abscesses, and cholangitis.
- *Pneumonia*: ExPEC is generally the third or fourth most commonly isolated GNB in hospital-acquired pneumonia and can be a common cause of pneumonia in pts residing in long-term-care facilities; see Chap. 141 for more details.
- *Meningitis*: E. coli is one of the two leading causes of neonatal meningitis (the other being group B *Streptococcus)*. Strains with the K1 capsular serotype are generally involved.
- *Cellulitis/musculoskeletal infection*: E. coli often contributes to infection of decubitus ulcers and diabetic lower-extremity ulcers; cellulitis; and burn-site or surgical-site infections. Hematogenously acquired osteomyelitis, particularly vertebral, is more commonly caused by E. coli than is generally appreciated. See Chap. 93 for more details.
- *Bacteremia*: E. coli is one of the two most common blood isolates of clinical significance. E. coli bacteremia can arise from primary infection at any site, but originates most commonly from the urinary tract (50–67% of episodes) and next most commonly from the abdomen (25% of episodes). E. coli bacteremia is typically associated with sepsis. Endovascular infections are rare but have been described.

Diagnosis

ExPEC grows readily on standard media under either aerobic or anaerobic conditions. More than 90% of strains ferment lactose and are indole positive.

TREATMENT   Extraintestinal Infections Caused by *E. coli*

- Rates of resistance to ampicillin, first-generation cephalosporins, trimethoprim-sulfamethoxazole (TMP-SMX), and fluoroquinolones are increasing. ESBLs are increasingly common in *E. coli*.
- Carbapenems and amikacin are the most predictably active agents overall, but carbapenemase-producing strains are on the rise.
- It is important to use the most appropriate narrower-spectrum agent whenever possible and to avoid treating colonized but uninfected pts, thus combating the increase in antibiotic resistance.

■ INFECTIONS CAUSED BY INTESTINAL PATHOGENIC *E. COLI*

Microbiology and Clinical Manifestations

At least five distinct pathotypes of intestinal pathogenic *E. coli* exist; see Chap. 91 for more details. As mentioned above, these strains are rarely encountered as part of the commensal flora in healthy individuals.

- *Shiga toxin–producing E. coli (STEC)/enterohemorrhagic E. coli (EHEC)*: In addition to diarrhea, STEC/EHEC infection results in the hemolytic-uremic syndrome in 2–8% of pts, particularly those who are very young or elderly.

- STEC/EHEC is associated with ingestion of contaminated food (e.g., undercooked ground beef, fresh produce) and water; person-to-person transmission (e.g., at day-care centers) is an important route for secondary spread.
- Disease can be caused by <10^2 colony-forming units (CFU) of STEC/EHEC.
- In contrast to the other pathotypes, STEC/EHEC (including *E. coli* O157:H7) causes infection more frequently in industrialized countries than in developing countries.

- *Enterotoxigenic E. coli (ETEC):* These strains are a major cause of endemic diarrhea among children residing in tropical and low-income countries and are the most common agent of traveler's diarrhea; 10^6–10^{10} CFU are needed to cause disease.
- *Enteropathogenic E. coli (EPEC):* EPEC is an important cause of diarrhea among infants in developing countries.
- *Enteroinvasive E. coli (EIEC):* EIEC, an uncommon cause of diarrhea, produces inflammatory colitis (stools containing mucus, blood, and inflammatory cells) similar to that caused by *Shigella* and primarily affects children and travelers in developing countries; 10^8–10^{10} CFU are needed to cause disease.
- *Enteroaggregative and diffusely adherent E. coli (EAEC):* Initially described in young children in developing countries, more recent studies indicate that EAEC may be a common cause of prolonged, watery diarrhea in all age groups in industrialized countries.

Diagnosis

Specific diagnosis is usually unnecessary except when STEC/EHEC is involved. To detect the latter, testing for Shiga toxins or toxin genes is more sensitive, specific, and rapid than screening for *E. coli* strains that do not ferment sorbitol followed by serotyping for O157.

TREATMENT   Intestinal Infections Caused by *E. coli*

- See Chap. 91 for more details. Replacement of water and electrolytes and avoidance of antibiotics in STEC/EHEC infection (since antibiotic use may increase the incidence of hemolytic-uremic syndrome) are indicated.

◼ *KLEBSIELLA* INFECTIONS

Epidemiology

K. pneumoniae colonizes the colon in 5–35% of healthy individuals and, from a medical standpoint, is the most important *Klebsiella* species. *K. oxytoca* primarily causes infections in long-term-care and hospital settings. *K. pneumoniae* subspecies *rhinoscleromatis*, which causes rhinoscleroma, and *K. pneumoniae* subspecies *ozaenae*, which causes chronic atrophic rhinitis, infect pts in tropical climates.

Clinical Manifestations

As in other GNB infections, the clinical presentation depends on the infected anatomic site.

- *Pneumonia*: *Klebsiella* is an uncommon cause of community-acquired pneumonia, which occurs primarily in pts with underlying disease (e.g., alcoholism, diabetes, chronic obstructive pulmonary disease) and among residents of long-term-care facilities and hospitalized pts.
  - The presentation is similar to that of pneumonia caused by other enteric GNB, with purulent sputum production and pulmonary infiltrates on CXR.
  - Infection can progress to pulmonary necrosis, pleural effusion, and empyema.
- *UTI*: *K. pneumoniae* causes 1–2% of cases of uncomplicated cystitis and 5–17% of cases of complicated UTI.
- *Abdominal infections*: *Klebsiella* causes a spectrum of disease similar to that of *E. coli*, but with less frequent occurrence. Hypervirulent variants that contain capsular serotype K1 or K2 have become more common in the past decade.
- *Bacteremia*: Bacteremia can arise from a primary infection at any site; infections of the urinary tract, respiratory tract, and abdomen (especially hepatic abscess) each account for 15–30% of episodes.
- *Other infections*: *Klebsiella* cellulitis or soft tissue infection most frequently affects devitalized tissue and immunocompromised hosts. *Klebsiella* can also cause endophthalmitis, nosocomial sinusitis, and osteomyelitis.

Diagnosis

Klebsiellae usually ferment lactose, although the subspecies *rhinoscleromatis* and *ozaenae* are nonfermenters and are indole negative.

TREATMENT   *Klebsiella* Infections

- Klebsiellae are resistant to ampicillin and ticarcillin.
  - Resistance to third-generation cephalosporins is increasing, as is the frequency of ESBL-containing isolates.
  - Fluoroquinolone resistance is increasing, especially among ESBL-containing strains.
- Empirical treatment of serious or health care–associated *Klebsiella* infections with amikacin or carbapenems is prudent; however, carbapenemase-producing strains are increasing in frequency. Optimal therapy for carbapenemase strains is unclear, but tigecycline, polymyxin B, and colistin are used most frequently on the basis of in vitro susceptibility profiles.

▇ *PROTEUS* INFECTIONS

Epidemiology

P. mirabilis is part of the normal flora in 50% of healthy people and causes 90% of *Proteus* infections. *P. vulgaris* and *P. penneri* are isolated primarily from pts in hospitals and long-term care facilities.

Clinical Manifestations

Most *Proteus* infections arise from the urinary tract. *Proteus* species account for 1–2% of uncomplicated UTIs, 5% of hospital-acquired UTIs, and 10–15% of complicated UTIs (especially those associated with urinary catheters).

- *Proteus* produces high levels of urease that result in alkalinization of urine and ultimately in formation of struvite and carbonate-apatite calculi.
- Other sites of infection are uncommon but include pneumonia, abdominal infections, soft tissue infections, and bacteremia.

Diagnosis

Proteus strains are typically lactose negative, produce H_2S, and exhibit swarming motility on agar plates. *P. mirabilis* is indole negative, whereas *P. vulgaris* and *P. penneri* are indole positive.

TREATMENT *Proteus* Infections

- *P. mirabilis* is susceptible to most agents except tetracycline, nitrofurantoin, polymyxin B, and tigecycline. Resistance to ampicillin, first-generation cephalosporins, and fluoroquinolones is increasing.
- *P. vulgaris* and *P. penneri* are more resistant; ~30% of *P. vulgaris* isolates have an inducible AmpC β-lactamase. Imipenem, fourth-generation cephalosporins, amikacin, and TMP-SMX exhibit excellent activity: 90–100% of *Proteus* isolates are susceptible.

■ INFECTIONS CAUSED BY OTHER GRAM-NEGATIVE ENTERIC PATHOGENS

- *Enterobacter* (e.g., *E. cloacae*, *E. aerogenes*), *Acinetobacter* (e.g., *A. baumannii*), *Serratia* (e.g., *S. marcescens*), and *Citrobacter* (e.g., *C. freundii*, *C. koseri*) usually cause nosocomial infections. Risk factors include immunosuppression, comorbid disease, prior antibiotic use, and ICU stays.
- Infections caused by *Morganella* (e.g., *M. morganii*) and *Providencia* (e.g., *P. stuartii*, *P. rettgeri*) resemble *Proteus* infections in terms of epidemiology, pathogenicity, and clinical manifestations but occur almost exclusively among persons in long-term-care facilities and, to a lesser degree, in hospitalized pts.

Clinical Manifestations

These organisms generally cause a spectrum of disease similar to that caused by other GNB, including pneumonia (particularly ventilator-associated), UTI (especially catheter-related), intravascular device–related infection, surgical-site infection, and abdominal infections.

- *Citrobacter*, *Morganella*, and *Providencia* infections are generally associated with UTIs.
- *Acinetobacter* has caused soft tissue and bone infections among soldiers with battlefield injuries and is a well-known pathogen in burn units.

| **TREATMENT** | Infections Caused by Other Gram-Negative Enteric Pathogens |

- Significant antibiotic resistance among these organisms makes therapy challenging.
  - Many of these organisms (e.g., *Serratia*, *Providencia*, *Acinetobacter*, *Citrobacter*, *Enterobacter*, *Morganella*) have a derepressible AmpC β-lactamase that results in resistance to third-generation cephalosporins, monobactams, and—in many cases—β-lactam/β-lactamase inhibitor combinations.
- Carbapenems and amikacin are most reliably active, and fourth-generation cephalosporins are active provided the organism does not express an ESBL. Susceptibility testing is essential. Some isolates may retain susceptibility only to colistin and polymyxin B.

■ *AEROMONAS* INFECTIONS

A. hydrophila causes >85% of *Aeromonas* infections. *Aeromonas* organisms proliferate in potable water, freshwater, and soil and are a putative cause of gastroenteritis. *Aeromonas* causes bacteremia and sepsis in infants and compromised hosts, especially those with cancer, hepatobiliary disease, trauma, or burns. The organisms can produce skin lesions similar to the ecthyma gangrenosum caused by *Pseudomonas aeruginosa*. *Aeromonas* causes nosocomial infections related to catheters, surgical incisions, and use of leeches.

| **TREATMENT** | *Aeromonas* Infections |

- *Aeromonas* is usually susceptible to fluoroquinolones (e.g., ciprofloxacin at a dosage of 500 mg PO q12h or 400 mg IV q12h), third-generation cephalosporins, carbapenems, and aminoglycosides.
- Susceptibility testing is critical to guide therapy since *Aeromonas* can produce various β-lactamases, including carbapenemases.

INFECTIONS DUE TO *PSEUDOMONAS AERUGINOSA* AND RELATED ORGANISMS

The pseudomonads make up a set of gram-negative organisms unable to ferment lactose. This group includes three medically important genera—*Pseudomonas*, *Burkholderia*, and *Stenotrophomonas*—that typically cause opportunistic disease.

■ *P. AERUGINOSA* INFECTIONS

Microbiology

P. aeruginosa is a motile gram-negative rod that commonly produces green or bluish pigment and may have a mucoid appearance (which is particularly common in isolates from pts with cystic fibrosis). *P. aeruginosa* differs from enteric GNB in that it has a positive reaction in the oxidase test and does not ferment lactose.

Epidemiology

Because *P. aeruginosa* is found in most moist environments (e.g., in soil, in tap water, and on countertops), people routinely come into contact with the organism. The many factors that predispose to *P. aeruginosa* infection include disruption of cutaneous or mucosal barriers (e.g., due to burns or trauma), immunosuppression (e.g., due to neutropenia, AIDS, or diabetes), and disruption of the normal bacterial flora (e.g., due to broad-spectrum antibiotic therapy).

- *P. aeruginosa* is no longer a major cause of life-threatening bacteremia among pts with neutropenia or burn injury.
- *P. aeruginosa* bacteremia is currently most common among pts in the ICU.

Clinical Manifestations

P. aeruginosa can infect virtually all sites in the body but has a strong predilection for the lungs.

- *Pneumonia*: *P. aeruginosa* is considered a major cause of ventilator-associated pneumonia, although colonization may be difficult to distinguish from true infection.
    - Clinically, most pts have a slowly progressive infiltrate, although progression is rapid in some cases. Infiltrates may become necrotic.
    - It is unclear whether an invasive procedure (e.g., bronchoalveolar lavage, protected-brush sampling of distal airways) is superior to tracheal aspiration in obtaining samples for culture.
    - Chronic respiratory infection with *P. aeruginosa* is associated with underlying or predisposing conditions (e.g., cystic fibrosis, bronchiectasis).
- *Bacteremia*: The presentation of *P. aeruginosa* bacteremia resembles that of sepsis in general.
    - Pathognomonic skin lesions (*ecthyma gangrenosum*) that at first are painful, reddish, and maculopapular and later become black and necrotic may develop in pts with marked neutropenia or with HIV infection.
    - Endovascular infections occur mostly in IV drug users and pts with prosthetic valves.
- *Bone and joint infections*: *P. aeruginosa* is an infrequent cause of bone and joint infections.
    - Injection drug use (associated with sternoclavicular joint infections and vertebral osteomyelitis) and UTIs in the elderly (associated with vertebral osteomyelitis) are risk factors.
    - *Pseudomonas* osteomyelitis of the foot most often follows puncture wounds through sneakers and most commonly affects children.
- *CNS infections*: CNS infections due to *P. aeruginosa* are relatively rare and are almost always secondary to a surgical procedure or head trauma.
- *Eye infections*: Keratitis and corneal ulcers can occur, usually resulting from trauma or surface injury by contact lenses. These infections are rapidly progressing entities that demand immediate therapeutic intervention. *P. aeruginosa* endophthalmitis secondary to bacteremia is a fulminant disease with severe pain, chemosis, decreased visual acuity, anterior uveitis, vitreous involvement, and panophthalmitis.

- *Ear infections*: In addition to mild swimmer's ear, *Pseudomonas* ear infections can result in malignant otitis externa, a life-threatening infection that presents as severe ear pain and decreased hearing.
  - Pts may develop cranial-nerve palsies or cavernous venous sinus thrombosis.
  - Most ear infections due to *P. aeruginosa* occur in elderly diabetic pts.
- *UTIs*: UTIs due to *P. aeruginosa* usually result from a foreign body in the urinary tract, an obstruction in the genitourinary system, or urinary tract instrumentation or surgery.
- *Skin and soft tissue infections*: *P. aeruginosa* can cause a variety of dermatitides, including pyoderma gangrenosum in neutropenic pts, folliculitis, and other papular or vesicular lesions. Multiple outbreaks have been linked to whirlpools, spas, and swimming pools.
- *Infections in pts with fever and neutropenia*: *P. aeruginosa* is always targeted in empirical treatment of these pts, given high rates of infection in the past and high associated mortality rates.
- *Infections in pts with AIDS*: *P. aeruginosa* infections in pts with AIDS can be fatal even though the clinical presentation is not particularly severe.
  - Pneumonia is the most common type of infection, with a high frequency of cavitary disease.
  - Since the advent of antiretroviral therapy, *P. aeruginosa* infection has declined in incidence among these pts but still occurs.

TREATMENT   *P. aeruginosa* **Infections**

- See Table 99-1 for antibiotic options and schedules.
- Several observational studies indicate that a single modern antipseudomonal β-lactam agent to which the isolate is sensitive is as efficacious as combination therapy. However, if—in the local environment—the susceptibility to first-line agents is <80%, empirical combination therapy should be administered until isolate-specific susceptibility data are available.

■ INFECTIONS CAUSED BY BACTERIA RELATED TO *PSEUDOMONAS* SPECIES

Stenotrophomonas maltophilia

S. maltophilia is an opportunistic pathogen. Most infections occur in the setting of prior broad-spectrum antimicrobial therapy that has eradicated the normal flora in immunocompromised pts.

- *S. maltophilia* causes pneumonia, especially ventilator-associated pneumonia, with or without bacteremia.
- Central venous line infection (most often in cancer pts) and ecthyma gangrenosum in neutropenic pts have been described.

Burkholderia cepacia

This organism can colonize airways during broad-spectrum antimicrobial treatment and is a cause of ventilator-associated pneumonia, catheter-associated infection, and wound infection.

- *B. cepacia* is recognized as an antibiotic-resistant nosocomial pathogen in ICU pts.
- *B. cepacia* can cause a rapidly fatal syndrome of respiratory distress and septicemia (the "cepacia syndrome") in pts with cystic fibrosis.

TREATMENT ▸ *S. maltophilia* and *B. cepacia* Infections

Intrinsic resistance to many antibiotics limits treatment. See Table 99-1 for recommended antibiotic regimens.

Miscellaneous Organisms

Melioidosis is endemic to Southeast Asia and is caused by *B. pseudomallei*. Glanders is associated with close contact with horses or other equines and is caused by *B. mallei*. These diseases present as acute or chronic pulmonary or extrapulmonary suppurative illnesses or as acute septicemia.

LEGIONELLA INFECTIONS

Microbiology

Legionellaceae are intracellular aerobic gram-negative bacilli that grow on buffered charcoal yeast extract (BCYE) agar. *L. pneumophila* causes 80–90% of cases of human *Legionella* disease and includes 16 serogroups; serogroups 1, 4, and 6 are most common.

Epidemiology

- *Legionella* is found in fresh water and human-constructed water sources. Outbreaks have been traced to drinking water systems and rarely to cooling towers.
- The organisms are transmitted to individuals primarily via aspiration but can also be transmitted by aerosolization and direct instillation into the lungs during respiratory tract manipulations.
- *Legionella* is the fourth most common cause of community-acquired pneumonia, accounting for 2–9% of cases. It causes 10–50% of cases of nosocomial pneumonia if the hospital's water system is colonized with the organism.
- Pts who have chronic lung disease, who smoke, and/or who are elderly, immunosuppressed, or recently discharged from the hospital are at particularly high risk for disease.

Clinical Manifestations

Legionellosis manifests as either an acute, febrile, self-limited illness (Pontiac fever) or pneumonia (Legionnaires' disease).

- Pontiac fever is a flulike illness with a 24- to 48-h incubation period. Malaise, fatigue, and myalgias occur in 97% of cases. Fever and headaches are also very common, but pneumonia does not develop. The disease is self-limited and does not require antimicrobial treatment. Recovery takes place in a few days.

TABLE 99-1 ANTIBIOTIC TREATMENT OF INFECTIONS DUE TO *PSEUDOMONAS AERUGINOSA* **AND RELATED SPECIES**

Infection	Antibiotics and Dosages	Other Considerations
Bacteremia		
Nonneutropenic host	Monotherapy: Ceftazidime (2 g q8h IV) or cefepime (2 g q12h IV) Combination therapy: Piperacillin/tazobactam (3.375 g q4h IV) or imipenem (500 mg q6h IV) or meropenem (1 g q8h IV) or doripenem (500 mg q8h IV) *plus* Amikacin (7.5 mg/kg q12h or 15 mg/kg q24h IV)	Add an aminoglycoside for pts in shock and in regions or hospitals where rates of resistance to the primary β-lactam agents are high. Tobramycin may be used instead of amikacin (susceptibility permitting). The duration of therapy is at least 2 weeks.
Neutropenic host	Cefepime (2 g q8h IV) or any of the other agents listed above (except doripenem) in the above dosages	
Endocarditis	Antibiotic regimens as for bacteremia for 6–8 weeks	Resistance during therapy is common. Surgery is required for relapse.
Pneumonia	Drugs and dosages as for bacteremia, except that the available carbapenems should not be the sole primary drugs because of high rates of resistance during therapy	IDSA guidelines recommend the addition of an aminoglycoside or ciprofloxacin. The duration of therapy is 10–14 days.
Bone infection, malignant otitis externa	Cefepime or ceftazidime at the same dosages as for bacteremia; aminoglycosides not a necessary component of therapy; ciprofloxacin (500–750 mg q12h PO) may be used	Duration of therapy varies with the drug used (e.g., 6 weeks for a β-lactam agent; at least 3 months for oral therapy except in puncture-wound osteomyelitis, for which the duration should be 2–4 weeks).
CNS infection	Ceftazidime or cefepime (2 g q8h IV) or meropenem (1 g q8h IV)	Abscesses or other closed-space infections may require drainage. The duration of therapy is ≥2 weeks.

TABLE 99-1 ANTIBIOTIC TREATMENT OF INFECTIONS DUE TO *PSEUDOMONAS AERUGINOSA* AND RELATED SPECIES (CONTINUED)

Infection	Antibiotics and Dosages	Other Considerations
Eye infection		
Keratitis/ulcer	Topical therapy with tobramycin/ciprofloxacin/levofloxacin eyedrops	Use maximal strengths available or compounded by pharmacy.
Endophthalmitis	Ceftazidime or cefepime as for CNS infection *plus* Topical therapy	
UTI	Ciprofloxacin (500 mg q12h PO) or levofloxacin (750 mg q24h) or any aminoglycoside (total daily dose given once daily)	Relapse may occur if an obstruction or a foreign body is present.
Multidrug-resistant *P. aeruginosa* infection	Colistin (100 mg q12h IV) for the shortest possible period to obtain a clinical response	Doses used have varied. Dosage adjustment is required in renal failure. Inhaled colistin may be added for pneumonia (100 mg q12h).
Stenotrophomonas maltophilia infection	TMP-SMX (1600/320 mg q12h IV for 14 days) Ticarcillin/clavulanate (3.1 g q4h IV for 14 days)	Resistance to all agents is increasing. Levofloxacin may be an alternative, but there is little published clinical experience with this agent.
Burkholderia cepacia infection	Meropenem (1 g q8h IV for 14 days) TMP-SMX (1600/320 mg q12h IV for 14 days)	Resistance to both agents is increasing. Do not use them in combination because of possible antagonism.
Melioidosis, glanders	Ceftazidime (2 g q6h for 2 weeks) or meropenem (1 g q8h for 2 weeks) or imipenem (500 mg q6h for 2 weeks) *followed by* TMP-SMX (1600/320 mg q12h PO for 3 months)	

Abbreviations: IDSA, Infectious Diseases Society of America; TMP-SMX, trimethoprim-sulfamethoxazole.

- Legionnaires' disease is more severe than other atypical pneumonias and is more likely to result in ICU admission.
  - After a usual incubation period of 2–10 days, nonspecific symptoms (e.g., malaise, fatigue, headache, anorexia) develop and are followed by a cough that is usually mild and only slightly productive. Chest pain can be prominent.
  - Radiologic findings are nonspecific, but pleural effusions are present in 28–63% of pts on hospital admission.
  - Legionnaires' disease is not readily distinguishable from pneumonia of other etiologies based on clinical manifestations, but diarrhea, confusion, temperatures >39°C, hyponatremia, increased aminotransferase levels, hematuria, hypophosphatemia, and elevated creatine phosphokinase levels are documented more frequently than in other pneumonias.
  - Extrapulmonary infection results from hematogenous dissemination and most commonly affects the heart (e.g., myocarditis, pericarditis).

Diagnosis

The use of *Legionella* testing—especially the *Legionella* urinary antigen test—is recommended for all pts with community-acquired pneumonia.

- Sputum or bronchoscopy specimens can be subjected to direct fluorescent antibody (DFA) staining and culture.
  - DFA testing is rapid and specific but is less sensitive than culture.
  - Cultures on BCYE media (with antibiotics to suppress competing flora) require 3–5 days to become positive.
- Serologic confirmation requires comparison of acute- and convalescent-phase samples. Detection of the necessary 4-fold rise in titers often requires 12 weeks.
- Urinary antigen testing is rapid, inexpensive, easy to perform, second only to culture in terms of sensitivity, and highly specific. It is useful only for *L. pneumophila* serogroup 1, which causes 80% of disease cases.
  - Urinary antigen is detectable 3 days after disease onset and generally disappears over 2 months, although positivity can be prolonged if the pt is receiving glucocorticoid therapy.
  - The test is not affected by antibiotic administration.

TREATMENT   *Legionella* Infections

- Newer macrolides (e.g., azithromycin at 500 mg/d PO, with consideration of doubling the first dose; or clarithromycin at 500 mg bid IV or PO) or fluoroquinolones (e.g., levofloxacin at 750 mg/d IV or 500 mg/d PO or moxifloxacin at 400 mg/d PO) are most effective.
  - Rifampin (100–600 mg bid) combined with either class of drug is recommended in severe cases.
  - Tetracyclines (doxycycline at 100 mg bid IV or PO) are alternatives.
- Immunocompetent hosts should receive 10–14 days of therapy, but immunocompromised hosts and pts with advanced disease should receive a 3-week course of treatment.
  - A 5- to 10-day course of azithromycin is adequate because of this drug's long half-life.
  - A clinical response usually occurs within 3–5 days after the initiation of parenteral therapy, at which point oral therapy can be substituted.

Prognosis

Mortality rates approach 80% among immunocompromised pts who do not receive timely therapy. Among immunocompetent hosts, mortality can approach 31% without treatment but ranges from 0 to 11% with appropriate and timely therapy. Fatigue, weakness, and neurologic symptoms can persist for >1 year.

> For a more detailed discussion, see Barlam TF, Kasper DL: Infections Due to the HACEK Group and Miscellaneous Gram-Negative Bacteria, Chap. 146, p. 1233; Sabria M, Yu VL: *Legionella* Infections, Chap. 147, p. 1236; Russo TA, Johnson JR: Diseases Caused by Gram-Negative Enteric Bacilli, Chap. 149, p. 1246; Paterson DL, Peleg AY: *Acinetobacter* Infections, Chap. 150, p. 1258; and Ramphal R: Infections Due to *Pseudomonas* Species and Related Organisms, Chap. 152, p. 1266, in HPIM-18.

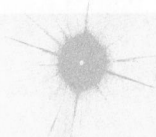

CHAPTER **100**
Infections Caused by Miscellaneous Gram-Negative Bacilli

BRUCELLOSIS

Microbiology

Brucellae are small, gram-negative, unencapsulated, nonsporulating, nonmotile rods or coccobacilli that can persist intracellularly. The genus *Brucella* includes four major clinically relevant species: *B. melitensis* (acquired by humans most commonly from sheep, goats, and camels), *B. suis* (from swine), *B. abortus* (from cattle or buffalo), and *B. canis* (from dogs).

Epidemiology

Brucellosis is transmitted via ingestion, inhalation, or mucosal or percutaneous exposure; the disease in humans is usually associated with exposure to infected animals or their products in either occupational settings (e.g., slaughterhouse work, farming) or domestic settings (e.g., consumption of contaminated foods, especially dairy products). The global prevalence of brucellosis is unknown because of difficulties in diagnosis and inadequacies in reporting systems.

Clinical Manifestations

Regardless of the specific infecting species, brucellosis often presents with one of three patterns: a febrile illness similar to but less severe than typhoid

TABLE 100-1 RADIOLOGY OF THE SPINE: DIFFERENTIATION OF BRUCELLOSIS FROM TUBERCULOSIS

	Brucellosis	Tuberculosis
Site	Lumbar and others	Dorsolumbar
Vertebrae	Multiple or contiguous	Contiguous
Discitis	Late	Early
Body	Intact until late	Morphology lost early
Canal compression	Rare	Common
Epiphysitis	Anterosuperior (Pom's sign)	General: upper and lower disk regions, central, subperiosteal
Osteophyte	Anterolateral (parrot beak)	Unusual
Deformity	Wedging uncommon	Anterior wedge, gibbus
Recovery	Sclerosis, whole body	Variable
Paravertebral abscess	Small, well-localized	Common and discrete loss, transverse process
Psoas abscess	Rare	More likely

fever; fever and acute monarthritis, typically of the hip or knee, in a young child (septic arthritis); or long-lasting fever, misery, and low-back or hip pain in an older man (vertebral osteomyelitis).

- An incubation period of 1 week to several months is followed by the development of undulating fever; sweats; increasing apathy, fatigue, and anorexia; and nonspecific symptoms such as headache, myalgias, and chills.
- *Brucella* infection can cause lymphadenopathy, hepatosplenomegaly, epididymoorchitis, neurologic involvement, and focal abscess.
- Given the persistent fever and similar symptoms, tuberculosis is the most important differential diagnosis (Table 100-1).

Diagnosis

Laboratory personnel must be alerted to the potential diagnosis to ensure that they take precautions to prevent occupational exposure.

- The organism is successfully cultured in 50–70% of cases. Cultures using the BACTEC systems usually become positive in 7–10 days and can be deemed negative at 3 weeks.
- PCR analysis of blood or tissue samples is more sensitive, faster, and safer than culture.
- Agglutination assays for IgM are positive early in infection. Single titers of ≥1:160 and ≥1:320 are diagnostic in nonendemic and endemic areas, respectively.

TREATMENT	Brucellosis

- The recommended regimen is streptomycin at a dosage of 0.75–1 g/d (or gentamicin at 5–6 mg/kg qd) for 14–21 days plus doxycycline at a dosage of 100 mg bid for 6 weeks.
  - Rifampin (600–900 mg/d) plus doxycycline (100 mg bid) for 6 weeks constitute an alternative regimen (the current World Health Organization [WHO] recommendation).
  - Significant neurologic disease requires at least 3–6 months of treatment, with ceftriaxone supplementation of a standard regimen.
  - Endocarditis requires a four-drug regimen (an aminoglycoside, rifampin, a tetracycline, and ceftriaxone or a fluoroquinolone) for at least 6 weeks.
  - Relapse rates range from 5 to >20% and depend on the specific antibiotic regimen used; pts should be monitored for at least 2 years.

TULAREMIA

Microbiology and Epidemiology

Tularemia is the only disease caused by *Francisella tularensis*, a small, gram-negative, aerobic bacillus that is a potential agent of bioterrorism (Chap. 33).

- Human infection occurs via interaction with biting or blood-sucking insects (especially ticks and tabanid flies in the spring and summer), wild or domestic animals (e.g., wild rabbits, squirrels), or the environment.
  - The organism gains entry into the skin or mucous membranes through bites or inapparent abrasions or is acquired via inhalation or ingestion.
  - As few as 10 organisms can result in infection when injected into the skin or inhaled.
- More than half of U.S. cases occur in Arkansas, Oklahoma, South Dakota, and Missouri.

Clinical Manifestations

After an incubation period of 2–10 days, tularemia generally starts with an acute onset of fever, chills, headache, and myalgias. The *ulceroglandular/glandular* forms of tularemia affect 75–85% of pts, but several other syndromes involving systemic manifestations can occur.

- *Ulceroglandular/glandular tularemia*: The hallmark of ulceroglandular tularemia is an indurated, erythematous, nonhealing ulcer lasting 1–3 weeks that begins as a pruritic or tender lesion, ulcerates, has sharply demarcated edges and a yellow exudate, and develops a black base.
  - Inguinal/femoral lymphadenopathy is most common in adults; nodes can become fluctuant and drain spontaneously.
  - In glandular tularemia (5–10% of cases), no primary skin lesion is apparent.

- *Oculoglandular tularemia*: In 1% of pts, infection of the conjunctiva—usually by contact with contaminated fingers—results in purulent conjunctivitis with regional lymphadenopathy and debilitating pain. Painful preauricular lymphadenopathy distinguishes tularemia from other diseases.
- *Oropharyngeal and GI tularemia*: Acquired through oral inoculation (via contaminated foods or fingers), the infection can present as pharyngitis and cervical adenopathy, intestinal ulcerations, mesenteric lymphadenopathy, diarrhea, nausea, vomiting, and abdominal pain.
- *Pulmonary tularemia*: Infection is acquired via inhalation or via hematogenous spread from ulceroglandular or typhoidal tularemia. Pts present with signs and symptoms similar to those of pneumonia of other etiologies (e.g., nonproductive cough, dyspnea, pleuritic chest pain, CXR with bilateral patchy or lobar infiltrates or cavitary lesions).
- *Typhoidal tularemia*: Due to pharyngeal or GI inoculation or to bacteremic disease, typhoidal tularemia consists of fever and signs of sepsis, generally without skin lesions or lymphadenopathy. This form is the result of a large inoculum or a preexisting compromising condition.

Diagnosis

The diagnosis of tularemia is most frequently confirmed by serology, although up to 30% of pts infected for 3 weeks have negative results in serologic tests.

- Cultures are positive in only 10% of cases; organisms in culture pose a significant risk to laboratory personnel.
- PCR has been used to detect *F. tularensis* DNA in clinical specimens, mainly for ulceroglandular disease.

TREATMENT Tularemia

- Gentamicin (2.5 mg/kg IV bid for 7–10 days) is considered the drug of choice; pts who defervesce within the first 48–72 h of treatment may receive a 5- to 7-day course.
  - Streptomycin (1 g IM q12h for 10 days) is also effective, but tobramycin is not.
  - Doxycycline is another alternative, but it must be given for at least 14 days because it is only bacteriostatic against *F. tularensis*.
  - Healing of skin lesions and lymph nodes may take 1–2 weeks. Late lymph-node suppuration can occur, with sterile necrotic tissue.

PLAGUE

Epidemiology

Yersinia pestis causes plague, a systemic zoonosis that primarily affects small rodents in rural areas of Africa (where 80% of all human cases worldwide occur), Asia, and the Americas. As the rodent population succumbs to disease, fleas (the arthropod vector) search for a new host and can transmit the bacteria to humans.

- In addition to fleabites, direct contact with infected tissues or airborne droplets can cause human infections. Given the possibility of airborne transmission, *Y. pestis* is a potential agent of bioterrorism (Chap. 33).
- There are a median of 7 cases per year in the U.S., most of them occurring near the "Four Corners" (the junction point of New Mexico, Arizona, Colorado, and Utah) and further west in California, southern Oregon, and western Nevada.

Clinical Manifestations

Worldwide, bubonic plague accounts for 80–95% of all plague cases, with primary septicemic plague occurring in 10–20% of cases and primary pulmonary plague in only a small minority of cases.

- *Bubonic plague*: After an incubation period of 2–6 days, the onset of bubonic plague is sudden and is characterized by fever (>38°C), malaise, myalgia, dizziness, and increasing pain due to progressive lymphadenitis in the regional lymph nodes near the fleabite or other inoculation site.
  - The tender, swollen lymph node (bubo) has a boggy consistency with an underlying hard core when palpated.
  - With treatment, fever resolves within 2–5 days; without treatment, infection can disseminate and cause serious illness (e.g., secondary pneumonic plague, meningitis).
- *Primary septicemic plague*: Pts present with gram-negative septicemia not preceded by lymphadenopathy. Persons >40 years old are at greater risk, although this form of the disease can occur in all age groups.
- *Pneumonic plague*: After a short incubation period averaging a few hours to 3 days, pts experience a sudden onset of fever, nonspecific signs and symptoms (e.g., headache, myalgias, vomiting), and respiratory manifestations (e.g., cough, chest pain, sputum production with hemoptysis).
  - Pneumonitis that is initially segmental can progress to lobar pneumonia and then to bilateral lung involvement.
  - The mortality rate is nearly 100% without treatment and is still >50% with effective treatment.

Diagnosis

The WHO recommends an initial presumptive diagnosis followed by confirmation in a reference laboratory.

- The appropriate specimens for diagnosis of bubonic, pneumonic, and septicemic plague are bubo aspirate (after injection of 1 mL of normal saline), bronchoalveolar lavage fluid or sputum, and blood, respectively. Gram's, Wayson, or Wright-Giemsa staining of these samples may reveal bipolar gram-negative rods.
- Given the potential risk to laboratory workers, culture of *Y. pestis* should be performed only at reference laboratories, which use direct immunofluorescence, PCR, and/or specific bacteriophage lysis as confirmatory tests for identification. The optimal growth temperature is 25–29°C.
- In the absence of other positive diagnostic testing, a serologic diagnosis can be made.

TREATMENT   Plague

- Streptomycin (1g IM q12h) or gentamicin (5 mg/kg IV q24h) is the drug of choice. Doxycycline (200 mg/d PO/IV in 1 or 2 doses) and chloramphenicol (12.5 mg/kg PO/IV q6h) are alternative agents.
- For pts who are hospitalized with pneumonic plague or in whom this disease is suspected, respiratory droplet precautions should be implemented until treatment has been given for at least 48 h.
- Postexposure antimicrobial prophylaxis lasting 7 days is recommended after household, hospital, or other close (<2 m) contact with persons with untreated pneumonic plague. Doxycycline (200 mg/d PO/IV in 1 or 2 doses), ciprofloxacin (1 g PO q12h), or TMP-SMX (320 mg of the TMP component PO q12h) are effective agents for prophylaxis.

BARTONELLA INFECTIONS

- *Bartonella* species are fastidious, facultative intracellular, gram-negative bacteria that cause an array of infectious disease syndromes in humans.
- Most *Bartonella* species have successfully adapted to survival in specific domestic or wild mammals, creating a reservoir for human infection. The exceptions are *B. bacilliformis* and *B. quintana,* which are not zoonotic.
- Clinical presentation generally depends on both the infecting *Bartonella* species and the immune status of the infected individual.
- Therapy for syndromes caused by *Bartonella* is summarized in Table 100-2.

■ CAT-SCRATCH DISEASE (CSD)

Microbiology and Epidemiology

B. henselae is the principal etiologic agent of CSD, although other *Bartonella* species may rarely be involved. Consistent with the disease's name, contact (being scratched, bitten, or licked) with apparently healthy cats, and especially with kittens, is the primary source of infection. Adults are affected nearly as frequently as children. In the U.S., the estimated incidence is ~10 cases per 100,000 population.

Clinical Manifestations

Of pts with CSD, 85–90% have typical disease consisting of a localized lesion (papule, vesicle, or nodule) at the site of inoculation with subsequent painful regional lymphadenopathy ≥1–3 weeks after cat contact.

- Axillary and epitrochlear nodes are most commonly involved and suppurate in 10–15% of cases.
- Low-grade fever, malaise, and anorexia develop in ~50% of pts.
- Atypical disease involves extranodal manifestations (e.g., fever of unknown origin, ophthalmologic manifestations, neurologic involvement, osteomyelitis).
- In immunocompetent pts, the disease resolves spontaneously without treatment, although its resolution takes weeks or months.

TABLE 100-2 ANTIMICROBIAL THERAPY FOR DISEASE CAUSED BY *BARTONELLA* SPECIES IN ADULTS

Disease	Antimicrobial Therapy
Typical cat-scratch disease (CSD)	Not routinely indicated; for pts with extensive lymphadenopathy, consider azithromycin (500 mg PO on day 1, then 250 mg PO qd for 4 days)
CSD retinitis	Doxycycline (100 mg PO bid) *plus* rifampin (300 mg PO bid) for 4–6 weeks
Other atypical CSD manifestations[a]	As per retinitis, with treatment duration individualized
Trench fever or chronic *B. quintana* bacteremia	Gentamicin (3 mg/kg IV qd for 14 days) *plus* doxycycline (200 mg PO qd or 100 mg PO bid for 6 weeks)
Suspected *Bartonella* endocarditis	Gentamicin[b] (1 mg/kg IV q8h for ≥14 days) *plus* doxycycline (100 mg PO/IV bid for 6 weeks[c]) *plus* ceftriaxone (2 g IV qd for 6 weeks)
Confirmed *Bartonella* endocarditis	As for suspected *Bartonella* endocarditis *minus* ceftriaxone
Bacillary angiomatosis	Erythromycin[d] (500 mg PO qid for 3 months) *or* Doxycycline (100 mg PO bid for 3 months)
Bacillary peliosis	Erythromycin[d] (500 mg PO qid for 4 months) *or* Doxycycline (100 mg PO bid for 4 months)
Bartonellosis (Carrión's disease)	
Oroya fever	Chloramphenicol (500 mg PO/IV qid for 14 days) *plus* another antibiotic (β-lactam preferred) *or* Ciprofloxacin (500 mg PO bid for 10 days)
Verruga peruana	Rifampin (10 mg/kg PO qd, to a maximum of 600 mg/d, for 14 days) *or* Streptomycin (15–20 mg/kg IM qd for 10 days)

[a]Data on treatment efficacy for encephalitis and hepatosplenic CSD are lacking. Therapy similar to that given for retinitis is reasonable.

[b]Some experts recommend gentamicin at 3 mg/kg IV qd. If gentamicin is contraindicated, rifampin (300 mg PO bid) can be added to doxycycline for documented *Bartonella* endocarditis.

[c]Some experts recommend extending oral doxycycline therapy for 3–6 months.

[d]Other macrolides are probably effective and may be substituted for erythromycin or doxycycline.

Source: Recommendations are modified from Rolain JM et al: Recommendations for treatment of human infections caused by *Bartonella* species. Antimicrob Agents Chemother 48:1921, 2004.

Diagnosis

Serologic testing is most commonly used but is variably sensitive and specific. It is noteworthy that seroconversion may take a few weeks. *Bartonella* species are difficult to culture, but PCR analysis of lymph node tissue, pus, or the primary inoculation lesion is highly sensitive and specific.

◼ BACILLARY ANGIOMATOSIS AND PELIOSIS

Bacillary angiomatosis is caused by *B. henselae* and *B. quintana*, while peliosis is caused only by the former species. These diseases occur most often in HIV-infected pts with CD4+ T cell counts of <100/μL.

- Pts with bacillary angiomatosis present with one or more painless skin lesions that may be tan, red, or purple in color. Subcutaneous masses or nodules, ulcerated plaques, and verrucous growths also occur. *B. quintana* is also associated with lytic bone lesions, primarily in the long bones.
- Peliosis is an angioproliferative disorder characterized by blood-filled cystic structures that affects primarily the liver but also the spleen and lymph nodes. Hypodense hepatic areas are usually evident on imaging.
- Both diseases are diagnosed on histologic grounds. Blood cultures may be positive.

◼ TRENCH FEVER

- Trench fever (*5-day fever*) is caused by *B. quintana*, which is spread by the human body louse among its only animal reservoir: humans.
- Much less common today than in the trenches of World War I, the disease now primarily affects homeless people.
- After a usual incubation period of 15–25 days, disease classically ranges from a mild febrile illness to a recurrent or protracted and debilitating disease. Fever is often periodic, with episodes of 4–5 days separated by ~5-day afebrile periods.
- Diagnosis requires identification of *B. quintana* in blood cultures.
- Untreated, the disease usually lasts 4–6 weeks. Death is rare.

◼ *BARTONELLA* ENDOCARDITIS

Bartonella species (typically *B quintana* or *B. henselae*) are an important cause of culture-negative endocarditis. The disease's manifestations are similar to those of subacute endocarditis of any etiology (Chap. 89). Even if incubated for prolonged periods (up to 6 weeks), blood cultures are positive in only ~25% of cases. Serologic or PCR testing for *Bartonella* in cardiac valve tissue can help establish the diagnosis in pts with negative blood cultures.

◼ BARTONELLOSIS (CARRIÓN'S DISEASE)

Bartonellosis is a biphasic disease caused by *B. bacilliformis,* which is transmitted by a sandfly vector found in the Andes valleys of Peru, Ecuador, and Colombia.

- *Oroya fever* is the initial, bacteremic, systemic form, and *verruga peruana* is its late-onset, eruptive manifestation.

- Oroya fever may present as a nonspecific bacteremic febrile illness without anemia or as acute, severe hemolytic anemia with hepatomegaly and jaundice of rapid onset.
  - In verruga peruana, red, hemangioma-like, cutaneous vascular lesions of various sizes appear either weeks to months after systemic illness or with no previous suggestive history. The lesions persist for months up to 1 year.
- In systemic illness, Giemsa-stained blood films show typical intraerythrocytic bacilli, and blood and bone marrow cultures are positive. Serologic assays may be helpful. Biopsy may be required to confirm the diagnosis of verruga peruana.

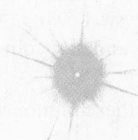

For a more detailed discussion, see Corbel MJ, Beeching NJ: Brucellosis, Chap. 157, p. 1296; Jacobs RF, Schutze GE: Tularemia, Chap. 158, p. 1301; Prentice MB: Plague and Other *Yersinia* Infections, Chap. 159, p. 1305; and Giladi M, Ephros M: *Bartonella* Infections, Including Cat-Scratch Disease, Chap. 160, p. 1314, in HPIM-18.

CHAPTER **101**
Anaerobic Infections

DEFINITIONS

- *Anaerobic bacteria:* require reduced oxygen tension for growth; do not grow on the surface of solid media in 10% CO_2 in air
- *Microaerophilic bacteria:* grow in an atmosphere of 10% CO_2 in air or under anaerobic or aerobic conditions, but grow best if only a small amount of atmospheric oxygen is present
- *Facultative bacteria:* grow in the presence or absence of oxygen

TETANUS

Microbiology, Epidemiology, and Pathogenesis

Tetanus is characterized by increased muscle tone and spasms caused by tetanospasmin ("tetanus toxin"), a toxin produced by *Clostridium tetani.*

- *C. tetani* is a spore-forming, anaerobic gram-positive rod that is ubiquitous in soil and whose spores are highly resilient.
- Worldwide, tetanus is a common disease because of low rates of vaccination. In 2006, ~290,000 people—most of them in Southeast Asia and Africa—died of tetanus; maternal and neonatal infections accounted for ~60% of these deaths. In contrast, only 28 cases were reported in the United States in 2007.
- After spores contaminate wounds (typically puncture wounds or, in the case of neonates, the umbilical stump) and reach a suitable anaerobic environment (e.g., devitalized tissue), organisms proliferate and release toxin.

- The toxin blocks release of inhibitory neurotransmitters (glycine and γ-aminobutyric acid) in presynaptic terminals, and rigidity results from an increased resting firing rate of the α-motor neurons.
- A toxin dose as low as 2.5 mg/kg can be fatal.

Clinical Manifestations

C. tetani can cause a usually mild local disease confined to the muscles near the wound or a more severe generalized disease (e.g., neonatal disease).

- If the cranial nerves are involved in localized cephalic tetanus, the pt may aspirate or develop airway obstruction due to pharyngeal or laryngeal muscle spasm. This situation is associated with a poor prognosis.
- The early symptoms of generalized tetanus often include trismus (lockjaw), muscle pain and stiffness, back pain, and difficulty swallowing. As the disease progresses, painful muscle spasms develop and can sometimes be strong enough to cause crush fractures.
  - Without ventilatory support, respiratory failure is the commonest cause of death in tetanus.
  - Autonomic disturbance (e.g., labile blood pressure; GI stasis; increased tracheal secretions; acute, high-output renal failure) is maximal during the second week of severe tetanus, and death due to cardiovascular events becomes the major risk.

Diagnosis

The diagnosis is made on clinical grounds. Culture of *C. tetani* from a wound provides supportive evidence.

TREATMENT   Tetanus

- The mainstays of early treatment are the elimination of ongoing toxin production and the neutralization of circulating toxin.
  - The entry wound should be identified, cleaned, and debrided of necrotic material in order to remove anaerobic foci of infection and prevent further toxin production.
  - Metronidazole (400 mg rectally or 500 mg IV q6h for 7 days) is the preferred antibiotic. Penicillin (100,000–200,000 IU/kg qd) is an alternative but theoretically may increase spasms.
  - Antitoxin should be given as early as possible.
  - Standard treatment consists of a single IM dose of tetanus immune globulin (TIG; 3000–6000 IU) or equine antitoxin (10,000–20,000 IU). However, there is evidence that intrathecal TIG (50–1500 IU) inhibits disease progression and leads to a better outcome than IM-administered TIG.
- TIG is preferred as it is less likely to cause an anaphylactoid reaction.
- Monitoring and supportive care in a calm, quiet environment are important because light and noise can trigger spasms.
  - Spasms are controlled by heavy sedation with benzodiazepines, chlorpromazine, and/or phenobarbital; magnesium sulfate can also be used as a muscle relaxant. The doses required to control spasms also cause

respiratory depression; thus it is difficult to control spasms adequately in settings without mechanical ventilation.

- Cardiovascular instability in severe tetanus is notoriously difficult to treat; increased sedation (e.g., with magnesium sulfate or morphine) or administration of short-acting agents that work specifically on the cardiovascular system (e.g., esmolol, calcium antagonists, inotropes) may be required.

• Recovery from tetanus may take 4–6 weeks. Because natural disease does not induce immunity, recovering pts should be immunized.

Prevention

Vaccination effectively prevents disease.

• "Catch-up" vaccination schedules recommend a three-dose primary course followed by two further doses for unimmunized adolescents. For persons who have received a complete primary course in childhood but no further boosters, two doses at least 4 weeks apart are recommended.

• Individuals sustaining tetanus-prone wounds should be immunized if their vaccination status is incomplete or unknown or if their last booster was given >10 years earlier. Pts sustaining wounds not classified as clean or minor should also undergo passive immunization with TIG.

Prognosis

A shorter incubation period (time from wound to first symptom) or onset period (time from first symptom to first generalized spasm) is associated with worse outcome.

BOTULISM

Microbiology, Epidemiology, and Pathogenesis

Botulism is a paralytic disease caused by neurotoxins elaborated by *Clostridium botulinum*, an anaerobic spore-forming gram-positive bacterium, as well as a few other toxigenic *Clostridium* species.

• Botulism is caused by the toxin's inhibition of acetylcholine release at the neuromuscular junction through an enzymatic mechanism.

- *C. botulinum* toxin types A, B, E, and (rarely) F cause human disease, with toxin type A causing the most severe syndrome.
- Toxin type E is associated with foods of aquatic origin.

• Transmission is usually due to consumption of foods contaminated with botulinum toxin, but contamination of wounds with spores also can result in disease.

- Most U.S. food-borne cases are associated with home-canned food.
- Infant botulism is the most common form of the disease in the United States, with ~80–100 cases reported annually.

• Toxin is heat-labile (inactivated when heated for 10 min at 100°C), and spores are heat-resistant (inactivated at 116°–121°C or with steam sterilizers or pressure cookers); these properties underscore the importance of properly heating foods.

- Botulinum toxin is the most toxic substance known and thus is of concern as a potential weapon of bioterrorism (Chap. 33).

Clinical Manifestations

Botulism occurs naturally as four syndromes: (1) food-borne illness; (2) wound infection; (3) infant botulism; and (4) adult intestinal toxemia, which is similar to infant botulism. The disease presents as symmetric cranial nerve palsies (diplopia, dysarthria, dysphonia, ptosis, and/or dysphagia) followed by symmetric descending flaccid paralysis that may progress to respiratory arrest and death.

- *Food-borne botulism* occurs 18–36 h after ingestion of food contaminated with toxin and ranges in severity from mild to fatal (within 24 h). Nausea, vomiting, and abdominal pain may precede or follow the onset of paralysis; constipation due to paralytic ileus is nearly universal. Fever is usually absent.
- *Wound botulism* occurs when spores contaminate wounds (e.g., in black-tar heroin users) and germinate. The clinical syndrome is indistinguishable from food-borne botulism except that GI symptoms are generally absent.
- In *infant botulism* and *adult intestinal toxemia*, spores germinate in the intestine and produce toxin, which is absorbed and causes illness. This form in infants has been associated with contaminated honey; thus honey should not be fed to children <12 months of age. Adult pts typically have some anatomic or functional bowel abnormality or have a bowel flora disrupted by recent antibiotic use.

Diagnosis

The clinical symptoms suggest the diagnosis. The definitive test is the demonstration of the toxin in clinical specimens (serum, stool, gastric aspirates, wound material) with a mouse bioassay (i.e., paralysis in a mouse after injection with the clinical sample).

- The results may not be available for up to 48 h, so clinical decisions (e.g., to administer botulinum antitoxin) need to be made in their absence.
- This test may yield a negative result even if the pt has botulism; additional tests may be necessary to rule out other conditions.

TREATMENT   Botulism

- The mainstays of treatment are meticulous supportive care and immediate administration of botulinum antitoxin—the only specific treatment.
  - Adults are given an equine antitoxin available through the CDC (770-488-7100); infant botulism is treated with a human-origin antitoxin (licensed as BabyBIG®) available through the California Department of Public Health (510-231-7600).
  - In wound botulism, suspect wounds and abscesses should be cleaned, debrided, and drained promptly, and antimicrobial therapy (e.g., penicillins) should be guided by clinical judgment, as its clinical efficacy has not been established.

Prognosis

Toxin binding is irreversible, but nerve terminals do regenerate. In the United States, 95% of pts recover fully, but this process may take many months.

OTHER CLOSTRIDIAL INFECTIONS

Microbiology and Pathogenesis

Clostridia are pleomorphic, gram-positive, spore-forming organisms. Most species are obligate anaerobes; some (e.g., *C. septicum*, *C. tertium*) can grow—but not sporulate—in air.

- In humans, clostridia reside in the GI and female genital tracts and on the oral mucosa.
- Clostridial species produce more protein toxins than any other bacterial genus; the *C. perfringens* epsilon toxin is among the most lethal and is considered a potential agent of bioterrorism (Chap. 33).

Epidemiology and Clinical Manifestations

Life-threatening clostridial infections range from intoxications (e.g., food poisoning, tetanus) to necrotizing enteritis/colitis, bacteremia, myonecrosis, and toxic shock syndrome (TSS).

- *Clostridial wound contamination*: Of open traumatic wounds, 30–80% are contaminated with clostridial species. Diagnosis and treatment of clostridial infection should be based on clinical signs and symptoms, given that clostridia are isolated with equal frequency from both suppurative and well-healing wounds.
- *Polymicrobial infections involving clostridia*: Clostridial species can be involved in infection throughout the body; 66% of intraabdominal infections related to compromised mucosal integrity involve clostridia (most commonly *C. ramosum*, *C. perfringens*, and *C. bifermentans*).
- *Enteric clostridial infections*: Disease ranges from food-borne illnesses and antibiotic-associated colitis (Chap. 91) to extensive necrosis of the intestine (e.g., *enteritis necroticans* and *necrotizing enterocolitis*, which are due to toxigenic *C. perfringens* type C and type A, respectively).
- *Clostridial bacteremia*: *C. perfringens* causes 79% of clostridial bacteremias; when associated with myonecrosis, clostridial bacteremia has a grave prognosis.
  - *C. septicum* is also commonly associated with bacteremia (<5% of cases). More than 50% of pts with *C. septicum* bacteremia have a GI anomaly or an underlying malignancy. Neutropenia (of any origin) is also associated with clostridial bloodstream infection.
    - Pts with clostridial bacteremia—particularly that due to *C. septicum*—require immediate treatment, as infection can metastasize and cause spontaneous myonecrosis.
- *Clostridial skin and soft-tissue infections*: Necrotizing clostridial soft-tissue infections are rapidly progressive and are characterized by marked tissue destruction, gas in the tissues, and shock. Most pts develop severe pain, crepitus, brawny induration with rapid progression to skin sloughing, violaceous bullae, and marked tachycardia.

– *C. perfringens myonecrosis (gas gangrene)* is accompanied by bacteremia, hypotension, and multiorgan failure and is invariably fatal if untreated.

• If due to trauma, gas gangrene has an incubation period of 6 h to <4 days. Disease initially presents as excruciating pain at the affected site and the development of a foul-smelling wound containing a thin serosanguineous discharge and gas bubbles.

• Spontaneous gas gangrene results from hematogenous seeding of normal muscle with toxigenic clostridia from a GI source. Confusion, extreme pain in the absence of trauma, and fever should heighten suspicion.

– *TSS*: Endometrial clostridial infection (particularly with *C. sordellii*) is usually related to pregnancy and proceeds rapidly to TSS and death.

• Systemic manifestations, including edema, effusions, profound leukocytosis (50,000–200,000/μL), and hemoconcentration (Hct of 75–80%), are followed by the rapid onset of hypotension and multiple-organ failure.

• Fever is usually absent.

– Other clostridial skin and soft-tissue infections include crepitant cellulitis (involving subcutaneous or retroperitoneal tissues in diabetic pts), cellulitis and abscess formation due to *C. histolyticum*, and endophthalmitis due to *C. sordellii* or *C. perfringens*.

Diagnosis

Isolation of clostridia from clinical sites does not in itself indicate severe disease. Clinical findings and presentation must also be taken into account.

TREATMENT **Other Clostridial Infections**

Table 101-1 lists treatment regimens for clostridial infections.

MIXED ANAEROBIC INFECTIONS

Microbiology, Epidemiology, and Pathogenesis

Nonsporulating anaerobic bacteria are important components of the normal flora of mucosal surfaces of the mouth, lower GI tract, skin, and female genital tract and contribute to physiologic, metabolic, and immunologic functions of the host.

• Most clinically relevant anaerobes are relatively aerotolerant and can survive for as long as 72 h in the presence of low levels of oxygen.

– Clinically relevant anaerobes include gram-positive cocci (e.g., *Peptostreptococcus* species), gram-positive rods (e.g., spore-forming clostridia and *Propionibacterium acnes*), and gram-negative bacilli (e.g., the *B. fragilis* group in the normal bowel flora, *Fusobacterium* species in the oral cavity and GI tract, *Prevotella* species in the oral cavity and female genital tract, and *Porphyromonas* species in the oral flora).

• Infections caused by anaerobes are typically polymicrobial (including at least one anaerobic organism and sometimes involving microaerophilic

TABLE 101-1 TREATMENT OF CLOSTRIDIAL INFECTIONS

Condition	Antibiotic Treatment	Penicillin Allergy	Adjunctive Treatment/Note
Wound contamination	None	—	—
Polymicrobial anaerobic infections involving clostridia (e.g., abdominal wall, gynecologic)	Ampicillin (2 g IV q4h) *plus* Clindamycin (600–900 mg IV q6–8h) *plus* Ciprofloxacin (400 mg IV q6–8 h)	Vancomycin (1 g IV q12h) *plus* Metronidazole (500 mg IV q6h) *plus* Ciprofloxacin (400 mg IV q6–8h)	Empirical therapy should be initiated. Therapy should be based on Gram's stain and culture results and on sensitivity data when available. Add gram-negative coverage if indicated.
Clostridial sepsis	Penicillin (3–4 mU IV q4–6h) *plus* Clindamycin (600–900 mg IV q6–8h)	Clindamycin alone *or* Metronidazole *or* Vancomycin As for polymicrobial anaerobic infections (see above)	Transient bacteremia without signs of systemic toxicity may be clinically insignificant.
Gas gangrene	Penicillin G (4 mU IV q4–6 h) *plus* Clindamycin (600–900 mg IV q6–8h)	Cefoxitin (2 g IV q6h) *plus* Clindamycin (600–900 mg IV q6–8h)	Emergent surgical exploration and thorough debridement are extremely important. Hyperbaric oxygen therapy may be considered after surgery and antibiotic treatment have been initiated.

and facultative bacteria) and occur when organisms penetrate a previously sterile site that has a reduced oxidation-reduction potential—e.g., from tissue ischemia, trauma, surgery, perforated viscus, shock, or aspiration. Bacterial synergy, bacterial virulence factors, and mechanisms of abscess formation are factors involved in the pathogenesis of anaerobic infections.

- Anaerobes account for 0.5–12% of all cases of bacteremia, with *B. fragilis* isolated in 35–80% of these cases.

Clinical Manifestations

The clinical presentation of anaerobic infections depends, in part, on the anatomic location affected.

- *Mouth, head, and neck infections*: Odontogenic infections (e.g., dental caries, periodontal disease, gingivitis) are common, can spread locally, and may be life-threatening.

  – Acute necrotizing ulcerative gingivitis (trench mouth, Vincent's stomatitis) is associated with bleeding tender gums, foul breath, and ulceration with gray exudates, often affecting malnourished children, pts with leukemia, or pts with a debilitating illness. Widespread destruction of bone and soft tissue can develop. Lesions heal but leave disfiguring defects.

  – Acute necrotizing infection of the pharynx is associated with ulcerative gingivitis. Pts have a sore throat, foul breath, fever, a choking sensation, and tonsillar pillars that are swollen, red, ulcerated, and covered with a gray membrane. Aspiration of infected material can lead to a lung abscess.

  – Peripharyngeal infections include peritonsillar abscess (*quinsy*; caused by a mixed flora including anaerobes and group A streptococci) and submandibular space infection (*Ludwig's angina*), which arises from the second and third molars in 80% of cases and is associated with swelling (which can lead to respiratory obstruction), pain, trismus, and displacement of the tongue.

  – Chronic sinusitis and otitis (Chap. 64) are commonly due to anaerobes.

  – Complications of anaerobic mouth, head, and neck infections include Lemierre's syndrome, osteomyelitis, CNS infections (e.g., brain abscess, epidural abscess, subdural empyema), mediastinitis, pleuro-pulmonary infections, and hematogenous dissemination.

    • Lemierre's syndrome, which is typically due to *Fusobacterium necrophorum*, is an acute oropharyngeal infection with secondary septic thrombophlebitis of the internal jugular vein and frequent metastasis, most commonly to the lung.

    • Pleuropulmonary infections include aspiration pneumonia (which is difficult to distinguish from chemical pneumonitis due to aspiration of gastric juices), necrotizing pneumonitis, lung abscesses, and empyema. Bacterial aspiration pneumonia is associated with a depressed gag reflex, impaired swallowing, or altered mental status; anaerobic lung abscess usually arises from a dental source.

- *Intraabdominal infections*: See Chap. 90.

- *Pelvic infections*: See Chap. 92 for more details. Anaerobes, typically in combination with coliforms, are isolated from most women with genital tract infections (e.g., Bartholin gland abscess, salpingitis, tuboovarian abscess, endometritis) that are not caused by a sexually transmitted pathogen. The major anaerobic pathogens are *Bacteroides fragilis*, *Prevotella* species (*bivia, disiens, melaninogenica*), anaerobic cocci, and *Clostridium* species.

- *Skin and soft tissue infections*: See Chap. 93 for more details. These infections most frequently occur at sites prone to contamination with feces or with upper airway secretions.

TABLE 101-2 TREATMENT OF SERIOUS INFECTIONS DUE TO COMMONLY ENCOUNTERED ANAEROBIC GRAM-NEGATIVE RODS

First-Line Therapy	Dose	Schedule[a]
Metronidazole[b]	500 mg	q6h
Ticarcillin/clavulanic acid	3.1 g	q4h
Piperacillin/tazobactam	3.375 g	q6h
Imipenem	0.5 g	q6h
Meropenem	1.0 g	q8h

[a]See disease-specific chapters in HPIM-18 for recommendations on duration of therapy.
[b]Should generally be used in conjunction with drugs active against aerobic or facultative organisms.
Note: All drugs are given by the IV route.

- *Bone and joint infections*: Anaerobic bone and joint infections usually occur adjacent to soft tissue infections. Actinomycosis is the leading cause of anaerobic bone infections worldwide; *Fusobacterium* species are the most common anaerobic cause of septic arthritis.

Diagnosis

The three critical steps in successfully culturing anaerobic bacteria from clinical samples are (1) proper specimen collection, with avoidance of contamination by normal flora; (2) rapid specimen transport to the microbiology laboratory in anaerobic transport media; and (3) proper specimen handling. A foul odor is often indicative (and nearly pathognomonic) of an anaerobic infection.

TREATMENT Mixed Anaerobic Infections

- Appropriate treatment requires antibiotic administration (Table 101-2), surgical resection or debridement of devitalized tissues, and drainage.
  - Given that most infections involving anaerobes also include aerobic organisms, therapeutic regimens should include agents active against both classes of organisms.
  - Infections above the diaphragm usually reflect the orodental flora, which includes many organisms that produce β-lactamase. Accordingly, the recommended regimens include clindamycin, a β-lactam/β-lactamase inhibitor combination, or metronidazole in combination with a drug active against microaerophilic and aerobic streptococci.
  - Infections below the diaphragm must be treated with agents active against *Bacteroides* species, such as metronidazole, β-lactam/β-lactamase inhibitor combinations, or carbapenems. Treatment should also cover the aerobic gram-negative flora, including enterococci (e.g., ampicillin or vancomycin) when indicated.
- Pts with anaerobic infections that fail to respond to treatment or that relapse should be reassessed, with consideration of additional surgical drainage or debridement. Superinfection with resistant gram-negative facultative or aerobic bacteria should also be considered.

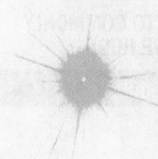

For a more detailed discussion, see Thwaites CL, Yen LM: Tetanus, Chap. 140, p. 1197; Sobel J, Maslanka S: Botulism, Chap. 141, p. 1200; Bryant AE, Stevens DL: Gas Gangrene and Other Clostridial Infections, Chap. 142, p. 1204; and Kasper DL, Cohen-Poradosu R: Infections Due to Mixed Anaerobic Organisms, Chap. 164, p. 1331, in HPIM-18.

CHAPTER 102
Nocardiosis and Actinomycosis

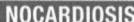

NOCARDIOSIS

Microbiology

Nocardiae are branching, beaded, gram-positive filaments that usually give positive results with modified acid-fast stains. These saprophytic aerobic actinomycetes are common in soil.

- Nine species or species complexes are most commonly associated with human disease.
- Speciation of nocardiae is precluded in most clinical laboratories because it is nearly impossible without molecular phylogenetic techniques.
- *Nocardia brasiliensis* is most often associated with localized skin lesions.

Epidemiology

Nocardiosis occurs worldwide and has an incidence of ~0.375 cases per 100,000 persons in Western countries. The risk of disease is greater than usual among persons who have deficient cell-mediated immunity—e.g., that associated with lymphoma, transplantation, glucocorticoid therapy, or HIV infection with <250 CD4+ T cells/μL.

Pathogenesis

Pneumonia and disseminated disease follow inhalation of fragmented bacterial mycelia.

- Nocardiosis causes abscesses with neutrophilic infiltration and necrosis.
- Organisms have multiple mechanisms for surviving within phagocytes.

Clinical Manifestations

- *Respiratory tract disease*: Pneumonia is usually subacute, presenting over days to weeks, but can be acute in immunocompromised pts.

  - A prominent cough productive of small amounts of thick purulent sputum, fever, anorexia, weight loss, and malaise are common; dyspnea, hemoptysis, and pleuritic chest pain are less common.
  - CXR may demonstrate single or multiple nodular infiltrates of varying sizes that tend to cavitate. Empyema is noted in one-quarter of cases.
  - Extrapulmonary disease is documented in >50% of cases.

- *Extrapulmonary disease*: In 20% of cases of disseminated disease, lung disease is absent.
  - Nocardial dissemination manifests as subacute abscesses in brain (most commonly), skin, kidneys, bone, and/or muscle.
  - Brain abscesses are usually supratentorial, are often multiloculated, can be single or multiple, and tend to burrow into ventricles or extend into the subarachnoid space.
  - Meningitis is uncommon, and nocardiae are difficult to recover from CSF.
- *Disease following transcutaneous inoculation*: usually presents as cellulitis, lymphocutaneous disease, or actinomycetoma
  - *Cellulitis* presents 1–3 weeks after a break in the skin (often with contamination by soil).
    - The firm, tender, erythematous, warm, and nonfluctuant lesions may involve underlying structures, but dissemination is rare.
    - *N. brasiliensis* and species in the *N. otitidiscaviarum* complex are most common in cellulitis.
  - *Lymphocutaneous* disease resembles sporotrichosis and presents as a pyodermatous nodule at the inoculation site, with central ulceration and purulent or honey-colored discharge.
    - Subcutaneous nodules often appear along lymphatics that drain the primary lesion.
  - *Actinomycetoma* progresses from a nodular swelling at the site of local trauma (typically on the feet or hands, although other sites can be affected) to fistula formation; dissemination is rare.
    - The discharge is serous or purulent and can contain granules consisting of masses of mycelia.
    - Lesions, which spread slowly along fascial planes to involve adjacent skin and SC tissue and bone, can cause extensive deformity after months or years.
- *Eye disease*: Endophthalmitis can occur after eye surgery or during disseminated disease.

Diagnosis

- Sputum or pus should be examined microscopically and by culture for the presence of nocardiae. In pts with nocardial pneumonia, sputum smears are often negative, and bronchoscopy may be needed to obtain adequate specimens.
  - Cultures take 2–4 weeks to yield the organism. To maximize the likelihood of isolation, the laboratory should be alerted if nocardiosis is being considered.
  - Sputum cultures positive for nocardiae should be assumed to reflect disease in immunocompromised hosts, but may represent colonization in immunocompetent pts.
- Discharge from lesions suspected to be an actinomycetoma should be examined for granules, the appearance of which can help differentiate this diagnosis from eumycetoma (cases involving fungi) and botryomycosis (cases involving cocci or bacilli).
  - Granules from actinomycetomas consist of fine filaments (0.5–1 μm wide) radiating from a central core.

- In contrast, granules from eumycetoma cases have broader filaments (2–5 μm wide) encased in a matrix, and those of botryomycosis are loose masses of bacteria.
- Brain imaging should be considered in pts with pulmonary or disseminated disease.

TREATMENT Nocardiosis

- Sulfonamides are the empirical drugs of choice, and trimethoprim-sulfamethoxazole (TMP-SMX; 10–20 mg of TMP/kg qd and 50–100 mg of SMX/kg qd initially, with later reduction to 5 and 25 mg/kg qd, respectively) may be more effective than sulfonamides alone.
  - Susceptibility testing, particularly in severe cases or cases failing to improve, can guide alternative treatments and should be performed at reference labs (e.g., the Mycobacteria/Nocardia Laboratory at the University of Texas Health Science Center; phone, 903-877-7685).
  - Alternative oral agents that are often effective include minocycline, linezolid (whose long-term use is complicated by side effects), amoxicillin/clavulanic acid, and fluoroquinolones.
  - Effective parenteral agents include amikacin, ceftriaxone, cefotaxime, and imipenem.
- Pts with severe disease are initially treated with a combination of TMP-SMX, amikacin, and either ceftriaxone or imipenem. After definite clinical improvement, the regimen can usually be simplified to a single oral agent.
- Surgical management of nocardial infections is similar to that of other bacterial diseases.
  - Brain abscesses that are large or unresponsive to antibiotics should be aspirated.
  - Medical therapy is generally sufficient for actinomycetomas.
- Relapse is common.
  - Long courses of therapy are required (Table 102-1).
  - Pts should be followed for at least 6 months after therapy is complete.

ACTINOMYCOSIS

Microbiology

Actinomycosis is caused by anaerobic or microaerophilic bacteria, primarily of the genus *Actinomyces* (e.g., *A. israelii, A. naeslundii, A. odontolyticus*), that colonize the mouth, colon, and vagina. Most infections are polymicrobial, but the role of other species in the pathogenesis of the disease is unclear.

Epidemiology

Actinomycosis is associated with poor dental hygiene, prolonged use of intrauterine contraceptive devices (IUCDs), and treatment with bisphosphonates.

TABLE 102-1 TREATMENT DURATION FOR NOCARDIOSIS

Disease	Duration
Pulmonary or systemic	
Intact host defenses	6–12 months
Deficient host defenses	12 months[a]
CNS disease	12 months[b]
Cellulitis, lymphocutaneous syndrome	2 months
Osteomyelitis, arthritis, laryngitis, sinusitis	4 months
Actinomycetoma	6–12 months after clinical cure
Keratitis	Topical: until apparent cure
	Systemic: until 2–4 months after apparent cure

[a]In some pts with AIDS and CD4+ T lymphocyte counts of <200/μL or with chronic granulomatous disease, therapy for pulmonary or systemic disease must be continued indefinitely.
[b]If all apparent diseased CNS tissue has been excised, the duration of therapy may be reduced to 6 months.

Pathogenesis

After disruption of the mucosal barrier, resident *Actinomyces* can infect locally and spread contiguously in a slow progressive manner, ignoring tissue planes. The hallmark of actinomycosis is the development of single or multiple indurated lesions with fibrotic walls often described as "wooden." Central necrosis of lesions with neutrophils and sulfur granules is virtually diagnostic of the disease.

Clinical Manifestations

- *Oral-cervicofacial disease*: Infection starts as a soft-tissue swelling, abscess, or mass, often at the angle of the jaw, with occasional contiguous extension to the brain, cervical spine, or thorax. Pain, fever, and leukocytosis are variable. Radiation therapy and particularly bisphosphonate treatment are associated with actinomycosis of the maxilla and mandible.
- *Thoracic disease*: The pulmonary parenchyma and/or pleural space is usually involved. Chest pain, fever, and weight loss are common.
  - Radiographic studies demonstrate a mass lesion or pneumonia. Cavitary disease or hilar adenopathy may occur, and >50% of pts have pleural thickening, effusion, or empyema.
  - Lesions cross fissures or pleura and may involve the mediastinum, contiguous bone, or the chest wall. In the absence of these findings, the disease is often mistaken for a neoplasm or for pneumonia.
- *Abdominal disease*: The diagnosis is challenging given that it may not present clinically until months or years after the initial event (e.g., appendicitis, diverticulitis, bowel surgery) and that any abdominal organ or region can be involved.

- The disease usually presents as an abscess, mass, or lesion fixed to underlying tissue and is often mistaken for cancer.
- Sinus tracts to the abdominal wall, perianal region, or other organs may develop and mimic inflammatory bowel disease. Recurrent disease or a wound or fistula that fails to heal suggests actinomycosis.

- *Pelvic disease*: Pelvic actinomycosis is often associated with IUCDs that have been in place for >1 year. The presentation is indolent and may follow removal of the device.
  - Pts have fever, weight loss, abdominal pain, and abnormal vaginal bleeding or discharge. Endometritis progresses to pelvic masses or tuboovarian abscess.
  - When there are no symptoms and *Actinomyces*-like organisms are identified on Papanicolaou-stained specimens, the pt should undergo close follow-up but the IUCD should be not removed.
- *Miscellaneous sites*: Actinomycosis can involve musculoskeletal tissue, soft tissue, or (rarely) the CNS. Hematogenous dissemination, most commonly to the lungs and liver, can occur.

Diagnosis

Actinomycosis should be considered when a chronic progressive process with mass-like features crosses tissue boundaries, a sinus tract develops, and/or the pt has evidence of a refractory or relapsing infection despite short courses of antibiotics.

- Aspirations, biopsies, or surgical excision may be required to obtain material for diagnosis.
- Microscopic identification of sulfur granules (an in vivo matrix of bacteria, calcium phosphate, and host material) in pus or tissues establishes the diagnosis.
- Cultures usually require 5–7 days to become positive but may take 2–4 weeks; even a single antibiotic dose can affect the yield of cultures.

TREATMENT Actinomycosis

- For serious infection and bulky disease, IV therapy for 2–6 weeks (usually with penicillin, 18–24 million units IV daily) followed by oral therapy for 6–12 months (e.g., with penicillin or ampicillin) is suggested.
  - Less extensive disease, particularly that involving the oral-cervicofacial region, may be cured with a shorter course.
  - If treatment is extended beyond the point of resolution of measurable disease (as quantified by CT or MRI), relapse is minimized.
- Suitable alternative agents include the tetracyclines (e.g., doxycycline or minocycline, 100 mg PO/IV q12h) or clindamycin (900 mg IV q8h or 300–450 mg PO q6h).

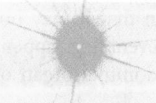

For a more detailed discussion, see Filice GA: Nocardiosis, Chap. 162, p. 1322; and Russo TA: Actinomycosis, Chap. 163, p. 1326, in HPIM-18.

CHAPTER **103**
Tuberculosis and Other Mycobacterial Infections

TUBERCULOSIS
■ MICROBIOLOGY

Tuberculosis (TB) is caused by organisms of the *Mycobacterium tuberculosis* complex, which includes *M. tuberculosis*, the most common and important agent of human mycobacterial disease, and *M. bovis*, which (like several other mycobacterial species) is acquired via ingestion of unpasteurized milk. *M. tuberculosis* is a thin aerobic bacillus that is neutral on Gram's staining but that, once stained, is acid-fast; i.e., it cannot be decolorized by acid alcohol because of the cell wall's high content of mycolic acids and other lipids.

■ EPIDEMIOLOGY

Approximately 9.4 million new cases of TB occurred worldwide in 2009, with ~1.7 million TB-related deaths in 2008—mostly in low-income countries. Globally, TB rates are stable or falling.

- In the United States, TB primarily affects HIV-infected adults, immigrants, the elderly, and disadvantaged/marginalized populations.
- Multidrug-resistant (MDR; resistant to at least isoniazid and rifampin) and extensively drug-resistant (XDR; resistant to isoniazid, rifampin, fluoroquinolones, and either amikacin, kanamycin, or capreomycin) isolates of *M. tuberculosis* are increasing in frequency; ~440,000 cases of MDR-TB may have emerged in 2008, of which ~10% were probably XDR.
- Disease from a pt with pulmonary TB is spread by droplet nuclei that are aerosolized by coughing, sneezing, or speaking.
  - Droplets <5–10 μm in diameter may be suspended in air for several hours.
  - Transmission is determined by the intimacy and duration of contact with a pt with TB, the degree of infectiousness of the pt, and the shared environment.
  - Pts with cavitary or laryngeal disease are most infectious, with as many as 10^5–10^7 acid-fast bacilli (AFB)/mL of sputum.
- Risk factors for development of active disease after *M. tuberculosis* infection include recent acquisition (within the preceding year), comorbidity (e.g., HIV disease, diabetes, silicosis, immunosuppression, gastrectomy), malnutrition, tobacco smoking, and presence of fibrotic lesions.

■ PATHOGENESIS

AFB that reach alveoli are ingested by macrophages. The bacilli impair phagosome maturation, multiply, lyse the macrophages, and spread to regional lymph nodes, from which they may disseminate throughout the body. These initial stages of infection are generally asymptomatic and induce cellular and humoral immunity.

- About 2–4 weeks after infection, a tissue-damaging response resulting from delayed-type hypersensitivity [the basis for tuberculin skin testing (TST)] destroys nonactivated macrophages that contain multiplying bacilli, and a macrophage-activating response activates cells capable of killing AFB. A granuloma forms at the site of the primary lesion and at sites of dissemination. The lesions can then either heal by fibrosis or undergo further evolution. Despite "healing," viable bacilli can remain dormant within macrophages or in necrotic material for years.
- Cell-mediated immunity confers partial protection against TB. Cytokines secreted by alveolar macrophages contribute to disease manifestations, granuloma formation, and mycobacterial killing.

■ CLINICAL MANIFESTATIONS

TB is classified as pulmonary, extrapulmonary, or both.

Pulmonary TB

TB is limited to the lungs in >80% of HIV-negative pts. Primary disease may cause no or mild symptoms (fever and occasional pleuritic chest pain) in contrast to the prolonged disease course that is common in postprimary or adult-type disease.

- Primary disease is frequently located in the middle and lower lobes. The primary lesion usually heals spontaneously, and a calcified nodule (Ghon lesion) remains.
  - Transient hilar and paratracheal lymphadenopathy is common.
  - In immunosuppressed pts and children, primary disease may progress rapidly to significant clinical disease, with cavitation, pleural effusions, and hematogenous dissemination (miliary disease).
- Adult-type disease presents initially with nonspecific and insidious symptoms, such as diurnal fever, night sweats, weight loss, anorexia, malaise, and weakness.
  - As the disease progresses, pts develop cough and purulent sputum production, often with blood streaking. Extensive cavitation may develop, with occasional massive hemoptysis following erosion of a vessel located in the wall of a cavity.
  - Disease is usually localized to the apical and posterior segments of the upper lobes and the superior segments of the lower lobes.

Extrapulmonary TB

Any site in the body can be involved, but the most commonly affected sites are (in order of frequency) the lymph nodes, pleura, genitourinary tract, bones and joints, meninges, peritoneum, and pericardium. Up to two-thirds of HIV-infected pts with TB have extrapulmonary disease.

- *Lymphadenitis* occurs in 35% of extrapulmonary TB cases, especially among HIV-infected pts. Painless swelling of cervical and supraclavicular nodes (scrofula) is typical.
  - Nodes are discrete early on but can develop into a matted nontender mass with a fistulous tract.
  - Fine-needle aspiration or surgical-excision biopsy of the node is required for diagnosis. Cultures are positive in 70–80% of cases.

- *Pleural involvement* is common and results from a hypersensitivity response to mycobacterial antigens or contiguous spread of parenchymal inflammation.
  - Fluid is straw-colored and exudative, with protein levels >50% of those in serum, normal to low glucose levels, a usual pH of ~7.3 (occasionally <7.2), and pleocytosis (500–6000 cells/μL). The pleural concentration of adenosine deaminase, if low, virtually excludes TB.
  - Pleural biopsy is often required for diagnosis, with up to 80% of biopsy cultures positive. Direct smears and cultures of pleural fluid are less sensitive.
  - Empyema is an uncommon complication of pulmonary TB and results from rupture of a cavity with many bacilli into the pleural space. In these cases, direct smears and cultures are often positive, and surgical drainage is usually required in addition to chemotherapy.
- In *genitourinary disease*, local symptoms predominate (e.g., frequency, dysuria, hematuria, abdominal or flank pain), and up to 75% of pts have a CXR demonstrating previous or concomitant pulmonary disease. Disease is occasionally identified only after severe destructive lesions of the kidneys have developed.
  - In >90% of cases, urinalysis shows pyuria and hematuria with negative bacterial cultures.
  - Mycobacterial culture of three morning urine specimens is diagnostic in 90% of cases.
- Weight-bearing joints (spine, hips, and knees) are the most common sites of *skeletal disease*.
  - Spinal TB (Pott's disease) often involves two or more adjacent vertebral bodies; in adults, lower thoracic/upper lumbar vertebrae are usually affected. Disease spreads to adjacent vertebral bodies, later affecting the intervertebral disk and causing collapse of vertebral bodies in advanced disease (kyphosis, gibbus). Paravertebral cold abscesses may form.
- *Meningitis* occurs most often in young children and HIV-seropositive pts. Disease typically evolves over 1–2 weeks and often involves paresis of cranial nerves (particularly of ocular nerves). The ultimate evolution is toward coma, with hydrocephalus and intracranial hypertension.
  - CSF can have a high lymphocyte count, an elevated protein level, and a low glucose concentration. Cultures are positive in 80% of cases. PCR is ~80% sensitive but gives a false-positive result 10% of the time.
  - Neurologic sequelae are seen in ~25% of treated pts; adjunctive glucocorticoids enhance survival among pts >14 years of age, but do not reduce the frequency of neurologic sequelae.
- *Gastrointestinal disease* can affect any portion of the GI tract (with the terminal ileum and cecum most commonly involved), causing abdominal pain, obstruction, hematochezia, and often a palpable mass. TB peritonitis can occur after spread of the organism from ruptured lymph nodes and intraabdominal organs; peritoneal biopsy is usually required for diagnosis.

- *Pericarditis* is characterized by an acute or subacute onset of fever, dull retrosternal pain, and sometimes a friction rub. Effusion is common. Chronic constrictive pericarditis is a potentially fatal complication, even in treated pts. Adjunctive glucocorticoids remain controversial; no conclusive data demonstrate a benefit.
- *Miliary disease* arises from hematogenous spread of *M. tuberculosis* throughout the body. Symptoms are nonspecific, and small (1- to 2-mm) granulomas may develop in many organs. Hepatomegaly, splenomegaly, lymphadenopathy, and choroidal tubercles of the eye may occur.

HIV-Associated TB

The manifestations of TB vary with the stage of HIV infection. When cell-mediated immunity is only partly compromised, pulmonary TB presents as typical upper-lobe cavitary disease. In late HIV infection, a primary TB–like pattern may be evident, with diffuse interstitial or miliary infiltrates, little or no cavitation, and intrathoracic lymphadenopathy.

- Extrapulmonary disease occurs frequently; common forms include lymphadenitis, meningitis, pleuritis, pericarditis, mycobacteremia, and disseminated disease.
- Immune reconstitution inflammatory syndrome (IRIS), which may occur 1–3 months after initiation of antiretroviral therapy, may exacerbate the signs and symptoms of TB.

■ DIAGNOSIS

The key to diagnosis is a high index of suspicion.

- AFB microscopy of diagnostic specimens—i.e., light microscopy of specimens stained with Ziehl-Neelsen basic fuchsin dyes or fluorescence microscopy of samples stained with auramine-rhodamine—can provide a presumptive diagnosis. In suspected pulmonary TB, 2 or 3 sputum samples should be examined.
- Definitive diagnosis requires growth of *M. tuberculosis* in culture or identification of the organism's DNA in clinical samples.
    - Liquid media and speciation by molecular methods have decreased the time required for diagnostic confirmation to 2–3 weeks (from 4–8 weeks).
    - Nucleic acid amplification is useful not only for rapid confirmation of TB in AFB-positive specimens but also for diagnosis of AFB-negative pulmonary and extrapulmonary TB.
- Drug susceptibility can be assessed via indirect testing on solid media (which takes ≥8 weeks), direct testing in liquid media (which takes ~3 weeks), or PCR (which can provide results within hours).
- TST is of limited value in active disease because of low sensitivity and specificity but is the most widely used screening test for latent TB infection.
- Interferon γ release assays (IGRAs) measure the release of interferon γ by T cells after stimulation with TB-specific antigens and are more specific for *M. tuberculosis* than is TST.
    - In low-incidence settings, IGRAs may be more sensitive than TST.
    - In high TB- and/or HIV-burden settings, the performance of IGRAs has varied greatly.

TREATMENT Tuberculosis

DRUGS

First-Line Agents

- *Rifampin*: Rifampin is the most important and potent antituberculous agent. The standard dosage in adults is 600 mg/d.
  - The drug distributes well throughout body tissues, including inflamed meninges. It turns body fluids (e.g., urine, saliva, tears) red-orange and is excreted through bile and the enterohepatic circulation.
  - Rifampin is usually well tolerated; adverse events are infrequent and generally mild.
  - Of note, rifampin is a potent inducer of the hepatic cytochrome P450 system and decreases the half-life of many other drugs.
- *Isoniazid*: Isoniazid is a critical drug for active and latent TB disease. The usual adult dosage is 300 mg/d or 900 mg twice per week.
  - Isoniazid is distributed well throughout the body and infected tissues, including CSF and caseous granulomas.
  - The most important toxicities are hepatotoxicity and peripheral neuropathy.
    - Isoniazid-associated hepatitis is idiosyncratic and increases with age and alcohol use and in the postpartum period.
    - Because peripheral neuropathy can result from interference with pyridoxine metabolism, pyridoxine (25–50 mg/d) should be given to pts with other risk factors for neuropathy, such as diabetes, alcohol abuse, or malnutrition.
- *Ethambutol*: The least potent first-line agent, ethambutol is synergistic with the other drugs in the standard first-line regimen. Ethambutol is usually given at a dosage of 15 mg/kg daily.
  - The drug is distributed throughout the body but reaches only low levels in CSF.
  - This agent can cause dose-dependent optic neuritis, producing central scotoma and impairing both visual acuity and the ability to see green.
- *Pyrazinamide*: The usual dosage is 15–30 mg/kg daily (maximum, 2 g/d). The drug distributes well throughout the body, including the CSF.
- Hyperuricemia that can be managed conservatively is common.
- Clinical gout is rare.

Other Effective Agents

- *Streptomycin*: The usual adult dose is 0.5–1.0 g IM daily or 5 times per week. Streptomycin causes ototoxicity (primarily vestibulotoxicity) but is less nephrotoxic than other aminoglycosides.
- *Rifabutin*: Rifabutin has fewer drug interactions than rifampin and is active in vitro against some rifampin-resistant strains of *M. tuberculosis*. Rifabutin reaches tissue concentrations 5 to 10 times higher than those in plasma and has a much longer half-life than rifampin. The drug is well tolerated, and its adverse effects are dose related.

- *Rifapentine*: Rifapentine is similar to rifampin but can be given once or twice weekly. This drug is not approved for the treatment of HIV-infected pts because of elevated rates of relapse.

Second-Line Agents

- *Fluoroquinolones*: Levofloxacin, gatifloxacin (no longer marketed in the United States because of its severe toxicity), and moxifloxacin have solid, broad antimycobacterial activity. Ciprofloxacin is no longer recommended for treatment of TB because of poor efficacy.
- Other agents are used uncommonly but may be needed in disease caused by resistant strains of *M. tuberculosis*.

REGIMENS

See Table 103-1.

- During the initial phase, the majority of tubercle bacilli are killed, symptoms resolve, and usually the pt becomes noninfectious. The continuation phase is required to eliminate persisting mycobacteria and prevent relapse.
- Nonadherence to the regimen is the most important impediment to cure. Directly observed treatment (especially during the initial 2 months) and fixed drug-combination products should be used if possible.
- Bacteriologic evaluation is the preferred method of monitoring response to treatment.
  - Virtually all pts should have negative sputum cultures after 3 months of treatment. If the culture remains positive, treatment failure and drug resistance should be suspected.
  - With extrapulmonary TB, bacteriologic monitoring may not be feasible. In these cases, the response to treatment must be assessed clinically and radiographically.
- Drug resistance may be either primary (i.e., present in a strain prior to therapy) or acquired (i.e., arising during treatment because of an inadequate regimen or noncompliance).
- Close monitoring for drug toxicity should take place during treatment and should include baseline LFTs and monthly questioning about possible hepatitis symptoms. High-risk pts (e.g., older pts, pts who use alcohol daily) should have LFT values monitored during treatment.

  For pts with symptomatic hepatitis and those with marked (five- to sixfold) elevations in serum levels of aspartate aminotransferase, treatment should be stopped and drugs reintroduced one at a time after liver function has returned to normal.
- Three important considerations are relevant to TB treatment in HIV-infected pts: an increased frequency of paradoxical reactions, interactions between antiretroviral agents and rifamycins, and development of rifampin monoresistance with widely spaced intermittent treatments.

TABLE 103-1 RECOMMENDED REGIMENS FOR TREATMENT OF TB

Indication	Initial Phase		Continuation Phase	
	Duration, Months	Drugs	Duration, Months	Drugs
New smear- or culture-positive cases	2	HRZE[a,b]	4	HR[a,c,d]
New culture-negative cases	2	HRZE[a]	4	HR[a]
Pregnancy	2	HRE[e]	7	HR
Relapses and treatment default (pending susceptibility testing)	3	HRZES[f]	5	HRE
Failures[g]	—	—	—	—
Resistance (or intolerance) to H	Throughout (6)	RZE[h]		
Resistance (or intolerance) to R	Throughout (12–18)	HZEQ[i]		
Resistance to H + R	Throughout (at least 20 months)	ZEQ + S (or another injectable agent[j])		
Resistance to all first-line drugs	Throughout (at least 20 months)	1 injectable agent[j] + 3 of these 4: ethionamide, cycloserine, Q, PAS		
Intolerance to Z	2	HRE	7	HR

[a]All drugs can be given daily or intermittently (three times weekly throughout). A twice-weekly regimen after 2–8 weeks of daily therapy during the initial phase is sometimes used, although it is not recommended by the WHO.

[b]Streptomycin can be used in place of ethambutol but is no longer considered a first-line drug by the ATS/IDSA/CDC.

[c]The continuation phase should be extended to 7 months for pts with cavitary pulmonary TB who remain sputum culture–positive after the initial phase of treatment.

[d]HIV-negative pts with noncavitary pulmonary TB who have negative sputum AFB smears after the initial phase of treatment can be given once-weekly rifapentine/isoniazid in the continuation phase.

[e]The 6-month regimen with pyrazinamide can probably be used safely during pregnancy and is recommended by the WHO and the International Union Against Tuberculosis and Lung Disease. If pyrazinamide is not included in the initial treatment regimen, the minimal duration of therapy is 9 months.

[f]Streptomycin should be discontinued after 2 months. Drug susceptibility results will determine the best regimen option.

[a]The regimen is tailored according to the results of drug susceptibility tests. The availability of rapid molecular methods to identify drug resistance allows initiation of a proper regimen at the start of treatment.

[b]A fluoroquinolone may strengthen the regimen for pts with extensive disease.

[c]Streptomycin for the initial 2 months may strengthen the regimen for pts with extensive disease.

[d]Amikacin, kanamycin, or capreomycin. All these agents should be used for at least 6 months and for 4 months after culture conversion. If susceptibility is confirmed, streptomycin could be used as the injectable agent.

Abbreviations: E, ethambutol; H, isoniazid; PAS, para-aminosalicylic acid; Q, a quinolone antibiotic; R, rifampin; S, streptomycin; Z, pyrazinamide.

■ PREVENTION

- *Vaccination*: An attenuated strain of *M. bovis*, bacille Calmette-Guérin (BCG), protects infants and young children from serious forms of TB (e.g., meningitis and miliary disease) and is recommended for routine use in countries with high TB prevalence.
- *Treatment of latent infection*: Candidates for chemoprophylaxis are identified by TST or IGRA. Positive skin tests are determined by reaction size and risk group (Table 103-2). Drug treatment should be considered for pts with evidence of latent infection (Table 103-3). Isoniazid should not be given to persons with active liver disease.

LEPROSY

■ MICROBIOLOGY AND EPIDEMIOLOGY

Leprosy is a nonfatal chronic infectious disease caused by *M. leprae*, an obligate intracellular bacterial species indistinguishable microscopically from other mycobacteria. The organism is confined to humans, armadillos (in some locales), and sphagnum moss.

- *M. leprae* cannot yet be cultured in vitro. The organism has a doubling time in mice of 2 weeks (compared with 20 min for *Escherichia coli* and 1 day for *M. tuberculosis*).
- Leprosy, which is associated with poverty and rural residence, is a disease of the developing world; its global prevalence is difficult to assess and is variously estimated at 0.6–8 million.
  - More than 80% of the world's cases occur in a few countries: India, China, Myanmar, Indonesia, Nepal, Brazil, Nigeria, and Madagascar.
  - In the U.S., ~4000 people have leprosy and 100–200 new cases are reported annually.
- The route of transmission is uncertain but may be via nasal droplets, contact with infected soil, or insect vectors.

■ CLINICAL MANIFESTATIONS

The spectrum from polar tuberculoid (TT) to polar lepromatous (LL) disease is associated with an evolution from asymmetric localized macules and plaques to nodular and indurated symmetric generalized skin manifestations, an increasing bacterial load, and loss of *M. leprae*–specific cellular immunity. Prognosis, complications, and intensity of antimicrobial therapy depend on where a pt presents on the clinical spectrum. The incubation period ranges from 2 to 40 years but is usually 5–7 years.

TABLE 103-2 TUBERCULIN REACTION SIZE AND TREATMENT OF LATENT TB INFECTION

Risk Group	Tuberculin Reaction Size, mm
HIV-infected pts or pts receiving immunosuppressive therapy	≥5
Close contacts of TB pts	≥5[a]
Pts with fibrotic lesions on CXR	≥5
Recently infected pts (≤2 years)	≥10
Pts with high-risk medical conditions[b]	≥10
Low-risk persons[c]	≥15

[a]Tuberculin-negative contacts, especially children, should receive prophylaxis for 2–3 months after contact ends and should then undergo repeat TST. Those whose results remain negative should discontinue prophylaxis. HIV-infected contacts should receive a full course of treatment regardless of TST results.

[b]Including diabetes mellitus, some hematologic and reticuloendothelial diseases, injection drug use (with HIV seronegativity), end-stage renal disease, and clinical situations associated with rapid weight loss.

[c]Except for employment purposes where longitudinal TST screening is anticipated, TST is not indicated for these low-risk persons. A decision to treat should be based on individual risk/benefit considerations.

Tuberculoid Leprosy (TL)

At the less severe end of the disease spectrum, TL results in symptoms confined to the skin and peripheral nerves.

- One or several hypopigmented macules or plaques with sharp margins that are hypesthetic and have lost sweat glands and hair follicles are present. AFB are few or absent.
- There is asymmetric enlargement of one or several peripheral nerves—most often the ulnar, posterior auricular, peroneal, and posterior tibial nerves—associated with hypesthesia and myopathy.

Lepromatous Leprosy (LL)

Pts develop symmetrically distributed skin nodules, raised plaques, and diffuse dermal infiltration that can cause leonine facies, loss of eyebrows and lashes, pendulous earlobes, and dry scaling.

- Numerous bacilli are present in skin (up to 10^9/g), nerves, and all organs except the lungs and CNS.
- Nerve enlargement and damage are usually symmetric and are due to bacillary invasion.

■ COMPLICATIONS

- *Reactional states*: These common, immunologically mediated inflammatory states cause considerable morbidity. Erythema nodosum leprosum—characterized by painful erythematous papules that resolve spontaneously in ~1 week—occurs in ~50% of pts near the LL end of the disease spectrum within 2 years of initiation of therapy.

TABLE 103-3 REVISED DRUG REGIMENS FOR TREATMENT OF LATENT TUBERCULOSIS INFECTION (LTBI) IN ADULTS

Drug	Interval and Duration	Comments[a]	Rating[b] (Evidence[c]) HIV-Negative	HIV-Infected
Isoniazid	Daily for 9 months[d,e]	In HIV-infected pts, isoniazid may be administered concurrently with nucleoside reverse transcriptase inhibitors, protease inhibitors, or NNRTIs.	A (II)	A (II)
	Twice weekly for 9 months[d,e]	DOT must be used with twice-weekly dosing.	B (II)	B (II)
	Daily for 6 months[e]	Regimen is not indicated for HIV-infected pts, those with fibrotic lesions on CXR, or children.	B (I)	C (I)
	Twice weekly for 6 months[e]	DOT must be used with twice-weekly dosing.	B (II)	C (I)
Rifampin[f]	Daily for 4 months	Regimen is used for contacts of pts with isoniazid-resistant, rifampin-susceptible TB. In HIV-infected pts, most protease inhibitors and delavirdine should not be administered concurrently with rifampin. Rifabutin, with appropriate dose adjustments, can be used with protease inhibitors (saquinavir should be augmented with ritonavir) and NNRTIs (except delavirdine). Clinicians should consult Web-based updates for the latest specific recommendations.	B (II)	B (III)

658

Rifampin plus pyrazinamide	Daily for 2 months	Regimen generally should not be offered for treatment of LTBI in either HIV-infected or HIV-negative pts.	D (II)
	Twice weekly for 2–3 months		D (III)

[a]Information on interactions with HIV-related drugs is updated frequently and is available at *www.aidsinfo.nih.gov/guidelines.*

[b]Strength of the recommendation: A. Both strong evidence of efficacy and substantial clinical benefit support recommendation for use. Should always be offered. B. Moderate evidence for efficacy or strong evidence for efficacy but only limited clinical benefit supports recommendation for use. Should generally be offered. C. Evidence for efficacy is insufficient to support a recommendation for or against use, or evidence for efficacy might not outweigh adverse consequences (e.g., drug toxicity, drug interactions) or cost of the treatment or alternative approaches. Optional. D. Moderate evidence for lack of efficacy or for adverse outcome supports a recommendation against use. Should generally not be offered. E. Good evidence for lack of efficacy or for adverse outcome supports a recommendation against use. Should never be offered.

[c]Quality of evidence supporting the recommendation: I. Evidence from at least one properly randomized controlled trial. II. Evidence from at least one well-designed clinical trial without randomization, from cohort or case-controlled analytic studies (preferably from more than one center), from multiple time-series studies, or from dramatic results in uncontrolled experiments. III. Evidence from opinions of respected authorities based on clinical experience, descriptive studies, or reports of expert committees.

[d]Recommended regimen for persons age <18 years.

[e]Recommended regimen for pregnant women.

[f]The substitution of rifapentine for rifampin is not recommended because rifapentine's safety and effectiveness have not been established for pts with LTBI.

Abbreviations: DOT, directly observed therapy; NNRTIs, nonnucleoside reverse transcriptase inhibitors.

Source: Adapted from CDC: Targeted tuberculin testing and treatment of latent tuberculosis infection. MMWR Recomm Rep 49:RR-6, 2000.

- *Extremities*: Neuropathy results in insensitivity and affects fine touch, pain, and heat receptors. The loss of distal digits in leprosy is a consequence of insensitivity, trauma, secondary infection, and—in lepromatous pts—a poorly understood and sometimes profound osteolytic process.
- *Eyes*: Owing to cranial nerve palsies, lagophthalmos and corneal insensitivity may complicate leprosy, resulting in trauma, secondary infection, and (without treatment) corneal ulcerations and opacities. Leprosy is a major cause of blindness in low-income countries.
- *Nerve abscesses*: Pts with leprosy can develop abscesses of nerves (most commonly the ulnar) and require urgent surgical decompression to prevent irreversible sequelae.

■ DIAGNOSIS

In TL, the advancing edge of a skin lesion should be biopsied. In LL, biopsy of even normal-appearing skin often yields positive results. Serology, skin testing, and PCR of the skin offer little diagnostic assistance.

TREATMENT   Leprosy

DRUGS

- Rifampin (600 mg daily or monthly) is the only agent bactericidal against *M. leprae*. See the preceding section on *M. tuberculosis* for more details on rifampin.
- Monotherapy with dapsone (50–100 mg/d) results in only a 2.5% resistance-related relapse rate.
  - A decrease in hemoglobin levels of ~1 g/dL is a common adverse effect; the sulfone syndrome (high fever, anemia, exfoliative dermatitis, and a mononucleosis-type blood picture) occurs rarely.
  - G6PD deficiency must be ruled out before therapy to avoid hemolytic anemia.
- Clofazimine (50–100 mg/d, 100 mg 3 times per week, or 300 mg monthly) is a phenazine iminoquinone dye that is weakly active against *M. leprae*. Adverse effects include red-black skin discoloration.

REGIMENS

Given the unreliability of skin smears and the lack of accessibility to histopathology in many countries in which leprosy is endemic, treatment regimens are based on the number of lesions present.

- *Paucibacillary disease* in adults (<6 skin lesions) is treated with dapsone (100 mg/d) and rifampin (600 mg monthly, supervised) for 6 months or with dapsone (100 mg/d) for 5 years. For a single lesion, a single dose of rifampin (600 mg), ofloxacin (400 mg), and minocycline (100 mg) is recommended.
- *Multibacillary disease* in adults (≥6 skin lesions) is treated with dapsone (100 mg/d) plus clofazimine (50 mg/d)—unsupervised—in addition to rifampin (600 mg monthly) plus clofazimine (300 mg monthly)—supervised—for 1–2 years.

- Some experts prefer rifampin (600 mg/d) for 3 years and dapsone (100 mg/d) for life.
- Relapse can occur years later; prolonged follow-up is needed.
- *Reactional states*
  - Lesions at risk for ulceration or in cosmetically important areas can be treated with glucocorticoids (40–60 mg/d for at least 3 months).
  - If erythema nodosum leprosum is present and persists despite two short courses of steroids (40–60 mg/d for 1–2 weeks), thalidomide (100–300 mg nightly) should be given. Because of thalidomide's teratogenicity, its use is strictly regulated.

INFECTIONS WITH NONTUBERCULOUS MYCOBACTERIA (NTM)

Mycobacteria other than those of the *M. tuberculosis* complex and *M. leprae* are referred to as *nontuberculous* or *atypical* mycobacteria and are ubiquitous in soil and water.

■ MICROBIOLOGY

NTM are broadly differentiated into rapidly and slowly growing forms (<7 days and ≥7 days, respectively). *M. abscessus*, *M. fortuitum*, and *M. chelonae* are examples of rapid growers; species such as *M. avium* and *M. intracellulare* (the *M. avium* complex, or MAC), *M. kansasii*, *M. ulcerans*, and *M. marinum* are slow growers.

■ EPIDEMIOLOGY

Most NTM cause disease in humans only rarely unless some aspect of host defense is impaired (as in bronchiectasis) or breached (as by inoculation— e.g., during liposuction or trauma). The bulk of nontuberculous mycobacterial disease in North America is due to *M. kansasii*, MAC organisms, and *M. abscessus*.

■ CLINICAL MANIFESTATIONS

Although there are many NTM species, the clinical presentations they cause can be broadly categorized by the organ system(s) affected.

- *Disseminated disease* is now quite rare; even pts with advanced HIV infection do not often develop disseminated NTM infection, given improved treatment of HIV infection and effective antimycobacterial prophylaxis.
  - Organisms typically spread from the bowel to the bone marrow and bloodstream, but disease is indolent, and it can take weeks or months for the pt to present for medical attention with malaise, fever, weight loss, organomegaly, and lymphadenopathy.
  - A child with involvement of ≥2 organ systems and no iatrogenic cause should be evaluated for defects in the interferon γ/interleukin-12 pathway.
- *Pulmonary disease* represents the most common NTM infection in industrialized countries. MAC organisms are most commonly involved in North America. Pts present with months or years of throat clearing,

nagging cough, and slowly progressive fatigue. *M. kansasii* can cause a TB-like syndrome, with hemoptysis, chest pain, and cavitary lung disease.

- Isolated *cervical lymphadenopathy* is the most common NTM infection among young children in North America and is most frequently caused by MAC organisms. The nodes are typically firm and painless and develop in the absence of systemic symptoms.

- *Skin and soft tissue disease* usually requires a break in the skin for introduction of the organism. Different NTM species are associated with specific exposures.

  – *M. fortuitum* is linked to pedicure bath–associated infections, particularly if skin abrasion (e.g., during leg shaving) has immediately preceded the pedicure.

  – Rapidly growing NTM are associated with outbreaks of infection acquired via skin contamination from surgical instruments (especially in cosmetic surgery), injections, and other procedures. These infections are typically accompanied by painful, erythematous, draining subcutaneous nodules, usually without associated fever or systemic symptoms.

  – *M. marinum* can be acquired from fish tanks, swimming pools, barnacles, and fish scales. Pts typically develop papules or ulcers ("fish-tank granuloma") that can progress to tendonitis and tender nodules on the arm in a pattern similar to that caused by *Sporothrix schenckii*. Lesions appear days or weeks after acquisition of the organism.

  – *M. ulcerans* is a waterborne organism found primarily in tropical areas, especially in Africa. Skin lesions are typically painless, clean ulcers that slough and can cause osteomyelitis.

■ DIAGNOSIS

Similar to *M. tuberculosis*, NTM can be detected on acid-fast or fluorochrome smears of clinical samples and can be cultured on mycobacterial medium. Isolation of NTM from a clinical specimen may reflect colonization and requires an assessment of the organism's clinical significance.

- Isolation of NTM from blood specimens is clear evidence of disease; many NTM species require special media and will not grow in standard blood culture medium.

- The American Thoracic Society has published guidelines for the diagnosis of pulmonary NTM disease that require the growth of NTM from 2 of 3 sputum samples, a positive bronchoalveolar lavage sample, or a pulmonary parenchyma biopsy sample with granulomatous inflammation or mycobacteria found on section and NTM in culture. Although these guidelines are specific to MAC, *M. abscessus,* and *M. kansasii*, they probably apply to other NTM as well.

- The only antibiotic susceptibility assessment indicated is testing of MAC organisms for susceptibility to clarithromycin and of *M. kansasii* for susceptibility to rifampin.

TREATMENT	Infections with NTM

Since NTM disease evolves over a long period, it is rarely necessary to begin treatment on an emergency basis before identifying the infecting species.

- MAC infection requires multidrug therapy with a macrolide (clarithromycin or azithromycin), ethambutol, and a rifamycin (rifampin or rifabutin). Therapy is prolonged, generally continuing for 12 months after culture conversion; typically, a course lasts for at least 18 months.
- *M. kansasii* lung disease is similar to TB in many ways and is also effectively treated with isoniazid (300 mg/d), rifampin (600 mg/d), and ethambutol (15 mg/kg per day).
- Extrapulmonary disease due to rapidly growing NTM is often treated successfully with a macrolide and another drug (with the choice based on in vitro susceptibility). Pulmonary disease due to *M. abscessus* is difficult to cure and often requires repeated courses that include a macrolide along with an IV-administered agent such as amikacin, a carbapenem, cefoxitin, or tigecycline.
- *M. marinum* infection is effectively treated with any combination of a macrolide, ethambutol, and a rifamycin for 1–2 months after clinical resolution of isolated soft-tissue disease; tendon and bone involvement may require longer courses in light of clinical evolution.
- Treatment of infections caused by other NTM is less well defined, but macrolides and aminoglycosides are usually effective, with other agents added as indicated.

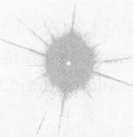

For a more detailed discussion, see Raviglione MC, O'Brien RJ: Tuberculosis, Chap. 165, p. 1340; Gelber RH: Leprosy, Chap. 166, p. 1359; Holland SM: Nontuberculous Mycobacterial Infections, Chap. 167, p. 1367; and O'Donnell MR, Saukkonen JJ: Antimycobacterial Agents, Chap. 168, p. 1371, in HPIM-18.

Chapter **104**

Lyme Disease and Other Nonsyphilitic Spirochetal Infections

LYME BORRELIOSIS

Microbiology and Epidemiology

Borrelia burgdorferi, the causative agent of Lyme disease, is a fastidious microaerophilic spirochete. The human infection Lyme borreliosis is caused primarily by three pathogenic genospecies: *B. burgdorferi sensu stricto* (hereafter referred to as *B. burgdorferi*), *Borrelia garinii*, and *Borrelia afzelii*.

- *B. burgdorferi* is the sole cause of Lyme borreliosis in the United States; all three genospecies are found in Europe, and the latter two species occur in Asia.

- Lyme disease is the most common vector-borne illness in the United States, with >25,000 cases each year.
  - *Ixodes* ticks transmit the disease.
  - *I. scapularis*, which also transmits babesiosis and anaplasmosis, is found in northeastern and midwestern states; *I. pacificus* is found in western states.
- The white-footed mouse is the preferred host for larval and nymphal ticks. Adult ticks prefer the white-tailed deer as host.
- Nymphal ticks transmit the disease to humans during the early summer months after feeding for ≥24 h.

Clinical Manifestations

Lyme disease usually begins with *erythema migrans* (EM; stage 1, localized infection) before disseminating (stage 2) or causing persistent infection (stage 3).

- *Stage 1 (localized infection)*: After an incubation period of 3–32 days, EM develops at the site of the tick bite (commonly the thigh, groin, or axilla) in 80% of pts.
  - The classic presentation is a red macule that expands slowly to form an annular lesion with a bright red outer border and central clearing. Central erythema, induration, necrosis, vesicular changes, or many red rings within an outer ring are also possible.
  - Most pts do not remember the preceding tick bite.
- *Stage 2 (disseminated infection)*: Given that some pts do not notice EM, many pts present within days or weeks after infection with secondary annular skin lesions, nonspecific systemic symptoms, neurologic deficits, or cardiac manifestations due to hematogenous spread.
  - Nonspecific symptoms include severe headache, mild neck stiffness, fever, chills, migratory musculoskeletal pain, arthralgias, malaise, and fatigue. These symptoms subside within a few weeks, even in untreated pts.
  - Neurologic deficits occur in ~15% of pts and may include meningitis; encephalitis; cranial neuritis, including bilateral facial palsy; motor or sensory radiculoneuropathy; mononeuritis multiplex; ataxia; or myelitis. Lymphocytic pleocytosis (~100 cells/μL) is found in CSF, often along with elevated protein levels and normal or slightly low glucose concentrations.
  - Cardiac involvement occurs in ~8% of pts. Atrioventricular (AV) block of fluctuating degree is most common, but acute myopericarditis is possible. Cardiac involvement usually lasts for only a few weeks but may recur.
- *Stage 3 (persistent infection)*: ~60% of untreated pts in the United States develop frank arthritis, usually consisting of intermittent attacks of oligoarticular arthritis in large joints (especially the knees) that last for weeks or months.
  - Joint-fluid cell counts range from 500 to 110,000/μL (average, 25,000/μL); the majority of the cells are neutrophils.
  - Arthritis can persist despite eradication of spirochetes.

- Chronic neurologic involvement (e.g., subtle encephalopathy affecting memory, mood, or sleep; peripheral neuropathy) is less common. In Europe, severe encephalomyelitis is seen with *B. garinii* infection.
- Acrodermatitis chronica atrophicans, a late skin manifestation, is seen in Europe and Asia and is associated with *B. afzelii* infection.

- *Chronic Lyme disease*: For months or years afterward, a small percentage of pts have pain, neurocognitive manifestations, or fatigue symptoms—a syndrome indistinguishable from chronic fatigue syndrome. There is no evidence that these symptoms are caused by active infection.

Diagnosis

Serologic evidence combined with a compatible clinical picture is the usual basis for diagnosis.

- Only 20–30% of pts have positive serologic results in acute-phase samples, whereas 70–80% have positive results in convalescent-phase samples obtained 2–4 weeks later. Of note, serologic tests do not discriminate between active and past disease.
  - Serologic analysis consisting of a two-step approach (ELISA screening with western blot confirmation for cases with positive or equivocal results) is recommended only for pts with at least an intermediate pretest likelihood of having Lyme disease.
  - IgM and IgG testing should be done in the first 2 months of illness, after which IgG testing alone is adequate.
  - CDC-adopted criteria dictate that the IgM western blot must show at least 2 of 3 defined bands and that the IgG western blot must show at least 5 of 10 defined bands to be considered positive.
- PCR is most useful for joint fluid, is less sensitive for CSF, and has little or no utility for plasma or urine.
- Although culture of the organism is possible, it is reserved primarily for research settings.

TREATMENT	Lyme Borreliosis

- Doxycycline (100 mg bid) is the agent of choice for men and non-pregnant women with localized or disseminated infection and is also effective against anaplasmosis (Chap. 105).
  - Amoxicillin (500 mg tid), cefuroxime (500 mg bid), erythromycin (250 mg qid), and newer macrolides—preferred in that order—are alternative agents.
  - Except in cases of neurologic disease and third-degree AV block, the drug can usually be taken by mouth.
  - More than 90% of pts have good outcomes with a 14-day course of treatment for localized infection or a 21-day course for disseminated infection.
- For pts with objective neurologic abnormalities (with the possible exception of isolated facial palsy), IV treatment with ceftriaxone for 14–28 days should be given. Cefotaxime or penicillin is an alternative.

- Pts with high-degree AV block (PR interval, >0.3 s) should receive IV therapy for at least part of the course; cardiac monitoring is recommended.
- Pts with Lyme arthritis should be treated with 30 days of oral doxycycline or amoxicillin.
  - For pts who do not respond to oral agents, re-treatment with IV ceftriaxone for 28 days is appropriate.
  - If joint inflammation persists after therapy but PCR testing for *B. burgdorferi* DNA in joint fluid gives negative results, anti-inflammatory agents or synovectomy may be successful.
- For pts diagnosed with chronic Lyme disease, no data demonstrate that additional antibiotic therapy is helpful.

Prophylaxis

The risk of infection with *B. burgdorferi* after a recognized tick bite is so low that antibiotic prophylaxis is not routinely indicated. However, if an attached, engorged *I. scapularis* nymph is found or if follow-up will be difficult, a single 200-mg dose of doxycycline, given within 72 h of the tick bite, effectively prevents the disease.

Prognosis

Early treatment results in an excellent prognosis. Most pts recover with minimal or no residual deficits.

ENDEMIC TREPONEMATOSES

Microbiology and Epidemiology

The endemic treponematoses—yaws (*Treponema pallidum* subspecies *pertenue*), endemic syphilis (*T. pallidum* subspecies *endemicum*), and pinta (*T. carateum*)—are nonvenereal chronic diseases acquired during childhood and caused by organisms closely related to the agent of syphilis, *T. pallidum* subspecies *pallidum*.

- Disease is transmitted by direct contact.
- The most recent WHO estimate (1997) suggested that there are 460,000 new cases per year and a prevalence of 2.5 million infected persons.
- Disease is limited to people in rural areas of developing nations and recent émigrés from these regions.

Clinical Manifestations

The major clinical distinctions made between venereal syphilis and the nonvenereal treponematoses are the apparent lack of congenital transmission and of CNS involvement in the nonvenereal infections. However, these distinctions may not be entirely accurate.

- *Yaws* is characterized by the development of one or more primary lesions ("mother yaw") followed by multiple disseminated skin lesions.
  - 3–4 weeks after acquisition of the organism, the pt develops a papule that ultimately enlarges, is associated with regional lymphadenopathy, and heals spontaneously within 6 months.

- Late gummatous lesions of the skin and long bones affect 10% of untreated persons and are similar to the destructive lesions of leprosy and leishmaniasis.

• *Endemic syphilis* is initially localized to mucocutaneous and mucosal surfaces. Pts develop an intraoral papule, which is followed by mucous patches on the oral mucosa and mucocutaneous lesions resembling the condylomata lata of secondary syphilis. Destructive gummas, osteitis, and gangosa (destruction of the nose, maxilla, palate, and pharynx) are more common in endemic syphilis than in late yaws.

• *Pinta* is the most benign of the treponemal infections in that it does not cause destructive lesions or involve tissues other than the skin. The disease has three stages that are characterized by marked changes in skin color.

Diagnosis

Diagnosis is based on clinical presentation, dark-field microscopy of scrapings from lesions, and serologic testing (as for venereal syphilis).

TREATMENT Endemic Treponematoses

Benzathine penicillin (1.2 million units for adults, 600,000 units for children <10 years of age) is the treatment of choice. Doxycycline is probably an effective alternative.

LEPTOSPIROSIS

Microbiology and Epidemiology

Leptospires are spirochetal organisms that cause an important zoonosis with a broad spectrum of clinical manifestations.

• The organisms are small enough to pass through filters used to sterilize culture medium.

• The most important sources of transmission to humans are rats, dogs, cattle, and pigs. Transmission can occur during contact with urine and other excreta (e.g., placenta, products of parturition) from infected animals or during exposure to contaminated environments.

• Only ~50–100 cases in the U.S. are passively reported annually to the CDC, but these numbers are likely to represent significant underestimates given that leptospirosis is not a notifiable disease.

Clinical Manifestations

After an average incubation period of 5–14 days, infection by *Leptospira* results in a subclinical infection, an undifferentiated febrile illness, or Weil's disease (the most severe form).

• Leptospirosis is a biphasic illness. The initial *leptospiremic* phase lasts 3–10 days and is characterized by fever. After another 3–10 days (the *immune* phase), some pts experience a return of fever, headache, and other systemic symptoms in association with the clearance of leptospires from the blood.

- Only the initial phase is responsive to antibiotic therapy.
- Nonspecific physical findings may include conjunctival suffusion, nonexudative pharyngeal erythema, muscle tenderness, rales on

lung auscultation, jaundice, meningismus, and hypo- or areflexia (particularly in the legs).

- *Weil's disease* is characterized by variable combinations of jaundice, acute renal injury, hypotension, and hemorrhage—most commonly involving the lungs. Cardiac involvement (e.g., myocarditis), severe myalgias (occasionally mimicking acute abdomen), rash, and neurologic findings (e.g., aseptic meningitis) are common.

Diagnosis

A high index of suspicion prompting elicitation of a detailed exposure history is critical and guides confirmatory testing.

- Serologic assays are the diagnostic mainstay in leptospirosis. The microscopic agglutination test is the gold standard and typically is performed only in reference laboratories, such as the CDC. Most other serologic tests use a saprophytic leptospire as the antigen and provide nonspecific results.
- Definitive diagnosis rests on demonstration of the organism by culture isolation (which takes weeks), detection of nucleic acids or antigen in body fluids (a method typically limited to research settings), or immunohistochemical visualization in tissue.
  - Leptospires can be cultured from blood and CSF during the first 7–10 days of illness.
  - Urine cultures are positive in the second week of illness and can remain positive for months or years despite antibiotic therapy.

TREATMENT   Leptospirosis

- Prompt initiation of antibiotics probably shortens the course of severe leptospirosis and prevents the progression of mild disease.
- For mild disease, oral doxycycline is the drug of choice. Azithromycin may also be effective.
- For severe disease, parenteral treatment with penicillin, ceftriaxone, or cefotaxime should be given. From a pragmatic viewpoint, severe leptospiral disease frequently requires empirical initiation of broad-spectrum parenteral therapy before the diagnosis is confirmed.

RELAPSING FEVER

Microbiology

Borrelia recurrentis causes louse-borne relapsing fever (LBRF) and is transmitted from person to person by the body louse. In this disease, spirochetes are introduced when the louse is crushed (e.g., by scratching) and the insect's infected hemolymph contaminates the skin. Tick-borne relapsing fever (TBRF), a zoonosis usually transmitted via the bite of various *Ornithodoros* ticks, is caused by multiple *Borrelia* species.

Epidemiology

TBRF is endemic in the western United States, southern British Columbia, the plateau regions of Mexico, Central and South America, the Mediterranean, Central Asia, and much of Africa. Only 13 counties have accounted for

~50% of all U.S. cases. Little is known about the epidemiology of LBRF, but it is well described in East Africa.

Clinical Manifestations

Symptoms are similar, although not identical, in the two types of relapsing fever.

- In addition to fever, pts commonly develop headaches, myalgias, chills, nausea/vomiting, and arthralgias.
  - Jaundice; CNS involvement; petechiae on the trunk, extremities, and mucous membranes; epistaxis; and blood-tinged sputum are more likely in LBRF.
  - Neurologic findings (e.g., meningitis, focal deficits, paralysis, altered sensorium) may occur in 10–30% of cases and are more common in LBRF.
- For TBRF and LBRF, the mean incubation periods are 7 and 8 days, respectively; the average durations of the first episode are 3 and 5.5 days, respectively; and the average times between the first episode and the first relapse are 7 and 9 days, respectively. Relapsing febrile episodes are typically of shorter duration than the first episode.

Diagnosis

Laboratory confirmation is made by the detection or isolation of spirochetes from blood during a febrile episode. Microscopic examination of Wright- or Giemsa-stained thick or thin blood smears or buffy coat analysis is most common.

- PCR techniques offer greater sensitivity but are limited to research settings.
- Serologic confirmation of TBRF is possible but is hampered by lack of standardization. An ELISA or an indirect fluorescent antibody assay can be performed; if positive, the results of these tests are confirmed with an immunoblot.

TREATMENT Relapsing Fever

- One dose of doxycycline (100 mg) or erythromycin (500 mg) is effective for LBRF; a 7- to 10-day course of either antibiotic is recommended for TBRF. Monitoring the pt for a Jarisch-Herxheimer reaction (an acute exacerbation of symptoms including hypotension, tachycardia, and marked elevation of body temperature) for the first 12 h after the first dose of antibiotic is recommended.
- If CSF pleocytosis is detected in the setting of meningitis or encephalitis, the pt should be treated with parenteral antibiotics.

Prognosis

LBRF has a fatality rate of 5% for treated pts; the rate is much lower for pts with TBRF.

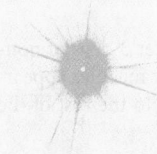

For a more detailed discussion, see Lukehart SA: Endemic Treponematoses, Chap. 170, p. 1389; Vinetz JM: Leptospirosis, Chap. 171, p. 1392; Dworkin MS: Relapsing Fever, Chap. 172, p. 1397; and Steere AC: Lyme Borreliosis, Chap. 173, p. 1401, in HPIM-18. For a discussion of syphilis, see Chap. 92 in this manual.

CHAPTER 105
Rickettsial Diseases

Microbiology

Rickettsiae are obligate intracellular gram-negative coccobacilli and short bacilli usually transmitted by tick, mite, flea, or louse vectors. Except in the case of louse-borne typhus, humans are incidental hosts.

Clinical Manifestations

The clinical manifestations of all the acute rickettsial presentations are similar during the first 5 days and consist of nonspecific symptoms: fever, headache, and myalgias with or without nausea, vomiting, and cough. As the course progresses, clinical manifestations—including occurrence of a macular, maculopapular, or vesicular rash; eschar; pneumonitis; and meningoencephalitis—vary from one disease to another. (See Table 105-1 and details below.)

TICK- AND MITE-BORNE SPOTTED FEVERS

■ ROCKY MOUNTAIN SPOTTED FEVER (RMSF)

Epidemiology

Caused by *R. rickettsii*, RMSF has the highest case-fatality rate of all rickettsial diseases.

- In the United States, the prevalence is highest in the south-central and southeastern states. Most cases occur between May and September.
- A rare presentation of fulminant RMSF is seen most often in male black pts with G6PD deficiency.
- RMSF is transmitted by different ticks in different geographic areas—e.g., the American dog tick (*Dermacentor variabilis*) transmits RMSF in the eastern two-thirds of the United States and in California, and the Rocky Mountain wood tick (*D. andersoni*) transmits RMSF in the western U.S.

Pathogenesis

Rickettsiae are inoculated by the tick after ≥6 h of feeding, spread lympho-hematogenously, and infect numerous foci of contiguous endothelial cells. Increased vascular permeability, with edema, hypovolemia, and ischemia, causes tissue and organ injury.

Clinical Manifestations

The incubation period is ~1 week (range, 2–14 days). After 3 days of non-specific symptoms, half of pts have a rash characterized by macules appearing on the wrists and ankles and subsequently spreading to the rest of the extremities and the trunk.

TABLE 105-1 FEATURES OF SELECTED RICKETTSIAL INFECTIONS

Disease	Organism	Transmission	Geographic Range	Incubation Period, Days	Duration, Days	Rash, %	Eschar, %	Lymphade-nopathy[a]
Rocky Mountain spotted fever	*Rickettsia rickettsii*	Tick bite: *Dermacentor andersoni, D. variabilis*	United States	2–14	10–20	90	<1	+
		Amblyomma cajennense, A. aureolatum	Central/South America					
		Rhipicephalus sanguineus	Mexico, Brazil, United States					
Mediterranean spotted fever	*R. conorii*	Tick bite: *R. sanguineus, R. pumilio*	Southern Europe, Africa, Middle East, Central Asia	5–7	7–14	97	50	+
Maculatum disease	*R. parkeri*	*A. maculatum*	United States, South America	2–10	?	88	94	++
African tick-bite fever	*R. africae*	Tick bite: *A. hebraeum, A. variegatum*	Sub-Saharan Africa, West Indies	4–10	?	50	90	++++
Rickettsialpox	*R. akari*	Mite bite: *Liponyssoides sanguineus*	United States, Ukraine, Turkey, Mexico, Croatia	10–17	3–11	100	90	+++
Tick-borne lymphadenopathy	*R. slovaca*	Tick bite: *Dermacentor marginatus, D. reticularis*	Europe	7–9	17–180	5	100	++++
Flea-borne spotted fever	*R. felis*	Flea (mechanism undetermined): *Ctenocephalides felis*	Worldwide	8–16	8–16	80	15	—

(continued)

671

TABLE 105-1 FEATURES OF SELECTED RICKETTSIAL INFECTIONS (CONTINUED)

Disease	Organism	Transmission	Geographic Range	Incubation Period, Days	Duration, Days	Rash, %	Eschar, %	Lymphade-nopathy[a]
Epidemic typhus	R. prowazekii	Louse feces: Pediculus humanus corporis; fleas and lice of flying squirrels; or recrudescence	Worldwide	7–14	10–18	80	None	—
Murine typhus	R. typhi	Flea feces: Xenopsylla cheopis, C. felis, others	Worldwide	8–16	9–18	80	None	—
Human monocytotropic ehrlichiosis	Ehrlichia chaffeensis	Tick bite: Amblyomma americanum, D. variabilis	United States	1–21	3–21	26	None	++
Ewingii ehrlichiosis	E. ewingii	Tick bite: A. americanum	United States				None	
Human granulocytotropic anaplasmosis	Anaplasma phagocytophilum	Tick bite: Ixodes scapularis, I. ricinus, I. pacificus, I. persulcatus	United States, Europe, Asia	4–8	3–14	Rare	None	—
Scrub typhus	Orientia tsutsugamushi	Mite bite: Leptotrombidium deliense, others	Asia, Australia, New Guinea, Pacific Islands	9–18	6–21	50	35	+++
Q fever	Coxiella burnetii	Inhalation of aerosols of infected parturition material (sheep, dogs, others), ingestion of infected milk or milk products	Worldwide	3–30	5–57	<1	None	—

[a]++++, severe; +++, marked; ++, moderate; +, present in a small portion of cases; —, not a noted feature.

- Lesions ultimately become petechial in 41–59% of pts, appearing on or after day 6 of illness in ~74% of all cases that include a rash. The palms and soles become involved after day 5 in 43% of pts but do not become involved at all in 18–64%.
- Pts may develop hypovolemia, prerenal azotemia, hypotension, non-cardiogenic pulmonary edema, renal failure, hepatic injury, and cardiac involvement with dysrhythmias. Bleeding is a rare but potentially life-threatening consequence of severe vascular damage.
- CNS involvement—manifesting as encephalitis, focal neurologic deficits, or meningoencephalitis—is an important determinant of outcome. In meningoencephalitis, CSF is notable for pleocytosis with a mononuclear cell or neutrophil predominance, increased protein levels, and normal glucose levels.
- Laboratory findings may include increased plasma levels of acute-phase reactants such as C-reactive protein, hypoalbuminemia, hyponatremia, and elevated levels of creatine kinase.

Prognosis

Without treatment, the pt usually dies in 8–15 days; fulminant RMSF can result in death within 5 days. The mortality rate is 3–5% despite the availability of effective antibiotics, mostly because of delayed diagnosis. Survivors of RMSF usually return to their previous state of health.

Diagnosis

Within the first 3 days, diagnosis is difficult, since only 3% of pts have the classic triad of fever, rash, and known history of tick exposure. When the rash appears, the diagnosis should be considered.

- Immunohistologic examination of a cutaneous biopsy sample from a rash lesion is the only useful diagnostic test during acute illness, with a sensitivity of 70% and a specificity of 100%.
- Serology, most commonly the indirect immunofluorescence assay (IFA), is usually positive 7–10 days after disease onset, and a diagnostic titer of ≥1:64 is usually documented.

TREATMENT   Rocky Mountain Spotted Fever

- Doxycycline (100 mg bid PO or IV) is the treatment of choice for both children and adults but not for pregnant women and pts allergic to this drug, who should receive chloramphenicol.
- Treatment is given until the pt is afebrile and has been improving for 2 or 3 days.

■ OTHER TICK-BORNE SPOTTED FEVERS

- *R. conorii* causes disease in southern Europe, Africa, and Asia. The name for *R. conorii* infection varies by region (e.g., Mediterranean spotted fever, Kenya tick typhus).
  - Disease is characterized by high fever, rash, and—in most locales—an inoculation eschar (*tâche noire*) at the site of the tick bite.

- A severe form of disease with a mortality rate of ~50% occurs in pts with diabetes, alcoholism, or heart failure.
- *R. africae* causes African tick-bite fever, which occurs in sub-Saharan Africa and the Caribbean and is the rickettsiosis most frequently imported into Europe and North America.
- Tick-borne spotted fever is diagnosed on the basis of clinical and epidemiologic findings; the diagnosis is confirmed by serology or detection of rickettsiae.
- Doxycycline (100 mg PO bid for 1–5 days), ciprofloxacin (750 mg bid PO for 5 days), or chloramphenicol (500 mg qid PO for 7–10 days) is effective for treatment.

◼ RICKETTSIALPOX

Epidemiology

Rickettsialpox is caused by *R. akari* and is maintained by mice and their mites. Recognized principally in New York City, rickettsialpox has been reported in other urban and rural locations in the United States as well as in Ukraine, Croatia, Mexico, and Turkey.

Clinical Manifestations

A papule forms at the site of the mite bite and develops a central vesicle that becomes a painless black-crusted eschar surrounded by an erythematous halo. Lymph nodes draining the region of the eschar enlarge.

- After an incubation period of 10–17 days, malaise, chills, fever, headache, and myalgia mark disease onset.
- A macular rash appears on day 2–6 of illness and evolves sequentially into papules, vesicles, and crusts that heal without scarring.
- If untreated, fever lasts 6–10 days.

TREATMENT	**Rickettsialpox**

Doxycycline is the drug of choice for treatment.

FLEA- AND LOUSE-BORNE TYPHUS GROUP RICKETTSIOSES
◼ ENDEMIC MURINE TYPHUS (FLEA-BORNE)

Etiology and Epidemiology

Caused by *R. typhi*, endemic murine typhus has a rat reservoir and is transmitted by fleas.

- Humans become infected when *Rickettsia*-laden flea feces are scratched into pruritic bite lesions; less often, the flea bite itself transmits the organisms or aerosolized rickettsiae from flea feces are inhaled.
- In the United States, endemic typhus occurs mainly in southern Texas and southern California; globally, it occurs in warm (often coastal) areas throughout the tropics and subtropics.
- Flea bites often are not recalled by pts, but exposure to animals such as cats, opossums, raccoons, skunks, and rats is reported by ~40%.

- Risk factors for severe disease include older age, underlying disease, and treatment with a sulfonamide drug.

Clinical Manifestations

Prodromal symptoms 1–3 days before the abrupt onset of chills and fever include headache, myalgia, arthralgia, nausea, and malaise; nausea and vomiting are nearly universal early in illness.

- Rash is apparent at presentation (usually ~4 days after symptom onset) in 13% of pts; 2 days later, half of the remaining pts develop a maculopapular rash that involves the trunk more than the extremities, is seldom petechial, and rarely involves the face, palms, or soles.
- Pulmonary disease is common, causing a hacking, nonproductive cough in 35% of pts. Almost one-fourth of pts who undergo CXR have pulmonary densities due to interstitial pneumonia, pulmonary edema, and pleural effusions.
- Laboratory abnormalities include anemia, leukopenia early in the course, leukocytosis late in the course, thrombocytopenia, hyponatremia, hypoalbuminemia, mildly increased hepatic aminotransferase levels, and prerenal azotemia.
- Complications may include respiratory failure, hematemesis, cerebral hemorrhage, and hemolysis.
- The duration of untreated disease averages 12 days (range, 9–18 days).

Diagnosis

The diagnosis can be based on culture, PCR, cross-adsorption serologic studies of acute- and convalescent-phase sera, or immunohistology, but most pts are treated empirically.

TREATMENT Endemic Murine Typhus (Flea-Borne)

Doxycycline (100 mg bid for 7–15 days) is effective. Ciprofloxacin provides an alternative if doxycycline is contraindicated.

■ EPIDEMIC TYPHUS (LOUSE-BORNE)

Etiology and Epidemiology

Epidemic typhus is caused by *R. prowazekii* and is transmitted by the human body louse. Eastern flying squirrels and their lice and fleas maintain *R. prowazekii* in a zoonotic cycle.

- The louse lives in clothing under poor hygienic conditions, particularly in colder climates and classically at times of war or natural disaster.
- Lice feed on pts with epidemic typhus and then defecate the organism into the bite at their next meal. The pt autoinoculates the organism while scratching.
- *Brill-Zinsser disease* is a recrudescent and mild form of epidemic typhus whose occurrence years after acute illness suggests that *R. prowazekii* remains dormant in the host, with reactivation when immunity wanes.

Clinical Manifestations

Epidemic typhus presents abruptly with the onset of high fevers, prostration, severe headache, cough, and severe myalgias. Photophobia with conjunctival injection and eye pain is also common.

- A rash appears on the upper trunk around the fifth day of illness and spreads to involve all body-surface areas except the face, palms, and soles.
- Confusion and coma, skin necrosis, and gangrene of the digits are noted in severe cases.
- Untreated, the disease is fatal in 7–40% of cases. Pts develop renal failure, multiorgan involvement, and prominent neurologic manifestations.

Diagnosis

Epidemic typhus is sometimes misdiagnosed as typhoid fever. The diagnosis can be based on serology, immunohistochemistry, or detection of the organism in a louse found on a pt. Cross-adsorption IFA can distinguish *R. prowazekii* from *R. typhi*.

> **TREATMENT**   Epidemic Typhus (Louse-Borne)
>
> Doxycycline (100 mg bid) is given until 2 or 3 days after the pt has defervesced, although a one-time dose of 200 mg has proved effective under epidemic conditions.

■ SCRUB TYPHUS

- *Orientia tsutsugamushi*, the agent of scrub typhus, is transmitted by larval mites or chiggers in environments with heavy scrub vegetation.
- Disease occurs during the wet season. It is endemic in eastern and southern Asia, northern Australia, and the Pacific islands.
- The classic case description includes an eschar at the site of chigger feeding, regional lymphadenopathy, and maculopapular rash—signs rarely seen in indigenous pts; Westerners commonly do not present with all three findings. Severe cases include encephalitis and interstitial pneumonia.
- Scrub typhus can be diagnosed by serologic assays (IFA, indirect immunoperoxidase, and enzyme immunoassays); PCR analysis of eschars and blood is also effective.
- A 7- to 15-day course of doxycycline (100 mg bid) or chloramphenicol (500 mg qid) or a 3-day course of azithromycin (500 mg qd) is effective.

EHRLICHIOSES AND ANAPLASMOSIS

Two distinct *Ehrlichia* species and one *Anaplasma* species—all obligately intracellular organisms—are transmitted by ticks to humans and cause infections that can be severe and prevalent.

■ HUMAN MONOCYTOTROPIC EHRLICHIOSIS (HME)

Etiology and Epidemiology

HME is caused by *Ehrlichia chaffeensis* and, in the United States, generally occurs in southeastern, south-central, and mid-Atlantic states. The incidence can be as high as 414 cases per 100,000 population.

- *E. chaffeensis* is transmitted by the Lone Star tick (*A. americanum*), and white-tailed deer are the major reservoir.
- Most pts are male; the median age of pts is 53 years.
- *E. ewingii* causes an illness similar to, but less severe than, that due to *E. chaffeensis*.

Clinical Manifestations

Clinical findings are nonspecific and include fever (96%), headache (72%), myalgia (68%), and malaise (77%). Nausea, vomiting, diarrhea, cough, rash, and confusion may be noted.

- The median incubation period is 8 days.
- Disease can be severe: up to 62% of pts are hospitalized and ~3% die. Complications include a toxic shock–like syndrome, respiratory distress, meningoencephalitis, fulminant infection, and hemorrhage.
- Leukopenia (61%), thrombocytopenia (73%), and elevated serum aminotransferase levels (84%) are common.

Diagnosis

Because HME can be fatal, empirical antibiotic therapy based on clinical diagnosis is required. PCR testing before initiation of antibiotic therapy or retrospective serodiagnosis to detect increased antibody titers can be performed. Morulae are seen in <10% of peripheral-blood smears.

Treatment

Treatment with doxycycline (100 mg PO/IV bid) or tetracycline (250–500 mg PO q6h) is effective and should be continued for 3–5 days after defervescence.

■ HUMAN GRANULOCYTOTROPIC ANAPLASMOSIS (HGA)

Etiology and Epidemiology

HGA is caused by *Anaplasma phagocytophilum* and, in the U.S., occurs mainly in northeastern and upper midwestern states.

- The geographic distribution is similar to that of Lyme disease and *Babesia microti* infection, given the shared *I. scapularis* tick vector.
- HGA incidence peaks in May through July, but the disease can occur year-round.

Clinical Manifestations

Given high seroprevalence rates in endemic areas, it appears that most people develop subclinical infections.

- After an incubation period of 4–8 days, pts develop fever (91%), myalgia (77%), headache (77%), and malaise (94%).
- Severe complications—respiratory insufficiency, a toxic shock–like syndrome, and opportunistic infections—occur most often in elderly pts.
- On laboratory examination, pts are found to have leukopenia, thrombocytopenia, and elevated serum aminotransferase levels.

Diagnosis

HGA should be considered in pts with influenza-like illness during May through December and in pts with atypical severe presentations of Lyme disease.

- Peripheral-blood films may reveal morulae in neutrophils in 20–75% of infections.
- PCR testing before antibiotic therapy or retrospective serologic testing demonstrating a ≥4-fold rise in antibody titer can confirm the diagnosis.

Treatment

Doxycycline (100 mg PO bid) is effective, and most pts defervesce within 24–48 h. Pregnant women and children <8 years old may be treated with rifampin.

■ PREVENTION

HME and HGA are prevented by avoidance of ticks in endemic areas, use of protective clothing and tick repellents, careful tick searches after exposures, and prompt removal of attached ticks.

Q FEVER

Microbiology

Coxiella burnetii—the etiologic agent of Q fever—is a small, pleomorphic coccobacillus with a gram-negative cell wall that exists intracellularly.

Epidemiology and Pathogenesis

A worldwide disease, Q fever is a zoonosis. Cattle, sheep, and goats are responsible for most cases of human infection; many other animals can serve as vectors of transmission or as reservoirs of disease.

- *C. burnetii* localizes to the uterus and mammary glands of infected female mammals. It is reactivated in pregnancy and is found at high concentrations in the placenta. At parturition, the organism is dispersed as an aerosol, and infection usually follows inhalation.
- Abattoir workers, veterinarians, farmers, and other persons who have contact with infected animals, and particularly with newborn animals or infected products of conception, are at risk.
- In the U.S., there are 28–54 cases per year; in Australia, there are 30 cases per 1 million population per year.

Clinical Manifestations

The specific presentation of acute Q fever differs geographically (e.g., pneumonia in Nova Scotia and granulomatous hepatitis in Marseille); chronic Q fever almost always implies endocarditis.

- *Acute Q fever:* After an incubation period of 3–30 days, pts may present with flulike syndromes, prolonged fever, pneumonia, hepatitis, pericarditis, myocarditis, meningoencephalitis, and infection during pregnancy.
  - Symptoms are often nonspecific (e.g., fever, fatigue, headache, chills, sweats, nausea, vomiting, diarrhea, cough, and occasionally rash).
  - Multiple rounded opacities on CXR in pts in endemic areas are highly suggestive of Q fever pneumonia.
  - The WBC count is usually normal, but thrombocytopenia occurs. During recovery, reactive thrombocytosis can develop.

- Prolonged fatigue, along with a constellation of nonspecific symptoms (e.g., headaches, myalgias, arthralgias), can follow Q fever (post–Q fever fatigue syndrome).
- *Chronic Q fever:* Pts with *C. burnetii* endocarditis typically have prior valvular heart disease, immunosuppression, or chronic renal failure.
  - Fever is absent or low grade; pts may be ill for >1 year before diagnosis.
  - Valvular vegetations are best seen with transesophageal echocardiography rather than transthoracic echocardiography, which identifies vegetations in only 12% of cases. The vegetations differ from those in bacterial endocarditis of other etiologies and manifest as endothelium-covered nodules on the valve.
  - The disease should be suspected in all pts with culture-negative endocarditis.
  - Although *C. burnetii* can be isolated by a shell-vial technique, most laboratories are not permitted to attempt isolation because of the organism's highly contagious nature. PCR testing of tissue or biopsy specimens can be used, but serology is the most common diagnostic tool; IFA is the method of choice.

TREATMENT   Q Fever

- Acute Q fever is treated with doxycycline (100 mg bid for 14 days).
  - Quinolones are also efficacious.
  - If Q fever is diagnosed during pregnancy, trimethoprim-sulfamethoxazole should be administered up to term.
- The currently recommended treatment for chronic Q fever is doxycycline (100 mg bid) and hydroxychloroquine (200 mg tid; plasma concentrations maintained at 0.8–1.2 µg/mL) for 18 months.
  - In vitro, hydroxychloroquine renders doxycycline bactericidal against *C. burnetii*.
  - The minimal inhibitory concentration (MIC) of doxycycline for the pt's isolate should be determined and serum levels monitored, with a goal of a serum level–to–doxycycline MIC ratio of ≥1.
  - Pts should be advised about photosensitivity and retinal toxicity risks with treatment.
  - Pts who cannot receive doxycycline-hydroxychloroquine should be treated with at least two agents active against *C. burnetii*. The combination of rifampin (300 mg once daily) plus doxycycline (100 mg bid) or ciprofloxacin (750 mg bid) has been used with success.
  - Treatment should be given for at least 3 years and discontinued only if phase I IgA and IgG antibody titers are ≤1:50 and ≤1:200, respectively.

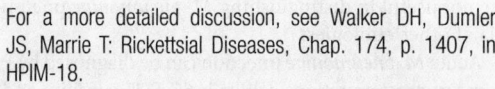

For a more detailed discussion, see Walker DH, Dumler JS, Marrie T: Rickettsial Diseases, Chap. 174, p. 1407, in HPIM-18.

CHAPTER **106**
Mycoplasma Infections

With a size of only 150–350 nm, mycoplasmas are the smallest free-living organisms. Genome sequence data from many different *Mycoplasma* species have helped define the minimal set of genes necessary for cellular life. Lacking a cell wall and bounded only by a plasma membrane, mycoplasmas colonize mucosal surfaces of the respiratory and urogenital tracts.

■ *M. PNEUMONIAE*

Epidemiology

M. pneumoniae occurs worldwide with no seasonal pattern. Infection causes upper respiratory tract disease ~20 times more frequently than pneumonia.

- Infection is acquired by inhalation of aerosols, with an incubation period of 2–4 weeks.
- *M. pneumoniae* accounts for ~23% of cases of community-acquired pneumonia in adults.

Clinical Manifestations

M. pneumoniae is often grouped with *Chlamydia pneumoniae* and *Legionella* species as the most important causes of "atypical" community-acquired pneumonia. The clinical presentation does not help distinguish *M. pneumoniae* pneumonia from that of any other bacterial etiology.

- Acute *M. pneumoniae* infection manifests as a nonspecific upper respiratory syndrome with pharyngitis, tracheobronchitis, and/or wheezing.
- Pneumonia develops in 3–13% of infected pts. The most common presenting symptom is a nonproductive cough. Headache, malaise, chills, and fever are common.
- On physical exam, ~80% of pts have wheezes or rales.
- Symptoms usually resolve in 2–3 weeks, and appropriate antimicrobial therapy significantly shortens the duration of clinical illness.
- Infection uncommonly results in critical illness and rarely causes death.
- Extrapulmonary manifestations of *M. pneumoniae* infection are relatively uncommon but include skin eruptions (e.g., erythema multiforme major, rashes), neurologic manifestations (e.g., encephalitis, Guillain-Barré syndrome, acute demyelinating encephalomyelitis), septic arthritis (particularly in pts with hypogammaglobulinemia), and hematologic manifestations (e.g., hemolytic anemia, coagulopathies).

Diagnosis

Clinical findings, nonmicrobiologic laboratory tests, and chest radiography are not useful in distinguishing *M. pneumoniae* pneumonia from pneumonia of other etiologies.

- Acute *M. pneumoniae* infection can be diagnosed by PCR analysis of respiratory tract secretions, which is 65–90% sensitive and 90–100% specific.

- *M. pneumoniae* culture (which requires special medium) is not recommended for routine diagnosis as its sensitivity is ≤60% and growth of the organism can take weeks.
- Serologic testing for IgM and IgG antibodies to *M. pneumoniae* requires acute- and convalescent-phase samples and is therefore less useful for diagnosis of active infections. Moreover, IgM antibodies to *M. pneumoniae* can persist for up to 1 year after acute infection.
- Measurement of cold agglutinin titers is no longer recommended for the diagnosis of *M. pneumoniae* infection because the findings are nonspecific.

TREATMENT ▸ *M. pneumoniae* Infections

- Antibiotic options include macrolides (azithromycin, 500 mg PO for 1 day followed by 250 mg for 4 days), tetracyclines (doxycycline, 100 mg PO bid for 10–14 days), and respiratory fluoroquinolones (levofloxacin, 500–750 mg PO qd for 10–14 days).
- Ciprofloxacin and ofloxacin are *not* recommended because of their high minimal inhibitory concentrations against *M. pneumoniae*.

■ **UROGENITAL MYCOPLASMAS**

See Chap. 92.

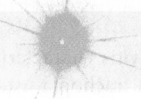 For a more detailed discussion, see Hardy RD: Infections Due to Mycoplasmas, Chap. 175, p. 1417, in HPIM-18.

CHAPTER **107**
Chlamydial Infections

■ **MICROBIOLOGY**

- Chlamydiae are obligate intracellular bacteria, possess both DNA and RNA (a characteristic that distinguishes them from viruses), and have a cell wall similar to that of gram-negative bacteria.
- These organisms have a complex reproductive cycle and exist in two forms.
    - The *elementary body* (the infective form) is adapted for extracellular survival, while the *reticulate body* is adapted for intracellular survival and multiplication.
    - Within 18–24 h after infection of the cell, reticulate bodies have replicated and begin to condense into elementary bodies that are released to infect other cells or people.
- Three chlamydial species infect humans: *Chlamydia trachomatis*, *C. psittaci*, and *C. pneumoniae*.

- CF tests and enzyme immunoassays that detect lipopolysaccharide identify chlamydiae only to the genus level.
- The microimmunofluorescence (MIF) test can differentiate among the three species.

C. TRACHOMATIS INFECTIONS

■ GENITAL INFECTIONS, INCLUDING LYMPHOGRANULOMA VENEREUM

See Chap. 92.

■ TRACHOMA AND ADULT INCLUSION CONJUNCTIVITIS (AIC)

Etiology

- Trachoma is a chronic conjunctivitis caused by *C. trachomatis* serovars A, B, Ba, and C. Transmission occurs through contact with ocular discharge from infected pts, which can also be transferred by flies.
- AIC is an acute eye infection in adults exposed to infected genital secretions and in their newborns. This infection is caused by sexually transmitted *C. trachomatis* strains, usually serovars D through K.

Epidemiology

Trachoma is a leading cause of preventable infectious blindness, with ~6 million pts having been affected. In the hyperendemic regions of northern and sub-Saharan Africa, the Middle East, and parts of Asia, the prevalence of trachoma is ~100% by the third year of life. Reinfection and persistent infection are common.

Clinical Manifestations

Both trachoma and AIC present clinically as conjunctivitis characterized by small lymphoid follicles in the conjunctiva, although trachoma usually starts insidiously before 2 years of age.

- With progression, there is inflammatory leukocytic infiltration and superficial vascularization (pannus formation) of the cornea.
  - Scarring eventually distorts the eyelids, turning lashes inward and abrading the eyeball (trichiasis and entropion).
  - The corneal epithelium eventually ulcerates, with subsequent scarring and blindness.
  - Destruction of goblet cells, lacrimal ducts, and glands causes dry-eye syndrome (xerosis), with resultant corneal opacity and secondary bacterial corneal ulcers.
- AIC is an acute unilateral follicular conjunctivitis with preauricular lymphadenopathy and presents similarly to acute conjunctivitis due to adenovirus or HSV.
  - Corneal inflammation is evidenced by discrete opacities, punctate epithelial erosions, and superficial corneal vascularization.
  - Left untreated, the disease may persist for 6 weeks to 2 years.

Diagnosis

Clinical diagnosis is based on the presence of two of the following signs: lymphoid follicles on the upper tarsal conjunctiva, typical conjunctival scarring, vascular pannus, or limbal follicles.

- Intracytoplasmic chlamydial inclusions are found in 10–60% of Giemsa-stained conjunctival smears from children with severe inflammation.
- However, chlamydial nucleic acid amplification tests are more sensitive in detecting infection.

> **TREATMENT** Trachoma/AIC

- AIC responds to azithromycin (a single 1-g oral dose) or doxycycline (100 mg PO bid for 7 days). Treatment of sexual partners is needed to prevent ocular reinfection and chlamydial genital disease.

C. PSITTACI INFECTIONS

Etiology and Epidemiology

Most avian species can harbor *C. psittaci*, but psittacine birds (e.g., parrots, parakeets) are most often infected; human infections are uncommon and occur only as a zoonosis.

- Exposure is greatest in poultry workers and in owners of pet birds.
- Present in nasal secretions, excreta, tissues, and feathers of infected birds, *C. psittaci* is transmitted to humans by direct contact with infected birds or by inhalation of aerosols. Transmission from person to person has never been documented.
- As a result of quarantine of imported birds and improved veterinary-hygienic measures, outbreaks and sporadic cases of psittacosis are now rare, with fewer than 50 confirmed cases reported in the U.S. each year.

Clinical Manifestations

Psittacosis in humans can range in severity from asymptomatic or mild infections to acute primary atypical pneumonia (which can be fatal in 10% of untreated cases) to severe chronic pneumonia.

- After an incubation period of >5–19 days, pts present with fever, chills, muscular aches and pains, severe headaches, hepatomegaly and/or splenomegaly, and gastrointestinal symptoms.
- Cardiac complications may include endocarditis and myocarditis.

Diagnosis

This diagnosis is confirmed by serologic studies.

- The gold standard is the MIF test.
- Any antibody titer >1:16 or a 4-fold rise between paired acute- and convalescent-phase serum samples, in combination with a clinically compatible syndrome, can be used to diagnose psittacosis.

> **TREATMENT** *C. psittaci* Infections

- Tetracycline (250 mg PO qid for 3 weeks) is the antibiotic of choice.
- Erythromycin (500 mg PO qid) is an alternative agent.

C. PNEUMONIAE INFECTIONS

Epidemiology

C. pneumoniae is a common cause of human respiratory diseases, primarily in young adults.

- Seroprevalence rates of 40–70% demonstrate that *C. pneumoniae* is widespread worldwide. Seropositivity is first detected at school age and then increases by ~10% per decade.
- The role of *C. pneumoniae* in atherosclerotic disease has long been discussed, but large-scale treatment studies have cast doubts on the etiologic role of this organism in this disease.

Clinical Manifestations

The clinical spectrum of *C. pneumoniae* infection includes acute pharyngitis, sinusitis, bronchitis, and pneumonia.

- Pneumonia due to *C. pneumoniae* resembles that due to *Mycoplasma pneumoniae*. Pts have antecedent upper respiratory tract symptoms, fever, nonproductive cough, minimal findings on auscultation, small segmental infiltrates on chest x-ray, and no leukocytosis.
  - Primary infection is more severe than reinfection.
  - Elderly pts can have severe disease.

Diagnosis

Serology is the most clinically useful means for diagnosing *C. pneumoniae* infection.

- The diagnosis of acute *C. pneumoniae* infection requires demonstration of a 4-fold rise in titer between acute- and convalescent-phase serum samples.
- Culture of the organism is difficult and is not routinely attempted. PCR assays for *C. pneumoniae* are currently available only for research purposes.

> **TREATMENT** *C. pneumoniae* Infections
>
> - Erythromycin or tetracycline (2 g/d for 10–14 days) is recommended.
> - Other macrolides (e.g., azithromycin) or quinolones (e.g., levofloxacin) are alternative agents.

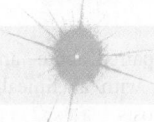

For a more detailed discussion, see Gaydos CA, Quinn TC: Chlamydial Infections, Chap. 176, p. 1421, in HPIM-18.

CHAPTER **108**
Herpesvirus Infections

■ MICROBIOLOGY AND PATHOGENESIS

The herpes simplex viruses HSV-1 and HSV-2 are linear, double-stranded DNA viruses that share ~50% sequence homology. Exposure to HSV at mucosal surfaces or abraded skin sites permits viral entry and replication in cells of the epidermis and dermis prior to infection of neuronal cells and development of a latent infection in ganglia.

- Reactivation occurs when normal viral gene expression resumes, with reappearance of the virus on mucosal surfaces.
- Both antibody-mediated and cell-mediated immunity (including type-specific immunity) are clinically important.

■ EPIDEMIOLOGY

HSV-1 is acquired more frequently and at an earlier age than HSV-2. More than 90% of adults have antibodies to HSV-1 by the fifth decade of life. Antibodies to HSV-2 usually are not detected until adolescence and correlate with sexual activity; in the United States, 15–20% of the population has antibody to HSV-2.

- HSV is transmitted by contact with active lesions or with virus shed from mucocutaneous surfaces by asymptomatic persons.
- HSV reactivation is very common: HSV-2 is shed on a median of 25% of days by infected pts, with 29% of genital reactivation episodes lasting <6 h.
- The large reservoir of unidentified carriers and the frequent asymptomatic reactivation of HSV-2 have fostered the continued spread of HSV throughout the world.

■ CLINICAL MANIFESTATIONS

Both viral subtypes can cause indistinguishable genital and oral-facial infections. Overall, genital HSV-2 is twice as likely to reactivate as genital HSV-1, and HSV-2 infection recurs 8–10 times more often. In contrast, oral-labial HSV-1 infection recurs more frequently than oral-labial HSV-2 infection. The incubation period for primary infection with either virus is 1–26 days (median, 6–8 days).

Oral-Facial Infections

Primary HSV-1 infection results in gingivostomatitis, pharyngitis, and up to 2 weeks of fever, malaise, myalgia, inability to eat, and cervical adenopathy, with lesions on the palate, gingiva, tongue, lip, face, posterior pharynx, and/or tonsillar pillars and occasional exudative pharyngitis.

- Reactivation of HSV from the trigeminal ganglia is associated with asymptomatic viral excretion in the saliva, intraoral mucosal ulcerations, or ulcers on the vermilion border of the lip or external facial skin.

- 50–70% of pts undergoing trigeminal nerve-root decompression and 10–15% of pts undergoing dental extraction develop oral-labial herpes a median of 3 days after the procedure.
- Reactivation of HSV-1 or VZV in the mandibular portion of the facial nerve causes flaccid paralysis (Bell's palsy).
- Immunosuppressed pts can have a severe infection that extends into the mucosa and skin, causing friability, necrosis, bleeding, pain, and inability to eat or drink.
- Pts with atopic dermatitis may also develop severe oral-facial HSV infection (eczema herpeticum), with extensive skin lesions and occasional visceral dissemination.
- HSV infection is the precipitating event in ~75% of cases of erythema multiforme.

Genital Infections (see Chap. 92)

First-episode primary genital herpes is characterized by fever, headache, malaise, and myalgias. Pain, itching, dysuria, vaginal and urethral discharge, and tender inguinal lymphadenopathy are the predominant local symptoms.
- Pts with prior HSV-1 infection have milder cases.
- Reactivation infections are often subclinical or can cause genital lesions or urethritis with dysuria.
- Even without a history of rectal intercourse, perianal lesions can occur as a result of latency established in the sacral dermatome from prior genital tract infection.

Whitlow

In HSV infection of the finger, pts experience an abrupt onset of edema, erythema, pain, and vesicular or pustular lesions of the fingertips that are often confused with the lesions of pyogenic bacterial infection. Fever, lymphadenitis, and epitrochlear and axillary lymphadenopathy are common.

Herpes Gladiatorum

HSV infection caused by trauma to the skin during wrestling can occur anywhere on the body but commonly affects the thorax, ears, face, and hands.

Eye Infections

HSV is the most frequent cause of corneal blindness in the United States.
- HSV keratitis presents with acute onset of pain, blurred vision, chemosis, conjunctivitis, and dendritic corneal lesions. Topical glucocorticoids may exacerbate disease. Recurrences are common.
- Other manifestations include chorioretinitis and acute necrotizing retinitis.

Central and Peripheral Nervous System Infections

In the United States, HSV causes 10–20% of all cases of sporadic viral encephalitis, and 95% of these cases are due to HSV-1 (either primary or reactivated infection). The estimated annual incidence is 2.3 cases per 1 million persons.

- Pts present with an acute onset of fever and focal neurologic symptoms and signs, especially in the temporal lobe. In severe cases, RBCs can be found in the CSF as a result of hemorrhagic necrosis.
- Given the potential severity of infection, antiviral treatment should be started empirically until the diagnosis is confirmed or an alternative diagnosis is made.
- HSV meningitis, which is usually seen in association with primary genital HSV infection, is an acute self-limited disease manifested by headache, fever, and mild photophobia and lasting 2–7 days.
  - Of cases of aseptic meningitis, 3–15% are due to HSV.
  - HSV is the most common cause of recurrent lymphocytic meningitis (Mollaret's meningitis).
- Autonomic dysfunction caused by either HSV or VZV most commonly affects the sacral region, resulting in numbness, tingling of the buttocks or perineal areas, urinary retention, constipation, and impotence.
  - Symptoms take days or weeks to resolve.
  - In rare instances, transverse myelitis or Guillain-Barré syndrome follows HSV infection.

Visceral Infections

HSV infection of visceral organs usually results from viremia; multiple-organ involvement is common, but occasionally only the esophagus, lung, or liver is affected.

- In HSV esophagitis, pts present with odynophagia, dysphagia, substernal pain, weight loss, and multiple oval ulcerations on an erythematous base. Detection of HSV is necessary to distinguish this entity from esophagitis of other etiologies (e.g., *Candida esophagitis*).
- HSV pneumonitis is rare except among severely immunocompromised pts and results in focal necrotizing pneumonitis with a mortality rate of >80%.
- Hepatic HSV infection occurs primarily in immunocompromised pts and is associated with fever, abrupt elevations of bilirubin and serum aminotransferase levels, and leukopenia (<4000 WBCs/μL).

Neonatal Infections

The frequency of visceral and/or CNS infection is highest among HSV-infected infants <6 weeks of age; the mortality rate without therapy is 65%.

- Infection is usually acquired perinatally from contact with infected genital secretions during delivery.
- More than two-thirds of cases are due to HSV-2. The risk is elevated by 10-fold for infants born to a mother who has recently acquired HSV.

■ DIAGNOSIS

Microscopic evaluation, viral culture, serology, and PCR are all clinically useful for diagnosing HSV infection.

- Regardless of the detection method, the sensitivity is greater for vesicular rather than ulcerative mucosal lesions, in primary rather than recurrent disease, and in immunocompromised rather than immunocompetent pts.
- PCR is most sensitive for detection of HSV and should be used whenever possible.
- A Tzanck smear (Giemsa-stained scrapings from the base of lesions) to detect giant cells or intranuclear inclusions characteristic of both HSV and VZV infections has a low level of sensitivity; its use requires clinicians skilled in this technique.
- Serologic tests can be used to demonstrate prior exposure to HSV; no reliable IgM detection method for defining acute HSV infection is available.

TREATMENT Infections with Herpes Simplex Viruses

- Table 108-1 details antiviral chemotherapy for HSV infection.
  - All antiviral agents licensed for use against HSV inhibit the viral DNA polymerase.
  - Acyclovir can crystallize in the renal parenchyma, causing transient renal insufficiency; this drug should be given over the course of 1 h to a well-hydrated pt.
  - Acyclovir-resistant strains of HSV are rare but have been identified, primarily in immunocompromised pts. In general, these isolates are also resistant to valacyclovir and famciclovir, which have similar mechanisms of action.

■ PREVENTION

The use of barrier forms of contraception, especially condoms, decreases the likelihood of HSV transmission, particularly during asymptomatic viral excretion. Chronic daily therapy with valacyclovir can also be partially effective in reducing acquisition of HSV-2, particularly among susceptible women.

VARICELLA-ZOSTER VIRUS

■ MICROBIOLOGY AND PATHOGENESIS

VZV—a double-stranded DNA virus in the family Herpesviridae—has a pathogenic cycle similar to that of HSV. Primary infection is transmitted by the respiratory route. The virus replicates and causes viremia, which is reflected by the diffuse and scattered skin lesions in varicella; it then establishes latency in the dorsal root ganglia and can reactivate through unknown mechanisms at a later time.

■ EPIDEMIOLOGY AND CLINICAL MANIFESTATIONS

VZV causes two distinct entities: primary infection (varicella or chickenpox) and reactivation infection (herpes zoster or shingles). Humans are the only known reservoir for VZV.

Chickenpox

Pts present with fever, malaise, and rash characterized by maculopapules, vesicles, and scabs in various stages of evolution. The skin lesions are small,

TABLE 108-1 ANTIVIRAL CHEMOTHERAPY FOR HSV INFECTION

I. Mucocutaneous HSV infections

A. *Infections in immunosuppressed pts*

1. *Acute symptomatic first or recurrent episodes:* IV acyclovir (5 mg/kg q8h) or oral acyclovir (400 mg qid), famciclovir (500 mg bid or tid), or valacyclovir (500 mg bid) is effective. Treatment duration may vary from 7 to 14 days.

2. *Suppression of reactivation disease (genital or oral-labial):* IV acyclovir (5 mg/kg q8h) or oral valacyclovir (500 mg bid) or acyclovir (400–800 mg 3–5 times per day) prevents recurrences during the 30-day period immediately after transplantation. Longer-term HSV suppression is often used for pts with continued immunosuppression. In bone marrow and renal transplant recipients, oral valacyclovir (2 g/d) is also effective in reducing CMV infection. Oral valacyclovir at a dose of 4 g/d has been associated with thrombotic thrombocytopenic purpura after extended use in HIV-positive pts. In HIV-infected pts, oral acyclovir (400–800 mg bid), valacyclovir (500 mg bid), or famciclovir (500 mg bid) is effective in reducing clinical and subclinical reactivations of HSV-1 and HSV-2.

B. *Infections in immunocompetent pts*

1. *Genital herpes*

a. *First episodes:* Oral acyclovir (200 mg 5 times per day or 400 mg tid), valacyclovir (1 g bid), or famciclovir (250 mg bid) for 7–14 days is effective. IV acyclovir (5 mg/kg q8h for 5 days) is given for severe disease or neurologic complications such as aseptic meningitis.

b. *Symptomatic recurrent genital herpes:* Short-course (1- to 3-day) regimens are preferred because of low cost, likelihood of adherence, and convenience. Oral acyclovir (800 mg tid for 2 days), valacyclovir (500 mg bid for 3 days), or famciclovir (750 or 1000 mg bid for 1 day, a 1500-mg single dose, or 500 mg stat followed by 250 mg q12h for 3 days) effectively shortens lesion duration. Other options include oral acyclovir (200 mg 5 times per day), valacyclovir (500 mg bid), and famciclovir (125 mg bid for 5 days).

c. *Suppression of recurrent genital herpes:* Oral acyclovir (400–800 mg bid) or valacyclovir (500 mg daily) is given. Pts with >9 episodes per year should take oral valacyclovir (1 g daily or 500 mg bid) or famciclovir (250 mg bid or 500 mg bid).

2. *Oral-labial HSV infections*

a. *First episode:* Oral acyclovir (200 mg) is given 4 or 5 times per day; an oral acyclovir suspension can be used (600 mg/m^2 qid). Oral famciclovir (250 mg bid) or valacyclovir (1 g bid) has been used clinically.

b. *Recurrent episodes:* If initiated at prodrome onset, single-dose or 1-day therapy effectively reduces pain and speeds healing. Regimens include oral famciclovir (a 1500-mg single dose or 750 mg bid for 1 day) or valacyclovir (a 2-g single dose or 2 g bid for 1 day). Self-initiated therapy with 6-times-daily topical penciclovir cream effectively speeds healing of oral-labial HSV lesions. Topical acyclovir cream also speeds healing.

(continued)

TABLE 108-1 ANTIVIRAL CHEMOTHERAPY FOR HSV INFECTION (CONTINUED)

I. Mucocutaneous HSV infections (continued)

    c. *Suppression of reactivation of oral-labial HSV:* If started before exposure and continued for the duration of exposure (usually 5–10 days), oral acyclovir (400 mg bid) prevents reactivation of recurrent oral-labial HSV infection associated with severe sun exposure.

    3. *Surgical prophylaxis of oral or genital HSV infection:* Several surgical procedures, such as laser skin resurfacing, trigeminal nerve-root decompression, and lumbar disk surgery, have been associated with HSV reactivation. IV acyclovir (3–5 mg/kg q8h) or oral acyclovir (800 mg bid), valacyclovir (500 mg bid), or famciclovir (250 mg bid) effectively reduces reactivation. Therapy should be initiated 48 h before surgery and continued for 3–7 days.

    4. *Herpetic whitlow:* Oral acyclovir (200 mg) is given 5 times daily for 7–10 days (alternative: 400 mg tid).

    5. *HSV proctitis:* Oral acyclovir (400 mg 5 times per day) is useful in shortening the course of infection. In immunosuppressed pts or in pts with severe infection, IV acyclovir (5 mg/kg q8h) may be useful.

    6. *Herpetic eye infections:* In acute keratitis, topical trifluorothymidine, vidarabine, idoxuridine, acyclovir, penciclovir, and interferon are all beneficial. Debridement may be required. Topical steroids may worsen disease.

II. CNS HSV infections

    A. *HSV encephalitis:* IV acyclovir (10 mg/kg q8h; 30 mg/kg per day) is given for 10 days or until HSV DNA is no longer detected in CSF.

    B. *HSV aseptic meningitis:* No studies of systemic antiviral chemotherapy exist. If therapy is given, IV acyclovir (15–30 mg/kg per day) should be used.

    C. *Autonomic radiculopathy:* No studies are available. Most authorities recommend a trial of IV acyclovir.

III. Neonatal HSV infections: Oral acyclovir (60 mg/kg per day, divided into 3 doses) is given. The recommended duration of treatment is 21 days. Monitoring for relapse should be undertaken, and some authorities recommend continued suppression with oral acyclovir suspension for 3–4 months.

IV. Visceral HSV infections

    A. *HSV esophagitis:* IV acyclovir (15 mg/kg per day) is given. In some pts with milder forms of immunosuppression, oral therapy with valacyclovir or famciclovir is effective.

    B. *HSV pneumonitis:* No controlled studies exist. IV acyclovir (15 mg/kg per day) should be considered.

V. Disseminated HSV infections: No controlled studies exist. IV acyclovir (5 mg/kg q8h) should be tried. Adjustments for renal insufficiency may be needed. No definite evidence indicates that therapy will decrease the risk of death.

VI. Erythema multiforme associated with HSV: Anecdotal observations suggest that oral acyclovir (400 mg bid or tid) or valacyclovir (500 mg bid) will suppress erythema multiforme.

VII. Infections due to acyclovir-resistant HSV: IV foscarnet (40 mg/kg IV q8h) should be given until lesions heal. The optimal duration of therapy and the usefulness of its continuation to suppress lesions are unclear. Some pts may benefit from cutaneous application of trifluorothymidine or 5% cidofovir gel.

with an erythematous base of 5–10 mm, and appear in successive crops over 2–4 days. Severity varies from person to person, but older pts tend to have more severe disease.

- In immunocompetent hosts, the disease is benign and lasts 3–5 days. In contrast, immunocompromised pts have numerous slower-healing lesions (often with a hemorrhagic base) and are more likely to develop visceral complications that, if not treated, are fatal in 15% of cases.
- The incubation period ranges from 10 to 21 days but is usually 14–17 days. Pts are infectious for 48 h before onset of rash and remain infectious until all vesicles have crusted.
- The virus is highly contagious, with an attack rate of 90% among susceptible persons. Historically, children 5–9 years old accounted for half of all cases; vaccination has dramatically changed the epidemiology of infection and has caused a significant decrease in the annualized incidence of chickenpox.
- Complications of varicella include bacterial superinfection of the skin, CNS involvement, pneumonia, myocarditis, and hepatic involvement.
  - Bacterial superinfection is usually caused by *Streptococcus pyogenes* or *Staphylococcus aureus*.
  - CNS involvement, usually manifesting as acute cerebellar ataxia and meningeal irritation ~21 days after the onset of rash, runs a benign course. Aseptic meningitis, encephalitis, transverse myelitis, Guillain-Barré syndrome, or Reye's syndrome (which mandates the avoidance of aspirin administration to children) can occur. There is no specific therapy other than supportive care.
  - VZV pneumonia is the most serious complication and develops more frequently among adults (occurring in up to 20% of cases) than among children. The onset comes 3–5 days into illness, with tachypnea, cough, dyspnea, fever, cyanosis, pleuritic chest pain, and hemoptysis. CXR shows nodular infiltrates and interstitial pneumonitis. Resolution of pneumonitis parallels improvement of the skin rash.

Herpes Zoster (Shingles)

Herpes zoster represents a reactivation of VZV from dorsal root ganglia and usually manifests as a unilateral vesicular eruption within a dermatome, often associated with severe pain.

- Dermatomal pain may precede lesions by 48–72 h, and dermatomes T3 to L3 are most frequently involved.
- The usual duration of disease is 7–10 days, but it may take as long as 2–4 weeks for the skin to return to normal.
- With ~1.2 million cases each year in the U.S., the incidence is highest among pts ≥60 years of age.
- Pts with herpes zoster can transmit infection to seronegative individuals, with consequent chickenpox.
- Complications include zoster ophthalmicus (which can lead to blindness), Ramsay Hunt syndrome (characterized by pain and vesicles in the external auditory canal, loss of taste in the anterior two-thirds of the tongue, and ipsilateral facial palsy), and postherpetic neuralgia (pain persisting for months after resolution of cutaneous disease).

- Immunocompromised pts—particularly those with Hodgkin's disease and non-Hodgkin's lymphoma—are at greatest risk for severe zoster and progressive disease. Cutaneous dissemination occurs in 40% of these pts and increases the risk for other complications (pneumonitis, meningoencephalitis, hepatitis).

◼ DIAGNOSIS

Definitive diagnosis requires isolation of VZV in culture, detection of VZV by molecular means (PCR, immunofluorescent staining of cells from the lesion base), or serology (seroconversion or a ≥4-fold rise in antibody titer between convalescent- and acute-phase serum specimens).

TREATMENT   Varicella-Zoster Virus Infections

- *Chickenpox:* Antiviral therapy can be helpful if started within 24 h of symptoms.
  - For children <12 years of age, acyclovir (20 mg/kg PO q6h) is recommended.
  - For adolescents and adults, acyclovir (800 mg PO five times daily), valacyclovir (1 g PO tid), or famciclovir (250 mg PO tid) for 5–7 days is recommended.
  - Good hygiene, meticulous skin care, and antipruritic drugs are important to relieve symptoms and prevent bacterial superinfection of skin lesions.
- *Zoster:* Lesions heal more quickly with antiviral treatment.
  - Acyclovir (800 mg PO five times daily for 7–10 days), famciclovir (500 mg PO tid for 7 days), or valacyclovir (1 g PO tid for 5–7 days) is recommended.
  - One study also showed twofold faster resolution of postherpetic neuralgia with famciclovir.
- *VZV infection in severely immunocompromised pts:* Severely immunocompromised pts should receive acyclovir, at least at the outset (10 mg/kg IV q8h for 7 days), for chickenpox and herpes zoster to reduce the risk of visceral complications, although this regimen does not speed the healing or relieve the pain of skin lesions.
  - Low-risk immunocompromised pts can be treated with oral valacyclovir or famciclovir.
  - If feasible, immunosuppression should be decreased during concomitant acyclovir administration.
- *Zoster ophthalmicus:* Antiviral treatment, analgesics for severe pain, and consultation with an ophthalmologist are required.
- *Postherpetic neuralgia:* Gabapentin, amitriptyline, lidocaine patches, and fluphenazine may relieve pain and can be given along with routine analgesic agents. Prednisone (given along with antiviral therapy at a dosage of 60 mg/d for the first week of zoster, with the dose then tapered by 50% weekly over the next 2 weeks) can accelerate quality-of-life improvements, including a return to usual activity; prednisone treatment is indicated only for healthy elderly persons with moderate or severe pain at presentation.

■ **PREVENTION**

Three methods are used for the prevention of VZV infections.

- *Active immunization:* For all children and seronegative adults, two doses of a live attenuated varicella vaccine are recommended. Irrespective of serologic status, pts >60 years old should receive a vaccine with 18 times the viral content of varicella vaccine; zoster vaccine reduces the incidence of zoster and postherpetic neuralgia.
- *Passive immunization:* Varicella-zoster immune globulin (VZIg) can be given to VZV-susceptible hosts within 96 h of a significant exposure if the risk of complications from varicella is high (e.g., immunocompromised pts, pregnant women, premature infants, neonates whose mothers had chickenpox onset within 5 days before or 2 days after delivery). VZIg is available under an investigational new drug protocol from FFF Enterprises (800-843-7477).
- *Antiviral treatment:* Seven days after intense exposure, antiviral prophylaxis can be given to high-risk pts who are ineligible for vaccine or for whom the 96-h window after direct contact has passed. This intervention may lessen illness severity.

HUMAN HERPESVIRUS (HHV) TYPES 6, 7, AND 8

- HHV-6 causes exanthem subitum (roseola infantum, a common childhood febrile illness with rash) and 20–30% of febrile seizures without rash in infancy.
  - In older age groups, HHV-6 has been associated with mononucleosis syndromes; focal encephalitis; and (in immunocompromised hosts) pneumonitis, syncytial giant-cell hepatitis, and disseminated disease.
  - More than 80% of adults are seropositive for HHV-6.
- HHV-7 is frequently acquired during childhood, and infections typically manifest as fever and seizures. The virus is commonly present in saliva.
- HHV-8 infection in healthy children can present as fever and rash; in immunocompromised pts, primary infection may present as fever, splenomegaly, pancytopenia, and rapid-onset Kaposi's sarcoma.
  - HHV-8 is associated with Kaposi's sarcoma, body cavity–based lymphoma in AIDS pts, and multicentric Castleman's disease.
  - Unlike other herpesvirus infections, HHV-8 infection is much more common in some geographic areas (e.g., central and southern Africa) than in others (North America, Asia, northern Europe).
  - The virus appears to be sexually spread and may also be transmitted in saliva, by organ transplantation, and through IV drug use.

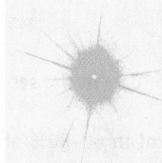

For a more detailed discussion, see Baden LR, Dolin R: Antiviral Chemotherapy, Excluding Antiretroviral Drugs, Chap. 178, p. 1442; Corey L: Herpes Simplex Virus Infections, Chap. 179, p. 1453; Whitley RJ: Varicella-Zoster Virus Infections, Chap. 180, p. 1462; and Hirsch MS: Cytomegalovirus and Human Herpesvirus Types 6, 7, and 8, Chap. 182, p. 1471, in HPIM-18.

CHAPTER **109**
Cytomegalovirus and Epstein-Barr Virus Infections

■ CYTOMEGALOVIRUS (CMV)

Microbiology

CMV is a herpesvirus, has double-stranded DNA, and renders infected cells 2–4 times the size of surrounding cells. These cytomegalic cells contain an eccentrically placed intranuclear inclusion surrounded by a clear halo, with an "owl's-eye" appearance.

Epidemiology

CMV disease is found worldwide. Perinatal and early childhood infections are common; ~1% of U.S. newborns are infected.
- The virus can be spread in breast milk, saliva, feces, and urine.
- Transmission requires repeated or prolonged contact as opposed to casual contact. Sexual transmission is common among adolescents and adults, and CMV has been identified in semen and cervical secretions.
- Latent CMV infection persists throughout life unless reactivation is triggered by depressed cell-mediated immunity (e.g., in transplant recipients or HIV-infected pts).

Pathogenesis

Primary CMV infection is associated with a vigorous T lymphocyte response; activated CD8+ T cells predominate among atypical lymphocytes.
- Latent infection occurs in multiple cell types and various organs. Chronic antigen stimulation in the presence of immunosuppression (e.g., in the transplantation setting) and certain immunosuppressive agents (e.g., antithymocyte globulin) promote CMV reactivation.
- CMV disease increases the risk of infection with opportunistic pathogens by depressing T lymphocyte responsiveness.

Clinical Manifestations

The most common presentation is CMV mononucleosis in immunocompetent pts, but disease can be more severe in immunocompromised pts (including newborns).

Congenital CMV Infection

Cytomegalic inclusion disease occurs in ~5% of infected fetuses in the setting of primary maternal CMV infection in pregnancy.
- Petechiae, hepatosplenomegaly, and jaundice are present in 60–80% of cases; microcephaly with or without cerebral calcifications, intrauterine growth retardation, prematurity, and chorioretinitis are less common.

- Laboratory findings include elevated values in LFTs, thrombocytopenia, conjugated hyperbilirubinemia, hemolysis, and increased CSF protein levels.
- The mortality rate is 20–30% among infants with severe disease; survivors have intellectual or hearing difficulties.

Perinatal CMV Infection

Perinatal infection with CMV is acquired by breast-feeding or contact with infected maternal secretions (e.g., in the birth canal). Although most pts are asymptomatic, disease similar to—but less severe than—congenital CMV can occur.

CMV Mononucleosis

Symptoms last 2–6 weeks and include high fevers, profound fatigue and malaise, myalgias, headache, and splenomegaly; in contrast to EBV infection, exudative pharyngitis and cervical lymphadenopathy are rare in CMV infection.

- Laboratory findings include relative lymphocytosis with >10% atypical lymphocytes, transaminitis, and immunologic abnormalities (e.g., the presence of cryoglobulins, rheumatoid factor, or cold agglutinins).
- The incubation period ranges from 20 to 60 days.
- Recovery is generally complete, but postviral asthenia can persist for months.

CMV Infection in the Immunocompromised Host

CMV is the most common and important viral pathogen complicating organ transplantation, with the greatest risk of infection at 1–4 months after transplantation. HIV-infected pts with CD4+ T cell counts of <50–100/μL also are at risk for severe CMV disease.

- Primary CMV infection (including reinfection with a new, donor-derived strain) is more likely than reactivation to cause severe disease with high viral loads.
  - Reactivation infection is common but less important clinically.
  - The transplanted organ is at particular risk; e.g., CMV pneumonitis tends to follow lung transplantation.
  - The risk of severe disease is reduced by antiviral prophylaxis or pre-emptive therapy.
- Pts present initially with prolonged fever, malaise, anorexia, fatigue, night sweats, and arthralgias or myalgias but can ultimately have multi-organ involvement.
  - Respiratory involvement is evidenced by tachypnea, hypoxia, unproductive cough, and chest radiographs demonstrating bilateral interstitial or reticulonodular infiltrates.
  - GI involvement often includes hepatitis and ulcer formation.
  - CMV encephalitis, particularly in HIV-infected pts, can occur as either progressive dementia or ventriculoencephalitis characterized by cranial nerve deficits, disorientation, and lethargy.
  - CMV retinitis is an important cause of blindness in pts with advanced AIDS.

Diagnosis

Diagnosis requires isolation of CMV or detection of its antigens or DNA in appropriate clinical specimens in conjunction with a compatible clinical syndrome. Immunofluorescence assays for CMV antigens (pp65), PCR, viral culture, and serology are all useful means of detection.

TREATMENT Cytomegalovirus Infections

- When possible, seronegative donors should be used for seronegative transplant recipients.
- Ganciclovir (5 mg/kg IV bid for 14–21 days followed by 5 mg/kg IV qd) or valganciclovir (the oral prodrug of ganciclovir; 900 mg PO bid for 14–21 days followed by 900 mg PO qd) produces response rates of 70–90% among HIV-infected pts with CMV retinitis or colitis.
  - In severe infections, ganciclovir is often combined with CMV immune globulin.
  - Neutropenia is an adverse reaction to ganciclovir treatment that may require administration of colony-stimulating factors.
  - Prophylactic or suppressive treatment can be given to high-risk transplant recipients (those who are seropositive before transplantation or culture positive without symptoms afterward).
  - Resistance to ganciclovir is common among pts treated for >3 months and is usually related to mutations in the CMV *UL97* gene.
  - For CMV retinitis, ganciclovir can be administered via a slow-release pellet sutured into the eye, but this intervention does not provide treatment for the contralateral eye or for systemic disease.
- Foscarnet (180 mg/kg qd divided into 2 or 3 doses for 2 weeks, followed by 90–120 mg/kg IV qd) inhibits CMV DNA polymerase and is active against most ganciclovir-resistant CMV isolates. The primary adverse events include electrolyte disturbances and renal dysfunction.
- Cidofovir (5 mg/kg IV per week for 2 weeks followed by 3–5 mg/kg IV every 2 weeks) is a nucleotide analogue that is also effective against CMV; however, it can cause severe nephrotoxicity by proximal tubular cell injury. The use of saline hydration and probenecid reduces this adverse effect.
- CMV immune or hyperimmune globulin may reduce the risk of CMV disease in seronegative renal transplant recipients and prevent congenital CMV infection in infants born to women with primary CMV infection during pregnancy.

■ EPSTEIN-BARR VIRUS (EBV)

Epidemiology

EBV is a DNA virus in the family Herpesviridae that infects >90% of persons by adulthood.

- Infectious mononucleosis (IM) is a disease of young adults and is more common in areas with higher standards of hygiene; infection occurs at a younger age in areas with deficient standards of hygiene.

- EBV is spread by contact with oral secretions (e.g., by transfer of saliva during kissing) and is shed in oropharyngeal secretions by >90% of asymptomatic seropositive individuals.

Pathogenesis

EBV infects the epithelium of the oropharynx and salivary glands as well as B cells in tonsillar crypts prior to a period of viremia.

- There is polyclonal activation of B cells, and memory B cells form the reservoir for EBV. Reactive T cells proliferate, with up to 40% of CD8+ T cells directed against EBV antigens during acute infection.
- Cellular immunity is more important than humoral immunity in controlling infection. If T cell immunity is compromised, EBV-infected B cells may proliferate—a step toward neoplastic transformation.

Clinical Manifestations

The nature of disease depends on the pt's age and immune status: young children typically develop asymptomatic infections or mild pharyngitis, adolescents and adults develop an IM syndrome, and immunocompromised pts can develop lymphoproliferative disease.

- In IM, a prodrome of fatigue, malaise, and myalgia may last for 1–2 weeks before the onset of fever, exudative pharyngitis, and lymphadenopathy with tender, symmetric, and movable nodes; splenomegaly is more prominent in the second or third week.
  - The incubation period is ~4–6 weeks.
  - Most pts treated with ampicillin develop a rash that does not represent a true penicillin allergy.
  - Illness lasts for 2–4 months, but malaise and difficulty with concentration can persist for months longer. EBV is not, however, a cause of chronic fatigue syndrome.
  - Lymphocytosis occurs in the second or third week, with >10% atypical lymphocytes (enlarged cells with abundant cytoplasm and vacuoles); abnormal liver function is common.
  - Complications include CNS disease (e.g., meningitis, encephalitis), Coombs-positive autoimmune hemolytic anemia, splenic rupture, and upper airway obstruction due to hypertrophy of lymphoid tissue.
- Lymphoproliferative disease—i.e., infiltration of lymph nodes and multiple organs by proliferating EBV-infected B cells—occurs in pts with deficient cellular immunity (e.g., pts with AIDS, those with severe combined immunodeficiency, and those receiving immunosuppressive medications). Pts develop fever and lymphadenopathy or GI symptoms.
- Oral hairy leukoplakia—raised, white, corrugated, EBV DNA–containing lesions on the tongue—is an early manifestation of infection with HIV in adults.
- EBV-associated malignancies include Burkitt's lymphoma (~90% of cases in Africa and ~15% of cases in the U.S.), anaplastic nasopharyngeal carcinoma in southern China, Hodgkin's disease (especially the mixed-cellularity type), and CNS lymphoma (especially HIV-related).

TABLE 109-1 SEROLOGIC FEATURES OF EBV-ASSOCIATED DISEASES

		Result in Indicated Test				
		Anti-VCA		Anti-EA		
Condition	Heterophile	IgM	IgG	EA-D	EA-R	Anti-EBNA
Acute infectious mononucleosis	+	+	++	+	−	−
Convalescence	±	−	+	−	±	+
Past infection	−	−	+	−	−	+
Reactivation with immunodeficiency	−	−	++	+	+	±
Burkitt's lymphoma	−	−	+++	±	++	+
Nasopharyngeal carcinoma	−	−	+++	++	±	+

Abbreviations: EA, early antigen; EA-D antibody, antibody to early antigen in diffuse pattern in nucleus and cytoplasm of infected cells; EA-R antibody, antibody to early antigen restricted to the cytoplasm; EBNA, Epstein-Barr nuclear antigen; VCA, viral capsid antigen.
Source: Adapted from Okano M et al: Clin Microbiol Rev 1:300, 1988.

Diagnosis

Serologic testing is the mainstay of diagnostic assessment. PCR analysis can be useful in monitoring EBV DNA levels in blood from pts with lympho-proliferative disease.

- Heterophile antibodies (Table 109-1) form the basis of most rapid testing, which assesses the ability of serum to agglutinate sheep, horse, or cow erythrocytes after adsorption with guinea pig kidney.
  - The antibodies can persist for up to 1 year after infection.
  - The monospot test for heterophile antibodies is ~75% sensitive and ~90% specific in comparison with EBV-specific serologies.
  - Pts <5 years old and elderly pts usually do not develop heterophile antibodies.
- EBV-specific antibody testing (Table 109-1) can be used in heterophile-negative pts and pts with atypical disease. Antibodies to viral capsid antigen occur in >90% of cases, with elevated IgM titers present only during the first 2–3 months of disease.
- Antibodies to Epstein-Barr nuclear antigen are not detected until 3–6 weeks after symptom onset and then persist for life.

TREATMENT Epstein-Barr Virus Infections

- IM is treated with supportive measures, including rest and analgesia.
  - Excessive physical activity should be avoided in the first month of illness to reduce the possibility of splenic rupture, which necessitates splenectomy.

- Administration of glucocorticoids may be indicated for some complications of IM; e.g., these agents may be given to prevent airway obstruction or to treat autoimmune hemolytic anemia.
- Antiviral therapy (e.g., with acyclovir) is generally not effective for IM but is effective for oral hairy leukoplakia.

• Treatment of posttransplantation EBV lymphoproliferative syndrome is generally directed toward reduction of immunosuppression, although other treatments—e.g., with interferon α, antibody to CD20 (rituximab), and donor lymphocyte infusions—have been used with varying success.

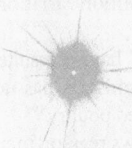

For a more detailed discussion, see Baden LR, Dolin R: Antiviral Chemotherapy, Excluding Antiretroviral Drugs, Chap. 178, p. 1442; Cohen JI: Epstein-Barr Virus Infections, Including Infectious Mononucleosis, Chap. 181, p. 1467; and Hirsch MS: Cytomegalovirus and Human Herpesvirus Types 6, 7, and 8, Chap. 182, p. 1471, in HPIM-18.

CHAPTER **110**
Influenza and Other Viral Respiratory Diseases

INFLUENZA

Microbiology and Pathogenesis

Influenza A, B, and C viruses are RNA viruses and members of the family Orthomyxoviridae with different nucleoprotein (NP) and matrix (M) protein antigens. Influenza A and B viruses are major human pathogens and are morphologically similar; influenza B infection is associated with less severe disease than influenza A infection, and influenza C virus causes subclinical disease.

• Influenza A viruses are subtyped by surface hemagglutinin (H) and neuraminidase (N) antigens.

- Virus attaches to sialic acid cell receptors via the hemagglutinin. Neuraminidase degrades the receptor and plays a role in the release of virus from infected cells after replication has occurred.
- Antibodies to the H antigen are the major determinants of immunity, while antibodies to the N antigen limit viral spread and contribute to reduction of the infection.

• Influenza is acquired from aerosolized respiratory secretions of acutely ill individuals and possibly by hand-to-hand contact or other personal or fomite contact. Viral shedding usually stops 2–5 days after disease onset.

Epidemiology

Influenza outbreaks occur each year but vary in extent and severity. Influenza A epidemics occur almost exclusively during the winter months in temperate climates but occur year-round in the tropics. These epidemics begin abruptly, peak over 2–3 weeks, last 2–3 months, and then subside rapidly.

- Global pandemics (the most recent of which took place in 2009 and was due to an A/H1N1 virus) occur, by definition, at multiple locations; they carry high attack rates (10–20% of the general population), extend beyond normal seasonality patterns, and are due in part to the propensity of the H and N antigens to undergo periodic antigenic variation.

  – Major changes (which are restricted to influenza A viruses) are called *antigenic shifts* and are associated with pandemics. Minor variations are called *antigenic drifts*.

  – The avian influenza strain A/H5N1, first detected in 1997, has not resulted in a pandemic because efficient person-to-person transmission has not occurred; infection is linked to direct contact with infected poultry.

- The segmented genome of influenza A and B viruses allows reassortment of strains between different animal species. The pandemic A/H1N1 virus of 2009–2010 represented a quadruple reassortment among swine, avian, and human influenza viruses.

- Interpandemic outbreaks of influenza are associated with economic costs exceeding $87 billion in the U.S. Chronic cardiopulmonary disease and old age are the most prominent risk factors for severe illness.

Clinical Manifestations

Influenza has a wide spectrum of clinical presentations, ranging from a mild illness resembling the common cold to severe prostration with relatively few respiratory symptoms. The classic description involves the abrupt onset of headache, fever, chills, myalgia, and malaise in the setting of respiratory symptoms (e.g., cough, sore throat).

- Pts typically defervesce within 2–3 days, but respiratory symptoms accompanied by substernal pain can persist for ≥1 week. Postinfluenzal asthenia may persist for weeks, particularly in the elderly.

- Complications of influenza (pneumonia and extrapulmonary manifestations) are more common among pts >64 years old, pregnant women, and pts with chronic disorders (e.g., cardiopulmonary disease, diabetes, renal diseases, hemoglobinopathies, or immunosuppression).

  – *Pneumonia*: Primary influenza pneumonia is the least common but most severe of the pneumonic complications, most often affecting pts with mitral stenosis and pregnant women. Pts have progressive pulmonary disease and high titers of virus in respiratory secretions.

    • *Secondary bacterial pneumonia* is usually due to *Streptococcus pneumoniae*, *Staphylococcus aureus*, or *Haemophilus influenzae* and presents as the reappearance of fever and respiratory symptoms after 2–3 days of clinical improvement.

    • The most common pneumonic complication involves aspects of viral and bacterial pneumonia.

  – *Extrapulmonary complications*: Reye's syndrome, myositis, rhabdomyolysis, myoglobinuria, and CNS disease (e.g., encephalitis, transverse myelitis, Guillain-Barré syndrome) can occur as complications of influenza infection.

- Reye's syndrome is a serious complication in children that is associated with influenza B virus (and less commonly with influenza A virus), varicella-zoster virus, and aspirin therapy for the antecedent viral infection.

Laboratory Findings

Most commonly, a laboratory diagnosis is made with a rapid test that detects viral antigens from throat swabs, nasopharyngeal washes, or sputum. These tests are relatively specific but variably sensitive.

- Reverse-transcription PCR of respiratory samples is most sensitive and specific for detecting influenza. Viral culture is also possible and gives a positive result within 48–72 h.
- Serologic testing requires the availability of acute- and convalescent-phase sera and is useful only retrospectively.

TREATMENT Influenza

- See Table 110-1 for specific treatment of influenza.
  - Antiviral agents have been tested in healthy adults with uncomplicated influenza but not in the treatment or prevention of complications associated with influenza.
  - If started within 2 days of illness due to a susceptible virus, the neuraminidase inhibitors (oseltamivir and zanamivir) and the adamantane agents (amantadine and rimantadine) reduce the duration of signs and symptoms by 1–1.5 days and ~50%, respectively.
  - IV formulations of neuraminidase inhibitors (peramivir and zanamivir) are currently in clinical trials but may be accessed through the FDA's Emergency Investigational New Drug (E-IND) application procedures.
  - Zanamivir may exacerbate bronchospasm in asthmatic pts, while oseltamivir has been associated with nausea and vomiting (reactions whose incidence is reduced if the drug is given with food) and with neuropsychiatric side effects in children.
  - Amantadine causes mild CNS side effects (e.g., jitteriness, anxiety, insomnia, difficulty concentrating) in ~5–10% of pts; rimantadine has fewer CNS side effects.
- For uncomplicated influenza in individuals at low risk for complications, symptom-based rather than antiviral therapy may be considered.

Prophylaxis

Annual vaccination with either an inactivated or a live attenuated vaccine is the main public health measure for prevention of influenza.

- Vaccine strains are generated from influenza A and B viruses that have circulated during the previous influenza season and whose circulation during the upcoming season is predicted.
  - For inactivated vaccines, 50–80% protection against influenza is expected if the vaccine virus and the currently circulating viruses are closely related.

TABLE 110-1 ANTIVIRAL MEDICATIONS FOR TREATMENT AND PROPHYLAXIS OF INFLUENZA

Antiviral Drug	Age Group (Years)		
	Children (≤12)	13–64	≥65
Oseltamivir			
Treatment, influenza A and B	Age 1–12, dose varies by weight[a]	75 mg PO bid	75 mg PO bid
Prophylaxis, influenza A and B	Age 1–12, dose varies by weight[b]	75 PO qd	75 mg PO qd
Zanamivir			
Treatment, influenza A and B	Age 7–12, 10 mg bid by inhalation	10 mg bid by inhalation	10 mg bid by inhalation
Prophylaxis, influenza A and B	Age 5–12, 10 mg qd by inhalation	10 mg qd by inhalation	10 mg qd by inhalation
Amantadine[c]			
Treatment, influenza A	Age 1–9, 5 mg/kg in 2 divided doses, up to 150 mg/d	Age ≥10, 100 mg PO bid	≤100 mg/d
Prophylaxis, influenza A	Age 1–9, 5 mg/kg in 2 divided doses, up to 150 mg/d	Age ≥10, 100 mg PO bid	≤100 mg/d
Rimantadine[c]			
Treatment, influenza A	Not approved	100 mg PO bid	100–200 mg/d
Prophylaxis, influenza A	Age 1–9, 5 mg/kg in 2 divided doses, up to 150 mg/d	Age ≥10, 100 mg PO bid	100–200 mg/d

[a]<15 kg: 30 mg bid; >15–23 kg: 45 mg bid; >23–40 kg: 60 mg bid; >40 kg: 75 mg bid. For children <1 year of age, see www.cdc.gov/h1n1flu/recommendations.htm.
[b]<15 kg: 30 mg qd; >15–23 kg: 45 mg qd; >23–40 kg: 60 mg qd; >40 kg: 75 mg qd. For children <1 year of age, see www.cdc.gov/h1n1flu/recommendations.htm.
[c]Amantadine and rimantadine are not currently recommended (2009–2010) because of widespread resistance among influenza A viruses. Their use may be reconsidered if viral susceptibility is reestablished.

- Influenza vaccination is currently recommended for all individuals >6 months of age.
- Chemoprophylaxis against influenza (see Table 110-1 for regimens) should be reserved for individuals at high risk of complications who have had close contact with a pt sick with influenza. Chemoprophylaxis can be administered simultaneously with inactivated—but not with live—vaccine.

OTHER COMMON VIRAL RESPIRATORY INFECTIONS

Acute viral respiratory illnesses account for ≥50% of all acute illnesses; adults have 3–4 cases per person per year. Clinical presentations for viral infections are generally not specific enough to allow an etiologic diagnosis, and viral illnesses are typically grouped into clinical syndromes (e.g., the "common cold," pharyngitis, tracheitis, pneumonia). This section will cover the six major groups of respiratory viruses; see Table 110-2 for an overview and Chap. 64 for additional details on viral respiratory infections.

◼ RHINOVIRUSES

Microbiology

Rhinoviruses are nonenveloped, single-stranded RNA viruses in the family Picornaviridae that together are the major cause of the "common cold" (up to 50% of cases).

Epidemiology

Rhinoviruses are spread by direct contact with infected secretions, usually respiratory droplets.

Clinical Manifestations

After an incubation period of 1–2 days, pts develop rhinorrhea, sneezing, nasal congestion, and sore throat that lasts 4–9 days. Fever and other systemic symptoms are unusual.

- Severe disease, including fatal pneumonia, is rare but has been described in immunocompromised pts, particularly bone marrow transplant recipients.

Diagnosis

An etiologic diagnosis usually is not attempted, given that the disease is generally mild and self-limited. PCR and tissue culture methods are available.

Treatment

Treatment is limited to symptom relief (e.g., with antihistamines, decongestants).

◼ CORONAVIRUSES

Microbiology

Coronaviruses are pleomorphic, single-stranded RNA viruses.

Epidemiology and Clinical Manifestations

Coronaviruses often result in the common cold (accounting for 10–35% of cases) with symptoms similar to those caused by rhinoviruses.

- Compared with rhinoviruses, the incubation period for coronaviruses is slightly longer (3 days) and the duration of illness is slightly shorter (6–7 days).
- In 2002–2003, a coronavirus-induced severe acute respiratory syndrome (SARS) developed in >8000 pts in 28 countries (with 90% of cases in China and Hong Kong) and was associated with a ~9.5% case-fatality rate; no cases were reported in 2005–2009.

TABLE 110-2 ILLNESSES ASSOCIATED WITH RESPIRATORY VIRUSES

| Virus | Frequency of Respiratory Syndromes | | |
	Most Frequent	Occasional	Infrequent
Rhinoviruses	Common cold	Exacerbation of chronic bronchitis and asthma	Pneumonia in children
Coronaviruses[a]	Common cold	Exacerbation of chronic bronchitis and asthma	Pneumonia and bronchiolitis
Human respiratory syncytial virus	Pneumonia and bronchiolitis in young children	Common cold in adults	Pneumonia in elderly and immunosuppressed pts
Parainfluenza viruses	Croup and lower respiratory tract disease in young children	Pharyngitis and common cold	Tracheobronchitis in adults; lower respiratory tract disease in immunosuppressed pts
Adenoviruses	Common cold and pharyngitis in children	Outbreaks of acute respiratory disease in military recruits[b]	Pneumonia in children; lower respiratory tract and disseminated disease in immunosuppressed pts
Influenza A viruses	Influenza[c]	Pneumonia and excess mortality in high-risk pts	Pneumonia in healthy individuals
Influenza B viruses	Influenza[c]	Rhinitis or pharyngitis alone	Pneumonia
Enteroviruses	Acute undifferentiated febrile illnesses[d]	Rhinitis or pharyngitis alone	Pneumonia
Herpes simplex viruses	Gingivostomatitis in children; pharyngotonsillitis in adults	Tracheitis and pneumonia in immunocompromised pts	Disseminated infection in immunocompromised pts
Human metapneumoviruses	Upper and lower respiratory tract disease in children	Upper respiratory tract illness in adults	Pneumonia in elderly and immunosuppressed pts

[a]SARS-associated coronavirus (SARS-CoV) caused epidemics of pneumonia from November 2002 to July 2003 (see text).
[b]Serotypes 4 and 7.
[c]Fever, cough, myalgia, malaise.
[d]May or may not have a respiratory component.

- SARS has an incubation period of 2–7 days, after which pts develop fever, malaise, headache, myalgias, and then (1–2 days later) a nonproductive cough and dyspnea.
- Respiratory function may worsen in the second week of illness and can progress to ARDS and multiorgan dysfunction.

Diagnosis

Laboratory diagnosis of coronavirus-induced colds is rarely required, but ELISA, immunofluorescence, and RT-PCR assays can detect the virus in clinical specimens.

- The coronavirus associated with SARS (SARS-CoV) can be detected by RT-PCR or viral culture from respiratory samples and serum early in illness and from urine and stool later on.
- SARS is also associated with lymphopenia (mostly CD4+ cells) in 50% of cases.

TREATMENT   Coronaviruses

- For the common cold, no treatment beyond symptom relief is generally needed.
- For SARS, aggressive supportive care is most important. No specific therapy (e.g., ribavirin, glucocorticoids) has been established as efficacious.

■ HUMAN RESPIRATORY SYNCYTIAL VIRUS

Microbiology

Human respiratory syncytial virus (HRSV) is an enveloped, single-stranded RNA virus and a member of the family Paramyxoviridae.

Epidemiology

With an attack rate approaching 100% among susceptible individuals, HRSV is a major respiratory pathogen among young children (particularly those 2–3 months of age) and the foremost cause of lower respiratory disease among infants.

- HRSV accounts for 20–25% of hospital admissions of young children for pneumonia and for up to 75% of cases of bronchiolitis in this age group.
- The virus is transmitted efficiently via contact with contaminated fingers or fomites and by spread of coarse aerosols. The incubation period is ~4–6 days.

Clinical Manifestations

Infants typically develop rhinorrhea, low-grade fever, cough, and wheezing; 20–40% of infections result in lower tract disease, including pneumonia, bronchiolitis, and tracheobronchitis.

- In adults, HRSV typically presents as the common cold, but it can cause lower respiratory tract disease with fever, including severe pneumonia in elderly or immunosuppressed pts. HRSV pneumonia has a case-fatality rate of 20–80% among transplant pts.

Diagnosis

Rapid viral diagnosis is available by immunofluorescence, ELISA, or RT-PCR of nasopharyngeal washes, aspirates, or (less satisfactorily) swabs.

TREATMENT Human Respiratory Syncytial Virus

- Treatment is symptom-based for upper tract disease and mild lower tract disease.
- For severe lower tract disease, intubation and ventilatory assistance should be given as needed.
  - Aerosolized ribavirin has a demonstrated modest beneficial effect for infants with severe HRSV pneumonia, but its efficacy in older children and adults (including immunocompromised pts) has not been established.
  - No benefit has been found in any pt population for IV immunoglobulin (IVIg), immunoglobulin with high titers of antibody to HRSV (RSVIg), or a monoclonal IgG antibody to HRSV (palivizumab).

Prevention

Monthly administration of palivizumab is approved for prophylaxis in children <2 years of age who have bronchopulmonary dysplasia or cyanotic heart disease or who were born prematurely. In settings with high transmission rates (e.g., pediatric wards), contact precautions are useful to limit spread of the virus.

■ HUMAN METAPNEUMOVIRUS

Microbiology

Human metapneumovirus (HMPV) is a pleomorphic, single-stranded RNA virus of the family Paramyxoviridae.

Epidemiology

HMPV accounts for 1–5% of childhood upper respiratory tract infections and for 2–4% of acute respiratory illnesses in ambulatory adults.

Clinical Manifestations

Disease manifestations are similar to those caused by HRSV.

Diagnosis

Diagnosis is made by immunofluorescence, PCR, or tissue culture of nasal aspirates or respiratory secretions.

Treatment

Treatment is primarily supportive and symptom-based.

■ PARAINFLUENZA VIRUS

Microbiology and Epidemiology

This enveloped, single-stranded RNA virus of the family Paramyxoviridae ranks second only to HRSV as a cause of lower respiratory tract disease among young children and is the most common cause of croup (laryngo-tracheobronchitis).

Clinical Manifestations

Infections are milder among older children and adults, but severe, prolonged, and fatal infection has been reported among pts with severe immunosuppression, including transplant recipients.

Diagnosis

Tissue culture, rapid testing with immunofluorescence or ELISA (both of which are less sensitive), or PCR of respiratory tract secretions, throat swabs, or nasopharyngeal washings can detect the virus.

Treatment

Treatment of upper respiratory tract disease is symptom-based. Humidified air may be helpful for mild cases of croup.

- For cases of croup with respiratory distress, intermittent racemic epinephrine and glucocorticoids are beneficial.
- Anecdotal reports describe the use of ribavirin (particularly in immunosuppressed pts), but its clinical utility is still unclear.

■ ADENOVIRUSES

Microbiology and Epidemiology

Adenoviruses are double-stranded DNA viruses that cause ~10% of acute respiratory infections among children and <2% of respiratory illnesses among civilian adults. Some serotypes are associated with outbreaks among military recruits. Transmission takes place primarily from fall to spring via inhalation of aerosolized virus, through inoculation of the conjunctival sacs, and probably via the fecal-oral route.

Clinical Manifestations

In children, adenovirus causes acute upper and lower respiratory tract infections and outbreaks of pharyngoconjunctival fever (a syndrome of fever, bilateral conjunctivitis, sore throat, and cervical adenopathy typically due to types 3 and 7).

- In adults, adenovirus types 4 and 7 cause an acute respiratory disease consisting of a prominent sore throat, fever on the second or third day of illness, cough, coryza, and regional adenopathy. Pharyngeal edema and tonsillar hypertrophy with little or no exudate may be seen.
- In addition to respiratory disease, adenovirus can cause diarrheal illness, hemorrhagic cystitis, and epidemic keratoconjunctivitis. In pts who have received a solid-organ transplant, adenovirus can affect the transplanted organ and disseminate to other organs.

Diagnosis

Definitive diagnosis can be made by isolation of the virus in tissue culture; by rapid testing (with immunofluorescence or ELISA) of nasopharyngeal aspirates, conjunctival or respiratory secretions, urine, or stool; or by PCR testing.

Treatment

Treatment is supportive. Ribavirin and cidofovir exhibit in vitro activity against adenovirus and therefore are used occasionally in disseminated adenovirus infections, but definitive efficacy data are not available.

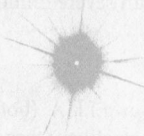

> For a more detailed discussion, see Baden LR, Dolin R: Antiviral Chemotherapy, Excluding Antiretroviral Drugs, Chap. 178, p. 1442; Dolin R: Common Viral Respiratory Infections, Chap. 186, p. 1485; and Dolin R: Influenza, Chap. 187, p. 1493, in HPIM-18.

CHAPTER **111**
Rubeola, Rubella, Mumps, and Parvovirus Infections

■ MEASLES (RUBEOLA)

Definition and Microbiology

Measles is a highly contagious disease that is characterized by a prodromal illness of fever, cough, coryza, and conjunctivitis followed by a generalized maculopapular rash. Measles is caused by a nonsegmented, single-stranded, negative-sense RNA virus of the genus *Morbillivirus* and the family Paramyxoviridae.

Epidemiology

Humans are the only reservoir for measles virus; unvaccinated infants who have lost maternal antibodies account for the bulk of susceptible individuals. However, as measles vaccine coverage increases, the age distribution of the disease shifts upward: in the United States, adolescents and adults are the most likely age groups to acquire measles.

- Routine administration of the measles vaccine has markedly reduced worldwide mortality due to measles; in 2008, there were ~164,000 deaths.
- Pts are contagious for several days before and after the rash appears. The virus is spread primarily via respiratory droplets over short distances. Secondary attack rates among susceptible contacts are >90%.

Clinical Manifestations

Approximately 10 days after infection with measles virus, pts develop fever and malaise, followed by cough, coryza, and conjunctivitis; the characteristic rash occurs 14 days after infection.

- An erythematous, nonpruritic, maculopapular rash begins at the hairline and behind the ears, spreads down the trunk and limbs to include the palms and soles, can become confluent, and begins to fade (in the same order of progression) by day 4.

- Koplik's spots are pathognomonic for measles and consist of bluish-white dots ~1 mm in diameter surrounded by erythema. They appear on the buccal mucosa ~2 days before the rash appears and fade with the onset of rash.
- Pts with impaired cellular immunity may not develop a rash and have a higher case-fatality rate than those with intact immunity.
- Complications include giant-cell pneumonitis, secondary bacterial infection of the respiratory tract (e.g., otitis media, bronchopneumonia), and CNS disorders.
  - Postmeasles encephalitis occurs within 2 weeks of rash onset in ~1 in 1000 cases and is characterized by fever, seizures, and a variety of neurologic abnormalities.
  - Measles inclusion-body encephalitis (MIBE) and subacute sclerosing panencephalitis (SSPE) occur months to years after acute infection and are caused by persistent measles virus infection.
    - MIBE is a fatal complication that primarily affects pts with defects in cellular immunity.
    - SSPE is a progressive disease characterized by seizures and deterioration of cognitive and motor functions, with death occurring 5–15 years after measles virus infection.

Diagnosis

The characteristic rash and pathognomonic Koplik's spots permit a clinical diagnosis.

- Serologic testing is the most common method of laboratory diagnosis. Measles-specific IgM is usually detectable within 1–3 days of rash onset.
- Viral culture and reverse-transcription PCR analysis of clinical specimens are used occasionally to detect measles.

TREATMENT ▶ **Measles**

- Supportive care is the mainstay of treatment, as there is no specific antiviral therapy for measles. Prompt antibiotic therapy for pts with secondary bacterial infections helps reduce morbidity and mortality risks.
- Vitamin A (for children ≥12 months: 200,000 IU daily for 2 days) is recommended by the World Health Organization (WHO) for all children with measles.

Prevention

In the U.S., children are routinely immunized with two doses of a live attenuated vaccine containing measles, mumps, and rubella (MMR) antigens.

- Vaccine-induced immunity lasts for at least several decades; rates of secondary vaccine failure 10–15 years after immunization are ~5%. In contrast, natural infection leads to life-long immunity.
- Administration of immunoglobulin within 6 days of exposure, which can prevent or modify the disease in immunocompetent persons, is recommended for children <1 year old, immunocompromised pts, and pregnant

women. A dose of 0.25 mL/kg is given to healthy pts and a dose of 0.5 mL/kg to immunocompromised hosts, with a maximal dose of 15 mL.

■ RUBELLA (GERMAN MEASLES)

Microbiology and Epidemiology

Rubella is a contagious infectious disease caused by a single-stranded, enveloped RNA virus in the family Togaviridae and the genus *Rubivirus*.

- In 2007, there were ~165,000 cases of rubella worldwide, although this figure is probably an underestimate because of poor reporting. Since 2004, rubella has not been an endemic disease in the U.S.
- Virus is spread via respiratory droplets, and primary implantation and replication occur in the nasopharynx. Placental infection can lead to chronic infection of virtually all fetal organs, which sometimes persists for up to 1 year after birth.

Clinical Manifestations

While acquired rubella infection is generally benign, congenital rubella infection can be more severe.

- *Acquired infection*: With an incubation period of 14 days, acquired rubella is characterized by a generalized maculopapular rash that lasts for ≤3 days; ~50% of infections are subclinical.
  - Occipital and/or postauricular lymphadenopathy may occur during the second week after exposure.
  - In older children and adults, the rash may be preceded by a 1- to 5-day prodrome consisting of low-grade fever, malaise, and upper respiratory symptoms.
  - Arthralgias and arthritis are common among adults, particularly women.
- *Congenital infection*: Congenital rubella infection can lead to a number of physical defects, usually involving the eyes (e.g., cataracts), ears (e.g., deafness), and heart (e.g., pulmonary arterial stenosis).
  - Up to 90% of women infected with rubella virus during the first 11 weeks of pregnancy will deliver an infant with congenital rubella.
  - The congenital rubella rate is 20% for maternal infections acquired during the first 20 weeks of pregnancy.

Diagnosis

Given the difficulty of diagnosing rubella clinically, serologic testing (for the presence of IgM or a ≥4-fold rise in IgG titer) is generally used for diagnosis.

- If the IgM sample taken within the first 4 days of rash is negative but clinical suspicion remains, testing should be repeated; IgM antibody titers are generally positive for up to 6 weeks.
- Congenital rubella can be diagnosed by detection of IgM antibodies, although titers may be negative during the first month; by isolation of the virus from throat swabs, urine, or CSF; and/or by an IgG titer that does not decline at the expected rate of a twofold dilution per month.
- In the U.S., screening of pregnant women for rubella IgG antibodies is part of routine prenatal care; seronegative women should be vaccinated postpartum.

Treatment

Symptom-based treatment for various manifestations, such as fever and arthralgia, is appropriate. No rubella-specific therapies are available.

Prevention

As of 2008, 66% of countries holding membership in the WHO had recommended inclusion of a rubella-containing vaccine in the routine childhood vaccination schedule. One dose induces seroconversion in ≥95% of persons >1 year of age and provides long-term (potentially life-long) immunity.

- Pregnant women should not receive the vaccine, and pregnancy should be avoided for at least 28 days after vaccination.
- Immunoglobulin does not prevent rubella virus infection after exposure and therefore is not recommended as routine postexposure prophylaxis.

■ MUMPS

Definition and Microbiology

Mumps is an acute systemic communicable viral infection whose most distinctive feature is swelling of one or both parotid glands. It is caused by mumps virus, a negative-strand nonsegmented RNA paramyxovirus.

Epidemiology

The estimated annual global incidence of mumps is 100–1000 cases per 100,000 population in countries without national mumps vaccination programs. In the U.S., there were <300 cases in 2001 because levels of childhood vaccination are high.

- The incubation period of mumps is ~19 days, and humans are the only natural hosts.
- Mumps virus is transmitted by respiratory secretions and fomites. Pts are contagious from 1 week before to 1 week after symptom onset and are most contagious 1–2 days before symptom onset.

Clinical Manifestations

Up to half of infections are asymptomatic or lead to nonspecific respiratory symptoms. Unilateral or bilateral parotitis lasting >2 days is present in 70–90% of symptomatic infections.

- A prodrome involving low-grade fever, malaise, myalgia, headache, and anorexia may precede the development of parotitis and last for 1–7 days.
  - Pts with parotitis typically have difficulty eating, swallowing, and/or talking and may have an earache.
  - Glandular swelling disappears within 1 week.
- Epididymo-orchitis is the second most common manifestation of mumps, developing in 15–30% of cases in postpubertal males.
  - Orchitis, characterized by a painful, tender, and enlarged testis, is bilateral in 10–30% of cases and resolves within 1 week.
  - Oophoritis (manifested by lower abdominal pain and vomiting) occurs in ~5% of women with mumps.
  - Sterility after mumps is rare.

- Symptomatic CNS disease (e.g., aseptic meningitis) occurs in <10% of pts and is usually self-limited.
  - In CSF pleocytosis, neutrophils often predominate in the first 24 h before being replaced by lymphocytes on the second day.
  - Cranial nerve palsies occasionally lead to permanent sequelae, particularly deafness.
- Other, less common manifestations of mumps include pancreatitis, myocarditis, thyroiditis, nephritis, and arthritis. Mumps in pregnancy does not appear to lead to premature birth, low birth weight, or fetal malformations.

Diagnosis

Laboratory diagnosis is generally based on detection of viral antigens or RNA in clinical samples (e.g., throat swab, CSF, urine, seminal fluid) via immunofluorescence or reverse-transcription PCR. Serologic assays are of limited utility since IgM is detected in <20% of cases in immunized pts and IgG titers often exhibit little fluctuation between acute- and convalescent-phase samples.

Treatment

Mumps is generally a benign, self-resolving illness in which symptom-based and supportive therapies are most helpful.

Prevention

Current U.S. recommendations are for a two-dose vaccination schedule, with the first dose at ≥1 year old and the second dose at least 1 month after the first. Outbreaks, such as those occurring in 2006 in the U.S., the United Kingdom, and Canada, demonstrate that vaccine-induced immunity is not life-long.

■ PARVOVIRUS INFECTION

Microbiology

Parvovirus B19 (B19V), a nonenveloped single-strand DNA virus of the family Parvoviridae, is the only member of this family shown definitively to be a human pathogen.

Epidemiology

B19V exclusively infects humans, is endemic worldwide, and is transmitted via the respiratory route. By the age of 15 years, ≥50% of children are seropositive. Of elderly pts, >90% have detectable antibody.

Pathogenesis

B19V replicates in erythroid progenitors, which are among the few cells that express the B19V receptor, blood group P antigen (globoside). Infection leads to high-titer viremia and arrest of erythropoiesis. When an IgM and IgG antibody response is mounted, normal erythropoiesis resumes.

Clinical Manifestations

Most B19V infections are asymptomatic or are associated with only a mild nonspecific illness.

- *Erythema infectiosum (fifth disease)*: The main manifestation of symptomatic B19V disease, erythema infectiosum presents as a low-grade fever ~7–10 days after exposure and a facial "slapped-cheek" rash (more common among children) a few days later. Two or three days after the facial rash develops, a lacy, reticular macular rash may spread to the extremities.
- *Polyarthropathy syndrome*: Arthralgias, typically symmetric and affecting the small joints of the hands and occasionally the ankles, knees, and wrists, occur in ~50% of adults (more commonly women). Most cases resolve in a few weeks, but some persist for months.
- *Transient aplastic crisis (TAC)*: Pts with chronic hemolytic conditions (e.g., hemoglobinopathies, autoimmune hemolytic anemia) can develop aplastic crisis with B19V infection that can be life-threatening. Pts display symptoms associated with severe anemia.
- *Pure red-cell aplasia/chronic anemia*: Immunosuppressed pts can develop persistent anemia with reticulocytopenia, high levels of B19V DNA in serum, and absent or low levels of B19V IgG. B19V occasionally causes a hemophagocytic syndrome.
- *Hydrops fetalis*: B19V infection during pregnancy can lead to hydrops fetalis and/or fetal loss. The risk of transplacental fetal infection is ~30%, and the risk of fetal loss (which occurs predominantly early in the second trimester) is ~9%. The risk of congenital infection is <1%.

Diagnosis

Diagnosis in immunocompetent pts generally relies on detection of B19V-specific IgM antibodies, which can be detected coincident with the rash in erythema infectiosum or by day 3 of TAC.

- B19V-specific IgG is detectable by the seventh day of illness and persists for life.
- Detection of B19V DNA via quantitative PCR should be used to diagnose early TAC or chronic anemia. In acute infection, the viremia load can be >10^{12} B19V DNA IU/mL of serum; pts with TAC or chronic anemia generally have >10^5 B19V IU/mL.

TREATMENT	Parvovirus Infection

- Treatment of B19V infection is generally supportive as no specific therapy exists. TAC should be treated with transfusions as needed.
- In pts receiving immunosuppressive agents, treatment should be reduced to the extent feasible to allow an immune response. IV immunoglobulin (400 mg/kg daily for 5–10 days) may cure or ameliorate persistent B19V infection in immunosuppressed pts.

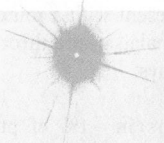

For a more detailed discussion, see Brown KE: Parvovirus Infections, Chap. 184, p. 1478; Moss WJ: Measles (Rubeola), Chap. 192, p. 1600; Zimmerman LA, Reef SE: Rubella (German Measles), Chap. 193, p. 1605; and Rubin S, Carbone KM: Mumps, Chap. 194, p. 1608, in HPIM-18.

CHAPTER **112**
Enteroviral Infections

■ **MICROBIOLOGY**

- Enteroviruses are so named because of their ability to multiply in the GI tract, but they do not typically cause gastroenteritis.
- Enteroviruses encompass 96 human serotypes: 3 serotypes of poliovirus, 21 serotypes of coxsackievirus A, 6 serotypes of coxsackievirus B, 28 serotypes of echovirus, enteroviruses 68–71, and 34 new enteroviruses (beginning with enterovirus 73) that have been identified by molecular techniques. In the United States, coxsackievirus B1 and echoviruses 18, 9, and 6 account for ~50% of all enteroviral infections.

■ **PATHOGENESIS**

- Studies of poliovirus infection form the basis of our understanding of enteroviral pathogenesis.
- After ingestion, poliovirus infects GI tract mucosal epithelial cells, spreads to regional lymph nodes, causes viremia, and replicates in the reticuloendothelial system; in some cases, a second round of viremia occurs.
- Virus gains access to the CNS either via the bloodstream or via direct spread from neural pathways.
- Virus is present in blood for 3–5 days. It is shed from the oropharynx for up to 3 weeks and from the GI tract for up to 12 weeks after infection; hypogammaglobulinemic pts can shed virus for up to 20 years.
- Infection is controlled by humoral and secretory immunity in the GI tract.

■ **EPIDEMIOLOGY**

- Enteroviruses cause disease worldwide, especially in areas with crowded conditions and poor hygiene.
- Infants and young children are most often infected and are the most frequent shedders.
- Transmission takes place mainly by the fecal-oral route, but airborne transmission and placental transmission have been described.
- The incubation period ranges from 2 to 14 days but usually is <1 week in duration. Pts are most infectious shortly before and after the onset of symptoms.

■ **CLINICAL MANIFESTATIONS**

Poliovirus

After an incubation period of 3–6 days, ~5% of pts present with a minor illness (abortive poliomyelitis) characterized by fever, malaise, sore throat, myalgias, and headache that usually resolves within 3 days.

- *Asymptomatic infection*: >90% of all infections
- *Aseptic meningitis (nonparalytic poliomyelitis)*: occurs in ~1% of pts. Examination of CSF reveals normal glucose and protein concentrations and lymphocytic pleocytosis (with PMNs sometimes predominating early).

- *Paralytic disease:* the least common form; presents ≥1 day after aseptic meningitis as severe back, neck, and muscle pain as well as a gradual development of motor weakness.
  - The weakness is usually asymmetric and proximal and is most common in the legs; the arms and the abdominal, thoracic, and bulbar muscles are other frequently involved sites.
  - Paralysis generally occurs only during the febrile phase.
  - Physical examination reveals weakness, fasciculations, decreased muscle tone, and reduced or absent reflexes in affected areas; hyperreflexia may precede the loss of reflexes. Bulbar paralysis is associated with dysphagia, difficulty handling secretions, or dysphonia.
  - Respiratory insufficiency due to aspiration or neurologic involvement may develop. Severe medullary infection may lead to circulatory collapse.
  - Most pts recover some function, but around two-thirds have residual neurologic sequelae.
- *Vaccine-associated poliomyelitis:* The risk of acquiring poliomyelitis after vaccination with the live oral vaccine is estimated to be 1 case per 2.5 million doses and is ~2000 times higher among immunodeficient persons.
- *Postpolio syndrome:* new weakness 20–40 years after poliomyelitis. Onset is insidious, progression is slow, and plateau periods can last 1–10 years.

Other Enteroviruses

In the United States, 5–10 million cases of symptomatic enteroviral disease other than poliomyelitis occur each year. More than 50% of nonpoliovirus enteroviral infections are subclinical.

- *Nonspecific febrile illness (summer grippe):* Pts present with acute-onset fever, malaise, and headache, with occasional upper respiratory symptoms.
  - Disease resolves within a week.
  - Disease frequently occurs during the summer and early fall.
- *Generalized disease of the newborn:* Neonates, typically within the first week of life, present with an illness resembling bacterial sepsis, with fever, irritability, and lethargy.
  - Myocarditis, hypotension, hepatitis, DIC, meningitis, and pneumonia are complications.
  - A history of a recent flu-like illness in the mother should prompt consideration of this disease.
- *Aseptic meningitis and encephalitis:* Enteroviruses cause 90% of cases of aseptic meningitis among children and young adults in which an etiologic agent can be identified; 10–35% of cases of viral encephalitis are due to enteroviruses.
  - Pts have an acute onset of fever, chills, headache, photophobia, nausea, and vomiting, with meningismus on examination. Diarrhea, rashes, myalgias, pleurodynia, myocarditis, and herpangina may occur. Encephalitis is much less common and is usually mild, with an excellent prognosis in healthy hosts.
  - CSF examination reveals pleocytosis, with PMNs sometimes predominating early but a shift to lymphocyte predominance within 24 h. Total

cell counts usually do not exceed 1000/μL. CSF glucose and protein levels are typically normal.

– Symptoms resolve within 1 week, but CSF abnormalities persist longer.

- *Pleurodynia (Bornholm disease)*: Pts have an acute onset of fever associated with spasms of pleuritic chest pain (more common among adults) or upper abdominal pain (more common among children) that typically last 15–30 min. Fever subsides when pain resolves.

  – Coxsackievirus B is the most common cause.

  – Disease lasts for a few days and can be treated with NSAIDs and heat application to the affected muscles.

- *Myocarditis and pericarditis*: Enteroviruses (e.g., coxsackievirus B) cause up to one-third of cases of acute myocarditis. Pts have upper respiratory symptoms followed by fever, chest pain, dyspnea, arrhythmias, and occasionally heart failure.

  – Disease occurs most often in newborns (who are most severely ill), adolescents, and young adults.

  – A pericardial friction rub, ST-segment and T-wave abnormalities on electrocardiography, and elevated serum levels of myocardial enzymes can be present.

  – Up to 10% of pts develop chronic dilated cardiomyopathy.

- *Exanthems*: Enteroviral infection is the leading cause of exanthems among children in the summer and fall. Echoviruses 9 and 16 are common causes.

- *Hand-foot-and-mouth disease*: generally due to coxsackievirus A16 and enterovirus 71. Pts present with fever, anorexia, and malaise, which are followed by sore throat and vesicles on the buccal mucosa, tongue, and dorsum or palms of the hands and occasionally on the palate, uvula, tonsillar pillars, or feet.

  – The disease is highly infectious, with attack rates of almost 100% among young children. Symptoms resolve within a week.

  – A Taiwan epidemic of enterovirus 71 infection in 1998 was associated with CNS disease, myocarditis, and pulmonary hemorrhage. Deaths occurred primarily among children ≤5 years old.

- *Herpangina*: usually caused by coxsackievirus A infection. Pts develop fever, sore throat, odynophagia, and grayish-white papulovesicular lesions on an erythematous base that ulcerate and are concentrated in the posterior portion of the mouth.

  – Lesions can persist for weeks.

  – In contrast to herpes simplex stomatitis, enteroviral herpangina is not associated with gingivitis.

- *Acute hemorrhagic conjunctivitis*: associated with enterovirus 70 and coxsackievirus A24. Pts experience an acute onset of severe eye pain, blurred vision, photophobia, and watery eye discharge; edema, chemosis, and subconjunctival hemorrhage are evident. Symptoms resolve within 10 days.

■ DIAGNOSIS

- Enterovirus can be isolated from throat or rectal swabs, stool, and/or normally sterile body fluids.

- Positive results for normally sterile body fluids, such as CSF and serum, reflect disease.
- However, stool and throat cultures may simply reflect colonization.
- In general, serotyping is not clinically useful.
- PCR detects all serotypes that infect humans, with high sensitivity (70–100%) and specificity (>80%).
  - PCR of CSF is less likely to be positive if pts present ≥3 days after meningitis onset or with enterovirus 71 infection.
  - PCR of serum is also useful in disseminated disease.

TREATMENT Enteroviral Infections

- Most enteroviral illness resolves spontaneously, but immunoglobulin may be helpful in pts with γ globulin defects and chronic infection.
- Glucocorticoids are contraindicated.

■ PREVENTION AND ERADICATION

- Hand hygiene, use of gowns and gloves, and enteric precautions (for 7 days after disease onset) prevent nosocomial transmission of enteroviruses during epidemics.
- The availability of poliovirus vaccines and the implementation of polio eradication programs have largely eliminated disease due to wild-type poliovirus; of 1781 cases in 2009, ~80% were from Nigeria, India, Pakistan, and Afghanistan. Outbreaks and sporadic disease due to vaccine-derived poliovirus occur.
- Both oral poliovirus vaccine (OPV) and inactivated poliovirus vaccine (IPV) induce IgG and IgA antibodies that persist for at least 5 years.
  - Most developing countries, particularly those with persistent wild-type poliomyelitis, use OPV because of its lower cost and ease of administration.
  - The suboptimal seroconversion rate among children in low-income countries, even after multiple doses of OPV, contributes to difficulties in eradication.
- Most industrialized countries have adopted all-IPV childhood vaccination programs.
  - Unvaccinated adults in the United States do not need routine poliovirus vaccination, but should receive three doses of IPV (the second dose 1–2 months after the first and the final dose 6–12 months later) if they are traveling to polio-endemic areas or might be exposed to wild-type poliovirus in their communities or workplaces.
  - Adults at increased risk of exposure who have received their primary vaccination series should receive a single dose of IPV.

For a more detailed discussion, see Cohen JI: Enteroviruses and Reoviruses, Chap. 191, p. 1593, in HPIM-18.

CHAPTER **113**
Insect- and Animal-Borne Viral Infections

■ RABIES

Microbiology

Rabies is a zoonosis generally transmitted to humans by the bite of a rabid animal and caused by rabies virus—a nonsegmented, negative sense, single-stranded RNA virus in the family Rhabdoviridae. Each animal reservoir harbors distinct rabies virus variants.

Epidemiology

Worldwide, canine rabies causes ~55,000 human deaths each year, most of them in Asia and Africa.

- Endemic canine rabies has been eliminated in the United States and most other resource-rich countries but persists in bats, raccoons, skunks, and foxes. In 2008, there were 6841 confirmed animal cases of rabies in the U.S.
- Bats (especially silver-haired and eastern pipistrelle bats) cause most human cases in North America, although there may be no known history of a bat bite or other bat exposure.

Pathogenesis

The incubation period can range from a few days to >1 year but is usually 20–90 days. During most of this period, rabies virus is present at or close to the site of the bite.

- The virus binds to postsynaptic nicotinic acetylcholine receptors and spreads centripetally along peripheral nerves toward the CNS at a rate up to ~250 mm/d. Establishment of CNS infection is followed by centrifugal spread along peripheral nerves to other tissues, including salivary glands—hence the excretion of virus in the saliva of rabid animals.
- The most characteristic pathologic CNS finding is the *Negri body*—an eosinophilic cytoplasmic inclusion that is composed of rabies virus proteins and viral RNA and is found primarily within Purkinje cells of the cerebellum and in pyramidal neurons of the hippocampus.

Clinical Manifestations

Rabies usually presents as atypical encephalitis with preservation of consciousness; the disease may be difficult to recognize after the onset of coma. This disease, which usually leads to death despite aggressive therapy, has three phases.

- *Prodrome*: Pts have fever, headache, malaise, nausea, vomiting, and anxiety or agitation lasting 2–10 days. Paresthesias, pain, or pruritus near

the site of exposure (which has usually healed at this point) is found in 50–80% of cases and strongly suggests rabies.
• *Acute neurologic phase*: Pts present with the encephalitic (furious) form of rabies in 80% of cases and with the paralytic form in 20%.
  – *Encephalitic form*: Pts develop symptoms common to other viral encephalitides (e.g., fever, confusion, hallucinations, combativeness, and seizures) that last 2–10 days. Autonomic dysfunction is common and includes hypersalivation, gooseflesh, cardiac arrhythmia, and/or priapism.
    • A distinguishing feature of rabies is prominent early brainstem dysfunction resulting in hydrophobia and aerophobia (involuntary, painful contraction of the diaphragm and the accessory respiratory, laryngeal, and pharyngeal muscles in response to swallowing liquid or exposure to a draft of air).
    • Hypersalivation and pharyngeal dysfunction produce characteristic foaming at the mouth.
    • Death usually occurs within days of brainstem involvement. With aggressive supportive care, late complications include cardiopulmonary failure, disturbances of water balance (syndrome of inappropriate antidiuretic hormone secretion or diabetes insipidus), and GI hemorrhage.
  – *Paralytic form*: For unknown reasons, muscle weakness predominates but cardinal features of rabies encephalitis (hyperexcitability, hydrophobia, aerophobia) are lacking. Muscle weakness usually begins in the bitten extremity and proceeds to quadriparesis.
• *Coma and death*: Even with aggressive supportive measures, recovery is rare. Death usually occurs within 2 weeks.

Diagnosis

In North America, the diagnosis is often considered relatively late in the clinical course. Rabies should be considered for pts with acute atypical encephalitis or acute flaccid paralysis (including those in whom Guillain-Barré syndrome is suspected).
• Most routine laboratory tests in rabies are normal or nonspecific; it is important to test for alternative, potentially treatable diagnoses.
• Negative antemortem rabies-specific laboratory tests never exclude a diagnosis of rabies, and tests may need to be repeated after an interval for diagnostic confirmation.
  – In a previously unimmunized pt, serum neutralizing antibodies to rabies virus are diagnostic, but these antibodies may not be present until late in the disease course. The presence of rabies virus–specific antibodies in CSF suggests rabies encephalitis, regardless of immunization status.
  – Reverse-transcription PCR (RT-PCR) can detect virus in fresh saliva samples, CSF, and skin and brain tissues.
  – Direct fluorescent antibody testing is highly sensitive and specific and can be applied to brain tissue or skin biopsy samples from the nape of the neck (where virus is found in cutaneous nerves at the base of hair follicles).

TREATMENT	Rabies

Management is palliative and supportive. There is no established treatment for rabies.

Prevention

Rabies is almost uniformly fatal but is nearly always preventable with appropriate postexposure prophylaxis during the incubation period. Only 7 pts have survived infection with rabies virus, and only 1 of these pts had not received rabies vaccine before disease onset.

- An algorithm for rabies postexposure prophylaxis is depicted in Fig. 113-1.
  - Local wound care (e.g., thorough washing, debridement of devitalized tissue) can greatly reduce the risk of rabies.
  - All previously unvaccinated pts should receive human rabies immune globulin (RIG, 20 IU/kg; 40 IU/kg for equine RIG) no later than 7 days after the first vaccine dose. The entire dose should be infiltrated at the site of the bite; if not anatomically feasible, the residual RIG should be given IM at a distant site.
  - Inactivated rabies vaccine should be given as soon as possible (1 mL IM in the deltoid region) and repeated on days 3, 7, and 14 for previously unvaccinated pts; previously vaccinated pts require booster doses only on days 0 and 3.
- Preexposure prophylaxis is occasionally given to persons at high risk (including certain travelers to rabies-endemic areas). A primary vaccine schedule is given on days 0, 7, and 21 or 28.

■ INFECTIONS CAUSED BY ARTHROPOD- AND RODENT-BORNE VIRUSES

Microbiology and Pathogenesis

Most zoonotic viruses only incidentally infect and produce disease in humans; only a few agents are regularly spread among humans by arthropods.

- The Arenaviridae, Bunyaviridae, and Flaviviridae—all RNA viruses—are among the major families of arthropod- and rodent-borne viruses.
- Arthropod-borne viruses infect the vector after a blood meal from a viremic vertebrate; after spreading throughout the vector and ultimately reaching the salivary glands, the viruses can be transmitted to another vertebrate during a blood meal.
- Humans become infected with rodent-borne viruses by inhalation of aerosols containing the viruses and through close contact with chronically infected rodents and their excreta.

Clinical Manifestations

Infection is usually subclinical; when disease does occur, it generally does so in one of four occasionally overlapping clinical syndromes: fever and myalgia, encephalitis, arthritis and rash, or hemorrhagic fever (HF).

Fever and Myalgia This is the most common syndrome associated with zoonotic viruses. Typically, pts have an acute onset of fever, severe myalgia,

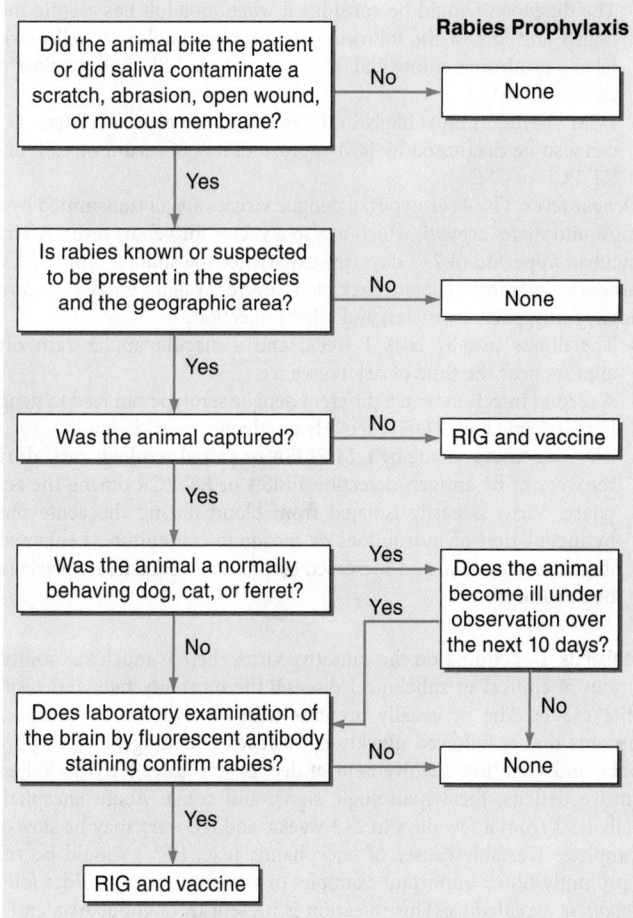

Rabies Prophylaxis

Did the animal bite the patient or did saliva contaminate a scratch, abrasion, open wound, or mucous membrane? → **No** → None

↓ Yes

Is rabies known or suspected to be present in the species and the geographic area? → **No** → None

↓ Yes

Was the animal captured? → **No** → RIG and vaccine

↓ Yes

Was the animal a normally behaving dog, cat, or ferret? → **Yes** → Does the animal become ill under observation over the next 10 days?

→ Yes

↓ No

Does laboratory examination of the brain by fluorescent antibody staining confirm rabies? ← **Yes**

Does the animal become ill under observation over the next 10 days? → **No** → None

Does laboratory examination of the brain by fluorescent antibody staining confirm rabies? → **No** → None

↓ Yes

RIG and vaccine

FIGURE 113-1 Algorithm for rabies postexposure prophylaxis. RIG, rabies immune globulin. *[From L Corey, in* Harrison's Principles of Internal Medicine, *15th ed. E Braunwald et al (eds): New York, McGraw-Hill, 2001, adapted with permission.]*

malaise, and headache. Complete recovery after 2–5 days of illness is usual. Important examples include the following.

- *Lymphocytic choriomeningitis (LCM)*: This infection is transmitted from chronically infected mice and pet hamsters via aerosols of excreta and secreta. About one-fourth of infected pts have a 3- to 6-day febrile phase, a brief remission, and then recurrent fever, headache, nausea, vomiting, and meningeal signs lasting ~1 week.
  - Other manifestations include transient alopecia, arthritis, pharyngitis, cough, maculopapular rash, and orchitis.
  - Pregnant women can have mild infection yet pass on the virus to the fetus, who can develop hydrocephalus and chorioretinitis.

- The diagnosis should be considered when an adult has aseptic meningitis and any of the following: autumn seasonality, a well-marked febrile prodrome, a low CSF glucose level, or CSF mononuclear cell counts >1000/μL.
- LCM viremia is most likely in the initial febrile phase of illness. LCM can also be diagnosed by IgM-capture ELISA of serum or CSF or by RT-PCR of CSF.

- *Dengue fever*: The 4 serotypes of dengue viruses are all transmitted by the mosquito *Aedes aegypti*, which is also a vector for yellow fever. After an incubation period of 2–7 days, pts experience the sudden onset of fever, headache, retroorbital pain, back pain, severe myalgia (*break-bone fever*), adenopathy, palatal vesicles, and scleral injection.
  - The illness usually lasts 1 week, and a maculopapular rash often appears near the time of defervescence.
  - A second infection with a different dengue serotype can lead to dengue hemorrhagic fever (DHF; see "Hemorrhagic Fever," below).
  - The diagnosis is made by IgM ELISA or paired serologic tests during recovery or by antigen-detection ELISA or RT-PCR during the acute phase. Virus is easily isolated from blood during the acute phase by inoculation of mosquitoes or mosquito cell culture. Leukopenia, thrombocytopenia, and increased serum aminotransferase levels may be documented.

Encephalitis Depending on the causative virus, there is much variability in the ratio of clinical to subclinical disease, the mortality rate, and residua (Table 113-1). The pt usually presents with a prodrome of nonspecific symptoms that is followed quickly by headache, meningeal signs, photophobia, and vomiting; involvement of deeper structures leads to lethargy, cognitive deficits, focal neurologic signs, and coma. Acute encephalitis usually lasts from a few days to 2–3 weeks, and recovery may be slow and incomplete. Treatable causes of encephalitis (e.g., HSV) should be ruled out promptly. Some important examples of arboviral encephalitides follow.

- *Japanese encephalitis*: This infection is present throughout Asia and the western Pacific islands. Spinal and motor neuron disease can be documented in addition to encephalitis. An effective vaccine (ideally given on days 0, 7, and 30) is available and is indicated for summer travelers to rural Asia, where the risk can be as high as 2.1 cases per 10,000 per week.
- *West Nile encephalitis*: Usually a mild or asymptomatic disease, West Nile virus infection can cause aseptic meningitis or encephalitis and is present throughout the Western Hemisphere. Encephalitis, serious sequelae, and death are more common among elderly pts, diabetic and hypertensive pts, and pts with previous CNS disease. Unusual clinical features include chorioretinitis and flaccid paralysis.
- *Eastern equine encephalitis (EEE)*: EEE occurs primarily within endemic swampy foci along the eastern coast of the United States during the summer and early fall. EEE is one of the most severe arboviral diseases and is characterized by rapid onset, rapid progression, high mortality risk, and frequent residua. PMN-predominant pleocytosis of the CSF within the first 3 days of disease is common.

TABLE 113-1 PROMINENT FEATURES OF ARBOVIRAL ENCEPHALITIS

Virus	Natural Cycle	Incubation Period, Days	Annual No. of Cases	Case-to-Infection Ratio	Age of Cases	Case-Fatality Rate, %	Residua
La Crosse	*Aedes triseriatus*–chipmunk (transovarial component in mosquito also important)	~3–7	70 (U.S.)	<1:1000	<15 years	<0.5	Recurrent seizures in ~10%; severe deficits in rare cases; decreased school performance and behavioral change suspected in small proportion
St. Louis	*Culex tarsalis,* *C. pipiens,* *C. quinquefasciatus*–birds	4–21	85, with hundreds to thousands in epidemic years (U.S.)	<1:200	Milder cases in the young; more severe cases in adults >40 years old, particularly the elderly	7	Common in the elderly
Japanese	*Culex tritaeniorhynchus*–birds	5–15	>25,000	1:200–300	All ages; children in highly endemic areas	20–50	Common (approximately half of cases); may be severe
West Nile	*Culex* mosquitoes–birds	3–6	?	Very low	Mainly the elderly	5–10	Uncommon
Central European	*Ixodes ricinus*–rodents, insectivores	7–14	Thousands	1:12	All ages; milder in children	1–5	20%

(continued)

TABLE 113-1 PROMINENT FEATURES OF ARBOVIRAL ENCEPHALITIS (CONTINUED)

Virus	Natural Cycle	Incubation Period, Days	Annual No. of Cases	Case-to-Infection Ratio	Age of Cases	Case-Fatality Rate, %	Residua
Russian spring-summer	*I. persulcatus*–rodents, insectivores	7–14	Hundreds	—	All ages; milder in children	20	Approximately half of cases; often severe; limb-girdle paralysis
Powassan	*I. cookei*–wild mammals	~10	~1 (U.S.)	—	All ages; some predilection for children	~10	Common (approximately half of cases)
Eastern equine	*Culiseta melanura*–birds	~5–10	5 (U.S.)	1:40 (adult) 1:17 (child)	All ages; predilection for children	50–75	Common
Western equine	*Culex tarsalis*–birds	~5–10	~20 (U.S.)	1:1000 (adult) 1:50 (child) 1:1 (infant)	All ages; predilection for children <2 years old (increased mortality among elderly)	3–7	Common only among infants <1 year old
Venezuelan equine (epidemic)	Unknown (multiple mosquito species and horses in epidemics)	1–5	?	1:250 (adult) ~1:25 (child)	All ages; predilection for children	~10	—

Arthritis and Rash Alphaviruses are common causes of true arthritis accompanied by a febrile illness and maculopapular rash. Examples include the following.

- *Sindbis virus*: Found in northern Europe and the independent states of the former Soviet Union, this virus causes a maculopapular rash that often vesiculates on the trunk and extremities. The arthritis of this condition is multiarticular, migratory, and incapacitating, with resolution of the acute phase in a few days; joint pains may persist for months or years.
- *Chikungunya virus*: Found in rural Africa and Asia, this virus results in the abrupt onset of fever, severe arthralgias, migratory polyarthritis mainly affecting small joints, and a rash that begins coincident with defervescence at day 2–3 of illness.
- *Ross River virus*: A cause of epidemic polyarthritis in Australia and the eastern Pacific Islands, this virus causes rash and persistent joint involvement, typically in the absence of other constitutional symptoms. Because of joint pain, only ~50% and 10% of pts can resume normal activities at 4 weeks and 3 months, respectively.

Hemorrhagic Fever The viral HF syndrome is a constellation of findings based on vascular instability and decreased vascular integrity. All HF syndromes begin with the abrupt onset of fever and myalgia and can progress to severe prostration, headache, dizziness, photophobia, abdominal and/or chest pain, anorexia, and GI disturbances. On initial physical examination, there is conjunctival suffusion, muscular or abdominal tenderness to palpation, hypotension, petechiae, and periorbital edema. Laboratory examination usually reveals elevated serum aminotransferase levels, proteinuria, and hemoconcentration. Shock, multifocal bleeding, and CNS involvement (encephalopathy, coma, convulsions) are poor prognostic signs. Early recognition is important; appropriate supportive measures and, in some cases, virus-specific therapy can be instituted.

- *Lassa fever*: Endemic and epidemic in West Africa, Lassa fever, which is caused by a rodent-borne virus, has a more gradual onset than other HF syndromes. Bleeding is evident in 15–30% of cases. A maculopapular rash is often noted in light-skinned pts with Lassa fever.
  - Pregnant women have higher mortality rates, and the fetal death rate is 92% in the last trimester.
  - Pts with high-level viremia or a serum aspartate aminotransferase level of >150 IU/mL are at an elevated risk of death, and the administration of ribavirin (32 mg/kg IV × 1 dose, followed by 16 mg/kg q6h for 4 days and then 8 mg/kg q8h for 6 days), which appears to reduce this risk, should be considered.
- *South American HF syndromes* (Argentine, Bolivian, Venezuelan, Brazilian): These syndromes resemble Lassa fever; however, thrombocytopenia, bleeding, and CNS dysfunction are common.
  - Passive antibody treatment for Argentine HF is effective, and an effective vaccine exists.
  - Ribavirin is likely to be effective in all South American HF syndromes.
- *Rift Valley fever*: Although Rift Valley fever virus typically causes fever and myalgia, HF can occur with prominent liver involvement, renal failure, and probably disseminated intravascular coagulation (DIC).

- Retinal vasculitis can occur in ~10% of otherwise mild infections, and pts' vision can be permanently impaired.
- There is no proven therapy for Rift Valley fever. A live attenuated vaccine is in trials.

- *HF with renal syndrome*: This entity is most often caused in Europe by Puumala virus (rodent reservoir, the bank vole) and in Asia by Hantaan virus (rodent reservoir, the striped field mouse).
  - Severe cases of HF with renal syndrome caused by Hantaan virus evolve in identifiable stages: the *febrile* stage with myalgia, lasting 3 or 4 days; the *hypotensive* stage, often associated with shock and lasting from a few hours to 48 h; the *oliguric* stage with renal failure, lasting 3–10 days; and the *polyuric* stage with diuresis and hyposthenuria.
  - Infections with Puumala virus result in a much-attenuated picture but the same general presentation.
  - IgM-capture ELISA is positive within 2 days of admission and confirms the diagnosis.
  - The mainstay of therapy is expectant management of shock and renal failure. Ribavirin may reduce rates of mortality and morbidity in severe cases if treatment is begun within the first 4 days of illness.

- *Hantavirus pulmonary syndrome (HPS)*: After a prodrome of ~3–4 days, pts enter a cardiopulmonary phase marked by tachycardia, tachypnea, and mild hypotension. Over the next few hours, the illness may rapidly progress to severe hypoxemia and respiratory failure; the mortality rate is ~30–40% with good management. Pts surviving the first 2 days of hospitalization usually recover with no residua.
  - The disease is linked to rodent exposure. Sin Nombre virus infects the deer mouse and is the most important virus causing HPS in the United States.
  - Thrombocytopenia (an important early clue), hemoconcentration, proteinuria, and hypoalbuminemia are typical.
  - IgM testing of acute-phase serum may give positive results, even during the prodromal stage, and can confirm the diagnosis. RT-PCR of blood clots or tissue usually gives a positive result in the first 7–9 days of illness.
  - Treatment is nonspecific and requires intensive respiratory management and other supportive measures.

- *Yellow fever*: A former cause of major epidemics, yellow fever causes a typical HF syndrome with prominent hepatic necrosis, most commonly in urban South America and Africa. Pts are viremic for 3–4 days and can have jaundice, hemorrhage, black vomit, anuria, and terminal delirium. Vaccination of visitors to endemic areas and control of the mosquito vector *A. aegypti* prevent disease.

- *Dengue hemorrhagic fever (DHF)/dengue shock syndrome (DSS)*: Previous infection with a heterologous dengue virus serotype may elicit nonprotective antibodies and enhanced disease if pts are reinfected. In mild cases, lethargy, thrombocytopenia, and hemoconcentration occur 2–5 days after typical dengue fever, usually at the time of defervescence. In severe cases, frank shock occurs, with cyanosis, hepatomegaly, ascites and pleural effusions, and GI bleeding.

- The risk decreases considerably after age 12; DHF/DSS is more common among females than among males, more severe among whites than among blacks, and more common among well-nourished than among malnourished persons.
- With good care, the overall mortality rate is as low as 1%. Control of *A. aegypti*, the mosquito vector, is the key to control of the disease.

■ EBOLA AND MARBURG VIRUS INFECTIONS

Microbiology

The family Filoviridae contains two genera, *Marburgvirus* and *Ebolavirus*, that consist of negative-sense, single-stranded RNA viruses. *Ebolavirus* has 5 species named for their original site of recognition.

- With the exception of Reston virus (an Ebola virus), all Filoviridae are African viruses that cause severe disease with high mortality rates.
- Both Marburg virus and Ebola virus are biosafety level 4 pathogens because of the high mortality rate from infection and the aerosol infectivity of the agents.

Epidemiology

Marburg virus was first identified in 1967; in 2004–2005, a Marburg virus epidemic occurred in Angola, with >250 cases and a case-fatality rate of 90%. Ebola virus was first identified in 1976 and has been associated with several epidemics of severe HF; the mortality rate ranges from 50 to 90%, depending on the species.

- Human-to-human transmission occurs, but epidemiologic studies have failed to yield evidence for an important role (like that documented in Ebola disease in monkeys) of airborne particles in human Ebola disease.
- The reservoir is unknown, but speculation currently centers on bats.

Pathogenesis

Both viruses replicate well in virtually all cell types, and viral replication is associated with cellular necrosis. Acute infection is associated with high levels of circulating virus and viral antigen. Fatal cases are associated with the lack of an antibody response, but clinical recovery is probably mediated by the cellular immune response since convalescent-phase plasma is not protective.

Clinical Manifestations

After a 7- to 10-day incubation period, pts experience an abrupt onset of fever, severe headache, myalgia, nausea, vomiting, diarrhea, prostration, and depressed mentation.

- A maculopapular rash may appear at day 5–7 and is followed by desquamation. Bleeding may occur at this time and is apparent from any mucosal site and into the skin.
- The fever may break after 10–12 days, and the pt may eventually recover.
- Recrudescence and secondary bacterial infection may occur.
- Leukopenia is common early on and is followed by neutrophilia. Thrombocytopenia, transaminitis, and jaundice are common.

Diagnosis

High concentrations of virus in blood can be documented by antigen-detection ELISA, virus isolation, or RT-PCR. Antibodies can be detected in recovering pts.

TREATMENT Ebola and Marburg Virus Infections

- No virus-specific therapy is available, and supportive measures may not be as useful as had been hoped.
- Studies in rhesus monkeys suggest that treatment with an inhibitor of factor VIIa/tissue factor or with activated protein C may improve survival rates.
- Barrier nursing precautions can greatly decrease the spread of filoviruses.

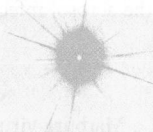

For a more detailed discussion, see Jackson AC: Rabies and Other Rhabdovirus Infections, Chap. 195, p. 1611; Peters CJ: Infections Caused by Arthropod- and Rodent-Borne Viruses, Chap. 196, p. 1617; and Peters CJ: Ebola and Marburg Viruses, Chap. 197, p. 1633, in HPIM-18.

CHAPTER **114**
HIV Infection and AIDS

■ **DEFINITION**

AIDS was originally defined empirically by the Centers for Disease Control and Prevention (CDC) as "the presence of a reliably diagnosed disease that is at least moderately indicative of an underlying defect in cell-mediated immunity." Following the recognition of the causative virus, HIV, and the development of sensitive and specific tests for HIV infection, the definition of AIDS has undergone substantial revision. The current surveillance definition categorizes HIV-infected persons on the basis of clinical conditions associated with HIV infection and CD4+ T lymphocyte counts (Tables 189-1, and 189-2, pp. 1506 and 1507, in HPIM-18). From a practical standpoint, the clinician should view HIV disease as a spectrum of disorders ranging from primary infection, with or without the acute HIV syndrome, to the asymptomatic infected state, to advanced disease.

■ **ETIOLOGY AND TRANSMISSION**

AIDS is caused by infection with the human retroviruses HIV-1 or -2. HIV-1 is the most common cause worldwide. These viruses are passed through sexual contact; through transfusion of contaminated blood or blood products; through sharing of contaminated needles and syringes among injection drug users; intrapartum or perinatally from mother to infant; or via breast milk. There is no evidence that the virus can be passed through casual or family contact or by insects such as mosquitoes. There is a definite, though small, occupational risk of infection for health care workers and laboratory personnel who work with HIV-infected specimens. The risk of transmission of HIV from an infected health care worker to his or her pts through invasive procedures is extremely low.

■ EPIDEMIOLOGY

As of January 1, 2010, an estimated 1,108,611 cumulative cases of AIDS had been diagnosed in the United States; there have been approximately 600,000 deaths due to AIDS. However, the death rate from AIDS has decreased substantially in the past 10 years primarily due to the increased use of potent antiretroviral drugs. As of January 1, 2010, an estimated 1.1 million HIV-infected persons were living in the United States; approximately 21% of these individuals are unaware that they are infected. An estimated 56,000 individuals are newly infected each year in the United States; this figure has remained stable for at least 15 years (Fig. 189-12, p. 1518, in HPIM-18). Among adults and adolescents newly diagnosed with HIV infection in 2009, ~76% were men and ~24% were women. Of new HIV/AIDS diagnoses among men, ~75% were due to male-to-male sexual contact, ~14% to heterosexual contact, and ~8% to injection drug use. Among women, ~85% were due to heterosexual contact and ~15% to injection drug use (Figs. 189-13 and 189-14, p. 1519, in HPIM-18). HIV infection/AIDS is a global pandemic, especially in developing countries. At the end of 2009, the estimated number of cases of HIV infection worldwide was ~33.3 million, two-thirds of which were in sub-Saharan Africa; ~50% of cases were in women and 2.5 million were in children. In 2009 there were 2.6 million new HIV infections worldwide and 1.8 million deaths (Fig. 189-10, p. 1517, in HPIM-18).

■ PATHOPHYSIOLOGY AND IMMUNOPATHOGENESIS

The hallmark of HIV disease is a profound immunodeficiency resulting from a progressive quantitative and qualitative deficiency of the subset of T lymphocytes referred to as *helper T cells*. This subset of T cells is defined phenotypically by the expression on the cell surface of the CD4 molecule, which serves as the primary cellular receptor for HIV. A co-receptor must be present with CD4 for efficient entry of HIV-1 into target cells. The two major co-receptors for HIV-1 are the chemokine receptors CCR5 and CXCR4. The CD4+ T lymphocyte and CD4+ monocyte lineage are the principal cellular targets of HIV.

Primary Infection

Following initial transmission, the virus infects CD4+ cells, probably T lymphocytes, monocytes, or bone marrow–derived dendritic cells. Both during this initial stage and later in infection, the lymphoid system is a major site for the establishment and propagation of HIV infection. The gut-associated lymphoid tissue (GALT) plays a major role in the establishment of infection and in the early depletion of memory CD4+ T cells.

Essentially all pts undergo a viremic stage during primary infection; in some pts this is associated with the "acute retroviral syndrome," a mononucleosis-like illness (see below). This phase is important in disseminating virus to lymphoid and other organs throughout the body, and it is ultimately contained partially by the development of an HIV-specific immune response.

Establishment of Chronic and Persistent Infection

Despite the robust immune response that is mounted following primary infection, the virus is not cleared from the body. Instead, a chronic infection develops that persists for a median time of 10 years before the untreated pt becomes clinically ill. During this period of what appears to be clinical latency, the number of CD4+ T cells gradually declines, but few, if any, clinical signs and symptoms may be evident. However, active viral replication can almost always be detected by measurable plasma viremia and the demonstration of virus replication in lymphoid tissue. The level of steady-state viremia (referred to as the *viral set point*) at ~6 months to 1 year post-infection has important prognostic implications for the progression of HIV disease; individuals with a low viral set point at 6 months to 1 year after infection progress to AIDS more slowly than do those whose set point is very high at this time (Fig. 189-22, p. 1524, in HPIM-18).

Advanced HIV Disease

In untreated pts or in pts in whom therapy has not controlled viral replication (see below), after some period of time (often years), CD4+ T cell counts will fall below a critical level (~200/μL) and pts become highly susceptible to opportunistic disease. The presence of a CD4+ T cell count of <200/μL or an AIDS-defining opportunistic disease establishes a diagnosis of AIDS. Control of plasma viremia by effective antiretroviral therapy, particularly maintaining the plasma viral load consistently at <50 copies of RNA per mL, even in individuals with low CD4+ T cell counts, has dramatically increased survival in these pts, including those whose CD4+ T cell counts may not increase significantly as a result of therapy.

■ IMMUNE ABNORMALITIES IN HIV DISEASE

A broad range of immune abnormalities has been documented in HIV-infected pts, resulting in varying degrees of immunodeficiency. These include both quantitative and qualitative defects in lymphocytes, and qualitative defects in monocyte/macrophage and natural killer (NK) cell function. Autoimmune phenomena also have been observed in HIV-infected individuals.

■ IMMUNE RESPONSE TO HIV INFECTION

Both humoral and cellular immune responses to HIV develop soon after primary infection (see summary in Table 189-6, p. 1535, and Fig. 189-26, p. 1536, in HPIM-18). Humoral responses include antibodies with HIV binding and neutralizing activity, as well as antibodies participating in antibody-dependent cellular cytotoxicity (ADCC). Cellular immune responses include the generation of HIV-specific CD4+ and CD8+ T lymphocytes, as well as NK cells and mononuclear cells mediating ADCC. CD8+ T lymphocytes may also suppress HIV replication in a noncytolytic, non-MHC-restricted manner. This effect is mediated by soluble factors such as the CC-chemokines RANTES, MIP-1α, and MIP-1β. For the most part, the natural immune response to HIV is not adequate. Broadly reacting neutralizing antibodies against HIV are not easily generated in infected individuals, and eradication of the virus from infected individuals by naturally occurring immune responses has not been reported.

■ DIAGNOSIS OF HIV INFECTION

Laboratory diagnosis of HIV infection depends on the demonstration of anti-HIV antibodies and/or the detection of HIV or one of its components.

The standard screening test for HIV infection is the detection of anti-HIV antibodies using an enzyme immunoassay (EIA). This test is highly sensitive (>99.5%) and is quite specific. Most commercial EIA kits are able to detect antibodies to both HIV-1 and -2. Western blot is the most commonly used confirmatory test and detects antibodies to HIV antigens of specific molecular weights. Antibodies to HIV begin to appear within 2 weeks of infection, and the period of time between initial infection and the development of detectable antibodies is rarely >3 months. The HIV p24 antigen can be measured using an EIA-type capture assay. Plasma p24 antigen levels rise during the first few weeks following infection, prior to the appearance of anti-HIV antibodies. A guideline for the use of these serologic tests in the diagnosis of HIV infection is depicted in Fig. 114-1.

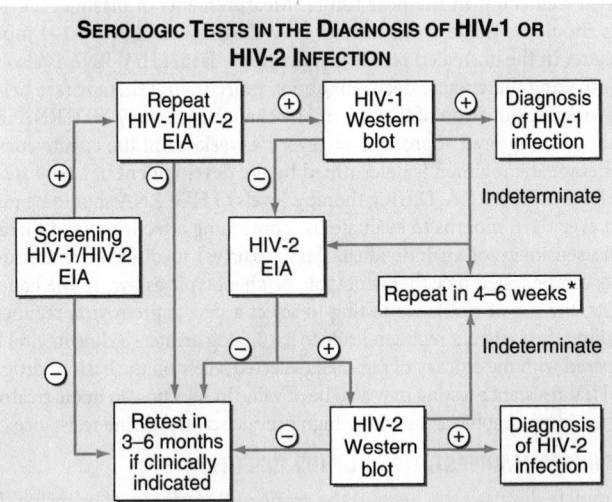

FIGURE 114-1 Algorithm for the use of serologic tests in the diagnosis of HIV-1 or HIV-2 infection. *Stable indeterminate Western blot 4–6 weeks later makes HIV infection unlikely. However, it should be repeated twice at 3-month intervals to rule out HIV infection. Alternatively, one may test for HIV-1 p24 antigen or HIV RNA. EIA, enzyme immunoassay.

HIV can be cultured directly from tissue, peripheral blood cells, or plasma, but this is most commonly done in a research setting. HIV genetic material can be detected using reverse transcriptase PCR (RT-PCR), branched DNA (bDNA), or nucleic acid sequence–based assay (NASBA). These tests are useful in pts with a positive or indeterminate EIA and an indeterminate Western blot. They turn positive early in infection and will usually be positive in pts in whom serologic testing may be unreliable (such as those with hypogammaglobulinemia).

▮ LABORATORY MONITORING OF PTS WITH HIV INFECTION

Measurement of the CD4+ T cell count and level of plasma HIV RNA are important parts of the routine evaluation and monitoring of HIV-infected individuals. The CD4+ T cell count is a generally accepted indicator of the immunologic competence of the pt with HIV infection, and there is a close relationship between the CD4+ T cell count and the clinical manifestations of AIDS (Fig. 189-32, p. 1541, in HPIM-18). Pts with CD4+ T cell counts <200/μL are at higher risk of infection with *Pneumocystis jiroveci*. Once the count declines to <50/μL, pts are also at higher risk for developing CMV disease and infection with *Mycobacterium avium intracellulare*. Pts should have their CD4+ T cell count measured at the time of diagnosis and every 3–6 months thereafter. (Measurements may be done more frequently in pts with declining counts.) According to DHHS practice guidelines, a CD4+ T cell count <500/μL is a clear indication to initiate antiretroviral therapy. While the CD4+ T cell count provides information on the current immunologic status of the pt, the HIV RNA level predicts what will happen to the CD4+ T cell count in the near future. Measurements of plasma HIV RNA levels should be made at the time of HIV diagnosis and every 3–4 months thereafter in the untreated pt. Measurement of plasma HIV RNA is also useful in making therapeutic decisions about antiretroviral therapy (see below). Following the initiation of therapy or any change in therapy, HIV RNA levels should be monitored approximately every 4 weeks until the effectiveness of the therapeutic regimen is determined by the development of a new steady-state level of HIV RNA. During therapy, levels of HIV RNA should be monitored every 3–6 months to evaluate the continuing effectiveness of therapy.

The sensitivity of an individual's HIV virus(es) to different antiretroviral agents can be tested by either genotypic or phenotypic assays. In the hands of experts, the use of resistance testing to select a new antiretroviral regimen in pts failing their current regimen leads to a ~0.5-log greater decline in viral load compared with the efficacy of regimens selected solely on the basis of drug history. HIV resistance testing may also be of value in selecting an initial treatment regimen in geographic areas with a high prevalence of baseline resistance.

▮ CLINICAL MANIFESTATIONS OF HIV INFECTION

A complete discussion is beyond the scope of this chapter. The major clinical features of the various stages of HIV infection are summarized below (see also Chap. 189, HPIM-18).

Acute HIV (Retroviral) Syndrome

Approximately 50–70% of infected individuals experience an acute syndrome following primary infection. The acute syndrome follows infection

TABLE 114-1 CLINICAL FINDINGS IN THE ACUTE HIV SYNDROME

General	Neurologic
Fever	Meningitis
Pharyngitis	Encephalitis
Lymphadenopathy	Peripheral neuropathy
Headache/retroorbital pain	Myelopathy
Arthralgias/myalgias	Dermatologic
Lethargy/malaise	Erythematous maculopapular rash
Anorexia/weight loss	Mucocutaneous ulceration
Nausea/vomiting/diarrhea	

Source: From B Tindall, DA Cooper: AIDS 5:1, 1991.

by 3–6 weeks. It can have multiple clinical features (Table 114-1), lasts 1–2 weeks, and resolves spontaneously as an immune response to HIV develops and the viral load diminishes from its peak levels. Most pts will then enter a phase of clinical latency, although an occasional pt will experience rapidly progressive immunologic and clinical deterioration.

Asymptomatic Infection

The length of time between HIV infection and development of disease in untreated individuals varies greatly, but the median is estimated to be 10 years. HIV disease with active viral replication usually progresses during this asymptomatic period, and CD4+ T cell counts fall. The rate of disease progression is directly correlated with plasma HIV RNA levels. Pts with high levels of HIV RNA progress to symptomatic disease faster than do those with low levels of HIV RNA.

Symptomatic Disease

Symptoms of HIV disease can develop at any time during the course of HIV infection. In general, the spectrum of illness changes as the CD4+ T cell count declines. The more severe and life-threatening complications of HIV infection occur in pts with CD4+ T cell counts <200/µL. Overall, the clinical spectrum of HIV disease is constantly changing as pts live longer and new and better approaches to treatment and prophylaxis of opportunistic infections are developed. In addition, a variety of neurologic, cardiovascular, renal, metabolic, and hepatic problems are increasingly seen in pts with HIV infection and may be a direct consequence of HIV infection. The key element to treating symptomatic complications of HIV disease, whether primary or secondary, is achieving good control of HIV replication through the use of combination antiretroviral therapy and instituting primary and secondary prophylaxis as indicated. Major clinical syndromes seen in the symptomatic stage of HIV infection are summarized below.

- *Persistent generalized lymphadenopathy*: Palpable adenopathy at two or more extrainguinal sites that persists for >3 months without explanation other than HIV infection. Many pts will go on to disease progression.

- *Constitutional symptoms*: Fever persisting for >1 month, involuntary weight loss of >10% of baseline, diarrhea for >1 month in absence of explainable cause.

- *Neurologic disease*: Most common is HIV-associated neurocognitive disease (HAND); other neurologic complications include opportunistic infections, primary CNS lymphoma, CNS Kaposi's sarcoma, aseptic meningitis, myelopathy, peripheral neuropathy, and myopathy.

- *Secondary infectious diseases*: Common secondary infectious agents include *P. jiroveci* (pneumonia), CMV (chorioretinitis, colitis, pneumonitis, adrenalitis), *Candida albicans* (oral thrush, esophagitis), *M. avium intracellulare* (localized or disseminated infection), *M. tuberculosis* (pulmonary or disseminated), *Cryptococcus neoformans* (meningitis, disseminated disease), *Toxoplasma gondii* (encephalitis, intracerebral mass lesion), herpes simplex virus (severe mucocutaneous lesions, esophagitis), diarrhea due to *Cryptosporidium* spp. or *Isospora belli* (diarrhea), JC virus (progressive multifocal leukoencephalopathy), bacterial pathogens (pneumonia, sinusitis, skin).

- *Secondary neoplasms*: Kaposi's sarcoma (cutaneous and visceral, more fulminant course than in non-HIV-infected pts), lymphoma (primarily B cell, may be CNS or systemic).

- *Other diseases*: A variety of organ-specific syndromes can be seen in HIV-infected pts, either as primary manifestations of the HIV infection or as complications of treatment. Diseases commonly associated with aging are also seen with an increased frequency in pts with HIV infection.

TREATMENT HIV Infection (See also Chap. 189, HPIM-18)

General principles of pt management include counseling, psychosocial support, and screening for infections and other conditions and require comprehensive knowledge of the disease processes associated with HIV infection.

ANTIRETROVIRAL THERAPY (SEE Table 114-2**)** The cornerstone of medical management of HIV infection is combination antiretroviral therapy, or cART. Suppression of HIV replication is an important component in prolonging life as well as in improving the quality of life of pts with HIV infection. However, several important questions related to the treatment of HIV disease lack definitive answers. Among them are questions regarding when antiretroviral therapy should be started, what the best cART regimen is, when a given regimen should be changed, and which drugs in a regimen should be changed when a change is made. The drugs that are currently licensed for the treatment of HIV infection are listed in Table 114-2. These drugs fall into four main categories: those that inhibit the viral reverse transcriptase enzyme, those that inhibit the viral protease enzyme, those that inhibit viral entry, and those that inhibit the viral integrase. There are numerous drug-drug interactions that must be taken into consideration when using these medications.

TABLE 114-2 ANTIRETROVIRAL DRUGS COMMONLY USED IN THE TREATMENT OF HIV INFECTION

Drug	Status	Indication	Dose in Combination	Supporting Data	Toxicity
Nucleoside or nucleotide reverse transcriptase inhibitors					
Zidovudine (AZT, azidothymidine, Retrovir, 3'azido-3'-deoxythymidine)	Licensed	Treatment of HIV infection in combination with other antiretroviral agents	200 mg q8h or 300 mg bid	19 vs 1 death in original placebo-controlled trial in 281 pts with AIDS or ARC. Decreased progression to AIDS in pts with CD4+ T cell counts <500/μL, $n = 2051$.	Anemia, granulocytopenia, myopathy, lactic acidosis, hepatomegaly with steatosis, headache, nausea
		Prevention of maternal-fetal HIV transmission		In pregnant women with CD4+ T cell count ≥200/μL, AZT PO beginning at weeks 14–34 of gestation plus IV drug during labor and delivery plus PO AZT to infant for 6-week decreased transmission of HIV by 67.5% (from 25.5% to 8.3%), $n = 363$	
Lamivudine (Epivir, 2'3'-dideoxy-3'-thiacytidine, 3TC)	Licensed	In combination with other antiretroviral agents for the treatment of HIV infection	150 mg bid 300 mg qd	Superior to AZT alone with respect to changes in CD4 counts in 495 pts who were zidovudine-naïve and 477 pts who were zidovudine-experienced. Overall CD4+ T cell counts for the zidovudine group were at baseline by 24 weeks, while in the group treated with zidovudine plus lamivudine, they were 10–50 cells/μL above baseline. 54% decrease in progression to AIDS/death compared with AZT alone.	Hepatotoxicity

(continued)

TABLE 114-2 ANTIRETROVIRAL DRUGS COMMONLY USED IN THE TREATMENT OF HIV INFECTION (CONTINUED)

Drug	Status	Indication	Dose in Combination	Supporting Data	Toxicity
Nucleoside or nucleotide reverse transcriptase inhibitors					
Emtricitabine (FTC, Emtriva)	Licensed	In combination with other antiretroviral agents for the treatment of HIV infection	200 mg qd	Comparable to d4T in combination with ddI and efavirenz in 571 treatment-naïve pts. Similar to 3TC in combination with AZT or d4T + NNRT1 or PI in 440 pts doing well for at least 12 weeks on a 3TC regimen.	Hepatotoxicity
Abacavir (Ziagen)	Licensed	For treatment of HIV infection in combination with other antiretroviral agents	300 mg bid	Abacavir + AZT + 3TC equivalent to indinavir + AZT + 3TC with regard to viral load suppression (~60% in each group with <400 HIV RNA copies/mL plasma) and CD4 cell increase (~100/µL in each group) at 24 weeks	Hypersensitivity reaction (can be fatal); fever, rash, nausea, vomiting, malaise or fatigue, and loss of appetite
Tenofovir (Viread)	Licensed	For use in combination with other antiretroviral agents when treatment is indicated	300 mg qd	Reduction of ~0.6 log in HIV-1 RNA levels when added to background regimen in treatment-experienced pts	Potential for renal toxicity
Nonnucleoside reverse transcriptase inhibitors					
Nevirapine (Viramune)	Licensed	In combination with other antiretroviral agents for treatment of progressive HIV infection	200 mg/d × 14 days, then 200 mg bid	Increases in CD4+ T cell count, decrease in HIV RNA when used in combination with nucleosides	Skin rash, hepatotoxicity

Drug	Status	Indication	Dose	Clinical data	Adverse effects
Efavirenz (Sustiva)	Licensed	For treatment of HIV infection in combination with other antiretroviral agents	600 mg qhs	Efavirenz + AZT + 3TC comparable to indinavir + AZT + 3TC with regard to viral load suppression (a higher percentage of the efavirenz group achieved viral load <50 copies/mL; however, the discontinuation rate in the indinavir group was unexpectedly high, accounting for most treatment "failures"); CD4 cell increase (~140/µL in each group) at 24 weeks.	Rash, dysphoria, elevated liver function tests, drowsiness, abnormal dreams, depression
Etravirine (Intelence)	Licensed	In combination with other antiretroviral agents in treatment-experienced adult pts who have evidence of viral replication and HIV-1 strains resistant to an NNRTI inhibitor and other antiretroviral agents	200 mg bid (or twice daily)	At 24 weeks in treatment-experienced pts with 1 or more NNRTI mutations and 3 or more PI mutations at screening, 74% of pts randomized to etravirine + background had HIV levels <400 copies/mL compared to 51.5% of pts randomized to background regimen + placebo. All subjects received darunavir/ritonavir as part of their background regimen. CD4+ T cell counts increased by 81 cells/mL in the etravirine arm and 64 cells/mL in the placebo arm.	Skin rash

(continued)

737

TABLE 114-2 ANTIRETROVIRAL DRUGS COMMONLY USED IN THE TREATMENT OF HIV INFECTION (CONTINUED)

Drug	Status	Indication	Dose in Combination	Supporting Data	Toxicity
Protease inhibitors					
Fosamprenavir (Lexiva)	Licensed	In combination with other antiretroviral agents for treatment of HIV infection	1400 mg bid or 700 mg + 100 mg ritonavir bid or 1400 mg + 200 mg ritonavir qd	In treatment-naïve pts, amprenavir + AZT + 3TC superior to AZT + 3TC with regard to viral load suppression (53% vs 11% with <400 HIV RNA copies/mL plasma at 24 weeks). CD4+ T cell responses similar between treatment groups. In treatment-experienced pts, amprenavir + NRTIs similar to indinavir + NRTIs with regard to viral load suppression (43% vs 53% with <400 HIV RNA copies/mL plasma at 24 weeks). CD4+ T cell responses superior in the indinavir + NRTIs group.	Nausea, vomiting, diarrhea, rash, oral paresthesias, elevated liver function tests, hyperglycemia, fat redistribution, lipid abnormalities, headache, nephrolithiasis
Lopinavir/ritonavir (Kaletra)	Licensed	For treatment of HIV infection in combination with other antiretroviral agents	400 mg/100 mg bid	In treatment-naïve pts, lopinavir/ritonavir + d4T + 3TC superior to nelfinavir + d4T + 3TC with regard to viral load suppression (79% vs 64% with <400 HIV RNA copies/μL at 40 weeks). CD4+ T cell increases similar in both groups.	Diarrhea, hyperglycemia, fat redistribution, lipid abnormalities
Atazanavir (Reyataz)	Licensed	For treatment of HIV infection in combination with other antiretroviral agents	400 mg qd or 300 mg qd + ritonavir 100 mg qd when given with efavirenz	Comparable to efavirenz when given in combination with AZT + 3TC in treatment-naïve pts. Comparable to nelfinavir when given in combination with d4T + 3TC in a study of 467 treatment-naïve pts.	Hyperbilirubinemia, PR prolongation, nausea, vomiting, hyperglycemia, fat maldistribution

738

Darunavir (Prezista)	Licensed	In combination with 100 mg ritonavir for combination therapy in treatment-experienced adults	600 mg + 100 mg ritonavir twice daily with food	At 24 weeks, pts with prior extensive exposure to antiretrovirals treated with a new combination including darunavir showed a −1.89-log change in HIV RNA levels and a 92-cell increase in CD4+ T cells compared with −0.48 log and 17 cells in the control arm.	Diarrhea, nausea, headache

Entry inhibitors

Maraviroc (Selzentry)	Licensed	In combination with other antiretroviral agents in treatment-experienced adults infected with only CCR5-tropic HIV-1 that is resistant to multiple antiretroviral agents	150–600 mg bid depending on concomitant medications (see text)	At 24 weeks, among 635 pts with CCR5-tropic virus and HIV-1 RNA >5000 copies/mL despite at least 6 months of prior therapy with at least one agent from 3 of the 4 antiretroviral drug classes, 61% of pts randomized to maraviroc achieved HIV RNA levels <400 copies/mL compared with 28% of pts randomized to placebo	Hepatotoxicity, nasopharyngitis, fever, cough, rash, abdominal pain, dizziness, fever, musculoskeletal symptoms

Integrase inhibitor

Raltegravir (Isentress)	Licensed	In combination with other antiretroviral agents in treatment experienced pts with evidence of ongoing HIV-1 replication	400 mg bid	At 24 weeks, among 436 pts with three-class drug resistance, 76% of pts randomized to receive raltegravir achieved HIV RNA levels <400 copies/mL compared with 41% of pts randomized to receive placebo	Nausea, rash

Abbreviations: ARC, AIDS-related complex; NRTIs, nonnucleoside reverse transcriptase inhibitors.

Nucleoside/Nucleotide Analogues These agents act by causing premature DNA-chain termination during the reverse transcription of viral RNA to proviral DNA and should be used in combination with other antiretroviral agents. The most common usage is together with another nucleoside/nucleotide analogue and a nonnucleoside reverse transcriptase inhibitor or a protease inhibitor (see below).

Nonnucleoside Reverse Transcriptase Inhibitors These agents interfere with the function of HIV-1 reverse transcriptase by binding to regions outside the active site and causing conformational changes in the enzyme that render it inactive. These agents are very potent; however, when they are used as monotherapy, they result in the rapid emergence of drug-resistant mutants. Five members of this class, *nevirapine, delavirdine, efavirenz, etravirine, and rilpivirine* are currently available for clinical use. These drugs are licensed for use in combination with other antiretrovirals.

Protease Inhibitors These drugs are potent and selective inhibitors of the HIV-1 protease enzyme and are active in the nanomolar range. Unfortunately, as in the case of the nonnucleoside reverse transcriptase inhibitors, this potency is accompanied by the rapid emergence of resistant isolates when these drugs are used as monotherapy. Thus, the protease inhibitors should be used only in combination with other antiretroviral drugs.

HIV Entry Inhibitors These agents act by interfering with the binding of HIV to its receptor or co-receptor or by interfering with the process of fusion. A variety of small molecules that bind to HIV-1 co-receptors are currently in clinical trials. The first drugs in this class to be licensed are the fusion inhibitor *enfuvirtide* and the entry inhibitor *maraviroc*.

HIV Integrase Inhibitors These drugs interfere with the integration of proviral DNA into the host cell genome. The first agent in this class, *raltegravir*, was approved in 2007 for use in treatment-experienced pts.

CHOICE OF ANTIRETROVIRAL TREATMENT STRATEGY The large number of available antiretroviral agents makes the subject of antiretroviral therapy one of the more complicated in the management of HIV-infected pts.

The principles of therapy for HIV infection have been articulated by a panel sponsored by the U.S. Department of Health and Human Services (Table 114-3). Treatment decisions must take into account the fact that one is dealing with a chronic infection and that complete eradication of HIV infection has not been achieved with currently available cART regimens. Thus, therapeutic decisions must take into account the balance between risks and benefits. At present a reasonable course of action is to initiate antiretroviral therapy in anyone with the acute HIV syndrome; pts with symptomatic disease; pts with evidence of renal disease; pts with asymptomatic infection and CD4+ counts <500/μL; and pts with hepatitis B infection when hepatitis B treatment is indicated, to avoid

TABLE 114-3 PRINCIPLES OF THERAPY OF HIV INFECTION

1. Ongoing HIV replication leads to immune system damage and progression to AIDS.

2. Plasma HIV RNA levels indicate the magnitude of HIV replication and the rate of CD4+ T cell destruction. CD4+ T cell counts indicate the current level of competence of the immune system.

3. Rates of disease progression differ among individuals, and treatment decisions should be individualized based on plasma HIV RNA levels and CD4+ T cell counts.

4. Maximal suppression of viral replication is a goal of therapy; the greater the suppression the less likely the appearance of drug-resistant quasi-species.

5. The most effective therapeutic strategies involve the simultaneous initiation of combinations of effective anti-HIV drugs with which the pt has not been previously treated and that are not cross-resistant with antiretroviral agents that the pt has already received.

6. The antiretroviral drugs used in combination regimens should be used according to optimum schedules and dosages.

7. The number of available drugs is limited. Any decisions on antiretroviral therapy have a long-term impact on future options for the pt.

8. Women should receive optimal antiretroviral therapy regardless of pregnancy status.

9. The same principles apply to children and adults. The treatment of HIV-infected children involves unique pharmacologic, virologic, and immunologic considerations.

10. Compliance is an important part of ensuring maximal effect from a given regimen. The simpler the regimen, the easier it is for the pt to be compliant.

Source: Modified from *Principles of Therapy of HIV Infection*, USPHS, and the Henry J. Kaiser Family Foundation.

development of resistant strains of HIV. In addition, one may wish to administer a 4-week course of therapy to uninfected individuals immediately following a high-risk exposure to HIV (see below). Some experts favor treating all pts with HIV infection with cART while awaiting the results of randomized, controlled trials.

When the decision to initiate therapy is made, the physician must decide which drugs to use in the initial regimen. The two options for initial therapy most commonly in use today are (1) two nucleoside/nucleotide analogues (one of which is usually tenofovir or abacavir, and the other of which is usually lamivudine or emtricitabine) combined with a protease inhibitor; or (2) two nucleoside/nucleotide analogues and a nonnucleoside reverse transcriptase inhibitor. There are no clear data at present on which to base a distinction between these two approaches.

TABLE 114-4 INDICATIONS FOR CHANGING ANTIRETROVIRAL THERAPY IN PTS WITH HIV INFECTION[a]

Less than a 1-log drop in plasma HIV RNA by 4 weeks following the initiation of therapy

A reproducible significant increase (defined as 3-fold or greater) from the nadir of plasma HIV RNA level not attributable to intercurrent infection, vaccination, or test methodology

Persistently declining CD4+ T cell numbers

Clinical deterioration

Side effects

---

[a]Generally speaking, a change should involve the initiation of at least 2 drugs felt to be effective in the given pt. The exception to this is when change is being made to manage toxicity, in which case a single substitution is reasonable.
Source: Guidelines for the Use of Antiretroviral Agents in HIV-Infected Adults and Adolescents, USPHS.

Following the initiation of therapy, one should expect a 1-log (tenfold) reduction in plasma HIV RNA within 1–2 months; eventually a decline in plasma HIV RNA to <50 copies/mL; and a rise in CD4+ T cell count of 100–150/μL during the first year. Failure to achieve and maintain an HIV RNA level <50 copies/mL is an indication to consider a change in therapy. Other reasons for changing therapy are listed in Table 114-4. When changing therapy because of treatment failure, it is important to attempt to provide a regimen with at least two new drugs. In the pt in whom a change is made for reasons of drug toxicity, a simple replacement of one drug is reasonable.

Treatment of Secondary Infections and Neoplasms Specific for each infection and neoplasm (see Chap. 189, in HPIM-18).

Prophylaxis against Secondary Infections

(See also Table 189-10, pp. 1544–1546, in HPIM-18)

Primary prophylaxis is clearly indicated for *P. jiroveci* pneumonia (especially when CD4+ T cell counts fall to <200 cells/μL), for *M. avium* complex infections in pts with CD4+ T cell counts <50 cells/μL, and for *M. tuberculosis* infections in pts with a positive PPD or anergy if at high risk of TB. Vaccination with the influenza and pneumococcal polysaccharide vaccines is generally recommended for all pts and may need to be repeated in pts with CD4+ T cell counts <200/μL when their counts increase to >200/μL (Table 189-10, pp. 1544–1546, in HPIM-18). Secondary prophylaxis, when available, is indicated for virtually every infection experienced by HIV-infected pts until they have significant immunologic recovery.

■ HIV AND THE HEALTH CARE WORKER

There is a small but definite risk to health care workers of acquiring HIV infection via needle stick exposures, large mucosal surface exposures, or exposure of open wounds to HIV-infected secretions or blood products.

The risk of HIV transmission after a skin puncture by an object contaminated with blood from a person with documented HIV infection is ~0.3%, compared with a 20–30% risk for hepatitis B infection from a similar incident. Postexposure prophylaxis appears to be effective in decreasing the likelihood of acquisition of infection through accidental exposure in the health care setting. In this regard, a U.S. Public Health Service working group has recommended that chemoprophylaxis be given as soon as possible after occupational exposure. While the precise regimen remains a subject of debate, the U.S. Public Health Service guidelines recommend (1) a combination of two nucleoside analogue reverse transcriptase inhibitors given for 4 weeks for routine exposures, or (2) a combination of two nucleoside analogue reverse transcriptase inhibitors plus a third drug given for 4 weeks for high-risk or otherwise complicated exposures. Most clinicians administer the latter regimen in all cases in which a decision to treat is made. Regardless of which regimen is used, treatment should be initiated as soon as possible after exposure.

Prevention of exposure is the best strategy and includes following universal precautions and proper handling of needles and other potentially contaminated objects.

Transmission of TB is another potential risk for all health care workers, including those dealing with HIV-infected pts. All workers should know their PPD status, which should be checked yearly.

■ VACCINES

A recent clinical trial conducted in Thailand demonstrated moderate (31% effective) protection against acquisition of HIV infection. However, this modest degree of efficacy does not justify deployment of the vaccine; active investigation continues in the pursuit of a safe and effective vaccine against HIV.

■ PREVENTION

Education, counseling, and behavior modification along with the consistent and correct use of condoms in risk situations remain the cornerstones of HIV prevention efforts. Avoidance of shared needle use by IDUs is critical. If possible, breast-feeding should be avoided by HIV-positive women, as the virus can be transmitted to infants via this route. In societies where withholding of breast-feeding is not feasible, treatment of the mother, if possible, greatly decreases the chances of transmission. Recent studies have demonstrated the important role of medically supervised adult male circumcision in the prevention of acquisition of heterosexually transmitted HIV infection. In addition, antiretroviral-containing vaginal gels, as well as pre-exposure prophylaxis in men who have sex with men and in heterosexual men and women practicing risk behavior, have proved to be effective means of prevention when the regimens are adhered to. Finally, treatment of the HIV-infected partner in heterosexual discordant couples has proved highly effective in preventing transmission of HIV to the uninfected partner.

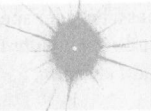

For a more detailed discussion, see Fauci AS, Lane HC: Human Immunodeficiency Virus Disease: AIDS and Related Disorders, Chap. 189, p. 1506, in HPIM-18.

CHAPTER **115**
Fungal Infections

■ GENERAL CONSIDERATIONS

- *Yeasts* (e.g., *Candida, Cryptococcus*) appear microscopically as round, budding forms; *molds* (e.g., *Aspergillus, Rhizopus*) appear as filamentous forms called *hyphae*; and *dimorphic fungi* (e.g., *Histoplasma*) are spherical in tissue but appear as molds in the environment.
  - *Endemic* fungi (e.g., *Coccidioides*) are not part of the normal human microbial flora and infect hosts preferentially by inhalation.
  - *Opportunistic* fungi (e.g., *Candida* and *Aspergillus*) invade the host from normal sites of colonization (e.g., mucous membranes or the GI tract).
- Definitive diagnosis of any fungal infection requires histopathologic identification of the fungus invading tissue and evidence of an accompanying inflammatory response.

■ ANTIFUNGAL AGENTS

Amphotericin B (AmB)

AmB is the broadest-spectrum antifungal agent but has significant toxicities, including nephrotoxicity, fever, chills, and nausea.

- AmB has fungicidal activity and is available only for parenteral administration.
- Lipid formulations lack nephrotoxicity and infusion reactions; whether there is a clinically significant difference in efficacy between the deoxycholate and lipid formulations remains controversial.

Azoles

The azoles' mechanism of action is inhibition of ergosterol synthesis in the fungal cell wall, resulting in fungistatic activity. Azoles have little or no nephrotoxicity and are available in oral preparations.

- *Fluconazole*: Fluconazole is available in both oral and IV formulations, has a long half-life, and penetrates into most body fluids, including ocular fluids and CSF.
  - Toxicity is minimal but includes (usually reversible) hepatotoxicity and—at high doses—alopecia, muscle weakness, dry mouth, and metallic taste.
  - Fluconazole is useful for coccidioidal and cryptococcal meningitis and for candidemia, but it is notably ineffective against aspergillosis or mucormycosis.
  - It is effective as fungal prophylaxis in bone-marrow and high-risk liver transplant recipients.
- *Voriconazole*: Available in oral and IV formulations, voriconazole is considered the first-line agent against *Aspergillus* and has a broader spectrum than fluconazole against *Candida* species (including *C. glabrata* and *C. krusei*). It is also active against *Scedosporium* and *Fusarium*.

– Disadvantages of voriconazole (compared to fluconazole) include multiple drug interactions, hepatotoxicity, skin rashes (including photosensitivity), visual disturbances, and the need to monitor drug levels.
– As it is metabolized completely by the liver, dose adjustments are required in pts with liver failure. Dose adjustments for renal insufficiency are not required, but the parenteral formulation should be avoided in pts with severe renal insufficiency given the presence of cyclodextrin.

• *Itraconazole*: Available in oral and IV formulations, itraconazole is the drug of choice for mild to moderate blastomycosis and histoplasmosis. It is approved by the U.S. Food and Drug Administration (FDA) for use in febrile neutropenic pts. Disadvantages of itraconazole include its poor penetration into CSF, the use of cyclodextrin in both the oral suspension and the IV preparation, the variable absorption of the drug in capsule form, and the need for monitoring of blood levels in pts taking capsules for disseminated mycoses.

• *Posaconazole*: Approved for prophylaxis of aspergillosis and candidiasis in high-risk immunocompromised pts, posaconazole is also effective against fluconazole-resistant *Candida* isolates and may be useful as salvage therapy for some other fungal infections.

Echinocandins

The echinocandins, including caspofungin, anidulafungin, and micafungin, act by inhibiting the β-1,3-glucan synthase that is necessary for fungal cell wall synthesis. These agents are considered fungicidal for *Candida* and fungistatic for *Aspergillus*.

• Among the safest antifungal agents, echinocandins offer broad-spectrum fungicidal activity against all *Candida* species, and caspofungin has been efficacious as salvage therapy for aspergillosis.

• If anidulafungin or micafungin is used in combination with cyclosporine, no dose adjustment is needed for either drug.

Flucytosine

Flucytosine has excellent CSF penetration, but development of resistance has led to its almost always being used in combination with AmB (e.g., for cryptococcal meningitis). Adverse effects include bone marrow suppression.

Griseofulvin and Terbinafine

Griseofulvin is used primarily for ringworm infection. Terbinafine is used for onychomycosis and ringworm and is as effective as itraconazole.

Topical Agents

Many drug classes are used for topical treatment of common fungal skin infections: azoles (e.g., clotrimazole, miconazole), polyene agents (e.g., nystatin), and other classes (e.g., ciclopirox olamine, terbinafine).

■ CANDIDIASIS

Microbiology and Epidemiology

Candida is a small, thin-walled, ovoid yeast that reproduces by budding and occurs in three forms in tissue: blastospores, pseudohyphae, and hyphae.

- *Candida* is ubiquitous in nature and inhabits the GI tract, the female genital tract, and the skin. Dissemination probably results from fungal entry into the bloodstream from mucosal surfaces after the organisms have multiplied to large numbers as a result of bacterial suppression by antibacterial drugs.
- *C. albicans* is common, but non-*albicans* species (e.g., *C. glabrata*, *C. krusei*, *C. parapsilosis*, *C. tropicalis*) now cause ~50% of all cases of candidemia and disseminated candidiasis.
  - *Candida* species represent the fourth most common blood-culture isolate from hospitalized pts in the United States.
  - Pts with a compromised immune system, pts with indwelling catheters, pts with severe burns, and neonates of low birth weight are at risk for hematogenous dissemination.

Clinical Manifestations

The severity of candidal infections ranges from mild to life-threatening, with deep organ infections being at the more severe end of the spectrum.

- *Mucocutaneous candidiasis*: *Thrush* is characterized by white, adherent, painless, discrete or confluent patches in the mouth, tongue, or esophagus.
  - *Vulvovaginal candidiasis* presents with pruritus, pain, and a vaginal discharge that may contain whitish "curds."
  - Other cutaneous infections include paronychia, balanitis, and intertrigo (erythematous irritation with pustules in skin folds).
  - *Chronic mucocutaneous candidiasis* is a heterogeneous infection of hair, nails, skin, and mucous membranes that persists despite therapy and is associated with a dysfunctional immune system.
- *Deeply invasive candidiasis*: These infections are most commonly due to hematogenous seeding of organs during candidemia, but they can also be due to contiguous spread of organisms after disruption of normal anatomic barriers (e.g., kidney infection associated with an indwelling urinary catheter).
  - Nearly any organ can be infected, but the brain, chorioretina, heart, and kidneys are most commonly involved. Except in neutropenic pts, the liver and spleen are less often infected.
  - Skin involvement manifests as macronodular lesions.
  - Chorioretinal or skin involvement predicts a high probability of abscess formation in deep organs from generalized hematogenous seeding.

Diagnosis

The most challenging aspect of diagnosis is determining which pts have hematogenously disseminated disease; recovery of *Candida* from sputum, urine, or peritoneal catheters may reflect colonization rather than deep infection.

- The diagnosis of *Candida* infection is established by visualization of pseudohyphae or hyphae in the presence of inflammation in appropriate clinical samples.
- The β-glucan test has a negative predictive value of ~90% and can help exclude disseminated disease.

TREATMENT	Candidiasis

- *Mucocutaneous* Candida *infection*: Azoles are the preferred agents; nystatin is an alternative.
  - Topical applications are appropriate when possible.
  - Oral therapy can be used for vulvovaginal infections (fluconazole, 150 mg PO as a single dose) and esophageal infections (fluconazole, 100–200 mg/d; or itraconazole, 200 mg/d).
- *Candidemia and suspected disseminated candidiasis*: All pts with candidemia should be treated with a systemic antifungal agent for at least 2 weeks after the last positive blood culture.
  - Lipid formulations of AmB, echinocandins, and fluconazole or voriconazole are all effective; no agent within a given class is clearly superior to the others.
  - The choice of antifungal drug depends on local epidemiology and susceptibility profiles.
  - Neutropenic or hemodynamically unstable pts should be treated with broader-spectrum agents (e.g., AmB, echinocandins) until the pathogen is specifically identified and a clinical response assessed.
  - Fluconazole is the preferred agent for nonneutropenic, hemodynamically stable pts when azole resistance is not considered likely.
  - When possible, foreign materials (e.g., catheters) should be removed or replaced.
  - All pts with candidemia should undergo an ophthalmologic exam because of high rates of *Candida* endophthalmitis, which may require partial vitrectomy.
  - *Candida* endocarditis should be treated with valve removal and long-term antifungal administration (see Chap. 89).
  - *Candida* meningitis is often treated with a polyene plus flucytosine.
  - Successful treatment of *Candida*-infected prosthetic material (e.g., an artificial joint) nearly always requires removal of the infected material followed by long-term antifungal therapy.

Prevention

Allogeneic stem-cell and high-risk liver transplant recipients typically receive prophylaxis with fluconazole (400 mg/d). Some centers also use antifungal prophylaxis for neutropenic pts.

■ ASPERGILLOSIS

Microbiology and Epidemiology

Aspergillus is a mold with septate hyphae that branch at 45° angles and have vast numbers of conidia (spores). It has a worldwide distribution and typically grows in decomposing plant materials and in bedding. *A. fumigatus* is responsible for most cases of invasive aspergillosis, almost all cases of chronic aspergillosis, and most allergic syndromes.

- Inhalation is common; only intense exposures cause disease in healthy, immunocompetent individuals.
- The primary risk factors for invasive aspergillosis are profound neutropenia and glucocorticoid use.
- Pts with chronic pulmonary aspergillosis have a wide spectrum of underlying pulmonary diseases (e.g., tuberculosis, sarcoidosis).

Clinical Manifestations

More than 80% of invasive disease cases involve the lungs; in pts who are significantly immunocompromised, virtually any organ can be affected.

- *Invasive pulmonary aspergillosis*: Pts can be asymptomatic or can present with fever, cough, chest discomfort, hemoptysis, and shortness of breath.
  - Acute and subacute forms have courses of ≤1 month and 1–3 months, respectively.
  - Early diagnosis requires a high index of suspicion, screening for circulating antigen (in leukemia), and urgent CT of the chest.
- *Invasive sinusitis*: Pts have fever, nasal or facial discomfort, and nasal discharge. The sinuses are involved in 5–10% of cases of invasive aspergillosis; sinus involvement is especially likely in leukemic pts and hematopoietic stem-cell transplant recipients.
- *Disseminated aspergillosis*: *Aspergillus* disseminates from lung to brain, skin, thyroid, bone, and other organs, after which pts develop skin lesions and deteriorate clinically over 1–3 days, with fever and signs of mild sepsis. Blood cultures are usually negative.
  - *Cerebral aspergillosis*: Single or multiple lesions, hemorrhagic infarction, and cerebral abscess are common. The presentation can be acute or subacute, with mood changes, focal signs, seizures, and a decline in mental status. MRI is the most useful investigation.
  - *Cutaneous aspergillosis*: Dissemination of *Aspergillus* occasionally results in cutaneous features, usually an erythematous or purplish nontender area that progresses to a necrotic eschar.
- *Chronic pulmonary aspergillosis*: Pts develop one or more cavities that expand over months or years, with pulmonary symptoms, fatigue, and weight loss. Pericavitary infiltrates and multiple cavities are typical. Without treatment, pulmonary fibrosis can develop.
- *Aspergilloma*: A fungal ball occurs in up to 20% of residual chest cavities ≥2.5 cm in diameter. Life-threatening hemoptysis may occur.
- *Chronic sinusitis*: Pts develop one of three presentations: a sinus aspergilloma in the maxillary sinus, chronic invasive sinusitis that is slowly destructive, or chronic granulomatous sinusitis.
- *Allergic bronchopulmonary aspergillosis (ABPA)*: A hypersensitivity reaction leads to bronchial plugging, coughing fits, and dyspnea, primarily affecting asthmatics and pts with cystic fibrosis. Total IgE levels are usually >1000 IU/mL.

Diagnosis

Culture, molecular diagnosis, antigen detection, and histopathology usually confirm the diagnosis; ~40% of cases of invasive aspergillosis are diagnosed only at autopsy.

- Culture may be falsely positive (e.g., in pts with airway colonization) or falsely negative; only 10–30% of pts with invasive *Aspergillus* have a positive culture at any time.
- Galactomannan antigen testing of serum from high-risk pts is best done prospectively, as positive results precede clinical disease; false-positive results can occur (e.g., due to certain β-lactam/β-lactamase inhibitor antibiotic combinations).
- A *halo sign* on high-resolution thoracic CT scan (a localized ground-glass appearance representing hemorrhagic infarction surrounding a nodule) suggests the diagnosis.

TREATMENT   Aspergillosis

- See Table 115-1 for recommended treatments and doses.
  - The duration of treatment for pts with invasive aspergillosis varies from ~3 months to years, depending on the host and the response.
  - Chronic cavitary pulmonary aspergillosis probably requires treatment for life.
- Surgical treatment is important for some forms of aspergillosis (e.g., maxillary sinus fungal ball; single aspergilloma; invasive disease of bone, heart valve, brain, or sinuses).

Outcome

Invasive aspergillosis is curable if immune reconstitution occurs, whereas allergic and chronic forms are not. The overall mortality rate is ~50% with treatment, but the disease is uniformly fatal without therapy.

■ CRYPTOCOCCOSIS

Microbiology and Epidemiology

Cryptococcus is a yeast-like fungus. *C. neoformans* and *C. gattii* are pathogenic for humans and can cause cryptococcosis; most clinical laboratories do not routinely distinguish between these species.

- Worldwide, there are ~1 million cases of cryptococcosis, with >600,000 deaths annually.
- Cryptococcosis is rare in the absence of impaired immunity.
- *C. neoformans* is found in soil contaminated with pigeon droppings, whereas *C. gattii* is associated with eucalyptus trees. Most cases are acquired via inhalation, which results in pulmonary infection.

Clinical Manifestations

The clinical manifestations of cryptococcosis reflect the site of fungal infection, which usually involves the CNS and/or the lungs.

- CNS involvement most commonly presents as chronic meningoencephalitis, with headache, fever, lethargy, sensory and memory deficits, cranial nerve paresis, visual deficits, and meningismus (absent in some cases) lasting for weeks.

TABLE 115-1 TREATMENT OF ASPERGILLOSIS

Indication[b]	Primary Treatment	Evidence Level[a]	Precautions	Secondary Treatment	Comments
Invasive[b]	Voriconazole	AI	Drug interactions (especially with rifampin), renal failure (IV only)	AmB, caspofungin, posaconazole, micafungin	As primary therapy, voriconazole carries 20% more responses than AmB. If azole prophylaxis fails, it is unclear whether a class change is required for therapy.
Prophylaxis	Posaconazole, itraconazole solution	AI	Diarrhea and vomiting with itraconazole, vincristine interaction	Micafungin, aerosolized AmB	Some centers monitor plasma levels of itraconazole and posaconazole.
ABPA	Itraconazole	AI	Some glucocorticoid interactions, including with inhaled formulations	Voriconazole, posaconazole	Long-term therapy is helpful in most pts. No evidence indicates whether therapy modifies progression to bronchiectasis/fibrosis.
Single aspergilloma	Surgery	BII	Multicavity disease: poor outcome of surgery; medical therapy preferable	Itraconazole, voriconazole, intracavity AmB	Single large cavities with an aspergilloma are best resected.
Chronic pulmonary[b]	Itraconazole, voriconazole	BII	Poor absorption of capsules with proton pump inhibitors or H$_2$ blockers	Posaconazole, IV AmB, IV micafungin	Resistance may emerge during treatment, especially if plasma drug levels are subtherapeutic.

[a]Evidence levels are those used in treatment guidelines [Walsh TJ et al: Treatment of aspergillosis: Clinical practice guidelines of the Infectious Diseases Society of America (IDSA): Clin Infect Dis 46:327, 2008].

[b]An infectious disease consultation is appropriate for these pts.

Note: The oral dose is usually 200 mg bid for voriconazole and itraconazole and 400 mg bid for posaconazole. The IV dose of voriconazole is 6 mg/kg twice at 12-h intervals (loading doses) followed by 4 mg/kg q12h. Plasma monitoring is helpful in optimizing the dosage. Caspofungin is given as a single loading dose of 70 mg and then at 50 mg/d; some authorities use 70 mg/d for pts weighing >80 kg, and lower doses are required with hepatic dysfunction. Micafungin is given as 50 mg/d for prophylaxis and as at least 150 mg/d for treatment; this drug has not yet been approved by the FDA for this indication. AmB deoxycholate is given at a daily dose of 1 mg/kg if tolerated. Several strategies are available for minimizing renal dysfunction. Lipid-associated AmB is given at 3 mg/kg (AmBisome) or 5 mg/kg (Abelcet). Different regimens are available for aerosolized AmB, but none is FDA approved. **Other** considerations that may alter dose selection or route include age; concomitant medications; renal, hepatic, or intestinal dysfunction; and drug tolerability.

- Pulmonary cryptococcosis is generally asymptomatic but can present as cough, increased sputum production, and chest pain. *Cryptococcomas* are granulomatous pulmonary masses associated with *C. gattii* infections.
- Skin lesions are common in pts with disseminated cryptococcosis and can be highly variable, including papules, plaques, purpura, vesicles, tumor-like lesions, and rashes.

Diagnosis

Diagnosis requires the demonstration of *C. neoformans* in normally sterile tissue (e.g., positive cultures of CSF or blood).

- India ink smear of CSF is a useful rapid diagnostic technique, but may yield negative results in pts with a low fungal burden.
- Cryptococcal antigen testing of CSF and/or serum provides strong presumptive evidence for cryptococcosis; these tests are often negative in pulmonary cryptococcosis.

TREATMENT Cryptococcosis

- Immunocompetent pts
  - Pulmonary cryptococcosis should be treated with fluconazole (200–400 mg/d) for 3–6 months.
  - Extrapulmonary cryptococcosis may initially require AmB (0.5–1.0 mg/kg daily for 4–6 weeks).
  - CNS disease should be treated with an induction phase of AmB (0.5–1.0 mg/kg daily) followed by prolonged consolidation therapy with fluconazole (400 mg/d).
  - Meningoencephalitis is treated with AmB (0.5–1.0 mg/kg) plus flucytosine (100 mg/kg) daily for 6–10 weeks or with the same drugs at the same dosages for 2 weeks followed by fluconazole (400 mg/d) for 10 weeks.
- Immunosuppressed pts are treated with the same initial regimens except that maintenance therapy with fluconazole is given for a prolonged period (sometimes throughout life) to prevent relapse.
  - HIV-infected pts with CNS involvement are typically treated with AmB (0.7–1.0 mg/kg daily) plus flucytosine (100 mg/kg qd) for at least 2 weeks followed by fluconazole (400 mg/d) for 10 weeks and then by lifelong maintenance therapy with fluconazole (200 mg/d).
  - An alternative regimen involves fluconazole (400–800 mg/d) plus flucytosine (100 mg/kg qd) for 6–10 weeks followed by fluconazole (200 mg/d) as maintenance therapy.

■ MUCORMYCOSIS

Microbiology and Epidemiology

Mucormycosis is caused by fungi of the order Mucorales, most commonly *Rhizopus oryzae*; despite the name of the disease, *Mucor* species are only rarely the cause.

- Mucorales have characteristic wide (≥6- to 30-μm), thick-walled, ribbon-like, aseptate hyphal elements that branch at right angles.
- These ubiquitous environmental fungi primarily affect pts with diabetes, defects in phagocytic function (e.g., associated with neutropenia or glucocorticoid therapy), and deferoxamine treatment for iron overload syndromes.

Clinical Manifestations

Mucormycosis is highly invasive and relentlessly progressive, with a mortality rate of >40%. The disease is usually categorized by the anatomic site involved.

- *Rhinocerebral mucormycosis*: In this, the most common form of the disease, pts initially have nonspecific symptoms that include eye or facial pain and facial numbness followed by the onset of conjunctival suffusion, blurry vision, and soft tissue swelling.
  - If untreated, the infection can spread from the ethmoid sinus to the orbit, affecting extraocular muscle function and being associated with proptosis and chemosis.
  - The visual appearance of infected tissue may progress from normal to erythematous to violaceous to a black necrotic eschar.
- *Pulmonary mucormycosis*: In this second most common manifestation, pts typically present with fever, dyspnea, cough, and chest pain. Angioinvasion results in necrosis, cavitation, and/or hemoptysis. Differentiation from aspergillosis is critical as treatment regimens differ; the presence of ≥10 pulmonary nodules, pleural effusion, or concomitant sinusitis makes mucormycosis more likely.
- *Cutaneous mucormycosis*: Caused by external implantation or hematogenous dissemination, necrotizing fasciitis due to mucormycosis has a mortality rate of ~80%.
- *Hematogenously disseminated mucormycosis*: Infection can disseminate from any primary site of infection to any organ, but most commonly metastasizes to the brain (with a mortality rate of ~100%).

Diagnosis

Although definitive diagnosis requires a positive culture from a sterile site, a positive culture from a nonsterile site [e.g., sputum or bronchoalveolar lavage (BAL) fluid] in a pt with a consistent clinical history should prompt treatment pending confirmation of the diagnosis.

- The fact that only ~50% of pts have positive cultures is due, in part, to the organisms' being killed by the tissue homogenization required for preparation of culture.
- The laboratory should be notified that mucormycosis is being considered so that tissue sections instead of tissue homogenates can be cultured.

TREATMENT **Mucormycosis**

- The successful treatment of mucormycosis requires four steps: (1) early diagnosis; (2) reversal of underlying predisposing risk factors, if possible; (3) surgical debridement; and (4) prompt antifungal therapy.

- AmB (AmB deoxycholate, 1–1.5 mg/kg qd; or liposomal AmB, 5–10 mg/kg qd) is the preferred antifungal agent for treatment of mucormycosis.
  - Limited retrospective data suggest that combinations of echinocandins and liposomal AmB may be more effective.
  - Although posaconazole has in vitro activity against Mucorales, few clinical data support its use.
  - Initial clinical trials suggest that liposomal AmB combined with deferasirox (an iron chelator that is fungicidal for clinical isolates of Mucorales; 20 mg/kg PO qd for 2–4 weeks) results in improved survival rates.
  - Treatment should be continued until (1) resolution of clinical signs and symptoms of infection; (2) resolution or stabilization of residual radiographic signs of disease on serial imaging; and (3) resolution of underlying immunosuppression.

■ HISTOPLASMOSIS

Microbiology and Epidemiology

Histoplasma capsulatum, a dimorphic fungus, causes histoplasmosis.

- Mycelia are infectious and have microconidial and macroconidial forms. Microconidia are inhaled, reach the alveoli, and are transformed into yeasts with occasional narrow budding. A granulomatous reaction results; in pts with impaired cellular immunity, infection may disseminate.
- Histoplasmosis is the most prevalent endemic mycosis in North America and is also found in Central and South America, Africa, and Asia. In the United States, histoplasmosis is endemic in the Ohio and Mississippi river valleys.
- The fungus is found in soil, particularly that enriched by droppings of birds and bats.

Clinical Manifestations

Depending on the intensity of exposure, the immune status of the exposed individual, and the underlying lung architecture of the host, disease can range from asymptomatic to life-threatening.

- Immunocompetent pts usually have asymptomatic or mild and self-limited disease.
  - 1–4 weeks after exposure, some pts develop a flu-like illness with fever, chills, sweats, headache, myalgia, anorexia, cough, dyspnea, and chest pain. 5–10% of pts with acute histoplasmosis develop arthralgia or arthritis, often associated with erythema nodosum.
  - Hilar or mediastinal lymphadenopathy may occur and can cause vascular or tracheoesophageal compression.
- Immunocompromised pts are more likely to develop progressive disseminated histoplasmosis (PDH).
  - The clinical spectrum ranges from a rapidly fatal course with diffuse interstitial or reticulonodular lung infiltrates, shock, and multiorgan

failure to a subacute course with focal organ involvement, hepatosplenomegaly, fever, and weight loss.
  – Meningitis, oral mucosal ulcerations, GI ulcerations, and adrenal insufficiency can occur.
• Chronic cavitary histoplasmosis most often affects smokers with structural lung disease (e.g., emphysema) and presents as productive cough, dyspnea, low-grade fever, night sweats, and weight loss.

Diagnosis

Fungal culture remains the gold standard, but cultures are often negative in less severe cases and may take up to 1 month to become positive.
• In PDH, the culture yield is highest for BAL fluid, bone marrow aspirate, and blood; cultures of sputum or bronchial washings are usually positive in chronic pulmonary histoplasmosis.
• Fungal stains of cytopathology or biopsy materials may be helpful in diagnosing PDH.
• *Histoplasma* antigen assay of body fluids (e.g., blood, urine, CSF, BAL fluid) is useful in diagnosing PDH or acute disease and in monitoring the response to treatment.
• Serology can be helpful in diagnosis but requires ≥1 month for antibody production.

TREATMENT   Histoplasmosis

• See Table 115-2 for treatment recommendations.
  – Fibrosing mediastinitis, which represents a chronic fibrotic reaction to past mediastinal histoplasmosis rather than an active infection, does not respond to antifungal therapy.

■ COCCIDIOIDOMYCOSIS

Microbiology and Epidemiology

Coccidioidomycosis is caused by the two species of the dimorphic soil-dwelling fungus *Coccidioides*: *C. immitis* and *C. posadasii*. These organisms exist as branching, filamentous molds.
• Coccidioidomycosis is confined to the Western Hemisphere between the latitudes of 40°N and 40°S. The disease is highly endemic in California, Arizona, and other areas of the southwestern United States; northern Mexico and localized regions in Central and South America also account for cases of infection.
• Direct exposure to soil harboring *Coccidioides* increases risk, but infection, which results from inhalation of airborne arthroconidia, can occur without overt soil exposure and may be related to other climatic factors (e.g., periods of dryness after rainy seasons).

Clinical Manifestations

60% of infected pts are asymptomatic; the remaining 40% have primarily pulmonary disease characterized by fever, cough, and pleuritic chest pain.

TABLE 115-2 RECOMMENDATIONS FOR THE TREATMENT OF HISTOPLASMOSIS

Type of Histoplasmosis	Treatment Recommendations	Comments
Acute pulmonary, moderate to severe illness with diffuse infiltrates and/or hypoxemia	Lipid AmB (3–5 mg/kg per day) ± glucocorticoids for 1–2 weeks; then itraconazole (200 mg bid) for 12 weeks. Monitor renal and hepatic function.	Pts with mild cases usually recover without therapy, but itraconazole should be considered if the pt's condition has not improved after 1 month.
Chronic/cavitary pulmonary	Itraconazole (200 mg qd or bid) for at least 12 months. Monitor hepatic function.	Continue treatment until radiographic findings show no further improvement. Monitor for relapse after treatment is stopped.
Progressive disseminated	Lipid AmB (3–5 mg/kg per day) for 1–2 weeks; then itraconazole (200 mg bid) for at least 12 months. Monitor renal and hepatic function.	Liposomal AmB is preferred, but the AmB lipid complex may be used because of cost. Chronic maintenance therapy may be necessary if the degree of immunosuppression cannot be reduced.
CNS	Liposomal AmB (5 mg/kg per day) for 4–6 weeks; then itraconazole (200 mg bid or tid) for at least 12 months. Monitor renal and hepatic function.	A longer course of lipid AmB is recommended because of the high risk of relapse. Itraconazole should be continued until CSF or CT abnormalities clear.

- Primary pulmonary infection is sometimes associated with erythema nodosum, erythema multiforme, arthralgias, and arthritis.
  - A history of night sweats, profound fatigue, eosinophilia, and hilar or mediastinal lymphadenopathy suggests the disease.
  - Pneumonic complications include pulmonary nodules (resembling pulmonary malignancies) and pulmonary cavities (a thin-walled lesion in a bronchus that is associated with cough, hemoptysis, and pleuritic chest pain).
- Disseminated infection affects <1% of infected pts, most commonly pts with depressed cellular immunity and pregnant women.

   – Common sites for dissemination include bone, skin, joint, soft tissue, and meninges.

   – Pts with meningitis present with persistent headache, lethargy, confusion, mild to moderate nuchal rigidity, and CSF with lymphocytic pleocytosis and profound hypoglycorrhachia. The mortality rate is ~100% without treatment.

Diagnosis

Serology and culture are the primary means of diagnosis. Alert the laboratory of the possible diagnosis to avoid exposure.

- Tube-precipitin (TP) and complement-fixation (CF) assays, immunodiffusion, and an EIA are available to detect IgM and IgG antibodies.
  - TP antibody does not gauge disease progression and is not found in CSF.
  - Rising CF titers in serum are associated with clinical progression, and CF antibody in CSF indicates meningitis.
  - EIA frequently yields false-positive results.
- Examination of sputum or other respiratory fluids after Papanicolaou or Gomori methenamine silver staining reveals spherules in many pts with pulmonary disease.

TREATMENT   Coccidioidomycosis

- The vast majority of pts with coccidioidomycosis do not require treatment. Exceptions include the following:
  - Pts with focal primary pneumonia *and* underlying cellular immunodeficiency or prolonged symptoms (symptoms persisting for ≥2 months, night sweats occurring for >3 weeks, weight loss of >10%, a serum CF antibody titer of >1:16, and extensive pulmonary involvement apparent on CXR) should be treated with fluconazole (≥400 mg/d) or itraconazole (400–600 mg/d).
  - Pts with diffuse pulmonary disease are often treated initially with AmB (deoxycholate, 0.7–1 mg/kg IV qd; liposomal, 5 mg/kg IV qd), with a switch to prolonged therapy with a triazole once clinical improvement occurs.
  - Pts with chronic pulmonary disease or disseminated infection are treated with prolonged triazole therapy (i.e., for ≥1 year). Relapse occurs in 15–30% of individuals once therapy is discontinued.
  - Pts with meningitis require lifelong triazole therapy; fluconazole is the drug of choice. If triazole therapy fails, intrathecal or intraventricular AmB may be used. Relapse occurs in 80% of pts when therapy is stopped.

■ BLASTOMYCOSIS

Microbiology and Epidemiology

Blastomyces dermatitidis is a dimorphic fungus that is found in the southeastern and south-central states bordering the Mississippi and Ohio river basins, in areas of the United States and Canada bordering the Great Lakes and the St. Lawrence River, and in Africa. Infection is caused by inhalation of *Blastomyces* from moist soil rich in organic debris.

Clinical Manifestations

Acute pulmonary infection can present as abrupt-onset fever, chills, pleuritic chest pain, myalgias, and arthralgias. However, most pts with pulmonary blastomycosis have chronic indolent pneumonia with fever, weight loss, productive cough, and hemoptysis. Skin disease is common and can present as verrucous (more common) or ulcerative lesions. Blastomycosis can include osteomyelitis in one-fourth of infections and CNS disease in ~40% of pts with AIDS.

Diagnosis

Smears of clinical samples or cultures of sputum, pus, or tissue are required for diagnosis. Antigen detection in urine and serum may assist in diagnosing infection and in monitoring pts during therapy.

TREATMENT	Blastomycosis

- Every pt should be treated because of the high risk of dissemination.
  - For immunocompetent pts with nonsevere disease that does not involve the CNS, itraconazole (200–400 mg/d for 6–12 months) is recommended.
  - Immunocompetent pts with severe disease or CNS manifestations should be treated initially with AmB (deoxycholate, 0.7–1 mg/kg IV qd; liposomal, 3–5 mg/kg IV qd); once their clinical condition improves, they can be switched to itraconazole (or, for those with CNS disease, fluconazole, 800 mg/d).
  - Immunocompromised pts with any form of infection should be treated initially with AmB, with a switch to a triazole, as above, once clinical improvement has occurred.

◼ *MALASSEZIA* INFECTION

Malassezia species are components of the normal skin flora and can cause tinea (pityriasis) versicolor, round scaly patches of hypo- or hyperpigmented skin on the neck, chest, or upper arms. *M. furfur* causes catheter-related fungemia in premature neonates receiving IV lipids by central venous catheter. Topical creams and lotions for 2 weeks are effective in treating superficial *Malassezia* infections; fungemia caused by *Malassezia* species is treated with AmB or fluconazole, prompt removal of the catheter, and discontinuation of the lipid infusion.

◼ SPOROTRICHOSIS

Microbiology and Epidemiology

Sporothrix schenckii is a dimorphic fungus found worldwide in soil, on plants, and on animals. Infection, which results from inoculation of the organism into the skin, is most common among people who participate in landscaping, gardening, or tree farming.

Clinical Manifestations

Lymphocutaneous sporotrichosis involves secondary lesions (papules that are not very painful and often ulcerate) developing along lymphatic channels proximally from the initial site of inoculation. Other presentations include a fixed lesion (verrucous or ulcerative) at the initial site of inoculation without lymphatic spread, osteoarticular disease (chronic synovitis or septic arthritis in alcoholics), pulmonary disease (most common among pts with chronic obstructive pulmonary disease), and disseminated disease (numerous skin lesions with occasional spread to visceral organs in immunocompromised pts).

Diagnosis

Culture of material from a skin lesion or histopathologic examination of a skin biopsy sample can confirm the diagnosis.

TREATMENT Sporotrichosis

- Cutaneous and lymphocutaneous sporotrichosis is treated with itraconazole (200 mg/d) for 2–4 weeks *after* the lesions have resolved.
- For extracutaneous disease, itraconazole (200 mg bid for 12 months) can be given, but initial therapy with liposomal AmB (3–5 mg/kg qd) is more effective for life-threatening pulmonary disease or disseminated infection.

■ PARACOCCIDIOIDOMYCOSIS

Paracoccidioidomycosis (South American blastomycosis) is caused by *Paracoccidioides brasiliensis*, a dimorphic fungus acquired by inhalation from environmental sources. Acute infection occurs in young or immunocompromised pts and manifests as disseminated infection of the reticuloendothelial system. Chronic infection accounts for 90% of cases and presents primarily as progressive pulmonary disease with occasional ulcerative and nodular mucocutaneous lesions in the nose and mouth. Diagnosis relies on culture of the organism. Itraconazole (100–200 mg/d for 6–12 months) is effective, but AmB may be required for seriously ill pts.

■ PENICILLIOSIS

Penicillium marneffei is a leading cause of opportunistic infection in pts with immunocompromise (e.g., due to AIDS) in Southeast Asia and is acquired by spore inhalation. Clinical manifestations are similar to those of disseminated histoplasmosis, with fever, fatigue, weight loss, lymphadenopathy, hepatomegaly, and skin lesions resembling molluscum contagiosum. The organism grows readily in culture and produces a distinctive red pigment. AmB is the initial treatment of choice for severely ill pts; less severe disease may be treated with itraconazole (400 mg/d for 12 weeks).

Suppressive therapy with itraconazole (200 mg/d) may be indicated for pts with HIV infection or AIDS.

■ FUSARIOSIS

Fusarium species are found worldwide in soil and on plants; inhalation, ingestion, and direct inoculation of spores can cause disease, particularly disseminated disease in immunocompromised pts. Fusariosis is angioinvasive and has clinical manifestations similar to those of aspergillosis. One difference is that painful, nodular or necrotic skin lesions are extremely common with disseminated fusariosis. Blood cultures are positive in 50% of cases; the organism is difficult to differentiate from *Aspergillus* in tissue. *Fusarium* species are often resistant to antifungal agents; liposomal AmB (≥5 mg/kg qd), voriconazole (200–400 mg bid), or posaconazole (400 mg bid) is recommended. Even with treatment, mortality rates are ~50%.

■ SCEDOSPORIOSIS

Pseudallescheria boydii, Scedosporium apiospermum, and *S. prolificans* are molds that are angioinvasive, causing pneumonia and widespread dissemination with abscesses (including brain abscess) in immunocompromised hosts. Most disseminated infections are fatal. These organisms are resistant to AmB, echinocandins, and some azoles, but some infections have been cured with voriconazole.

■ DERMATOPHYTOSIS

See Chap. 66.

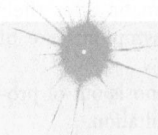

For a more detailed discussion, see Edwards JE Jr: Diagnosis and Treatment of Fungal Infections, Chap. 198, p. 1637; Hage CA, Wheat LJ: Histoplasmosis, Chap. 199, p. 1640; Ampel NM: Coccidioidomycosis, Chap. 200, p. 1643; Chapman SW, Sullivan DC: Blastomycosis, Chap. 201, p. 1646; Casadevall A: Cryptococcosis, Chap. 202, p. 1648; Edwards JE Jr: Candidiasis, Chap. 203, p. 1651; Denning DW: Aspergillosis, Chap. 204, p. 1655; Spellberg B, Ibrahim AS: Mucormycosis, Chap. 205, p. 1661; and Kauffman CA: Superficial Mycoses and Less Common Systemic Mycoses, Chap. 206, p. 1665, in HPIM-18.

CHAPTER **116**
Pneumocystis Infections

Pneumocystis, an opportunistic fungal pulmonary pathogen, is an important cause of pneumonia in immunocompromised hosts.

■ MICROBIOLOGY

• *P. jirovecii* infects humans, whereas *P. carinii*—the original species described—infects rats.

- In contrast to most fungi, *Pneumocystis* lacks ergosterol and thus is not susceptible to antifungal drugs that inhibit ergosterol synthesis.
- Developmental stages include the small trophic form, the cyst, and the intermediate precyst stage.

◼ EPIDEMIOLOGY

- *Pneumocystis* is found worldwide, and most healthy children have been exposed to the organism by 3–4 years of age.
- Both airborne transmission and person-to-person transmission have been demonstrated; the cyst is the transmissible form.
- Defects in cellular and humoral immunity (including immunosuppressive medications) predispose to *Pneumocystis* pneumonia. The risk in HIV-infected pts rises dramatically when CD4+ T cell counts fall below 200/µL.

◼ PATHOGENESIS

- The organisms are inhaled and attach tightly to type I cells in alveoli, although they remain extracellular.
- On histology, alveoli are seen to be filled with foamy, vacuolated exudates.
- Severe disease may cause interstitial edema, fibrosis, and hyaline membrane formation.

◼ CLINICAL MANIFESTATIONS

- Pts develop dyspnea, fever, and nonproductive cough.
  - HIV-infected pts are usually ill for several weeks or longer with subtle manifestations.
  - Pts without HIV infection often become symptomatic after their glucocorticoid dose has been tapered, and their symptoms are of shorter duration.
- Physical exam reveals tachypnea, tachycardia, and cyanosis out of proportion to the few abnormalities present on chest auscultation.
- Nonspecific laboratory findings include elevated serum concentrations of lactate dehydrogenase and β-D-glucan, a component of the fungal cell wall.
- CXR classically reveals bilateral diffuse infiltrates beginning in the perihilar regions. Other findings (e.g., nodular densities, cavitary lesions) have been described.
- Rare cases of disseminated infection have been described, generally involving lymph nodes, spleen, liver, and bone marrow.

◼ DIAGNOSIS

- Histopathologic staining makes the definitive diagnosis.
  - Cell-wall stains (e.g., methenamine silver) are used for *Pneumocystis* cysts and Wright-Giemsa stains for the nuclei of all developmental stages.
  - Immunofluorescence with monoclonal antibodies increases diagnostic sensitivity.
- DNA amplification by PCR is most sensitive but may not distinguish colonization from infection.
- Proper specimens are key.
  - Fiberoptic bronchoscopy with bronchoalveolar lavage remains the mainstay of diagnosis.

- Sputum induction and oral washes are noninvasive options that are gaining popularity.
- Transbronchial biopsy and open lung biopsy are used only when a diagnosis cannot be made by bronchoalveolar lavage.

TREATMENT *Pneumocystis* Infections

- Trimethoprim-sulfamethoxazole (TMP-SMX) is the drug of choice for all pts. For doses and adverse effects of TMP-SMX and alternative regimens, see Table 116-1.
- For mild to moderate cases (a Pao_2 >70 mmHg or a $PAo_2 - Pao_2$ gradient <35 mmHg on room air), alternatives include TMP plus dapsone and clindamycin plus primaquine. Atovaquone is less effective than TMP-SMX but is better tolerated.

TABLE 116-1 TREATMENT OF PNEUMOCYSTOSIS

Drug(s), Dose, Route	Adverse Effects
First choice[a]	
TMP-SMX (TMP: 5 mg/kg; SMX: 25 mg/kg[b]) q6–8h PO or IV	Fever, rash, cytopenias, hepatitis, hyperkalemia, GI disturbances
Other agents[a]	
TMP, 5 mg/kg q6–8h; plus dapsone, 100 mg qd PO	Hemolysis (G6PD deficiency), methemoglobinemia, fever, rash, GI disturbances
Atovaquone, 750 mg bid PO	Rash, fever, GI and hepatic disturbances
Clindamycin, 300–450 mg q6h PO or 600 mg q6–8h IV; plus primaquine, 15–30 mg qd PO	Hemolysis (G6PD deficiency), methemoglobinemia, rash, colitis, neutropenia
Pentamidine, 3–4 mg/kg qd IV	Hypotension, azotemia, cardiac arrhythmias, pancreatitis, dysglycemias, hypocalcemia, neutropenia, hepatitis
Trimetrexate, 45 mg/m² qd IV; plus leucovorin,[c] 20 mg/kg q6h PO or IV	Cytopenias, peripheral neuropathy, hepatic disturbances
Adjunctive agent	
Prednisone, 40 mg bid × 5 d, 40 mg qd × 5 d, 20 mg qd × 11 d; PO or IV	Immunosuppression, peptic ulcer, hyperglycemia, mood changes, hypertension

[a]Therapy is administered for 14 days to non-HIV-infected pts and for 21 days to HIV-infected pts.
[b]Equivalent of 2 double-strength (DS) tablets. (One DS tablet contains 160 mg of TMP and 800 mg of SMX.)
[c]Leucovorin prevents bone marrow toxicity from trimetrexate.

- For moderate to severe cases (a Pao_2 ≤70 mmHg or a $PAo_2 - Pao_2$ gradient ≥35 mmHg), alternatives include IV pentamidine, IV clindamycin plus primaquine (potentially more effective than pentamidine), and trimetrexate plus leucovorin.
- Adjunctive administration of tapering doses of glucocorticoids to HIV-infected pts with moderate to severe disease reduces the risk of respiratory function deterioration shortly after initiation of treatment. Use of glucocorticoids in other pts remains to be evaluated.

■ PROGNOSIS
- Therapy is most effective if started early, before there is extensive alveolar damage.
- The mortality rate among HIV-infected pts is 0–15%.
- The risk of early death remains high among people who need mechanical ventilation (60%) and among non-HIV-infected pts (40%).

■ PREVENTION
- Prophylaxis is indicated for HIV-infected pts with CD4+ T cell counts <200/µL or a history of oropharyngeal candidiasis and for any pt with a

TABLE 116-2 PROPHYLAXIS OF PNEUMOCYSTOSIS[a]

Drug(s), Dose, Route	Comments
First choice	
TMP-SMX, 1 DS tablet or 1 SS tablet qd PO[b]	TMP-SMX can be safely reintroduced for treatment of some pts who have had mild to moderate side effects.
Other agents	
Dapsone, 50 mg bid or 100 mg qd PO	—
Dapsone, 50 mg qd PO; plus pyrimethamine, 50 mg weekly PO; plus leucovorin, 25 mg weekly PO	Leucovorin prevents bone marrow toxicity from pyrimethamine.
Dapsone, 200 mg weekly PO; plus pyrimethamine, 75 mg weekly PO; plus leucovorin, 25 mg weekly PO	Leucovorin prevents bone marrow toxicity from pyrimethamine.
Pentamidine, 300 mg monthly via Respirgard II nebulizer	Adverse reactions include cough and bronchospasm.
Atovaquone, 1500 mg qd PO	—
TMP-SMX, 1 DS tablet three times weekly PO	TMP-SMX can be safely reintroduced for treatment of some pts who have had mild to moderate side effects.

[a]For list of adverse effects, see Table 116-1.
[b]One DS tablet contains 160 mg of TMP and 800 mg of SMX.
Abbreviations: DS, double-strength; SS, single-strength.

history of *Pneumocystis* pneumonia. Guidelines for other compromised hosts are less clear.

- In HIV infection, once CD4+ counts have risen to >200/µL and have remained above that cutoff for ≥3 months, prophylaxis may be stopped.
- For prophylactic regimens, see Table 116-2. TMP-SMX is the drug of choice for both primary and secondary prophylaxis and also protects against toxoplasmosis and some bacterial infections.

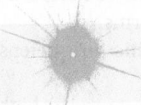

For a more detailed discussion, see Smulian AG, Walzer PD: *Pneumocystis* Infections, Chap. 207, p. 1671, in HPIM-18.

CHAPTER **117**
Protozoal Infections

MALARIA

Microbiology

Five major species of *Plasmodium* cause nearly all cases of human disease: *P. falciparum, P. vivax, P. ovale, P. malariae,* and *P. knowlesi.*

- *P. falciparum*, the cause of most cases of severe disease and most deaths, predominates in Africa, New Guinea, and Hispaniola.
- *P. vivax* is more common in Central America.
- *P. falciparum* and *P. vivax* are equally prevalent in South America, the Indian subcontinent, eastern Asia, and Oceania.
- *P. ovale* is unusual outside of Africa, where it makes up ~1% of isolates.
- *P. malariae* is found in most areas (especially throughout sub-Saharan Africa) but is less common.
- *P. knowlesi* (the monkey malaria parasite) can reliably be identified only by molecular techniques and is present in Borneo and Southeast Asia.

Epidemiology

Malaria is the most important parasitic disease in humans, causing ~1 million deaths each year.

Pathogenesis

After introduction of *sporozoites* into the bloodstream by female anopheline mosquitoes, the parasite travels to the liver and reproduces asexually to form *merozoites* that infect RBCs. The merozoites transform into *trophozoites*, feed on intracellular proteins (principally hemoglobin), multiply 6- to 20-fold every 48–72 h, and cause the RBCs to rupture, releasing daughter merozoites. The process then repeats.

- Some parasites develop into long-lived sexual forms called *gametocytes*, which can be taken up by another female anopheline mosquito, allowing transmission.

- In *P. vivax* or *P. ovale* infection, dormant forms called *hypnozoites* remain in liver cells and may cause disease 3 weeks to >1 year later.
- RBCs infected with *P. falciparum* may exhibit *cytoadherence* (attachment to venular and capillary endothelium), *rosetting* (adherence to uninfected RBCs), and *agglutination* (adherence to other infected RBCs). The result is sequestration of *P. falciparum* in vital organs, with consequent under-estimation (through parasitemia determinations) of parasite numbers in the body. Sequestration is central to the pathogenesis of falciparum malaria but is not evident in the other three "benign" forms.
- In nonimmune individuals, infection triggers nonspecific host defense mechanisms such as increased splenic filtration.
  - With repeated exposure to malaria, pts develop resistance to high-level parasitemia and disease but not to infection.
  - Hemoglobinopathies (e.g., sickle cell disease, ovalocytosis, thalassemia) and G6PD deficiency are more common in endemic areas and protect against death from malaria.

Clinical Manifestations

Pts initially develop nonspecific symptoms (e.g., headache, fatigue, myalgias) that are followed by fever.

- Febrile paroxysms at regular intervals are unusual and suggest infection with *P. vivax* or *P. ovale*.
- Splenomegaly, hepatomegaly, mild anemia, and jaundice may develop.
- The diagnosis of severe falciparum malaria requires ≥1 of the following: impaired consciousness/coma, severe normocytic anemia, renal failure, pulmonary edema, ARDS, circulatory shock, DIC, spontaneous bleeding, acidosis, hemoglobinuria, jaundice, repeated generalized convulsions, and a parasitemia level of >5%.
  - Cerebral malaria manifests as diffuse symmetric encephalopathy, typically without focal neurologic signs.
  - Coma is an ominous sign associated with mortality rates of ~20%.
- Pregnant women have unusually severe illness. Premature labor, fetal distress, stillbirth, and delivery of low-birth-weight infants are common.
- Tropical splenomegaly (hyperreactive malarial splenomegaly) may result as a chronic complication of malaria and is characterized by massive splenomegaly, hepatomegaly, and an abnormal immunologic response to infection.

Diagnosis

Although antibody-based diagnostic tests are being used with increasing frequency, demonstration of asexual forms of the parasite on peripheral-blood smears is required for diagnosis.

- Thick and thin smears should be examined; thick smears and the less sensitive thin smears detect parasitemia levels as low as 0.001% and ~0.05%, respectively.
- If the level of clinical suspicion is high and smears are initially negative, they should be repeated q12–24h for 2 days.
- Other laboratory findings generally include normochromic, normocytic anemia; elevated inflammatory markers; and thrombocytopenia ($\sim10^5/\mu L$).

TREATMENT ▶ Malaria

- See Table 117-1 for treatment regimens. IV artesunate is approved by the U.S. Food and Drug Administration for emergency use against severe malaria through the CDC [Malaria Hotline: 770-488-7788; Emergency Operations Center (after hours): 770-488-7100].
- Pts receiving quinidine should undergo cardiac monitoring; a total plasma level of >8 μg/mL, increased QT intervals (>0.6 s), or QRS widening by >25% is an indication for slowing the infusion rate.
- Exchange transfusions can be considered for severely ill pts, although indications for their use are not yet agreed upon.
- All pts with severe malaria should receive a continuous infusion of dextrose. Unconscious pts should have blood glucose levels measured q4–6h.
- Parasite counts and hematocrits for pts with severe malaria and pts with uncomplicated disease should be measured q6–12h and q24h, respectively.
- Primaquine (0.5 mg of base/kg for 14 days) eradicates persistent liver stages and prevents relapse in *P. vivax* or *P. ovale* infection. G6PD deficiency must be ruled out before treatment.

Personal Protection Measures

Measures that can protect persons against infection include avoidance of mosquito exposure, with particular caution at peak feeding times (dusk and dawn); use of insect repellents containing DEET (10–35%) or (if DEET is unacceptable) picaridin (7%); suitable clothing; and insecticide-impregnated bed nets.

Chemoprophylaxis

See Table 117-2 for prophylaxis options.

- Mefloquine is the only drug advised for pregnant women traveling to areas with drug-resistant malaria and is generally considered safe in the second and third trimesters; data regarding use in the first trimester, although limited, are reassuring.

BABESIOSIS

Microbiology

Babesiosis is caused by intraerythrocytic protozoa of the genus *Babesia*. *B. microti* is the etiologic agent in the northeastern United States, and *B. duncani* is responsible for disease on the West Coast. *B. divergens* causes disease in Europe. The deer tick (*Ixodes scapularis*) transmits *B. microti*; the vectors of transmission for the other *Babesia* species are unknown.

Epidemiology

In the United States, infections occur most frequently along the northeastern coast. In 2009, >700 cases were reported in the U.S.; this number is probably

TABLE 117-1 REGIMENS FOR THE TREATMENT OF MALARIA

Type of Disease or Treatment	Regimen(s)
Uncomplicated malaria	
Known chloroquine-sensitive strains of *Plasmodium vivax*, *P. malariae*, *P. ovale*, *P. knowlesi*, *P. falciparum*[a]	Chloroquine (10 mg of base/kg stat followed by 5 mg/kg at 12, 24, and 36 h or by 10 mg/kg at 24 h and 5 mg/kg at 48 h) *or* Amodiaquine (10–12 mg of base/kg qd for 3 days)
Radical treatment for *P. vivax* or *P. ovale* infection	In addition to chloroquine or amodiaquine as detailed above, primaquine (0.5 mg of base/kg qd) should be given for 14 days to prevent relapse. In mild G6PD deficiency, 0.75 mg of base/kg should be given once weekly for 6–8 weeks. Primaquine should not be given in severe G6PD deficiency.
Sensitive *P. falciparum* malaria[b]	Artesunate[c] (4 mg/kg qd for 3 days) plus sulfadoxine (25 mg/kg)/pyrimethamine (1.25 mg/kg) as a single dose *or* Artesunate[c] (4 mg/kg qd for 3 days) plus amodiaquine (10 mg of base/kg qd for 3 days)[d]
Multidrug-resistant *P. falciparum* malaria	Either artemether-lumefantrine[c] (1.5/9 mg/kg bid for 3 days with food) *or* Artesunate[c] (4 mg/kg qd for 3 days) *plus* Mefloquine (25 mg of base/kg—either 8 mg/kg qd for 3 days or 15 mg/kg on day 2 and then 10 mg/kg on day 3)[d]
Second-line treatment/treatment of imported malaria	Either artesunate[c] (2 mg/kg qd for 7 days) or quinine (10 mg of salt/kg tid for 7 days) *plus 1 of the following 3:* 1. Tetracycline[e] (4 mg/kg qid for 7 days) 2. Doxycycline[e] (3 mg/kg qd for 7 days) 3. Clindamycin (10 mg/kg bid for 7 days) *or* Atovaquone-proguanil (20/8 mg/kg qd for 3 days with food)

TABLE 117-1 REGIMENS FOR THE TREATMENT OF MALARIA (CONTINUED)

Type of Disease or Treatment	Regimen(s)
Severe falciparum malaria[f]	Artesunate[c] (2.4 mg/kg stat IV followed by 2.4 mg/kg at 12 and 24 h and then daily if necessary)[g] *or, if unavailable, one of the following:*
	Artemether[c] (3.2 mg/kg stat IM followed by 1.6 mg/kg qd)
	or
	Quinine dihydrochloride (20 mg of salt/kg[h] infused over 4 h, followed by 10 mg of salt/kg infused over 2–8 h q8h[i])
	or
	Quinidine (10 mg of base/kg[h] infused over 1–2 h, followed by 1.2 mg of base/kg per hour[i] with electrocardiographic monitoring)

[a]Very few areas now have chloroquine-sensitive *P. falciparum* malaria (see Fig. 210-2 in HPIM-18).
[b]In areas where the partner drug to artesunate is known to be effective.
[c]Artemisinin derivatives are not readily available in some temperate countries.
[d]Fixed-dose coformulated combinations are available. The World Health Organization now recommends artemisinin combination regimens as first-line therapy for falciparum malaria in all tropical countries and advocates use of fixed-dose combinations.
[e]Tetracycline and doxycycline should not be given to pregnant women or to children <8 years of age.
[f]Oral treatment should be substituted as soon as the pt recovers sufficiently to take fluids by mouth.
[g]Artesunate is the drug of choice when available. The data from large studies in Southeast Asia showed a 35% lower mortality rate than with quinine, and very large studies in Africa showed a 22.5% lower mortality rate than with quinine.
[h]A loading dose should not be given if therapeutic doses of quinine or quinidine have definitely been administered in the previous 24 h. Some authorities recommend a lower dose of quinidine.
[i]Infusions can be given in 0.9% saline and 5–10% dextrose in water. Infusion rates for quinine and quinidine should be carefully controlled.

an underestimate, given that most pts experience a mild and self-limiting disease and may not seek medical attention.

Clinical Manifestations

Most pts develop a mild illness, but immunosuppressed pts may have more severe disease.

- After an incubation period of 1–6 weeks, pts gradually develop fevers, fatigue, and weakness. Other symptoms may include chills, sweats, myalgias, arthralgias, headache, and—less often—neck stiffness, shortness of breath, and abdominal pain.

TABLE 117-2 DRUGS USED IN THE PROPHYLAXIS OF MALARIA

Drug	Usage	Adult Dose	Pediatric Dose	Comments
Atovaquone/proguanil (Malarone)	Prophylaxis in areas with chloroquine- or mefloquine-resistant *Plasmodium falciparum*	1 adult tablet PO[a]	5–8 kg: ½ pediatric tablet[b] daily ≥8–10 kg: ¾ pediatric tablet daily ≥10–20 kg: 1 pediatric tablet daily ≥20–30 kg: 2 pediatric tablets daily ≥30–40 kg: 3 pediatric tablets daily ≥40 kg: 1 adult tablet daily	Begin 1–2 days before travel to malarious areas. Take daily at the same time each day while in the malarious areas and for 7 days after leaving such areas. Atovaquone-proguanil is contraindicated in persons with severe renal impairment (creatinine clearance rate <30 mL/min). In the absence of data, it is not recommended for children weighing <5 kg, pregnant women, or women breast-feeding infants weighing <5 kg. Atovaquone/proguanil should be taken with food or a milky drink.
Chloroquine phosphate (Aralen and generic)	Prophylaxis, restricted to areas with chloroquine-sensitive *P. falciparum*[c] or *P. vivax* only	300 mg of base (500 mg of salt) PO once weekly	5 mg/kg of base (8.3 mg of salt/kg) PO once weekly, up to maximal adult dose of 300 mg of base	Begin 1–2 weeks before travel to malarious areas. Take weekly on the same day of the week while in the malarious areas and for 4 weeks after leaving such areas. Chloroquine phosphate may exacerbate psoriasis.
Doxycycline (many brand names and generic)	Prophylaxis in areas with chloroquine- or mefloquine-resistant *P. falciparum*[c]	100 mg PO qd	≥8 years of age: 2 mg/kg, up to adult dose	Begin 1–2 days before travel to malarious areas. Take daily at the same time each day while in the malarious areas and for 4 weeks after leaving such areas. Doxycycline is contraindicated for children <8 years of age and for pregnant women.

Hydroxychloroquine sulfate (Plaquenil)	An alternative to chloroquine for primary prophylaxis, restricted to areas with chloroquine-sensitive *P. falciparum*[c] or *P. vivax* only	310 mg of base (400 mg of salt/ kg) PO once weekly	5 mg of base/kg (6.5 mg of salt/ kg) PO once weekly, up to maximal adult dose of 310 mg of base	Begin 1–2 weeks before travel to malarious areas. Take weekly on the same day of the week while in the malarious areas and for 4 weeks after leaving such areas. Hydroxychloroquine may exacerbate psoriasis.
Mefloquine (Lariam and generic)	Prophylaxis in areas with chloroquine-resistant *P. falciparum*[c]	228 mg of base (250 mg of salt) PO once weekly	228 mg of base/kg (5 mg of salt/kg) PO once weekly ≤9 kg: 4.6 mg of base/kg (5 mg of salt/kg) 10–19 kg: ¼ tablet once weekly 20–30 kg: ½ tablet once weekly 31–45 kg: ¾ tablet once weekly ≥46 kg: 1 tablet once weekly	Begin 1–2 weeks before travel to malarious areas. Take weekly on the same day of the week while in the malarious areas and for 4 weeks after leaving such areas. Mefloquine is contraindicated in persons allergic to this drug or related compounds (e.g., quinine and quinidine) and in persons with active or recent depression, generalized anxiety disorder, psychosis, schizophrenia, other major psychiatric disorders, or seizures. Use with caution in persons with psychiatric disturbances or a history of depression. Mefloquine is not recommended for persons with cardiac conduction abnormalities.
Primaquine	For prevention of malaria in areas with mainly *P. vivax*	30 mg of base (52.6 mg of salt) PO qd	0.5 mg of base/kg (0.8 mg of salt/kg) PO qd, up to adult dose; should be taken with food	Begin 1–2 days before travel to malarious areas. Take daily at the same day while in the malarious areas and for 7 days after leaving such areas. Primaquine is contraindicated in persons with G6PD deficiency. It is also contraindicated during pregnancy and in lactation unless the infant being breast-fed has a documented normal G6PD level.

(continued)

769

TABLE 117-2 DRUGS USED IN THE PROPHYLAXIS OF MALARIA (CONTINUED)

Drug	Usage	Adult Dose	Pediatric Dose	Comments
Primaquine	Used for presumptive therapy to decrease risk of relapses of *P. vivax* and *P. ovale* (terminal prophylaxis)	30 mg of base (52.6 mg of salt) PO qd for 14 days after departure from the malarious area	0.5 mg of base/kg (0.8 mg of salt/kg), up to adult dose, PO qd for 14 days after departure from the malarious area	This therapy is indicated for persons who have had prolonged exposure to *P. vivax* and/or *P. ovale*. It is contraindicated in persons with G6PD deficiency as well as during pregnancy and in lactation unless the infant being breast-fed has a documented normal G6PD level.

[a]An adult tablet contains 250 mg of atovaquone and 100 mg of proguanil hydrochloride.

[b]A pediatric tablet contains 62.5 mg of atovaquone and 25 mg of proguanil hydrochloride.

[c]Very few areas now have chloroquine-sensitive malaria (see Fig. 210-2 in HPIM-18).

Source: CDC: *wwwnc.cdc.gov/travel/yellowbook/2012/chapter-3-infectious-diseases-related-to-travel/malaria.htm#1939*

- Severe babesiosis is associated with parasitemia levels of >4%.
  - Risk factors include an age of >50 years, male gender, asplenia, HIV infection/AIDS, malignancy, and immunosuppression.
  - Complications include respiratory failure, DIC, CHF, and renal failure.
  - The fatality rate is 5% among all hospitalized pts and 20% among immunocompromised pts.

Diagnosis

Giemsa-stained thin smears identify intraerythrocytic *Babesia* parasites, which appear round or pear-shaped.

- Ring forms resembling *P. falciparum* but without pigment are most common.
- Tetrads ("Maltese crosses")—formed by four budding merozoites—are pathognomonic for *B. microti* and other small *Babesia* species.
- PCR and serology can also be used for diagnostic purposes.

TREATMENT Babesiosis

- Mild illness should be treated with atovaquone (750 mg PO q12h) plus azithromycin (500–1000 mg/d PO on day 1 followed by 250 mg/d PO) for 7–10 days.
  - Clindamycin plus quinine is equally effective but not as well tolerated.
  - Treatment should be given only if *Babesia* is detected on blood smear, regardless of serology or PCR results.
- Severe disease should be treated with clindamycin (300–600 mg q6h IV or 600 mg q8h PO) plus quinine (650 mg q6–8h PO) for 7–10 days.
  - Consider exchange transfusion in cases with high-level parasitemia (>10%); hemoglobin levels of ≤10 g/dL; or pulmonary, hepatic, or renal compromise.
  - Immunocompromised pts generally need longer courses of treatment (e.g., 6 weeks), with at least 2 weeks of therapy after parasites are no longer detected on blood smear.
- *B. duncani* and *B. divergens* infections can be treated with IV clindamycin and quinine for 7–10 days.

LEISHMANIASIS

Microbiology

Leishmania species are extracellular, flagellated promastigotes while dwelling in their sandfly vector, but are obligate intracellular, nonflagellated amastigotes while living in vertebrate hosts, including humans.

- Organisms of the *L. donovani* complex usually cause visceral leishmaniasis and are present in Asia, the Middle East, the horn of Africa, the Mediterranean, and Central and South America.
- *L. tropica*, *L. major*, and *L. aethiopica* cause Old World cutaneous leishmaniasis and are present in Asia and in northern and sub-Saharan Africa.
- The *L. mexicana* complex causes New World cutaneous leishmaniasis and is present in Central America and northern South America.

Epidemiology

Roughly 2 million cases of leishmaniasis occur annually worldwide, of which 1–1.5 million are cutaneous and 500,000 are visceral.

Clinical Manifestations

Visceral Leishmaniasis (kala-azar): Pts most commonly present with an abrupt onset of moderate- to high-grade fever associated with rigor and chills.

- Splenomegaly, hepatomegaly, and (except in the Indian subcontinent) lymphadenopathy are common.
- Leukopenia, anemia, thrombocytopenia, a polyclonal increase in serum immunoglobulins, and hepatic transaminitis are common.
- Up to 50% of pts in India, East Africa, and the Sudan may develop hypopigmented skin lesions (post–kala-azar dermal leishmaniasis) concurrent with or after cure of visceral leishmaniasis. In some cases, these pts may require unusually long treatment courses.

Cutaneous Leishmaniasis: After an incubation period of days or weeks, papular lesions progress to nodules that ulcerate over weeks or months. Lesions usually heal spontaneously after 2–15 months.

- The margins of the ulcer are raised and indurated, and the base of the ulcer is usually painless.
- Disease due to *L. tropica* may involve *leishmaniasis recidivans:* development of new scaly, erythematous papules in the area of a healed sore.

Mucosal Leishmaniasis: This disfiguring sequela of New World cutaneous leishmaniasis results from dissemination of parasites from the skin to the naso-oropharyngeal mucosa.

- Disease may occur 1–5 years after the initial cutaneous episode.
- Persistent nasal congestion and bleeding are followed by progressive ulcerative destruction.
- These lesions do not resolve spontaneously.

Diagnosis

- *Visceral leishmaniasis:* Identification of amastigotes in smears of tissue aspirates is the gold standard for diagnosis.
  - The sensitivity of splenic smears is >95%, but splenic aspiration may be very dangerous; smears of bone marrow and lymph node aspirates have sensitivities of 60–85% and 50%, respectively.
  - Several serologic techniques, including a rapid test, are available and offer good sensitivity.
- *Cutaneous and mucosal leishmaniasis:* Diagnosis is made by microscopy, culture, or PCR examination of aspirates and biopsy specimens from skin lesions and lymph nodes.

TREATMENT   Leishmaniasis

- *Visceral leishmaniasis:* The pentavalent antimonial (Sb^V) compounds sodium stibogluconate and meglumine antimoniate (20 mg/kg per day IV or IM for 28–30 days) are the first-line therapeutic agents.

- Amphotericin B (AmB; either deoxycholate or a lipid formulation) is recommended in areas with Sb^V resistance (e.g., northeastern India) or if initial Sb^V therapy fails.
- Paromomycin and the oral agent miltefosine have been approved for treatment of visceral leishmaniasis in India.
- Liposomal AmB is the drug of choice for HIV-infected pts.
- *Cutaneous leishmaniasis*: Although lesions generally self-resolve, treatment may be needed if lesions spread or persist.
  - Topical agents can be effective for a few small lesions. Systemic treatment is needed for multiple lesions; lesions on the face, hands, or joints; and lesions of New World cutaneous leishmaniasis.
  - Administration of Sb^V (20 mg/kg daily for 20 days) constitutes the most effective treatment. Exceptions include disease due to *L. guyanensis* (pentamidine isethionate preferred) or *L. aethiopica* (paromomycin preferred).
- *Mucosal leishmaniasis*: Sb^V (20 mg/kg for 30 days) is recommended.
  - Pts require long-term follow-up, and neither relapse nor failure of therapy is uncommon.
  - AmB and potentially miltefosine can be used in cases of relapse or therapy failure.

TRYPANOSOMIASIS

◼ CHAGAS' DISEASE

Microbiology and Pathology

Trypanosoma cruzi causes Chagas' disease (American trypanosomiasis) and is transmitted among mammalian hosts by hematophagous reduviid bugs. Organisms disseminate through the lymphatics and the bloodstream, often parasitizing muscles particularly heavily.

Epidemiology

T. cruzi is found exclusively in the Americas and causes disease mostly among the poor in rural areas of Mexico and Central and South America. An estimated 8 million people are chronically infected, with 14,000 deaths annually.

Clinical Manifestations

An indurated area of erythema and swelling (the *chagoma*) with local lymphadenopathy generally precedes malaise, fever, anorexia, and edema of the face and lower extremities.

- *Romaña's sign*—unilateral painless edema of the palpebrae and periocular tissues—occurs when the conjunctiva is the portal of entry.
- Acute disease resolves spontaneously within 4–8 weeks, and pts enter an asymptomatic phase of chronic infection.
- Symptomatic chronic disease becomes apparent years or even decades after the initial infection.
  - Cardiac symptoms are common and include rhythm disturbances, segmental or dilated cardiomyopathy, and thromboembolism.

- Pts can develop megaesophagus and suffer from dysphagia, odynophagia, chest pain, and regurgitation.
- Megacolon may develop, leading to abdominal pain, chronic constipation, fecaloma formation, obstruction, and volvulus.

Diagnosis

Microscopic examination of fresh anticoagulated blood, the buffy coat, or blood smears may reveal organisms in cases of acute Chagas' disease. Serology has no diagnostic role in acute disease. Chronic Chagas' disease is diagnosed by detection of specific IgG antibodies. Given the frequency of false-positive results, a positive result should be confirmed by at least two assays.

TREATMENT Chagas' Disease

- Only two drugs—nifurtimox and benznidazole—are available to treat Chagas' disease; neither is entirely effective.
  - Nifurtimox (8–10 mg/kg qd in 4 divided oral doses for 90–120 days) reduces symptom duration, parasitemia level, and mortality rate but offers a parasitologic cure in only ~70% of cases.
  - Benznidazole (5 mg/kg qd in 2 or 3 divided doses for 60 days) is the drug of choice in Latin America and may provide parasitologic cure rates as high as 90%.
  - Both drugs have a number of side effects.
- Treatment of chronic Chagas' disease is controversial; no adequate studies demonstrate efficacy. However, a panel of experts convened by the CDC recommends that pts <50 years old with presumably longstanding *T. cruzi* infection be offered treatment.

◼ SLEEPING SICKNESS

Microbiology and Epidemiology

Sleeping sickness (human African trypanosomiasis, HAT) is caused by parasites of the *T. brucei* complex and is transmitted via tsetse flies.

- *T. b. rhodesiense* causes the East African form and *T. b. gambiense* the West African form; these two forms are epidemiologically and clinically distinct illnesses.
- Humans are the only reservoir for *T. b. gambiense*; infection occurs primarily in rural populations and rarely develops in tourists. *T. b. rhodesiense* has reservoirs in antelope and cattle; tourists can be infected when visiting areas where infected game and vectors are present.
- HAT was nearly eradicated in the mid-1960s but resurged in the 1990s. There were an estimated 50,000–70,000 new cases in 2004.

Clinical Manifestations

A trypanosomal chancre develops ~1 week after the bite of an infected tsetse fly. A systemic febrile illness without involvement of the CNS (stage I disease) then evolves as the parasites disseminate through the bloodstream and lymphatics.

- Bouts of high-grade fever lasting several days are separated by afebrile periods. Malaise, headache, arthralgias, hepatosplenomegaly, and other nonspecific manifestations can develop.
- Lymphadenopathy with discrete, rubbery, nontender nodes is prominent in *T. b. gambiense* disease. Enlargement of nodes of the posterior cervical triangle (*Winterbottom's sign*) is a classic manifestation.
- With CNS invasion (stage II disease), pts develop progressive indifference and daytime somnolence, a state that sometimes alternates with restlessness and insomnia. Extrapyramidal signs may include choreiform movements, tremors, and fasciculations; ataxia is common.
- Disease due to *T. b. rhodesiense* is more acute and, if untreated, can lead to death in weeks to months; in contrast, disease due to *T. b. gambiense* can smolder for months or years.

Diagnosis

Examination of fluid from the chancre, thin or thick blood smears, buffy coats, lymph node aspirates, bone marrow biopsy specimens, or CSF samples can reveal the parasite.

- Parasitemia is more likely in stage I disease than in stage II disease and in pts infected with *T. b. rhodesiense* rather than *T. b. gambiense.*
- CSF should be examined whenever the diagnosis is being considered. Increased opening pressure, increased protein level, and increased mononuclear cell counts are common.

TREATMENT   Sleeping Sickness

Stage I disease
- *T. b. rhodesiense*: suramin (a test dose of 100–200 mg followed by 20 mg/kg IV on days 1, 5, 12, 18, and 26)
  - Hypersensitivity reactions and renal damage are the most important side effects.
  - A urinalysis should be done before each dose. Treatment should be discontinued if there is hematuria or increasing proteinuria or if casts are present in the sediment.
- *T. b. gambiense*: pentamidine (4 mg/kg daily IM or IV for 10 days)
  - Serious adverse reactions include nephrotoxicity, abnormal liver function, neutropenia, hypoglycemia, and sterile abscesses.
  - Suramin is an alternative agent.

Stage II disease
- *T. b. rhodesiense*: melarsoprol (2–3.6 mg/kg daily in 3 divided doses for 3 days; 1 week later, 3.6 mg/kg per day in 3 divided doses for 3 days; 1 week later, the latter course repeated). To reduce melarsoprol-induced encephalopathy, administer prednisolone (1 mg/kg up to 40 mg daily, starting 1–2 days before the first dose of melarsoprol and continuing through the last dose).
- *T. b. gambiense*: Eflornithine (100 mg/kg IV qid for 2 weeks) is the first-line agent. Melarsoprol (2.2 mg/kg qd IV for 10 days) is an alternative.

TOXOPLASMOSIS

Microbiology and Epidemiology

Toxoplasmosis is caused by the intracellular parasite *Toxoplasma gondii*; cats and their prey are the definitive hosts. The primary route of transmission to humans is ingestion of tissue cysts from contaminated soil, food (e.g., undercooked meat), or water.

- Roughly one-third of women who contract *T. gondii* during pregnancy transmit the parasite to the fetus, with a 65% risk of transmission if the maternal infection is acquired during the third trimester.
- In the United States and most European countries, seroconversion rates increase with age and exposure; 10–67% of persons >50 years old are seropositive.

Pathogenesis

Both humoral and cellular immunity are important, but subclinical infection commonly persists for the pt's lifetime. Immunocompromised hosts lack factors required to control infection; the consequences are progressive focal destruction and organ failure.

Clinical Manifestations

Disease in immunocompetent hosts is usually asymptomatic (80–90% of cases) and self-limited and does not require therapy. In contrast, immunocompromised pts, including newborns, can develop severe infections typically involving the CNS.

- In the minority of immunocompetent pts who develop symptoms of acute infection, cervical lymphadenopathy is the most common finding; nodes are nontender and discrete. Generalized lymphadenopathy, fever <40°C, headache, malaise, and fatigue occur in 20–40% of pts. Clinical disease usually resolves within several weeks, although lymphadenopathy may persist for several months.
- Immunocompromised pts develop acute toxoplasmosis through reactivation of latent infection in 95% of cases; the remainder of cases are due to new acquisition of parasites.
  - CNS findings include encephalopathy, meningoencephalitis, and mass lesions. Pts may develop changes in mental status (75%), fever (10–72%), seizures (33%), headaches (56%), and focal neurologic findings (60%). The brainstem, basal ganglia, pituitary gland, and corticomedullary junction are most often involved.
  - Multiple organs (e.g., lungs, GI tract, skin, eyes, heart, liver) can be affected. *Toxoplasma* pneumonia is often confused with *Pneumocystis* pneumonia because of an overlapping pt population and similar clinical presentations (i.e., fever, dyspnea, and nonproductive cough rapidly progressing to respiratory failure).
- Congenital infection, which affects 400–4000 infants each year in the U.S., may initially be asymptomatic but can result in reactivation and clinical disease (e.g., chorioretinitis) decades later.
- *Toxoplasma* causes ~35% of all cases of chorioretinitis in the U.S. and Europe, most of which are thought to be due to congenital infection.

Blurred vision, macular involvement with loss of central vision, scotoma, photophobia, and eye pain are manifestations of infection. On examination, yellow-white cotton-like patches with indistinct margins of hyperemia are seen. Older lesions appear as white plaques with distinct borders and black spots.

Diagnosis

Culture of the parasite is difficult and can be done only at specialized laboratories. However, serology is the primary method of diagnosis.

- Results of IgM, IgG, and antibody avidity levels can be combined to help determine when infection may have occurred. (Of note, IgM can persist for >1 year.) These tests, along with a more extensive panel of serologic tests, can be performed at the *Toxoplasma* reference lab at the Palo Alto Medical Foundation (www.pamf.org/serology/clinicianguide.html).
- In immunocompromised pts, a presumptive clinical diagnosis can be based on clinical presentation, history of exposure (e.g., a positive IgG result), and radiologic evaluation. Radiologic studies demonstrate bilateral contrast-enhancing lesions, typically in the basal ganglia and corticomedullary junction. These lesions can be difficult to distinguish from CNS lymphoma, although the latter more frequently consists of only a single lesion. A brain biopsy may be required for definitive diagnosis.
- Congenital toxoplasmosis is diagnosed by PCR of amniotic fluid (to detect the B1 gene of the parasite) and by the persistence of IgG antibody or a positive IgM titer after the first week of life; IgG antibody determinations should be repeated every 2 months.
- Ocular toxoplasmosis is diagnosed by the detection of typical lesions on ophthalmologic examination and the demonstration of a positive IgG titer in serum or ocular fluids.

TREATMENT   Toxoplasmosis

- Immunocompetent pts with only lymphadenopathy do not require treatment unless they have persistent, severe symptoms.
- Immunocompromised pts should receive pyrimethamine plus sulfadiazine. In resource-poor settings, trimethoprim-sulfamethoxazole (TMP-SMX; one double-strength tablet daily) is an effective alternative.
  - Either dapsone plus pyrimethamine or atovaquone with or without pyrimethamine is an alternative for pts who cannot take TMP-SMX.
- Congenital infection is treated daily for 1 year with oral pyrimethamine (1 mg/kg), sulfadiazine (100 mg/kg), and folinic acid.
- Ocular toxoplasmosis is treated with pyrimethamine and either sulfadiazine or clindamycin for 1 month.

Chemoprophylaxis

The risk of disease is very high among AIDS pts who are seropositive for *T. gondii* and have a CD4+ T lymphocyte count of <100/μL. TMP-SMX (one double-strength tablet daily) should be given to these pts as prophylaxis against both *Pneumocystis* pneumonia and toxoplasmosis. Primary or secondary prophylaxis can be stopped if, after institution of antiretroviral treatment, the CD4+ T lymphocyte count is >200/μL for 3 months.

Personal Protection Measures

Toxoplasma infection can be prevented by the avoidance of undercooked meats and oocyst-contaminated materials (e.g., a cat's litter box).

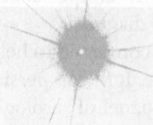

For a more detailed discussion, see Reed SL, Davis CE: Laboratory Diagnosis of Parasitic Infections, Chap. e25; Moore TA: Pharmacology of Agents Used to Treat Parasitic Infections, Chap. e26; and White NJ, Breman JG: Atlas of Blood Smears of Malaria and Babesiosis, Chap. e27; Moore TA: Agents Used to Treat Parasitic Infections, Chap. 208, p. 1675; White NJ, Breman JG: Malaria, Chap. 210, p. 1688; Vannier E, Gelfand JA: Babesiosis, Chap. 211, p. 1706; Sundar S: Leishmaniasis, Chap. 212, p. 1709; Kirchhoff LV, Rassi A Jr: Trypanosomiasis, Chap. 213, p. 1716; and Kim K, Kasper LH: *Toxoplasma* Infections, Chap. 214, p. 1722, in HPIM-18.

CHAPTER **118**
Helminthic Infections and Ectoparasite Infestations

HELMINTHS

■ NEMATODES

The nematodes, or roundworms, that are of medical significance can be broadly classified as either tissue or intestinal parasites.

Tissue Nematode Infections

With the exception of trichinellosis, these infections are due to invasive larval stages that do not reach maturity in humans.

Trichinellosis

Microbiology and Epidemiology Eight species of *Trichinella* cause human infection; two—*T. spiralis* and *T. pseudospiralis*—are found worldwide.

- Infection results when humans ingest meat (usually pork) that contains encysted *Trichinella* larvae.
  - The larvae invade the small-bowel mucosa.
  - After 1 week, female worms release new larvae that migrate to striated muscle via the circulation and encyst.
- The host immune response has little effect on muscle-dwelling larvae.
- About 12 cases of trichinellosis are reported annually in the United States.

Clinical Manifestations Most light infections (<10 larvae per gram of muscle) are asymptomatic. A burden of >50 larvae per gram can cause fatal disease.

- In the first week of infection, large numbers of parasites invading the gut usually cause diarrhea, abdominal pain, constipation, nausea, and/or vomiting.
- In the second week of infection, pts develop symptoms related to larval migration and muscle invasion: hypersensitivity reactions with fever and hypereosinophilia; periorbital and facial edema; and hemorrhages in conjunctivae, retina, and nail beds. Deaths are usually due to myocarditis with arrhythmias or heart failure.
- 2–3 weeks after infection, larval encystment in muscle causes myositis, myalgias, muscle edema, and weakness (especially in extraocular muscles; the biceps; and muscles of the jaw, neck, lower back, and diaphragm).
- Symptoms peak at 3 weeks; convalescence is prolonged.

Diagnosis Eosinophilia develops in >90% of pts, peaking at a level of >50% at 2–4 weeks after infection.

- An increase in parasite-specific antibody titers after the third week of infection confirms the diagnosis.
- Detection of larvae by microscopic examination of ≥1 g of fresh muscle tissue (i.e., not routine histopathologic sections) also confirms the diagnosis. Yields are highest near tendon insertions.

> **TREATMENT** Trichinellosis
>
> - Mebendazole (200–400 mg tid for 3 days; then 400 mg tid for 8–14 days) or albendazole (400 mg bid for 8–14 days) is active against enteric-stage parasites; the efficacy of these drugs against encysted larvae is inconclusive.
> - Glucocorticoids (e.g., prednisone at 1 mg/kg daily for 5 days) may reduce severe myositis and myocarditis.

Prevention Cooking pork until it is no longer pink or freezing it at –15°C for 3 weeks kills larvae and prevents infection by most *Trichinella* species.

Visceral and Ocular Larva Migrans

Microbiology and Epidemiology Humans are an incidental host for nematodes that cause visceral larva migrans. Most cases are caused by the canine ascarid *Toxocara canis*. Infection results when humans—most often preschool children—ingest soil contaminated by puppy feces that contain infective *T. canis* eggs. Larvae penetrate the intestinal mucosa and disseminate hematogenously to a wide variety of organs (e.g., liver, lungs, CNS), provoking intense eosinophilic granulomatous responses.

Clinical Manifestations Symptomatic infections result in fever, malaise, anorexia, weight loss, cough, wheezing, rashes, hepatosplenomegaly, and profound eosinophilia (up to 90%). Ocular disease usually develops in older children or young adults and includes an eosinophilic mass that mimics retinoblastoma, endophthalmitis, uveitis, and/or chorioretinitis.

Diagnosis The clinical diagnosis can be confirmed by an ELISA for toxocaral antibodies. Stool examination for eggs is ineffective because larvae do not develop into adult worms in humans.

TREATMENT > Visceral and Ocular Larva Migrans

- The vast majority of *Toxocara* infections are self-limited and resolve without specific therapy.
- For pts with severe disease, glucocorticoids can reduce inflammatory complications.
- Antihelminthic drugs, including mebendazole and albendazole, have not been shown to alter the course of larva migrans.
- Ocular disease can be treated with albendazole (800 mg bid) and glucocorticoids for 5–20 days.

Cutaneous Larva Migrans This disease is caused by larvae of animal hookworms, usually the dog and cat hookworm *Ancylostoma braziliense*. Larvae in contaminated soil penetrate human skin; intensely pruritic, erythematous lesions form along the tracks of larval migration and advance several centimeters each day. Ivermectin (a single dose of 200 μg/kg) or albendazole (200 mg bid for 3 days) can relieve the symptoms of this self-limited infestation.

Intestinal Nematode Infections

Intestinal nematodes infect >1 billion persons worldwide, most commonly in regions with poor sanitation and particularly in developing countries in the tropics or subtropics. Because most helminthic parasites do not self-replicate, clinical disease (as opposed to asymptomatic infection) generally develops only with prolonged residence in an endemic area and is typically related to infection intensity.

Ascariasis

Microbiology Ascariasis is caused by *Ascaris lumbricoides*, the largest intestinal nematode, which reaches lengths up to 40 cm.
- Humans—primarily younger children—are infected by ingestion of fecally contaminated soil that contains ascarid eggs.
- Larvae hatch in the intestine, invade the mucosa, migrate to the lungs, break into the alveoli, ascend the bronchial tree, are swallowed, mature in the small intestine, and produce up to 240,000 eggs per day that pass in the feces.

Clinical Manifestations Most infections have a low worm burden and are asymptomatic. During lung migration of the parasite (~9–12 days after egg ingestion), pts may develop a cough and substernal discomfort, occasionally with dyspnea or blood-tinged sputum, fever, and eosinophilia.

- Eosinophilic pneumonitis (Löffler's syndrome) may be evident.
- Heavy infections with numerous entangled worms can occasionally cause pain, small-bowel obstruction, perforation, volvulus, biliary obstruction and colic, or pancreatitis.

Laboratory Findings *Ascaris* eggs (65 by 45 μm) can be found in fecal samples. Adult worms can pass in the stool or through the mouth.

> **TREATMENT** Ascariasis
>
> A single dose of albendazole (400 mg), mebendazole (500 mg), or ivermectin (150–200 μg/kg) is effective. Pyrantel pamoate (a single dose of 11 mg/kg; maximal dose, 1 g) is safe in pregnancy.

Hookworm

Microbiology Two hookworm species, *Ancylostoma duodenale* and *Necator americanus*, cause human infections. Infectious larvae present in soil penetrate the skin, reach the lungs via the bloodstream, invade the alveoli, ascend the airways, are swallowed, reach the small intestine, mature into adult worms, attach to the mucosa, and suck blood (0.2 mL/d per *Ancylostoma* adult) and interstitial fluid.

Clinical Manifestations Most infections are asymptomatic. Chronic infection causes iron deficiency and—in marginally nourished persons—progressive anemia and hypoproteinemia, weakness, and shortness of breath. Larvae may cause pruritic rash ("ground itch") at the site of skin penetration as well as serpiginous tracks of subcutaneous migration (similar to those of cutaneous larva migrans).

Laboratory Findings Hookworm eggs (40 by 60 μm) can be found in the feces. Stool concentration may be needed for the diagnosis of light infections.

> **TREATMENT** Hookworm
>
> - Albendazole (400 mg once), mebendazole (500 mg once), or pyrantel pamoate (11 mg/kg daily for 3 days) is effective. Nutritional support, iron replacement, and deworming are undertaken as needed.

Strongyloidiasis

Microbiology and Epidemiology Unlike other helminths, *Strongyloides stercoralis* can replicate in the human host, permitting ongoing cycles of autoinfection from endogenously produced larvae.

- Infection results when filariform larvae in fecally contaminated soil penetrate the skin or mucous membranes.
  - Larvae travel through the bloodstream to the lungs, break through into alveolar spaces, ascend the bronchial tree, are swallowed, reach the small intestine, mature into adult worms, and penetrate the mucosa of the proximal small bowel; eggs hatch in the intestinal mucosa.

   – Rhabditiform larvae can pass with the feces into the soil or can develop into filariform larvae that penetrate the colonic wall or **peri**-anal skin and enter the circulation to establish ongoing autoinfection.
- Autoinfection is constrained by unknown factors of the host immune system, disruption of which (e.g., by glucocorticoid therapy) can lead to hyperinfection.

Clinical Features Uncomplicated disease is associated with mild cutaneous and/or abdominal manifestations such as recurrent urticaria, *larva currens* (a pathognomonic serpiginous, pruritic, erythematous eruption along the course of larval migration that may advance up to 10 cm/h), abdominal pain, nausea, diarrhea, bleeding, and weight loss.
- Disseminated disease involves tissues outside the GI tract and lungs, including the CNS, peritoneum, liver, and kidney.
  - Gram-negative sepsis, pneumonia, or meningitis can complicate or dominate the clinical course.
  - Disease can be fatal in pts given glucocorticoids; disseminated infection is uncommon among pts with HIV-1 infection.
- Fluctuating eosinophilia is common in uncomplicated disease but is uncommon in disseminated disease.

Diagnosis A single stool examination detects rhabditiform larvae (~250 µm long) in about one-third of uncomplicated infections. Duodenojejunal contents can be sampled if stool examinations are repeatedly negative.
- Antibodies can be detected by ELISA.
- In disseminated infection, filariform larvae can be found in stool or at sites of larval migration (e.g., sputum, bronchoalveolar lavage fluid, surgical drainage fluid).

TREATMENT   Strongyloidiasis

- Ivermectin (200 µg/kg daily for 2 days) is more effective than albendazole (400 mg daily for 3 days). Asymptomatic pts should be treated, given the potential for later fatal hyperinfection.
- Disseminated disease should be treated with ivermectin for ≥5–7 days (or until the parasites are eradicated).

Enterobiasis

Microbiology and Epidemiology Enterobiasis (pinworm) is caused by *Enterobius vermicularis* and affects ~40 million people in the U.S. (primarily children).
- Gravid female worms migrate nocturnally from the cecum to the perianal region, each releasing up to 10,000 immature eggs that become infective within hours.
- Autoinfection and person-to-person transmission result from perianal scratching and transport of infective eggs to the mouth.

Clinical Manifestations Perianal pruritus is the cardinal symptom and is often worst at night. Eosinophilia is uncommon.

Diagnosis Eggs (55 by 25 μm and flattened on one side) are detected by microscopic examination of cellulose acetate tape applied to the perianal region in the morning.

TREATMENT Enterobiasis

- One dose of mebendazole (100 mg), albendazole (400 mg), or pyrantel pamoate (11 mg/kg; maximum, 1 g) is given, with the same treatment repeated after 2 weeks. Household members should also be treated to avoid reservoirs of potential reinfection.

Filarial and Related Infections

Filarial worms, which infect more than 170 million people worldwide, are nematodes that dwell in the SC tissue and lymphatics. Usually, infection is established only with repeated and prolonged exposures to infective larvae; however, filarial disease is characteristically more intense and acute in newly exposed individuals than in natives of endemic areas.

- Filarial parasites have a complex life cycle, including infective larval stages carried by insects and adult worms that reside in humans.
  - The offspring of adults are microfilariae (200–250 μm long, 5–7 μm wide) that either circulate in the blood or migrate through the skin.
  - Microfilariae are ingested by the arthropod vector and develop over 1–2 weeks into new infective larvae.
- A *Rickettsia*-like endosymbiont, *Wolbachia*, is found in all stages of *Brugia*, *Wuchereria*, *Mansonella*, and *Onchocerca* and has become a target for antifilarial chemotherapy.

Lymphatic Filariasis

Microbiology Lymphatic filariasis is caused by *Wuchereria bancrofti* (most commonly), *Brugia malayi*, or *B. timori*, which can reside in and cause inflammatory damage to lymphatic channels or lymph nodes.

Clinical Manifestations Subclinical microfilaremia, hydrocele, acute adenolymphangitis (ADL), and chronic lymphatic disease are the main clinical presentations.

- ADL is associated with high fever, lymphatic inflammation, and transient local edema. Both the upper and lower extremities can be involved in both bancroftian and brugian filariasis, but *W. bancrofti* almost exclusively affects genital lymphatics.
- ADL may progress to more chronic lymphatic obstruction and elephantiasis with brawny edema, thickening of the SC tissues, and hyperkeratosis. Superinfection is a problem.

Diagnosis Detection of the parasite is difficult, but microfilariae can be found in peripheral blood, hydrocele fluid, and occasionally other body fluids.

- Timing of blood collection is critical and should be based on the periodicity of the microfilariae in the endemic region involved (primarily nocturnal in many regions).

- Two assays are available to detect *W. bancrofti* circulating antigens, and a PCR has been developed to detect DNA of both *W. bancrofti* and *B. malayi* in the blood.
- High-frequency ultrasound (with Doppler techniques) of the scrotum or the female breast can identify motile adult worms.
- The presence of antifilarial antibody supports the diagnosis, but cross-reactivity with other helminthic infections makes interpretation of this finding difficult.

TREATMENT Lymphatic Filariasis

- Pts with active lymphatic filariasis (defined by microfilaremia, antigen positivity, or adult worms on ultrasound) should be treated with diethylcarbamazine (DEC; 6 mg/kg daily for 12 days). Albendazole (400 mg bid for 21 days), albendazole and DEC both given daily for 7 days, and doxycycline (100 mg bid for 4–6 weeks) are alternative regimens with macrofilaricidal efficacy.
- A single dose of albendazole (400 mg) combined with DEC (6 mg/kg) or ivermectin (200 μg/kg) has sustained microfilaricidal activity and is used in lymphatic filariasis eradication campaigns.
- For pts with chronic lymphatic filariasis, treatment regimens should focus on hygiene, prevention of secondary bacterial infections, and physiotherapy. Drug treatment should be reserved for individuals with evidence of active infection.

Onchocerciasis

Microbiology and Epidemiology Onchocerciasis ("river blindness") is caused by *Onchocerca volvulus*, which infects 37 million people worldwide and is transmitted by the bite of an infected blackfly near free-flowing rivers and streams.

- Larvae deposited by the blackfly develop into adult worms (females and males are ~40–60 cm and ~3–6 cm in length, respectively) that are found in SC nodules (*onchocercomata*). About 7 months to 3 years after infection, the gravid female releases microfilariae that migrate out of the nodules and concentrate in the dermis.
- In contrast to lymphatic filariasis, onchocerciasis is characterized by microfilarial induction of inflammation.

Clinical Manifestations Onchocerciasis most commonly presents as dermatologic manifestations (an intensely pruritic papular rash or firm nontender onchocercomata), but visual impairment is the most serious complication in pts with moderate or heavy infections.

- Conjunctivitis with photophobia is an early ocular finding.
- Sclerosing keratitis (the leading cause of onchocercal blindness in Africa, affecting 1–5% of pts), anterior uveitis, iridocyclitis, and secondary glaucoma due to pupillary deformities are more serious ocular complications.

Diagnosis A definitive diagnosis is based on the finding of an adult worm in an excised nodule or of microfilariae in a skin snip.

- Specific antibody assays and PCR to detect onchocercal DNA are available in reference laboratories.
- Eosinophilia and elevated serum IgE levels are common but nonspecific.

TREATMENT Onchocerciasis

- Ivermectin (a single dose of 150 μg/kg), given yearly or semiannually, is microfilaricidal and is the mainstay of treatment.
  - In African regions where *O. volvulus* is co-endemic with *Loa loa*, ivermectin is contraindicated because of the risk of severe post-treatment encephalopathy.
  - Doxycycline therapy for 6 weeks is macrofilaristatic, rendering adult female worms sterile for long periods, and also targets the *Wolbachia* endosymbiont.
- Nodules on the head should be excised to avoid ocular infection.

■ TREMATODES

- The trematodes, or flatworms, may be classified according to the tissues invaded by the adult flukes: blood, biliary tree, intestines, and lungs.
- The life cycle involves a definitive mammalian host (e.g., humans), in which adult worms produce eggs through sexual reproduction, and an intermediate host (e.g., snails), in which miracidial forms undergo asexual reproduction to form cercariae. Worms do not multiply within the definitive host.
- Human infection results from either direct penetration of intact skin or ingestion.
- Infections with trematodes that migrate through or reside in host tissues are associated with a moderate to high degree of peripheral-blood eosinophilia.

Schistosomiasis

Microbiology and Epidemiology Five species cause human schistosomiasis: the intestinal species *Schistosoma mansoni*, *S. japonicum*, *S. mekongi*, and *S. intercalatum* and the urinary species *S. haematobium*.

- After infective cercariae penetrate intact skin, they mature into schistosomula and migrate through venous or lymphatic vessels to the lungs and ultimately the liver parenchyma. Sexually mature worms migrate to the veins of the bladder and ureters (*S. haematobium*) or the mesentery (*S. mansoni*, *S. japonicum*, *S. mekongi*, *S. intercalatum*) and deposit eggs.
  - Some mature ova are extruded into the intestinal or urinary lumina, from which they may be voided and ultimately may reach water and perpetuate the life cycle.
  - The persistence of ova in tissues leads to a granulomatous host response and fibrosis.
- These blood flukes infect 200–300 million persons in South America, the Caribbean, Africa, the Middle East, and Southeast Asia.

Clinical Manifestations Schistosomiasis occurs in three stages that vary by species, intensity of infection, and host factors.

- *Cercarial invasion*, most often with *S. mansoni* and *S. japonicum* infections, causes a pruritic maculopapular rash ("swimmers' itch") 2–3 days later.
- *Acute schistosomiasis* (Katayama fever) presents 4–8 weeks after skin invasion as a serum sickness–like illness characterized by fever, generalized lymphadenopathy, hepatosplenomegaly, and significant eosinophilia.
- *Chronic schistosomiasis* causes manifestations that depend primarily on the schistosome species.
  - Intestinal species cause colicky abdominal pain, bloody diarrhea, anemia, hepatosplenomegaly, portal hypertension, and esophageal varices with bleeding.
  - Urinary species cause dysuria, frequency, hematuria, obstruction with hydroureter and hydronephrosis, fibrosis of bladder granulomas, and late development of squamous cell carcinoma of the bladder.
  - Pulmonary disease (e.g., endarteritis obliterans, pulmonary hypertension, cor pulmonale) and CNS disease (e.g., Jacksonian epilepsy, transverse myelitis) can occur and are due to granulomas and fibrosis.

Diagnosis Diagnosis is based on geographic history, clinical presentation, and presence of schistosome ova in excreta.
- Serologic assays for schistosomal antibodies (available through the CDC in the U.S.) may yield positive results before eggs are seen in excreta.
- Infection may also be diagnosed by examination of tissue samples, typically from rectal biopsies.

TREATMENT Schistosomiasis

- Because antischistosomal therapy has no significant impact on maturing worms, supportive measures and the consideration of glucocorticoid treatment constitute initial management for acute schistosomiasis.
  - After the acute critical phase has resolved, a single day of treatment with praziquantel (20 mg/kg bid for *S. mansoni*, *S. intercalatum*, and *S. haematobium* infections; 20 mg/kg tid for *S. japonicum* and *S. mekongi* infections) results in parasitologic cure in ~85% of cases and reduces egg counts by >90%.
  - Late established manifestations, such as fibrosis, do not improve with treatment.

Prevention Travelers to endemic regions should avoid contact with all freshwater bodies.

Liver (Biliary) Flukes
- Clonorchiasis (due to *Clonorchis sinensis*) and opisthorchiasis (due to *Opisthorchis viverrini* and *O. felineus*) occur in Southeast Asia and Eastern Europe.
  - Infection is acquired by ingestion of contaminated raw freshwater fish; larvae travel through the ampulla of Vater and mature in biliary canaliculi.
  - Most infected individuals are asymptomatic; chronic or repeated infection causes cholangitis, cholangiohepatitis, and biliary obstruction and is associated with cholangiocarcinoma.

- Therapy for acute infection consists of praziquantel administration (25 mg/kg tid for 1 day).
- Fascioliasis (due to *Fasciola hepatica* and *F. gigantica*) is endemic in sheep-raising countries and has a worldwide prevalence of 17 million cases.
  - Infection is acquired by ingestion of contaminated aquatic plants (e.g., watercress).
  - Acute disease develops 1–2 weeks after infection and causes fever, right-upper-quadrant pain, hepatomegaly, and eosinophilia. Chronic infection is infrequently associated with bile duct obstruction and biliary cirrhosis.
  - For treatment, triclabendazole is given as a single dose of 10 mg/kg.
- Stool ova and parasite (O & P) examination diagnoses infection with liver flukes.

Lung Flukes Infection with *Paragonimus* spp. is acquired by ingestion of contaminated crayfish and freshwater crabs.

- Acute infection causes lung hemorrhage, necrosis with cyst formation, and parenchymal eosinophilic infiltrates. A productive cough with brownish or bloody sputum, in association with peripheral-blood eosinophilia, is the usual presentation in pts with heavy infection.
  - In chronic cases, bronchitis or bronchiectasis may predominate.
  - CNS disease can also occur and can result in seizures.
- The diagnosis is made by O & P examination of sputum or stool; serology can be helpful.
- Praziquantel (25 mg/kg tid for 2 days) is the recommended therapy.

■ CESTODES

The cestodes, or tapeworms, are segmented worms that can be classified into two groups according to whether humans are the definitive or the intermediate hosts. The tapeworm attaches to intestinal mucosa via sucking cups or hooks located on the scolex. Proglottids (segments) form behind the scolex and constitute the bulk of the tapeworm.

Taeniasis Saginata and Taeniasis Asiatica

Microbiology Humans are the definitive host for *Taenia saginata*, the beef tapeworm, and *T. asiatica*, the swine tapeworm, which inhabit the upper jejunum. Eggs are excreted in feces and ingested by cattle or other herbivores (*T. saginata*) or pigs (*T. asiatica*); larvae encyst (cysticerci) in the striated muscles of these animals. When humans ingest raw or undercooked meat, the cysticerci mature into adult worms in ~2 months.

Clinical Manifestations Pts become aware of the infection by noting passage of motile proglottids in their feces. They may experience perianal discomfort, mild abdominal pain, nausea, change in appetite, weakness, and weight loss.

Diagnosis The diagnosis is made by detection of eggs or proglottids in the stool; eggs may be detected in the perianal area by the cellophane-tape test (as in pinworm infection). Eosinophilia and elevated IgE levels may occur.

TREATMENT   Taeniasis Saginata and Taeniasis Asiatica

TREATMENT   Taeniasis Saginata and Taeniasis Asiatica

Praziquantel is given in a single dose of 10 mg/kg.

Taeniasis Solium and Cysticercosis

Microbiology and Pathogenesis   Humans are the definitive host and pigs the usual intermediate host for *T. solium*, the pork tapeworm.
- The disease has two forms, which depend on the form of parasite ingested.
  - By ingesting undercooked pork containing cysticerci, humans develop intestinal tapeworms and a disease similar to taeniasis saginata.
  - If humans ingest *T. solium* eggs (e.g., as a result of close contact with a tapeworm carrier or via autoinfection), they develop cysticercosis due to larvae penetrating the intestinal wall and migrating to many tissues.

Clinical Manifestations   Intestinal infections are generally asymptomatic except for fecal passage of proglottids. The presentation of cysticercosis depends on the number and location of cysticerci as well as the extent of associated inflammatory responses or scarring.
- Cysticerci can be found anywhere in the body but most often are detected in the brain, skeletal muscle, SC tissue, or eye.
- Neurologic manifestations are most common and include seizures (due to inflammation surrounding cysticerci in the brain), hydrocephalus (from obstruction of CSF flow by cysticerci and accompanying inflammation or by arachnoiditis), and signs of increased intracranial pressure (e.g., headache, nausea, vomiting, changes in vision).

Diagnosis   Intestinal infection is diagnosed by detection of eggs or proglottids in stool. A consensus conference has delineated criteria for the diagnosis of cysticercosis (Table 118-1). Findings on neuroimaging include cystic lesions with or without enhancement, one or more nodular calcifications, or focal enhancing lesions.

TREATMENT   Taeniasis Solium and Cysticercosis

- Intestinal infections respond to a single dose of praziquantel (10 mg/kg), but this treatment may evoke an inflammatory response in the CNS if there is cryptic cysticercosis.
- Neurocysticercosis can be treated with albendazole (15 mg/kg per day for 8–28 days) or praziquantel (50–100 mg/kg daily in 3 divided doses for 15–30 days).
  - Given the potential for an inflammatory response to treatment, pts should be carefully monitored and high-dose glucocorticoids should be used during treatment.
  - Since glucocorticoids induce praziquantel metabolism, cimetidine should be given with praziquantel to inhibit this effect.
  - Supportive measures include antiepileptic administration and treatment of hydrocephalus as indicated.

TABLE 118-1 DIAGNOSTIC CRITERIA FOR HUMAN CYSTICERCOSIS[a]

1. Absolute criteria
   a. Demonstration of cysticerci by histologic or microscopic examination of biopsy material
   b. Visualization of the parasite in the eye by funduscopy
   c. Neuroradiologic demonstration of cystic lesions containing a characteristic scolex

2. Major criteria
   a. Neuroradiologic lesions suggestive of neurocysticercosis
   b. Demonstration of antibodies to cysticerci in serum by enzyme-linked immunoelectrotransfer blot
   c. Resolution of intracranial cystic lesions spontaneously or after therapy with albendazole or praziquantel alone

3. Minor criteria
   a. Lesions compatible with neurocysticercosis detected by neuroimaging studies
   b. Clinical manifestations suggestive of neurocysticercosis
   c. Demonstration of antibodies to cysticerci or cysticercal antigen in CSF by ELISA
   d. Evidence of cysticercosis outside the CNS (e.g., cigar-shaped soft tissue calcifications)

4. Epidemiologic criteria
   a. Residence in a cysticercosis-endemic area
   b. Frequent travel to a cysticercosis-endemic area
   c. Household contact with an individual infected with *Taenia solium*

[a]Diagnosis is confirmed by either one absolute criterion or a combination of two major criteria, one minor criterion, and one epidemiologic criterion. A probable diagnosis is supported by the fulfillment of (1) one major criterion plus two minor criteria; (2) one major criterion plus one minor criterion and one epidemiologic criterion; or (3) three minor criteria plus one epidemiologic criterion.
Source: Modified from Del Brutto OH et al: Proposed diagnostic criteria for neurocysticercosis. Neurology 57:177, 2001.

Echinococcosis

Microbiology and Epidemiology Humans are an intermediate host for *Echinococcus* larvae and acquire echinococcal disease by ingesting eggs spread by canine feces (for *E. granulosus*).

- After ingestion, embryos escape from the eggs, penetrate the intestinal mucosa, enter the portal circulation, and are carried to many organs but particularly the liver and lungs. Larvae develop into fluid-filled unilocular hydatid cysts within which daughter cysts develop, as do germinating cystic structures (*brood capsules*). Cysts expand over years.
- Disease is prevalent on all continents, particularly in areas where livestock is raised in association with dogs.

- *E. multilocularis,* found in arctic or subarctic regions, is similar, but wild canines (e.g., foxes) are the definitive hosts and rodents are the intermediate hosts. The parasite is multilocular, and vesicles progressively invade host tissue.

Clinical Manifestations Expanding cysts exert the effects of space-occupying lesions, causing symptoms in the affected organ (usually liver and lung); the liver is involved in two-thirds of *E. granulosus* infections and ~100% of *E. multilocularis* infections.

- Pts with hepatic disease most commonly present with abdominal pain or a palpable mass in the right upper quadrant. Compression of a bile duct may mimic biliary disease, and rupture or leakage from a hydatid cyst may cause fever, pruritus, urticaria, eosinophilia, or anaphylaxis.
- Pulmonary cysts may rupture into the bronchial tree or the peritoneal cavity and cause cough, salty phlegm, chest pain, or hemoptysis.
- Rupture of cysts may result in multifocal dissemination.
- *E. multilocularis* disease may present as a hepatic tumor, with destruction of the liver and extension into adjoining (e.g., lungs, kidneys) or distant (e.g., brain, spleen) organs.

Diagnosis Radiographic imaging is important in detecting and evaluating echinococcal cysts.

- Daughter cysts within a larger cyst are pathognomonic of *E. granulosus.* Eggshell or mural calcification on CT is also indicative of *E. granulosus* infections.
- Serologic testing yields positive results in ~90% of pts with hepatic disease, but results can be negative in up to half of pts with lung cysts.
- Aspiration of cysts usually is not attempted because leakage of cyst fluid can cause dissemination or anaphylactic reactions.

TREATMENT Echinococcosis

- Therapy is based on considerations of the size, location, and manifestations of cysts and the overall health of the pt. Ultrasound staging is recommended for *E. granulosus* infection.
- For some uncomplicated lesions, PAIR [*p*ercutaneous *a*spiration, *i*nfusion of scolicidal agents (95% ethanol or hypertonic saline), and *r*easpiration] is recommended.
  - Albendazole (7.5 mg/kg bid for 4 days before the procedure and for at least 4 weeks afterward) is given for prophylaxis of secondary peritoneal echinococcosis due to inadvertent spillage of fluid during this treatment.
  - PAIR is contraindicated for superficial cysts, for cysts with multiple thick internal septal divisions, and for cysts communicating with the biliary tree.
- Surgical resection is the treatment of choice for complicated *E. granulosus* cysts.
  - Albendazole should also be given prophylactically, as just described. Praziquantel (50 mg/kg daily for 2 weeks) may hasten the death of protoscolices.

- Medical therapy alone with albendazole for 12 weeks to 6 months results in cure in ~30% of cases and in clinical improvement in another 50%.
- *E. multilocularis* infection is treated surgically, and albendazole is given for at least 2 years after presumptively curative surgery. If surgery is not curative, albendazole should be continued indefinitely.

Diphyllobothriasis *Diphyllobothrium latum*, the longest tapeworm (up to 25 m), attaches to the ileal and occasionally the jejunal mucosa. Humans are infected by consumption of infected raw or smoked fish. Symptoms are rare and usually mild, but infection, particularly in Scandinavia, can cause vitamin B_{12} deficiency because the tapeworm absorbs large amounts of vitamin B_{12} and interferes with ileal B_{12} absorption. Up to 2% of infected pts, especially the elderly, have megaloblastic anemia resembling pernicious anemia and can suffer neurologic sequelae due to B_{12} deficiency. The diagnosis is made by detection of eggs in the stool. Praziquantel (5–10 mg/kg once) is highly effective.

ECTOPARASITES

Ectoparasites are arthropods or helminths that infest the skin of other animals, from which they derive sustenance and shelter. These organisms can inflict direct injury, elicit hypersensitivity, or inoculate toxins or pathogens.

Scabies

Etiology and Epidemiology Scabies is caused by the human itch mite *Sarcoptes scabiei* and infests ~300 million people worldwide.

- Gravid female mites burrow beneath the stratum corneum, deposit eggs that mature in 2 weeks, and emerge as adults to reinvade the same or another host.
- Scabies transmission is facilitated by intimate contact with an infested person and by crowding, uncleanliness, or contact with multiple sexual partners.

Clinical Manifestations Itching, which is due to a sensitization reaction against excreta of the mite, is worst at night and after a hot shower. Burrows appear as dark wavy lines (≤15 mm in length), with most lesions located between the fingers or on the volar wrists, elbows, and penis. Norwegian or crusted scabies—hyperinfestation with thousands of mites—is associated with glucocorticoid use and immunodeficiency diseases.

Diagnosis Scrapings from unroofed burrows reveal the mite, its eggs, or fecal pellets.

TREATMENT	Scabies

- Permethrin cream (5%) should be applied thinly behind the ears and from the neck down after bathing and removed 8 h later with soap and water. A dose of ivermectin (200 μg/kg) is also effective but has not yet been approved by the U.S. Food and Drug Administration for scabies treatment.

- For crusted scabies, first a keratolytic agent (e.g., 6% salicylic acid) and then scabicides are applied to the scalp, face, and ears in addition to the rest of the body. Two doses of ivermectin, separated by an interval of 1–2 weeks, may be required for pts with crusted scabies.
- Itching and hypersensitivity may persist for weeks or months in scabies and should be managed with symptom-based treatment. Bedding and clothing should be washed in hot water and dried in a heated dryer, and close contacts (regardless of symptoms) should be treated to prevent reinfestations.

Pediculiasis

Etiology and Epidemiology Nymphs and adults of human lice—*Pediculus capitis* (the head louse), *P. humanus* (the body louse), and *Pthirus pubis* (the pubic louse)—feed at least once a day and ingest human blood exclusively. The saliva of these lice produces an irritating rash in sensitized persons. Eggs are cemented firmly to hair or clothing, and empty eggs (nits) remain affixed for months after hatching. Lice are generally transmitted from person to person. Head lice are transmitted among schoolchildren and body lice among disaster victims and indigent people; pubic lice are usually transmitted sexually. The body louse is a vector for the transmission of diseases such as louse-borne typhus, relapsing fever, and trench fever.

Diagnosis The diagnosis can be suspected if nits are detected, but confirmatory measures should include the demonstration of a live louse.

TREATMENT Pediculiasis

- If live lice are found, treatment with 1% permethrin (two 10-min applications 10 days apart) is usually adequate. If this course fails, treatment for ≤12 h with 0.5% malathion may be indicated. Eyelid infestations should be treated with petrolatum applied for 3–4 days.
- Body lice usually are eliminated by bathing and by changing to laundered clothes.
  - Pediculicides applied from head to foot may be needed in hirsute pts to remove body lice.
  - Clothes and bedding should be deloused by placement in a hot dryer for 30 minutes or by heat pressing.

Myiasis In this infestation, maggots invade living or necrotic tissue or body cavities and produce clinical syndromes that vary with the species of fly. Certain flies are attracted to blood and pus, and newly hatched larvae enter wounds or diseased skin. Treatment consists of maggot removal and tissue debridement.

Leech Infestations Medicinal leeches can reduce venous congestion in surgical flaps or replanted body parts. Pts occasionally develop sepsis from *Aeromonas hydrophila*, which colonizes the gullets of commercially available leeches.

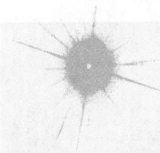

For a more detailed discussion, see Reed SL, Davis CE: Laboratory Diagnosis of Parasitic Infections, Chap. e25; Moore TA: Pharmacology of Agents Used to Treat Parasitic Infections, Chap. e26; and Moore TA: Agents Used to Treat Parasitic Infections, Chap. 208, p. 1675; Weller PF: Trichinellosis and Other Tissue Nematode Infections, Chap. 216, p. 1735; Weller PF, Nutman TB: Intestinal Nematode Infections, Chap. 217, p. 1739; Nutman TB, Weller PF: Filarial and Related Infections, Chap. 218, p. 1745; Mahmoud AAF: Schistosomiasis and Other Trematode Infections, Chap. 219, p. 1752; White AC Jr, Weller PF: Cestode Infections, Chap. 220, p. 1759; and Pollack RJ: Ectoparasite Infestations and Arthropod Bites and Stings, Chap. 397, p. 3576, in HPIM-18.

CHAPTER **119**
Physical Examination of the Heart

General examination of a pt with suspected heart disease should include vital signs (respiratory rate, pulse, blood pressure) and observation of skin color (e.g., cyanosis, pallor), clubbing, edema, evidence of decreased perfusion (cool and diaphoretic skin), and hypertensive changes in optic fundi. Examine abdomen for evidence of hepatomegaly, ascites, or abdominal aortic aneurysm. An ankle-brachial index (systolic bp at ankle divided by arm systolic bp) <0.9 indicates lower extremity arterial obstructive disease. Important findings on cardiovascular examination include:

CAROTID ARTERY PULSE (FIG. 119-1)

- *Pulsus parvus:* Weak upstroke due to decreased stroke volume (hypovolemia, LV failure, aortic or mitral stenosis).
- *Pulsus tardus:* Delayed upstroke (aortic stenosis).
- *Bounding (hyperkinetic) pulse:* Hyperkinetic circulation, aortic regurgitation, patent ductus arteriosus, marked vasodilatation.
- *Pulsus bisferiens:* Double systolic pulsation (aortic regurgitation, hypertrophic cardiomyopathy).
- *Pulsus alternans:* Regular alteration in pulse pressure amplitude (severe LV dysfunction).
- *Pulsus paradoxus:* Exaggerated inspiratory fall (>10 mmHg) in systolic bp (pericardial tamponade, severe obstructive lung disease).

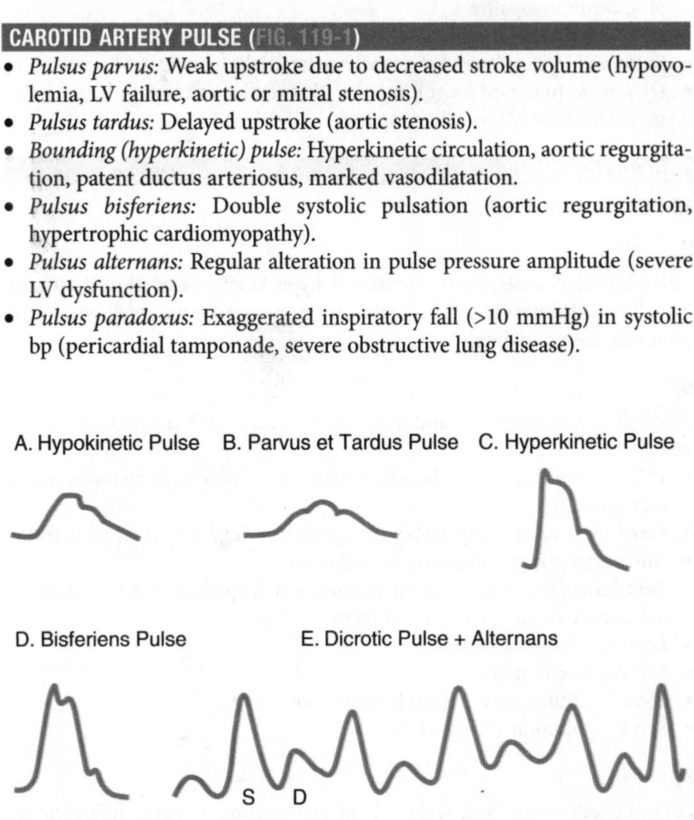

A. Hypokinetic Pulse   B. Parvus et Tardus Pulse   C. Hyperkinetic Pulse

D. Bisferiens Pulse   E. Dicrotic Pulse + Alternans

FIGURE 119-1 Carotid artery pulse patterns.

JUGULAR VENOUS PULSATION (JVP)

Jugular venous distention develops in right-sided heart failure, constrictive pericarditis, pericardial tamponade, obstruction of superior vena cava. JVP normally falls with inspiration but may rise (Kussmaul sign) in constrictive pericarditis. Abnormalities in examination include:

- *Large "a" wave:* Tricuspid stenosis (TS), pulmonic stenosis, AV dissociation (right atrium contracts against closed tricuspid valve).
- *Large "v" wave:* Tricuspid regurgitation, atrial septal defect.
- *Steep "y" descent:* Constrictive pericarditis.
- *Slow "y" descent:* Tricuspid stenosis.

PRECORDIAL PALPATION

Cardiac apical impulse is normally localized at the fifth intercostal space, midclavicular line. Abnormalities include:

- *Forceful apical thrust:* Left ventricular hypertrophy.
- *Lateral and downward displacement of apex impulse:* Left ventricular dilatation.
- *Prominent presystolic impulse:* Hypertension, aortic stenosis, hypertrophic cardiomyopathy.
- *Double systolic apical impulse:* Hypertrophic cardiomyopathy.
- *Sustained "lift" at lower left sternal border:* Right ventricular hypertrophy.
- *Dyskinetic (outward bulge) impulse:* Ventricular aneurysm, large dyskinetic area post MI, cardiomyopathy.

AUSCULTATION

■ HEART SOUNDS (FIG. 119-2)

S_1

Loud: Mitral stenosis, short PR interval, hyperkinetic heart, thin chest wall.
Soft: Long PR interval, heart failure, mitral regurgitation, thick chest wall, pulmonary emphysema.

S_2

Normally A_2 precedes P_2 and splitting increases with inspiration; abnormalities include:

- *Widened* splitting: Right bundle branch block, pulmonic stenosis, mitral regurgitation.
- *Fixed* splitting (no respiratory change in splitting): Atrial septal defect.
- *Narrow* splitting: Pulmonary hypertension.
- *Paradoxical* splitting (splitting narrows with inspiration): Aortic stenosis, left bundle branch block, heart failure.
- *Loud A_2:* Systemic hypertension.
- *Soft A_2:* Aortic stenosis (AS).
- *Loud P_2:* Pulmonary arterial hypertension.
- *Soft P_2:* Pulmonic stenosis (PS).

S_3

Low-pitched, heard best with bell of stethoscope at apex, following S_2; normal in children; after age 30–35, indicates LV failure or volume overload.

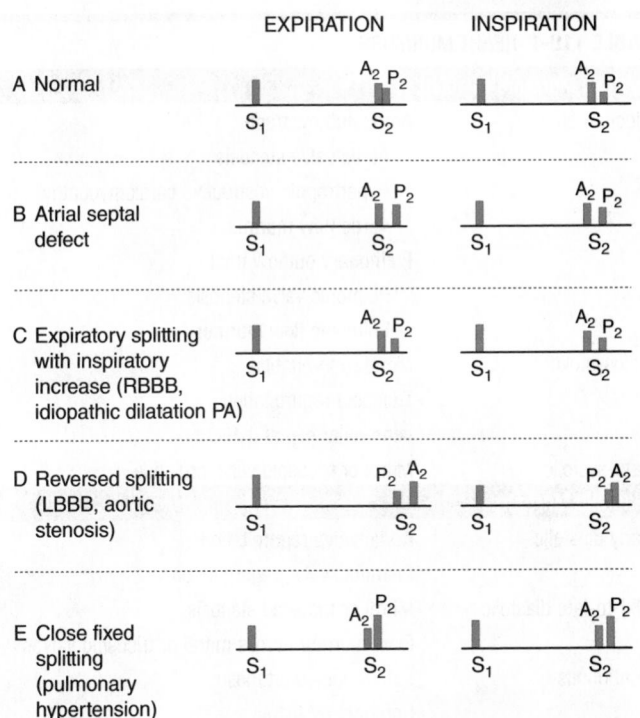

FIGURE 119-2 Heart sounds. **A.** Normal. S1, first heart sound; S2, second heart sound; A2, aortic component of the second heart sound; P2, pulmonic component of the second heart sound. **B.** Atrial septal defect with fixed splitting of S2. **C.** Physiologic but wide splitting of S2 with right bundle branch block. **D.** Reversed or paradoxical splitting of S2 with left bundle branch block. **E.** Narrow splitting of S2 with pulmonary hypertension. *(From NO Fowler: Diagnosis of Heart Disease. New York, Springer-Verlag, 1991, p 31.)*

S_4

Low-pitched, heard best with bell at apex, preceding S_1; reflects atrial contraction into a noncompliant ventricle; found in AS, hypertension, hypertrophic cardiomyopathy, and coronary artery disease (CAD).

Opening Snap (OS)

High-pitched; follows S_2 (by 0.06–0.12 s), heard at lower left sternal border and apex in mitral stenosis (MS); the more severe the MS, the shorter the S_2–OS interval.

Ejection Clicks

High-pitched sounds following S_1; observed in dilatation of aortic root or pulmonary artery, congenital AS (loudest at apex) or PS (upper left sternal border); the latter decreases with inspiration.

TABLE 119-1 HEART MURMURS

Systolic Murmurs	
Ejection-type	Aortic outflow tract
	Aortic valve stenosis
	Hypertrophic obstructive cardiomyopathy
	Aortic flow murmur
	Pulmonary outflow tract
	Pulmonic valve stenosis
	Pulmonic flow murmur
Holosystolic	Mitral regurgitation
	Tricuspid regurgitation
	Ventricular septal defect
Late-systolic	Mitral or tricuspid valve prolapse
Diastolic Murmurs	
Early diastolic	Aortic valve regurgitation
	Pulmonic valve regurgitation
Mid-to-late diastolic	Mitral or tricuspid stenosis
	Flow murmur across mitral or tricuspid valves
Continuous	Patent ductus arteriosus
	Coronary AV fistula
	Ruptured sinus of Valsalva aneurysm

Midsystolic Clicks

At lower left sternal border and apex, often followed by late systolic murmur in mitral valve prolapse.

■ **HEART MURMURS (TABLES 119-1 AND 119-2, FIG. 119-3)**

Systolic Murmurs

May be "crescendo-decrescendo" ejection type, pansystolic, or late systolic; right-sided murmurs (e.g., tricuspid regurgitation) typically increase with inspiration.

Diastolic Murmurs

- *Early diastolic murmurs:* Begin immediately after S_2, are high-pitched, and are usually caused by aortic or pulmonary regurgitation.
- *Mid-to-late diastolic murmurs:* Low-pitched, heard best with bell of stethoscope; observed in MS or TS; less commonly due to atrial myxoma.
- *Continuous murmurs:* Present in systole and diastole (envelops S_2); found in patent ductus arteriosus and sometimes in coarctation of aorta; less common causes are systemic or coronary AV fistula, aortopulmonary septal defect, ruptured aneurysm of sinus of Valsalva.

TABLE 119-2 EFFECTS OF PHYSIOLOGIC AND PHARMACOLOGIC INTERVENTIONS ON THE INTENSITY OF HEART MURMURS AND SOUNDS

Respiration

Systolic murmurs due to TR or pulmonic blood flow through a normal or stenotic valve and diastolic murmurs of TS or PR generally increase with inspiration, as do right-sided S_3 and S_4. Left-sided murmurs and sounds usually are louder during expiration, as is the pulmonic ejection sound.

Valsalva Maneuver

Most murmurs decrease in length and intensity. Two exceptions are the systolic murmur of HCM, which usually becomes much louder, and that of MVP, which becomes longer and often louder. Following release of the Valsalva maneuver, right-sided murmurs tend to return to control intensity earlier than left-sided murmurs.

After VPB or AF

Murmurs originating at normal or stenotic semilunar valves increase in the cardiac cycle following a VPB or in the cycle after a long cycle length in AF. By contrast, systolic murmurs due to AV valve regurgitation either do not change, diminish (papillary muscle dysfunction), or become shorter (MVP).

Positional Changes

With *standing*, most murmurs diminish, two exceptions being the murmur of HCM, which becomes louder, and that of MVP, which lengthens and often is intensified. With *squatting*, most murmurs become louder, but those of HCM and MVP usually soften and may disappear. Passive leg raising usually produces the same results.

Exercise

Murmurs due to blood flow across normal or obstructed valves (e.g., PS, MS) become louder with both isotonic and submaximal isometric (handgrip) exercise. Murmurs of MR, VSD, and AR also increase with handgrip exercise. However, the murmur of HCM often decreases with near maximum handgrip exercise. Left-sided S_4 and S_3 are often accentuated by exercise, particularly when due to ischemic heart disease.

Abbreviations: AF, atrial fibrillation; AR, aortic regurgitation; HCM, hypertrophic cardiomyopathy; HOCM, hypertrophic obstructive cardiomyopathy; MR, mitral regurgitation; MS, mitral stenosis; MVP, mitral valve prolapse; PES, pulmonic ejection sound; PR, pulmonic regurgitation; PS, pulmonic stenosis; TR, tricuspid regurgitation; TS, tricuspid stenosis; VPB, ventricular premature beat; VSD, ventricular septal defect.

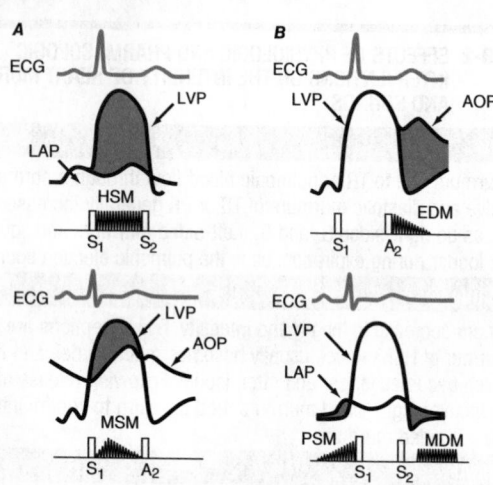

FIGURE 119-3 A. Schematic representation of ECG, aortic pressure (AOP), left ventricular pressure (LVP), and left atrial pressure (LAP). The gray areas indicated a transvalvular pressure difference during systole. HSM, holosystolic murmur; MSM, midsystolic murmur. **B.** Graphic representation of ECG, aortic pressure (AOP), left ventricular pressure (LVP), and left atrial pressure (LAP) with gray areas indicating transvalvular diastolic pressure difference. EDM, early diastolic murmur; PSM, presystolic murmur; MDM, middiastolic murmur.

For a more detailed discussion, see O'Gara P, Loscalzo J: Physical Examination of the Cardiovascular System, Chap. 227, p. 1821, in HPIM-18.

CHAPTER **120**
Electrocardiography

STANDARD APPROACH TO THE ECG

Normally, standardization is 1.0 mV per 10 mm, and paper speed is 25 mm/s (each horizontal small box = 0.04 s).

Heart Rate

Beats/min = 300 divided by the number of *large* boxes (each 5 mm apart) between consecutive QRS complexes. For faster heart rates, divide 1500 by number of *small* boxes (1 mm apart) between each QRS.

Rhythm

Sinus rhythm is present if every P wave is followed by a QRS, PR interval ≥0.12 s, every QRS is preceded by a P wave, and the P wave is upright in leads I, II, and III. Arrhythmias are discussed in Chaps. 131 and 132.

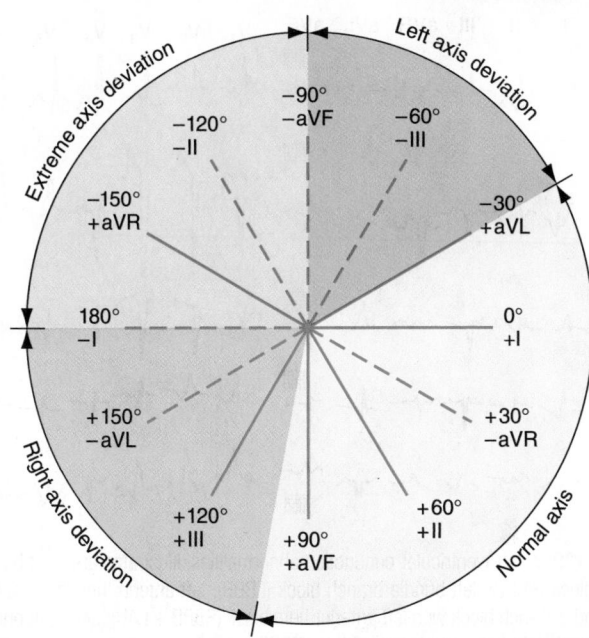

FIGURE 120-1 Electrocardiographic lead systems: The hexaxial frontal plane reference system to estimate electrical axis. Determine leads in which QRS deflections are maximum and minimum. For example, a maximum positive QRS in I which is isoelectric in aVF is oriented to 0°. Normal axis ranges from −30° to +90°. An axis > +90° is right-axis deviation and <30° is left-axis deviation.

Mean Axis

If QRS is primarily positive in limb leads I and II, then axis is *normal*. Otherwise, find limb lead in which QRS is most isoelectric (R = S). The mean axis is perpendicular to that lead (Fig. 120-1). If the QRS complex is *positive* in that perpendicular lead, then mean axis is in the direction of that lead; if *negative*, then mean axis points directly away from that lead.

Left-axis deviation (more negative than −30°) occurs in diffuse left ventricular disease, inferior MI; also in left anterior hemiblock (small R, deep S in leads II, III, and aVF).

Right-axis deviation (>90°) occurs in right ventricular hypertrophy (R > S in V_1) and left posterior hemiblock (small Q and tall R in leads II, III, and aVF). Mild right-axis deviation is seen in thin, healthy individuals (up to 110°).

■ INTERVALS (NORMAL VALUES IN PARENTHESES)

PR (0.12–0.20 s)

- *Short:* (1) preexcitation syndrome (look for slurred QRS upstroke due to "delta" wave), (2) nodal rhythm (inverted P in aVF).
- *Long:* first-degree AV block (Chap. 131).

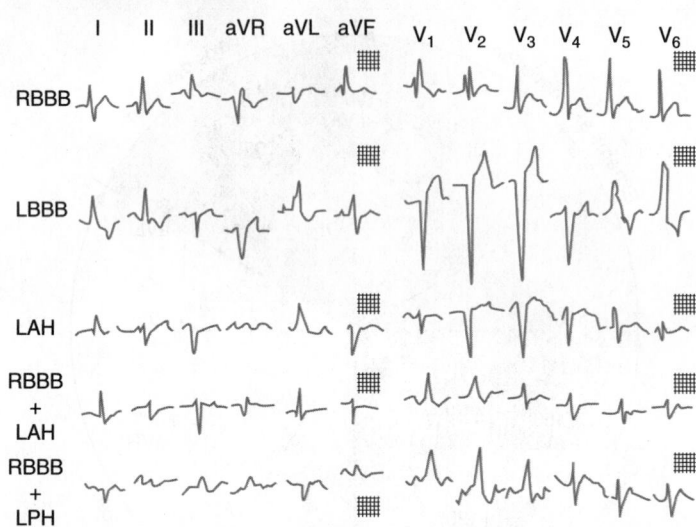

FIGURE 120-2 Intraventricular conduction abnormalities. Illustrated are right bundle branch block (RBBB); left bundle branch block (LBBB); left anterior hemiblock (LAH); right bundle branch block with left anterior hemiblock (RBBB + LAH); and right bundle branch block with left posterior hemiblock (RBBB + LPH).

QRS (0.06–0.10 s)

Widened: (1) ventricular premature beats, (2) bundle branch blocks: *right* (RsR' in V_1, deep S in V_6) and *left* [RR' in V_6 (Fig. 120-2)], (3) toxic levels of certain drugs (e.g., flecainide, propafenone, quinidine), (4) severe hypokalemia.

QT (<50% of RR interval; corrected QT ≤0.44 s)

Prolonged: congenital, hypokalemia, hypocalcemia, drugs (e.g., class IA and class III antiarrhythmics, tricyclics).

■ HYPERTROPHY

- *Right atrium:* P wave ≥2.5 mm in lead II.
- *Left atrium:* P biphasic (positive, then negative) in V_1, with terminal negative force wider than 0.04 s.
- *Right ventricle:* R > S in V_1 and R in V_1 > 5 mm; deep S in V_6; right-axis deviation.
- *Left ventricle:* S in V_1 plus R in V_5 or V_6 ≥35 mm or R in aVL >11 mm.

Infarction (Figs. 120-3 and 120-4)

Following acute ST-segment elevation MI without successful reperfusion: *Pathologic Q waves* (≥0.04 s and ≥25% of total QRS height) in leads shown in Table 120-1; acute *non-ST-segment elevation MI* shows ST-T changes in these leads without Q-wave development. A number of conditions (other than acute MI) can cause Q waves (Table 120-2).

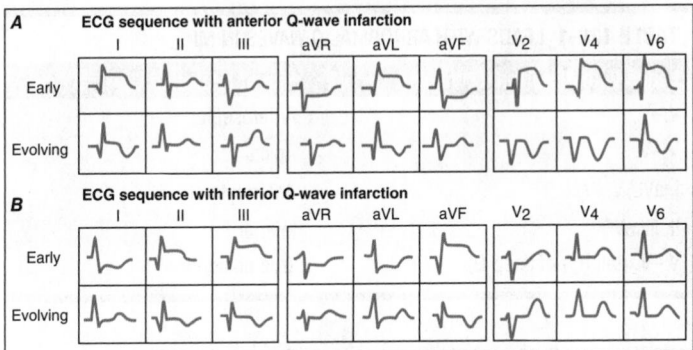

FIGURE 120-3 Sequence of depolarization and repolarization changes with **A.** acute anterior and **B.** acute inferior wall Q-wave infarctions. With anterior infarcts, ST elevation in leads I, aVL, and the precordial leads may be accompanied by reciprocal ST depressions in leads II, III, and aVF. Conversely, acute inferior (or posterior) infarcts may be associated with reciprocal ST depressions in leads V_1 to V_3. (*After AL Goldberger: Clinical Electrocardiography: A Simplified Approach, 7th ed. St. Louis, Mosby/Elsevier, 2006.*)

◼ ST-T WAVES

- *ST elevation:* Acute MI, coronary spasm, pericarditis (concave upward) (see Fig. 125-1 and Table 125-2), LV aneurysm, Brugada pattern (RBBB with ST elevation in V_1–V_2).
- *ST depression:* Digitalis effect, strain (due to ventricular hypertrophy), ischemia, or nontransmural MI.

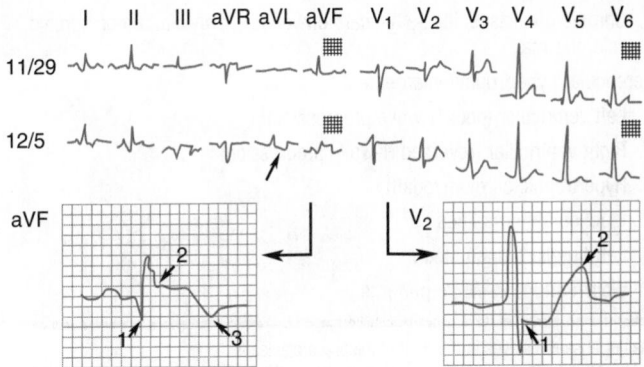

FIGURE 120-4 Acute inferior wall myocardial infarction. The ECG of 11/29 shows minor nonspecific ST-segment and T-wave changes. On 12/5 an acute myocardial infarction occurred. There are pathologic Q waves **1**, ST-segment elevation **2**, and terminal T-wave inversion **3** in leads II, III, and aVF indicating the location of the infarct on the inferior wall. Reciprocal changes in aVL (small arrow). Increasing R-wave voltage with ST depression and increased voltage of the T wave in V_2 are characteristic of true posterior wall extension of the inferior infarction. (*Reproduced from R.J. Myerburg: HPIM-12.*)

TABLE 120-1 LEADS WITH ABNORMAL Q WAVES IN MI

Leads with Abnormal Q Waves	Site of Infarction
V_1–V_2	Anteroseptal
V_3–V_4	Apical
I, aVL, V_5–V_6	Anterolateral
II, III, aVF	Inferior
V_1–V_2 (tall R, *not* deep Q)	True posterior

- *Tall peaked T*: Hyperkalemia; acute MI ("hyperacute T").
- *Inverted T*: Non-Q-wave MI, ventricular "strain" pattern, drug effect (e.g., digitalis), hypokalemia, hypocalcemia, increased intracranial pressure (e.g., subarachnoid bleed).

TABLE 120-2 DIFFERENTIAL DIAGNOSIS OF Q WAVES (WITH SELECTED EXAMPLES)

Physiologic or positional factors

1. Normal variant "septal" Q waves
2. Normal variant Q waves in V_1 to V_2, aVL, III, and aVF
3. Left pneumothorax or dextrocardia

Myocardial injury or infiltration

1. Acute processes: myocardial ischemia or infarction, myocarditis, hyperkalemia
2. Chronic processes: idiopathic cardiomyopathy, amyloid, tumor, sarcoid, scleroderma

Ventricular hypertrophy/enlargement

1. Left ventricular (poor R-wave progression)[a]
2. Right ventricular (reversed R-wave progression)
3. Hypertrophic cardiomyopathy

Conduction abnormalities

1. Left bundle branch block
2. Wolff-Parkinson-White patterns

[a]Small or absent R waves in the right to midprecordial leads.
Source: After AL Goldberger: *Myocardial Infarction: Electrocardiographic Differential Diagnosis,* 4th ed. St. Louis, Mosby-Year Book, 1991.

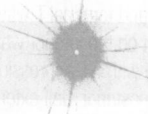

For a more detailed discussion, see Goldberger AL: Electrocardiography, Chap. 228, p. 1831 in HPIM-18.

CHAPTER **121**
Noninvasive Examination of the Heart

ECHOCARDIOGRAPHY (TABLE 121-1 AND FIG. 121-1)

Visualizes heart in real time with ultrasound; Doppler recordings noninvasively assess hemodynamics and abnormal flow patterns. Imaging may be compromised in pts with chronic obstructive lung disease, thick chest wall, or narrow intercostal spaces.

Chamber Size and Ventricular Performance

Assessment of atrial and ventricular dimensions, global and regional systolic wall motion abnormalities, ventricular hypertrophy/infiltration, evaluation for pulmonary hypertension: RV systolic pressure (RVSP) is calculated from maximum velocity of tricuspid regurgitation (TR):

$$RVSP = 4 \times (TR\ velocity)^2 + RA\ pressure$$

(RA pressure is same as JVP estimated by physical exam.) In absence of RV outflow obstruction, RVSP = pulmonary artery systolic pressure.

LV diastolic function is assessed by transmitral Doppler (see Fig. 229-9, p. 1844, in HPIM-18) and Doppler tissue imaging, which measures velocity of myocardial relaxation.

Valvular Abnormalities

Thickness, mobility, calcification, and regurgitation of each cardiac valve can be assessed. Severity of valvular stenosis is calculated by Doppler

TABLE 121-1 CLINICAL USES OF ECHOCARDIOGRAPHY

2-D Echo	Transesophageal Echocardiography
Cardiac chambers: size, hypertrophy, wall motion abnormalities	Superior to 2-D echo to identify: Infective endocarditis
Valves: morphology and motion	Cardiac source of embolism
Pericardium: effusion, tamponade	Prosthetic valve dysfunction
Aorta: aneurysm, dissection	Aortic dissection
Assess intracardiac masses	
Doppler Echocardiography	**Stress Echocardiography**
Valvular stenosis and regurgitation	Assess myocardial ischemia and viability
Intracardiac shunts	
Diastolic filling/dysfunction	
Approximate intracardiac pressures	

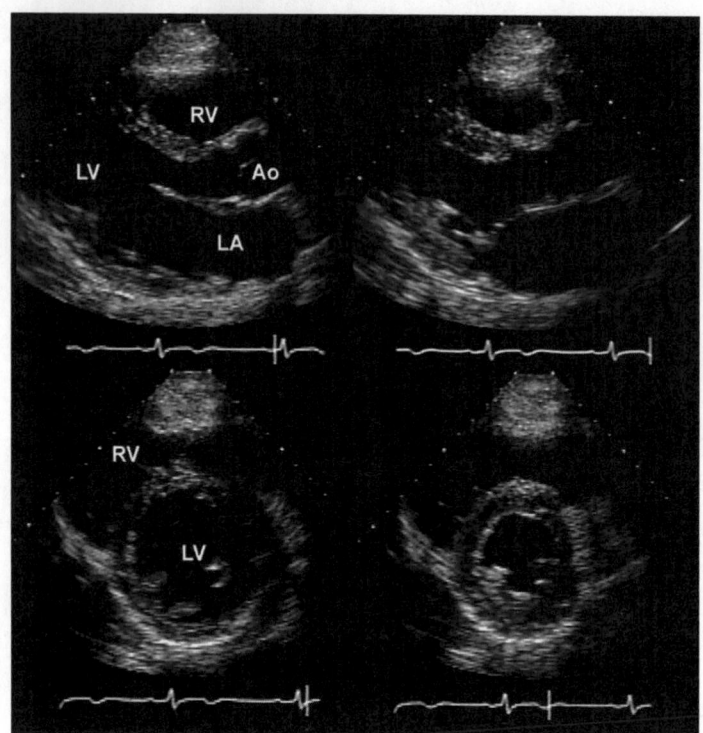

FIGURE 121-1 Two-dimensional echocardiographic still-frame images of a normal heart. *Upper:* Parasternal long axis view during systole and diastole (*left*) and systole (*right*). During systole, there is thickening of the myocardium and reduction in the size of the left ventricle (LV). The valve leaflets are thin and open widely. *Lower:* Parasternal short axis view during diastole (*left*) and systole (*right*) demonstrating a decrease in the left ventricular cavity size during systole as well as an increase in wall thickness. LA, left atrium; RV, right ventricle; Ao, aorta. (*Reproduced from R.J. Myerburg: HPIM-12.*)

[peak gradient $= 4 \times$ (peak velocity)^2]. Structural lesions (e.g., flail leaflet, vegetation) resulting in regurgitation may be identified, and Doppler (Fig. 121-2) estimates severity of regurgitation.

Pericardial Disease

Echo is noninvasive modality of choice to rapidly identify pericardial effusion and assess its hemodynamic significance; in tamponade there is diastolic RA and RV collapse, dilatation of IVC, exaggerated respiratory alterations in transvalvular Doppler velocities. Actual thickness of pericardium (e.g., in suspected constrictive pericarditis) is better measured by CT or MRI.

Intracardiac Masses

May visualize atrial or ventricular thrombus, intracardiac tumors, and valvular vegetations. Yield of identifying cardiac source of embolism is *low*

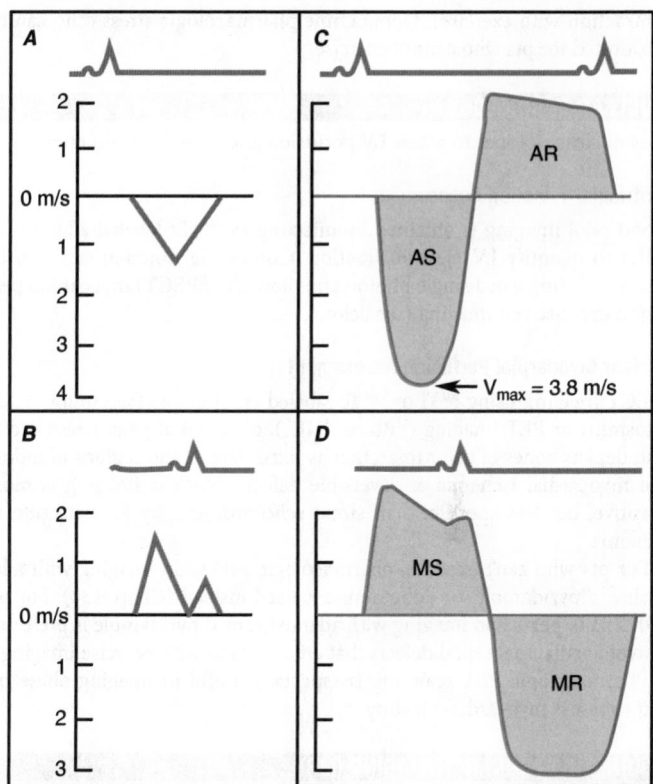

FIGURE 121-2 Schematic presentation of normal Doppler flow across the aortic **A.** and mitral valves **B.** Abnormal continuous wave Doppler profiles: **C.** Aortic stenosis (AS) [peak transaortic gradient $= 4 \times V_{max}^2 = 4 \times (3.8)^2 = 58$ mmHg] and regurgitation (AR). **D.** Mitral stenosis (MS) and regurgitation (MR).

in absence of cardiac history or physical findings. Transesophageal echocardiography (TEE) is more sensitive than standard transthoracic study for masses <1 cm in diameter.

Aortic Disease

Aneurysm and dissection of the aorta may be evaluated and complications (aortic regurgitation, tamponade) assessed (Chap. 134) by standard transthoracic echo. TEE is more sensitive and specific for aortic dissection.

Congenital Heart Disease (See Chap. 122)

Echo, Doppler, and contrast echo (rapid IV injection of agitated saline) are useful to identify congenital lesions and shunts.

Stress Echocardiography

Echo performed prior to, and after, treadmill or bicycle exercise identifies regions of prior MI and inducible myocardial ischemia (↓ regional contraction with exercise). Dobutamine pharmacologic stress echo can be substituted for pts who cannot exercise.

NUCLEAR CARDIOLOGY

Uses nuclear isotopes to assess LV perfusion and contractile function.

Ventricular Function Assessment

Blood pool imaging is obtained by injecting IV ^{99m}Tc-labeled albumin or RBCs to quantify LV ejection fraction. Contractile function can also be assessed during gated single photon emission CT (SPECT) myocardial perfusion exercise test imaging (see below).

Nuclear Myocardial Perfusion Assessment

SPECT imaging using ^{201}Tl or ^{99m}Tc-labeled compounds (sestamibi or tetrofosmin) or PET imaging (^{82}Rb or ^{13}NH$_3$), obtained at peak stress and at rest, depicts zones of prior infarction as fixed defects and regions of inducible myocardial ischemia as reversible defects. Nuclear imaging is more sensitive, but less specific, than stress echocardiography for detection of ischemia.

For pts who can't exercise, pharmacologic perfusion imaging with adenosine, dipyridamole, or dobutamine is used instead (Chap. 130). For pts with LBBB, perfusion imaging with adenosine or dipyridamole is preferred to avoid artifactual septal defects that are common with exercise imaging.

Pharmacologic PET scanning is especially useful in imaging obese pts and to assess myocardial viability.

MAGNETIC RESONANCE IMAGING (MRI)

Delineates cardiac structures with high resolution without ionizing radiation. Excellent technique to characterize intracardiac masses, the pericardium, great vessels, and anatomic relationships in congenital heart disease. MRI with delayed gadolinium enhancement (avoid in pts with renal insufficiency) differentiates ischemic from nonischemic cardiomyopathy and is useful in assessing myocardial viability. Pharmacologic stress testing with MR identifies significant CAD and detects subendocardial ischemia with higher sensitivity than SPECT imaging.

COMPUTED TOMOGRAPHY (CT)

Provides high-resolution images of cardiac structures and detects coronary calcification in atherosclerosis with high sensitivity (but low specificity). CT angiography delineates abnormalities of the great vessels, including aortic aneurysms and dissection, and pulmonary embolism. It is useful for assessment of pericardial thickness and calcification, cardiac masses, and arrhythmogenic RV cardiomyopathy. Multislice spiral CT provides high-resolution images of coronary anatomy. It is most useful in evaluation of suspected coronary anatomic anomalies and to exclude high-grade coronary stenoses in pts with chest pain and intermediate pretest probability of coronary artery disease. Its greatest accuracy is in detection of left main and proximal LAD and circumflex disease.

TABLE 121-2 SELECTION OF IMAGING TESTS

	Echo	Nuclear	CT[a]	MRI[b]
LV Size/function	Initial modality of choice Low cost, portable Provides ancillary structural and hemodynamic information	Available from gated SPECT stress imaging	Best resolution High cost	Best resolution High cost
Valve disease	Initial modality of choice Valve motion Doppler hemodynamics			Visualize valve motion Delineate abnormal flow
Pericardial disease	Pericardial effusion Doppler hemodynamics		Pericardial thickening	Pericardial thickening
Aortic disease	TEE rapid diagnosis of acute dissection[c]		Image entire aorta Acute aneurysm Aortic dissection	Image entire aorta Aortic aneurysm Chronic dissection
Cardiac masses	TTE—large intracardiac masses TEE—smaller intracardiac masses[c]		Extracardiac masses Myocardial masses	Extracardiac masses Myocardial masses

[a]Contrast required.
[b]Relative contraindication: pacemakers, metallic objects, claustrophobic.
[c]When not seen on TTE.

Abbreviations: Echo, echocardiography; SPECT, single photon emission CT; TEE, transesophageal echocardiography; TTE, transthoracic echocardiogram.

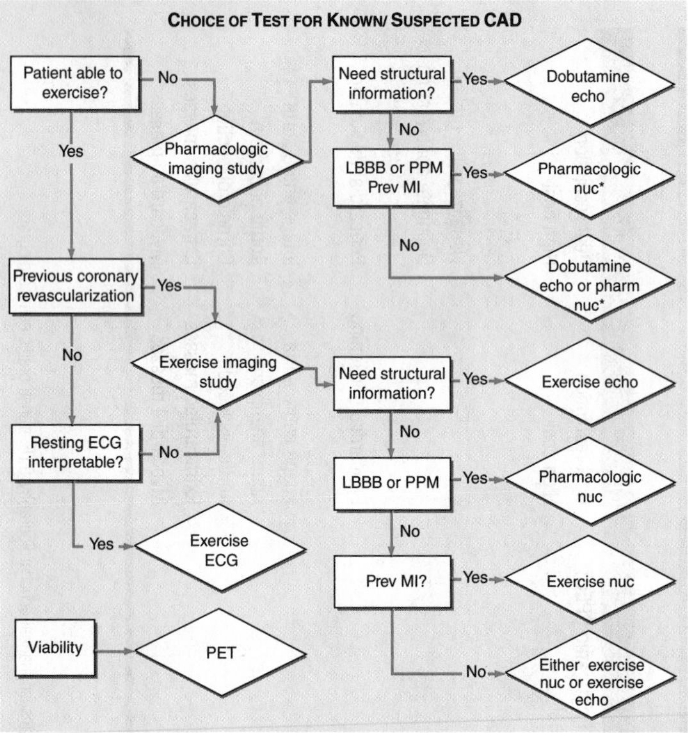

CHOICE OF TEST FOR KNOWN/ SUSPECTED CAD

FIGURE 121-3 Flow diagram showing selection of initial stress test in a pt with chest pain. LBBB, left bundle branch block; Prev MI-Reg ischemia, previous MI with a need to detect regional ischemia; Nuc, SPECT nuclear imaging study; Pharm, pharmacologic. *Consider PET if morbidly obese or female with large/dense breasts.

Table 121-2 summarizes key diagnostic features of the noninvasive imaging modalities. Figure 121-3 provides an algorithm for diagnostic imaging assessment of suspected CAD.

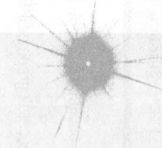

For a more detailed discussion, see Nishimura RA, Chareonthaitawee P, Martinez M: Noninvasive Cardiac Imaging: Echocardiography, Nuclear Cardiology, and MRI/CT Imaging, Chap. 229, p. 1840 in HPIM-18.

CHAPTER **122**
Congenital Heart Disease in the Adult

■ ATRIAL SEPTAL DEFECT (ASD)

Most common is *ostium secundum* ASD, located at mid interatrial septum. *Sinus venosus* type ASD involves the high atrial septum and may be associated with anomalous pulmonary venous drainage to the right heart. *Ostium primum* ASDs (e.g., typical of Down syndrome) appear at lower atrial septum, adjacent to atrioventricular (AV) valves.

History

Usually asymptomatic until third or fourth decades, when exertional dyspnea, fatigue, and palpitations may occur. Onset of symptoms may be associated with development of pulmonary hypertension (see below).

Physical Examination

Prominent right ventricular (RV) impulse, wide fixed splitting of S_2, systolic murmur from flow across pulmonic valve, diastolic flow rumble across tricuspid valve, prominent jugular venous *v* wave.

ECG

Incomplete RBBB (rSR' in right precordial leads) common. Left axis deviation frequently present with ostium primum defect. Ectopic atrial pacemaker or first degree AV block occur in sinus venosus defects.

CXR

Increased pulmonary vascular markings, prominence of right atrium (RA), RV, and main pulmonary artery (LA enlargement *not* usually present).

Echocardiogram

RA, RV, and pulmonary artery enlargement; Doppler shows abnormal turbulent transatrial flow. Echo contrast (agitated saline injection into peripheral systemic vein) may visualize transatrial shunt. Transesophageal echo usually diagnostic if transthoracic echo is ambiguous.

> **TREATMENT** Atrial Septal Defect
>
> In the absence of contraindications an ASD with pulmonary-to-systemic flow ratio (PF:SF) >2.0:1.0 should be repaired surgically or by percutaneous transcatheter closure. Surgery is contraindicated with significant pulmonary hypertension and PF:SF <1.2:1.0. Medical management includes antiarrhythmic therapy for associated atrial fibrillation or supraventricular tachycardia (Chap. 132) and standard therapy for symptoms of heart failure (Chap. 133).

■ VENTRICULAR SEPTAL DEFECT (VSD)

Congenital VSDs may close spontaneously during childhood. Symptoms relate to size of the defect and pulmonary vascular resistance.

History

CHF may develop in infancy. Adults may be asymptomatic or develop fatigue and reduced exercise tolerance.

Physical Examination

Systolic thrill and holosystolic murmur at lower left sternal border, loud P_2, S_3; diastolic flow murmur across mitral valve.

ECG

Normal with small defects. Large shunts result in LA and LV enlargement.

CXR

Enlargement of main pulmonary artery, LA, and LV, with increased pulmonary vascular markings.

Echocardiogram

LA and LV enlargement; defect may be directly visualized. Color Doppler demonstrates flow across the defect.

> **TREATMENT**   Ventricular Septal Defect
>
> Fatigue and mild dyspnea are treated with diuretics and afterload reduction (Chap. 133). Surgical closure is indicated if PF:SF >1.5:1 in absence of very high pulmonary vascular resistance.

■ PATENT DUCTUS ARTERIOSUS (PDA)

Abnormal communication between the descending aorta and pulmonary artery; associated with birth at high altitudes and maternal rubella.

History

Asymptomatic or fatigue and dyspnea on exertion.

Physical Examination

Hyperactive LV impulse; loud continuous "machinery" murmur at upper left sternal border. If pulmonary hypertension develops, diastolic component of the murmur may disappear.

ECG

LV hypertrophy is common; RV hypertrophy if pulmonary hypertension develops.

CXR

Increased pulmonary vascular markings: enlarged main pulmonary artery, LV, ascending aorta; occasionally, calcification of ductus.

Echocardiography

Hyperdynamic, enlarged LV; the PDA can often be visualized on two-dimensional echo; Doppler demonstrates abnormal flow through it.

> **TREATMENT** Patent Ductus Arteriosus
>
> In absence of pulmonary hypertension, PDA should be surgically ligated or divided to prevent infective endocarditis, LV dysfunction, and pulmonary hypertension. Transcatheter device closure is frequently possible.

■ PROGRESSION TO PULMONARY HYPERTENSION (PHT)

Pts with large, uncorrected left-to-right shunts (e.g., ASD, VSD, or PDA) may develop progressive, irreversible PHT with reverse shunting of desaturated blood into the arterial circulation (right-to-left direction), resulting in *Eisenmenger syndrome*. Fatigue, lightheadedness, and chest pain due to RV ischemia are common, accompanied by cyanosis, clubbing of digits, loud P_2, murmur of pulmonary valve regurgitation, and signs of RV failure. ECG and echocardiogram show RV hypertrophy. Therapeutic options are limited and include pulmonary artery vasodilators and consideration of single lung transplant with repair of the cardiac defect, or heart-lung transplantation.

ACYANOTIC CONGENITAL HEART LESIONS WITHOUT A SHUNT

■ PULMONIC STENOSIS (PS)

A transpulmonary valve gradient < 30 mmHg indicates mild PS, 30–50 mmHg is moderate PS, and >50 mmHg is considered severe PS. Mild to moderate PS rarely causes symptoms, and progression tends not to occur. Pts with higher gradients may manifest dyspnea, fatigue, light-headedness, chest pain (RV ischemia).

Physical Examination

Jugular venous distention with prominent *a* wave, RV parasternal impulse, wide splitting of S_2 with soft P_2, ejection click followed by "diamond-shaped" systolic murmur at upper left sternal border, right-sided S_4.

ECG

Normal in mild PS; RA and RV enlargement in advanced PS.

CXR

Often shows poststenotic dilatation of the pulmonary artery and RV enlargement.

Echocardiography

RV hypertrophy and systolic "doming" of the pulmonic valve. Doppler accurately measures transvalvular gradient.

> **TREATMENT** Pulmonic Stenosis
>
> Symptomatic or severe stenosis requires balloon valvuloplasty or surgical correction.

■ **CONGENITALLY BICUSPID AORTIC VALVE**

One of the most common congenital heart malformations (up to 1.4% of the population); rarely results in childhood aortic stenosis (AS), but is a cause of AS and/or regurgitation later in life. May go undetected in early life or suspected by the presence of a systolic ejection click; often identified during echocardiography that was obtained for another reason. See Chap. 123 for typical history, physical findings, and treatment of subsequent clinical aortic valve disease.

■ **COARCTATION OF THE AORTA**

Aortic constriction just distal to the origin of the left subclavian artery is a surgically correctable form of hypertension (Chap. 126). Usually asymptomatic, but may cause headache, fatigue, or claudication of lower extremities. Often accompanied by bicuspid aortic valve.

Physical Examination

Hypertension in upper extremities; delayed femoral pulses with decreased pressure in lower extremities. Pulsatile collateral arteries can be palpated in the intercostal spaces. Systolic (and sometimes also diastolic) murmur is best heard over the mid-upper back at left interscapular space.

ECG

LV hypertrophy.

CXR

Notching of the ribs due to collateral arteries; "figure 3" appearance of distal aortic arch.

Echocardiography

Can delineate site and length of coarctation, and Doppler determines the pressure gradient across it. MR or CT angiography also visualizes the site of coarctation and can identify associated collateral vessel formation.

TREATMENT   Coarctation of the Aorta

Surgical correction (or percutaneous transcatheter stent dilation in selected pts), although hypertension may persist. Recoarctation after surgical repair may be amenable to percutaneous balloon dilatation.

COMPLEX CONGENITAL HEART LESIONS

Such lesions are often accompanied by cyanosis. Examples include:

■ **TETRALOGY OF FALLOT**

The four main components are (1) malaligned VSD, (2) obstruction to RV outflow, (3) aorta that overrides the VSD, and (4) RV hypertrophy (RVH). Degree of RV outflow obstruction largely determines clinical presentation; when severe, the large right-to-left shunt causes cyanosis and systemic hypoxemia. *ECG* shows RVH. *CXR* demonstrates "boot-shaped" heart with prominent RV. *Echocardiography* delineates VSD, overriding aorta, and RVH and quantitates degree of RV outflow obstruction.

■ COMPLETE TRANSPOSITION OF THE GREAT ARTERIES

Accounts for 10% of pts with cyanotic congenital heart disease. Aorta and pulmonary artery arise abnormally from the right and left ventricles respectively, creating two separate parallel circulations; a communication must exist between the two sides (ASD, PDA, or VSD) to sustain life. Development of RV dysfunction and heart failure are common by the third decade. *Echocardiography* reveals the aberrant anatomy.

■ EBSTEIN ANOMALY

Abnormal downward placement of tricuspid valve within the RV; tricuspid regurgitation, hypoplasia of RV, and a right-to-left shunt are common. *Echocardiography* shows apical displacement of tricuspid septal leaflet, abnormal RV size, and quantitates degree of tricuspid regurgitation.

ENDOCARDITIS PROPHYLAXIS IN CONGENITAL HEART DISEASE

American Heart Association 2007 Guidelines recommend antibiotic prophylaxis only in specific pts with congenital heart disease, i.e., those who are to undergo a dental procedure associated with bacteremia who have:

1. Unrepaired cyanotic congenital heart disease (e.g., tetralogy of Fallot)
2. Repaired congenital heart disease with residual defects adjacent to site of a prosthetic patch or transcatheter device
3. A history of complete repair of congenital defects with prosthetic material or a transcatheter device within the previous 6 months.

> For a more detailed discussion, see Child JS, Aboulhosn J: Congenital Heart Disease in the Adult, Chap. 236, p. 1920, in HPIM-18.

CHAPTER **123**
Valvular Heart Disease

■ MITRAL STENOSIS (MS)

Etiology

Most commonly rheumatic, although history of acute rheumatic fever is now uncommon; congenital MS is rare cause, observed primarily in infants.

History

Symptoms most commonly begin in the fourth decade, but MS often causes severe disability at earlier ages in developing nations. Principal symptoms are dyspnea and pulmonary edema precipitated by exertion, excitement, fever, anemia, paroxysmal tachycardia, pregnancy, sexual intercourse, etc.

Physical Examination

Right ventricular lift; palpable S_1; opening snap (OS) follows A_2 by 0.06–0.12 s; OS–A_2 interval inversely proportional to severity of obstruction. Diastolic rumbling murmur with presystolic accentuation in sinus rhythm. Duration of murmur correlates with severity of obstruction.

Complications

Hemoptysis, pulmonary embolism, pulmonary infection, systemic embolization; endocarditis is uncommon in pure MS.

Laboratory ECG

Typically shows atrial fibrillation (AF) or left atrial (LA) enlargement when sinus rhythm is present. Right-axis deviation and RV hypertrophy in the presence of pulmonary hypertension.

CXR

Shows LA and RV enlargement and Kerley B lines.

Echocardiogram

Most useful noninvasive test; shows inadequate separation, calcification and thickening of valve leaflets and subvalvular apparatus, and LA enlargement. Doppler flow recordings provide estimation of transvalvular gradient, mitral valve area, and degree of pulmonary hypertension (Chap. 121).

TREATMENT	Mitral Stenosis (See Fig. 123-1)

At-risk pts should receive prophylaxis for recurrent rheumatic fever (penicillin V 250–500 mg PO bid or benzathine penicillin G 1–2 M units IM monthly). In the presence of dyspnea, sodium restriction and oral diuretic therapy; beta blockers, digitalis, or rate-limiting calcium channel antagonists (i.e., verapamil or diltiazem) to slow ventricular rate in AF. Warfarin (with target INR 2.0–3.0) for pts with AF and/or history of systemic and pulmonic emboli. For AF of recent onset, consider reversion (chemical or electrical) to sinus rhythm, ideally after ≥3 weeks of anticoagulation. Mitral valvotomy in the presence of symptoms and mitral orifice ≤ ~1.5 cm². In uncomplicated MS, percutaneous balloon valvuloplasty is the procedure of choice; if not feasible, then open surgical valvotomy (Fig. 123-1).

■ MITRAL REGURGITATION (MR)

Etiology

Mitral valve prolapse (see below), rheumatic heart disease, ischemic heart disease with papillary muscle dysfunction, LV dilatation of any cause, mitral annular calcification, hypertrophic cardiomyopathy, infective endocarditis, congenital.

Clinical Manifestations

Fatigue, weakness, and exertional dyspnea. Physical examination: sharp upstroke of arterial pulse, LV lift, S_1 diminished: wide splitting of S_2; S_3; loud

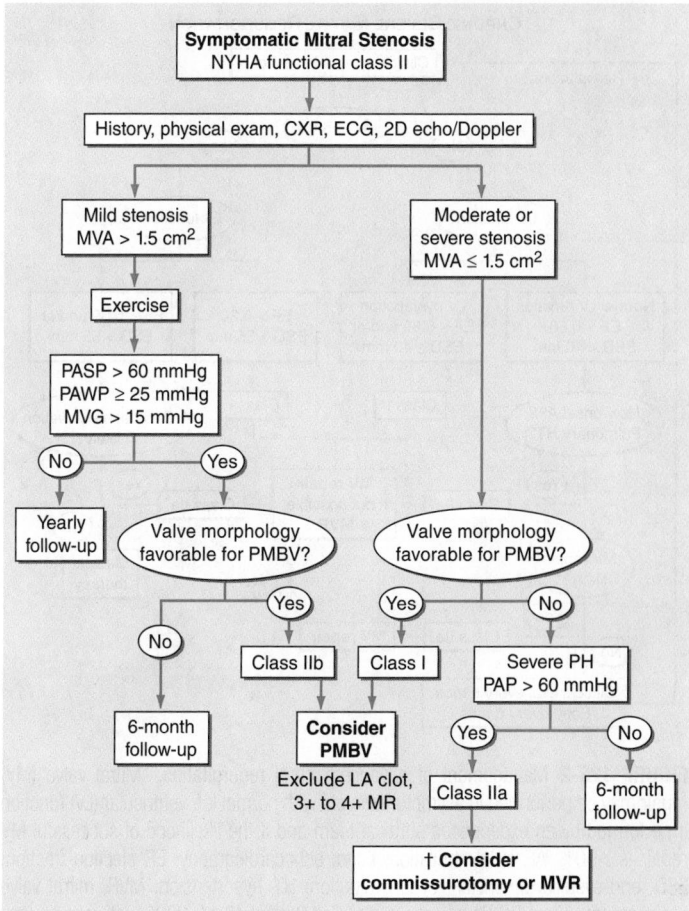

FIGURE 123-1 Management of mitral stenosis (MS). †There is controversy as to whether pts with severe MS (MVA <1.0 cm²) and severe pulmonary hypertension (PH) (PASP >60 mmHg) should undergo percutaneous mitral balloon valvotomy (PMBV) or mitral valve replacement (MVR) to prevent right ventricular failure. CXR, chest x-ray; ECG, electrocardiogram; echo, echocardiography; LA, left atrial; MR, mitral regurgitation; MVA, mitral valve area; MVG, mean mitral valve pressure gradient; NYHA, New York Heart Association; PASP, pulmonary artery systolic pressure; PAWP, pulmonary artery wedge pressure; 2D, 2-dimensional. *(From RO Bonow et al: J Am Coll Cardiol 48:e1, 2006; with permission.)*

holosystolic murmur and often a brief early-mid-diastolic murmur due to increased transvalvular flow.

Echocardiogram

Enlarged LA, hyperdynamic LV, identifies mechanism of MR; Doppler analysis helpful in diagnosis and assessment of severity of MR and degree of pulmonary hypertension.

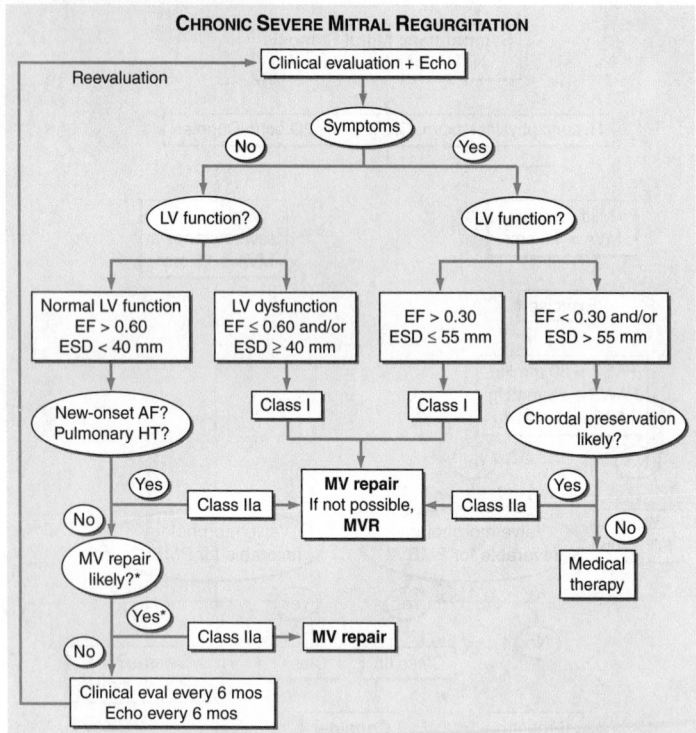

FIGURE 123-2 Management of advanced mitral regurgitation. *Mitral valve (MV) repair may be performed in asymptomatic pts with normal left ventricular (LV) function if performed by an experienced surgical team and if the likelihood of successful MV repair is >90%. AF, atrial fibrillation; Echo, echocardiography; EF, ejection fraction; ESD, end-systolic dimension; eval, evaluation; HT, hypertension; MVR, mitral valve replacement. *(From RO Bonow et al: J Am Coll Cardiol 48:e1, 2006; with permission.)*

TREATMENT   Mitral Regurgitation (See Fig. 123-2)

For severe/decompensated MR, treat as for heart failure (Chap. 133). IV vasodilators (e.g., nitroprusside) are beneficial for acute, severe MR. Anticoagulation is indicated in the presence of atrial fibrillation. Surgical treatment, either valve repair or replacement, is appropriate if pt has symptoms or evidence of progressive LV dysfunction [LV ejection fraction (LVEF) ≤60% or end-systolic LV diameter by echo ≥40 mm]. Operation should be carried out before development of chronic heart failure symptoms.

MITRAL VALVE PROLAPSE (MVP)

Etiology

Most commonly idiopathic; may accompany rheumatic fever, ischemic heart disease, atrial septal defect, Marfan syndrome, Ehlers-Danlos syndrome.

Pathology

Redundant mitral valve tissue with myxedematous degeneration and elongated chordae tendineae.

Clinical Manifestations

More common in females. Most pts are asymptomatic and remain so. Most common symptoms are vague chest pain and supraventricular and ventricular arrhythmias. Most important complication is severe MR resulting in LV failure. Rarely, systemic emboli from platelet-fibrin deposits on valve. Sudden death is a very rare complication.

Physical Examination

Mid or late systolic click(s) followed by late systolic murmur at the apex; exaggeration by Valsalva maneuver, reduced by squatting and isometric exercise (Chap. 119).

Echocardiogram

Shows posterior displacement of one or both mitral leaflets late in systole.

TREATMENT ▸ **Mitral Valve Prolapse**

Asymptomatic pts should be reassured. Beta blockers may lessen chest discomfort and palpitations. Prophylaxis for infective endocarditis is indicated only if prior history of endocarditis. Valve repair or replacement for pts with severe mitral regurgitation; aspirin or anticoagulants for pts with history of TIA or embolization.

■ AORTIC STENOSIS (AS)

Etiologies

Most common are (1) degenerative calcification of a congenitally bicuspid valve, (2) chronic deterioration of a trileaflet valve, and (3) rheumatic disease (almost always associated with rheumatic *mitral* disease).

Symptoms

Exertional dyspnea, angina, and syncope are cardinal symptoms; they occur late, after years of obstruction and aortic valve area ≤ 1.0 cm^2.

Physical Examination

Weak and delayed (parvus et tardus) arterial pulses with carotid thrill. Double apical impulse (palpable S$_4$); A$_2$ soft or absent; S$_4$ common. Diamond-shaped systolic murmur $\geq$ grade 3/6, often with systolic thrill. Murmur is typically loudest at second right intercostal space, with radiation to carotids and sometimes to the apex (*Gallavardin effect*).

ECG

Often shows LV hypertrophy, but not useful for predicting gradient.

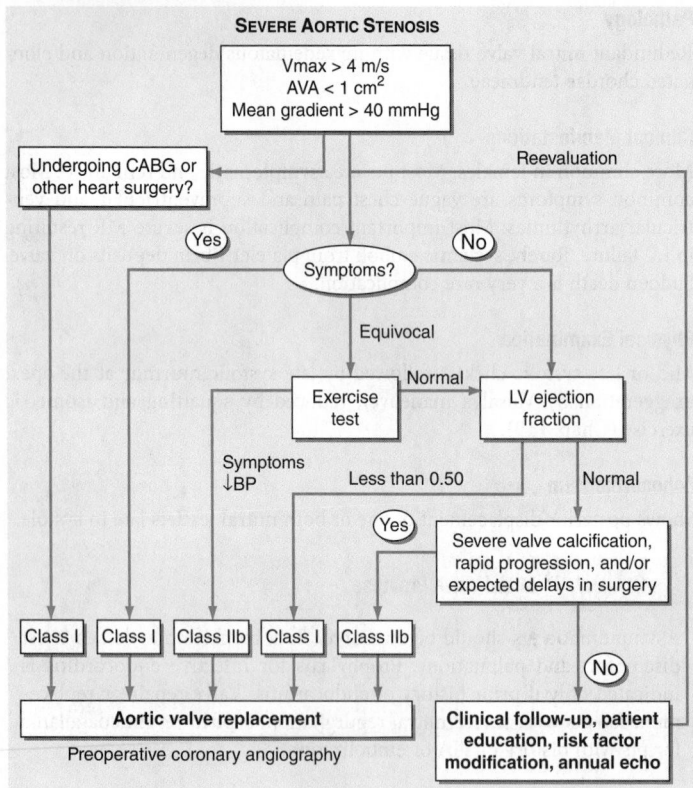

FIGURE 123-3 Algorithm for the management of aortic stenosis (AS). AVA, aortic valve area; BP, blood pressure; CABG, coronary artery bypass graft surgery; LV, left ventricle; Vmax, maximal velocity across aortic valve by Doppler echocardiography. *(Modified from CM Otto: J Am Coll Cardiol 47:2141, 2006.)*

Echocardiogram

Shows LV hypertrophy, calcification and thickening of aortic valve cusps with reduced systolic opening. Dilatation and reduced contraction of LV indicate poor prognosis. Doppler quantitates systolic gradient and allows calculation of valve area.

TREATMENT Aortic Stenosis (See Fig. 123-3)

Avoid strenuous activity in severe AS, even in asymptomatic phase. Treat heart failure in standard fashion (Chap. 133), but use vasodilators with caution in pts with advanced disease. Valve replacement is indicated in adults with symptoms resulting from AS and hemodynamic evidence of severe obstruction. Transcatheter aortic valve implantation (TAVI) is an investigational approach for pts at excessive surgical risk that has demonstrated favorable results.

■ AORTIC REGURGITATION (AR)

Etiology

Valvular: Rheumatic (especially if rheumatic mitral disease is present), bicuspid valve, endocarditis. *Dilated aortic root:* dilatation due to cystic medial necrosis, aortic dissection, ankylosing spondylitis, syphilis. Three-fourths of pts are male.

Clinical Manifestations

Exertional dyspnea and awareness of forceful heartbeat, angina pectoris, and signs of LV failure. Wide pulse pressure, water hammer pulse, capillary pulsations (Quincke's sign), A_2 soft or absent, S_3 common. Blowing, decrescendo diastolic murmur along left sternal border (along right sternal border with aortic dilatation). May be accompanied by systolic murmur of augmented blood flow.

Laboratory ECG and CXR

LV enlargement.

Echocardiogram

LA enlargement, LV enlargement, high-frequency diastolic fluttering of mitral valve. Failure of coaptation of aortic valve leaflets may be present. Doppler studies useful in detection and quantification of AR.

> **TREATMENT** Aortic Regurgitation
>
> Standard therapy for LV failure (Chap. 133). Vasodilators (long-acting nifedipine or ACE inhibitors) are recommended if hypertension present. Surgical valve replacement should be carried out in pts with severe AR when symptoms develop or in asymptomatic pts with LV dysfunction (LVEF <50%, LV end-systolic volume >55 mL/m², end-systolic diameter >55 mm, or LV diastolic dimension >75 mm) by imaging studies.

■ TRICUSPID STENOSIS (TS)

Etiology

Usually rheumatic; most common in females; almost invariably associated with MS.

Clinical Manifestations

Hepatomegaly, ascites, edema, jaundice, jugular venous distention with slow *y* descent (Chap. 119). Diastolic rumbling murmur along left sternal border increased by inspiration with loud presystolic component. Right atrial and superior vena caval enlargement on chest x-ray. Doppler echocardiography demonstrates thickened valve and impaired separation of leaflets and provides estimate of transvalvular gradient.

> **TREATMENT** **Tricuspid Stenosis**
>
> In severe TS, surgical relief is indicated, with valvular repair or replacement.

■ TRICUSPID REGURGITATION (TR)

Etiology
Usually functional and secondary to marked RV dilatation of any cause and often associated with pulmonary hypertension.

Clinical Manifestations
Severe RV failure, with edema, hepatomegaly, and prominent *v* waves in jugular venous pulse with rapid *y* descent (Chap. 119). Systolic murmur along lower left sternal edge is increased by inspiration. Doppler echocardiography confirms diagnosis and estimates severity.

> **TREATMENT** **Tricuspid Regurgitation**
>
> Intensive diuretic therapy when right-sided heart failure signs are present. In severe cases (in absence of severe pulmonary hypertension), surgical treatment consists of tricuspid annuloplasty or valve replacement.

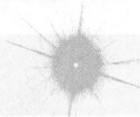

For a more detailed discussion, see O'Gara P, Loscalzo J: Valvular Heart Disease, Chap. 237, p. 1929, in HPIM-18.

CHAPTER **124**
Cardiomyopathies and Myocarditis

Cardiomyopathies are primary diseases of heart muscle. Table 124-1 summarizes distinguishing presenting features of the three major types of cardiomyopathy. Table 124-2 details the comprehensive initial evaluation of suspected cardiomyopathies.

■ DILATED CARDIOMYOPATHY (CMP)

Symmetrically dilated left ventricle (LV), with poor systolic contractile function; right ventricle (RV) commonly involved.

TABLE 124-1 PRESENTATION WITH SYMPTOMATIC CARDIOMYOPATHY

	Dilated	Restrictive	Hypertrophic
Ejection fraction (normal >55%)	Usually <30% when symptoms severe	25–50%	>60%
Left ventricular diastolic dimension (normal <55 mm)	≥60 mm	<60 mm (may be decreased)	Often decreased
Left ventricular wall thickness	Decreased	Normal or increased	Markedly increased
Atrial size	Increased	Increased; may be massive	Increased; related to abnormal
Valvular regurgitation	Related to annular dilation; mitral appears earlier, during decompensation; tricuspid regurgitation in late stages	Related to endocardial involvement; frequent mitral and tricuspid regurgitation, rarely severe	Related to valve-septum interaction; mitral regurgitation
Common first symptoms	Exertional intolerance	Exertional intolerance, fluid retention early	Exertional intolerance; may have chest pain
Congestive symptoms*	Left before right, except right prominent in young adults	Right often dominates	Left-sided congestion may develop late
Arrhythmia	Ventricular tachyarrhythmia; conduction block in Chagas' disease, and some families. Atrial fibrillation.	Ventricular uncommon except in sarcoidosis conduction block in sarcoidosis and amyloidosis. Atrial fibrillation.	Ventricular tachyarrhythmias; atrial fibrillation

*Left-sided symptoms of pulmonary congestion: dyspnea on exertion, orthopnea, paroxysmal nocturnal dyspnea. Right-sided symptoms of systemic versus congestion: discomfort on bending, hepatic and abdominal distention, peripheral edema.

Etiology

Approximately one-third of pts have a familial form, including those cases due to mutations in genes encoding sarcomeric proteins. Other causes include previous myocarditis, toxins [ethanol, certain antineoplastic agents (doxorubicin, trastuzumab, imatinib mesylate)], connective tissue disorders, muscular dystrophies, "peripartum." Impaired LV function owing to severe coronary disease/infarction or chronic aortic/mitral regurgitation may behave similarly.

TABLE 124-2 INITIAL EVALUATION OF CARDIOMYOPATHY

Clinical Evaluation

Thorough history and physical examination to identify cardiac and noncardiac disorders[a]

Detailed family history of heart failure, cardiomyopathy, skeletal myopathy, conduction disorders and tachyarrhythmias, sudden death

History of alcohol, illicit drugs, chemotherapy or radiation therapy[a]

Assessment of ability to perform routine and desired activities[a]

Assessment of volume status, orthostatic blood pressure, body mass index[a]

Laboratory Evaluation

Electrocardiogram[a]

Chest radiograph[a]

Two-dimensional and Doppler echocardiogram[a]

Chemistry:

    Serum sodium,[a] potassium,[a] calcium,[a] magnesium[a]

    Fasting glucose (glycohemoglobin in DM)

    Creatinine, [a] blood urea nitrogen[a]

    Albumin,[a] total protein,[a] liver function tests[a]

    Lipid profile

    Thyroid-stimulating hormone[a]

    Serum iron, transferrin saturation

    Urinalysis

    Creatine kinase

Hematology:

    Hemoglobin/hematocrit[a]

    White blood cell count with differential,[a] including eosinophils

    Erythrocyte sedimentation rate

Initial Evaluation Only in Pts Selected for Possible Specific Diagnosis

Titers for infection in presence of clinical suspicion:

    Acute viral (coxsackievirus virus, echovirus, influenza virus)

    Human immunodeficiency virus,

    Chagas' disease, Lyme disease, toxoplasmosis

Catheterization with coronary angiography in pts with angina who are candidates for intervention[a]

Serologies for active rheumatologic disease

Endomyocardial biopsy including sample for electron microscopy when suspecting specific diagnosis with therapeutic implications

Screening for sleep-disordered breathing

[a]Level I Recommendations from ACC/AHA Practice Guidelines for Chronic Heart Failure in the adult.
Source: From SA Hunt et al: Circulation 112: 2005.

Symptoms

Congestive heart failure (Chap. 133); tachyarrhythmias and peripheral emboli from LV mural thrombus occur.

Physical Examination

Jugular venous distention (JVD), rales, diffuse and dyskinetic LV apex, S_3, hepatomegaly, peripheral edema; murmurs of mitral and tricuspid regurgitation are common.

Laboratory ECG

Left bundle branch block and ST-T-wave abnormalities common.

CXR

Cardiomegaly, pulmonary vascular redistribution, pulmonary effusions common.

Echocardiogram, CT, and Cardiac MRI

LV and RV enlargement with globally impaired contraction. *Regional* wall motion abnormalities suggest coronary artery disease rather than primary cardiomyopathy.

B-Type Natriuretic Peptide (BNP)

Level elevated in heart failure/cardiomyopathy but not in pts with dyspnea due to lung disease.

TREATMENT Dilated Cardiomyopathy

Standard therapy of heart failure (Chap. 133): Diuretic for volume overload, vasodilator therapy with ACE inhibitor (preferred), angiotensin receptor blocker or hydralazine-nitrate combination shown to limit disease progression and improve longevity. Add beta blocker in most pts. Add spironolactone for pts with advanced heart failure. Consider chronic anticoagulation with warfarin if accompanying atrial fibrillation (AF), prior embolism, or recent large anterior MI. Antiarrhythmic drugs (e.g., amiodarone or dofetilide) may be useful to maintain sinus rhythm in pts with AF. Consider implanted cardioverter defibrillator for pts with ≥ class III heart failure and LVEF <35%. For those with persistent class III–IV heart failure, LVEF <35%, and QRS duration >120 ms, consider biventricular pacing. Possible trial of immunosuppressive drugs, if active myocarditis present on RV biopsy (controversial as long-term efficacy has not been demonstrated). In selected pts, consider cardiac transplantation.

■ RESTRICTIVE CARDIOMYOPATHY

Increased myocardial stiffness impairs ventricular relaxation; diastolic ventricular pressures are elevated. Etiologies include infiltrative disease (amyloid, sarcoid, hemochromatosis, eosinophilic disorders), endomyocardial fibrosis, Fabry's disease, and prior mediastinal irradiation.

Symptoms

Are of heart failure, although right-sided heart failure often predominates, with peripheral edema and ascites.

Physical Examination

Predominantly signs of right-sided heart failure: JVD, hepatomegaly, peripheral edema, murmur of tricuspid regurgitation. Left-sided S_4 is common.

Laboratory ECG

Low limb lead voltage, sinus tachycardia, ST-T-wave abnormalities.

CXR

Mild LV enlargement.

Echocardiogram, CT, Cardiac MRI

Bilateral atrial enlargement; increased ventricular thickness ("speckled pattern") in infiltrative disease, especially amyloidosis. Systolic function is usually normal but may be mildly reduced.

Cardiac Catheterization

Increased LV and RV diastolic pressures with "dip and plateau" pattern; RV biopsy useful in detecting infiltrative disease (rectal or fat pad biopsy useful in diagnosis of amyloidosis).

    Note: Must distinguish restrictive cardiomyopathy from constrictive pericarditis, which is surgically correctable. Thickening of pericardium in pericarditis usually apparent in CT or MRI.

TREATMENT	**Restrictive Cardiomyopathy**

Salt restriction and diuretics ameliorate pulmonary and systemic congestion; digitalis is not indicated unless systolic function is impaired or atrial arrhythmias are present. *Note:* Increased sensitivity to digitalis in amyloidosis. Anticoagulation often indicated, particularly in pts with eosinophilic endomyocarditis. For specific therapy of hemochromatosis and sarcoidosis, see Chaps. 357 and 329, respectively, in HPIM-18.

■ HYPERTROPHIC CARDIOMYOPATHY

Marked LV hypertrophy; often asymmetric, without underlying hypertension or valvular disease. Systolic function is usually normal; increased LV stiffness results in elevated diastolic filling pressures. Typically results from mutations in sarcomeric proteins (autosomal dominant transmission).

Symptoms

Secondary to elevated diastolic pressure, dynamic LV outflow obstruction (if present), and arrhythmias; dyspnea on exertion, angina, and presyncope; sudden death may occur.

Physical Examination

Brisk carotid upstroke with pulsus bisferiens; S_4, harsh systolic murmur along left sternal border, blowing murmur of mitral regurgitation at apex; murmur changes with Valsalva and other maneuvers (Chap. 119).

Laboratory ECG

LV hypertrophy with prominent "septal" Q waves in leads I, aVL, V_{5-6}. Periods of atrial fibrillation or ventricular tachycardia are often detected by Holter monitor.

Echocardiogram

LV hypertrophy, often with asymmetric involvement, especially of the septum or apex; LV contractile function typically excellent with small end-systolic volume. If LV outflow tract obstruction is present, systolic anterior motion (SAM) of mitral valve and midsystolic partial closure of aortic valve are present. Doppler shows early systolic accelerated blood flow through LV outflow tract.

TREATMENT Hypertrophic Cardiomyopathy

Strenuous exercise should be avoided. Beta blockers, verapamil, or disopyramide used individually to reduce symptoms. Digoxin, other inotropes, diuretics, and vasodilators are generally *contraindicated*. Endocarditis antibiotic prophylaxis (Chap. 89) is necessary only in pts with a prior history of endocarditis. Antiarrhythmic agents, especially amiodarone, may suppress atrial and ventricular arrhythmias. However, consider implantable cardioverter defibrillator for pts with high-risk profile, e.g., history of syncope or aborted cardiac arrest, nonsustained ventricular tachycardia, marked LVH (>3 cm), exertional hypotension, or family history of sudden death. In selected pts, LV outflow gradient can be reduced by controlled septal infarction by ethanol injection into the septal artery. Surgical myectomy may be useful in pts refractory to medical therapy.

■ MYOCARDITIS

Inflammation of the myocardium that may progress to chronic dilated cardiomyopathy, most commonly due to acute viral infection (e.g., parvovirus B19, coxsackievirus, adenovirus, Epstein-Barr virus). Myocarditis may also develop in pts with HIV infection, hepatitis C or Lyme disease. Chagas' disease is a common cause of myocarditis in endemic areas, typically Central and South America.

History

Fever, fatigue, palpitations; if LV dysfunction develops, symptoms of heart failure are present. Viral myocarditis may be preceded by URI.

Physical Examination

Fever, tachycardia, soft S_1; S_3 common.

Laboratory

CK-MB isoenzyme and cardiac troponins may be elevated in absence of MI. Convalescent antiviral antibody titers may rise.

ECG

Transient ST-T-wave abnormalities.

CXR

Cardiomegaly

Echocardiogram, Cardiac MRI

Depressed LV function; pericardial effusion present if accompanying pericarditis present. MRI demonstrates mid-wall gadolinium enhancement.

TREATMENT   **Myocarditis**

Rest; treat as heart failure (Chap. 133); efficacy of immunosuppressive therapy (e.g., steroids) has not been demonstrated except in isolated conditions such as sarcoidosis and giant cell myocarditis. In fulminant cases, cardiac transplantation may be indicated.

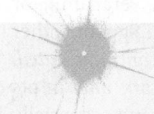

For a more detailed discussion, see Stevenson LW, Loscalzo J: Cardiomyopathy and Myocarditis, Chap. 238, p. 1951, in HPIM-18.

CHAPTER **125**
Pericardial Disease

◼ ACUTE PERICARDITIS

Etiologies (See Table 125-1)

History

Chest pain, which may be intense, mimicking acute MI, but characteristically sharp, pleuritic, and positional (relieved by leaning forward); fever and palpitations are common. Typical pain may not be present in slowly developing pericarditis (e.g., tuberculous, post-irradiation, neoplastic, uremic).

Physical Examination

Rapid or irregular pulse, coarse pericardial friction rub, which may vary in intensity and is loudest with pt sitting forward.

Laboratory ECG (See Table 125-2 and Fig. 125-1)

Diffuse ST elevation (concave upward) usually present in all leads except aVR and V_1; PR-segment depression (and/or PR elevation in lead aVR)

TABLE 125-1 MOST COMMON CAUSES OF PERICARDITIS

"Idiopathic"
Infections (particularly viral)
Acute myocardial infarction
Neoplasms
Mediastinal radiation therapy
Chronic renal failure
Connective tissue disease (e.g., rheumatoid arthritis, SLE)
Drug reaction (e.g., procainamide, hydralazine)
Post–cardiac injury (i.e., weeks following heart surgery or myocardial infarction)

may be present; *days* later (unlike acute MI), ST returns to baseline and T-wave inversion develops. Atrial premature beats and atrial fibrillation may appear. Differentiate from ECG of early repolarization (ER) (ratio of ST elevation/T wave height <0.25 in ER, but >0.25 in pericarditis).

CXR

Symmetrically increased size of cardiac silhouette if large (>250 mL) pericardial effusion is present.

Echocardiogram

Most readily available test for detection of pericardial effusion, which commonly accompanies acute pericarditis.

TABLE 125-2 ECG IN ACUTE PERICARDITIS VS ACUTE ST-ELEVATION MI

ST-Segment Elevation	ECG Lead Involvement	Evolution of ST and T Waves	PR-Segment Depression
Pericarditis			
Concave upward	All leads involved except aVR and V_1	ST remains elevated for several days; after ST returns to baseline, T waves invert	Yes, in majority
Acute ST elevation MI			
Convex upward	ST elevation over infarcted region only; reciprocal ST depression in opposite leads	In absence of successful reperfusion therapies: T waves invert within hours, while ST still elevated; followed by Q-wave development	No

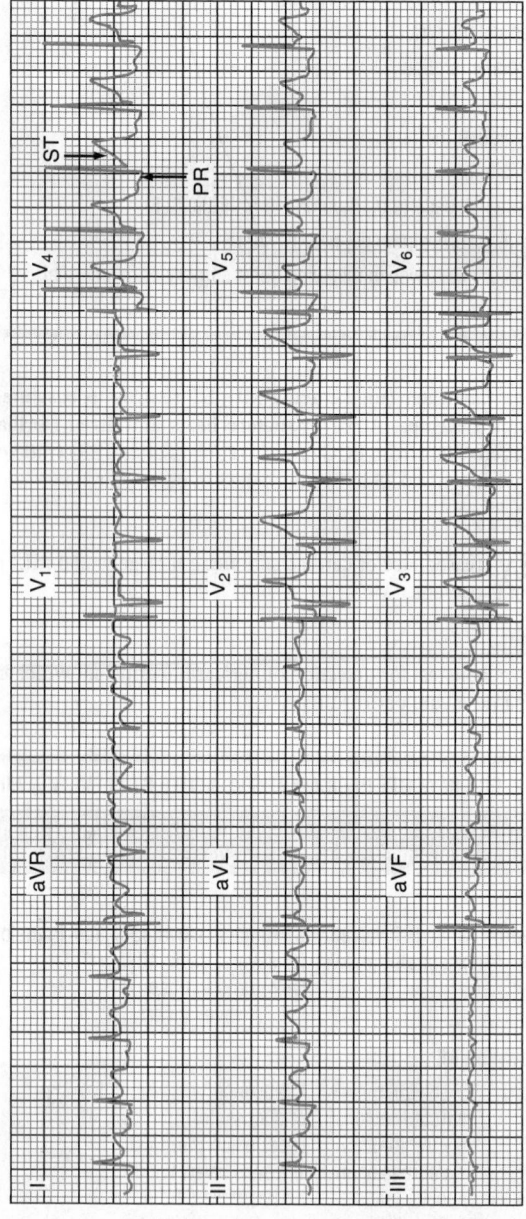

FIGURE 125-1 Electrocardiogram in acute pericarditis. Note diffuse ST-segment elevation and PR-segment depression.

TREATMENT ▶ Acute Pericarditis

Aspirin 650–975 mg qid or other NSAIDs (e.g., ibuprofen 400–600 mg tid or indomethacin 25–50 mg tid); addition of colchicine 0.6 mg bid may be beneficial and reduces frequency of recurrences. For *severe, refractory* pain, prednisone 40–80 mg/d can be used as last resort. Intractable, prolonged pain or frequently recurrent episodes may require pericardiectomy. Anticoagulants are relatively contraindicated in acute pericarditis because of risk of pericardial hemorrhage.

■ CARDIAC TAMPONADE

Life-threatening condition resulting from accumulation of pericardial fluid under pressure; impaired filling of cardiac chambers and decreased cardiac output.

Etiology

Previous pericarditis (most commonly metastatic tumor, uremia, viral or idiopathic pericarditis), cardiac trauma, or myocardial perforation during catheter or pacemaker placement.

History

Hypotension may develop suddenly; subacute symptoms include dyspnea, weakness, confusion.

Physical Examination

Tachycardia, hypotension, pulsus paradoxus (inspiratory fall in systolic blood pressure >10 mmHg), jugular venous distention with preserved x descent but loss of y descent; heart sounds distant. If tamponade develops subacutely, peripheral edema, hepatomegaly, and ascites may be present.

Laboratory ECG

Low limb lead voltage; large effusions may cause electrical alternans (alternating size of QRS complex due to swinging of heart).

CXR

Enlarged cardiac silhouette if large (>250 mL) effusion present.

Echocardiogram

Swinging motion of heart within large effusion; prominent respiratory alteration of RV dimension with RA and RV collapse during diastole. Doppler shows marked respiratory variation of transvalvular flow velocities.

Cardiac Catheterization

Confirms diagnosis; shows equalization of diastolic pressures in all four chambers; pericardial = RA pressure.

TREATMENT ▶ Cardiac Tamponade

Immediate pericardiocentesis and IV volume expansion.

■ CONSTRICTIVE PERICARDITIS

Condition in which a rigid pericardium impairs cardiac filling, causing elevation of systemic and pulmonary venous pressures, and decreased cardiac output. Results from healing and scar formation in some pts with previous pericarditis. Viral, tuberculosis (mostly in developing nations), previous cardiac surgery, collagen vascular disorders, uremia, neoplastic and radiation-associated pericarditis are potential causes.

History

Gradual onset of dyspnea, fatigue, pedal edema, abdominal swelling; symptoms of LV failure uncommon.

Physical Examination

Tachycardia, jugular venous distention (with prominent *y* descent) that increases further on inspiration (Kussmaul sign); hepatomegaly, ascites, peripheral edema are common; sharp diastolic sound, "pericardial knock" following S$_2$ sometimes present.

Laboratory ECG

Low limb lead voltage; atrial arrhythmias are common.

CXR

Rim of pericardial calcification is most common in tuberculous pericarditis.

Echocardiogram

Thickened pericardium, normal ventricular contraction; abrupt halt in ventricular filling in early diastole. Dilatation of IVC is common. Dramatic

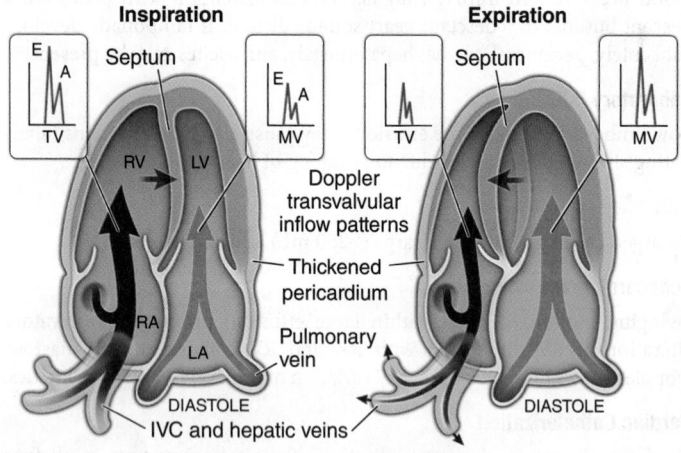

FIGURE 125-2 Constrictive pericarditis. Doppler schema of respirophasic changes in mitral and tricuspid inflow. Reciprocal patterns of ventricular filling are assessed on pulsed Doppler examination of mitral (MV) and tricuspid (TV) inflow. *(Courtesy of Bernard E. Bulwer, MD; with permission.)*

effects of respiration are typical: During inspiration the ventricular septum shifts to the left with prominent reduction of blood flow velocity across mitral valve; pattern reverses during expiration (Fig 125-2).

CT or MRI

More precise than echocardiogram for demonstrating thickened pericardium.

Cardiac Catheterization

Equalization of diastolic pressures in all chambers; ventricular pressure tracings show "dip and plateau" appearance. Differentiate from restrictive cardiomyopathy (Table 125-3).

| **TREATMENT** | **Constrictive Pericarditis** |

Surgical stripping of the pericardium. Progressive improvement ensues over several months.

TABLE 125-3 FEATURES THAT DIFFERENTIATE CONSTRICTIVE PERICARDITIS FROM RESTRICTIVE CARDIOMYOPATHY

	Constrictive Pericarditis	Restrictive Cardiomyopathy
Physical exam		
Kussmaul sign	Present	May be present
Pericardial knock	May be present	Absent
Chest X-ray		
Pericardial calcification	May be present	Absent
Echocardiography		
Thickened pericardium	Present	Absent
Thickened myocardium	Absent	Present
Exaggerated variation in transvalvular velocities	Present	Absent
CT or MRI		
Thickened pericardium	Present	Absent
Cardiac catheterization		
Equalized RV and LV diastolic pressures	Yes	Often LV > RV
Elevated PA systolic pressure	Uncommon	Usual
Effect of inspiration on systolic pressures	Discordant: LV↓, RV↑	Concordant: LV↓, RV↓
Endomyocardial biopsy	Normal	Usually abnormal (e.g., amyloid)

Abbreviations: LV, left ventricle; PA, pulmonary artery; RV, right ventricle.

If careful history and physical exam do not suggest etiology, the following may lead to diagnosis:

- Skin test and cultures for tuberculosis (Chap. 103)
- Serum albumin and urine protein measurement (nephrotic syndrome)
- Serum creatinine and BUN (renal failure)
- Thyroid function tests (myxedema)
- Antineutrophil antibodies (SLE and other collagen-vascular disease)
- Search for a primary tumor (especially lung and breast)

For a more detailed discussion, see Braunwald E: Pericardial Disease, Chap. 239, p. 1971, in HPIM-18.

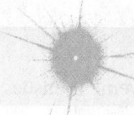

CHAPTER **126**
Hypertension

Definition

Chronic elevation in bp (systolic ≥140 mmHg or diastolic ≥90 mmHg); etiology unknown in 80–95% of pts ("essential hypertension"). Always consider a secondary correctable form of hypertension, especially in pts under age 30 or those who become hypertensive after 55. Isolated systolic hypertension (systolic ≥140, diastolic <90) most common in elderly pts, due to reduced vascular compliance.

■ SECONDARY HYPERTENSION

Renal Artery Stenosis (Renovascular Hypertension)

Due to either atherosclerosis (older men) or fibromuscular dysplasia (young women). Presents with recent onset of hypertension, refractory to usual antihypertensive therapy. Abdominal bruit is present in 50% of cases; often audible; mild hypokalemia due to activation of the renin-angiotensin-aldosterone system may be present.

Renal Parenchymal Disease

Elevated serum creatinine and/or abnormal urinalysis, containing protein, cells, or casts.

Coarctation of Aorta

Presents in children or young adults; constriction is usually present in aorta at origin of left subclavian artery. Exam shows diminished, delayed femoral pulsations; late systolic murmur loudest over the midback. CXR shows indentation of the aorta at the level of the coarctation and rib notching (due to development of collateral arterial flow).

Pheochromocytoma

A catecholamine-secreting tumor, typically of the adrenal medulla or extraadrenal paraganglion tissue, that presents as paroxysmal or sustained hypertension in young to middle-aged pts. Sudden episodes of headache, palpitations, and profuse diaphoresis are common. Associated findings include chronic weight loss, orthostatic *hypotension*, and impaired glucose tolerance. Pheochromocytomas may be localized to the bladder wall and may present with micturition-associated symptoms of catecholamine excess. Diagnosis is suggested by elevated plasma metanephrine level or urinary catecholamine metabolites in a 24-h urine collection (see below); the tumor is then localized by CT scan or MRI.

Hyperaldosteronism

Usually due to aldosterone-secreting adenoma or bilateral adrenal hyperplasia. Should be suspected when hypokalemia is present in a hypertensive pt off diuretics (Chap. 182).

Other Causes

Oral contraceptive usage, obstructive sleep apnea (Chap. 146), Cushing's and adrenogenital syndromes (Chap. 182), thyroid disease (Chap. 181), hyperparathyroidism, and acromegaly (Chap. 179). In pts with systolic hypertension and wide pulse pressure, consider thyrotoxicosis, aortic regurgitation (Chap. 123), and systemic AV fistula.

APPROACH TO THE PATIENT | **Hypertension**

History: Most pts are asymptomatic. Severe hypertension may lead to headache, dizziness, or blurred vision.

Clues to specific forms of secondary hypertension: Use of medications (e.g., birth control pills, glucocorticoids, decongestants, erythropoietin, NSAIDs, cyclosporine); paroxysms of headache, sweating, or tachycardia (pheochromocytoma); history of renal disease or abdominal trauma (renal hypertension); daytime somnolence and snoring (sleep apnea).

Physical examination: Measure bp with appropriate-sized cuff (large cuff for large arm). Measure bp in both arms as well as a leg (to evaluate for aortic coarctation). Signs of hypertension include retinal arteriolar changes (narrowing/nicking); left ventricular lift, loud A_2, S_4. Clues to secondary forms of hypertension include cushingoid appearance, thyromegaly, abdominal bruit (renal artery stenosis), delayed femoral pulses (coarctation of aorta).

Laboratory Workup

Screening tests for secondary hypertension: Should be carried out on all pts with documented hypertension: (1) serum creatinine, BUN, and urinalysis (renal parenchymal disease); (2) serum K measured off diuretics (hypokalemia prompts workup for hyperaldosteronism or renal artery stenosis); (3) CXR (rib notching or indentation of distal aortic arch in coarctation of the aorta); (4) ECG (LV hypertrophy suggests chronicity of hypertension); (5) other useful screening blood tests including CBC, glucose, lipid levels, calcium, uric acid; (6) thyroid-stimulating hormone if thyroid disease suspected.

Further workup: Indicated for specific diagnoses if screening tests are abnormal or bp is refractory to antihypertensive therapy: (1) *renal artery stenosis:* magnetic resonance angiography, captopril renogram, renal duplex ultrasound, digital subtraction angiography, renal arteriography; (2) *Cushing's syndrome:* dexamethasone suppression test (Chap. 182); (3) *pheochromocytoma:* 24-h urine collection for catecholamines, metanephrines, and vanillylmandelic acid and/or measurement of plasma metanephrine; (4) *primary hyperaldosteronism:* depressed plasma renin activity and hypersecretion of aldosterone, both of which fail to change with volume expansion; (5) *renal parenchymal disease* (Chap. 149).

TREATMENT Hypertension

Helpful lifestyle modifications include weight reduction (to attain BMI <25 kg/m²); sodium restriction; diet rich in fruits, vegetables, and low-fat dairy products; regular exercise; and moderation of alcohol consumption.

DRUG THERAPY OF ESSENTIAL HYPERTENSION (SEE TABLE 126-1 AND FIG. 126-1) Goal is to control hypertension with minimal side effects. A combination of medications with complementary actions is often required. First-line agents include diuretics, ACE inhibitors, angiotensin receptor antagonists, calcium channel antagonists, and beta blockers. On-treatment blood pressure goal is <135–140 systolic, <80–85 diastolic (<130/80 in pts with diabetes or chronic kidney disease).

Diuretics Should be cornerstone of most antihypertensive regimens. Thiazides preferred over loop diuretics because of longer duration of action; however, the latter are more potent when serum creatinine >2.5 mg/dL. Major side effects include hypokalemia, hyperglycemia, and hyperuricemia, which can be minimized by using low dosage (e.g., hydrochlorothiazide 6.25–50 mg qd). Diuretics are particularly effective in elderly and black pts. Prevention of hypokalemia is especially important in pts on digitalis glycosides.

ACE Inhibitors and Angiotensin II Receptor Blockers (ARBs) ACE inhibitors and ARBs are well tolerated with low frequency of side effects. May be used as monotherapy or in combination with a diuretic, calcium antagonist, or beta blocker. Side effects are uncommon and include angioedema (more common with ACE inhibitors than ARBs), hyperkalemia, and azotemia (particularly in pts with elevated baseline serum creatinine). A nonproductive cough may develop in the course of

TABLE 126-1 ORAL DRUGS COMMONLY USED IN TREATMENT OF HYPERTENSION

Drug Class	Examples	Usual Total Daily Dose (Dosing Frequency/Day)	Potential Adverse Effects
Diuretics			
Thiazides	Hydrochlorothiazide	6.25–50 mg (1–2)	Hypokalemia, hyperuricemia, hyperglycemia, ↑ cholesterol, ↑ triglycerides
Thiazide-like	Chlorthalidone	25–50 mg (1)	same as above
Loop diuretics	Furosemide	40–80 mg (2–3)	Hypokalemia, hyperuricemia
K⁺-retaining	Spironolactone	25–100 mg (1–2)	Hyperkalemia, gynecomastia
	Eplerenone	50–100 mg (1–2)	Hyperkalemia
	Amiloride	5–10 mg (1–2)	
	Triamterene	50–100 mg (1–2)	
Beta blockers			
β₁-selective	Atenolol	25–100 mg (1–2)	Bronchospasm, bradycardia, heart block, fatigue, sexual dysfunction, ↑ triglycerides, ↓ HDL
	Metoprolol	25–100 mg (1–2)	same as above
Nonselective	Propranolol	40–160 mg (2)	same as above
	Propranolol LA	60–180 mg (1)	same as above
Combined alpha/beta	Labetolol	200–800 mg (2)	Bronchospasm, bradycardia, heart block
	Carvedilol	12.5–50 mg (2)	

(continued)

TABLE 126-1 ORAL DRUGS COMMONLY USED IN TREATMENT OF HYPERTENSION (CONTINUED)

Drug Class	Examples	Usual Total Daily Dose (Dosing Frequency/Day)	Potential Adverse Effects
ACE inhibitors	Captopril	25–200 mg (2)	Cough, hyperkalemia, azotemia, angioedema
	Lisinopril	10–40 mg (1)	
	Ramipril	2.5–20 mg (1–2)	
Angiotensin II receptor blockers	Losartan	25–100 mg (1–2)	Hyperkalemia, azotemia
	Valsartan	80–320 mg (1)	
	Candesartan	2–32 mg (1–2)	
Calcium channel antagonists			
Dihydropyridines	Nifedipine long-acting	30–60 mg (1)	Edema, constipation
Nondihydropyridines	Verapamil long-acting	120–360 mg (1–2)	Edema, constipation, bradycardia, heart block
	Diltiazem long-acting	180–420 mg (1)	

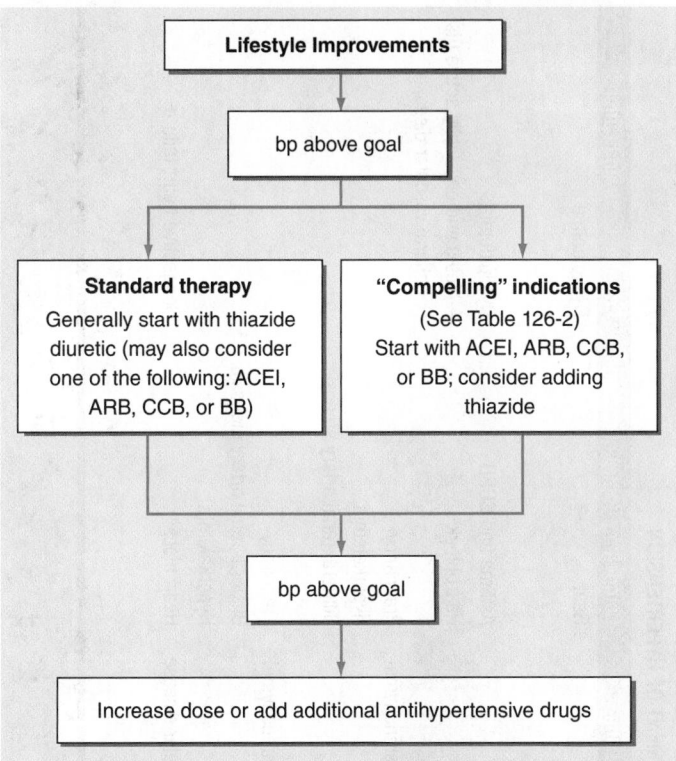

FIGURE 126-1 Initiation of therapy in pts with hypertension. ACEI, angiotensin-converting enzyme inhibitor; ARB, angiotensin receptor blocker; CCB, calcium channel blocker; BB, beta blocker.

therapy in up to 15% of pts on an ACE inhibitor, prompting substitution with an ARB (cough is not common side effect) or alternate antihypertensives. Note that renal function may deteriorate rapidly as a result of inhibition of the renin-angiotensin system in pts with bilateral renal artery stenosis.

Potassium supplements and potassium-sparing diuretics should be used cautiously with ACE inhibitors or ARBs to prevent hyperkalemia. If pt is intravascularly volume depleted, hold diuretics for 2–3 days prior to initiation of drug, which should then be administered at low dosage.

Calcium Antagonists Direct arteriolar vasodilators; all have negative inotropic effects (particularly verapamil) and should be used cautiously if LV dysfunction is present. Verapamil and, to a lesser extent, diltiazem can result in bradycardia and AV block, so combination with beta blockers is generally avoided. Use sustained-release formulations, as short-acting dihydropyridine calcium channel blockers may increase incidence of coronary events. Common side effects include peripheral edema and constipation.

TABLE 126-2 GUIDELINES FOR SELECTING INITIAL DRUG TREATMENT OF HYPERTENSION

Class of Drug	Compelling Indications	Possible Indications	Compelling Contraindications	Possible Contraindications
Diuretics	Heart failure Elderly pts Systolic hypertension		Gout	Dyslipidemia
Beta blockers	Angina After MI Tachyarrhythmias	Heart failure Pregnancy	Asthma and COPD Heart block[a]	Dyslipidemia Athletes and physically active pts Peripheral vascular disease
ACE inhibitors	Heart failure LV dysfunction After MI Diabetic nephropathy	Chronic renal parenchymal disease	Pregnancy Hyperkalemia Bilateral renal artery stenosis	
Angiotensin receptor blockers	ACE inhibitor cough Heart failure Diabetic nephropathy	Chronic renal parenchymal disease	Pregnancy Bilateral renal artery stenosis Hyperkalemia	
Calcium channel blockers	Angina Elderly pts Systolic hypertension	Peripheral vascular disease	Heart block[b]	Congestive heart failure[c]

[a]Grade 2 or 3 atrioventricular block.

[b]Grade 2 or 3 atrioventricular block with verapamil or diltiazem.

[c]Verapamil or diltiazem.

Abbreviations: ACE, angiotensin-converting enzyme; ARB, angiotensin receptor blocker; COPD, chronic obstructive pulmonary disease; LV, left ventricular; MI, myocardial infarction.

TABLE 126-3 USUAL INTRAVENOUS DOSES OF ANTIHYPERTENSIVE AGENTS USED IN HYPERTENSIVE EMERGENCIES[a]

Antihypertensive Agent	IV Dose
Nitroprusside	Initial 0.3 (mg/kg)/min; usual 2–4 (mg/kg)/min; maximum 10 (mg/kg)/min for 10 min
Nicardipine	Initial 5 mg/h; titrate by 2.5 mg/h at 5–15 min intervals; max 15 mg/h
Labetalol	2 mg/min up to 300 mg *or* 20 mg over 2 min, then 40–80 mg at 10-min intervals up to 300 mg total
Enalaprilat	Usual 0.625–1.25 mg over 5 min every 6–8 h; maximum 5 mg/dose
Esmolol	Initial 80–500 mg/kg over 1 min, then 50–300 (mg/kg)/min
Phentolamine	5–15 mg bolus
Nitroglycerin	Initial 5 mg/min, then titrate by 5 mg/min at 3–5 min intervals; if no response is seen at 20 mg/min, incremental increases of 10–20 mg/min may be used
Hydralazine	10–50 mg at 30-min intervals

[a]Constant blood pressure monitoring is required. Start with the lowest dose. Subsequent doses and intervals of administration should be adjusted according to the blood pressure response and duration of action of the specific agent.

If bp proves refractory to drug therapy, work up for secondary forms of hypertension, especially renal artery stenosis and pheochromocytoma.

Beta Blockers Particularly useful in young pts with "hyperkinetic" circulation. Begin with low dosage (e.g., metoprolol succinate 25–50 mg daily). Relative contraindications: bronchospasm, CHF, AV block, bradycardia, and "brittle" insulin-dependent diabetes.

Table 126-2 lists compelling indications for specific initial drug treatment.

SPECIAL CIRCUMSTANCES

Pregnancy Most commonly used antihypertensives include methyldopa (250–1000 mg PO bid-tid), labetalol (100–200 mg bid), and hydralazine (10–150 mg PO bid-tid). Calcium channel blockers (e.g., nifedipine, long-acting, 30–60 mg daily) also appear to be safe in pregnancy. Beta blockers should be used cautiously; fetal hypoglycemia and low birth weights have been reported. ACE inhibitors and ARBs are *contraindicated* in pregnancy.

Renal Disease Standard thiazide diuretics may not be effective. Consider metolazone, furosemide, or bumetanide, alone or in combination.

Diabetes Goal bp <130/80. Consider ACE inhibitors and angiotensin receptor blockers as first-line therapy to control bp and slow renal deterioration.

Malignant Hypertension   Defined as an abrupt increase in bp in pt with chronic hypertension or sudden onset of severe hypertension; a medical emergency. Immediate therapy is mandatory if there is evidence of cardiac decompensation (CHF, angina), encephalopathy (headache, seizures, visual disturbances), or deteriorating renal function. Inquire about use of cocaine, amphetamines, or monoamine oxidase inhibitors. Drugs to treat hypertensive crisis are listed in Table 126-3. Replace with PO antihypertensive as pt becomes asymptomatic and bp improves.

For a more detailed discussion, see Kotchen TA: Hypertensive Vascular Disease, Chap. 247, p. 2042, in HPIM-18.

CHAPTER **127**
Metabolic Syndrome

The *metabolic syndrome* (*insulin resistance syndrome, syndrome X*) is an important risk factor for cardiovascular disease and type 2 diabetes; it consists of a constellation of metabolic abnormalities that includes central obesity, insulin resistance, hypertension, dyslipidemia, and endothelial dysfunction. The prevalence of metabolic syndrome varies among ethnic groups; it increases with age, degree of obesity and propensity to type 2 diabetes. In the United States, 44% of persons over age 50 have the metabolic syndrome; women are affected in greater numbers than men.

ETIOLOGY

Overweight/obesity (especially central adiposity), sedentary lifestyle, increasing age, and lipodystrophy are all risk factors for the metabolic syndrome. The exact cause is not known and may be multifactorial. Insulin resistance is central to the development of the metabolic syndrome. Increased intracellular fatty acid metabolites contribute to insulin resistance by impairing insulin-signaling pathways and accumulating as triglycerides in skeletal and cardiac muscle, while stimulating hepatic glucose and triglyceride production. Excess adipose tissue leads to increased production of proinflammatory cytokines.

CLINICAL FEATURES

There are no specific symptoms of the metabolic syndrome. The major features include central obesity, hypertriglyceridemia, low HDL cholesterol, hyperglycemia, and hypertension (Table 127-1). Associated conditions include cardiovascular disease, type 2 diabetes, nonalcoholic fatty liver disease, hyperuricemia/gout, polycystic ovary syndrome, and obstructive sleep apnea.

TABLE 127-1 NCEP:ATPIII 2001 AND IDF CRITERIA FOR THE METABOLIC SYNDROME

NCEP:ATPIII 2001 Criteria
Three or more of the following:
Central obesity: Waist circumference >102 cm (M), >88 cm (F)
Hypertriglyceridemia: Triglycerides ≥150 mg/dL or specific medication
Low HDL cholesterol: <40 mg/dL (M) and <50 mg/dL (F) or specific medication
Hypertension: Blood pressure ≥130 mm systolic or ≥85 mm diastolic or specific medication
Fasting plasma glucose ≥100 mg/dL or specific medication or previously diagnosed type 2 diabetes

IDF Criteria		
Differ from NCEP: ATPIII 2001 criteria by more stringent and ethnicity-specific waist circumference limits. Other criteria are the same.		
Waist circumference:	Europid,	≥94 cm (M), ≥80 cm (F)
	Sub-Saharan African	
	Eastern and Middle Eastern	
	South Asian, Chinese	≥90 cm (M), ≥80 cm (F)
	South and Central American	
	Japanese	≥90 cm (M), ≥80 cm (F)

Abbreviations: HDL, high-density lipoprotein; IDF, International Diabetes Foundation; NCEP:ATPIII, National Cholesterol Education Program, Adult Treatment Panel III.

■ **DIAGNOSIS**

The diagnosis of the metabolic syndrome relies on satisfying the criteria listed in Table 127-1. Screening for associated conditions should be undertaken.

TREATMENT Metabolic Syndrome

Obesity is the driving force behind the metabolic syndrome. Thus, weight reduction is the primary approach to this disorder. In general, recommendations for weight loss include a combination of caloric restriction, increased physical activity, and behavior modification. Weight loss drugs (orlistat) or bariatric surgery are adjuncts that may be considered for obesity management (Chap. 183). Metformin or thiazolidinedione (pioglitazone) reduce insulin resistance. Hypertension (Chap. 126), impaired fasting glucose or diabetes (Chap. 184), and lipid abnormalities (Chap. 189) should be managed according to current guidelines. The antihypertensive regimen should include an angiotensin-converting enzyme (ACE) inhibitor or angiotensin receptor blocker when possible.

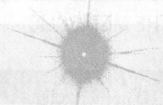

For a more detailed discussion, see Eckel RH: The Metabolic Syndrome, Chap. 242, p. 1992, in HPIM-18.

CHAPTER **128**
ST-Segment Elevation Myocardial Infarction (STEMI)

Early recognition and immediate treatment of acute MI are essential; diagnosis is based on characteristic history, ECG, and serum cardiac markers.

Symptoms

Chest pain similar to angina (Chap. 37) but more intense and persistent; not fully relieved by rest or nitroglycerin, often accompanied by nausea, sweating, apprehension. However, ~25% of MIs are clinically silent.

Physical Examination

Pallor, diaphoresis, tachycardia, S_4, dyskinetic cardiac impulse may be present. If CHF exists, rales and S_3 are present. Jugular venous distention is common in right ventricular infarction.

ECG

ST elevation, followed (if acute reperfusion is not achieved) by T-wave inversion, then Q-wave development over several hours (see Figs. 120-3 and 120-4).

Non-ST Elevation MI, or NSTEMI

ST depression followed by persistent ST-T-wave changes *without* Q-wave development. Comparison with old ECG helpful (see Chap. 129).

Cardiac Biomarkers

Cardiac-specific troponins T and I are highly specific for myocardial injury and are the preferred biochemical markers for diagnosis of acute MI. They remain elevated for 7–10 days. Creatine phosphokinase (CK) level rises within 4–8 h, peaks at 24 h, and returns to normal by 48–72 h. CK-MB isoenzyme is more specific for MI but may also be elevated with myocarditis or after electrical cardioversion. Total CK (but not CK-MB) rises (two- to threefold) after IM injection, vigorous exercise, or other skeletal muscle trauma. A ratio of CK-MB mass:CK activity ≥2.5 suggests acute MI. CK-MB peaks earlier (about 8 h) following acute reperfusion therapy (see below). Serum cardiac markers should be measured at presentation, 6–9 h later, and then at 12–24 h.

Noninvasive Imaging Techniques

Useful when diagnosis of MI is not clear. *Echocardiography* detects infarct-associated regional wall motion abnormalities (but cannot distinguish acute MI from a previous myocardial scar). Echo is also useful in detecting RV infarction, LV aneurysm, and LV thrombus. *Myocardial perfusion imaging* (thallium 201 or technetium 99m-sestamibi) is sensitive for regions of decreased perfusion, but is not specific for acute MI. *MRI with delayed gadolinium enhancement* accurately indicates regions of infarction, but is technically difficult to obtain in acutely ill pts.

TREATMENT STEMI

INITIAL THERAPY Initial goals are to (1) quickly identify if pt is candidate for reperfusion therapy, (2) relieve pain, and (3) prevent/treat arrhythmias and mechanical complications.

- Aspirin should be administered immediately (162–325 mg chewed at presentation, then 162–325 mg PO qd), unless pt is aspirin-intolerant.
- Perform targeted history, exam, and ECG to identify STEMI (>1 mm ST elevation in two contiguous limb leads, ≥2 mm ST elevation in two contiguous precordial leads, or new LBBB) and appropriateness of reperfusion therapy [percutaneous coronary intervention (PCI) or IV fibrinolytic agent], which reduces infarct size, LV dysfunction, and mortality.
- Primary PCI is generally more effective than fibrinolysis and is preferred at experienced centers capable of performing the procedure rapidly (Fig. 128-1), especially when diagnosis is in doubt, cardiogenic shock is present, bleeding risk is increased, or symptoms have been present for >3 h.
- Proceed with IV fibrinolysis if PCI is not available or if logistics would delay PCI >1 h longer than fibrinolysis could be initiated (Fig. 128-1). Door-to-needle time should be <30 min for maximum benefit. Ensure absence of contraindications (Fig. 128-2) before administering fibrinolytic agent. Those treated within 1–3 h benefit most; can still be useful up to 12 h if chest pain is persistent or ST remains elevated in leads that have not developed new Q waves. Complications include bleeding, reperfusion arrhythmias, and, in case of streptokinase (SK), allergic reactions. Enoxaparin or heparin [60 U/kg (maximum 4000 U), then 12 (U/kg)/h (maximum 1000 U/h)] should be initiated with fibrinolytic agents (Fig. 128-2); maintain activated partial thromboplastin time (aPTT) at 1.5–2.0 × control (~50–70 s).
- If chest pain or ST elevation persists >90 min after fibrinolysis, consider referral for rescue PCI. Coronary angiography after fibrinolysis should also be considered for pts with recurrent angina or high-risk features (Fig. 128-2) including extensive ST elevation, signs of heart failure (rales, S_3, jugular venous distension, LVEF ≤35%), or systolic BP <100 mmHg.

The initial management of NSTEMI (non-Q MI) is different (Chap. 129). In particular, fibrinolytic therapy should not be administered.

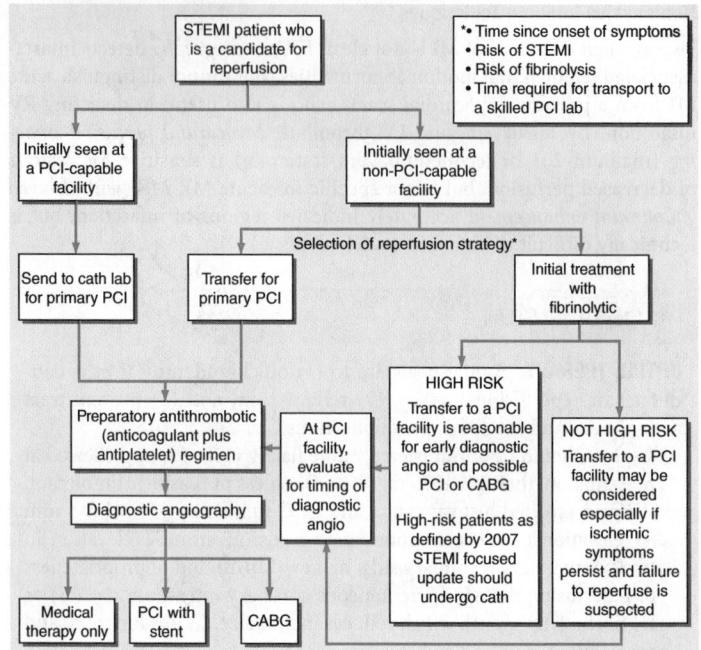

FIGURE 128-1 Reperfusion strategies in STEMI. *[Adapted from Kushner FG et al: 2009 focused update of the ACC/AHA Guidelines for the Management of Patients with ST-Elevation Myocardial Infarction (updating the 2004 guideline and 2007 focused update): A report of the American College of Cardiology Foundation/American Heart Association Task Force on Practice Guidelines. Circulation 120:2271, 2009.]*

ADDITIONAL STANDARD TREATMENT (Whether or not reperfusion therapy is undertaken):

- *Hospitalize in CCU* with continuous ECG monitoring.
- *IV line* for emergency arrhythmia treatment.
- *Pain control:* (1) Morphine sulfate 2–4 mg IV q5–10 min until pain is relieved or side effects develop [nausea, vomiting, respiratory depression (treat with naloxone 0.4–1.2 mg IV), hypotension (if bradycardic, treat with atropine 0.5 mg IV; otherwise use careful volume infusion)]; (2) nitroglycerin 0.3 mg SL if systolic bp >100 mmHg; for refractory pain: IV nitroglycerin (begin at 10 µg/min, titrate upward to maximum of 200 µg/min, monitoring bp closely); do not administer nitrates within 24 h of sildenafil or within 48 h of tadalafil (used for erectile dysfunction); (3) β-adrenergic antagonists (see below).
- *Oxygen:* 2–4 L/min by nasal cannula (if needed to maintain O_2 saturation >90%).
- Mild *sedation* (e.g., diazepam 5 mg, oxazepam 15–30 mg, or lorazepam 0.5–2 mg PO three to four times daily).
- *Soft diet* and stool softeners (e.g., docusate sodium 100–200 mg/d).

SELECTION CRITERIA

1. Acute chest discomfort characteristic of myocardial infarction
2. ECG criteria for ST-elevation MI (a, b, or c):
   a. ST elevation ≥ 0.1 mV (1 mm) in at least 2 leads of either:
      Inferior group: II, III, aVF
      Lateral group: I, aVL, V₅, V₆
   b. ST elevation ≥ 0.2 mV (1 mm) in at least 2 contiguous anterior leads (V₁–V₄)
   c. New LBBB
3. Primary PCI not available, or delay to PCI would be >1 h longer than initiation of fibrinolysis

ASSESS FOR CONTRAINDICATIONS

- Prior intracranial bleeding
- Intracranial malignancy or vascular malformation
- Ischemic stroke or head trauma in previous 3 months
- Aortic dissection
- Active bleeding (with exception of menses)
- Internal bleeding in previous 4 weeks
- Severe hypertension (systolic >180 or diastolic >110)
- Prolonged (>10 min) CPR chest compressions
- INR ≥ 2.0 on warfarin, or known bleeding diathesis
- Pregnancy

FIBRINOLYTIC DRUG	INTRAVENOUS DOSAGE
Streptokinase	1.5 million U over 60 min
Alteplase*	15-mg bolus, then 0.75 mg/kg (up to 50 mg) over 30 min, then 0.5 mg/kg (up to 35 mg) over 60 min
Reteplase*	10 U over 2 min; repeat same dose 30 min later
Tenecteplase*	Single bolus of 0.53 mg/kg over 10 sec.

*If alteplase, reteplase, or tenecteplase used, also administer IV heparin 60-U/kg bolus (maximum 4000 U) followed by 12 (U/kg)/h (maximum 1000 U/h), then adjusted to maintain aPTT at 1.5–2 x control (~50–70 s) for 48 h

SUBSEQUENT CORONARY ANGIOGRAPHY RESERVED FOR

- Failure of reperfusion (persistent chest pain or ST elevation after 90 min)
- Spontaneous recurrent ischemia during hospitalization
- High risk features: e.g., extensive ST elevation, heart failure, hypotension

FIGURE 128-2 Algorithm for fibrinolytic therapy of acute STEMI.

- β-*Adrenergic blockers* (Chap. 126) reduce myocardial O_2 consumption, limit infarct size, and reduce mortality. Especially useful in pts with hypertension, tachycardia, or persistent ischemic pain; contraindications include active CHF, systolic bp <95 mmHg, heart rate <50 beats/min, AV block, or history of bronchospasm. Consider IV (e.g., metoprolol 5 mg q2–5min to total dose of 15 mg) if pt is hypertensive. Otherwise, begin PO regimen (e.g., metoprolol tartrate 25–50 mg four times daily).

- *Anticoagulation/antiplatelet agents:* Pts who receive fibrinolytic therapy are begun on heparin and aspirin as indicated above. In absence of fibrinolytic therapy, administer aspirin, 160–325 mg qd, and low-dose heparin (5000 U SC q12h) or low-molecular-weight heparin (LMWH, e.g., enoxaparin 40 mg SC daily) for DVT prevention. Full-dose IV heparin (PTT 1.5-2 × control) or LMWH (e.g., enoxaparin 1 mg/kg SC q12h) followed by oral anticoagulants is recommended for pts with severe CHF, presence of ventricular thrombus by echocardiogram, or large dyskinetic region in acute anterior MI. If used, oral anticoagulants are continued for 3–6 months, then replaced by aspirin. The addition of a P2Y12 platelet receptor antagonist after STEMI (e.g., clopidogrel 75 mg daily) reduces future adverse cardiac events whether or not fibrinolysis or PCI are undertaken.
- *ACE inhibitors* reduce mortality in pts following acute MI and should be prescribed within 24 h of hospitalization for pts with STEMI—e.g., captopril (6.25 mg PO test dose advanced to 50 mg PO tid). ACE inhibitors should be continued indefinitely after discharge in pts with CHF or those with asymptomatic LV dysfunction (ejection fraction ≤40%); if pt is ACE inhibitor intolerant, use ARB (e.g., valsartan or candesartan).
- *Aldosterone antagonists (spironolactone or eplerenone 25–50 mg daily)* further reduce mortality in pts with LVEF ≤40% and either symptomatic heart failure or diabetes; do not use in pts with advanced renal insufficiency (e.g., creatinine ≥2.5 mg/dL) or hyperkalemia.
- *Serum magnesium* level should be measured and repleted if necessary to reduce risk of arrhythmias.

■ COMPLICATIONS

(For arrhythmias, see also Chaps. 131 and 132)

Ventricular Arrhythmias

Isolated ventricular premature beats (VPBs) occur frequently. Precipitating factors should be corrected [hypoxemia, acidosis, hypokalemia (maintain serum K^+ ~4.5 mmol/L), hypercalcemia, hypomagnesemia, CHF, arrhythmogenic drugs]. Routine beta blocker administration (see above) diminishes ventricular ectopy. Other in-hospital antiarrhythmic therapy should be reserved for pts with sustained ventricular arrhythmias.

Ventricular Tachycardia

If hemodynamically unstable, perform immediate electrical countershock (unsynchronized discharge of 200–300 J or 50% less if using biphasic device). If hemodynamically tolerated, use IV amiodarone (bolus of 150 mg over 10 min, then infusion of 1.0 mg/min for 6 h, then 0.5 mg/min).

Ventricular Fibrillation (VF)

VF requires immediate defibrillation (200–400 J). If unsuccessful, initiate cardiopulmonary resuscitation (CPR) and standard resuscitative measures (Chap. 11). Ventricular arrhythmias that appear several days or weeks following MI often reflect pump failure and may warrant invasive electrophysiologic study and implantation of a cardioverter defibrillator (ICD).

Accelerated Idioventricular Rhythm

Wide QRS complex, regular rhythm, rate 60–100 beats/min, is common and usually benign; if it causes hypotension, treat with atropine 0.6 mg IV.

Supraventricular Arrhythmias

Sinus tachycardia may result from heart failure, hypoxemia, pain, fever, pericarditis, hypovolemia, administered drugs. If no cause is identified, suppressive beta blocker therapy may be beneficial to reduce myocardial oxygen demand. Other *supraventricular arrhythmias* (paroxysmal supraventricular tachycardia, atrial flutter, and fibrillation) are often secondary to heart failure. If hemodynamically unstable, proceed with electrical cardioversion. In absence of acute heart failure, suppressive alternatives include beta blockers, verapamil, or diltiazem (Chap. 132).

Bradyarrhythmias and AV Block

(See Chap. 131) In *inferior MI*, usually represent heightened vagal tone or discrete AV nodal ischemia. If hemodynamically compromised (CHF, hypotension, emergence of ventricular arrhythmias), treat with atropine 0.5 mg IV q5min (up to 2 mg). If no response, use temporary external or transvenous pacemaker. Isoproterenol should be avoided. In *anterior MI*, AV conduction defects usually reflect extensive tissue necrosis. Consider temporary external or transvenous pacemaker for (1) complete heart block, (2) Mobitz type II block (Chap. 131), (3) new bifascicular block (LBBB, RBBB + left anterior hemiblock, RBBB + left posterior hemiblock), (4) any bradyarrhythmia associated with hypotension or CHF.

Heart Failure

CHF may result from systolic "pump" dysfunction, increased LV diastolic "stiffness," and/or acute mechanical complications.

Symptoms Dyspnea, orthopnea, tachycardia.

Examination Jugular venous distention, S_3 and S_4 gallop, pulmonary rales; systolic murmur if acute mitral regurgitation or ventricular septal defect (VSD) has developed.

TREATMENT   Heart Failure (See Chaps. 14 and 133)

Initial therapy includes diuretics (begin with furosemide 10–20 mg IV), inhaled O_2, and vasodilators, particularly nitrates [PO, topical, or IV (Chap. 133) unless pt is hypotensive (systolic bp <100 mmHg)]; digitalis is usually of little benefit in acute MI unless supraventricular arrhythmias are present. Diuretic, vasodilator, and inotropic therapy (Table 128-1) may be guided by invasive hemodynamic monitoring (Swan-Ganz pulmonary artery catheter, arterial line), particularly in pts

TABLE 128-1 IV VASODILATORS AND INOTROPIC DRUGS USED IN ACUTE MI

Drug	Usual Dosage Range	Comment
Nitroglycerin	5–100 µg/min	May improve coronary blood flow to ischemic myocardium
Nitroprusside	0.5–10 (µg/kg)/min	More potent vasodilator, but improves coronary blood flow less than nitroglycerin
		With therapy >24 h or in renal failure, watch for thiocyanate toxicity (blurred vision, tinnitus, delirium)
Dobutamine	2–20 (µg/kg)/min	Results in ↑ cardiac output, ↓ PCW, but does not raise bp
Dopamine	2–20 (µg/kg)/min	More appropriate than dobutamine if hypotensive
		Hemodynamic effect depends on dose: (µg/kg)/min
		<5: ↑ renal blood flow
		2.5–10: positive inotrope
		>10: vasoconstriction
Milrinone	50 µg/kg over 10 min, then 0.375–0.75 (µg/kg)/min	Ventricular arrhythmias may result

with accompanying hypotension (Table 128-2; Fig. 128-3). In acute MI, optimal pulmonary capillary wedge pressure (PCW) is 15–20 mmHg; in the absence of hypotension, PCW >20 mmHg is treated with diuretic plus vasodilator therapy [IV nitroglycerin (begin at 10 µg/min) or nitroprusside (begin at 0.5 µg/kg per min)] and titrated to optimize bp, PCW, and systemic vascular resistance (SVR).

$$SVR = \frac{(\text{mean arterial pressure} - \text{mean RA pressure}) \times 80}{\text{cardiac output}}$$

Normal SVR = 900 – 1350 dyne•s/cm^5. If PCW >20 mmHg and pt is hypotensive (Table 128-2 and Fig. 128-3), evaluate for VSD or acute mitral regurgitation, consider dobutamine [begin at 1–2 (µg/kg)/min], titrate upward to maximum of 10 (µg/kg)/min; beware of drug-induced tachycardia or ventricular ectopy.

After stabilization on parenteral vasodilator therapy, oral therapy follows with an ACE inhibitor or an ARB (Chap. 133). Consider addition of long-term aldosterone antagonist (spironolactone 25–50 mg daily or eplerenone 25–50 mg daily) to ACE inhibitor if LVEF ≤40% or symptomatic heart failure or diabetes are present—do not use if renal insufficiency or hyperkalemia are present.

TABLE 128-2 HEMODYNAMIC COMPLICATIONS IN ACUTE MI

Condition	Cardiac Index, (L/min)/m²	PCW, mmHg	Systolic bp, mmHg	Treatment
Uncomplicated	>2.5	≤18	>100	—
Hypovolemia	<2.5	<15	<100	Successive boluses of normal saline
				In setting of inferior wall MI, consider RV infarction (esp. if RA pressure >10)
Volume overload	>2.5	>20	>100	Diuretic (e.g., furosemide 10–20 mg IV)
				Nitroglycerin, topical paste or IV (Table 128-1)
LV failure	<2.5	>20	>100	Diuretic (e.g., furosemide 10–20 mg IV)
				IV nitroglycerin (or if hypertensive, use IV nitroprusside)
Severe LV failure	<2.5	>20	<100	If bp ≥90: IV dobutamine ± IV nitroglycerin or sodium nitroprusside
				If bp <90: IV dopamine
				If accompanied by pulmonary edema: attempt diuresis with IV furosemide; may be limited by hypotension
				If new systolic murmur present, consider acute VSD or mitral regurgitation
Cardiogenic shock	<2.2	>20	<90 with oliguria and confusion	IV dopamine
				Intraaortic balloon pump
				Reperfusion by PCI or CABG may be life-saving

Abbreviations: CABG, coronary artery bypass graft; LV, left ventricle; PCI, percutaneous coronary intervention; PCW, pulmonary capillary wedge pressure; RA, right atrium; RV, right ventricle; VSD, ventricular septal defect.

Cardiogenic Shock

(See Chap. 12) Severe LV failure with hypotension (bp <90 mmHg) *and* elevated PCW (>20 mmHg), accompanied by oliguria (<20 mL/h), peripheral vasoconstriction, dulled sensorium, and metabolic acidosis.

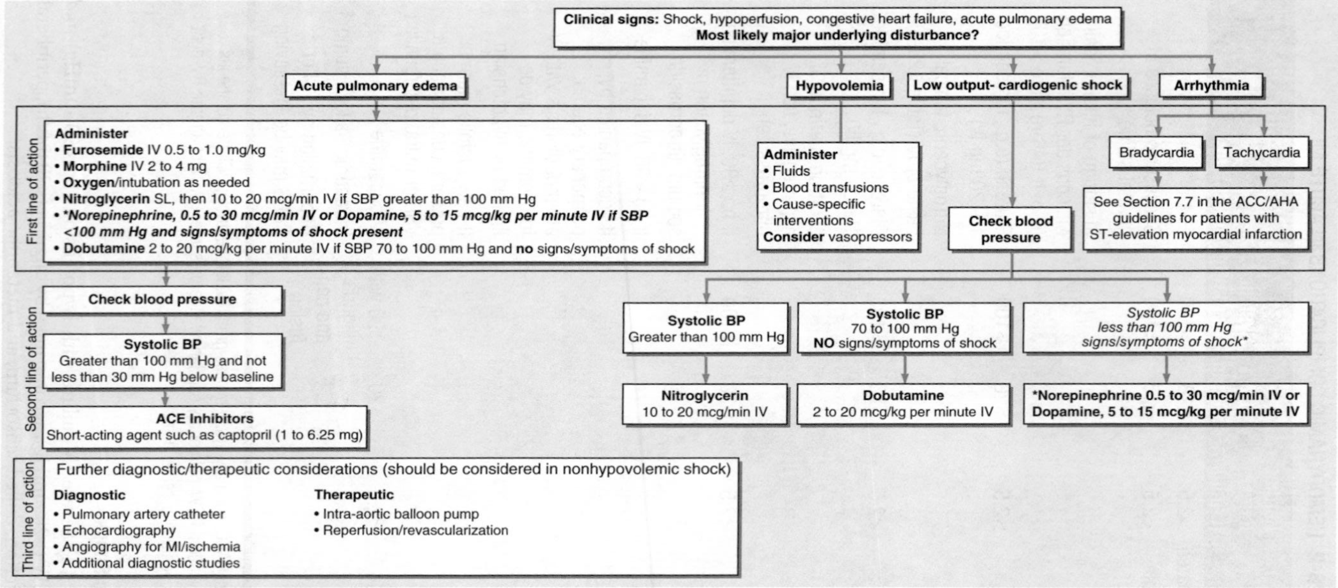
Clinical signs: Shock, hypoperfusion, congestive heart failure, acute pulmonary edema
Most likely major underlying disturbance?
Acute pulmonary edema
Hypovolemia
Low output- cardiogenic shock
Arrhythmia
First line of action
Administer
• Furosemide IV 0.5 to 1.0 mg/kg
• Morphine IV 2 to 4 mg
• Oxygen/intubation as needed
• Nitroglycerin SL, then 10 to 20 mcg/min IV if SBP greater than 100 mm Hg
• *Norepinephrine, 0.5 to 30 mcg/min IV or Dopamine, 5 to 15 mcg/kg per minute IV if SBP <100 mm Hg and signs/symptoms of shock present
• Dobutamine 2 to 20 mcg/kg per minute IV if SBP 70 to 100 mm Hg and no signs/symptoms of shock
Administer
• Fluids
• Blood transfusions
• Cause-specific interventions
Consider vasopressors
Check blood pressure
Bradycardia
Tachycardia
See Section 7.7 in the ACC/AHA guidelines for patients with ST-elevation myocardial infarction
Second line of action
Check blood pressure
Systolic BP
Greater than 100 mm Hg and not less than 30 mm Hg below baseline
ACE Inhibitors
Short-acting agent such as captopril (1 to 6.25 mg)
Systolic BP
Greater than 100 mm Hg
Systolic BP
70 to 100 mm Hg
NO signs/symptoms of shock
Systolic BP
less than 100 mm Hg
signs/symptoms of shock*
Nitroglycerin
10 to 20 mcg/min IV
Dobutamine
2 to 20 mcg/kg per minute IV
*Norepinephrine 0.5 to 30 mcg/min IV or Dopamine, 5 to 15 mcg/kg per minute IV
Third line of action
Further diagnostic/therapeutic considerations (should be considered in nonhypovolemic shock)
Diagnostic
• Pulmonary artery catheter
• Echocardiography
• Angiography for MI/ischemia
• Additional diagnostic studies
Therapeutic
• Intra-aortic balloon pump
• Reperfusion/revascularization

FIGURE 128-3 Emergency management of cardiogenic shock and pulmonary edema. ACE, angiotensin converting-enzyme; BP, blood pressure; MI, myocardial infarction. *[Modified from Guidelines 2000 for Cardiopulmonary Resuscitation and Emergency Cardiovascular Care. Part 7: The era of reperfusion: Section 1: Acute coronary syndromes (acute myocardial infarction). The American Heart Association in collaboration with the International Liaison Committee on Resuscitation. Circulation 102:I172, 2000.]*

TREATMENT Cardiogenic Shock (Fig. 128-3)

Swan-Ganz catheter and intraarterial bp monitoring are not always essential but may be helpful; aim for mean PCW of 18–20 mmHg with adjustment of volume (diuretics or infusion) as needed. Vasopressors [e.g., dopamine (Table 128-1)] and/or intraaortic balloon counterpulsation may be necessary to maintain systolic bp >90 mmHg and reduce PCW. Administer high concentration of O_2 by mask; if pulmonary edema coexists, consider bilateral positive airway pressure (BiPAP) or intubation and mechanical ventilation. Acute mechanical complications (see below) should be sought and promptly treated.

If cardiogenic shock develops within 36 h of acute STEMI, reperfusion by PCI or coronary artery bypass grafting (CABG) may markedly improve LV function.

Hypotension

May also result from *right ventricular MI*, which should be suspected in inferior or posterior MI, if jugular venous distention and elevation of right-heart pressures predominate (rales are typically absent and PCW may be normal); right-sided ECG leads typically show ST elevation, and echocardiography may confirm diagnosis. *Treatment* consists of volume infusion. Noncardiac causes of hypotension should be considered: hypovolemia, acute arrhythmia, or sepsis.

Acute Mechanical Complications

Ventricular septal rupture and acute mitral regurgitation due to papillary muscle ischemia/infarct develop during the first week following MI and are characterized by sudden onset of CHF and new systolic murmur. Echocardiography and Doppler interrogation can confirm presence of these complications. PCW tracings may show large *v* waves in either condition, but an oxygen "step-up" as the catheter is advanced from right atrium to right ventricle suggests septal rupture.

Acute medical therapy of these conditions includes vasodilator therapy (IV nitroprusside: begin at 10 μg/min and titrate to maintain systolic bp ~100 mmHg); intraaortic balloon pump may be required to maintain cardiac output. Mechanical correction is the definitive therapy. Acute ventricular free-wall rupture presents with sudden loss of bp, pulse, and consciousness, while ECG shows an intact rhythm (pulseless electrical activity); emergent surgical repair is crucial, and mortality is high.

Pericarditis

Characterized by *pleuritic, positional* pain and pericardial rub (Chap. 125); atrial arrhythmias are common; must be distinguished from recurrent angina. Often responds to aspirin, 650 mg PO qid. Anticoagulants should be avoided when pericarditis is suspected to avoid development of tamponade.

Ventricular Aneurysm

Localized "bulge" of LV chamber due to infarcted myocardium. *True aneurysms* consist of scar tissue and do not rupture. However, complications include CHF, ventricular arrhythmias, and thrombus formation. Typically an aneurysm is confirmed by echocardiography or by left ventriculography. The presence of thrombus within the aneurysm, or a large aneurysmal segment due to anterior MI, warrants oral anticoagulation with warfarin for 3–6 months.

Pseudoaneurysm is a form of cardiac rupture contained by a local area of pericardium and organized thrombus; direct communication with the LV cavity is present; surgical repair usually necessary to prevent rupture.

Recurrent Angina

Usually associated with transient ST-T wave changes; signals high incidence of reinfarction; when it occurs in early post-MI period, proceed directly to coronary arteriography, to identify those who would benefit from PCI or CABG.

■ SECONDARY PREVENTION

For pts who have not already undergone coronary angiography and PCI, submaximal exercise testing should be performed prior to or soon after discharge. A positive test in certain subgroups (angina at a low workload, a large region of provocable ischemia, or provocable ischemia with a reduced LVEF) suggests need for cardiac catheterization to evaluate myocardium at risk of recurrent infarction. *Beta blockers* (e.g., metoprolol, 25–200 mg daily) should be prescribed routinely for at least 2 years following acute MI, unless contraindications present (asthma, CHF, bradycardia, "brittle" diabetes). Continue oral antiplatelet agents (e.g., aspirin 81–325 mg daily, clopidogrel 75 mg daily) to reduce incidence of reinfarction. If LVEF ≤40%, an ACE inhibitor (e.g., captopril 6.25 mg PO tid, advanced to target dose of 50 mg PO tid) or ARB (if ACE inhibitor is not tolerated) should be used indefinitely. Consider addition of aldosterone antagonist (see "Heart Failure," above).

Modification of cardiac risk factors must be encouraged: discontinue smoking; control hypertension, diabetes, and serum lipids (typically atorvastatin 80 mg daily in immediate post-MI period—see Chap. 189); and pursue graduated exercise.

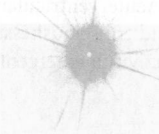

For a more detailed discussion, see Antman EM, Loscalzo J: ST-Segment Elevation Myocardial Infarction, Chap. 245, p. 2021; and Hochman JS, Ingbar DH: Cardiogenic Shock and Pulmonary Edema, Chap. 272, p. 2232, in HPIM-18.

CHAPTER **129**

Unstable Angina and Non-ST-Elevation Myocardial Infarction

Unstable angina (UA) and non-ST-elevation MI (NSTEMI) are acute coronary syndromes with similar mechanisms, clinical presentations, and treatment strategies.

Clinical Presentation

UA includes (1) new onset of severe angina, (2) angina at rest or with minimal activity, and (3) recent increase in frequency and intensity of chronic angina. NSTEMI is diagnosed when symptoms of UA are accompanied by evidence of myocardial necrosis (e.g., elevated cardiac biomarkers). Some pts with NSTEMI present with symptoms identical to STEMI—the two are differentiated by ECG (Chap. 128).

Physical Examination

May be normal or include diaphoresis, pale cool skin, tachycardia, S_4, basilar rales; if large region of ischemia, may demonstrate S_3, hypotension.

Electrocardiogram

Most commonly ST depression and/or T-wave inversion; unlike STEMI, there is no Q-wave development.

Cardiac Biomarkers

CK-MB and/or cardiac-specific troponins (more specific and sensitive markers of myocardial necrosis) are elevated in NSTEMI. Small troponin elevations may also occur in pts with CHF, myocarditis, or pulmonary embolism.

TREATMENT	Unstable Angina and Non-ST-Elevation Myocardial Infarction

First step is appropriate triage based on likelihood of coronary artery disease (CAD) and acute coronary syndrome (Fig. 129-1) as well as identification of higher-risk pts (Fig. 129-2). Pts with low likelihood of active ischemia are initially monitored by serial ECGs and serum cardiac biomarkers, and for recurrent chest discomfort; if these are negative, stress testing (or CT angiography if probability of CAD is low) can be used for further therapeutic planning.

Therapy of UA/NSTEMI is directed (1) against the inciting intracoronary thrombus, and (2) toward restoration of balance between myocardial oxygen supply and demand. Pts with the highest risk scores (Fig. 129-2) benefit the most from aggressive interventions.

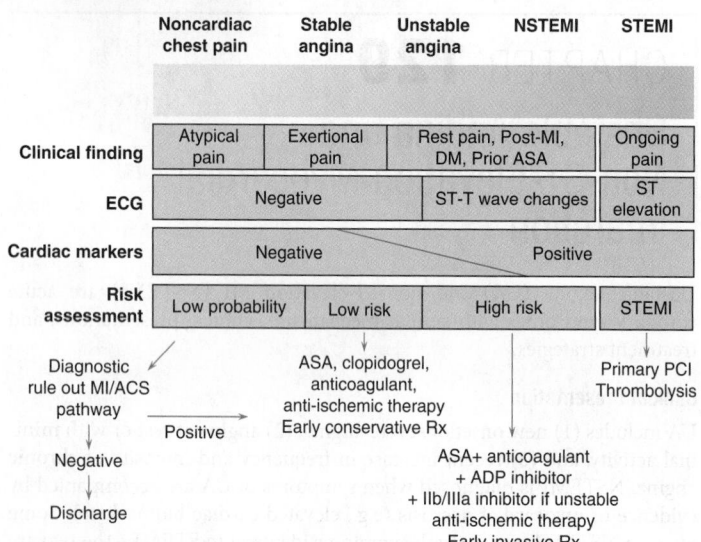

FIGURE 129-1 Algorithm for risk stratification and treatment of pts with suspected coronary artery disease. ACS, acute coronary syndrome; ASA, aspirin; DM, diabetes mellitus; ECG, electrocardiogram; LMWH, low-molecular-weight heparin; MI, myocardial infarction; PCI, percutaneous coronary intervention; Rx, treatment; STEMI, ST-segment elevation myocardial infarction. *[Adapted from CP Cannon, E Braunwald, in Braunwald's Heart Disease: A Textbook of Cardiovascular Medicine, 8th ed, P Libby et al (eds). Philadelphia, Saunders, 2008.]*

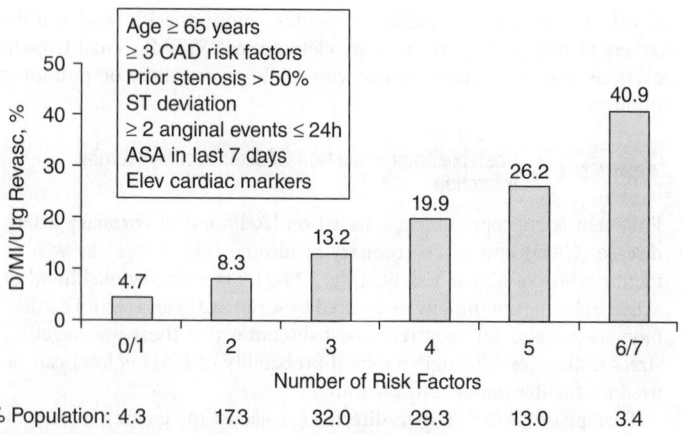

FIGURE 129-2 The TIMI Risk Score for UA/NSTEMI. The quantity of listed attributes correlates with risk of death, MI, or need for urgent revascularization over 14 days. *(Modified from E Antman et al: JAMA 284:835, 2000.)*

ANTITHROMBOTIC THERAPIES

- Aspirin (325 mg initially, then 75–325 mg/d).
- Platelet ADP receptor antagonist: Clopidogrel (300–600 mg PO load, then 75 mg/d) unless excessive risk of bleeding or immediate coronary artery bypass grafting (CABG) likely; alternatives include ticagrelor [180 mg PO, then 90 mg PO bid (chronic aspirin dose should not exceed 100 mg daily)] or prasugrel (60 mg PO, then 10 mg daily) if PCI is planned.
- Anticoagulant: Unfractionated heparin (UFH) [60 U/kg then 12 (U/kg)/h (maximum 1000 U/h)] to achieve aPTT 1.5–2.5 × control, *or* low-molecular-weight heparin (e.g., enoxaparin 1 mg/kg SC q12h), which is superior to UFH in reduction of future cardiac events. Alternatives include (1) the factor Xa inhibitor fondaparinux (2.5 mg SC daily), which is associated with lower bleeding risk, or (2) the direct thrombin inhibitor bivalirudin [0.1 mg/kg, then 0.25 (mg/kg)/h], which causes less bleeding in pts undergoing catheterization compared with UFH plus a GP IIb/IIIa inhibitor.
- For high-risk unstable pts who undergo PCI, consider an IV GP IIb/IIIa antagonist [e.g., tirofiban, 0.4 (μg/kg)/min × 30 min, then 0.1 (μg/kg)/min for 48–96 h; or eptifibatide, 180-μg/kg bolus, then 2.0 (μg/kg)/min for 72–96 h].

ANTI-ISCHEMIC THERAPIES

- Nitroglycerin 0.3–0.6 mg sublingually or by buccal spray. If chest discomfort persists after three doses given 5 min apart, consider IV nitroglycerin (5–10 μg/min, then increase by 10 μg/min every 3–5 min until symptoms relieved or systolic bp <100 mmHg). Do not use nitrates in pts with recent use of phosphodiesterase-5 inhibitors for erectile dysfunction (e.g., not within 24 h of sildenafil or within 48 h of tadalafil).
- Beta blockers (e.g., metoprolol 25–50 mg PO q6h) targeted to a heart rate of 50–60 beats/min. In pts with contraindications to beta blockers (e.g., bronchospasm), consider long-acting verapamil or diltiazem (Table 126-1).

ADDITIONAL RECOMMENDATIONS

- Admit to unit with continuous ECG monitoring, initially with bed rest.
- Consider morphine sulfate 2–5 mg IV q5–30min for refractory chest discomfort.
- Add HMG-CoA reductase inhibitor (initially at high dose, e.g., atorvastatin 80 mg daily) and consider ACE inhibitor (Chap. 128).

INVASIVE VS CONSERVATIVE STRATEGY   In highest-risk pts (Table 129-1), an early invasive strategy (coronary arteriography within ~48 h followed by percutaneous intervention or CABG) improves outcomes. In lower-risk pts, angiography can be deferred but should be pursued if myocardial ischemia recurs spontaneously (angina or ST deviations at rest or with minimal activity) or is provoked by stress testing.

TABLE 129-1 CLASS I RECOMMENDATIONS FOR USE OF AN EARLY INVASIVE STRATEGY

Recurrent angina/ischemia at rest or minimal exertion despite anti-ischemic therapy
Elevated cardiac TnI or TnT
New ST-segment depression
Recurrent ischemia with CHF or worsening mitral regurgitation
Positive stress test
LVEF <0.40
Hemodynamic instability or hypotension
Sustained ventricular tachycardia
PCI within previous 6 months, or prior CABG
High risk score

Abbreviations: CABG, coronary artery bypass grafting; LVEF, left ventricular ejection fraction; PCI, percutaneous coronary intervention; TnI, troponin I; TnT, troponin T.
Source: Modified from Anderson JL et al: J Am Coll Cardiol 50:e1, 2007.

LONG-TERM MANAGEMENT
- Stress importance of smoking cessation, achieving optimal weight, diet low in saturated and trans fats, regular exercise; these principles can be reinforced by encouraging pt to enter cardiac rehabilitation program.
- Continue aspirin, clopidogrel (or prasugrel or ticagrelor), beta blocker, statin, and ACE inhibitor or angiotensin receptor blocker (especially if hypertensive, or diabetic, or LV ejection fraction is reduced).

> For a more detailed discussion, see Cannon CP, Braunwald E: Unstable Angina and Non-ST-Elevation Myocardial Infarction, Chap. 244, p. 2015, in HPIM-18

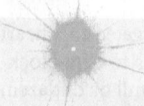

CHAPTER **130**
Chronic Stable Angina

■ ANGINA

Angina pectoris, the most common clinical manifestation of coronary artery disease (CAD), results from an imbalance between myocardial O_2 supply and demand, most often due to atherosclerotic coronary artery obstruction. Other major conditions that upset this balance and result in angina include aortic valve disease (Chap. 123), hypertrophic cardiomyopathy (Chap. 124), and coronary artery spasm (see below).

Symptoms

Angina is typically associated with exertion or emotional upset; relieved quickly by rest or nitroglycerin (Chap. 37). Major risk factors are cigarette smoking, hypertension, hypercholesterolemia (↑LDL fraction; ↓HDL), diabetes, obesity, and family history of CAD before age 55.

Physical Examination

Often normal; arterial bruits or retinal vascular abnormalities suggest generalized atherosclerosis; S_4 is common. During acute anginal episode, other signs may appear: loud S_3 or S_4, diaphoresis, rales, and a transient murmur of mitral regurgitation due to papillary muscle ischemia.

Laboratory ECG

May be normal between anginal episodes or show old infarction (Chap. 120). During angina, ST- and T-wave abnormalities typically appear (ST-segment depression reflects subendocardial ischemia; ST-segment elevation may reflect acute infarction or transient coronary artery spasm). Ventricular arrhythmias frequently accompany acute ischemia.

Stress Testing

Enhances diagnosis of CAD (Fig. 130-1). Exercise is performed on treadmill or bicycle until target heart rate is achieved or pt becomes symptomatic (chest pain, light-headedness, hypotension, marked dyspnea, ventricular tachycardia) or develops diagnostic ST-segment changes. Useful information includes duration of exercise achieved; peak heart rate and bp; depth, morphology, and persistence of ST-segment depression; and whether and at which level of exercise pain, hypotension, or ventricular arrhythmias develop. Exercise testing with radionuclide, echocardiographic, or magnetic resonance imaging increases sensitivity and specificity and is particularly useful if baseline ECG abnormalities prevent interpretation of test. *Note:* Exercise testing should not be performed in pts with acute MI, unstable angina, or severe aortic stenosis. If the pt is unable to exercise, pharmacologic stress with IV dipyridamole (or adenosine) or dobutamine can be performed in conjunction with radionuclide or echocardiographic imaging. (Table 130-1). Pts with LBBB on baseline ECG should be referred for adenosine or dipyridamole radionuclide imaging, which is most specific for diagnosis of CAD in this setting.

The prognostic utility of coronary calcium detection (by electron-beam or multidetector CT) in the diagnosis of CAD has not yet been fully characterized.

Some pts do not experience chest pain during ischemic episodes with exertion ("silent ischemia") but are identified by transient ST-T-wave abnormalities during stress (see below).

Coronary Arteriography

The definitive test for assessing severity of CAD; major indications are (1) angina refractory to medical therapy, (2) markedly positive exercise test (≥2-mm ST-segment depression, onset of ischemia at low workload, or ventricular tachycardia or hypotension with exercise) suggestive of left

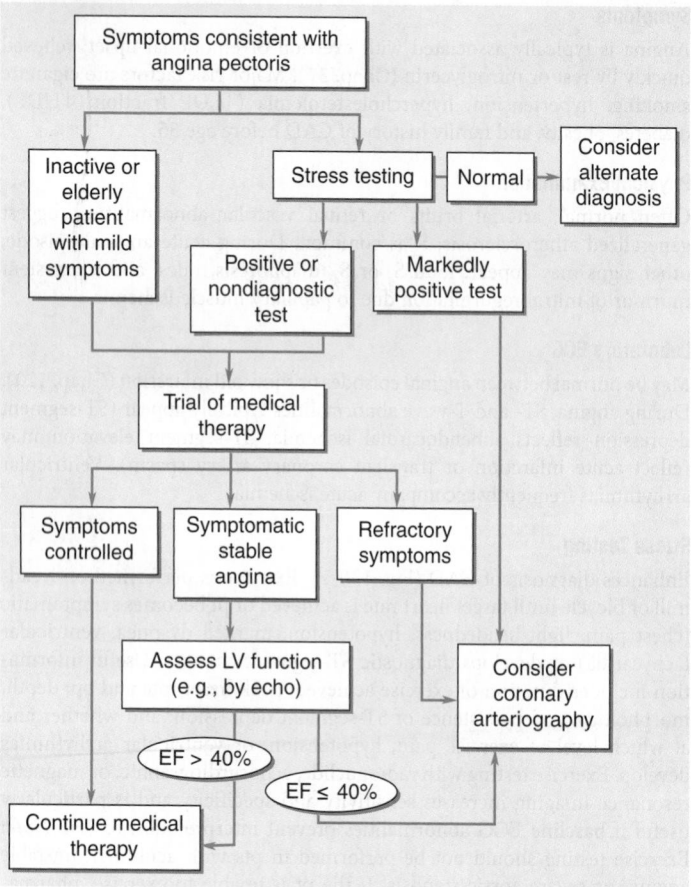

FIGURE 130-1 Role of exercise testing in management of CAD; EF, left ventricular ejection fraction. [*Modified from LS Lilly, in* Textbook of Primary Care Medicine, *3rd ed., J Nobel (ed.) St. Louis, Mosby, 2001, p. 552.*]

main or three-vessel disease, (3) recurrent angina or positive exercise test after MI, (4) to assess for coronary artery spasm, and (5) to evaluate pts with perplexing chest pain in whom noninvasive tests are not diagnostic.

The role of newer *noninvasive* coronary imaging techniques (CT and MR angiography) has not yet been defined.

TREATMENT   Chronic Stable Angina

GENERAL
- Identify and treat risk factors: mandatory cessation of smoking; treatment of diabetes, hypertension, and lipid disorders (Chap. 189); advocate a diet low in saturated fat and trans fats.

TABLE 130-1 STRESS TESTING RECOMMENDATIONS

Subgroup	Recommended Study
Pt able to exercise	
If baseline ST-T on ECG is normal	Standard exercise test (treadmill, bicycle, or arm ergometry)
If baseline ST-T impairs test interpretation (e.g., LVH with strain, digoxin)	Standard exercise test (above) combined with *either*
	Perfusion scintigraphy (thallium-201, ^{99m}Tc-sestamibi) *or*
	Echocardiography
Pt *not* able to exercise (regardless of baseline ST-T abnormality)	Pharmacologic stress test (IV dobutamine, dipyridamole, or adenosine) combined with imaging:
	Perfusion scintigraphy [thallium 201, ^{99m}Tc-sestamibi, or PET (rubidium-82 or N-13 ammonia)] *or*
	Echocardiography *or*
	Cardiac MRI
LBBB on baseline ECG	Adenosine (or dipyridamole) ^{99m}Tc-sestamibi or PET scintigraphy

- Correct exacerbating factors contributing to angina: morbid obesity, CHF, anemia, hyperthyroidism.
- Reassurance and pt education.

DRUG THERAPY Sublingual nitroglycerin (TNG 0.3–0.6 mg); may be repeated at 5-min intervals; warn pts of possible headache or light-headedness; teach prophylactic use of TNG prior to activity that regularly evokes angina. If chest pain persists for >10 min despite 2–3 TNG, pt should report promptly to nearest medical facility for evaluation of possible unstable angina or acute MI.

LONG-TERM ANGINA SUPPRESSION The following classes of drugs are used, frequently in combination.

Long-Acting Nitrates May be administered by many routes (Table 130-2); start at the lowest dose and frequency to limit tolerance and side effects of headache, light-headedness, tachycardia.

Beta Blockers (See Table 126-1) All have antianginal properties; β_1-selective agents are less likely to exacerbate airway or peripheral vascular disease. Dosage should be titrated to resting heart rate of 50–60 beats/min. *Contraindications* to beta blockers include CHF, AV block, bronchospasm, "brittle" diabetes. Side effects include fatigue, bronchospasm, depressed LV function, impotence, depression, and masking of hypoglycemia in diabetics.

TABLE 130-2 EXAMPLES OF COMMONLY USED NITRATES

	Usual Dose	Recommended Dosing Frequency
Short-acting agents		
Sublingual TNG	0.3–0.6 mg	As needed
Aerosol TNG	0.4 mg (1 inhalation)	As needed
Sublingual ISDN	2.5–10 mg	As needed
Long-acting agents		
ISDN		
Oral	5–30 mg	tid
Sustained-action	40 mg	bid (once in the A.M., then 7 h later)
TNG ointment (2%)	0.5–2	qid (with one 7- to 10-h nitrate-free interval)
TNG skin patches	0.1–0.6 mg/h	Apply in morning, remove at bedtime
ISMO		
Oral	20–40 mg	bid (once in the A.M., then 7 h later)
Sustained-action	30–240 mg	Daily

Abbreviations: TNG, nitroglycerin; ISDN, isosorbide dinitrate; ISMO, isosorbide mononitrate.

Calcium Antagonists (See Table 126-1)   Useful for stable and unstable angina, as well coronary vasospasm. Combination with other antianginal agents is beneficial, but verapamil should be administered cautiously to pts on beta blockers (additive effects on slowing heart rate). Use sustained-release, not short-acting, calcium antagonists; the latter are associated with increased coronary mortality.

Ranolazine   For pts who continue to experience stable angina despite the above standard medications, consider addition of ranolazine (500–1000 mg PO bid), which reduces anginal frequency and improves exercise capacity without affecting blood pressure or heart rate. Ranolazine is contraindicated in hepatic impairment, in pts with prolongation of the QT_c interval, or in combination with drugs that inhibit its metabolism (e.g., ketoconazole, macrolide antibiotics, HIV protease inhibitors, diltiazem, and verapamil).

Aspirin   75–325 mg/d reduces the incidence of MI in chronic stable angina, following MI, and in asymptomatic men. It is recommended in pts with CAD in the absence of contraindications (GI bleeding or allergy). Consider clopidogrel (75 mg/d) for aspirin-intolerant individuals.

The addition of an ACE inhibitor is recommended in pts with CAD and LV ejection fraction <40%, hypertension, diabetes, or chronic kidney disease.

MECHANICAL REVASCULARIZATION   Used in conjunction with, not as replacement for, risk factor modification and medical therapies.

Percutaneous Coronary Intervention (PCI)   Technique of balloon dilatation, usually with intracoronary stent implantation. Performed on anatomically suitable stenoses of native vessels and bypass grafts; more effective than medical therapy for relief of angina. Has not been shown to reduce risk of MI or death in chronic stable angina; should not be performed on asymptomatic or only mildly symptomatic individuals. With PCI initial relief of angina occurs in 95% of pts; however, restenosis develops in 30–45% following balloon dilatation alone, in ~20% after bare metal stenting, but in only <10% after drug-eluting stent (DES) implantation. Late stent thrombosis may occur rarely in pts with DES; it is diminished by prolonged antiplatelet therapy [aspirin indefinitely and clopidogrel (or alternate platelet ADP receptor antagonist) for a minimum of 12 months].

Coronary Artery Bypass Graft (CABG)   Appropriately used for angina refractory to medical therapy or when the latter is not tolerated (and when lesions are not amenable to PCI) or if severe CAD is present (e.g., left main, three-vessel disease with impaired LV function). In type 2 diabetics with multivessel CAD, CABG plus optimal medical therapy is superior to medical therapy alone in prevention of major coronary events.

The relative advantages of PCI and CABG are summarized in Table 130-3.

TABLE 130-3   COMPARISON OF REVASCULARIZATION PROCEDURES IN MULTIVESSEL DISEASE

Procedure	Advantages	Disadvantages
Percutaneous coronary revascularization	Less invasive	Restenosis requiring repeat procedure
	Shorter hospital stay	
	Lower initial cost	Possible incomplete revascularization
	Effective in relieving symptoms	Limited to specific anatomic subsets
Coronary artery bypass grafting	Lower rate of recurrent angina	Cost
		Risk of a repeat procedure due to late graft closure
	Ability to achieve complete revascularization	Morbidity and mortality of major surgery

Source: Modified from DP Faxon, in GA Beller (ed), Chronic Ischemic Heart Disease, in E Braunwald (series ed), *Atlas of Heart Disease*, Philadelphia, Current Medicine, 1994.

■ PRINZMETAL'S VARIANT ANGINA (CORONARY VASOSPASM)

Intermittent focal spasm of coronary artery; often associated with atherosclerotic lesion near site of spasm. Chest discomfort is similar to angina but more severe and occurs typically at rest, with transient ST-segment elevation. Acute infarction or malignant arrhythmias may develop during spasm-induced ischemia. Evaluation includes observation of ECG for transient ST elevation during discomfort; diagnosis confirmed at coronary angiography using provocative (e.g., IV acetylcholine) testing. Primary treatment consists of long-acting nitrates and calcium antagonists. Prognosis is better in pts with anatomically normal coronary arteries than in those with fixed coronary stenoses.

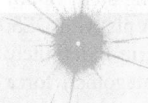

For a more detailed discussion, see Antman EM, Selwyn AP, Loscalzo J: Ischemic Heart Disease, Chap. 243, p. 1998, in HPIM-18.

CHAPTER **131**
Bradyarrhythmias

Bradyarrhythmias arise from (1) failure of impulse initiation (sinoatrial node dysfunction) or (2) impaired electrical conduction (e.g., AV conduction blocks).

■ SINOATRIAL (SA) NODE DYSFUNCTION

Etiologies are either *intrinsic* [degenerative, ischemic, inflammatory, infiltrative (e.g., senile amyloid), or rare mutations in sodium channel or pacemaker current genes] or *extrinsic* [e.g., drugs (beta blockers, Ca^{++} channel blockers, digoxin), autonomic dysfunction, hypothyroidism].

Symptoms are due to *bradycardia* (fatigue, weakness, lightheadedness, syncope) and/or episodes of associated *tachycardia* (e.g., rapid palpitations, angina) in pts with sick sinus syndrome (SSS).

Diagnosis

Examine ECG for evidence of sinus bradycardia (sinus rhythm at <60 beats/min) or failure of rate to increase with exercise, sinus pauses, or exit block. In pts with SSS, periods of tachycardia (i.e., atrial fibrillation/flutter) occur. Prolonged ECG monitoring (24-h Holter or 30-day loop event monitor) aids in identifying these abnormalities. Invasive electrophysiologic testing is rarely necessary to establish diagnosis.

TREATMENT Sinoatrial Node Dysfunction

Remove or treat extrinsic causes such as contributing drugs or hypothyroidism. Otherwise, symptoms of bradycardia respond to permanent pacemaker placement. In SSS, treat associated atrial fibrillation or flutter as indicated in Chap. 132.

■ **AV BLOCK**

Impaired conduction from atria to ventricles may be structural and permanent, or reversible (e.g., autonomic, metabolic, drug-related)—see Table 131-1.

TABLE 131-1 ETIOLOGIES OF ATRIOVENTRICULAR BLOCK

Autonomic	
Carotid sinus hypersensitivity	Vasovagal
Metabolic/Endocrine	
Hyperkalemia	Hypothyroidism
Hypermagnesemia	Adrenal insufficiency
Drug-Related	
Beta blockers	Adenosine
Calcium channel blockers	Antiarrhythmics (class I and III)
Digitalis	Lithium
Infectious	
Endocarditis	Tuberculosis
Lyme disease	Diphtheria
Chagas' disease	Toxoplasmosis
Syphilis	
Heritable/Congenital	
Congenital heart disease	Kearns-Sayre syndrome (OMIM #530000)
Maternal SLE	Myotonic dystrophy
Inflammatory	
SLE	MCTD
Rheumatoid arthritis	Scleroderma
Infiltrative	
Amyloidosis	Hemochromatosis
Sarcoidosis	
Neoplastic/Traumatic	
Lymphoma	Radiation
Mesothelioma	Catheter ablation
Melanoma	
Degenerative	
Lev disease	Lenègre disease
Coronary Artery Disease	
Acute MI	

Abbreviations: MCTD, mixed connective tissue disease; MI, myocardial infarction; OMIM, Online Mendelian Inheritance in Man (database); SLE, systemic lupus erythematosus.

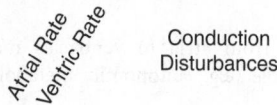

Conduction
Disturbances

A. First degree heart block

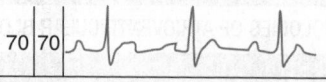

B. Second degree heart block

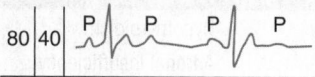

C. Third degree heart block
(complete H. B.)

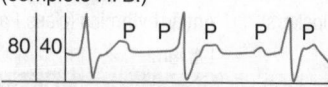

D. Wenckebach

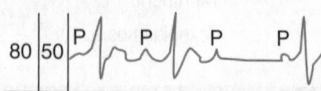

FIGURE 131-1 Bradyarrhythmias. (*Modified from BE Sobel, E Braunwald: HPIM-9, p. 1052.*)

First Degree (See Fig. 131-1A)

Prolonged, constant PR interval (>0.20 s). May be normal or secondary to increased vagal tone or drugs (e.g., beta blocker, diltiazem, verapamil, digoxin); treatment not usually required.

Second Degree (See Fig. 131-1B)

Mobitz I (Wenckebach)

Narrow QRS, progressive increase in PR interval until a ventricular beat is dropped, then sequence is repeated (Fig. 131-1D). Seen with drug intoxication (digitalis, beta blockers), increased vagal tone, inferior MI. Usually transient, no therapy required; if symptomatic, use atropine (0.6 mg IV, repeated × 3–4) or temporary pacemaker.

Mobitz II

Fixed PR interval with occasional dropped beats, in 2:1, 3:1, or 4:1 pattern; the QRS complex is usually wide. Seen with MI or degenerative conduction system disease; more serious than Mobitz I—may progress suddenly to complete AV block; permanent pacemaker is indicated.

Third Degree (Complete AV Block) (See Fig. 131-1C)

Complete failure of conduction from atria to ventricles; atria and ventricles depolarize independently. May occur with MI, digitalis toxicity, or degenerative conduction system disease. Permanent pacemaker is usually indicated, except when reversible (e.g., drug-related or appears only transiently in MI without associated bundle branch block).

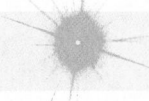

For a more detailed discussion, see Spragg DD, Tomaselli GF: The Bradyarrhythmias, Chap. 232, p. 1867, in HPIM-18.

CHAPTER **132**
Tachyarrhythmias

Tachyarrhythmias may appear in the presence or absence of structural heart disease; they are more serious in the former. Conditions that provoke arrhythmias include (1) myocardial ischemia, (2) heart failure, (3) hypoxemia, (4) hypercapnia, (5) hypotension, (6) electrolyte disturbances (e.g., hypokalemia and/or hypomagnesemia), (7) drug toxicity (digoxin, pharmacologic agents that prolong the QT interval), (8) caffeine consumption, (9) ethanol consumption.

Diagnosis

Examine ECG for evidence of ischemic changes (Chap. 120), prolonged or shortened QT interval, characteristics of Wolff-Parkinson-White (WPW) syndrome (see below), or ST elevation in leads V_1–V_3 typical of Brugada syndrome. See Fig. 132-1 and Table 132-1 for diagnosis of tachyarrhythmias; always identify atrial activity and relationship between P waves and QRS complexes. To aid the diagnosis:

- Obtain long rhythm strip of lead II, aVF, or V_1. P waves can be made more evident by intentionally doubling the ECG voltage.
- Place accessory ECG leads (e.g., right-sided chest leads) to help identify P waves. Record ECG during carotid sinus massage (Table 132-1). *Note:* Do not massage both carotids simultaneously.
- For intermittent symptoms, consider 24-h Holter monitor (if symptoms occur daily), a pt-activated or continuously recording event monitor over 2–4 weeks, or, if symptoms are very infrequent but severely symptomatic, an implanted loop monitor. A standard exercise test may be used to provoke arrhythmias for diagnostic purposes.

Tachyarrhythmias with wide QRS complex beats may represent ventricular tachycardia or supraventricular tachycardia with aberrant conduction. Factors favoring ventricular tachycardia include (1) AV dissociation, (2) QRS >0.14 s, (3) rightward and superior QRS axis, (4) no response to carotid sinus massage, (5) morphology of QRS unlike typical RBBB or LBBB, and similar to that of previous ventricular premature beats (Table 132-2).

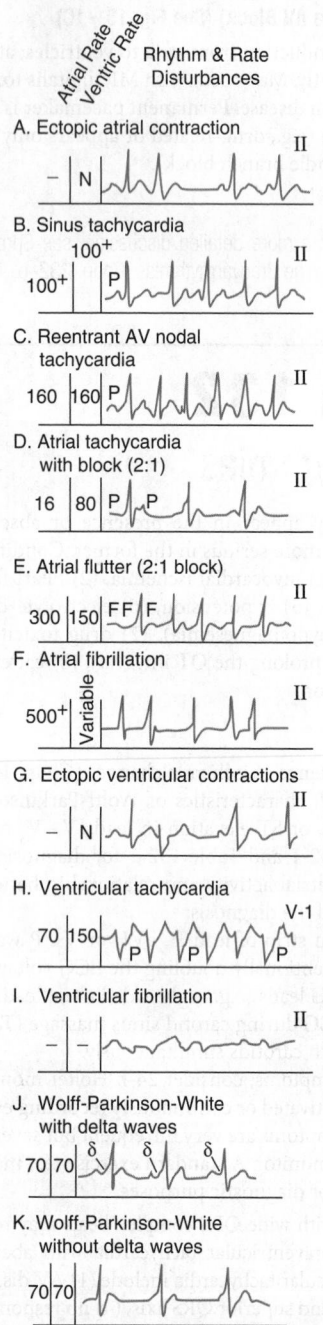

FIGURE 132-1 Tachyarrhythmias. *(Modified from BE Sobel, E Braunwald: HPIM-9, p. 1052.)*

TABLE 132-1 CLINICAL AND ELECTROCARDIOGRAPHIC FEATURES OF COMMON ARRHYTHMIAS

Rhythm	Example (Fig. 132-1)	Atrial Rate	Features	Carotid Sinus Massage	Precipitating Conditions	Initial Treatment
Narrow QRS complex						
Atrial premature beats	A	—	P wave abnormal; QRS width normal	—	Can be normal or due to anxiety, CHF, hypoxia, caffeine, abnormal electrolytes ($\downarrow$K$^+$, $\downarrow$Mg^{2+})	Remove precipitating cause; if symptomatic: beta blocker
Sinus tachycardia	B	100–160	Normal P wave contour	Rate gradually slows	Fever, anxiety, dehydration, pain, CHF, hyperthyroidism, COPD	Remove precipitating cause; if symptomatic: beta blocker
AV nodal tachycardia (reentrant)	C	120–250	Absent or retrograde P wave	Abruptly converts to sinus rhythm (or no effect)	Can occur in healthy individuals	Vagal maneuvers; if unsuccessful: adenosine, verapamil, beta blocker, cardioversion (100–200 J). To prevent recurrence: beta blocker, verapamil, diltiazem, digoxin, class IC agent, or catheter ablation
Atrial tachycardia	D	130–200	P contour different from sinus P wave; AV block may occur; automatic form shows "warm-up" in rate in first several beats	AV block may $\uparrow$	Digitalis toxicity; pulmonary disease; scars from prior cardiac surgery	If digitalis toxic: hold digoxin, correct [K$^+$] In absence of digoxin toxicity: slow rate with beta blocker, verapamil, or diltiazem; can attempt conversion with IV procainamide or amiodarone; if unsuccessful, proceed to cardioversion or catheter ablation

(continued)

869

TABLE 132-1   CLINICAL AND ELECTROCARDIOGRAPHIC FEATURES OF COMMON ARRHYTHMIAS (CONTINUED)

Rhythm	Example (Fig. 132-1)	Atrial Rate	Features	Carotid Sinus Massage	Precipitating Conditions	Initial Treatment
Atrial flutter	E	260–300	"Sawtooth" flutter waves; 2:1, 4:1 block	↑ AV block with ↓ventricular rate	Mitral valve disease, hypertension, pulmonary embolism, pericarditis, post–cardiac surgery; hyperthyroidism; obstructive lung disease, EtOH, idiopathic	1. Slow the ventricular rate: beta blocker, verapamil, diltiazem, or digoxin 2. Convert to NSR (after anticoagulation if chronic) electrically (50–100 J for atrial flutter, 100–200 J for atrial fibrillation) or chemically with IV ibutilide or oral class IC, III, or IA[a] agent
Atrial fibrillation	F	>350	No discrete P; irregularly spaced QRS	↓ Ventricular rate		Atrial flutter may respond to rapid atrial pacing, and radio frequency ablation highly effective to prevent recurrences
Multifocal atrial tachycardia		100–150	More than 3 different P wave shapes with varying PR intervals	No effect	Severe respiratory insufficiency	Treat underlying lung disease; verapamil may be used to slow ventricular rate; class IC agents or amiodarone may ↓ episodes

Wide QRS Complex					
Ventricular premature beats	G	Fully compensatory pause between normal beats	No effect	CAD, MI, CHF, hypoxia, hypokalemia, digitalis toxicity, prolonged QT interval (congenital or drug-related)	May not require therapy; if needed for symptomatic suppression, use beta blocker
Ventricular tachycardia	H	QRS rate 100–250; slightly irregular rate	No effect		If unstable: electrical conversion/defibrillation ($\geq$200 J monophasic, or 100 J biphasic) Otherwise: acute (IV): amiodarone, lidocaine, procainamide; chronic management: usually ICD Pts without structural heart disease (e.g., focal outflow tract ventricular tachycardia) may respond to beta blockers or verapamil
Accelerated idioventricular rhythm (AIVR)		Gradual onset and offset; QRS rate 40–120		Acute MI, cocaine, myocarditis	Usually none; for symptoms, use atropine or atrial pacing
Ventricular fibrillation	I	Erratic electrical activity only	No effect		Immediate defibrillation

(continued)

TABLE 132-1 CLINICAL AND ELECTROCARDIOGRAPHIC FEATURES OF COMMON ARRHYTHMIAS (CONTINUED)

Rhythm	Example (Fig. 132-1)	Atrial Rate	Features	Carotid Sinus Massage	Precipitating Conditions	Initial Treatment
Torsades de pointes			Ventricular tachycardia with sinusoidal oscillations of QRS height	No effect	Prolonged QT interval (congenital or drug-related)	IV magnesium (1- to 2-g bolus); overdrive pacing; isoproterenol for bradycardia-dependent torsades (unless CAD present); lidocaine Drugs that prolong QT interval are contraindicated
Supraventricular tachycardias with aberrant ventricular conduction			P wave typical of the supraventricular rhythm; wide QRS complex due to conduction through partially refractory pathways		Etiologies of the respective supraventricular rhythms listed above; atrial fibrillation with rapid, wide QRS may be due to preexcitation (WPW)	Same as treatment of respective supraventricular rhythm; if ventricular rate rapid (>200), treat as WPW (see text)

ªAntiarrhythmic drug groups listed in Table 132-3.

Abbreviations: CAD, coronary artery disease; EtOH, ethyl alcohol; ICD, implantable cardioverter defibrillator; NSR, normal sinus rhythm; COPD, chronic obstructive pulmonary disease; WPW, Wolff-Parkinson-White.

TABLE 132-2 WIDE COMPLEX TACHYCARDIA

ECG Criteria That Favor Ventricular Tachycardia

1. AV dissociation
2. QRS width: >0.14 s with RBBB configuration
   >0.16 s with LBBB configuration
3. QRS axis: Left axis deviation with RBBB morphology
   Extreme left axis deviation (northwest axis) with LBBB morphology
4. Concordance of QRS in precordial leads
5. Morphologic patterns of the QRS complex
   RBBB: Mono-or biphasic complex in V_1
   RS *(only with left axis deviation)* or QS in V_6

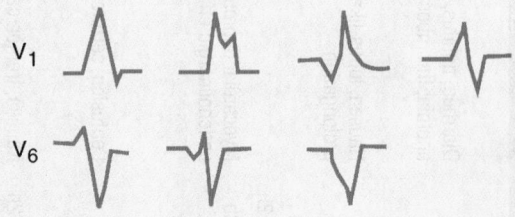

   LBBB: Broad R wave V_1 or $V_2 \geq 0.04$ s
   Onset of QRS to nadir of S wave in V_1 or V_2 of ≥ 0.07 s
   Notched downslope of S wave in V_1 or V_2
   Q wave in V_6

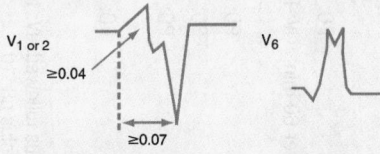

Abbreviations: AV, atrioventricular; BBB, bundle branch block.

TREATMENT Tachyarrhythmias (Tables 132-1 and 132-3)

Precipitating causes (listed above) should be corrected. If pt is hemodynamically compromised (angina, hypotension, CHF), proceed to immediate cardioversion.

Do not cardiovert sinus tachycardia; exercise caution if digitalis toxicity is suspected. Initiate drugs as indicated in the tables; follow ECG intervals (esp. QRS and QT). Reduce dosage for pts with hepatic or renal dysfunction as indicated in Table 132-3. Drug efficacy is confirmed

TABLE 132-3 ANTIARRHYTHMIC DRUGS

Drug	Loading Dose	Maintenance Dose	Side Effects	Excretion
Class IA				
Quinidine sulfate		PO: 200–400 mg q6h	Diarrhea, tinnitus, QT prolongation, hypotension, anemia, thrombocytopenia	Hepatic
Quinidine gluconate		PO: 324–628 mg q8h		Hepatic
Procainamide	IV: 15 mg/kg over 60 min	IV: 1–4 mg/min	Nausea, lupus-like syndrome, agranulocytosis, QT prolongation	Renal and hepatic
		PO: 500–1000 mg q4h		
Sustained-release		PO: 1000–2500 mg q12h		
Disopyramide		PO: 100–300 mg q6–8h	Myocardial depression, AV block, QT prolongation anticholinergic effects	Renal and hepatic
Sustained-release		PO: 200–400 mg q12h		
Class IB				
Lidocaine	IV: 1-mg/kg bolus followed by 0.5-mg/kg bolus q8–10 min to total 3 mg/kg	IV: 1–4 mg/min	Confusion, seizures, respiratory arrest	Hepatic
Mexiletine		PO: 150–300 mg q8–12h	Nausea, tremor, gait disturbance	Hepatic

	Dosing	Adverse Effects	Elimination
Class IC			
Flecainide	PO: 50–200 mg q12h	Nausea, exacerbation of ventricular arrhythmia, prolongation of PR and QRS intervals	Hepatic and renal
Propafenone	PO: 150–300 mg q8h		Hepatic
Class II			
Metoprolol	IV: 5–10 mg q5min × 3 PO: 25–100 mg q6h	CHF, bradycardia, AV block, bronchospasm	Hepatic
Esmolol	IV: 500 µg/kg over 1 min IV: 50 (µg/kg)/min		
Class III			
Amiodarone	PO: 800–1600 mg qd × 1–2 weeks, then 400–600 mg/d × 3 weeks IV: 150 mg over 10 min IV: 1 mg/min × 6 h, then 0.5 mg/min	Thyroid abnormalities, pulmonary fibrosis, hepatitis, bluish skin	Hepatic
Ibutilide	IV (≥60 kg): 1 mg over 10 min, can repeat after 10 min —	Torsades de pointes, hypotension, nausea	Hepatic
Dofetilide	PO: 125–500 µg bid	Torsades de pointes, headache, dizziness	Renal
Sotalol	PO: 80–160 mg q12h	Fatigue, bradycardia, exacerbation of ventricular arrhythmia	Renal
Dronedarone	PO: 400 mg q12h	Bradycardia, AV block, prolonged QT, exacerbation of heart failure, GI discomfort	Hepatic

(continued)

875

TABLE 132-3 ANTIARRHYTHMIC DRUGS (CONTINUED)

Drug	Loading Dose	Maintenance Dose	Side Effects	Excretion
Class IV				
Verapamil	IV: 2.5–10 mg over 3–5 min	IV: 2.5–10 mg/h PO: 80–120 mg q6–8 h	AV block, CHF, hypotension, constipation	Hepatic
Diltiazem	IV: 0.25 mg/kg over 3–5 min (maximum 20 mg)	IV: 5–15 mg/h PO: 30–60 mg q6h		Hepatic
Other				
Digoxin	IV, PO: 0.75–1.5 mg over 24 h	IV, PO: 0.125–0.25 mg qd	Nausea, AV block, ventricular and supraventricular arrhythmias	Renal
Adenosine	IV: 6-mg rapid bolus; if no effect then 12-mg bolus	—	Transient hypotension or atrial standstill	—

by ECG (or Holter) monitoring, stress testing, and, in special circumstances, invasive electrophysiologic study.

Antiarrhythmic agents all have potential toxic side effects, including provocation of ventricular arrhythmias, esp. in pts with LV dysfunction or history of sustained ventricular arrhythmias. Drug-induced QT prolongation and associated torsades de pointes ventricular tachycardia (Table 132-1) is most common with class IA and III agents; the drug should be discontinued if the QTc interval (QT divided by square root of RR interval) increases by >25%. Antiarrhythmic drugs should be avoided in pts with asymptomatic ventricular arrhythmias after MI, since mortality risk increases.

CHRONIC ATRIAL FIBRILLATION (AF) Evaluate potential underlying cause (e.g., thyrotoxicosis, mitral stenosis, excessive ethanol consumption, pulmonary embolism). Pts with risk factors for stroke (e.g., rheumatic mitral valve disease, history of cerebrovascular accident or transient ischemic attack, hypertension, diabetes, heart failure, age >75, left atrial diameter >5.0 cm) should receive anticoagulation with either warfarin (INR 2.0–3.0) or, for AF not associated with valvular disease, newer agents that do not require prothrombin time monitoring— e.g., dabigatran 150 mg bid [75 mg bid for creatinine clearance (CrCl) 30–50 mL/min; avoid if CrCl <30] or rivaroxaban 20 mg daily with the evening meal (15 mg daily for CrCl 15–50 mL/min; avoid if CrCl <15). Substitute aspirin, 325 mg/d, for pts without these risk factors or if contraindication to systemic anticoagulation exists.

Control ventricular rate (60–80 beats/min at rest, <100 beats/min with mild exercise) with beta blocker, calcium channel blocker (verapamil, diltiazem), or digoxin.

Consider cardioversion (100–200 J) after ≥3 weeks therapeutic anticoagulation, or acutely if no evidence of left atrial thrombus by transesophageal echo, especially if symptomatic despite rate control. Initiation of class IC, III, or IA agents prior to electrical cardioversion facilitates maintenance of sinus rhythm after successful procedure. Class IC (Table 132-3) drugs are preferred in pts without structural heart disease, and class III drugs are recommended in presence of left ventricular dysfunction or coronary artery disease (Fig. 132-2). Anticoagulation should be continued for a minimum of 3 weeks after successful cardioversion.

Catheter-based ablation (pulmonary vein isolation) can be considered for recurrent symptomatic AF refractory to pharmacologic measures.

■ PREEXCITATION SYNDROME (WPW)

Conduction occurs through an accessory pathway between atria and ventricles. Baseline ECG typically shows a short PR interval and slurred upstroke of the QRS ("delta" wave) (Fig. 132-1J). Associated tachyarrhythmias are of two types:

- Narrow QRS complex tachycardia (antegrade conduction through AV node). Treat cautiously with IV adenosine or beta blocker, verapamil, or diltiazem (Table 132-2).

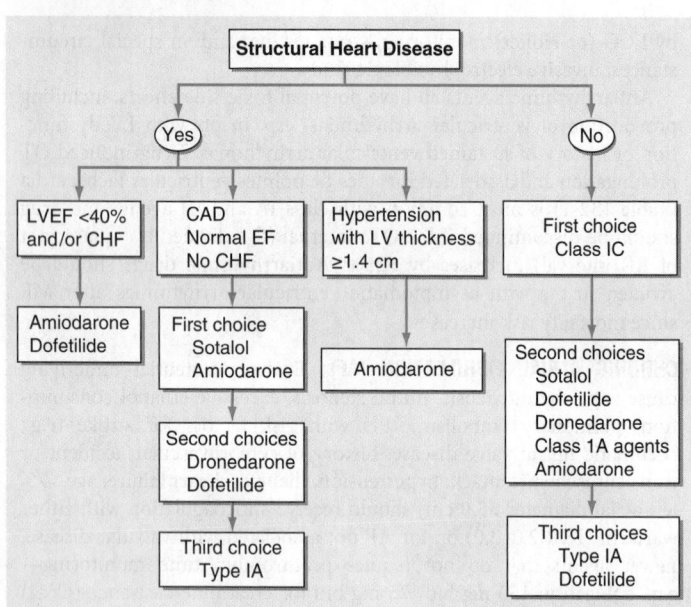

FIGURE 132-2 Recommendations for the selection of antiarrhythmic medications to prevent the recurrence of atrial fibrillation. See Table 132-3 for definition of class IA and IC drugs. An atrioventricular nodal blocking agent (i.e., beta blocker, calcium channel blocker, or digoxin) should be added to all class IC and IA agents as well as to dofetilide. LVEF, left ventricular ejection fraction; CHF, congestive heart failure; CAD, coronary artery disease; EF, ejection fraction.

- Wide QRS complex tachycardia (antegrade conduction through accessory pathway); may also be associated with AF with a very rapid (>250/min) ventricular rate, which can degenerate into VF. If hemodynamically compromised, immediate cardioversion is indicated; otherwise, treat with IV procainamide or ibutilide (Table 132-3), *not* digoxin, beta blocker, or verapamil.

Consider catheter ablation of accessory pathway for long-term prevention.

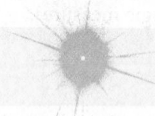

For a more detailed discussion, see Marchlinski F: The Tachyarrhythmias, Chap. 233, p. 1878, in HPIM-18.

CHAPTER **133**
Heart Failure and Cor Pulmonale

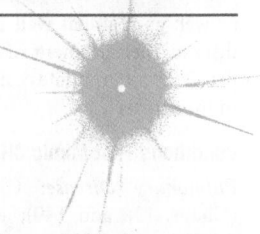

HEART FAILURE

Definition

Abnormality of cardiac structure and/or function resulting in clinical symptoms (e.g., dyspnea, fatigue) and signs (e.g., edema, rales), hospitalizations, poor quality of life, and shortened survival. It is important to identify the underlying nature of the cardiac disease and the factors that precipitate acute CHF.

Underlying Cardiac Disease

Includes (1) states that depress systolic ventricular function and ejection fraction (coronary artery disease, hypertension, dilated cardiomyopathy, valvular disease, congenital heart disease); and (2) states of heart failure with preserved ejection fraction (e.g., restrictive cardiomyopathies, hypertrophic cardiomyopathy, fibrosis, endomyocardial disorders), also termed *diastolic failure.*

Acute Precipitating Factors

Include (1) excessive Na^+ intake, (2) noncompliance with heart failure medications, (3) acute MI (may be silent), (4) exacerbation of hypertension, (5) acute arrhythmias, (6) infections and/or fever, (7) pulmonary embolism, (8) anemia, (9) thyrotoxicosis, (10) pregnancy, (11) acute myocarditis or infective endocarditis, and (12) certain drugs (e.g., nonsteroidal anti-inflammatory agents, verapamil).

Symptoms

Due to inadequate perfusion of peripheral tissues (fatigue, dyspnea) and elevated intracardiac filling pressures (orthopnea, paroxysmal nocturnal dyspnea, peripheral edema).

Physical Examination

Jugular venous distention, S_3, pulmonary congestion (rales, dullness over pleural effusion), peripheral edema, hepatomegaly, and ascites. Sinus tachycardia is common.

In pts with diastolic dysfunction, an S_4 is often present.

Laboratory

CXR may reveal cardiomegaly, pulmonary vascular redistribution, Kerley B lines, pleural effusions. Left ventricular contraction and diastolic dysfunction can be assessed by *echocardiography* with Doppler. In addition, echo can identify underlying valvular, pericardial, or congenital heart disease, as well as regional wall motion abnormalities typical of coronary artery disease. Measurement of B-type natriuretic peptide (BNP) or N-terminal pro-BNP differentiates cardiac from pulmonary causes of dyspnea (elevated in the former).

Conditions That Mimic CHF

Pulmonary Disease: Chronic bronchitis, emphysema, and asthma (Chaps. 138 and 140); assess for sputum production and abnormalities on CXR and pulmonary function tests. *Other Causes of Peripheral Edema*: Liver disease, varicose veins, and cyclic edema, none of which results in jugular venous distention. Edema due to renal dysfunction is often accompanied by elevated serum creatinine and abnormal urinalysis (Chap. 42).

TREATMENT   Heart Failure (See Fig. 133-1)

Aimed at symptomatic relief, prevention of adverse cardiac remodeling, and prolonging survival. Overview of treatment shown in Table 133-1; notably, ACE inhibitors and beta blockers are cornerstones of therapy in pts with impaired ejection fraction (EF). Once symptoms develop:

- *Control excess fluid retention*: (1) *Dietary sodium restriction* (eliminate salty foods, e.g., potato chips, canned soups, bacon, salt added at table); more stringent requirements (<2 g NaCl/d in advanced CHF. If dilutional hyponatremia present, restrict fluid intake (<1000 mL/d). (2) *Diuretics: Loop diuretics* [e.g., furosemide or torsemide (Table 133-2)] are most potent and, unlike thiazides, remain effective when GFR

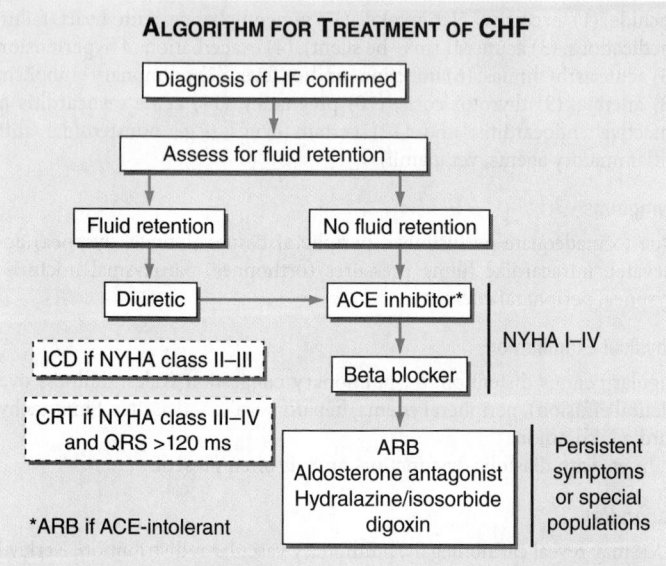

FIGURE 133-1 Treatment algorithm for chronic heart failure with reduced ejection fraction.

TABLE 133-1 THERAPY FOR HEART FAILURE

1. General measures
   a. Restrict salt intake
   b. Avoid antiarrhythmics for asymptomatic arrhythmias
   c. Avoid NSAIDs
   d. Immunize against influenza and pneumococcal pneumonia
2. Diuretics
   a. Use in volume-overloaded pts to achieve normal JVP and relief of edema
   b. Weigh daily to adjust dose
   c. For diuretic resistance, administer IV or use 2 diuretics in combination (e.g., furosemide plus metolazone)
   d. Low-dose dopamine to enhance renal flow
3. ACE inhibitor or angiotensin receptor blocker
   a. For all pts with LV systolic heart failure or asymptomatic LV dysfunction
   b. Contraindications: Serum K^+ >5.5, advanced renal failure (e.g., creatinine >3 mg/dL), bilateral renal artery stenosis, pregnancy
4. Beta blocker
   a. For pts with symptomatic or asymptomatic heart failure and LVEF <40%, combined with ACE inhibitor and diuretics
   b. Contraindications: Bronchospasm, symptomatic bradycardia or advanced heart block, unstable heart failure
5. Aldosterone antagonist
   a. Consider for class III–IV heart failure and LVEF <35%
   b. Avoid if K^+ >5.0 or creatinine >2.5 mg/dL
6. Digitalis
   a. For persistently symptomatic pts with systolic heart failure (especially if atrial fibrillation present) added to ACE inhibitor, diuretics, beta blocker
7. Other measures
   a. Consider combination of hydralazine and oral nitrate if not tolerant of ACE inhibitor/ARB
   b. Consider ventricular resynchronization (biventricular pacemaker) for pts with class III or IV heart failure, LVEF <35%, and QRS >120 ms
   c. Consider implantable cardioverter-defibrillator in pts with class II–III heart failure and ejection fraction <30–35%

<25 mL/min. Combine loop diuretic with thiazide or metolazone for augmented effect.

During diuresis, obtain daily weights, aiming for loss of 1–1.5 kg/d.

- *ACE inhibitors* (Table 133-2): Recommended as standard initial CHF therapy. They have been shown to prolong life in pts with symptomatic CHF. ACE inhibitors have also been shown to delay the onset of CHF

TABLE 133-2 DRUGS FOR THE TREATMENT OF CHRONIC HEART FAILURE (EF <40%)

	Initiating Dose	Maximal Dose
Diuretics		
Furosemide	20–40 mg qd or bid	400 mg/d[a]
Torsemide	10–20 mg qd bid	200 mg/d[a]
Bumetanide	0.5–1.0 mg qd or bid	10 mg/d[a]
Hydrochlorothiazide	25 mg qd	100 mg/d[a]
Metolazone	2.5–5.0 mg qd or bid	20 mg/d[a]
Angiotensin-converting enzyme inhibitors		
Captopril	6.25 mg tid	50 mg tid
Enalapril	2.5 mg bid	10 mg bid
Lisinopril	2.5–5.0 mg qd	20–35 mg qd
Ramipril	1.25–2.5 mg bid	2.5–5 mg bid
Trandolapril	0.5 mg qd	4 mg qd
Angiotensin receptor blockers		
Valsartan	40 mg bid	160 mg bid
Candesartan	4 mg qd	32 mg qd
Irbesartan	75 mg qd	300 mg qd[b]
Losartan	12.5 mg qd	50 mg qd
β receptor blockers		
Carvedilol	3.125 mg bid	25–50 mg bid
Bisoprolol	1.25 mg qd	10 mg qd
Metoprolol succinate CR	12.5–25 mg qd	Target dose 200 mg qd
Additional therapies		
Spironolactone	12.5–25 mg qd	25–50 mg qd
Eplerenone	25 mg qd	50 mg qd
Combination of hydralazine/ isosorbide dinitrate	10–25 mg/10 mg tid	75 mg/40 mg tid
Fixed dose of hydralazine/ isosorbide dinitrate	37.5 mg/20 mg (one tablet) tid	75 mg/40 mg (two tablets) tid
Digoxin	0.125 mg qd	≤0.375 mg/d[b]

[a]Dose must be titrated to reduce the pt's congestive symptoms.
[b]Target dose not established.

in pts with asymptomatic LV dysfunction and to lower mortality when begun soon after acute MI. ACE inhibitors may result in significant hypotension in pts who are volume depleted, so start at lowest dosage (e.g., captopril 6.25 mg PO tid). ARBs (Table 133-2) may be substituted if pt is intolerant of ACE inhibitor (e.g., because of cough or angioedema). Consider hydralazine plus an oral nitrate instead in pts who develop hyperkalemia or renal insufficiency on ACE inhibitor.

- *Beta blockers* (Table 133-2) administered in gradually augmented dosage improve symptoms and prolong survival in pts with heart failure and reduced EF <40%. After pt stabilized on ACE inhibitor and diuretic, begin at low dosage and increase gradually [e.g., carvedilol 3.125 mg bid, double q2weeks as tolerated to maximum of 25 mg bid (for weight <85 kg) or 50 mg bid (weight >85 kg)].

- Aldosterone antagonist therapy (*spironolactone* or *eplerenone* [Table 133-2]), added to standard therapy in pts with advanced heart failure reduces mortality. The diuretic properties may also be symptomatically beneficial, and such therapy should be considered in pts with class III/IV heart failure symptoms and LVEF <35%. Should be used cautiously when combined with ACE inhibitor or angiotensin receptor blocker (ARB) to avoid hyperkalemia.

- *Digoxin* is useful in heart failure due to (1) marked systolic dysfunction (LV dilatation, low EF, S_3) and (2) heart failure with atrial fibrillation (AF) and rapid ventricular rates. Unlike ACE inhibitors and beta blockers, digoxin does not prolong survival in heart failure pts but reduces hospitalizations. Not indicated in CHF due to pericardial disease, restrictive cardiomyopathy, or mitral stenosis (unless AF is present). Digoxin is contraindicated in hypertrophic cardiomyopathy and in pts with AV conduction blocks.
  - Digoxin dosing (0.125–0.25 mg qd) depends on age, weight, and renal function and can be guided by measurement of serum digoxin level (maintain level <1.0 ng/mL).
  - *Digitalis toxicity* may be precipitated by hypokalemia, hypoxemia, hypercalcemia, hypomagnesemia, hypothyroidism, or myocardial ischemia. Early signs of toxicity include anorexia, nausea, and lethargy. *Cardiac toxicity* includes ventricular extrasystoles and ventricular tachycardia and fibrillation; atrial tachycardia with block; sinus arrest and sinoatrial block; all degrees of AV block. *Chronic* digitalis intoxication may cause cachexia, gynecomastia, "yellow" vision, or confusion. At first sign of digitalis toxicity, discontinue the drug; maintain serum K^+ concentration between 4.0 and 5.0 mmol/L. Bradyarrhythmias and AV block may respond to atropine (0.6 mg IV); otherwise, a temporary pacemaker may be required. Antidigoxin antibodies are available for massive overdose.

- The combination of the oral vasodilators *hydralazine* (10–75 mg tid) and *isosorbide dinitrate* (10–40 mg tid) may be of benefit for chronic administration in pts intolerant of ACE inhibitors and ARBs and is also beneficial as part of standard therapy, along with ACE inhibitor and beta blocker, in African Americans with class II–IV heart failure.

- In sicker, hospitalized pts, IV vasodilator therapy (Table 133-3) is often necessary. *Nitroprusside* is a potent mixed vasodilator for pts with markedly elevated systemic vascular resistance. It is metabolized to thiocyanate, which is excreted via the kidneys. To avoid thiocyanate

TABLE 133-3 DRUGS FOR TREATMENT OF ACUTE HEART FAILURE

	Initiating Dose	Maximal Dose
Vasodilators		
Nitroglycerin	20 µg/min	40–400 µg/min
Nitroprusside	10 µg/min	30–350 µg/min
Nesiritide	Bolus 2 µg/kg	0.01–0.03 µg/kg per min[a]
Inotropes		
Dobutamine	1–2 µg/kg per min	2–10 µg/kg per min[b]
Milrinone	Bolus 50 µg/kg	0.1–0.75 µg/kg per min[b]
Dopamine	1–2 µg/kg per min	2–4 µg/kg per min[b]
Levosimendan	Bolus 12 µg/kg	0.1–0.2 µg/kg per min[c]
Vasoconstrictors		
Dopamine for hypotension	5 µg/kg per min	5–15 µg/kg per min
Epinephrine	0.5 µg/kg per min	50 µg/kg per min
Phenylephrine	0.3 µg/kg per min	3 µg/kg per min
Vasopressin	0.05 units/min	0.1–0.4 units/min

[a]Usually <4 (µg/kg)/min.
[b]Inotropes will also have vasodilatory properties.
[c]Approved outside of the United States for the management of acute heart failure.

toxicity (seizures, altered mental status, nausea), follow thiocyanate levels in pts with renal dysfunction or if administered for >2 days. IV *nesiritide* (Table 133-3), a purified preparation of BNP, is a vasodilator that reduces pulmonary capillary wedge pressure and dyspnea in pts with acutely decompensated CHF. It should be used only in pts with refractory heart failure.

IV inotropic agents (see Table 133-3) are administered to hospitalized pts for refractory symptoms or acute exacerbation of CHF to augment cardiac output. They are contraindicated in hypertrophic cardiomyopathy. *Dobutamine* augments cardiac output without significant peripheral vasoconstriction or tachycardia. *Dopamine* at low dosage [1–5 (µg/kg)/min] facilitates diuresis; at higher dosage [5–10 (µg/kg)/min] positive inotropic effects predominate; peripheral vasoconstriction is greatest at dosage >10 (µg/kg)/min. *Milrinone* [0.1–0.75 (µg/kg)/min after 50-µg/kg loading dose] is a nonsympathetic positive inotrope and vasodilator. The above vasodilators and inotropic agents may be used together for additive effect.

- The initial approach to treatment of acute decompensated heart failure can rely on the pt's hemodynamic profile (Fig. 133-2) based on clinical exam and, if necessary, invasive hemodynamic monitoring:
  - *Profile A "Warm and dry"*: Symptoms due to conditions other than heart failure (e.g., acute ischemia). Treat underlying condition.

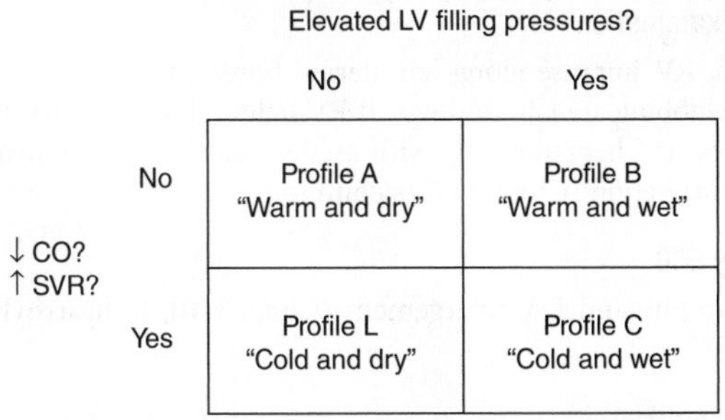

Elevated LV filling pressures?

FIGURE 133-2 Hemodynamic profiles in pts with acute heart failure. CO, cardiac output; LV, left ventricular; SVR, systemic vascular resistance. *(Modified from Grady et al: Circulation 102:2443, 2000.)*

- *Profile B "Warm and wet"*: Treat with diuretic and vasodilators.
- *Profile C "Cold and wet"*: Treat with IV vasodilators and inotropic agents.
- *Profile L "Cold and dry"*: If low filling pressure (PCW <12 mmHg) confirmed, consider trial of volume repletion.
- Consider implantable cardioverter defibrillator (ICD) prophylactically for chronic class II–III heart failure and LVEF <30–35%. Pts with an LVEF <35%, refractory CHF (NYHA class III–IV), and QRS >120 ms may be candidates for biventricular pacing (cardiac resynchronization therapy), typically in combination with an ICD. Pts with severe disease and <6 months expected survival, who meet stringent criteria, may be candidates for a ventricular assist device or cardiac transplantation.
- Pts with predominantly diastolic heart failure are treated with salt restriction and diuretics. Beta blockers and ACE inhibitors may be of benefit in blunting neurohormonal activation.

COR PULMONALE

RV enlargement resulting from *primary* lung disease; leads to RV hypertrophy and eventually to RV failure. Etiologies include:

- *Pulmonary parenchymal or airway disease* leading to hypoxemic vasoconstriction. Chronic obstructive lung disease (COPD), interstitial lung diseases, bronchiectasis, cystic fibrosis (Chaps. 140 and 143).
- *Conditions that occlude the pulmonary vasculature.* Recurrent pulmonary emboli, pulmonary arterial hypertension (PAH) (Chap. 136), vasculitis, sickle cell anemia.
- *Inadequate mechanical ventilation (chronic hypoventilation).* Kyphoscoliosis, neuromuscular disorders, marked obesity, sleep apnea (Chap. 146).

Symptoms

Depend on underlying disorder but include dyspnea, cough, fatigue, and sputum production (in parenchymal diseases).

Physical Examination

Tachypnea, RV impulse along left sternal border, loud P_2, right-sided S_4; cyanosis, clubbing are late findings. If RV failure develops, elevated jugular venous pressure, hepatomegaly with ascites, pedal edema; murmur of tricuspid regurgitation (Chap. 119) is common.

Laboratory ECG

RV hypertrophy and RA enlargement (Chap. 120); tachyarrhythmias are common.

Radiologic Studies

CXR shows RV and pulmonary artery enlargement; if PAH present, tapering of the pulmonary artery branches. Chest CT identifies emphysema, interstitial lung disease, and acute pulmonary embolism; V/Q scan is more reliable for diagnosis of chronic thromboemboli. Pulmonary function tests and ABGs characterize intrinsic pulmonary disease.

Echocardiogram

RV hypertrophy; LV function typically normal. RV systolic pressure can be estimated from Doppler measurement of tricuspid regurgitant flow. If imaging is difficult because of air in distended lungs, RV volume and wall thickness can be evaluated by MRI.

Right-Heart Catheterization

Can confirm presence of pulmonary hypertension and exclude left-heart failure as cause.

TREATMENT Cor Pulmonale

Aimed at underlying pulmonary disease and may include bronchodilators, antibiotics, oxygen administration, and noninvasive mechanical ventilation. For pts with PAH, pulmonary vasodilator therapy may be beneficial to reduce RV afterload (Chap. 136). See Chap. 142 for specific treatment of pulmonary embolism.

If RV failure is present, treat as heart failure, instituting low-sodium diet and diuretics; digoxin is of uncertain benefit and must be administered cautiously (toxicity increased due to hypoxemia, hypercapnia, acidosis). Loop diuretics must also be used with care to prevent significant metabolic alkalosis that blunts respiratory drive.

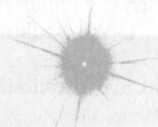

For a more detailed discussion, see Mann DL, Chakinala M: Heart Failure and Cor Pulmonale, Chap. 234, p. 1901, in HPIM-18.

CHAPTER **134**
Diseases of the Aorta

Abnormal dilatation of the abdominal or thoracic aorta; in ascending aorta most commonly secondary to cystic medial necrosis (e.g., familial, Marfan syndrome, Ehlers-Danlos syndrome type IV); aneurysms of descending thoracic and abdominal aorta are primarily atherosclerotic. Rare causes of aneurysms are infections (syphilitic, tuberculous, mycotic) and vasculitides (e.g., Takayasu's arteritis, giant cell arteritis).

History

May be clinically silent, but thoracic aortic aneurysms can result in deep, diffuse chest pain, dysphagia, hoarseness, hemoptysis, dry cough; abdominal aneurysms may result in abdominal pain or thromboemboli to the lower extremities.

Physical Examination

Abdominal aneurysms are often palpable, most commonly in periumbilical area. Pts with ascending thoracic aneurysms may show features of Marfan syndrome (Chap. 363, HPIM-18).

Laboratory

Suspect thoracic aneurysm by abnormal *CXR* (enlarged aortic silhouette) and confirm by *echocardiography*, *contrast CT*, or *MRI*. Confirm abdominal aneurysm by *abdominal plain film* (rim of calcification), *ultrasound*, *CT*, *MRI*, or *contrast aortography*. If clinically suspected, obtain serologic test for syphilis, especially if ascending thoracic aneurysm shows thin shell of calcification.

> **TREATMENT** Aortic Aneurysm
>
> Pharmacologic control of hypertension (Chap. 126) is essential, usually including a beta blocker. Preliminary studies suggest inhibition of the renin-angiotensin system (e.g., with the ARB losartan) may reduce rate of aortic dilation in Marfan syndrome via blockade of TGF-β signaling. Surgical resection for large aneurysms (ascending thoracic aortic aneurysms >5.5–6 cm, descending thoracic aortic aneurysms >6.5–7.0 cm, or abdominal aortic aneurysm >5.5 cm), for persistent pain despite bp control, or for evidence of rapid expansion. In pts with Marfan syndrome or bicuspid aortic valve, thoracic aortic aneurysms >5 cm usually warrant repair. Less invasive endovascular repair is an option for some pts with descending thoracic or abdominal aortic aneurysms.

Potentially life-threatening condition in which disruption or aortic intima allows dissection of blood into vessel wall; may involve ascending aorta

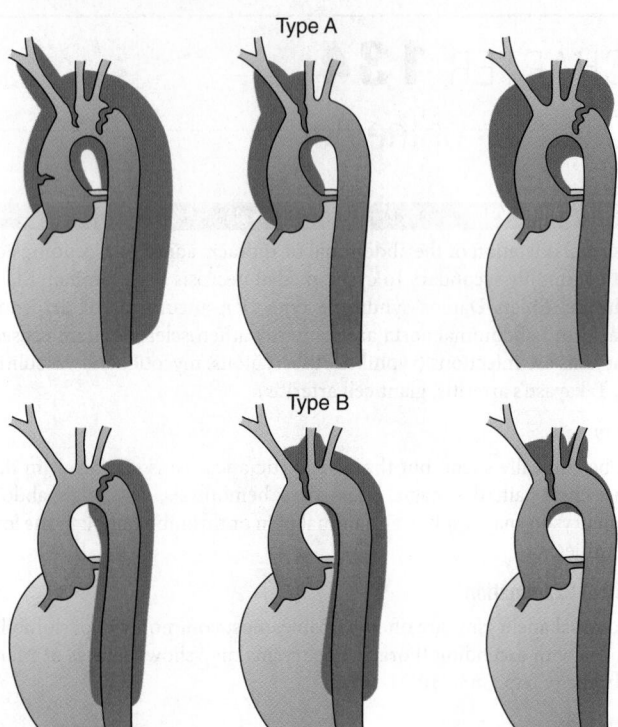

FIGURE 134-1 Classification of aortic dissections. Stanford classification: Top panels illustrate type A dissections that involve the ascending aorta independent of site of tear and distal extension; type B dissections (bottom panels) involve transverse and/or descending aorta without involvement of the ascending aorta. DeBakey classification: Type I dissection involves ascending to descending aorta (top left); type II dissection is limited to ascending or transverse aorta, without descending aorta (top center + top right); type III dissection involves descending aorta only (bottom left). *[From DC Miller, in RM Doroghazi, EE Slater (eds.),* Aortic Dissection. *New York, McGraw-Hill, 1983, with permission.]*

(type II), descending aorta (type III), or both (type I). Alternative classification: Type A—dissection involves ascending aorta; type B—limited to transverse and/or descending aorta. Involvement of the ascending aorta is most lethal form. Variant acute aortic syndromes include intramural hematoma without an intimal flap, and penetrating atherosclerotic ulcer.

Etiology

Ascending aortic dissection is associated with hypertension, cystic medial necrosis, Marfan and Ehlers-Danlos syndromes; descending dissections are commonly associated with atherosclerosis or hypertension. Incidence is increased in pts with coarctation of aorta, bicuspid aortic valve, and rarely in third trimester of pregnancy in otherwise normal women.

Symptoms

Sudden onset of severe anterior or posterior chest pain, with "ripping" quality; maximal pain may travel if dissection propagates. Additional symptoms relate to obstruction of aortic branches (stroke, MI), dyspnea (acute aortic regurgitation), or symptoms of low cardiac output due to cardiac tamponade (dissection into pericardial sac).

Physical Examination

Sinus tachycardia common; if cardiac tamponade develops, hypotension, pulsus paradoxus, and pericardial rub appear. Asymmetry of carotid or brachial pulses, aortic regurgitation, and neurologic abnormalities associated with interruption of carotid artery flow are possible findings.

Laboratory

CXR: Widening of mediastinum; dissection can be confirmed by *CT, MRI,* or *transesophageal echocardiography.* Aortography is rarely required, as sensitivity of these noninvasive techniques is >90%.

TREATMENT Aortic Dissection

Reduce cardiac contractility and treat hypertension to maintain systolic bp between 100 and 120 mmHg using IV agents (Table 134-1), e.g., sodium nitroprusside accompanied by a beta blocker (e.g., IV metoprolol, labetolol, or esmolol, aiming for heart rate of 60 beats per min), followed by oral therapy. If beta blocker contraindicated, consider IV verapamil or diltiazem (see Table 132-3). Avoid direct vasodilators (e.g., hydralazine) because they may increase shear stress. Ascending aortic dissection (type A) requires surgical repair emergently or, if pt can be stabilized with medications, semielectively. Descending aortic dissections are stabilized medically (maintain systolic bp between 110 and 120 mmHg) with oral antihypertensive agents (esp. beta blockers); surgical repair is not usually indicated unless continued pain or extension of dissection is observed (by serial MRI or CT performed every 6–12 months).

TABLE 134-1 TREATMENT OF AORTIC DISSECTION

Preferred Regimen	Dose
Sodium nitroprusside	20–400 µg/min IV
plus a beta blocker:	
Propranolol *or*	0.5 mg IV; then 1 mg q5min, to total of 0.15 mg/kg
Esmolol *or*	500 µg/kg IV over 1 min; then 50–200 (µg/kg)/min
Labetalol	20 mg IV over 2 min, then 40–80 mg q10–15min to max of 300 mg

OTHER ABNORMALITIES OF THE AORTA

Atherosclerotic Occlusive Disease of Abdominal Aorta

Particularly common in presence of diabetes mellitus or cigarette smoking. Symptoms include intermittent claudication of the buttocks and thighs and impotence (Leriche syndrome); femoral and other distal pulses are absent. Diagnosis is established by noninvasive leg pressure measurements and Doppler velocity analysis, and confirmed by MRI, CT, or aortography. Catheter-based endovascular treatment or aortic-femoral bypass surgery is required for symptomatic treatment.

Takayasu's ("Pulseless") Disease

Arteritis of aorta and major branches in young women. Anorexia, weight loss, fever, and night sweats occur. Localized symptoms relate to occlusion of aortic branches (cerebral ischemia, claudication, and loss of pulses in arms). ESR and C-reactive protein are increased; diagnosis confirmed by aortography. Glucocorticoid and immunosuppressive therapy may be beneficial.

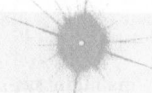

For a more detailed discussion, see Creager MA, Loscalzo J: Diseases of the Aorta, Chap. 248, p. 2060, in HPIM-18.

CHAPTER **135**
Peripheral Vascular Disease

Occlusive or inflammatory disease that develops within the peripheral arteries, veins, or lymphatics.

ARTERIOSCLEROSIS OF PERIPHERAL ARTERIES

History

Intermittent claudication is muscular cramping with exercise; quickly relieved by rest. Pain in buttocks and thighs suggests aortoiliac disease; calf muscle pain implies femoral or popliteal artery disease. More advanced arteriosclerotic obstruction results in pain at rest; painful ulcers of the feet (sometimes painless in diabetics) may result.

Physical Examination

Decreased peripheral pulses (ankle:brachial index <1.0; <0.5 with severe ischemia), blanching of affected limb with elevation, dependent rubor (redness). Ischemic ulcers or gangrene of toes may be present.

Laboratory

Segmental pressure measurements and Doppler ultrasound of peripheral pulses before and during exercise localizes stenoses; magnetic resonance angiography, computed tomographic angiography (CTA), or conventional arteriography is performed if mechanical revascularization (surgical or percutaneous) is planned.

TREATMENT Arteriosclerosis

Most pts can be managed medically with daily exercise program, careful foot care (especially in diabetics), treatment of hypercholesterolemia, and local debridement of ulcerations. Abstinence from cigarettes is mandatory. Antiplatelet therapy is indicated to reduce future cardiovascular events. Some, but not all, pts note symptomatic improvement with drug therapy (cilostazol or pentoxifylline). Pts with severe claudication, rest pain, or gangrene are candidates for revascularization (arterial reconstructive surgery or percutaneous transluminal angioplasty/stent placement).

OTHER CONDITIONS THAT IMPAIR PERIPHERAL ARTERIAL FLOW

Arterial Embolism

Results from thrombus or vegetation within the heart or aorta, or paradoxically from a venous thrombus through a right-to-left intracardiac shunt.

History

Sudden pain or numbness in an extremity in the absence of previous history of claudication.

Physical Examination

Absent pulse, pallor, and decreased temperature of limb distal to the occlusion. Lesion is identified by angiography.

TREATMENT Arterial Embolism

IV heparin is administered to prevent propagation of clot. For acute severe ischemia, immediate endovascular or surgical embolectomy is indicated. Thrombolytic therapy (e.g., tissue plasminogen activator, reteplase, or tenecteplase) may be effective for thrombus within atherosclerotic vessel or arterial bypass graft.

Atheroembolism

A subset of acute arterial occlusion due to embolization of fibrin, platelets, and cholesterol debris from more proximal atheromas or aneurysm; typically occurs after intraarterial instrumentation. Depending on location, may lead to stroke, renal insufficiency, or pain and tenderness in embolized tissue. Atheroembolism to lower extremities results in blue toe syndrome, which can progress to necrosis and gangrene. Treatment is supportive; for recurrent episodes, surgical intervention in the proximal atherosclerotic vessel or aneurysm may be required.

Vasospastic Disorders

Manifest by Raynaud's phenomenon in which cold exposure results in triphasic color response: blanching of the fingers, followed by cyanosis, then

TABLE 135-1 CLASSIFICATION OF RAYNAUD'S PHENOMENON

Primary or idiopathic Raynaud's phenomenon: Raynaud's disease

Secondary Raynaud's phenomenon

    Collagen vascular diseases: scleroderma, systemic lupus erythematosus, rheumatoid arthritis, dermatomyositis, polymyositis

    Arterial occlusive diseases: atherosclerosis of the extremities, thromboangiitis obliterans, acute arterial occlusion, thoracic outlet syndrome

    Pulmonary hypertension

    Neurologic disorders: intervertebral disk disease, syringomyelia, spinal cord tumors, stroke, poliomyelitis, carpal tunnel syndrome

    Blood dyscrasias: cold agglutinins, cryoglobulinemia, cryofibrinogenemia, myeloproliferative disorders, Waldenström's macroglobulinemia

    Trauma: vibration injury, hammer hand syndrome, electric shock, cold injury, typing, piano playing

    Drugs: ergot derivatives, methysergide, β-adrenergic receptor blockers, bleomycin, vinblastine, cisplatin

rubor. Usually a benign disorder. However, suspect an underlying disease (Table 135-1) if tissue necrosis occurs, if disease is unilateral, or if it develops after age 50.

TREATMENT   Vasospastic Disorders

Keep extremities warm. Tobacco use is contraindicated. Dihydropyridine calcium channel blockers (e.g., nifedipine XL 30–90 mg PO qd) or α_1-adrenergic antagonists (e.g., prazosin 1–5 mg tid) may be effective.

Thromboangiitis Obliterans (Buerger's Disease)

Occurs in young men who are heavy smokers and involves both upper and lower extremities; nonatheromatous inflammatory reaction develops in veins and small arteries, leading to superficial thrombophlebitis and arterial obstruction with ulceration or gangrene of digits. Arteriography shows smooth tapering lesions in distal vessels, often without proximal atherosclerotic disease. Abstinence from tobacco is essential.

VENOUS DISEASE

Superficial Thrombophlebitis

A benign disorder characterized by erythema, tenderness, and edema along involved vein. Conservative therapy includes local heat, elevation, and anti-inflammatory drugs such as aspirin. More serious conditions such as cellulitis or lymphangitis may mimic this, but these are associated with fever, chills, lymphadenopathy, and red superficial streaks along inflamed lymphatic channels.

TABLE 135-2 CONDITIONS ASSOCIATED WITH AN INCREASED RISK FOR DEVELOPMENT OF VENOUS THROMBOSIS

Surgery: Orthopedic, thoracic, abdominal, and genitourinary procedures

Neoplasms: Pancreas, lung, ovary, testes, urinary tract, breast, stomach

Trauma: Fractures of spine, pelvis, femur, tibia

Immobilization: Acute MI, CHF, stroke, postoperative convalescence

Pregnancy: Estrogen use (for replacement or contraception)

Hypercoagulable states: Resistance to activated protein C; prothrombin 20210A mutation; deficiencies of antithrombin III, protein C, or protein S; antiphospholipid antibodies; myeloproliferative disease; dysfibrinogenemia; DIC

Venulitis: Thromboangiitis obliterans, Behçet's disease, homocystinuria

Previous deep-vein thrombosis

Deep-Vein Thrombosis (DVT)

This is a more serious condition that may lead to pulmonary embolism (Chap. 142). Particularly common in pts on prolonged bed rest, those with chronic debilitating disease, and those with malignancies (Table 135-2).

History

Pain or tenderness in calf or thigh, usually unilateral; may be asymptomatic, with pulmonary embolism as primary presentation.

Physical Examination

Often normal; local swelling or tenderness to deep palpation may be present over affected vein.

Laboratory

D-Dimer testing is sensitive but not specific for diagnosis. Most helpful noninvasive testing is ultrasound imaging of the deep veins with Doppler interrogation [most sensitive for proximal (upper leg) DVT, less sensitive for calf DVT]. Invasive venography is rarely indicated. MRI may be useful for diagnosis of proximal DVT and DVT within the pelvic veins or in the superior or inferior vena cavae.

> **TREATMENT** Venous Disease
>
> Systemic anticoagulation with heparin [5000- to 10,000-U bolus, followed by continuous IV infusion to maintain aPTT at 2 × normal (or using a nomogram: 80-U/kg bolus followed by initial infusion of 18 (U/kg)/h)] or low-molecular-weight heparin (LMWH) (e.g., enoxaparin 1 mg/kg SC bid), followed by warfarin PO (overlap with heparin for at least 4–5 days and continue for at least 3 months if proximal deep veins involved). Adjust warfarin dose to maintain prothrombin time INR 2.0–3.0.

DVT can be prevented by early ambulation following surgery or with low-dose unfractionated heparin during prolonged bed rest (5000 U SC bid-tid) or LMWH (e.g., enoxaparin 40 mg SC daily), supplemented by pneumatic compression boots. Following knee or hip surgery, warfarin (INR 2.0–3.0) is an effective regimen. LMWHs are also effective in preventing DVT after general or orthopedic surgery.

Chronic Venous Insufficiency

Results from prior DVT or venous valvular incompetence and manifests as chronic dull ache in leg that worsens with prolonged standing, edema, and superficial varicosities. May lead to erythema, hyperpigmentation, and recurrent cellulitis; ulcers may appear at medial and lateral malleoli. Treatment includes graduated compression stockings and leg elevation.

LYMPHEDEMA

Chronic, painless edema, usually of the lower extremities; may be primary (inherited) or secondary to lymphatic damage or obstruction (e.g., recurrent lymphangitis, tumor, filariasis).

Physical Examination

Marked pitting edema in early stages; limb becomes indurated with *non*pitting edema chronically. Differentiate from chronic *venous* insufficiency, which displays hyperpigmentation, stasis dermatitis, and superficial venous varicosities.

Laboratory

Abdominal and pelvic ultrasound or CT or MRI to identify obstructing lesions. Lymphangiography or lymphoscintigraphy (rarely done) to confirm diagnosis. If *unilateral* edema, differentiate from DVT by noninvasive venous studies (above).

TREATMENT　Lymphedema

(1) Meticulous foot hygiene to prevent infection, (2) leg elevation, (3) compression stockings and/or pneumatic compression boots. Diuretics should be *avoided* to prevent intravascular volume depletion.

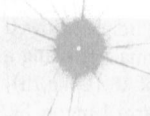

For a more detailed discussion, see Creager MA, Loscalzo J: Vascular Diseases of the Extremities, Chap. 249, p. 2066, in HPIM-18.

CHAPTER **136**
Pulmonary Hypertension

Definition
Elevation of pulmonary artery (PA) pressure due to pulmonary vascular or parenchymal disease, increased left heart filling pressures, or a combination. Table 136-1 lists etiologies by underlying categories.

Symptoms
Exertional dyspnea, fatigue, angina (due to RV ischemia), syncope, peripheral edema.

TABLE 136-1 CATEGORIES OF PULMONARY HYPERTENSION

1. Pulmonary Arterial Hypertension
Idiopathic
Collagen vascular diseases (e.g., CREST, scleroderma, SLE, RA)
Congenital systemic to pulmonary shunts (e.g., ventricular septal defect, patent ductus arteriosus, atrial septal defect)
Portal hypertension
HIV infection
Drugs or toxins (e.g., fenfluramines)
2. Pulmonary Venous Hypertension
LV systolic or diastolic dysfunction
Left-sided valvular disease
Pulmonary venous obstruction
3. Hypoxemic Lung Disease
Chronic obstructive lung disease
Interstitial lung disease
Sleep-disordered breathing
Chronic hypoventilation
4. Chronic Pulmonary Thromboembolic Disease
Chronic pulmonary embolism
Nonthrombotic pulmonary embolism (e.g., tumor or foreign material)
5. Miscellaneous
Sarcoidosis
Histiocytosis X
Schistosomiasis

Abbreviation: CREST, calcinosis, Raynaud's phenomenon, esophageal involvement, sclerodactyly, and telangiectasia (syndrome).

Physical Examination

Jugular venous distention, RV lift, increased P_2, right-sided S_4, tricuspid regurgitation. Peripheral cyanosis and edema are late manifestations.

Laboratory

CXR shows enlarged central PA. *ECG* may demonstrate RV hypertrophy and RA enlargement. *Echocardiogram* shows RV and RA enlargement; RV systolic pressure can be estimated from Doppler recording of tricuspid regurgitation (Chap. 120). *Pulmonary function tests* identify underlying obstructive or restrictive lung disease; impaired CO diffusion capacity is common. *Chest CT* identifies contributing interstitial lung disease or pulmonary thromboembolic disease. *ANA titer* is elevated in collagen vascular diseases. *HIV testing* should be performed in individuals at risk. *Cardiac catheterization* accurately assesses PA pressures, cardiac output, and pulmonary vascular resistance, and it identifies underlying congenital vascular shunts; during procedure, response to short-acting vasodilators can be assessed.

Figure 136-1 summarizes workup of pt with unexplained pulmonary hypertension.

◼ IDIOPATHIC PULMONARY ARTERIAL HYPERTENSION (PAH)

Uncommon (2 cases/million), very serious form of pulmonary hypertension. Most pts present in fourth and fifth decades, female » male predominance; up to 20% of cases are familial. Major symptom is dyspnea, often with insidious onset. Mean survival <3 years in absence of therapy.

Physical Examination

Prominent *a* wave in jugular venous pulse, right ventricular heave, narrowly split S_2 with accentuated P_2. Terminal course is characterized by signs of right-sided heart failure.

Laboratory

CXR: RV and central pulmonary arterial prominence. Pulmonary arteries taper sharply. *PFTs:* usually normal or mild restrictive defect. *ECG:* RV enlargement, right axis deviation, and RV hypertrophy. *Echocardiogram:* RA and RV enlargement and tricuspid regurgitation.

Differential Diagnosis

Other disorders of heart, lungs, and pulmonary vasculature must be considered. Lung function studies will identify chronic pulmonary disease causing pulmonary hypertension and cor pulmonale. Interstitial diseases (PFTs, CT scan) and hypoxic pulmonary hypertension (ABGs, Sao_2) should be excluded. Perfusion lung scan should be considered to exclude chronic pulmonary embolism (PE). Rarely, pulmonary hypertension is due to parasitic disease (schistosomiasis, filariasis). Cardiovascular disorders to be excluded include pulmonary artery and pulmonic valve stenosis, ventricular and atrial shunts with secondary pulmonary vascular disease (Eisenmenger syndrome), and clinically silent mitral stenosis.

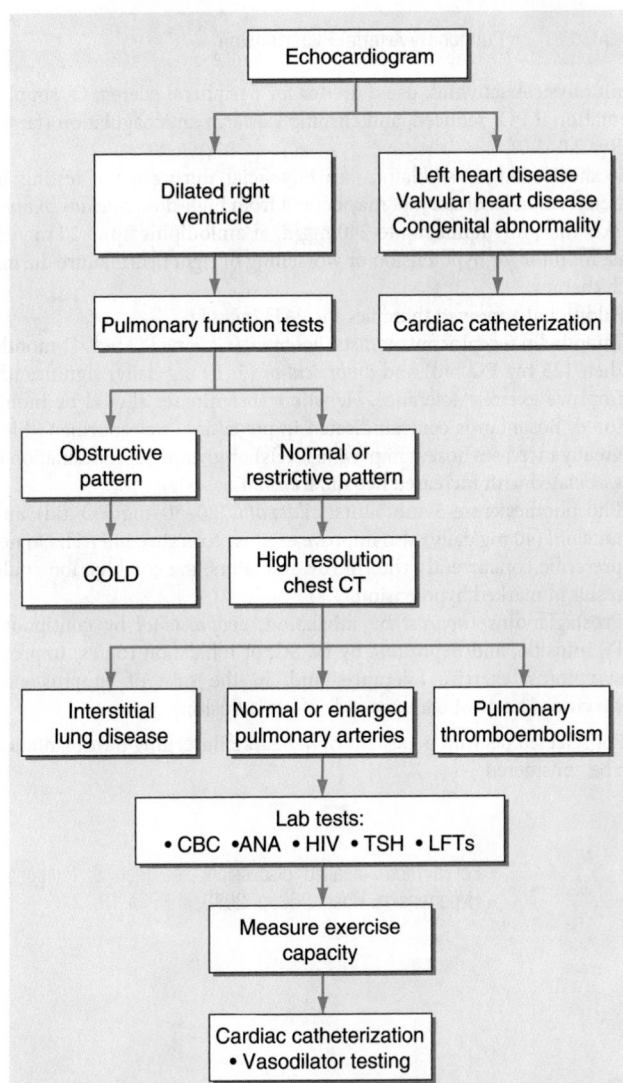

FIGURE 136-1 An algorithm for the workup of a pt with unexplained pulmonary hypertension. All potential etiologies and associated conditions must be investigated in a pt with clinical findings consistent with pulmonary hypertension. ANA, antinuclear antibodies; CBC, complete blood count; COLD, chronic obstructive lung disease; HIV, human immunodeficiency virus; LFTs, liver function tests; TSH, thyroid-stimulating hormone.

| TREATMENT | Pulmonary Arterial Hypertension |

Limit physical activities, use diuretics for peripheral edema, O_2 supplementation if PO_2 reduced, and chronic warfarin anticoagulation (target INR = 2.0–3.0).

If short-acting vasodilators are beneficial during acute testing in catheterization laboratory, pt may benefit from high-dose *calcium channel blocker* (e.g., nifedipine, up to 240 mg/d, or amlodipine up to 20 mg/d); must monitor for hypotension or worsening of right heart failure during such therapy.

Additional approved therapies for PAH include:

1. Endothelin receptor antagonists: *bosentan* (62.5 mg PO bid × 1 month, then 125 mg PO bid) and *ambrisentan* (5–10 mg daily) significantly improve exercise tolerance. Hepatic transaminases should be monitored. Bosentan is contraindicated in pts taking cyclosporine (which greatly increases bosentan plasma levels) or glyburide (combination is associated with increased hepatic transaminases).

2. Phosphodiesterase-5 inhibitors: *sildenafil* (20–80 mg PO tid) and *tadalafil* (40 mg daily) also improve exercise tolerance in PAH. Do not prescribe concurrently with nitrovasodilators; the combination could result in marked hypotension.

3. Prostaglandins (*iloprost* by inhalation, *epoprostenol* by continuous IV infusion, and *treprostinil* by IV, SC, or inhalation routes) improve symptoms, exercise tolerance, and, in the case of epoprostenol, survival. The most common side effect is flushing.

For selected pts with persistent right heart failure, lung transplantation can be considered.

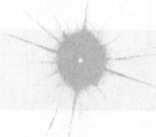

For a more detailed discussion, see Rich S: Pulmonary Hypertension, Chap. 250, p. 2076, in HPIM-18.

CHAPTER **137**
Respiratory Function and
Pulmonary Diagnostic
Procedures

RESPIRATORY FUNCTION

The major classes of lung diseases include obstructive lung diseases (e.g., asthma, chronic obstructive pulmonary disease, and bronchiectasis), restrictive lung diseases (e.g., interstitial lung diseases, chest wall abnormalities, and neuromuscular diseases), and vascular abnormalities (e.g., pulmonary thromboembolism and pulmonary arterial hypertension). The respiratory system includes not only the lungs but also the chest wall, pulmonary circulation, and central nervous system. There are three key types of respiratory system physiologic disturbances that occur in varying combinations in different lung diseases: ventilatory function, pulmonary circulation, and gas exchange.

Disturbances in Ventilatory Function

Ventilation involves the delivery of gas to the alveoli. Pulmonary function tests are used to assess ventilatory function. The classification of lung volumes, which are measured with pulmonary function testing, is shown in Fig. 137-1. Spirometry involves forced exhalation from total lung capacity

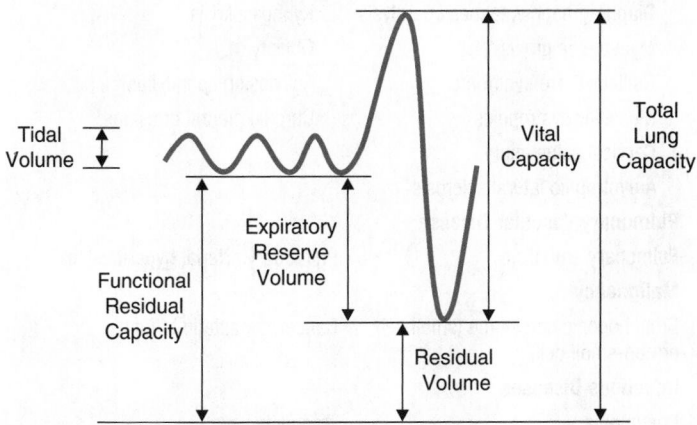

FIGURE 137-1 Spirogram of a slow vital capacity maneuver demonstrating various lung volumes.

899

(TLC) to residual volume (RV); key measurements from a spirogram are the forced expiratory volume in 1 s (FEV_1) and the forced vital capacity (FVC). Expiratory flow rates may be plotted against lung volumes to yield a flow-volume curve. Plateau of the inspiratory curve on the flow-volume loop suggests extrathoracic large airway obstruction, while plateau of the expiratory curve suggests intrathoracic large airway obstruction. Other lung volumes, including TLC and RV, are measured under static conditions using either helium dilution or body plethysmography. Lung volumes and flow rates are typically compared with population-based normal values that adjust for the age, height, sex, and race of the pt.

There are two major patterns of abnormal ventilatory function detected by pulmonary function testing: restrictive and obstructive (Tables 137-1 and 137-2). The presence of obstruction is determined by a reduced ratio

TABLE 137-1 COMMON RESPIRATORY DISEASES BY DIAGNOSTIC CATEGORIES

Obstructive	
Asthma	Bronchiectasis
Chronic obstructive pulmonary disease	Cystic fibrosis
	Bronchiolitis
Restrictive—Parenchymal	
Sarcoidosis	Pneumoconiosis
Idiopathic pulmonary fibrosis	Drug- or radiation-induced interstitial lung disease
Desquamative interstitial pneumonitis	Asbestosis
Restrictive—Extraparenchymal	
Neuromuscular	Chest wall
Diaphragmatic weakness/paralysis	Kyphoscoliosis
Myasthenia gravis	Obesity
Guillain-Barré syndrome	Ankylosing spondylitis
Muscular dystrophies	Chronic pleural effusions
Cervical spine injury	
Amyotrophic lateral sclerosis	
Pulmonary Vascular Disease	
Pulmonary embolism	Pulmonary arterial hypertension
Malignancy	
Bronchogenic carcinoma (small cell or non-small cell)	Cancer metastatic to lung
Infectious Diseases	
Pneumonia	Tracheitis
	Bronchitis

TABLE 137-2 ALTERATIONS IN VENTILATORY FUNCTION IN DIFFERENT PULMONARY DISEASE CATEGORIES

	TLC	RV	VC	FEV_1/FVC
Obstructive	N to ↑	↑	↓	↓
Restrictive				
Pulmonary parenchymal	↓	↓	↓	N to ↑
Extraparenchymal—neuromuscular weakness	↓	Variable	↓	Variable
Extraparenchymal—chest wall deformity	↓	Variable	↓	N

Abbreviation: N, normal; for other abbreviations, see text.

of FEV_1/FVC (with abnormal often defined using a threshold of <0.7), and the severity of airflow obstruction is determined by the level of reduction of FEV_1. With airflow obstruction, TLC may be normal or increased, and RV is typically elevated. With severe airflow obstruction, the FVC is often reduced.

The presence of a restrictive pattern is determined by a reduction in lung volumes, especially TLC. When pulmonary parenchymal processes cause restriction, RV is also decreased, but the FEV_1/FVC is normal. With extraparenchymal etiologies of restrictive ventilatory defects, such as neuromuscular weakness or chest wall abnormalities, the impact on RV and FEV_1/FVC is more variable. Weakness of the respiratory muscles can be assessed by measuring maximal inspiratory and expiratory pressures.

Disturbances in Pulmonary Circulation

The pulmonary vasculature normally handles the right ventricular output (~5 L/min) at a low pressure. Normal mean pulmonary artery pressure (PAP) is 15 mmHg. When cardiac output increases, pulmonary vascular resistance (PVR) normally falls, leading to only small increases in mean PAP.

Assessment of the pulmonary vasculature requires measuring pulmonary vascular pressures and cardiac output to derive PVR. PVR rises with hypoxemia (due to vasoconstriction), intraluminal thrombi (due to diminished cross-sectional area from obstruction), or destruction of small pulmonary vessels (due to scarring or loss of the alveolar walls).

All diseases of the respiratory system causing hypoxemia are capable of causing pulmonary hypertension. However, pts with prolonged hypoxemia related to chronic obstructive pulmonary disease, interstitial lung disease, chest wall disease, and obesity-hypoventilation/obstructive sleep apnea are particularly likely to develop pulmonary hypertension. When pulmonary vessels are directly affected, as with recurrent pulmonary emboli, the decrease in cross-sectional area of the pulmonary vasculature is the primary mechanism for increased PVR, rather than hypoxemia.

Disturbances in Gas Exchange

The primary functions of the respiratory system are to remove CO_2 from blood entering the pulmonary circulation and to provide O_2 to blood leaving the pulmonary circulation. Normal tidal volume is approximately 500 mL and normal respiratory rate is approximately 15 breaths/min, leading to a total minute ventilation of approximately 7.5 L/min. Because of anatomic dead space, alveolar ventilation is approximately 5 L/min. Gas exchange depends on alveolar ventilation rather than total minute ventilation.

Partial pressure of CO_2 in arterial blood ($Paco_2$) is directly proportional to the amount of CO_2 produced each minute ($\dot{V}co_2$) and inversely proportional to alveolar ventilation ($\dot{V}A$)

$$Paco_2 = 0.863 \times \dot{V}co_2 / \dot{V}A$$

Adequate movement of gas between alveoli and pulmonary capillaries by diffusion is required for normal gas exchange. Diffusion can be tested by measuring the diffusing capacity of the lung for a low (and safe) concentration of carbon monoxide ($Dlco$) during a 10-second breath-hold. $Dlco$ measurement is typically corrected for the pt's hemoglobin level. Diffusion abnormalities rarely result in arterial hypoxemia at rest but can cause hypoxemia with exercise. A restrictive ventilatory defect with reduced $Dlco$ suggests parenchymal lung disease. The pattern of normal spirometry, normal lung volumes, and reduced $Dlco$ is consistent with pulmonary vascular disease. Gas exchange is critically dependent on proper matching of ventilation and perfusion.

Assessment of gas exchange is commonly performed with arterial blood gases, which provide measurements of the partial pressures of O_2 and CO_2. The actual content of O_2 in blood is determined by both Po_2 and hemoglobin concentration. The alveolar-arterial O_2 difference [$(A - a)$ gradient] can provide useful information when assessing abnormalities in gas exchange. The normal $(A - a)$ gradient is <15 mmHg under age 30 but increases with aging. In order to calculate the $(A - a)$ gradient, the alveolar Po_2 ($Paco_2$) must be calculated:

$$Pao_2 = Fio_2 \times (PB - P_{H_2O}) - Paco_2/R$$

where Fio_2 = fractional concentration of inspired O_2 (0.21 while breathing room air), PB = barometric pressure (760 mmHg at sea level), P_{H_2O} = water vapor pressure (47 mmHg when air is saturated at 37°C), and R = respiratory quotient (the ratio of CO_2 production to O_2 consumption, usually assumed to be 0.8). Severe arterial hypoxemia rarely occurs purely due to alveolar hypoventilation while breathing air at sea level. The $(A - a)$ gradient is calculated by subtracting the measured Pao_2 from the calculated Pao_2.

Adequacy of CO_2 removal is reflected in the partial pressure of CO_2 measured in an arterial blood gas. Pulse oximetry is a valuable, widely used, and noninvasive tool to assess O_2 saturation, but it provides no information about $Paco_2$. Other limitations of pulse oximetry include relative insensitivity to oxygenation changes when Pao_2 is >60 mmHg, problems with obtaining an adequate signal when cutaneous perfusion is decreased, and inability to distinguish oxyhemoglobin from other forms of hemoglobin, such as carboxyhemoglobin and methemoglobin.

Mechanisms of Abnormal Respiratory Function

The four basic mechanisms of hypoxemia are (1) decrease in inspired Po_2, (2) hypoventilation, (3) shunt, and (4) ventilation/perfusion mismatch. Decrease in inspired Po_2 (e.g., at high altitude) and hypoventilation (characterized by an increased $Paco_2$) both lower arterial oxygenation by reducing alveolar oxygenation; thus, the $(A - a)$ gradient is normal. Shunting (e.g., intracardiac shunt) causes hypoxemia by bypassing the alveolar capillaries. Shunting is characterized by an elevated $(A - a)$ gradient and is relatively refractory to oxygenation improvement with supplemental O_2. Ventilation/perfusion mismatch is the most common cause of hypoxemia; it is associated with an elevated $(A - a)$ gradient, but supplemental O_2 corrects the hypoxemia by raising the O_2 content of blood from regions with low ventilation/perfusion ratios. An algorithm for approaching the hypoxemic pt is shown in Fig. 137-2.

Hypercapnia is caused by inadequate alveolar ventilation. Potential contributing factors include (1) increased CO_2 production, (2) decreased ventilatory drive, (3) malfunction of the respiratory pump or increased airway resistance, and (4) inefficiency of gas exchange (increased dead space or ventilation/perfusion mismatch).

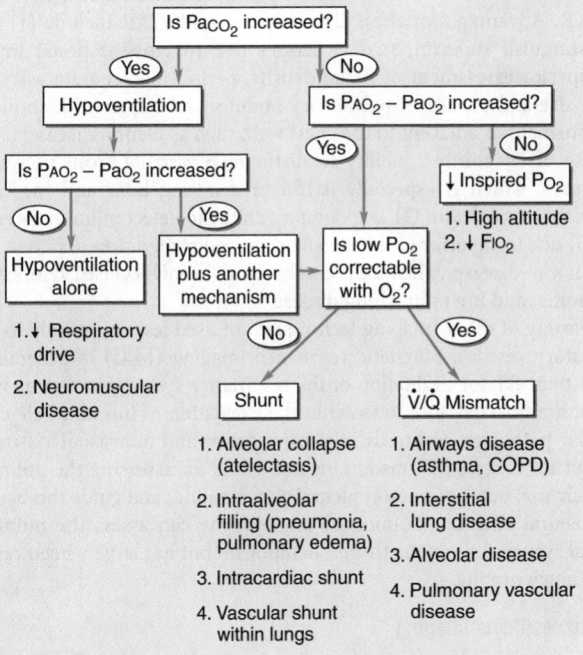

FIGURE 137-2 Flow diagram outlining the diagnostic approach to the pt with hypoxemia. COPD, chronic obstructive pulmonary disease. (*From SE Weinberger:* Principles of Pulmonary Medicine, *4th ed. Philadelphia, Saunders, 2004; with permission.*)

Although diffusion abnormalities rarely cause hypoxemia at rest, assessment of D$_{LCO}$ can be used to determine the functional integrity of the alveolar-capillary membrane. Diseases that solely affect the airways typically do not reduce the D$_{LCO}$. D$_{LCO}$ is reduced in interstitial lung disease, emphysema, and pulmonary vascular disease. D$_{LCO}$ can be elevated in alveolar hemorrhage, asthma, and congestive heart failure.

DIAGNOSTIC PROCEDURES

■ NONINVASIVE PROCEDURES

Radiographic Studies

The chest x-ray (CXR), generally including both posteroanterior and lateral views, is often the first diagnostic study in pts presenting with respiratory symptoms. With some exceptions (e.g., pneumothorax), the CXR pattern is usually not sufficiently specific to *establish* a diagnosis; instead, the CXR serves to *detect* disease, assess magnitude, and guide further diagnostic investigation. With diffuse lung disease, CXR can detect an alveolar, interstitial, or nodular pattern. CXR can also detect pleural effusion and pneumothorax, as well as abnormalities in the hila and mediastinum. Lateral decubitus views can be used to estimate the size of freely flowing pleural effusions.

Chest CT is widely used to clarify radiographic abnormalities detected by CXR. Advantages of chest CT compared with CXR include (1) ability to distinguish superimposed structures due to cross-sectional imaging; (2) superior assessment of tissue density, permitting accurate assessment of the size and density of pulmonary nodules and improved identification of abnormalities adjacent to the chest wall, such as pleural disease; (3) with the use of IV contrast, ability to distinguish vascular from nonvascular structures, which is especially useful in assessing hilar and mediastinal abnormalities; (4) with CT angiography, ability to detect pulmonary emboli; and (5) due to superior visible detail, improved recognition of parenchymal and airway diseases, including emphysema, bronchiectasis, lymphangitic carcinoma, and interstitial lung disease.

A variety of other imaging techniques are used less commonly to assess respiratory disease. Magnetic resonance imaging (MRI) is generally less useful than CT for evaluation of the respiratory system but can be helpful as a nonradioactive tool to assist in the evaluation of intrathoracic cardiovascular pathology and to distinguish vascular and nonvascular structures without IV contrast. Ultrasound is not useful for assessing the pulmonary parenchyma, but it can detect pleural abnormalities and guide thoracentesis of a pleural effusion. Pulmonary angiography can assess the pulmonary arterial system for venous thromboembolism but has largely been replaced by CT angiography.

Nuclear Medicine Imaging

Ventilation-perfusion lung scans can be used to assess for pulmonary thromboembolism but have also largely been replaced by CT angiography. Positron emission tomographic (PET) scanning assesses the uptake and metabolism of a radiolabeled glucose analogue. Because malignant lesions usually have increased metabolic activity, PET scanning, especially when combined with CT images in PET/CT, is useful to assess pulmonary nodules for potential malignancy and to stage lung cancer. PET studies are limited in assessing lesions <1 cm in diameter; false-negative screening for malignancy can result from lesions with low metabolic activity, such as bronchioloalveolar cell carcinoma. False-positive PET signals can be observed in inflammatory conditions such as pneumonia.

Sputum Exam

Sputum can be obtained by spontaneous expectoration or induced by inhalation of an irritating aerosol like hypertonic saline. Sputum is distinguished from saliva by the presence of bronchial epithelial cells and alveolar macrophages as opposed to squamous epithelial cells. Sputum exam should include gross inspection for blood, color, and odor, as well as Gram's stain and routine bacterial culture. Bacterial culture of expectorated sputum may be misleading due to contamination with oropharyngeal flora. Sputum samples can also be assessed for a variety of other pathogens, including mycobacteria, fungi, and viruses. Sputum samples induced by hypertonic saline can be stained for the presence of *Pneumocystis jiroveci*. Cytologic examination of sputum samples can be used as an initial screen for malignancy.

■ INVASIVE PROCEDURES

Bronchoscopy

Bronchoscopy is a procedure that provides direct visualization of the tracheobronchial tree, typically to the subsegmental level. The fiberoptic bronchoscope is used in most cases, but rigid bronchoscopy is valuable in specific circumstances, including massive hemorrhage and foreign body removal. Flexible fiberoptic bronchoscopy allows visualization of the airways; identification of endobronchial abnormalities, including tumors and sites of bleeding; and collection of diagnostic specimens by washing, brushing, biopsy, or lavage. Washing involves instilling sterile saline through the bronchoscope channel onto the surface of a lesion; part of the saline is suctioned back through the bronchoscope and processed for cytology and microorganisms. Bronchial brushings can be obtained from the surface of an endobronchial lesion or from a more distal mass or infiltrate (potentially with fluoroscopic guidance) for cytologic and microbiologic studies. Biopsy forceps can be used to obtain biopsies of endobronchial lesions or passed into peribronchial alveolar tissue (often with fluoroscopic guidance) to obtain transbronchial biopsies of more distal lung tissue. Transbronchial biopsy is particularly useful in diagnosing diffuse infectious processes, lymphangitic spread of cancer, and granulomatous diseases. Complications of transbronchial biopsy include hemorrhage and pneumothorax.

Bronchoalveolar lavage (BAL) is an adjunct to fiberoptic bronchoscopy, permitting collection of cells and fluid from distal air spaces. After wedging the bronchoscope in a subsegmental airway, saline is instilled and then suctioned back through the bronchoscope for analyses, which can include cytology, microbiology, and cell counts. BAL is especially useful in the diagnosis of *P. jiroveci* pneumonia and some other infections.

Additional bronchoscopic approaches to obtain tissue samples from locations adjacent to the trachea or large bronchi for cytologic assessment of malignancy include transbronchial needle aspiration (TBNA). TBNA can be supplemented with endobronchial ultrasound (EBUS), which can allow guided aspiration of hilar and mediastinal lymph nodes.

Percutaneous Needle Aspiration of the Lung

A needle can be inserted through the chest wall and into a pulmonary lesion to aspirate material for cytologic and microbiologic studies. Percutaneous needle aspiration is usually performed under CT guidance. Owing to the small size of the sample obtained, sampling error is a limitation of the procedure.

Thoracentesis

Thoracentesis should be performed as an early step in the evaluation of a pleural effusion of uncertain etiology. Analysis of pleural fluid can determine the etiology of the effusion (Chap. 144). Large-volume thoracentesis can be therapeutic by palliating dyspnea.

Mediastinoscopy

Tissue biopsy of mediastinal masses or lymph nodes is often required for cancer diagnosis and staging. Mediastinoscopy is performed from a suprasternal approach, and a rigid mediastinoscope is inserted—from which biopsies can be obtained. Lymph nodes in the aortopulmonary location typically require a parasternal mediastinotomy to provide access for biopsy.

Video-Assisted Thoracic Surgery

Video-assisted thoracic surgery (VATS), also known as thoracoscopy, is widely used for the diagnosis of pleural lesions as well as peripheral parenchymal infiltrates and nodules. VATS, which requires that the pt tolerate single lung ventilation during the procedure, involves passing a rigid scope with a camera through a trocar and into the pleural space; instruments can be inserted and manipulated through separate intercostal incisions. VATS has largely replaced "open biopsy," which requires a thoracotomy.

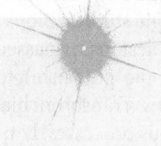

For a more detailed discussion, see Kritek P, Choi AMK: Approach to the Patient With Disease of the Respiratory System, Chap. 251, p. 2084, in HPIM-18; Naureckas ET, Solway J: Disturbances of Respiratory Function, Chap. 252, p. 2087, in HPIM-18; and Fuhlbrigge AL, Choi AMK: Diagnostic Procedures in Respiratory Disease, Chap. 253, p. 2094, in HPIM-18.

CHAPTER **138**
Asthma

Definition and Epidemiology

Asthma is a syndrome characterized by airflow obstruction that varies both spontaneously and with specific treatment. Chronic airway inflammation causes airway hyperresponsiveness to a variety of triggers, leading to airflow obstruction and respiratory symptoms including dyspnea and wheezing. Although asthmatics typically have periods of normal lung function with intermittent airflow obstruction, a subset of pts develop chronic airflow obstruction.

The prevalence of asthma has increased markedly over the past 30 years. In developed countries, approximately 10% of adults and 15% of children have asthma. Most asthmatics are atopic, and they often have allergic rhinitis and/or eczema. The majority of asthmatics have childhood-onset disease. Most asthmatics have atopy, and asthmatics often have atopic dermatitis (eczema) and/or allergic rhinitis. A minority of asthmatic pts do not have atopy (negative skin prick tests to common allergens and normal serum total IgE levels). These individuals, occasionally referred to as *intrinsic asthmatics*, often have adult-onset disease. Occupational asthma can result from a variety of chemicals, including toluene diisocyanate and trimellitic anhydride, and also can have an adult onset.

Asthmatics can develop increased airflow obstruction and respiratory symptoms in response to a variety of different triggers. Inhaled allergens can be potent asthma triggers for individuals with specific sensitivity to those agents. Viral upper respiratory infections (URIs) commonly trigger asthma exacerbations. β-Adrenergic blocking medications can markedly worsen asthma symptoms and should typically be avoided in asthmatics. Exercise often triggers increased asthma symptoms, which usually begin after exercise has ended. Other triggers of increased asthma symptoms include air pollution, cold air, occupational exposures, and stress.

Clinical Evaluation of the Patient History

Common respiratory symptoms in asthma include wheezing, dyspnea, and cough. These symptoms often vary widely within a particular individual, and they can change spontaneously or with age, season of the year, and treatment. Symptoms may be worse at night, and nocturnal awakenings are an indicator of inadequate asthma control. The severity of a pt's asthmatic symptoms, as well as the pt's need for systemic steroid treatment, hospitalization, and intensive care treatment, are important to ascertain. Types of asthmatic triggers for the particular pt, and their recent exposure to them, should be determined. Approximately 1–5% of asthmatics have sensitivity to aspirin and other cyclooxygenase inhibitors; they typically are nonatopic and have nasal polyps. Cigarette smoking leads to more hospital admissions and more rapid decline in lung function; smoking cessation is essential.

Physical Exam

It is important to assess for signs of respiratory distress, including tachypnea, use of accessory respiratory muscles, and cyanosis. On lung exam, there may be wheezing and rhonchi throughout the chest, typically more prominent in expiration than inspiration. Localized wheezing may indicate an endobronchial lesion. Evidence of allergic nasal, sinus, or skin disease should be assessed. When asthma is adequately controlled, the physical exam may be normal.

Pulmonary Function Tests

Spirometry often shows airflow obstruction, with a reduction in forced expiratory volume in 1 s (FEV_1) and FEV_1/forced vital capacity (FVC) ratio. However, spirometry may be normal, especially if asthma symptoms are adequately treated. Bronchodilator reversibility is demonstrated by an increase in FEV_1 by ≥200 mL and ≥12% from baseline FEV_1 15 min after a short-acting β agonist (often albuterol metered-dose inhaler two puffs or 180 μg). Many but not all asthmatics will demonstrate significant bronchodilator reversibility; optimal pharmacologic treatment may reduce bronchodilator reversibility. Airway hyperresponsiveness is characteristic of asthma; it can be assessed by exposure to direct bronchoconstrictors such as methacholine or histamine. Greater airway responsiveness is associated with increased asthmatic symptoms. The peak expiratory flow rate (PEF) can be used by the pt to track asthma control objectively at home. Measurement of lung volumes is not typically performed, but increases in total lung capacity and residual volume may be observed. The diffusing capacity for carbon monoxide is usually normal.

Other Laboratory Tests

Blood tests are usually not helpful. CBC may demonstrate eosinophilia. Specific IgE measurements for inhaled allergens (RAST) or allergy skin testing may assist in determining allergic triggers. Total serum IgE is markedly elevated in allergic bronchopulmonary aspergillosis (ABPA). Exhaled nitric oxide levels can provide an assessment of eosinophilic airway inflammation.

Radiographic Findings

Chest x-ray is usually normal. In acute exacerbations, pneumothorax may be identified. In ABPA, eosinophilic pulmonary infiltrates may be observed. Chest CT scan is not typically performed in routine asthma but may show central bronchiectasis in ABPA.

Differential Diagnosis

The differential diagnosis of asthma includes other disorders that can cause wheezing and dyspnea. Upper airway obstruction by tumor or laryngeal edema can mimic asthma, but stridor in the large airways is typically noted on physical examination. Localized wheezing in the chest may indicate an endobronchial tumor or foreign body. Congestive heart failure can cause wheezing but is typically accompanied by bibasilar crackles. Eosinophilic pneumonias and Churg-Strauss syndrome may present with wheezing.

Vocal cord dysfunction can mimic severe asthma and may require direct laryngoscopy to assess. When asthma involves chronic airflow obstruction, distinguishing it from chronic obstructive pulmonary disease (COPD) can be very difficult.

TREATMENT Chronic Asthma

If a specific inciting agent for asthmatic symptoms can be identified and eliminated, that is an optimal part of treatment. In most cases, pharmacologic therapy is required. The two major classes of drugs are bronchodilators, which provide rapid symptomatic relief by relaxing airway smooth muscle, and controllers, which limit the airway inflammatory process.

BRONCHODILATORS The most widely used class of bronchodilators is β_2-adrenergic agonists, which relax airway smooth muscle by activating β_2-adrenergic receptors. Two types of inhaled β_2 agonists are widely used in asthma treatment: short-acting (SABA) and long-acting (LABA). SABAs, which include albuterol, have rapid onset of action and last for up to 6 h. SABAs are effective rescue medications, but excessive use indicates inadequate asthma control. SABAs can prevent exercise-induced asthma if administered before exercise. LABAs, which include salmeterol and formoterol, have a slower onset of action but last for >12 h. LABAs have replaced regularly scheduled use of SABAs, but they do not control airway inflammation and should not be used without inhaled corticosteroid (ICS) therapy. Combinations of LABAs with ICS reduce asthma exacerbations and provide an excellent long-term treatment option for asthma severity of moderate persistent degree or greater.

Common side effects of β_2-adrenergic agonists include muscle tremors and palpitations. These side effects are more prominent with oral formulations, which should not generally be used. There have been ongoing concerns about mortality risks associated with β_2-adrenergic agonists, which have not been completely resolved. LABAs taken without concomitant inhaled steroid treatment may increase this risk.

Other available bronchodilator medications include anticholinergics and theophylline. Anticholinergics, which are available in short-acting and long-acting inhaled formulations, are commonly used in COPD. They appear to be considerably less effective than β_2-adrenergic agonists in asthma, and they are typically considered as an additional treatment option only if other asthma medications do not provide adequate asthma control. Theophylline may have both bronchodilator and anti-inflammatory effects; it is not widely used due to the potential toxicities associated with high plasma levels. Low doses of theophylline may have additive effects with ICS at levels below the standard therapeutic range, and this can be a useful treatment option for severe asthma.

CONTROLLER THERAPIES ICS are the most effective controller treatments for asthma. ICS are usually given twice daily; a variety of ICS medications are available. Although they do not provide immediate symptom relief, respiratory symptoms and lung function often begin to improve within several days of initiating treatment. ICS reduces exercise-induced symptoms, nocturnal symptoms, and acute exacerbations. ICS treatment typically leads to reductions in airway hyperresponsiveness.

ICS side effects include hoarseness and oral candidiasis; these effects may be minimized by use of a spacer device and by rinsing out the mouth after taking ICS.

Other available controller therapies for asthma include systemic corticosteroids. Although quite helpful in the management of acute asthma exacerbations, oral or IV steroid use should be avoided if at all possible in the chronic management of asthma due to multiple potential side effects. Antileukotrienes, such as montelukast and zafirlukast, may be quite beneficial in some pts. Cromolyn sodium and nedocromil sodium are not widely used due to their brief durations of action and typically modest effects. Omalizumab is a blocking antibody that neutralizes IgE; with SC injection, it appears to reduce acute asthma exacerbation frequency in severe asthmatics. However, it is expensive and considered only for highly selected pts with elevated total serum IgE levels and refractory asthma symptoms despite maximal inhaled bronchodilator and ICS therapy.

OVERALL TREATMENT APPROACH   In addition to limiting exposure to their environmental triggers for asthma, pts should receive stepwise therapy appropriate for their disease severity (Fig. 138-1). Asthmatics with mild intermittent symptoms are typically managed adequately with SABAs taken on an as-needed basis. Use of SABAs more than three times a week suggests that controller therapy, typically with an ICS twice per day, is required. If symptoms are not adequately controlled with ICS, LABAs can be added. If symptoms are still not adequately controlled, higher doses of ICS and/or alternative controller therapies should be considered.

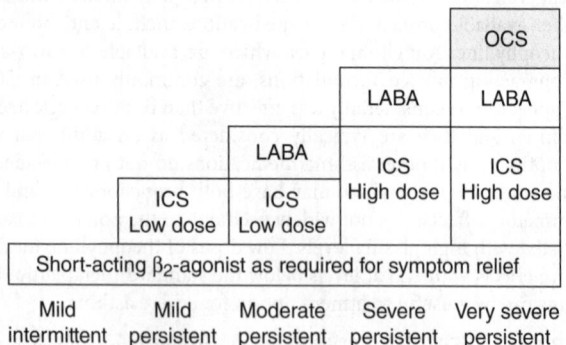

FIGURE 138-1 Step-wise approach to asthma therapy according to the severity of asthma and ability to control symptoms. ICS, inhaled corticosteroid; LABA, long-acting β_2 agonists; OCS, oral corticosteroid.

ASTHMA EXACERBATIONS

Clinical Features

Asthma exacerbations are periods of acute worsening of asthma symptoms that may be life-threatening. Exacerbations are commonly triggered by viral URIs, but other triggers also can be involved. Symptoms often include increased dyspnea, wheezing, and chest tightness. Physical examination can reveal pulsus paradoxus as well as tachypnea, tachycardia, and lung hyperinflation. Pulmonary function testing reveals a reduction in FEV_1 and PEF. Hypoxemia can result; Pco_2 is usually reduced due to hyperventilation. Normal or rising Pco_2 can signal impending respiratory failure.

> **TREATMENT** Asthma Exacerbations
>
> The mainstays of asthma exacerbation treatment are high doses of SABAs and systemic corticosteroids. SABAs may be administered by nebulizer or metered-dose inhaler with a spacer; very frequent dosing (q1h or more often) may be required initially. Inhaled anticholinergic bronchodilator medication can be added to the SABAs. IV corticosteroids, such as methylprednisolone (e.g., 80 mg IV q8h), may be used, although oral corticosteroids also may be used. Supplemental oxygen should be provided to maintain adequate oxygen saturation (>90%). If respiratory failure occurs, mechanical ventilation should be instituted, with care to minimize airway pressures and auto-PEEP. Because bacterial infections rarely trigger asthma exacerbations, antibiotics are not routinely administered unless there are signs of pneumonia.
>
> In an effort to treat asthma exacerbations before they become severe, asthma pts should receive written action plans with instructions for self-initiation of treatment based on respiratory symptoms and reductions in PEF.

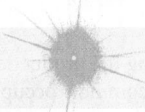

For a more detailed discussion, see Barnes PJ: Asthma, Chap. 254, p. 2102, in HPIM-18.

CHAPTER **139**
Environmental Lung Diseases

The susceptibility to develop many pulmonary diseases is influenced by environmental factors. This chapter will focus on occupational and toxic chemical exposures. However, a variety of nonoccupational indoor exposures such as environmental tobacco smoke exposure (lung cancer), radon gas (lung cancer), and biomass fuel cooking (chronic obstructive pulmonary disease [COPD]) also should be considered. Particle size is an important determinant of the impact of environmental exposures on the respiratory system. Particles >10 μm in diameter typically are captured by the upper airway. Particles 2.5–10 μm in diameter will likely deposit in the upper tracheobronchial tree, while smaller particles (including nanoparticles) will reach the alveoli. Water-soluble gases like ammonia are absorbed in the upper airways and produce irritative and bronchoconstrictive responses, while less water-soluble gases (e.g., phosgene) may reach the alveoli and cause a life-threatening acute chemical pneumonitis.

APPROACH TO THE PATIENT | **Environmental Lung Diseases**

Because there are many types of occupational lung disease (pneumoconiosis) that can mimic diseases not known to relate to environmental factors, obtaining a careful occupational history is essential. In addition to the types of occupation performed by the pt, the specific environmental exposures, use of protective respiratory devices, and ventilation of the work environment can provide key information. Assessing the temporal development of symptoms relative to the pt's work schedule also can be very useful.

The chest x-ray is helpful in the assessment of environmental lung disease, but it may over- or underestimate the functional impact of pneumoconioses. Pulmonary function tests should be used to assess the severity of impairment, but they typically do not suggest a specific diagnosis. Changes in spirometry before and after a work shift can provide strong evidence for bronchoconstriction in suspected occupational asthma. Some radiologic patterns are distinctive for certain occupational lung diseases; chest x-rays are widely used, and chest CT scans can provide more detailed evaluation.

OCCUPATIONAL EXPOSURES AND PULMONARY DISEASE

◼ INORGANIC DUSTS

Asbestos-Related Diseases

In addition to exposures to asbestos that may occur during the production of asbestos products (from mining to manufacturing), common occupational asbestos exposures occur in shipbuilding and other construction trades (e.g., pipefitting, boilermaking) and in the manufacture of safety garments and friction materials (e.g., brake and clutch linings). Along with worker exposure in these areas, bystander exposure (e.g., spouses) can be responsible for some asbestos-related lung diseases.

A range of respiratory diseases has been associated with asbestos exposure. Pleural plaques indicate that asbestos exposure has occurred, but they are typically not symptomatic. Interstitial lung disease, often referred to as asbestosis, is pathologically and radiologically similar to idiopathic pulmonary fibrosis; it is typically accompanied by a restrictive ventilatory defect with reduced diffusing capacity for carbon monoxide (DLCO) on pulmonary function testing. Asbestosis can develop after 10 years of exposure, and no specific therapy is available.

Benign pleural effusions can also occur from asbestos exposure. Lung cancer is clearly associated with asbestos exposure, but does not typically present for at least 15 years after initial exposure. The lung cancer risk increases multiplicatively with cigarette smoking. In addition, mesotheliomas (both pleural and peritoneal) are strongly associated with asbestos exposure, but they are not related to smoking. Relatively brief asbestos exposures may lead to mesotheliomas, which typically do not develop for decades after the initial exposure. Biopsy of pleural tissue, typically by thoracoscopic surgery, is required for diagnosing mesothelioma.

Silicosis

Silicosis results from exposure to free silica (crystalline quartz), which occurs in mining, stone cutting, abrasive industries (e.g., stone, clay, glass, and cement manufacturing), foundry work, and quarrying. Heavy exposures over relatively brief time periods (as little as 10 months) can cause acute silicosis—which is pathologically similar to pulmonary alveolar proteinosis and associated with a characteristic chest CT pattern known as "crazy paving." Acute silicosis can be severe and progressive; whole lung lavage may be of some therapeutic benefit.

Longer-term exposures can result in simple silicosis, with small rounded opacities in the upper lobes of the lungs. Calcification of hilar lymph nodes can give a characteristic "eggshell" appearance. Progressive nodular fibrosis can result in masses >1 cm in diameter in complicated silicosis. When such masses become very large, the term *progressive massive fibrosis* is used to describe the condition. Due to impaired cell-mediated immunity, silicosis pts are at increased risk of tuberculosis, atypical mycobacterial infections, and fungal infections. Silica may also be a lung carcinogen.

Coal Worker's Pneumoconiosis

Occupational exposure to coal dust predisposes to coal worker's pneumoconiosis (CWP), which is less common among coal workers in the western United States due to a lower risk from the bituminous coal found in that region. Simple CWP is defined radiologically by small nodular opacities and is not typically symptomatic; however, an increased risk of COPD may occur. The development of larger nodules (>1 cm in diameter), usually in the upper lobes, characterizes complicated CWP. Complicated CWP is often symptomatic and is associated with reduced pulmonary function and increased mortality.

Berylliosis

Beryllium exposure may occur in the manufacturing of alloys, ceramics, and electronic devices. Although acute beryllium exposure can rarely produce acute pneumonitis, a chronic granulomatous disease very similar to sarcoidosis is much more common. Radiologically, chronic beryllium disease, like sarcoidosis, is characterized by pulmonary nodules along septal lines. As in sarcoidosis, either a restrictive or obstructive ventilatory pattern with reduced DLco on pulmonary function testing can be seen. Bronchoscopy with transbronchial biopsy is typically required to diagnose chronic beryllium disease. The most effective way to distinguish chronic beryllium disease from sarcoidosis is to assess for delayed hypersensitivity to beryllium by performing a lymphocyte proliferation test using blood or bronchoalveolar lavage lymphocytes. Removal from further beryllium exposure is required, and corticosteroids may be beneficial.

■ ORGANIC DUSTS

Cotton Dust (Byssinosis)

Dust exposures occur in the production of yarns for textiles and rope-making. At the early stages of byssinosis, chest tightness occurs near the end of the first day of the workweek. In progressive cases, symptoms are present throughout the workweek. After at least 10 years of exposure, chronic airflow obstruction can develop. In symptomatic individuals, limiting further exposure is essential.

Grain Dust

Farmers and grain elevator operators are at risk for grain dust–related lung disease, which is similar to COPD. Symptoms include productive cough, wheezing, and dyspnea. Pulmonary function tests typically show airflow obstruction.

Farmer's Lung

Exposure to moldy hay containing spores of thermophilic actinomycetes can lead to the development of hypersensitivity pneumonitis. Within 8 h after exposure, the acute presentation of farmer's lung includes fever, cough, and dyspnea. With repeated exposures, chronic and patchy interstitial lung disease can develop.

Toxic Chemicals

Many toxic chemicals can affect the lung in the form of vapors and gases. For example, smoke inhalation can be lethal to firefighters and fire victims through a variety of mechanisms. Carbon monoxide poisoning can cause life-threatening hypoxemia. Combustion of plastics and polyurethanes can release toxic agents including cyanide. Occupational asthma can result from exposure to diisocyanates in polyurethanes and acid anhydrides in epoxides. Radon gas, released from earth materials and concentrated within buildings, is a risk factor for lung cancer.

PRINCIPLES OF MANAGEMENT

Treatment of environmental lung diseases typically involves limiting or avoiding exposures to the toxic substance. Chronic interstitial lung diseases (e.g., asbestosis, CWP) are not responsive to glucocorticoids, but acute organic dust exposures may respond to corticosteroids. Therapy of occupational asthma (e.g., diisocyanates) follows usual asthma guidelines (Chap. 138), and therapy of occupational COPD (e.g., byssinosis) follows usual COPD guidelines (Chap. 140).

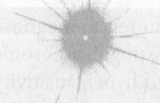

For a more detailed discussion, see Balmes JR, Speizer FE: Occupational and Environmental Lung Disease, Chap. 256, p. 2121, in HPIM-18.

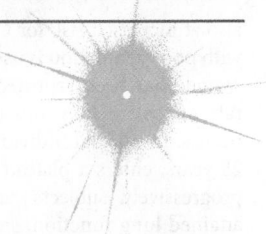

CHAPTER **140**
Chronic Obstructive Pulmonary Disease

DEFINITION AND EPIDEMIOLOGY

Chronic obstructive pulmonary disease (COPD) is a disease state characterized by chronic airflow obstruction; thus, pulmonary function testing is central to its diagnosis. The presence of airflow obstruction is determined by a reduced ratio of the forced expiratory volume in 1 s (FEV_1) to the forced vital capacity (FVC). Among individuals with a reduced FEV_1/FVC ratio, the severity of airflow obstruction is determined by the level of reduction in FEV_1 (Table 140-1): ≥80% is stage I, 50–80% is stage II, 30–50% is stage III, and <30% is stage IV. Cigarette smoking is the major environmental risk factor for COPD. The risk of COPD increases with cigarette smoking intensity, which is typically quantified as pack-years. (One pack of cigarettes smoked per day for 1 year equals 1 pack-year.) Individuals with airway hyperresponsiveness and certain occupational exposures (e.g., coal mining, gold mining, and cotton textiles) are likely

TABLE 140-1 GOLD CRITERIA FOR COPD SEVERITY

GOLD Stage	Severity	Symptoms	Spirometry
0	At risk	Chronic cough, sputum production	Normal
I	Mild	With or without chronic cough or sputum production	FEV_1/FVC <0.7 and FEV_1 ≥80% predicted
IIA	Moderate	With or without chronic cough or sputum production	FEV_1/FVC <0.7 and FEV_1 ≥50% but <80% predicted
III	Severe	With or without chronic cough or sputum production	FEV_1/FVC <0.7 and FEV_1 ≥30% but <50% predicted
IV	Very severe	With or without chronic cough or sputum production	FEV_1/FVC <0.7 and FEV_1 <30% predicted *or* FEV_1 <50% predicted with respiratory failure or signs of right heart failure

Abbreviation: GOLD, Global Initiative for Lung Disease.
Source: From RA Pauwels et al: *Am J Respir Crit Care Med* 163:1256, 2001; with permission.

also at increased risk for COPD. In countries in which biomass combustion with poor ventilation is used for cooking, an increased risk of COPD among women has been reported. COPD is a progressive disorder; however, the rate of loss of lung function often slows markedly if smoking cessation occurs. In normal individuals, FEV_1 reaches a lifetime peak at around age 25 years, enters a plateau phase, and subsequently declines gradually and progressively. Subjects can develop COPD by having reduced maximally attained lung function, shortened plateau phase, or accelerated decline in lung function.

Symptoms often occur only when COPD is advanced; thus, early detection requires spirometric testing. The Pao_2 typically remains near normal until the FEV_1 falls to <50% of the predicted value. Hypercarbia and pulmonary hypertension are most common after FEV_1 has fallen to <25% of predicted. COPD pts with similar FEV_1 values can vary markedly in their respiratory symptoms and functional impairment. COPD often includes periods of increased respiratory symptoms, such as dyspnea, cough, and phlegm production, which are known as exacerbations. Exacerbations are often triggered by bacterial and/or viral respiratory infections. These exacerbations become more common as COPD severity increases, but some individuals are much more susceptible to developing exacerbations than others with similar degrees of airflow obstruction.

CLINICAL MANIFESTATIONS

History

Subjects with COPD usually have smoked ≥20 pack-years of cigarettes. Common symptoms include cough and phlegm production; individuals with chronic productive cough for 3 months per year for the preceding 2 years have chronic bronchitis. However, chronic bronchitis without airflow obstruction is not included within COPD. Exertional dyspnea is a common and potentially disabling symptom in COPD pts. Exercise involving upper-body activity is especially difficult for severe COPD pts. Weight loss and cachexia are common in advanced disease. Hypoxemia and hypercarbia may result in fluid retention, morning headaches, sleep disruption, erythrocytosis, and cyanosis.

Exacerbations are more frequent as disease progresses and are most often triggered by respiratory infections, often with a bacterial component. The history of prior exacerbations is a strong predictor of future exacerbations.

Physical Findings

The physical examination may be normal until COPD is fairly advanced. As disease progresses, signs of hyperinflation may become more prominent, including barrel chest and poor diaphragmatic excursion. Expiratory wheezing may be observed, but it does not predict the severity of obstruction or response to therapy. Persistently localized wheezing and digital clubbing raise the possibility of lung cancer.

During COPD exacerbations, signs of respiratory distress may be prominent, including tachycardia, tachypnea, use of accessory muscles of respiration, and cyanosis.

Radiographic Findings

Plain chest x-ray may show hyperinflation, emphysema, and pulmonary hypertension. It is typically performed to exclude other disease processes during routine evaluation and to exclude pneumonia during exacerbations. Chest CT scanning has much greater sensitivity for detecting emphysema but is typically reserved for the evaluation of advanced disease when surgical options such as lung volume reduction and lung transplantation are being considered.

Pulmonary Function Tests

Objective documentation of airflow obstruction is essential for diagnosing COPD. Standardized staging of COPD is based on postbronchodilator spirometry. In COPD, the FEV_1/FVC ratio is reduced below 0.7. Despite prolonged expiratory efforts, subjects may not be able to achieve a plateau in their FVC. Increases in total lung capacity and residual volume, as well as reduced diffusing capacity for carbon monoxide, are typically seen in emphysema.

Laboratory Tests

α_1 Antitrypsin (α_1AT) testing, typically by measurement of the protein level in the bloodstream, is recommended to exclude severe α_1AT deficiency. Augmentation therapy (a weekly IV infusion) is available for individuals with severe α_1AT deficiency (e.g., PI Z). Pulse oximetry can determine the O_2 saturation. However, arterial blood gases remain useful to assess the severity of CO_2 retention as well as acid-base disorders. During acute exacerbations, arterial blood gases should be considered in pts with mental status changes, significant respiratory distress, very severe COPD, or a history of hypercarbia. Complete blood counts are useful in advanced disease to assess for erythrocytosis, which can occur secondary to hypoxemia, and anemia, which can worsen dyspnea.

TREATMENT COPD

OUTPATIENT MANAGEMENT

Smoking Cessation Elimination of tobacco smoking has been convincingly shown to reduce decline in pulmonary function and to prolong survival in pts with COPD. Although lung function does not typically improve substantially after smoking cessation, the rate of decline in FEV_1 often reverts to that of nonsmokers. Pharmacologic treatment to assist with smoking cessation is often beneficial. Use of nicotine replacement therapy (available as a transdermal patch, gum, nasal spray, and oral inhaler) can increase rates of smoking cessation; oral bupropion (150 mg bid after starting at 150 mg qd for 3 days) also produces significant benefit and can be combined successfully with nicotine replacement. Varenicline, a partial agonist for nicotinic acetylcholine receptors, also can promote smoking cessation. All adult, nonpregnant smokers without specific contraindications should be offered pharmacologic treatment to assist with smoking cessation.

Nonpharmacologic Treatment Pulmonary rehabilitation improves dyspnea and functional status and reduces hospitalizations. Annual influenza vaccinations are strongly recommended; in addition, pneumococcal vaccination is recommended.

Bronchodilators Although inhaled bronchodilator medications have not been proven to increase longevity in COPD, they may significantly reduce respiratory symptoms. Short- and long-acting β-adrenergic agonists, short- and long-acting anticholinergics, and theophylline derivatives all may be used. Although oral medications are associated with greater rates of adherence, inhaled medications generally have fewer side effects.

Pts with mild disease can usually be managed with an inhaled short-acting anticholinergic such as ipratropium or a short-acting β agonist such as albuterol. Combination therapy and long-acting β agonists and/or long-acting anticholinergics should be added in pts with severe disease. The narrow toxic-therapeutic ratio of theophylline compounds limits their use, and either low doses or regular monitoring of serum levels are required.

Corticosteroids Chronic systemic corticosteroid treatment is not recommended in COPD pts due to the risk of multiple complications, including osteoporosis, weight gain, cataracts, and diabetes mellitus. Although inhaled steroids have not been proven to reduce the rate of decline of FEV_1 in COPD, inhaled steroid medications reduce the frequency of exacerbations in individuals with severe COPD. Combinations of inhaled steroids and long-acting β agonists reduce COPD exacerbations and may reduce mortality—although that has not been conclusively shown.

Oxygen Long-term supplemental oxygen therapy has been shown to reduce symptoms and improve survival in COPD pts who are chronically hypoxemic. Documentation of the need for O_2 requires a measurement of Pao_2 or oxygen saturation (Sao_2) after a period of stability. Pts with a Pao_2 ≤55 mmHg or Sao_2 ≤88% should receive O_2 to raise the Sao_2 to ≥90%. O_2 is also indicated for pts with Pao_2 of 56–59 mmHg or Sao_2 ≤89% if associated with signs and symptoms of pulmonary hypertension or cor pulmonale. For individuals who meet these guidelines, continuous O_2 therapy is recommended because the number of hours per day of oxygen use is directly related to the mortality benefit. Supplemental oxygen may also be prescribed for selected COPD pts who desaturate only with exercise or during sleep, although the evidence for benefit is less compelling.

Surgical Options for Severe COPD Two main types of surgical options are available for end-stage COPD. Lung volume reduction surgery can reduce mortality and improve lung function in selected pts with upper lobe–predominant emphysema and low exercise capacity (after pulmonary rehabilitation). Individuals who meet the criteria for the high-risk group (FEV$_1$ <20% predicted and either a diffuse distribution of emphysema or lung carbon monoxide diffusing capacity <20% predicted) should not be considered for lung volume reduction surgery. Lung transplantation should be considered for COPD pts who have very severe chronic airflow obstruction and disability at a relatively young age despite maximal medical therapy.

MANAGEMENT OF COPD EXACERBATIONS COPD exacerbations are a major cause of morbidity and mortality. Critical decisions in management include whether hospitalization is required. Although there are no definitive guidelines to determine which COPD pts require hospitalization for an exacerbation, the development of respiratory acidosis, worsening hypoxemia, severe underlying COPD, pneumonia, or social situations without adequate home support for the treatment required should prompt consideration of hospitalization.

Key components of exacerbation treatment include bronchodilators, antibiotics, and short courses of systemic glucocorticoids.

Antibiotics Because bacterial infections often trigger COPD exacerbations, antibiotic therapy should be strongly considered, especially with increased sputum volume or change in sputum color. Common pathogens include *Streptococcus pneumoniae*, *Haemophilus influenzae*, and *Moraxella catarrhalis*. Antibiotic choice should depend on the local antibiotic sensitivity patterns, previous sputum culture results for a particular pt, and the severity of disease. Trimethoprim-sulfamethoxazole, doxycycline, and amoxicillin are reasonable choices for subjects with mild to moderate COPD; broader-spectrum antibiotics should be considered for subjects with more severe underlying COPD and/or more severe exacerbations.

Bronchodilators Bronchodilator therapy is essential during COPD exacerbations. Short-acting β-adrenergic agonists by inhalation (e.g., albuterol q1–2h) are used; addition of anticholinergics is likely of benefit (e.g., ipratropium q4–6h). Administration of bronchodilators by nebulizer is often used initially because it is easier to administer to pts in respiratory distress. Conversion to metered-dose inhaler administration can be successfully achieved with appropriate training of the pt and staff.

Glucocorticoids Systemic steroids hasten resolution of symptoms and reduce relapses and subsequent exacerbations for up to 6 months. Dosing is not well worked out, but 30–40 mg of prednisone daily (or IV equivalent) is standard, with a total course of 10–14 days. Hyperglycemia is the most commonly reported complication and should be monitored.

Oxygen Hypoxemia often worsens during COPD exacerbations. Supplemental O$_2$ should be administered to maintain Sao$_2$ ≥90%. Very high O$_2$ delivery can worsen hypercarbia, primarily due to increasing ventilation-perfusion mismatch. However, providing adequate O$_2$ to obtain saturation of ~90% is the key goal. Therefore, supplemental O$_2$ delivery should be focused on providing adequate oxygenation without providing unnecessarily high O_2 saturations. Pts may require use of supplemental O_2 after hospital discharge until the exacerbation completely resolves.

Ventilatory Support Numerous studies suggest that noninvasive mask ventilation [noninvasive ventilation (NIV)] can improve outcomes in acute COPD exacerbations with respiratory failure ($Paco_2$ >45 mmHg). Contraindications to NIV include cardiovascular instability, impaired mental status, inability to cooperate, copious secretions, craniofacial abnormalities or facial trauma, extreme obesity, or significant burns. Progressive hypercarbia, refractory hypoxemia, or alterations in mental status that compromise ability to comply with NIV therapy, hemodynamic instability, and respiratory arrest may necessitate endotracheal intubation for mechanical ventilation. Sufficient expiratory time is required to avoid the development of auto-PEEP.

> For a more detailed discussion, see Reilly JJ Jr., Silverman EK, Shapiro SD: Chronic Obstructive Pulmonary Disease, Chap. 260, p. 2151, in HPIM-18.

CHAPTER **141**
Pneumonia, Bronchiectasis, and Lung Abscess

PNEUMONIA

Pneumonia, an infection of the lung parenchyma, is classified as community-acquired (CAP) or health care–associated (HCAP). The HCAP category is subdivided into hospital-acquired pneumonia (HAP) and ventilator-associated pneumonia (VAP). HCAP is associated with hospitalization for ≥48 h, hospitalization for ≥2 days in the prior 3 months, residence in a nursing home or extended-care facility, antibiotic therapy in the preceding 3 months, chronic dialysis, home infusion therapy, home wound care, and contact with a family member who has a multidrug-resistant (MDR) infection.

PATHOPHYSIOLOGY

- Microorganisms gain access to the lower respiratory tract via micro-aspiration from the oropharynx (the most common route), inhalation of contaminated droplets, hematogenous spread, or contiguous extension from an infected pleural or mediastinal space.
- Before disease manifests, the size of the organism burden must overcome the ability of macrophages and other components of innate immunity (e.g., surfactant proteins A and D) to clear bacteria.

- Classic pneumonia (typified by that due to *Streptococcus pneumoniae*) presents as a lobar pattern and evolves through four phases characterized by changes in the alveoli:
  - *Edema:* Proteinaceous exudates are present in the alveoli.
  - *Red hepatization:* Erythrocytes and neutrophils are present in the intraalveolar exudate.
  - *Gray hepatization:* Neutrophils and fibrin deposition are abundant.
  - *Resolution:* Macrophages are the dominant cell type.
- In VAP, respiratory bronchiolitis can precede a radiologically apparent infiltrate.

COMMUNITY-ACQUIRED PNEUMONIA

Microbiology

Although many bacteria, viruses, fungi, and protozoa can cause CAP, most cases are caused by relatively few pathogens. In >50% of cases, a specific etiology is never determined.

- Typical bacterial pathogens include *S. pneumoniae, Haemophilus influenzae, Staphylococcus aureus*, and gram-negative bacteria such as *Klebsiella pneumoniae* and *Pseudomonas aeruginosa*.
- Atypical organisms include *Mycoplasma pneumoniae, Chlamydia pneumoniae, Legionella* species, and respiratory viruses (e.g., influenza viruses, adenoviruses, respiratory syncytial viruses).
  - A virus may be responsible for up to 18% of cases of CAP that require hospital admission.
  - 10–15% of CAP cases are polymicrobial and involve a combination of typical and atypical organisms.
- Involvement of anaerobes, which play a significant role in CAP only when aspiration precedes presentation by days or weeks, often results in significant empyemas.

Epidemiology

CAP affects ~4 million adults each year in the United States, 80% of whom are treated on an outpatient basis. CAP causes 45,000 deaths annually and is associated with an overall yearly cost of $9–10 billion.

- Incidence rates of CAP are highest at the extremes of age (i.e., <4 and >60 years).
- Risk factors for CAP include alcoholism, asthma, immunosuppression, institutionalization, and an age of ≥70 years (vs. 60–69 years).
- Many factors—e.g., tobacco smoking, chronic obstructive pulmonary disease, colonization with methicillin-resistant *S. aureus* (MRSA), recent hospitalization or antibiotic therapy—influence the types of pathogens that should be considered in the etiologic diagnosis.

Clinical Manifestations

Pts frequently have fever, chills, sweats, cough (either nonproductive or productive of mucoid, purulent, or blood-tinged sputum), pleuritic chest pain, and dyspnea.

- Other common symptoms include nausea, vomiting, diarrhea, fatigue, headache, myalgias, and arthralgias.
- Elderly pts may present atypically, with confusion but few other manifestations.
- Physical examination often reveals tachypnea; increased or decreased tactile fremitus; dull or flat percussion reflecting consolidation and pleural fluid, respectively; crackles; bronchial breath sounds; or a pleural friction rub.

Diagnosis

Both confirmation of the diagnosis and assessment of the likely etiology are required. Although no data have demonstrated that treatment directed at a specific pathogen is superior to empirical treatment, an etiologic diagnosis allows narrowing of the empirical regimen, identification of organisms with public safety implications (e.g., *Mycobacterium tuberculosis*, influenza virus), and monitoring of antibiotic susceptibility trends.

- *Chest radiography* is often required to differentiate CAP from other conditions, particularly since the sensitivity and specificity of physical exam findings for CAP are only 58% and 67%, respectively.
  - CT of the chest may be helpful for pts with suspected postobstructive pneumonia.
  - Some radiographic patterns suggest an etiology; e.g., pneumatoceles suggest *S. aureus*.
- *Sputum samples* must have >25 WBCs and <10 squamous epithelial cells per high-power field to be appropriate for culture. The sensitivity of sputum cultures is highly variable; in cases of proven bacteremic pneumococcal pneumonia, the yield of positive cultures from sputum samples is ≤50%.
- *Blood cultures* are positive in 5–14% of cases, most commonly yielding *S. pneumoniae*. Blood cultures are optional for most CAP pts, but should be performed for high-risk pts (e.g., pts with chronic liver disease or asplenia).
- *Urine antigen tests* for *S. pneumoniae* and *Legionella pneumophila* type 1 can be helpful.
- *Serology:* A fourfold rise in titer of specific IgM antibody can assist in the diagnosis of pneumonia due to some pathogens; however, the time required to obtain a final result makes serology of limited clinical utility.

TREATMENT   Community-Acquired Pneumonia

DECIDING WHETHER TO HOSPITALIZE PTS

- Two sets of criteria identify pts who will benefit from hospital care. It is not clear which set is superior, and application of each tool should be tempered by a consideration of factors relevant to the individual pt.
  - Pneumonia Severity Index (PSI): Points are given for 20 variables, including age, coexisting illness, and abnormal physical and laboratory findings. On this basis, pts are assigned to one of five classes of mortality risk.

– CURB-65: Five variables are included: confusion (C); urea >7 mmol/L (U); respiratory rate ≥30/min (R); blood pressure, systolic ≤90 mmHg or diastolic ≤60 mmHg (B); and age ≥65 years (65). Pts with a score of 0 can be treated at home, pts with a score of 2 should be hospitalized, and pts with a score of ≥3 may require management in the intensive care unit (ICU).

ANTIBIOTIC THERAPY

- For recommendations on empirical antibiotic treatment of CAP, see Table 141-1. U.S. guidelines always target *S. pneumoniae* and atypical pathogens. Retrospective data suggest that this approach lowers the mortality rate.
- Pts initially treated with IV antibiotics can be switched to oral agents when they can ingest and absorb drugs, are hemodynamically stable, and are improving clinically.
- CAP has historically been treated for 10–14 days, but a 5-day course of a fluoroquinolone is sufficient for cases of uncomplicated CAP. A longer course is required for pts with bacteremia, metastatic infection, or infection with a particularly virulent pathogen and in most cases of severe CAP.
- Fever and leukocytosis usually resolve within 2–4 days. Pts who have not responded to therapy by day 3 should be reevaluated, with consideration of alternative diagnoses, antibiotic resistance in the pathogen, and the possibility that the wrong drug is being given.

Complications

Common complications of severe CAP include respiratory failure, shock and multiorgan failure, coagulopathy, and exacerbation of comorbid disease. Metastatic infection (e.g., brain abscess, endocarditis) occurs rarely and requires immediate attention.

- Lung abscess may occur in association with aspiration or infection caused by single CAP pathogens [e.g., community-acquired MRSA (CA-MRSA) or *P. aeruginosa*]. Drainage should be established and proper antibiotics administered.
- Any significant pleural effusion should be tapped for diagnostic and therapeutic purposes. If the fluid has a pH <7, a glucose level <2.2 mmol/L, and a lactate dehydrogenase content >1000 U or if bacteria are seen or cultured, fluid should be drained; a chest tube is usually required.

Follow-Up

Chest x-ray abnormalities may require 4–12 weeks to clear. Pts should receive influenza and pneumococcal vaccines, as appropriate.

HEALTH CARE–ASSOCIATED PNEUMONIA (SEE ALSO CHAP. 87)

■ VENTILATOR-ASSOCIATED PNEUMONIA

Microbiology

Potential etiologic agents include MDR and non-MDR pathogens; the prominence of the various pathogens depends on the length of hospital stay at the time of infection.

TABLE 141-1 EMPIRICAL ANTIBIOTIC TREATMENT OF COMMUNITY-ACQUIRED PNEUMONIA

Outpatients

Previously healthy and no antibiotics in past 3 months

- A macrolide [clarithromycin (500 mg PO bid) or azithromycin (500 mg PO once, then 250 mg qd)] *or*
- Doxycycline (100 mg PO bid)

Comorbidities or antibiotics in past 3 months: select an alternative from a different class

- A respiratory fluoroquinolone [moxifloxacin (400 mg PO qd), gemifloxacin (320 mg PO qd), or levofloxacin (750 mg PO qd)] *or*
- A β-lactam [preferred: high-dose amoxicillin (1 g tid) or amoxicillin/clavulanate (2 g bid); alternatives: ceftriaxone (1–2 g IV qd), cefpodoxime (200 mg PO bid), or cefuroxime (500 mg PO bid)] *plus* a macrolide[a]

In regions with a high rate of "high-level" pneumococcal macrolide resistance,[b] consider alternatives listed above for pts with comorbidities.

Inpatients, Non-ICU

- A respiratory fluoroquinolone [moxifloxacin (400 mg PO or IV qd), gemifloxacin (320 mg PO qd), or levofloxacin (750 mg PO or IV qd)]
- A β-lactam[c] [cefotaxime (1–2 g IV q8h), ceftriaxone (1–2 g IV qd), ampicillin (1–2 g IV q4–6h), or ertapenem (1 g IV qd in selected pts)] *plus* a macrolide[d] [oral clarithromycin or azithromycin (as listed above for previously healthy pts) or IV azithromycin (1 g once, then 500 mg qd)]

Inpatients, ICU

- A β-lactam[e] [cefotaxime (1–2 g IV q8h), ceftriaxone (2 g IV qd), or ampicillin-sulbactam (2 g IV q8h)] *plus*
- Azithromycin or a fluoroquinolone (as listed above for inpatients, non-ICU)

Special Concerns

If *Pseudomonas* is a consideration

- An antipneumococcal, antipseudomonal β-lactam [piperacillin/tazobactam (4.5 g IV q6h), cefepime (1–2 g IV q12h), imipenem (500 mg IV q6h), or meropenem (1 g IV q8h)] *plus* either ciprofloxacin (400 mg IV q12h) or levofloxacin (750 mg IV qd)
- A β-lactam (as listed above) *plus* an aminoglycoside [amikacin (15 mg/kg qd) or tobramycin (1.7 mg/kg qd)] *plus* azithromycin
- A β-lactam (as listed above)[f] *plus* an aminoglycoside *plus* an antipneumococcal fluoroquinolone

If CA-MRSA is a consideration

- Add linezolid (600 mg IV q12h) or vancomycin (1 g IV q12h).

[a]Doxycycline (100 mg PO bid) is an alternative to the macrolide.
[b]MICs of >16 μg/mL in 25% of isolates.
[c]A respiratory fluoroquinolone should be used for penicillin-allergic pts.
[d]Doxycycline (100 mg IV q12h) is an alternative to the macrolide.
[e]For penicillin-allergic pts, use a respiratory fluoroquinolone and aztreonam (2 g IV q8h).
[f]For penicillin-allergic pts, substitute aztreonam.
Abbreviation: CA-MRSA, community-acquired methicillin-resistant *Staphylococcus aureus*.

Epidemiology, Pathogenesis, and Clinical Manifestations

Prevalence estimates of VAP are 6–52 cases per 100 pts, with the highest hazard ratio in the first 5 days of mechanical ventilation.

- Three factors important in the pathogenesis of VAP are colonization of the oropharynx with pathogenic microorganisms, aspiration of these organisms to the lower respiratory tract, and compromise of normal host defense mechanisms.
- Clinical manifestations are similar to those in other forms of pneumonia.

Diagnosis

Application of clinical criteria consistently results in overdiagnosis of VAP. Use of quantitative cultures to discriminate between colonization and true infection by determining bacterial burden may be helpful; the more distal in the respiratory tree the diagnostic sampling, the more specific the results.

TREATMENT	Ventilator-Associated Pneumonia

- See Table 141-2 for recommended options for empirical therapy for HCAP.
  - Higher mortality rates are associated with inappropriate initial empirical treatment.
  - Broad-spectrum treatment should be modified when a pathogen is identified.
  - Clinical improvement, if it occurs, is usually evident within 48–72 h of the initiation of antimicrobial treatment.
- Treatment failure in VAP is not uncommon, especially when MDR pathogens are involved; MRSA and *P. aeruginosa* are associated with high failure rates.
- VAP complications include prolongation of mechanical ventilation, increased length of ICU stay, and necrotizing pneumonia with pulmonary hemorrhage or bronchiectasis. VAP is associated with significant mortality risk.
- Strategies effective for the prevention of VAP are listed in Table 141-3.

◼ HOSPITAL-ACQUIRED PNEUMONIA

Less well studied than VAP, HAP more commonly involves non-MDR pathogens. Anaerobes may also be more commonly involved in non-VAP pts because of the increased risk of macroaspiration in pts who are not intubated.

◼ BRONCHIECTASIS

Etiology and Epidemiology

Bronchiectasis is an irreversible airway dilation that involves the lung in either a focal (due to obstruction) or a diffuse (due to a systemic or infectious process) manner. Bronchiectasis can arise from infectious or noninfectious causes.

- The epidemiology varies greatly with the underlying etiology; in general, the incidence of bronchiectasis increases with age and is higher among women than among men.
- 25–50% of pts with bronchiectasis have idiopathic disease.

TABLE 141-2 EMPIRICAL ANTIBIOTIC TREATMENT OF HEALTH CARE–ASSOCIATED PNEUMONIA

Pts without Risk Factors for MDR Pathogens

Ceftriaxone (2 g IV q24h) *or*

Moxifloxacin (400 mg IV q24h), ciprofloxacin (400 mg IV q8h), or levofloxacin (750 mg IV q24h) *or*

Ampicillin/sulbactam (3 g IV q6h) *or*

Ertapenem (1 g IV q24h)

Pts with Risk Factors for MDR Pathogens

1. A β-lactam:

    Ceftazidime (2 g IV q8h) or cefepime (2 g IV q8–12h) *or*

    Piperacillin/tazobactam (4.5 g IV q6h), imipenem (500 mg IV q6h or 1 g IV q8h), or meropenem (1 g IV q8h) *plus*

2. A second agent active against gram-negative bacterial pathogens:

    Gentamicin or tobramycin (7 mg/kg IV q24h) or amikacin (20 mg/kg IV q24h) *or*

    Ciprofloxacin (400 mg IV q8h) or levofloxacin (750 mg IV q24h) *plus*

3. An agent active against gram-positive bacterial pathogens:

    Linezolid (600 mg IV q12h) *or*

    Vancomycin (15 mg/kg, up to 1 g IV q12h)

Pathogenesis

The most widely cited mechanism of infectious bronchiectasis is the "vicious cycle hypothesis," in which susceptibility to infection and poor mucociliary clearance result in microbial colonization of the bronchial tree. Proposed mechanisms for noninfectious bronchiectasis include immune-mediated reactions that damage the bronchial wall and parenchymal distortion as a result of lung fibrosis (e.g., postradiation fibrosis or idiopathic pulmonary fibrosis).

Clinical Manifestations

Presenting pts typically have a persistent productive cough with ongoing production of thick, tenacious sputum.

- Physical exam usually reveals crackles and wheezing on lung auscultation and occasionally reveals digital clubbing.
- Acute exacerbations are associated with increased purulent-sputum production.

Diagnosis

The diagnosis of bronchiectasis is based on clinical presentation with consistent radiographic findings, such as parallel "tram tracks," a "signet-ring sign" (a cross-sectional area of the airway with a diameter at least 1.5 times that of the adjacent vessel), lack of bronchial tapering, bronchial wall thickening, or cysts emanating from the bronchial wall.

TABLE 141-3 PATHOGENIC MECHANISMS AND CORRESPONDING PREVENTION STRATEGIES FOR VENTILATOR-ASSOCIATED PNEUMONIA

Pathogenic Mechanism	Prevention Strategy
Oropharyngeal colonization with pathogenic bacteria	
Elimination of normal flora	Avoidance of prolonged antibiotic courses
Large-volume oropharyngeal aspiration around time of intubation	Short course of prophylactic antibiotics for comatose pts[a]
Gastroesophageal reflux	Postpyloric enteral feeding[b]; avoidance of high gastric residuals, prokinetic agents
Bacterial overgrowth of stomach	Prophylactic agents that raise gastric pH[b]; selective decontamination of digestive tract with nonabsorbable antibiotics[b]
Cross-infection from other colonized pts	Hand washing, especially with alcohol-based hand rub; intensive infection-control education[a]; isolation; proper cleaning of reusable equipment
Large-volume aspiration	Endotracheal intubation; avoidance of sedation; decompression of small-bowel obstruction
Microaspiration around endotracheal tube	
Endotracheal intubation	Noninvasive ventilation[a]
Prolonged duration of ventilation	Daily awakening from sedation,[a] weaning protocols[a]
Abnormal swallowing function	Early percutaneous tracheostomy[a]
Secretions pooled above endotracheal tube	Head of bed elevated[a]; continuous aspiration of subglottic secretions with specialized endotracheal tube[a]; avoidance of reintubation; minimization of sedation and pt transport
Altered lower respiratory host defenses	Tight glycemic control[b]; lowering of hemoglobin transfusion threshold; specialized enteral feeding formula

[a]Strategies demonstrated to be effective in at least one randomized controlled trial.
[b]Strategies with negative randomized trials or conflicting results.

| TREATMENT | Bronchiectasis |

Treatment of infectious bronchiectasis is directed at the control of active infection and at improvements in secretion clearance and bronchial hygiene.

- Acute exacerbations should be treated with a 7- to 10-day course of antibiotics targeting the causative or presumptive pathogen; *H. influenzae* and *P. aeruginosa* are isolated commonly.
- Hydration and mucolytic administration, aerosolization of bronchodilators and hyperosmolar agents (e.g., hypertonic saline), and chest physiotherapy can be used to enhance secretion clearance.
- For pts with ≥3 recurrences per year, suppressive antibiotic treatment to minimize the microbial load and reduce the frequency of exacerbations has been proposed.
- In select cases, surgery (including lung transplantation) should be considered.

■ LUNG ABSCESS

Microbiology

Lung abscess—infection of the lung that results in necrosis of the pulmonary parenchyma—can be caused by a variety of microorganisms. The etiology depends, in part, on the characteristics of the host.

- Previously healthy pts are at risk for infection with bacteria (e.g., *S. aureus*, *Streptococcus milleri*, *K. pneumoniae*, group A *Streptococcus*) and parasites (e.g., *Entamoeba histolytica*, *Paragonimus westermani*, *Strongyloides stercoralis*).
- Aspiration-prone pts are at risk for infection with anaerobic bacteria; *S. aureus*, *P. aeruginosa*, and *F. necrophorum* (embolic lesions); endemic fungi; and mycobacteria.
- Immunocompromised pts are susceptible to *M. tuberculosis*, *Nocardia asteroides*, *Rhodococcus equi*, *Legionella* species, Enterobacteriaceae, *Aspergillus* species, and *Cryptococcus* species.

Clinical Manifestations

Nonspecific lung abscesses—typically presumed to be due to anaerobic organisms—present as an indolent infection with fatigue, cough, sputum production, fever, weight loss, and anemia. Pts may have foul-smelling breath or evidence of periodontal infection with pyorrhea or gingivitis.

Diagnosis

A chest CT is the preferred radiographic study to precisely delineate the lesion.

- Sputum samples can be cultured to detect aerobic bacteria but are unreliable for culture of anaerobic bacteria.
- Pleural fluid or bronchoalveolar lavage specimens may be helpful if they are processed promptly and appropriately for anaerobic bacteria.

TREATMENT   Lung Abscess

Treatment depends on the presumed or established etiology.
- Most infections caused by anaerobic bacteria should be treated initially with clindamycin (600 mg IV qid). Any β-lactam/β-lactamase inhibitor combination is an alternative.
- A transition from parenteral to oral therapy is appropriate once pts become afebrile and improve clinically.
- Although the duration of therapy is arbitrary, continuation of oral treatment is recommended until imaging shows that chest lesions have cleared or have left a small, stable scar.
- Fever persisting for 5–7 days after antibiotics have been started suggests failure of therapy and a need to exclude factors such as obstruction, complicating empyema, and involvement of antibiotic-resistant bacteria.
  - Clinical improvement with decreased fever usually occurs within 3–5 days, with defervescence in 5–10 days.
  - Pts with fevers persisting for 7–14 days should undergo bronchoscopy or other diagnostic tests to better define anatomic changes and microbiologic findings.

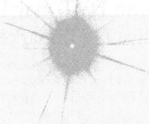

For a more detailed discussion, see Mandell LA, Wunderink R: Pneumonia, Chap. 257, p. 2130; and Baron RM, Bartlett JG: Bronchiectasis and Lung Abscess, Chap. 258, p. 2142, in HPIM-18.

CHAPTER **142**
Pulmonary Thromboembolism and Deep-Vein Thrombosis

DEFINITION AND NATURAL HISTORY

Venous thromboembolism includes both deep-vein thrombosis (DVT) and pulmonary thromboembolism (PE). DVT results from blood clot formation within large veins, usually in the legs. PE results from DVTs that have broken off and traveled to the pulmonary arterial circulation. About one-half of pts with pelvic vein or proximal leg DVT develop PE, which is often asymptomatic. Isolated calf vein thrombi have much lower risk of PE. Although DVTs are typically related to thrombus formation in the legs and/or pelvis, indwelling venous catheters have increased the occurrence of upper extremity DVT. In the absence of PE, the major complication of DVT is postphlebitic syndrome, which causes chronic leg swelling and discomfort due to damage to the venous valves of the affected leg. In its most severe form, postphlebitic syndrome causes skin ulceration. PE is often fatal, usually due to progressive right ventricular failure. Chronic thromboembolic pulmonary hypertension is another long-term complication of PE.

Some genetic risk factors, including factor V Leiden and the prothrombin G20210A mutation, have been identified, but they account for only a minority of venous thromboembolic disease. A variety of other risk factors have been identified, including immobilization during prolonged travel, cancer, obesity, smoking, surgery, trauma, pregnancy, oral contraceptives, and postmenopausal hormone replacement. Medical conditions that increase the risk of venous thromboembolism include cancer and antiphospholipid antibody syndrome.

CLINICAL EVALUATION

History

DVTs often present with progressive lower calf discomfort. For PE, dyspnea is the most common presenting symptom. Chest pain, cough, or hemoptysis can indicate pulmonary infarction with pleural irritation. Syncope can occur with massive PE.

Physical Examination

Tachypnea and tachycardia are common in PE. Low-grade fever, neck vein distention, and a loud P_2 on cardiac examination can be seen. Hypotension and cyanosis suggest massive PE. Physical examination with DVT may be notable only for mild calf tenderness. However, with massive DVT, marked thigh swelling and inguinal tenderness can be observed.

Laboratory Tests

Normal D-dimer level (<500 µg/mL by enzyme-linked immunosorbent assay) essentially rules out PE in pts with low-to-moderate likelihood of PE, although hospitalized pts often have elevated D-dimer levels due to other disease processes. Although hypoxemia and an increased alveolar-arterial O_2 gradient may be observed in PE, arterial blood gases are rarely useful in diagnosing PE. Elevated serum troponin, plasma heart-type fatty acid-binding protein, and brain natriuretic peptide levels are associated with increased risk of complications and mortality in PE. The electrocardiogram can show an S1Q3T3 sign in PE, but that finding is not frequently observed.

Imaging Studies

Venous ultrasonography can detect DVT by demonstrating loss of normal venous compressibility. When combined with Doppler imaging of venous flow, the detection of DVT by ultrasonography is excellent. For pts with nondiagnostic venous ultrasound studies, CT or MRI can be used to assess for DVT. Contrast phlebography is very rarely required. About one-half of pts with PE have no imaging evidence for DVT.

In PE, a normal chest x-ray (CXR) is common. Although not commonly observed, focal oligemia and peripheral wedge-shaped densities on CXR are well-established findings in PE. Chest CT with IV contrast has become the primary diagnostic imaging test for PE. Ventilation-perfusion lung scanning is primarily used for subjects unable to tolerate IV contrast. Transthoracic echocardiography is valuable to assess for right ventricular hypokinesis with moderate to large PE, but it is not typically useful for diagnosing the presence of a PE. Transesophageal echocardiography can be used to identify large central PE when IV contrast chest CT scans are not appropriate (e.g., renal failure or severe contrast allergy). With the advent of contrast chest CT scans for PE diagnosis, pulmonary angiography studies are rarely performed.

Integrated Diagnostic Approach

An integrated diagnostic approach that considers the clinical suspicion for DVT and PE is required. For individuals with a low clinical likelihood of DVT or with a low to moderate clinical likelihood of PE, the D-dimer level can be used to determine if further imaging studies are required. An algorithm for imaging studies in both DVT and PE is shown in Fig. 142-1. The differential diagnosis of DVT includes a ruptured Baker's cyst and cellulitis. The differential diagnosis of PE is broad and includes pneumonia, acute myocardial infarction, and aortic dissection.

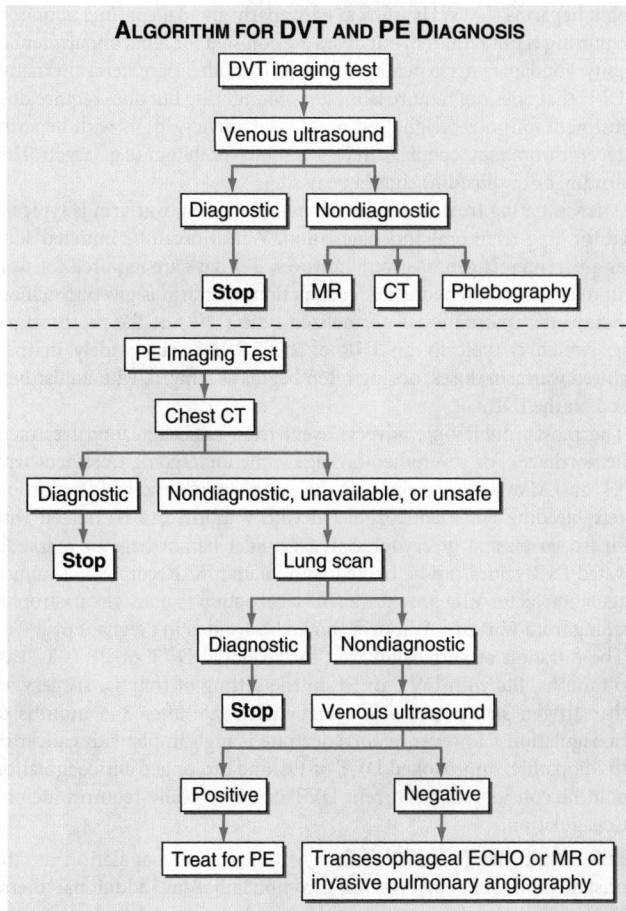

FIGURE 142-1 Imaging tests useful to diagnose DVT and PE. ECHO, echocardiogram.

TREATMENT Deep-Vein Thrombosis and Pulmonary Thromboembolism

ANTICOAGULATION Although anticoagulants do not dissolve existing clots in DVT or PE directly, they limit further thrombus formation and allow fibrinolysis to occur. In order to provide effective anticoagulation rapidly, parenteral anticoagulation is used for the initial treatment of venous thromboembolism. Traditionally, unfractionated heparin (UFH) has been used, with a target activated partial thromboplastin time (aPTT) of 2–3 times the upper limit of the normal laboratory value. UFH is typically administered with a bolus of 5000–10,000 U followed by a continuous infusion of approximately 1000 U/h. Frequent dosage adjustments are often required to achieve and maintain a therapeutic aPTT with UFH. Heparin-induced thrombocytopenia can occur with UFH. However, the short half-life of UFH remains a significant advantage.

Alternatives to UFH for acute anticoagulation include low-molecular-weight heparins (LMWHs) such as enoxaparin and dalteparin. Laboratory monitoring is not required, but doses are adjusted for renal impairment or obesity. Fondaparinux, a pentasaccharide, is another parenteral alternative to UFH that does not require laboratory monitoring but does require dose adjustment for body weight and renal insufficiency. In pts with heparin-induced thrombocytopenia, direct thrombin inhibitors (e.g., argatroban, lepirudin, or bivalirudin) should be used.

After initiating treatment with a parenteral agent, warfarin is typically used for long-term oral anticoagulation. Warfarin can be initiated soon after a parenteral agent is given; however, 5–7 days are required for warfarin to achieve therapeutic anticoagulation. Warfarin is given to achieve a therapeutic international normalized ratio (INR) of the prothrombin time, which is typically an INR of 2.0–3.0. Pts vary widely in their required warfarin doses; dosing often begins at 5 mg/d, with adjustment based on the INR.

The most troublesome adverse event from anticoagulation treatment is hemorrhage. For severe hemorrhage while undergoing treatment with UFH or LMWH, protamine can be given to reverse anticoagulation. Severe bleeding while anticoagulated with warfarin can be treated with fresh frozen plasma or cryoprecipitate; milder hemorrhage or markedly elevated INR values can be treated with vitamin K. Recombinant human coagulation factor VIIa provides an off-label option to manage catastrophic bleeding from warfarin. Warfarin should be avoided in pregnant pts.

The duration of anticoagulation for an initial DVT or PE is at least 3–6 months. Pts with DVT or PE in the setting of trauma, surgery, or high estrogen states have a low recurrence rate after 3–6 months of anticoagulation. However, recurrence rate is high in pts with cancer or with idiopathic, unprovoked DVT or PE, and prolonged anticoagulation should be considered. Recurrent DVT or PE typically requires lifelong anticoagulation.

OTHER TREATMENT MODALITIES Although anticoagulation is the mainstay of therapy for venous thromboembolism, additional therapeutic modalities also can be employed, based on risk stratification

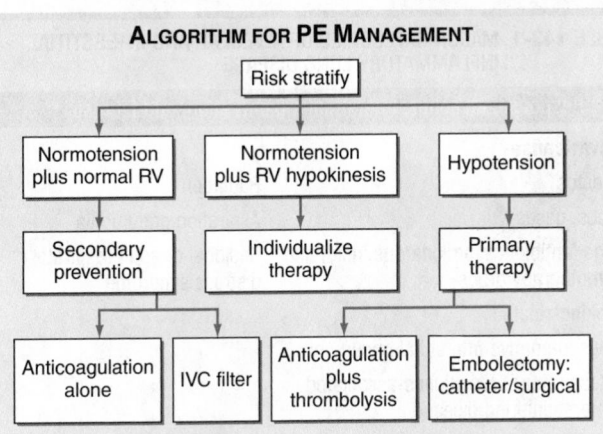

FIGURE 142-2 Acute management of pulmonary thromboembolism. IVC, inferior vena cava; RV, right ventricle.

(Fig. 142-2). Inferior vena cava filters can be used if thrombosis recurs despite adequate anticoagulation or if active bleeding precludes anticoagulation. Fibrinolytic therapy (often with tissue plasminogen activator) should be considered for PE causing right heart failure, although the risk of hemorrhage is significant. Surgical or catheter embolectomy also can be considered for massive PE.

If PE pts develop chronic thromboembolic pulmonary hypertension, surgical intervention (pulmonary thromboendarterectomy) can be performed. There is no effective therapy for postphlebitic syndrome.

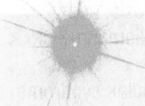

For a more detailed discussion, see Goldhaber SZ: Deep Venous Thrombosis and Pulmonary Thromboembolism, Chap. 262, p. 2170, in HPIM-18.

CHAPTER **143**
Interstitial Lung Disease

Interstitial lung diseases (ILDs) are a group of >200 disease entities characterized by diffuse parenchymal abnormalities. ILDs can be classified into two major groups: (1) diseases associated with predominant inflammation and fibrosis, and (2) diseases with predominantly granulomatous reaction in interstitial or vascular areas (Table 143-1). ILDs are nonmalignant and noninfectious, and they are typically chronic. The differential diagnosis of ILDs often includes infections (e.g., atypical mycobacteria, fungi) and

TABLE 143-1 MAJOR CATEGORIES OF ALVEOLAR AND INTERSTITIAL INFLAMMATORY LUNG DISEASE

Lung Response: Alveolitis, Interstitial Inflammation, and Fibrosis

Known cause

Asbestos

Fumes, gases

Drugs (antibiotics, amiodarone, gold) and chemotherapy drugs

Smoking-related

  Desquamative interstitial pneumonia

  Respiratory bronchiolitis-associated interstitial lung disease

  Langerhans cell granulomatosis (eosinophilic granulomatosis of the lung)

Radiation

Aspiration pneumonia

Residual of adult respiratory distress syndrome

Unknown cause

Idiopathic interstitial pneumonias

  Idiopathic pulmonary fibrosis (usual interstitial pneumonia)

  Acute interstitial pneumonia (diffuse alveolar damage)

  Cryptogenic organizing pneumonia (bronchiolitis obliterans with organizing pneumonia)

  Nonspecific interstitial pneumonia

Connective tissue diseases

  Systemic lupus erythematosus, rheumatoid arthritis, ankylosing spondylitis, systemic sclerosis, Sjögren's syndrome, polymyositis-dermatomyositis

Pulmonary hemorrhage syndromes

  Goodpasture's syndrome, idiopathic pulmonary hemosiderosis, isolated pulmonary capillaritis

Pulmonary alveolar proteinosis

Lymphocytic infiltrative disorders (lymphocytic interstitial pneumonitis associated with connective tissue disease)

Eosinophilic pneumonias

Lymphangioleiomyomatosis

Amyloidosis

Inherited diseases

  Tuberous sclerosis, neurofibromatosis, Niemann-Pick disease, Gaucher's disease, Hermansky-Pudlak syndrome

Gastrointestinal or liver diseases (Crohn's disease, primary biliary cirrhosis, chronic active hepatitis, ulcerative colitis)

Graft-versus-host disease (bone marrow transplantation; solid organ transplantation)

TABLE 143-1 MAJOR CATEGORIES OF ALVEOLAR AND INTERSTITIAL INFLAMMATORY LUNG DISEASE (CONTINUED)

Lung Response: Granulomatous	
Known cause	
Hypersensitivity pneumonitis (organic dusts)	Inorganic dusts: beryllium, silica
Unknown cause	
Sarcoidosis	Bronchocentric granulomatosis
Granulomatous vasculitides	Lymphomatoid granulomatosis
Granulomatosis with polyangiitis (Wegener's), allergic granulomatosis of Churg-Strauss	

malignancy (e.g., bronchioloalveolar cell carcinoma, lymphangitic carcinomatosis). One of the most common ILDs associated with a granulomatous reaction, sarcoidosis, is discussed in Chap. 177. Many ILDs are of unknown etiology; however, some ILDs are known to be associated with specific environmental exposures including asbestos, radiation therapy, and organic dusts.

APPROACH TO THE PATIENT Interstitial Lung Disease

History: Common presenting symptoms for pts with ILDs include dyspnea and nonproductive cough. Symptom onset and duration can assist in the differential diagnosis. Chronic symptoms (over months to years) are typically seen in most ILDs, including idiopathic pulmonary fibrosis (IPF), pneumoconioses, and pulmonary Langerhans cell histiocytosis (PLCH or eosinophilic granuloma). Subacute symptoms (over weeks to months) can also be observed in many ILDs, especially in sarcoidosis, drug-induced ILDs, cryptogenic organizing pneumonitis [COP, also known as bronchiolitis obliterans with organizing pneumonia (BOOP)], and alveolar hemorrhage syndromes. Acute presentations are uncommon for ILDs but are typically observed with acute interstitial pneumonia (AIP), and they can also occur with eosinophilic pneumonia and hypersensitivity pneumonitis. Sudden onset of dyspnea can indicate a pneumothorax, which occurs in PLCH and tuberous sclerosis/lymphangioleiomyomatosis. Fatigue and weight loss are common in all ILDs. Episodic presentations also are unusual, but they are more typical for eosinophilic pneumonia, hypersensitivity pneumonitis, and COP.

Age at presentation also can guide the differential diagnosis. IPF pts typically present at age >60, while sarcoidosis, PLCH, lymphangioleiomyomatosis (LAM), and connective tissue disease–related ILD often present between the ages of 20 and 40. LAM occurs exclusively in women, while ILD in rheumatoid arthritis (RA) typically occurs in men. Cigarette smoking is a risk factor for several ILDs including IPF, PLCH,

Goodpasture's syndrome, and respiratory bronchiolitis. Occupational exposures can be important risk factors for many types of hypersensitivity pneumonitis as well as pneumoconioses. Medical treatment with radiation and drugs also should be assessed.

Physical examination: Tachypnea and bibasilar end-inspiratory crackles are commonly observed in inflammatory ILDs, but they are less frequent in granulomatous ILDs. Clubbing of the digits is observed in some pts with advanced ILD.

Laboratory studies: Antinuclear antibodies and rheumatoid factor at low titers are observed in some IPF pts without a connective tissue disorder. Specific serum antibodies can confirm exposure to relevant antigens in hypersensitivity pneumonitis, but they do not prove causation.

Chest imaging: Chest x-ray (CXR) does not typically provide a specific diagnosis but often raises the possibility of ILD by demonstrating a bibasilar reticular pattern. Upper-lung-zone predominance of nodular opacities is noted in several ILDs, including PLCH, sarcoidosis, chronic hypersensitivity pneumonitis, and silicosis. High-resolution chest CT scans provide improved sensitivity for the early detection of ILDs and may be sufficiently specific to allow a diagnosis to be made in ILDs such as IPF, PLCH, and asbestosis. Honeycombing is indicative of advanced fibrosis.

Pulmonary function testing: Lung function measurements can assess the extent of pulmonary involvement in pts with ILD. Most ILDs produce a restrictive ventilatory defect with reduced total lung capacity. The forced expiratory volume in 1 s (FEV_1) and forced vital capacity (FVC) are typically reduced, but the ratio of FEV_1/FVC is usually normal to increased. Reduction in the diffusing capacity of the lung for carbon monoxide (D_{LCO}) is commonly observed. Cardiopulmonary exercise testing can be useful to detect exercise-induced hypoxemia.

Tissue and cellular examination: In order to provide a specific diagnosis and assess disease activity, lung biopsy is often required. Bronchoscopy with transbronchial biopsies can be diagnostic in some ILDs, including sarcoidosis and eosinophilic pneumonia. In addition, bronchoscopy can assist by excluding chronic infections or lymphangitic carcinomatosis. However, the more extensive tissue samples provided by open lung biopsies, often obtained by video-assisted thoracic surgery, are often required to establish a specific diagnosis. Evidence for diffuse end-stage disease, such as widespread honeycombing, or other major operative risks are relative contraindications to lung biopsy procedures.

PRINCIPLES OF MANAGEMENT

If a causative agent can be identified (e.g., thermophilic actinomyces in hypersensitivity pneumonitis), cessation of exposure to that agent is imperative. Because the response to treatment among different ILDs is so variable, identification of treatable causes is essential. Glucocorticoids can be highly effective for eosinophilic pneumonias, COP, hypersensitivity pneumonitis (HP), radiation pneumonitis, and drug-induced ILD. Prednisone at

0.5–1.0 mg/kg qd is commonly given for 4–12 weeks, followed by a gradual tapering dose. On the other hand, glucocorticoids are typically not beneficial in IPF. Smoking cessation is essential, especially for smoking-related ILDs such as PLCH and respiratory bronchiolitis.

Supportive therapeutic measures include providing supplemental O_2 for pts with significant hypoxemia (Pao_2 <55 mmHg at rest and/or with exercise). Pulmonary rehabilitation may also be beneficial. For young pts with end-stage ILD, lung transplantation should be considered.

SELECTED INDIVIDUAL ILDS

Idiopathic Pulmonary Fibrosis

IPF, which is also known as usual interstitial pneumonia (UIP), is the most common idiopathic interstitial pneumonia. Cigarette smoking is a risk factor for IPF. Common respiratory symptoms include exertional dyspnea and a nonproductive cough. Physical examination is notable for inspiratory crackles at the lung bases. Clubbing may occur. High-resolution chest CT scans show subpleural reticular opacities predominantly in the lower lung fields, which are associated with honeycombing in advanced disease. Pulmonary function tests reveal a restrictive ventilatory defect with reduced D_{LCO}. Surgical lung biopsy is usually required to confirm the diagnosis, although classic presentations may not require a biopsy. IPF can include acute exacerbations characterized by accelerated clinical deterioration over days to weeks. IPF is poorly responsive to available pharmacologic treatment.

Nonspecific Interstitial Pneumonia

Nonspecific interstitial pneumonia (NSIP) is a histologic pattern that can be observed in connective tissue disease, drug-induced ILD, and chronic HP. NSIP is a subacute restrictive process with similar presentation to IPF. High-resolution CT (HRCT) shows bilateral ground-glass opacities, and honeycombing is rare. Unlike IPF, NSIP pts have a good prognosis and typically respond well to systemic glucocorticoid treatment.

ILD Associated with Connective Tissue Disorders

Pulmonary manifestations may precede systemic manifestations of a connective tissue disorder. In addition to direct pulmonary involvement, it is necessary to consider complications of therapy (e.g., opportunistic infections), respiratory muscle weakness, esophageal dysfunction, and associated malignancies as contributors to pulmonary parenchymal abnormalities in pts with connective tissue disorders.

Progressive systemic sclerosis (scleroderma) commonly includes ILD as well as pulmonary vascular disease. Lung involvement tends to be highly resistant to available treatment.

In addition to pulmonary fibrosis (ILD), RA can involve a range of pulmonary complications, including pleural effusions, pulmonary nodules, and pulmonary vasculitis. ILD in RA pts is more common in men.

Systemic lupus erythematosus (SLE) also can involve a range of pulmonary complications, including pleural effusions, pulmonary vascular disease, pulmonary hemorrhage, and BOOP. Chronic, progressive ILD is not commonly observed.

Cryptogenic Organizing Pneumonia

When the BOOP pathologic pattern occurs without another primary pulmonary disorder, the term *cryptogenic organizing pneumonia (COP)* is used. COP may present with a flulike illness. Recurrent and migratory pulmonary opacities are common. Glucocorticoid therapy is often effective.

Desquamative Interstitial Pneumonia and Respiratory Bronchiolitis-Associated ILD

Desquamative interstitial pneumonia (DIP) includes extensive macrophage accumulation in intraalveolar spaces with minimal fibrosis. It is seen almost exclusively in cigarette smokers and improves with smoking cessation. Respiratory bronchiolitis-associated ILD is a subset of DIP that includes bronchial wall thickening, ground-glass opacities, and air trapping on HRCT; it also resolves in most pts after smoking cessation.

Pulmonary Alveolar Proteinosis

Pulmonary alveolar proteinosis (PAP) is a rare diffuse lung disease, with a male predominance, that involves the accumulation of lipoproteinaceous material in the distal airspaces, rather than a classic ILD. More common in males, PAP usually presents insidiously, with dyspnea, fatigue, weight loss, cough, and low-grade fever. Whole-lung lavage is often of therapeutic benefit.

Pulmonary Infiltrates with Eosinophilia

Several disorders are characterized by pulmonary infiltrates and peripheral blood eosinophilia. Tropical eosinophilia relates to parasitic infection; drug-induced eosinophilic pneumonias are more common in the United States. Löffler's syndrome typically includes migratory pulmonary infiltrates and minimal clinical symptoms. Acute eosinophilic pneumonia involves pulmonary infiltrates with severe hypoxemia. Chronic eosinophilic pneumonia is often in the differential diagnosis with other ILDs; it includes fever, cough, and weight loss, with a CXR notable for peripheral infiltrates. Eosinophilic pneumonias tend to be rapidly responsive to glucocorticoid therapy.

Alveolar Hemorrhage Syndromes

A variety of diseases can cause diffuse alveolar hemorrhage, including systemic vasculitic syndromes [e.g., granulomatosis with polyangiitis (Wegener's)], connective tissue diseases (e.g., SLE), and Goodpasture's syndrome. Although typically an acute process, recurrent episodes can lead to pulmonary fibrosis. Hemoptysis may not occur initially in one-third of cases. CXR typically shows patchy or diffuse alveolar opacities. The D$_{LCO}$ may be increased. High doses of IV methylprednisolone are typically required, followed by gradual tapering of systemic steroid doses. Plasmapheresis may be effective for Goodpasture's syndrome.

Pulmonary Langerhans Cell Histiocytosis

PLCH is a smoking-related diffuse lung disease that typically affects men 20 to 40 years of age. Presenting symptoms often include cough, dyspnea, chest pain, weight loss, and fever. Pneumothorax occurs in 25% of pts. High-resolution chest CT scan reveals upper-zone-predominant nodular opacities and thin-walled cysts, which are virtually diagnostic of this disorder. Smoking cessation is the key therapeutic intervention.

Hypersensitivity Pneumonitis

HP is an inflammatory lung disorder caused by repeated inhalation of an organic agent in a susceptible individual. Many organic agents have been implicated. Clinical presentations can be acute, with cough, fever, malaise, and dyspnea developing within 6–8 h after exposure; subacute, with cough and dyspnea that can become progressively worse over weeks; and chronic, which can appear similar to IPF. Peripheral blood eosinophilia is not observed. Serum precipitins can be measured as an indicator of an environmental exposure. Although helpful in implicating specific agents, the presence of a specific serum precipitin is not diagnostic since many exposed individuals without HP will have such precipitins; false-negative results can also occur. Diagnosis is made based on symptoms, physical findings, pulmonary function tests (restrictive or obstructive pattern), and radiographic studies (chest CT scans typically show ground-glass opacification in acute and subacute forms) that are consistent with HP; history of exposure to a recognized antigen; and presence of an antibody to that antigen. In some cases, lung biopsy (transbronchial or open lung) may be required to confirm the diagnosis. Treatment involves avoiding exposure to the causative antigen; systemic corticosteroids may be required in subacute or chronic HP.

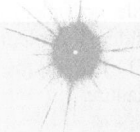

For a more detailed discussion, see King TE Jr: Interstitial Lung Diseases, Chap. 261, p. 2160; Gerke AK, Hunninghake GW: Hypersensitivity Pneumonitis and Pulmonary Infiltrates With Eosinophilia, Chap. 255, p. 2116, in HPIM-18.

CHAPTER **144**
Diseases of the Pleura and Mediastinum

PLEURAL EFFUSION

Etiology and Diagnostic Approach

Pleural effusion is defined as excess fluid accumulation in the pleural space. It can result from increased pleural fluid formation in the lung interstitium, parietal pleura, or peritoneal cavity, or from decreased pleural fluid removal by the parietal pleural lymphatics.

The two major classes of pleural effusions are transudates, which are caused by systemic influences on pleural fluid formation or resorption, and exudates, which are caused by local influences on pleural fluid formation and resorption. Common causes of transudative effusions are left ventricular heart failure, cirrhosis, and nephrotic syndrome. Common causes of exudative effusions are bacterial pneumonia, malignancy, viral infection, and pulmonary embolism. A more comprehensive list of the etiologies of transudative and exudative pleural effusions is provided in Table 144-1. Additional diagnostic procedures are indicated with exudative effusions to define the cause of the local disease.

Exudates fulfill at least one of the following three criteria: high pleural fluid/serum protein ratio (>0.5), pleural fluid lactate dehydrogenase (LDH) greater than two-thirds of the laboratory normal upper limit for serum LDH, or pleural/serum LDH ratio >0.6. Transudative effusions typically do not meet any of these criteria. However, these criteria misidentify about 25% of transudates as exudates. For exudative effusions, pleural fluid should also be tested for pH, glucose, white blood cell count with differential, microbiologic studies, cytology, and amylase. An algorithm for determining the etiology of a pleural effusion is presented in Fig. 144-1.

A subset of the most common types of pleural effusions is described in the following sections.

Transudative Pleural Effusions

Transudative pleural effusions related to left ventricular failure are often bilateral; if unilateral, right-sided effusions are more common than left-sided effusions. Thoracentesis is not always required to confirm the transudative nature of the pleural effusions if congestive heart failure is present; however, if the effusions are not comparable in size, if the pt is febrile, or if pleuritic chest pain is present, thoracentesis should be strongly considered. A pleural fluid N-terminal pro-brain natriuretic peptide (NT-proBNP) >1500 pg/mL is highly suggestive of an effusion related to congestive heart failure.

Parapneumonic Effusion/Empyema

Parapneumonic effusions are exudates that are associated with contiguous bacterial lung infections, including pneumonia and lung abscess. In the setting of pulmonary infections, the presence of free pleural fluid can be demonstrated with a lateral decubitus x-ray, chest CT scan, or ultrasound. If the pleural fluid is grossly purulent, it is referred to as an empyema.

Tube thoracostomy (i.e., chest tube) for management of parapneumonic effusions is likely indicated if any of the following applies (in descending order of importance): (1) gross pus is present, (2) Gram's stain or culture of pleural fluid is positive, (3) pleural fluid glucose is <3.3 mmol/L (<60 mg/dL), (4) pleural fluid pH is <7.20, or (5) there is loculated pleural fluid.

If chest tube drainage does not result in complete removal of pleural fluid, a fibrinolytic agent (e.g., tissue plasminogen activator 10 mg) can be instilled through the tube, or thoracoscopy can be performed to lyse adhesions. If these approaches are not effective, surgical decortication may be required.

Malignant Pleural Effusions

Metastatic cancer is a common cause of exudative pleural effusions. Tumors that frequently cause malignant effusions include lung cancer, breast cancer, and lymphoma. The pleural fluid glucose level may be markedly reduced. Cytologic examination of the pleural fluid is usually diagnostic. If cytologic examination of thoracentesis fluid is negative, thoracoscopy should be considered. Symptomatic relief of dyspnea can be provided by therapeutic thoracentesis. If the pleural fluid recurs, pleural sclerosis can be performed

TABLE 144-1 DIFFERENTIAL DIAGNOSES OF PLEURAL EFFUSIONS

Transudative Pleural Effusions

1. Congestive heart failure
2. Cirrhosis
3. Pulmonary embolism
4. Nephrotic syndrome
5. Peritoneal dialysis
6. Superior vena cava obstruction
7. Myxedema
8. Urinothorax

Exudative Pleural Effusions

1. Neoplastic diseases
   a. Metastatic disease
   b. Mesothelioma
2. Infectious diseases
   a. Bacterial infections
   b. Tuberculosis
   c. Fungal infections
   d. Viral infections
   e. Parasitic infections
3. Pulmonary embolism
4. Gastrointestinal disease
   a. Esophageal perforation
   b. Pancreatic disease
   c. Intraabdominal abscess
   d. Diaphragmatic hernia
   e. After abdominal surgery
   f. Endoscopic variceal sclerotherapy
   g. After liver transplant
5. Collagen-vascular diseases
   a. Rheumatoid pleuritis
   b. Systemic lupus erythematosus
   c. Drug-induced lupus
   d. Immunoblastic lymphadenopathy
   e. Sjögren's syndrome
   f. Granulomatosis with polyangiitis (Wegener's)
   g. Churg-Strauss syndrome
6. Post–coronary artery bypass surgery

(*continued*)

TABLE 144-1 DIFFERENTIAL DIAGNOSES OF PLEURAL EFFUSIONS (CONTINUED)

Exudative Pleural Effusions
7. Asbestos exposure
8. Sarcoidosis
9. Uremia
10. Meigs' syndrome
11. Yellow nail syndrome
12. Drug-induced pleural disease
a. Nitrofurantoin
b. Dantrolene
c. Methysergide
d. Bromocriptine
e. Procarbazine
f. Amiodarone
g. Dasatinib
13. Trapped lung
14. Radiation therapy
15. Post–cardiac injury syndrome
16. Hemothorax
17. Iatrogenic injury
18. Ovarian hyperstimulation syndrome
19. Pericardial disease
20. Chylothorax

with pleural abrasion via thoracoscopy or with instillation of a sclerosing agent, such as doxycycline, through a chest tube; alternatively, a small indwelling catheter can be placed.

Effusions Related to Pulmonary Thromboembolism

Pleural effusions in pulmonary thromboembolism are usually exudative but can be transudative. The presence of a pleural effusion does not alter the standard treatment for pulmonary embolism (Chap. 142). If the effusion increases in size during anticoagulation treatment, possible explanations include recurrent embolism, hemothorax, or empyema.

Tuberculous Pleuritis

Usually associated with primary tuberculosis (Tb) infection, tuberculous pleural effusions are exudative with predominant lymphocytosis. High levels of Tb markers in the pleural fluid, such as adenosine deaminase and interferon γ, are present. Mycobacterial cultures obtained from pleural fluid (low positive culture rate) or pleural biopsy (high positive culture rate with needle biopsy or thoracoscopy) can definitively confirm the diagnosis. Although

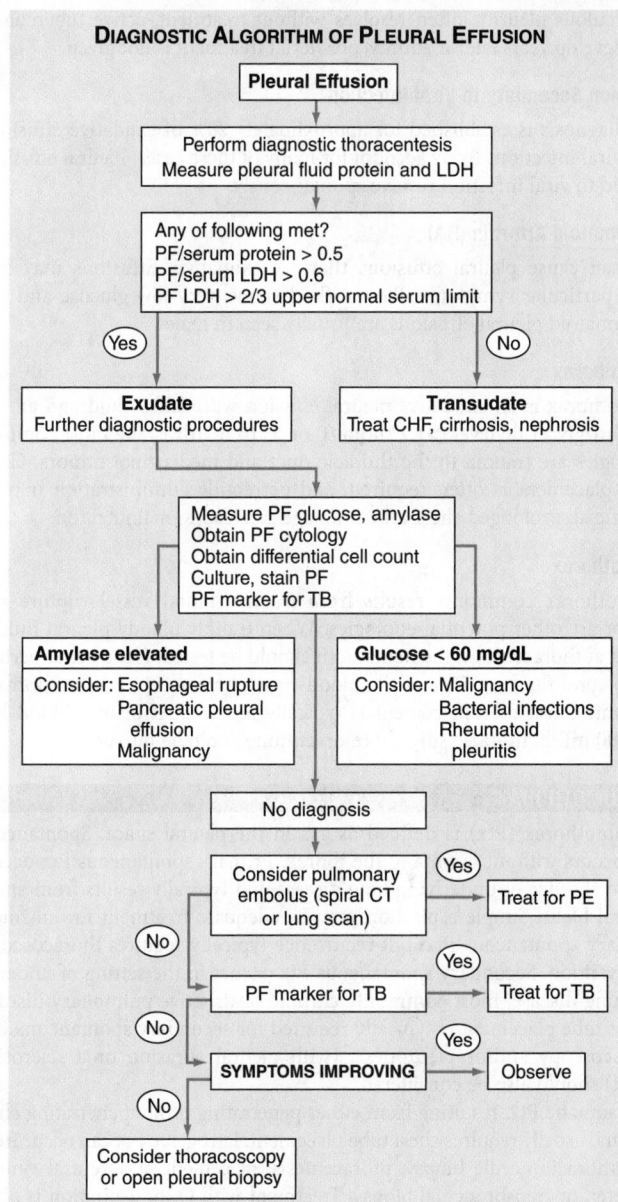

FIGURE 144-1 Approach to the diagnosis of pleural effusions. CHF, congestive heart failure; CT, computed tomography; LDH, lactate dehydrogenase; PE, pulmonary embolism; PF, pleural fluid; TB, tuberculosis.

tuberculous pleuritis often resolves without treatment, active tuberculosis can develop years later if antimycobacterial treatment is not given.

Effusion Secondary to Viral Infection

No diagnosis is established for approximately 20% of exudative effusions, and viral infections likely account for many of these cases. Pleural effusions related to viral infection resolve spontaneously.

Rheumatoid Arthritis (RA)

RA can cause pleural effusions that are exudative. Effusions may precede particular symptoms. Pleural fluid shows very low glucose and pH. Rheumatoid pleural effusions are usually seen in males.

Chylothorax

Chylothorax is an exudative pleural effusion with milky fluid and an elevated triglyceride level (>1.2 mmol/L or >110 mg/dL). The most common etiologies are trauma to the thoracic duct and mediastinal tumors. Chest tube placement is often required, and octreotide administration may be beneficial. Prolonged chest tube drainage can lead to malnutrition.

Hemothorax

Hemothorax commonly results from trauma; blood vessel rupture and tumor are other potential etiologies. When frankly bloody pleural fluid is noted at thoracentesis, the hematocrit should be tested. If the hematocrit of the pleural fluid is >50% of the bloodstream hematocrit, a hemothorax is present. Chest tube placement is typically required. If pleural blood loss is >200 mL/h, thoracic surgical intervention should be pursued.

PNEUMOTHORAX

Pneumothorax (Ptx) is defined as gas in the pleural space. Spontaneous Ptx occurs without trauma to the thorax. Primary spontaneous Ptx occurs in the absence of underlying lung disease and typically results from apical pleural blebs. Simple aspiration may be adequate treatment for an initial primary spontaneous Ptx, but recurrence typically requires thoracoscopic intervention. Secondary spontaneous Ptx occurs in the setting of underlying lung disease, most commonly chronic obstructive pulmonary disease. Chest tube placement is typically required for secondary spontaneous Ptx; thoracoscopy and/or pleurodesis (with pleural abrasion or a sclerosing agent) should also be considered.

Traumatic Ptx, resulting from either penetrating or nonpenetrating chest trauma, usually requires chest tube placement. Iatrogenic Ptx can occur from transthoracic needle biopsy, thoracentesis, placement of a central venous catheter, or transbronchial biopsy. Treatment with O_2 or aspiration is often adequate for iatrogenic Ptx, but chest tube placement may be required. Tension Ptx can result from trauma or mechanical ventilation. Positive pleural pressure in mechanical ventilation can rapidly lead to a tension Ptx with reduced cardiac output. Urgent treatment is required, either with a chest tube or, if not immediately available, with a large-bore needle inserted into the pleural space through the second anterior intercostal space.

MEDIASTINAL DISEASE

Mediastinitis

Mediastinitis can be an acute or chronic process. Acute mediastinitis can result from esophageal perforation or after cardiac surgery with median sternotomy. Esophageal perforation can occur spontaneously or iatrogenically; surgical exploration of the mediastinum, repair of the esophageal perforation, and drainage of the pleural space and mediastinum are required. Mediastinitis after median sternotomy typically presents with wound drainage and is diagnosed by mediastinal needle aspiration. Treatment requires immediate drainage, debridement, and IV antibiotics.

Chronic mediastinitis can cause a spectrum of disease ranging from granulomatous inflammation of lymph nodes to fibrosing mediastinitis. Chronic mediastinitis is commonly caused by Tb and histoplasmosis; other etiologies are also possible, including sarcoidosis and silicosis. Granulomatous mediastinal inflammation is usually asymptomatic. Fibrosing mediastinitis causes symptoms related to compression of mediastinal structures, such as the superior vena cava, esophagus, or large airways. Fibrosing mediastinitis is very difficult to treat.

Mediastinal Masses

Different types of mediastinal masses are found in the anterior, middle, and posterior mediastinal compartments. The most common mass lesions in the anterior mediastinum are thymomas, lymphomas, teratomas, and thyroid lesions. In the middle mediastinum, vascular masses, enlarged lymph nodes (e.g., metastatic cancer or granulomatous disease), and bronchogenic or pleuropericardial cysts are found. Posterior mediastinal masses include neurogenic tumors, gastroenteric cysts, and esophageal diverticula.

CT scans are invaluable for evaluating mediastinal masses. Barium swallow studies can assist in evaluating posterior mediastinal masses. Biopsy procedures are typically required to diagnose mediastinal masses; needle biopsy procedures (e.g., percutaneous or bronchoscopy), mediastinoscopy, and thoracoscopy are potential options.

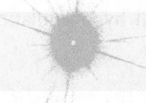
For a more detailed discussion, see Light RW: Disorders of the Pleura and Mediastinum, Chap. 263, p. 2178, in HPIM-18.

CHAPTER **145**
Disorders of Ventilation

DEFINITION

Ventilatory disorders, reflected by abnormalities in $Paco_2$, include alterations in CO_2 production, minute ventilation, or respiratory system dead space. Many diseases can cause acute elevations in CO_2 production; chronic ventilatory disorders relate to inappropriate minute ventilation or dead space fraction.

HYPOVENTILATION

■ ETIOLOGY

Chronic hypoventilation can result from parenchymal lung diseases, chest wall abnormalities (e.g., severe kyphoscoliosis), sleep-disordered breathing, neuromuscular diseases, and abnormal respiratory drive. Obesity-hypoventilation syndrome includes body mass index $\geq$30 kg/m^2; sleep-disordered breathing (typically obstructive sleep apnea); $Paco_2$ >45 mmHg; and Pao_2 <70 mmHg. Central hypoventilation syndrome is a rare disorder that includes a failure of the normal respiratory response to hypoxemia and/or hypercapnia.

■ CLINICAL ASSESSMENT

Key symptoms of hypoventilation can include exertional dyspnea, orthopnea, daytime somnolence, morning headache, and anxiety. Parenchymal lung diseases, such as chronic obstructive pulmonary disease and interstitial lung disease, often include dyspnea and cough. Sleep-disordered breathing includes daytime somnolence, snoring, and fragmented sleep. Orthopnea is common in neuromuscular disorders, although weakness of the extremities or other muscle groups often precedes respiratory system muscular weakness. Hypoventilation related to neuromuscular and chest wall disorders progresses from asymptomatic to nocturnal hypoventilation to daytime hypercapnia. Chronic narcotic use and hypothyroidism can lead to reduced respiratory drive.

Physical examination, chest radiographic studies (chest x-ray and possibly chest CT), and pulmonary function tests reveal most lung parenchymal and chest wall causes of hypoventilation. Measurement of maximal inspiratory and expiratory pressures can assess respiratory muscle strength. Polysomnography to assess for obstructive sleep apnea should also be considered. When pts have hypercapnia with normal pulmonary function, normal respiratory muscle strength, and normal alveolar-arterial Po_2 difference, respiratory drive abnormalities may be present, which can be revealed by polysomnography. Laboratory findings include increased $Paco_2$ and often reduced Pao_2 as well. Compensatory increases in plasma bicarbonate levels and normal pH are seen in chronic hypoventilation. Eventually, pulmonary hypertension and cor pulmonale can develop. In central hypoventilation syndrome, hypercapnia worsens substantially during sleep.

TREATMENT	Hypoventilation

In all forms of hypoventilation, supplemental oxygen should be given to correct hypoxemia. Obesity-hypoventilation is treated with weight reduction and continuous positive airway pressure (CPAP) during sleep. Some pts may require bilevel positive airway pressure (BiPAP).

Noninvasive positive pressure ventilation during sleep can provide ventilatory support and treat sleep apnea associated with neuromuscular disorders, chest wall disorders, and central hypoventilation. With progressive neuromuscular disorders, full-time mechanical ventilatory support is often required.

Pts with respiratory drive disorders may benefit from phrenic nerve pacing

HYPERVENTILATION

■ ETIOLOGY

Hyperventilation is caused by ventilation in excess of requirements based on CO_2 production, leading to a reduced $Paco_2$. Although anxiety can contribute to the initiation and progression of hyperventilation, hyperventilation is not always related to anxiety. Hyperventilation can precede systemic illnesses such as diabetic ketoacidosis.

■ CLINICAL ASSESSMENT

Symptoms of chronic hyperventilation can include dyspnea, paresthesias, headache, tetany, and atypical chest pain. Laboratory findings of chronic hyperventilation include a reduced $Paco_2$, but low serum bicarbonate level and near normal pH on arterial blood gas analysis.

> **TREATMENT** Hyperventilation
>
> Treatment of chronic hyperventilation is problematic. Identification of initiating factors and excluding alternative diagnoses can be helpful.

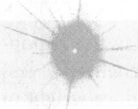

For a more detailed discussion, see McConville JF, Solway J: Disorders of Ventilation, Chap. 264, p. 2182, in HPIM-18.

CHAPTER **146**
Sleep Apnea

■ DEFINITION AND ETIOLOGY

Sleep apnea is defined by the presence of at least five episodes per hour of apnea (no airflow for ≥10 seconds) and/or hypopnea (reduction in airflow by at least 50% from baseline for ≥10 seconds). Obstructive sleep apnea/hypopnea syndrome (OSAHS) is the most common medical cause of daytime somnolence. OSAHS is caused by upper airway closure during inspiration, punctuated by brief arousals that terminate apneic episodes. Risk factors for OSAHS include obesity and anatomic shortening of the mandible or maxilla. Hypothyroidism and acromegaly are systemic diseases associated with OSAHS.

Central sleep apnea (CSA) is characterized by respiratory pauses during sleep related to absence of respiratory effort. CSA is commonly found in heart failure and stroke pts; spontaneous CSA is rare.

■ CLINICAL ASSESSMENT

Symptoms of OSAHS include daytime somnolence, impaired cognitive performance and driving skills, nocturnal choking, nocturia, and decreased libido. Loud snoring is typically reported by sleeping partners. Depression and hypertension are associated with OSAHS, and cardiovascular disease risk may be increased. Differential diagnosis of OSAHS includes insufficient amount of sleep, somnolence related to shift work, depression, drug effects (both stimulants and sedatives), narcolepsy, and idiopathic hypersomnolence.

Severity of somnolence can be assessed with the Epworth Sleepiness Score, although somnolent pts who don't fall asleep at inappropriate times may be missed with this questionnaire. Obtaining the sleep history from the pt's partner can be very helpful. Daytime somnolence may be seen in CSA as well as OSAHS.

Physical examination should include assessment of body mass index, jaw and upper airway structure, and blood pressure. Potentially related systemic illnesses, including acromegaly and hypothyroidism, should be considered.

Diagnostic testing often includes a polysomnogram in a sleep laboratory. However, limited sleep studies without neurophysiologic monitoring may be used for screening. Significant daytime somnolence with a negative limited screening study should be followed by a full polysomnogram. Many apneic events previously labeled as central apneas in polysomnographic studies may have been obstructive events despite lack of thoracoabdominal movement.

TREATMENT Sleep Apnea

Pts with significant daytime somnolence and >15 apneic and/or hypopneic events per hour clearly benefit from treatment; benefits are less compelling with milder degrees of OSAHS. Efforts to reduce weight in obese pts, to limit alcohol use, and to carefully withdraw sedative medications should be pursued.

The primary therapy for OSAHS is continuous positive airway pressure (CPAP). Selecting a comfortable mask delivery system and titrating the appropriate amount of CPAP are essential. Airway drying related to CPAP can be reduced by including a heated humidification component in the CPAP system. Alternative OSAHS therapies include mandibular repositioning splints (oral devices), which hold the jaw and tongue forward to widen the pharyngeal airway. Several types of surgical procedures have been used in OSAHS, including bariatric surgery in obese pts, tonsillectomy, jaw advancement surgery, and pharyngeal surgery. Tracheostomy is curative since it bypasses the upper airway obstruction site, but it is rarely used. No drugs have been proven to reduce apneic events; however, modafinil may reduce sleepiness.

Treatment of CSA involves managing any predisposing conditions, such as congestive heart failure. CPAP may be effective in some CSA pts.

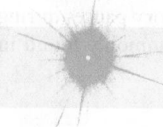

For a more detailed discussion, see Douglas NJ: Sleep Apnea, Chap. 265, p. 2186, in HPIM-18.

CHAPTER **147**
Approach to the Patient With Renal Disease

The approach to renal disease begins with recognition of particular syndromes on the basis of findings such as presence or absence of azotemia, proteinuria, hypertension, edema, abnormal urinalysis, electrolyte disorders, abnormal urine volumes, or infection (Table 147-1).

ACUTE RENAL INJURY (SEE CHAP. 148)

Clinical syndrome is characterized by a rapid, severe decrease in glomerular filtration rate (GFR) [rise in serum creatinine and blood urea nitrogen (BUN)], usually with reduced urine output. Extracellular fluid expansion leads to edema, hypertension, and occasionally acute pulmonary edema. Hyperkalemia, hyponatremia, and acidosis are common. Etiologies include ischemia; nephrotoxic injury due to drugs, toxins, or endogenous pigments; sepsis; severe renovascular disease; glomerulonephritis (GN); interstitial nephritis, particularly allergic interstitial nephritis due to medications; thrombotic microangiopathy; or conditions related to pregnancy. Prerenal failure and postrenal failure are potentially reversible causes.

Rapidly Progressive Glomerulonephritis

Defined as a >50% reduction in renal function, occurring over weeks to months. Broadly classified into three major subtypes on the basis of renal biopsy findings and pathophysiology: (1) immune complex–associated, e.g., in systemic lupus erythematosus (SLE); (2) "pauci-immune," associated with antineutrophil cytoplasmic antibodies (ANCA) specific for myeloperoxidase or proteinase-3; and (3) associated with anti–glomerular basement membrane (anti-GBM) antibodies, e.g., in Goodpasture's syndrome.

Pts are initially nonoliguric and may have recent flulike symptoms (myalgias, low-grade fevers, etc.); later, oliguric renal failure with uremic symptoms supervenes. Hypertension is common, particularly in poststreptococcal GN. Symptoms of associated disorders may be prominent, e.g., arthritis/arthralgias in SLE or vasculitis. Pulmonary manifestations in ANCA- and anti-GBM-associated rapidly progressive GN range from asymptomatic infiltrates to life-threatening pulmonary hemorrhage. Urinalysis typically shows hematuria, proteinuria, and red blood cell (RBC) casts; however, while highly specific for GN, RBC casts are not a particularly sensitive finding.

Acute Glomerulonephritis (See Chap. 152)

Often called nephritic syndrome, classically caused by poststreptococcal GN. An acute illness with sudden onset of hematuria, edema, hypertension, oliguria, and elevated BUN and creatinine. Mild pulmonary congestion

949

TABLE 147-1   INITIAL CLINICAL AND LABORATORY DATABASE FOR DEFINING MAJOR SYNDROMES IN NEPHROLOGY

Syndromes	Important Clues to Diagnosis	Common Findings
Acute or rapidly progressive renal failure	Anuria Oliguria Documented recent decline in GFR	Hypertension, pulmonary edema, peripheral edema, hematuria, proteinuria, pyuria
Acute nephritis	Hematuria, RBC casts Azotemia, oliguria Edema, hypertension	Proteinuria Pyuria Circulatory congestion
Chronic renal failure	Azotemia for >3 months Symptoms or signs of uremia Shrunken, echogenic kidneys on ultrasound Anemia, hyperparathyroidism	Hematuria, proteinuria Edema, hypertension Hyperkalemia, acidosis, hypocalcemia, anemia
Nephrotic syndrome	Proteinuria >3.5 g per 1.73 m^2 per 24 h Hypoalbuminemia Hyperlipidemia Lipiduria	Edema
Asymptomatic urinary abnormalities	Hematuria Proteinuria (below nephrotic range) Sterile pyuria, casts	
Urinary tract infection	Bacteriuria >10^5 colonies per mL Other infectious agent documented in urine Pyuria, leukocyte casts Frequency, urgency Bladder tenderness, flank tenderness	Hematuria Mild azotemia Mild proteinuria Fever
Renal tubule defects	Electrolyte (Na^+, K^+, Mg^{2+}, phosphate, or Ca^{2+}) or solute (glucose, uric acid, amino acid) disorders Polyuria, nocturia	Hematuria "Tubular" proteinuria Enuresis Electrolyte or acid-base disorders

TABLE 147-1 INITIAL CLINICAL AND LABORATORY DATABASE FOR DEFINING MAJOR SYNDROMES IN NEPHROLOGY (CONTINUED)

Syndromes	Important Clues to Diagnosis	Common Findings
	Symptoms or signs of renal osteodystrophy	
	Structurally abnormal kidneys, e.g., cysts	
Hypertension	Systolic/diastolic hypertension	Moderate proteinuria Azotemia
Nephrolithiasis	Previous history of stone passage or removal	Hematuria Pyuria
	Previous history of stone seen by x-ray	Frequency, urgency
	Renal colic	
Urinary tract obstruction	Azotemia, oliguria, anuria	Hematuria
	Polyuria, nocturia, urinary retention	Pyuria
	Slowing of urinary stream	Enuresis, dysuria
	Large prostate, large kidneys	
	Flank tenderness, full bladder after voiding	

Abbreviations: GFR, glomerular filtration rate; RBC, red blood cell.
Source: Modified from FL Coe, BM Brenner: HPIM-14.

may be present. An antecedent or concurrent infection or multisystem disease may be causative, or glomerular disease may exist alone. Hematuria, proteinuria, and pyuria are usually present, and RBC casts confirm the diagnosis. Serum complement may be decreased in certain conditions.

CHRONIC RENAL FAILURE (SEE CHAP. 149)

Progressive permanent loss of renal function over months to years does not cause symptoms of uremia until GFR is reduced to about 10–15% of normal. Hypertension and/or edema may occur early. Later, manifestations include anorexia, nausea, vomiting, dysgeusia, insomnia, weight loss, weakness, paresthesia, pruritus, bleeding, serositis (typically pericarditis), anemia, acidosis, hypocalcemia, hyperphosphatemia, and hyperkalemia. Common causes include diabetes mellitus, severe hypertension, glomerular disease, urinary tract obstruction, vascular disease, polycystic kidney disease, and interstitial nephritis. Indications of chronicity include longstanding azotemia, anemia, hyperphosphatemia, hypocalcemia, shrunken kidneys, renal osteodystrophy by x-ray, or findings on renal biopsy (extensive glomerular sclerosis, arteriosclerosis, and/or tubulointerstitial fibrosis).

NEPHROTIC SYNDROME (SEE CHAP. 152)

Defined as heavy albuminuria (>3.5 g/d in the adult) with or without edema, hypoalbuminemia, hyperlipidemia, and varying degrees of renal insufficiency. Can be idiopathic or due to drugs, infections, neoplasms, or multisystem or hereditary diseases. Complications include severe edema, thromboembolic events, infection, and protein malnutrition.

ASYMPTOMATIC URINARY ABNORMALITIES

Hematuria may be due to neoplasms, stones, infection at any level of the urinary tract, sickle cell disease, or analgesic abuse. Renal parenchymal causes are suggested by RBC casts, proteinuria, and/or dysmorphic RBCs in urine. Pattern of gross hematuria may be helpful in localizing site. Hematuria with minimal or low-grade proteinuria is most commonly due to thin basement membrane nephropathy or IgA nephropathy. Modest *proteinuria* may be an isolated finding due to fever, exertion, congestive heart failure (CHF), or upright posture; renal causes include early stages of diabetes nephropathy, amyloidosis, or other causes of glomerular disease. *Pyuria* can be caused by urinary tract infection (UTI), interstitial nephritis, GN, or renal transplant rejection. "Sterile" pyuria can be associated with UTI treated with antibiotics, cyclophosphamide therapy, pregnancy, genitourinary trauma, prostatitis, cystourethritis, tuberculosis and other mycobacterial infections, and fungal infection.

URINARY TRACT INFECTION (SEE CHAP. 154)

Generally defined as >10^5 bacteria per mL of urine. Levels between 10^2 and 10^5/mL may indicate infection but are usually due to poor sample collection, especially if mixed flora are present. Adults at risk are sexually active women or anyone with urinary tract obstruction, vesicoureteral reflux, bladder catheterization, neurogenic bladder (associated with diabetes mellitus), or primary neurologic diseases. Prostatitis, urethritis, and vaginitis may be distinguished by quantitative urine culture. Flank pain, nausea, vomiting, fever, and chills indicate kidney infection, i.e., pyelonephritis. UTI is a common cause of sepsis, especially in the elderly and institutionalized.

RENAL TUBULAR DEFECTS (SEE CHAP. 153)

Generally inherited, these include anatomic defects (polycystic kidneys, medullary cystic disease, medullary sponge kidney) detected in the evaluation of hematuria, flank pain, infection, or renal failure of unknown cause. Isolated or generalized defects of renal tubular salt, solute, acid, and water transport can also occur. The Fanconi syndrome is characterized by multiple defects in proximal tubular solute transport; cardinal features include generalized aminoaciduria, glycosuria with a normal serum glucose, and phosphaturia. The Fanconi syndrome can also encompass a proximal renal tubular acidosis, hypouricemia, hypokalemia, polyuria, hypovitaminosis D and hypocalcemia, and low-molecular-weight proteinuria. This syndrome can be hereditary (e.g., in Dent's disease and cystinosis) or acquired, the latter due to drugs (ifosfamide, tenofovir, valproic acid), toxins (aristolochic acid), heavy metals, multiple myeloma, or amyloidosis. Hereditary hypo-kalemic alkalosis is typically caused by defects in ion transport by the thick ascending limb (Bartter's syndrome) or the distal convoluted tubule (Gitelman's syndrome); similar acquired defects can occur after exposure to aminoglycosides or cisplatin. Nephrogenic diabetes insipidus and renal tubular acidosis are caused by defects in distal tubular water and acid transport, respectively; these also have both hereditary and acquired forms. Lithium, prescribed for bipolar disease and related psychiatric disorders, is a very common cause of acquired nephrogenic diabetes insipidus.

HYPERTENSION (SEE CHAP. 126)

Blood pressure >140/90 mmHg affects 20% of the U.S. adult population; when inadequately controlled, it is an important cause of cerebrovascular accident, myocardial infarction, and CHF, and can contribute to the devel-opment of renal failure. Hypertension is usually asymptomatic until cardiac, renal, or neurologic symptoms appear; retinopathy or left ventricular hypertrophy (S_4 heart sound, electrocardiographic or echocardiographic evidence) may be the only clinical sequelae. In most cases, hypertension is idiopathic and becomes evident between ages 25 and 45. Secondary hypertension is generally suggested by the following clinical scenarios: (1) severe or refractory hypertension, (2) a sudden increase in blood pressure over prior values, (3) onset prior to puberty, or (4) age <30 in a nonobese, non-African-American pt with a negative family history. Clinical clues may suggest specific causes. Hypokalemia suggests renovascular hypertension or primary hyperaldosteronism; paroxysmal hypertension with headache, diaphoresis, and palpitations can occur in pheochromocytoma.

NEPHROLITHIASIS (SEE CHAP. 156)

Causes colicky pain, UTI, hematuria, dysuria, or unexplained pyuria. Stones may be found on routine x-ray of kidneys, ureter, and bladder (KUB); however, noncontrast helical CT, with 5-mm CT cuts, will pick up stones not detected by KUB x-ray and will furthermore assess for the presence of obstruction. Most are radiopaque Ca stones and are associated with high levels of urinary Ca, and/or oxalate excretion, and/or low levels of urinary citrate excretion. Staghorn calculi are large, branching, radiopaque stones within the renal pelvis due to recurrent infection. Uric acid stones are radiolucent. Urinalysis may reveal hematuria, pyuria, or pathologic crystals.

URINARY TRACT OBSTRUCTION (SEE CHAP. 157)

Causes variable symptoms depending on the underlying etiology and whether obstruction is acute or chronic, unilateral or bilateral, and complete or partial. It is an important, reversible cause of unexplained renal failure. Upper tract obstruction may be silent or produce flank pain, hematuria, and renal infection. Bladder symptoms or prostatism may be present in lower tract obstruction. Functional consequences include polyuria, anuria, noctu-ria, acidosis, hyperkalemia, and hypertension. A flank or suprapubic mass may be found on physical exam; an obstructed, enlarged bladder is typically dull to percussion. An increased post-void residual urine volume can be confirmed with bedside bladder scan or by ultrasound.

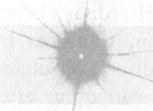

For a more detailed discussion, see Part 13: Disorders of the Kidney and Urinary Tract, p. 2279, in HPIM-18.

CHAPTER **148**
Acute Renal Failure

DEFINITION

Acute renal failure (ARF) or acute kidney injury (AKI), defined as a measurable increase in the serum creatinine (Cr) concentration [usually relative increase of 50% or absolute increase by 44–88 μmol/L (0.5–1.0 mg/dL)], occurs in ~5–7% of hospitalized pts. It is associated with a substantial increase in in-hospital mortality and morbidity. AKI can be anticipated in some clinical circumstances (e.g., after radiocontrast exposure or major surgery), and there are no specific pharmacologic therapies proven helpful at preventing or reversing the condition. Maintaining optimal renal perfusion and intravascular volume appears to be important in most clinical circumstances; important cofactors in AKI include hypovolemia and drugs that interfere with renal perfusion and/or glomerular filtration [nonsteroidal anti-inflammatory drugs (NSAIDs), angiotensin-converting enzyme (ACE) inhibitors, and angiotensin receptor blockers].

DIFFERENTIAL DIAGNOSIS

The separation into three broad categories (prerenal, intrinsic renal, and postrenal failure) is of considerable clinical utility (Table 148-1). *Prerenal failure* is most common among hospitalized pts. It may result from true volume depletion [e.g., diarrhea, vomiting, gastrointestinal (GI) or other hemorrhage] or "effective circulatory volume" depletion or "arterial underfilling," i.e., reduced renal perfusion in the setting of adequate or excess blood volume. Reduced renal perfusion may be seen in congestive heart failure (CHF) (due to reduced cardiac output and/or potent vasodilator therapy), hepatic cirrhosis (due most likely to peripheral vasodilation and arteriovenous shunting), nephrotic syndrome and other states of severe hypoproteinemia [total serum protein <54 g/L (<5.4 g/dL)], and renovascular disease (because of fixed stenosis at the level of the main renal artery or large branch vessels). Several drugs can reduce renal perfusion, most notably NSAIDs. ACE inhibitors and angiotensin II receptor antagonists may reduce glomerular filtration rate but do not tend to reduce renal perfusion.

Causes of *intrinsic renal failure* depend on the clinical setting. Among hospitalized pts, especially on surgical services or in intensive care units, acute tubular necrosis (ATN) is the most common diagnosis. A well-defined ischemic event or toxic exposure (e.g., aminoglycoside therapy)

TABLE 148-1 COMMON CAUSES OF ACUTE KIDNEY INJURY

Prerenal

Volume depletion

  Blood loss

  GI fluid loss (e.g., vomiting, diarrhea)

  Overzealous diuretic use

Volume overload with reduced renal perfusion

  Congestive heart failure

    Low-output with systolic dysfunction

    "High-output" (e.g., anemia, thyrotoxicosis)

  Hepatic cirrhosis

  Severe hypoproteinemia

Renovascular disease

Drugs

  NSAIDs, cyclosporine, ACE inhibitors, ARBs, cisplatin, aminoglycosides

Other

  Hypercalcemia, "third spacing" (e.g., pancreatitis, systemic inflammatory response), hepatorenal syndrome

Intrinsic

Acute tubular necrosis (ATN)

  Hypotension or shock, prolonged prerenal azotemia, postoperative sepsis syndrome, rhabdomyolysis, hemolysis, drugs

  Radiocontrast, aminoglycosides, cisplatin

Other tubulointerstitial disease

  Allergic interstitial nephritis

  Pyelonephritis (bilateral, or unilateral in single functional kidney)

  Heavy metal poisoning

Atheroembolic disease—after vascular procedures, thrombolysis, or anticoagulation

Glomerulonephritis

  1. ANCA-associated: granulomatosis with polyangiitis (Wegener's), idiopathic pauci-immune GN, PAN

  2. Anti-GBM disease; isolated or with pulmonary involvement (Goodpasture's syndrome)

  3. Immune complex–mediated

  Subacute bacterial endocarditis, SLE, cryoglobulinemia (with or without hepatitis C infection), postinfectious GN (classically poststreptococcal)

IgA nephropathy and Henoch-Schönlein purpura

Glomerular endotheliopathies

  Thrombotic microangiopathy, malignant hypertension, scleroderma, antiphospholipid syndrome, preeclampsia

(continued)

TABLE 148-1 COMMON CAUSES OF ACUTE KIDNEY INJURY (CONTINUED)

Postrenal (urinary tract obstruction)

Bladder neck obstruction, bladder calculi

Prostatic hypertrophy

Ureteral obstruction due to compression

    Pelvic or abdominal malignancy, retroperitoneal fibrosis

Nephrolithiasis

Papillary necrosis with obstruction

Abbreviations: ACE, angiotensin-converting enzyme; ANCA, antineutrophil cytoplasmic antibody; ARBs, angiotensin receptor blockers; GBM, glomerular basement membrane; GI, gastrointestinal; GN, glomerulonephritis; NSAIDs, nonsteroidal anti-inflammatory drugs; PAN, polyarteritis nodosa; SLE, systemic lupus erythematosus.

may lead to in-hospital ATN. Alternatively, pts may be admitted to the hospital with ATN associated with rhabdomyolysis; common predisposing factors include alcoholism, hypokalemia, and various drugs (e.g., statins). Allergic interstitial nephritis, usually due to antibiotics (e.g., penicillins, cephalosporins, sulfa drugs, quinolones, and rifampin), or NSAIDs, may also be responsible. Radiographic contrast dyes may cause AKI in pts with preexisting kidney disease; the risk is substantially higher in diabetics with chronic kidney disease. Coronary angiography, other vascular procedures, thrombolysis, or anticoagulation may lead to atheroemboli, which cause AKI due to both hemodynamic and inflammatory effects; livedo reticularis, embolic phenomena with preserved peripheral pulses, and eosinophilia are important clues to this diagnosis. Acute glomerulonephritis (Chap. 152) and thrombotic microangiopathies (Chap. 155) may also cause AKI. Thrombotic microangiopathies can be clinically subdivided into renal-limited forms [e.g., *Escherichia coli*–associated hemolytic uremic syndrome (HUS)] and systemic forms [e.g., thrombotic thrombocytopenic purpura (TTP)]. A variety of drugs can cause thrombotic microangiopathies, including calcineurin inhibitors (cyclosporine and tacrolimus), quinine, antiplatelet agents (e.g., ticlopidine), and chemotherapeutics (e.g., mitomycin C and gemcitabine). Important associated disorders in TTP include HIV infection, bone marrow transplantation, systemic lupus erythematosus (SLE), and antiphospholipid syndrome.

Postrenal failure is due to urinary tract obstruction, which is also more common among ambulatory rather than hospitalized pts. More common in men than women, it is most often caused by ureteral or urethral blockade. Occasionally, stones, sloughed renal papillae, or malignancy (primary or metastatic) may cause more proximal obstruction.

CHARACTERISTIC FINDINGS AND DIAGNOSTIC WORKUP

All pts with AKI manifest some degree of azotemia [increased blood urea nitrogen (BUN) and Cr]. Other clinical features depend on the etiology of renal disease. Pts with *prerenal azotemia* due to volume depletion usually demonstrate orthostatic hypotension, tachycardia, low jugular venous pressure, and dry mucous membranes. Pts with prerenal azotemia and CHF ("cardiorenal syndrome") may show jugular venous distention, an S_3 gallop, and peripheral and pulmonary edema. Therefore, the physical exam is critical in the workup of pts with prerenal AKI. In general, the BUN/Cr ratio tends to be high (>20:1), more so with volume depletion and CHF than with cirrhosis. The uric acid may also be disproportionately elevated in noncirrhotic prerenal states (due to increased proximal tubular absorption). Urine chemistries tend to show low urine [Na^+] (<10–20 mmol/L, <10 with hepatorenal syndrome) and a fractional excretion of sodium (FE_{Na}) of <1% (Table 148-2). The urinalysis (UA) typically shows hyaline and a few granular casts, without cells or cellular casts. Renal ultrasonography is usually normal.

Pts with *intrinsic renal disease* present with varying complaints. Glomerulonephritis (GN) is often accompanied by hypertension and mild to moderate edema (associated with Na retention and proteinuria, and sometimes with gross hematuria). An antecedent prodromal illness and/or prominent extrarenal symptoms and signs may occur if GN occurs in the context of a systemic illness, e.g., vasculitis or SLE; these may include hemoptysis or pulmonary hemorrhage (vasculitis and Goodpasture's syndrome), arthralgias/arthritis (vasculitis or SLE), serositis (SLE), and unexplained sinusitis (vasculitis). The urine chemistries may be indistinguishable from those in pts with prerenal failure; in fact, some pts with GN have renal hypoperfusion (due to glomerular inflammation and ischemia)

TABLE 148-2 URINE DIAGNOSTIC INDICES IN DIFFERENTIATION OF PRERENAL VERSUS INTRINSIC RENAL AZOTEMIA

	Typical Findings	
Diagnostic Index	Prerenal Azotemia	Intrinsic Renal Azotemia
Fractional excretion of sodium (%)[a] $U_{Na} \times P_{Cr}/P_{Na} \times U_{Cr} \times 100$	<1	>1
Urine sodium concentration (mmol/L)	<10	>20
Urine creatinine to plasma creatinine ratio	>40	>20
Urine urea nitrogen to plasma urea nitrogen ratio	>8	<3
Urine specific gravity	>1.018	<1.015
Urine osmolality (mosmol/kg H_2O)	>500	<300
Plasma BUN/creatinine ratio	>20	<10–15
Renal failure index $U_{Na}/U_{Cr}/P_{Cr}$	<1	>1
Urinary sediment	Hyaline casts	Muddy brown granular casts

[a]Most sensitive indices

Abbreviations: BUN, blood urea nitrogen; P_{Cr}, plasma creatinine concentration; P_{Na}, plasma sodium concentration; U_{Cr}, urine creatinine concentration; U_{Na}, urine sodium concentration.

with resultant hyperreninemia leading to acute volume expansion and hypertension. The urine sediment can be very helpful in these cases. Red blood cell (RBC), white blood cell (WBC), and cellular casts are characteristic of GN; RBC casts are rarely seen in other conditions (i.e., they are highly specific). In the setting of inflammatory nephritis (GN or interstitial nephritis, see below), there may be increased renal echogenicity on ultrasonography. Unlike pts with GN, pts with interstitial diseases are less likely to have hypertension or proteinuria; a notable exception is NSAID-associated acute interstitial nephritis, which can be accompanied by proteinuria due to an associated minimal-change glomerular lesion. Hematuria and pyuria may present on UA. The classic sediment finding in allergic interstitial nephritis is a predominance (>10%) of urinary eosinophils with Wright's or Hansel's stain; however, urinary eosinophils can be increased in several other causes of AKI. WBC casts may also be seen, particularly in cases of pyelonephritis.

The urinary sediment of pts with ischemic or toxic ATN will characteristically contain pigmented "muddy-brown" granular casts and casts containing tubular epithelial cells; free tubular epithelial cells can also be seen. The FE_{Na} is typically >1% in ATN, but may be <1% in pts with milder, nonoliguric ATN (e.g., from rhabdomyolysis) and in pts with underlying "prerenal" disorders, such as CHF or cirrhosis.

Pts with *postrenal* AKI due to urinary tract obstruction are usually less severely ill than pts with prerenal or intrinsic renal disease, and their presentation may be delayed until azotemia is markedly advanced [BUN >54 μmol/L (150 mg/dL), Cr >1060–1325 μmol/L (12–15 mg/dL)]. An associated impairment of urinary concentrating ability often "protects" the pt from complications of volume overload. Urinary electrolytes typically show a FE_{Na} >1%, and microscopic examination of the urinary sediment is usually bland. Ultrasonography is the key diagnostic tool. More than 90% of pts with postrenal AKI show obstruction of the urinary collection system on ultrasound (e.g., dilated ureter, calyces); false negatives include hyperacute obstruction and encasement of the ureter and/or kidney by tumor or of the ureter by retroperitoneal fibrosis, functionally obstructing urinary outflow without structural dilation.

TREATMENT Acute Renal Failure

Treatment should focus on providing etiology-specific supportive care. For example, pts with prerenal failure due to GI fluid loss may experience relatively rapid correction of AKI after the administration of IV fluid to expand volume. The same treatment in prerenal pts with CHF would be counterproductive; in this case, treatment of the underlying disease with vasodilators and/or inotropic agents would more likely be of benefit.

There are relatively few intrinsic renal causes of AKI for which there is safe and effective therapy. GN associated with vasculitis or SLE may respond to high-dose glucocorticoids and cytotoxic agents (e.g., cyclophosphamide); plasmapheresis and plasma exchange may be useful in other selected circumstances (e.g., Goodpasture's syndrome and HUS/TTP, respectively). Antibiotic therapy may be sufficient for the treatment of AKI associated with pyelonephritis or endocarditis. There are conflicting data regarding the utility of glucocorticoids in allergic interstitial nephritis. Many practitioners advocate their use with clinical evidence of progressive renal insufficiency despite discontinuation of the offending drug, or with biopsy evidence of potentially reversible, severe disease.

The treatment of urinary tract obstruction often involves consultation with a urologist. Interventions as simple as Foley catheter placement or as complicated as multiple ureteral stents and/or nephrostomy tubes may be required.

DIALYSIS FOR AKI AND RECOVERY OF RENAL FUNCTION Most cases of community- and hospital-acquired AKI resolve with conservative supportive measures, time, and patience. If nonprerenal AKI continues to progress, dialysis must be considered. The traditional indications for dialysis—volume overload refractory to diuretic agents; hyperkalemia; encephalopathy not otherwise explained; pericarditis, pleuritis, or other inflammatory serositis; and severe metabolic acidosis, compromising respiratory or circulatory function—can seriously compromise recovery from acute nonrenal illness. Therefore, dialysis should generally be provided in advance of these complications. The inability to provide requisite fluids for antibiotics, inotropes and other drugs, and/or nutrition should also be considered an indication for acute dialysis.

Dialytic options for AKI include (1) intermittent hemodialysis (IHD), (2) peritoneal dialysis (PD), and (3) continuous renal replacement therapy (CRRT, i.e., continuous arteriovenous or venovenous hemodiafiltration). Most pts are treated with IHD. It is unknown whether conventional thrice-weekly hemodialysis is sufficient or more frequent treatments are required. Few centers rely on PD for management of AKI (risks include infection associated with intraperitoneal catheter insertion and respiratory compromise due to abdominal distention). At some centers, CRRT is prescribed only in pts intolerant of IHD, usually because of hypotension; other centers use it as the modality of choice for pts in intensive care units. Hybrid hemodialysis techniques, such as slow low-efficiency dialysis (SLED), may be used in centers in which CRRT is not employed.

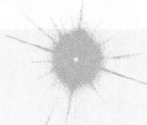

For a more detailed discussion, see Liu KD, Chertow GM: Dialysis in the Treatment of Acute Renal Failure, Chap. 281, p. 2322, in HPIM-18.

CHAPTER **149**
Chronic Kidney Disease and Uremia

EPIDEMIOLOGY

The prevalence of chronic kidney disease (CKD), generally defined as a long-standing, irreversible impairment of kidney function, is substantially greater than the number of pts with end-stage renal disease (ESRD), now ≥500,000 in the United States. There is a spectrum of disease related to decrements in renal function; clinical and therapeutic issues differ greatly depending on whether the glomerular filtration rate (GFR) reduction is moderate (stage 3 CKD, 30–59 mL/min per 1.73 m^2) (Table 52-1), severe (stage 4 CKD, 15–29 mL/min per 1.73 m^2), or "end-stage renal disease" (stage 5 CKD, <15 mL/min per 1.73 m^2). Dialysis is usually required once GFR <10 mL/min per 1.73 m^2. Common causes of CKD are outlined in Table 149-1.

DIFFERENTIAL DIAGNOSIS

The first step in the differential diagnosis of CKD is establishing its chronicity, i.e., disproving a major acute component. The two most common means of determining disease chronicity are the history and prior laboratory data (if available) and the renal ultrasound, which is used to measure kidney size. In general, kidneys that have shrunk (<10–11.5 cm, depending on body size) are more likely affected by chronic disease. While reasonably specific (few false positives), reduced kidney size is only a moderately sensitive marker for CKD, i.e., there are several relatively common conditions in which kidney disease may be chronic without any reduction in renal size. Diabetic nephropathy, HIV-associated nephropathy, and infiltrative diseases such as

TABLE 149-1 COMMON CAUSES OF CHRONIC RENAL FAILURE

Diabetic nephropathy
Hypertensive nephropathy[a]
Glomerulonephritis
Renovascular disease (ischemic nephropathy)
Polycystic kidney disease
Reflux nephropathy and other congenital renal diseases
Interstitial nephritis, including analgesic nephropathy
HIV-associated nephropathy
Transplant allograft failure ("chronic rejection")

[a]Often diagnosis of exclusion; very few pts undergo renal biopsy; may be occult renal disease with hypertension.

multiple myeloma may in fact be associated with relatively large kidneys despite chronicity. Renal biopsy, although rarely performed in pts with CKD, is a more reliable means of proving chronicity; a predominance of glomerulosclerosis or interstitial fibrosis argues strongly for chronic disease. Hyperphosphatemia, anemia, and other laboratory abnormalities are not reliable indicators in distinguishing acute from chronic disease.

Once chronicity has been established, clues from the physical exam, laboratory panel, and urine sediment evaluation can be used to determine etiology. A detailed history (Hx) will identify important comorbid conditions, such as diabetes, HIV seropositivity, or peripheral vascular disease. The family Hx is paramount in the workup of autosomal dominant polycystic kidney disease or hereditary nephritis (Alport's syndrome). An occupational Hx may reveal exposure to environmental toxins or culprit drugs (including over-the-counter agents, such as analgesics or Chinese herbs).

Physical exam may demonstrate abdominal masses (i.e., polycystic kidneys), diminished pulses or femoral/carotid bruits (i.e., atherosclerotic peripheral vascular disease), or abdominal or femoral bruits (i.e., renovascular disease). The Hx and exam may also yield important data regarding severity of disease. Excoriations (uremic pruritus), pallor (anemia), muscle wasting, and a nitrogenous fetor are all signs of advanced CKD, as are pericarditis, pleuritis, and asterixis, complications of particular concern that usually prompt the initiation of dialysis.

Laboratory Findings

Serum and urine laboratory findings typically provide additional information useful in determining the etiology and severity of CKD; serial studies determine the pace of progression and/or whether the renal failure is in fact acute. Heavy proteinuria (>3.5 g/d), hypoalbuminemia, hypercholesterolemia, and edema suggest nephrotic syndrome (Chap. 152). Diabetic nephropathy, membranous nephropathy, focal segmental glomerulosclerosis, minimal change disease, amyloid, and HIV-associated nephropathy are principal causes. Proteinuria may decrease slightly with decreasing GFR, but rarely to normal levels. Hyperkalemia and metabolic acidosis may complicate all forms of CKD eventually, but can be more prominent in pts with interstitial renal diseases. Serum and urine protein electrophoresis, in addition to serum free light chains, should be obtained in all pts >35 years of age with CKD to exclude paraproteinemia-associated renal disease. If underlying glomerulonephritis is suspected, autoimmune disorders such as lupus and infectious etiologies such as hepatitis B and C should be assessed. Serum concentrations of calcium, phosphate, vitamin D, and PTH should be measured to evaluate metabolic bone disease. Hemoglobin, vitamin B_{12}, folate, and iron studies should be measured to evaluate anemia.

THE UREMIC SYNDROME

The culprit toxin(s) responsible for the uremic syndrome remain elusive. The serum creatinine (Cr) is the most common laboratory surrogate of renal function. GFR can be estimated using serum Cr–based equations derived from the Modification of Diet in Renal Disease Study. This "eGFR" is now reported with serum Cr by most clinical laboratories in the

United States and is the basis for the National Kidney Foundation classification of chronic kidney disease (Table 52-1).

Uremic symptoms tend to develop with serum Cr >530–710 μmol/L (>6–8 mg/dL) or Cr_{Cl} <10 mL/min, although these values vary widely. Uremia is thus a clinical diagnosis made in pts with CKD. Symptoms of advanced uremia include anorexia, weight loss, dyspnea, fatigue, pruritus, sleep and taste disturbance, and confusion and other forms of encephalopathy. Key findings on physical exam include hypertension, jugular venous distention, pericardial and/or pleural friction rub, muscle wasting, asterixis, excoriations, and ecchymoses. Laboratory abnormalities may include hyperkalemia, hyperphosphatemia, metabolic acidosis, hypocalcemia, hyperuricemia, anemia, and hypoalbuminemia. Most of these abnormalities eventually resolve with initiation of dialysis or renal transplantation (Chaps. 150 and 151) or with appropriate drug therapies (see below).

TREATMENT Chronic Kidney Disease and Uremia

Hypertension complicates many forms of CKD and warrants aggressive treatment to reduce the risk of stroke and potentially to slow the progression of CKD (see below). Volume overload contributes to hypertension in many cases, and potent diuretic agents are frequently required. Anemia can be ameliorated with recombinant human erythropoietin (rHuEPO); current practice is to target a hemoglobin concentration of 100–110 g/L. Iron deficiency and/or other causes of anemia can reduce the response to rHuEPO and should be investigated if present. Iron supplementation is often required; many pts require parenteral iron therapy, since intestinal iron absorption is reduced in CKD.

Hyperphosphatemia can be controlled with judicious restriction of dietary phosphorus and the use of postprandial phosphate binders, either calcium-based salts (calcium carbonate or acetate) or nonabsorbed agents (e.g., sevelamer). Hyperkalemia should be controlled with dietary potassium restriction. Dialysis should be considered if the potassium is >6 mmol/L on repeated occasions. If these conditions cannot be conservatively controlled, dialysis should be instituted (Chap. 150). It is also advisable to begin dialysis if severe anorexia, weight loss, and/or hypoalbuminemia develop, as it has been definitively shown that outcomes for dialysis pts with malnutrition are particularly poor.

SLOWING PROGRESSION OF RENAL DISEASE Prospective clinical trials have explored the roles of blood pressure control and dietary protein restriction on the rate of progression of renal failure. Control of hypertension is of benefit, although angiotensin-converting enzyme (ACE) inhibitors and angiotensin receptor blockers (ARBs) may exert unique beneficial effects, most likely due to their effects on intrarenal hemodynamics. The effects of ACE inhibitors and ARBs are most pronounced in pts with diabetic nephropathy and in those without diabetes but with significant proteinuria (>1 g/d). Diuretics and other antihypertensive agents are often required, in addition to ACE inhibitors and ARBs, to optimize hypertension control and attenuate disease progression; diuretics may also help control serum $[K^+]$.

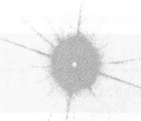

For a more detailed discussion, see Bargman JM, Skorecki K: Chronic Kidney Disease, Chap. 280, p. 2308, in HPIM-18.

CHAPTER **150**
Dialysis

OVERVIEW

The decision to initiate dialysis usually depends on a combination of the pt's symptoms, comorbid conditions, and laboratory parameters. Unless a living donor is identified, transplantation is deferred by necessity, due to the scarcity of cadaveric donor organs (median waiting time, 3–6 years at most transplant centers). Dialytic options include hemodialysis and peritoneal dialysis (PD). Roughly 85% of U.S. pts are started on hemodialysis.

Absolute indications for dialysis include severe volume overload refractory to diuretic agents, severe hyperkalemia and/or acidosis, encephalopathy not otherwise explained, and pericarditis or other serositis. Additional indications for dialysis include symptomatic uremia (Chap. 149) (e.g., intractable fatigue, anorexia, dysgeusia, nausea, vomiting, pruritus, difficulty maintaining attention and concentration) and protein-energy malnutrition/failure to thrive without other overt cause. No absolute serum creatinine, blood urea nitrogen, creatinine or urea clearance, or glomerular filtration rate (GFR) is used as an absolute cutoff for requiring dialysis, although most individuals experience, or will soon develop, symptoms and complications when the GFR is below ~10 mL/min. However, the "pre-emptive" initiation of dialysis in such pts, prior to the onset of clinical indications, does not improve outcomes in ESRD.

HEMODIALYSIS

This requires direct access to the circulation, either via a native arteriovenous fistula (the preferred method of vascular access), usually at the wrist (a "Brescia-Cimino" fistula); an arteriovenous graft, usually made of polytetrafluoroethylene; a large-bore intravenous catheter; or a subcutaneous device attached to intravascular catheters. Blood is pumped though hollow fibers of an artificial kidney (the "dialyzer") and bathed with a solution of favorable chemical composition (isotonic, free of urea and other nitrogenous compounds, and generally low in potassium). Dialysate [K^+] is varied from 0 to 4 mM, depending on predialysis [K^+] and the clinical setting. Dialysate [Ca^{2+}] is typically 2.5 mg/dL (1.25 mM), [HCO_3^-] typically 35 meq/L, and dialysate [Na^+] 140 mM; these can also be modified, depending on the clinical situation. Most pts undergo dialysis thrice weekly, usually for 3–4 h. The efficiency of dialysis is largely dependent on the duration of dialysis, blood flow rate, dialysate flow rate, and surface area of the dialyzer.

TABLE 150-1 COMPLICATIONS OF HEMODIALYSIS

Hypotension	Dialysis-related amyloidosis
Accelerated vascular disease	Protein-energy malnutrition
Rapid loss of residual renal function	Hemorrhage
Access thrombosis	Anaphylactoid reaction[a]
Access or catheter sepsis	

[a]Primarily with first use of "bioincompatible" modified cellulosic dialyzer membranes.

Complications of hemodialysis are outlined in Table 150-1. Many of these relate to the process of hemodialysis as an intense, intermittent therapy. In contrast to the native kidney or to PD, both major dialytic functions (i.e., clearance of solutes and fluid removal, or "ultrafiltration") are accomplished over relatively short time periods. The rapid flux of fluid can cause hypotension, even without a pt reaching "dry weight." Hemodialysis-related hypotension is common in diabetic pts whose neuropathy prevents the compensatory responses (vasoconstriction and tachycardia) to intravascular volume depletion. Occasionally, confusion or other central nervous system symptoms will occur. The dialysis "disequilibrium syndrome" refers to the development of headache, confusion, and rarely seizures, in association with rapid solute removal early in the pt's dialysis history, before adaptation to the procedure; this complication is largely avoided by an incremental induction of chronic dialytic therapy in uremic pts, starting with treatments of short duration, lower blood flows, and lower dialysate flow rates.

PERITONEAL DIALYSIS

PD does not require direct access to the circulation; rather, it obligates placement of a peritoneal catheter that allows infusion of a dialysate solution into the abdominal cavity; this allows transfer of solutes (i.e., urea, potassium, other uremic molecules) across the peritoneal membrane, which serves as the "artificial kidney." This solution is similar to that used for hemodialysis, except that it must be sterile, and it uses lactate, rather than bicarbonate, to provide base equivalents. PD is far less efficient at cleansing the bloodstream than hemodialysis and therefore requires a much longer duration of therapy. Pts generally have the choice of performing their own "exchanges" (2–3 L of dialysate, 4–5 times during daytime hours) or using an automated device at night. Compared with hemodialysis, PD offers the major advantages of (1) independence and flexibility, and (2) a more gentle hemodynamic profile.

Complications are outlined in Table 150-2. Peritonitis is the most important complication. The clinical presentation typically consists of abdominal pain and cloudy dialysate; peritoneal fluid leukocyte count is typically >100/μL, 50% neutrophils. In addition to the negative effects of the systemic inflammatory response, protein loss is magnified severalfold during the peritonitis episode. If severe or prolonged, an episode of peritonitis may prompt removal of the peritoneal catheter or even discontinuation of the modality (i.e., switch to hemodialysis). Gram-positive organisms (especially *Staphylococcus aureus* and other *Staphylococcus* spp.) predominate;

TABLE 150-2 COMPLICATIONS OF PERITONEAL DIALYSIS

Peritonitis	Dialysis-related amyloidosis
Hyperglycemia	Insufficient clearance due to vascular disease or other factors
Hypertriglyceridemia	Uremia secondary to loss of residual renal function
Obesity	
Hypoproteinemia	

Pseudomonas or fungal (usually *Candida*) infections tend to be more resistant to medical therapy and typically obligate catheter removal. Antibiotic administration may be intravenous or intraperitoneal when intensive therapy is required.

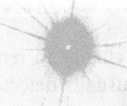

For a more detailed discussion, see Liu KD, Chertow GM: Dialysis in the Treatment of Renal Failure: Chap. 281, p. 2322, in HPIM-18.

CHAPTER **151**
Renal Transplantation

With the advent of more potent and well-tolerated immunosuppressive regimens and further improvements in short-term graft survival, renal transplantation remains the treatment of choice for most pts with end-stage renal disease. Results are best with living-related transplantation, in part because of optimized tissue matching and in part because waiting time can be minimized; ideally, these pts are transplanted prior to the onset of symptomatic uremia or indications for dialysis. Many centers now perform living-unrelated donor (e.g., spousal) transplants. Graft survival in these cases is far superior to that observed with cadaveric transplants, although less favorable than with living-related transplants. Factors that influence graft survival are outlined in Table 151-1. Pretransplant blood transfusion should be avoided, so as to reduce the likelihood of sensitization to incompatible HLA antigens; if transfusion is necessary, leukocyte-reduced irradiated blood is preferred. Contraindications to renal transplantation are outlined in Table 151-2. Overall, the current standard of care is that the pt should have >5 years of life expectancy to be eligible for a renal transplant, since the benefits of transplantation are only realized after a perioperative period in which the mortality rate is higher than in comparable pts on dialysis.

REJECTION

Immunologic rejection is the major hazard to the short-term success of renal transplantation. Rejection may be (1) hyperacute (immediate graft

TABLE 151-1 SOME FACTORS THAT INFLUENCE GRAFT SURVIVAL IN RENAL TRANSPLANTATION

HLA mismatch	↓
Presensitization (preformed antibodies)	↓
Very young or older donor age	↓
Female donor sex	↓
African-American donor race (compared with white)	↓
Older recipient age	↑
African-American recipient race (compared with white)	↓
Recipient diabetes as the cause of end-stage renal disease	↓
Prolonged cold ischemia time	↓
Hepatitis C infection	↓
Large recipient body size	↓

dysfunction due to presensitization) or (2) acute (sudden change in renal function occurring within weeks to months). Rejection is usually detected by a rise in serum creatinine but may also lead to hypertension, fever, reduced urine output, and occasionally graft tenderness. A percutaneous renal transplant biopsy confirms the diagnosis. Treatment usually consists

TABLE 151-2 CONTRAINDICATIONS TO RENAL TRANSPLANTATION

Absolute contraindications

Active glomerulonephritis

Active bacterial or other infection

Active or very recent malignancy

Overt AIDS[a]

Active hepatitis

Severe degrees of comorbidity (e.g., advanced atherosclerotic vascular disease)

Relative contraindications

Severe psychiatric disease

Moderately severe degrees of comorbidity

Hepatitis C infection with chronic hepatitis or cirrhosis

Noncompliance with dialysis or other medical therapy

Primary renal diseases

    Primary focal sclerosis with prior recurrence in transplant

    Multiple myeloma

    Amyloid

    Oxalosis

[a]Most centers consider overt AIDS a contraindication to transplantation; however, transplantation of HIV-positive pts is increasing in frequency.

of a "pulse" of methylprednisolone (500–1000 mg/d for 3 days). In refractory or particularly severe cases, 7–10 days of a monoclonal antibody directed at human T lymphocytes may be given.

IMMUNOSUPPRESSION

Maintenance immunosuppressive therapy usually consists of a three-drug regimen, with each drug targeted at a different stage in the immune response. The calcineurin inhibitors cyclosporine and tacrolimus are the cornerstones of immunosuppressive therapy. The most potent of orally available agents, calcineurin inhibitors have vastly improved short-term graft survival. Side effects of cyclosporine include hypertension, hyperkalemia, resting tremor, hirsutism, gingival hypertrophy, hyperlipidemia, hyperuricemia and gout, and a slowly progressive loss of renal function with characteristic histopathologic patterns (also seen in exposed recipients of heart and liver transplants). While the side effect profile of tacrolimus is generally similar to cyclosporine, there is a higher risk of hyperglycemia, a lower risk of hypertension, and occasional hair loss rather than hirsutism.

Prednisone is frequently used in conjunction with cyclosporine, at least for the first several months following successful graft function. Side effects of prednisone include hypertension, glucose intolerance, cushingoid features, osteoporosis, hyperlipidemia, acne, and depression and other mood disturbances.

Mycophenolate mofetil has proved more effective than azathioprine in combination therapy with calcineurin inhibitors and prednisone. The major side effects of mycophenolate mofetil are gastrointestinal (diarrhea is most common); leukopenia (and thrombocytopenia to a lesser extent) develops in a fraction of pts.

Sirolimus is a newer immunosuppressive agent often used in combination with other drugs, particularly when calcineurin inhibitors are reduced or eliminated. Side effects include hyperlipidemia and oral ulcers.

OTHER COMPLICATIONS

Infection and neoplasia are important complications of renal transplantation. Infection is common in the heavily immunosuppressed host (e.g., cadaveric transplant recipient with multiple episodes of rejection requiring steroid pulses or monoclonal antibody treatment). The culprit organism depends in part on characteristics of the donor and recipient and timing following transplantation (Table 151-3). In the first month, bacterial organisms predominate. After 1 month, there is a significant risk of systemic infection with cytomegalovirus (CMV), particularly in recipients without prior exposure whose donor was CMV positive. Prophylactic use of ganciclovir or valacyclovir can reduce the risk of CMV disease. Later on, there is a substantial risk of fungal and related infections, especially in pts who are unable to taper prednisone to <20–30 mg/d. Daily low-dose trimethoprim-sulfamethoxazole is effective at reducing the risk of *Pneumocystis carinii* infection.

The polyoma group of DNA viruses (BK, JC, SV40) can be activated by immunosuppression. Reactivation of BK is associated with a typical

TABLE 151-3 THE MOST COMMON OPPORTUNISTIC INFECTIONS IN RENAL TRANSPLANT RECIPIENTS

Peritransplant (<1 month)	Late (>6 months)
Wound infections	*Aspergillus*
Herpesvirus	*Nocardia*
Oral candidiasis	BK virus (polyoma)
Urinary tract infection	Herpes zoster
Early (1–6 months)	Hepatitis B
Pneumocystis carinii	Hepatitis C
Cytomegalovirus	
Legionella	
Listeria	
Hepatitis B	
Hepatitis C	

pattern of renal inflammation, BK nephropathy, which can lead to loss of the allograft; therapy typically involves reduction of immunosuppression to aid in clearance of the reactivated virus.

Epstein-Barr virus–associated lymphoproliferative disease is the most important neoplastic complication of renal transplantation, especially in pts who receive polyclonal (antilymphocyte globulin, used at some centers for induction of immunosuppression) or monoclonal antibody therapy. Non-Hodgkin's lymphoma and squamous cell carcinoma of the skin are also more common in this population.

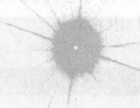

For a more detailed discussion, see Chandraker A, Milford EL, Sayegh MH: Transplantation in the Treatment of Renal Failure, Chap. 282, p. 2327, in HPIM-18.

CHAPTER **152**
Glomerular Diseases

ACUTE GLOMERULONEPHRITIS (GN)

Often called the "nephritic syndrome." Characterized by development, over days, of azotemia, hypertension, edema, hematuria, proteinuria, and sometimes oliguria. Salt and water retention are due to reduced glomerular filtration rate (GFR) and may result in circulatory congestion. Red blood cell (RBC) casts on urinalysis confirm diagnosis (Dx). Proteinuria is

TABLE 152-1 CAUSES OF ACUTE GLOMERULONEPHRITIS

I. Infectious diseases

   A. Poststreptococcal glomerulonephritis[a]

   B. Nonstreptococcal postinfectious glomerulonephritis

      1. Bacterial: infective endocarditis, "shunt nephritis," sepsis, pneumococcal pneumonia, typhoid fever, secondary syphilis, meningococcemia

      2. Viral: hepatitis B, infectious mononucleosis, mumps, measles, varicella, vaccinia, echovirus, and coxsackievirus

      3. Parasitic: malaria, toxoplasmosis

II. Multisystem diseases: SLE, vasculitis, Henoch-Schönlein purpura, Goodpasture's syndrome

III. Primary glomerular diseases: mesangiocapillary glomerulonephritis, Berger's disease (IgA nephropathy), "pure" mesangial proliferative glomerulonephritis

IV. Miscellaneous: Guillain-Barré syndrome, irradiation of Wilms' tumor, self-administered diphtheria-pertussis-tetanus vaccine, serum sickness

[a]Most common cause.

Abbreviation: SLE, systemic lupus erythematosus.

Source: RJ Glassock, BM Brenner: HPIM-13.

usually <3 g/d. Most forms of acute GN are mediated by humoral immune mechanisms. Clinical course depends on underlying lesion (Table 152-1).

Acute Poststreptococcal GN

This is the prototype and most common cause in childhood. Nephritis develops 1–3 weeks after pharyngeal or cutaneous infection with "nephritogenic" strains of group A β-hemolytic streptococci. Dx depends on a positive pharyngeal or skin culture (if available), positive titers for antistreptococcal antigens (ASO, anti-DNAse, or antihyaluronidase), and hypocomplementemia. Renal biopsy reveals diffuse proliferative GN. Treatment consists of correction of fluid and electrolyte imbalance. In most cases the disease is self-limited, although the prognosis is less favorable and urinary abnormalities are more likely to persist in adults.

Postinfectious GN

May follow other bacterial, viral, and parasitic infections. Examples are bacterial endocarditis, sepsis, hepatitis B, and pneumococcal pneumonia. Features are milder than with poststreptococcal GN. Control of primary infection usually produces resolution of GN.

RAPIDLY PROGRESSIVE GLOMERULONEPHRITIS

Defined as a subacute reduction in GFR of >50%, with evidence of a proliferative GN; causes overlap with those of acute GN (Table 152-2). Broadly classified into three major subtypes on the basis of renal biopsy

TABLE 152-2 CAUSES OF RAPIDLY PROGRESSIVE GLOMERULONEPHRITIS

I. Infectious diseases
  A. Poststreptococcal glomerulonephritis[a]
  B. Infective endocarditis
  C. Occult visceral sepsis
  D. Hepatitis B infection (with vasculitis and/or cryoglobulinemia)
  E. HIV infection
  F. Hepatitis C infection (with cryoglobulinemia, membranoproliferative glomerulonephritis)

II. Multisystem diseases
  A. Systemic lupus erythematosus
  B. Henoch-Schönlein purpura
  C. Systemic necrotizing vasculitis [including granulomatosis with polyangiitis (Wegener's)]
  D. Goodpasture's syndrome
  E. Essential mixed (IgG/IgM) cryoglobulinemia
  F. Malignancy
  G. Relapsing polychondritis
  H. Rheumatoid arthritis (with vasculitis)

III. Drugs
  A. Penicillamine
  B. Hydralazine
  C. Allopurinol (with vasculitis)
  D. Rifampin

IV. Idiopathic or primary glomerular disease
  A. Idiopathic crescentic glomerulonephritis
    1. Type I—with linear deposits of Ig (anti-GBM antibody–mediated)
    2. Type II—with granular deposits of Ig (immune complex–mediated)
    3. Type III—with few or no immune deposits of Ig ("pauci-immune")
    4. Antineutrophil cytoplasmic antibody–induced, forme fruste of vasculitis
    5. Immunotactoid glomerulonephritis
    6. Fibrillary glomerulonephritis
  B. Superimposed on another primary glomerular disease
    1. Mesangiocapillary (membranoproliferative) glomerulonephritis (especially type II)
    2. Membranous glomerulonephritis
    3. Berger's disease (IgA nephropathy)

[a]Most common cause.
Abbreviation: GBM, glomerular basement membrane.
Source: RJ Glassock, BM Brenner: HPIM-13.

findings and pathophysiology: (1) immune complex–associated, e.g., in systemic lupus erythematosus (SLE); (2) "pauci-immune," associated with antineutrophil cytoplasmic antibodies (ANCA); and (3) associated with anti–glomerular basement (anti-GBM) antibodies, e.g., in Goodpasture's syndrome. All three forms will typically have a proliferative, crescentic GN by light microscopy but differ in the results of the immunofluorescence and electron microscopy components of the renal biopsy.

SLE (Lupus)

Renal involvement is due to deposition of circulating immune complexes. Clinical features of SLE with or without renal involvement include arthralgias, "butterfly" skin rash, serositis, alopecia (hair loss), and central nervous system disease. Nephrotic syndrome with renal insufficiency is common. Renal biopsy reveals mesangial, focal, or diffuse GN and/or membranous nephropathy. Diffuse GN, the most common finding in renal biopsy series, is characterized by an active sediment, severe proteinuria, and progressive renal insufficiency and may have an ominous prognosis. Pts have a positive antinuclear antibody test, anti-dsDNA antibodies, and hypocomplementemia. Treatment includes glucocorticoids and cytotoxic agents. Oral or IV monthly cyclophosphamide is most commonly employed, typically for a period of 6 months; pts of childbearing age should first bank sperm and eggs. Mycophenolate mofetil is an alternative.

Antineutrophil Cytoplasmic Antibody (ANCA)–Associated, Pauci-Immune GN

May be renal-limited (idiopathic pauci-immune GN) or associated with systemic vasculitis [granulomatosis with polyangiitis (Wegener's) or microscopic polyarteritis nodosa]. Defining characteristic is the presence of circulating ANCA. These are detected by immunofluorescence of alcohol-fixed neutrophils; a "perinuclear" pattern (pANCA) is usually due to antibodies against myeloperoxidase (MPO), whereas a "cytoplasmic" pattern (cANCA) is almost always due to reactivity against proteinase-3 (PR3). Confirmatory enzyme-linked immunosorbent assay testing against the MPO and PR3 antigens is mandatory, since the pANCA pattern can be caused by antibodies against other neutrophil components, e.g., lactoferrin; these do not have the same consistent relationship to vasculitis and pauci-immune GN. The anti-MPO or anti-PR3 titer does not always correlate with disease activity.

Pts typically have a prodromal, "flulike" syndrome, which may encompass myalgias, fever, arthralgias, anorexia, and weight loss. There may be associated cutaneous, pulmonary, upper respiratory (sinusitis), or neurologic (mononeuritis monoplex) complications of associated systemic vasculitis. In particular, pulmonary necrotizing capillaritis can lead to hemoptysis and pulmonary hemorrhage.

Standard initial therapy for ANCA-associated rapidly progressive GN includes methylprednisolone and cyclophosphamide; more specific depletion of B cells by anti-CD20 antibody therapy with rituximab is an alternative. Some centers will also utilize plasmapheresis in the initial management of pts with a severe pulmonary-renal syndrome or to stave off dialysis in pts with severe renal impairment. Steroids are quickly tapered soon after the acute inflammation subsides; cyclophosphamide is continued until a stable remission is achieved, typically within 3–6 months. Pts must receive prophylaxis for *Pneumocystis carinii (jiroveci)* pneumonia (PCP) with trimethoprim-sulfamethoxazole, atovaquone, or dapsone. Some form of maintenance immunosuppression is standard, typically for 12–18 months after achievement of a stable remission; drugs include methotrexate, mycophenolate mofetil, and azathioprine.

Anti–Glomerular Basement Membrane Disease

Caused by antibodies against the α3 NCI (noncollagenous) domain of type IV collagen; circulating anti-GBM antibody and linear immunofluorescence on renal biopsy establish the Dx. Pts may have isolated GN; Goodpasture's syndrome encompasses GN and lung hemorrhage. Plasma exchange may produce remission; renal prognosis is worse in those who require dialytic support, with >50% crescents on renal biopsy, or creatinine >5–6 mg/dL. Severe lung hemorrhage is treated with IV glucocorticoids (e.g., 1 g/d × 3 days). Approximately 10–15% will also have ANCA against MPO, some with evidence of vasculitis, e.g., leukocytoclastic vasculitis in the skin.

Henoch-Schönlein Purpura

A generalized vasculitis causing IgA nephropathy, purpura, arthralgias, and abdominal pain; occurs mainly in children. Renal involvement is manifested by hematuria and proteinuria. Serum IgA is increased in half of pts. Renal biopsy is useful for prognosis. Treatment is symptomatic.

NEPHROTIC SYNDROME (NS)

Characterized by albuminuria (>3.5 g/d) and hypoalbuminemia (<30 g/L) and accompanied by edema, hyperlipidemia, and lipiduria. Protein excretion can be quantified by 24-h urine collection or by measurement of the urine protein:creatinine ratio or albumin:creatinine ratio on a random spot urine. The measurement of creatinine excretion helps define the adequacy of 24-h urine collections: daily creatinine excretion should be 20–25 mg/kg lean body weight in men and 15–20 mg/kg lean body weight in women. For random urine samples, the ratio of protein or albumin to creatinine in mg/dL approximates the 24-h urine protein excretion, since creatinine excretion is only slightly greater than 1000 mg/d per 1.73 m². A urine protein:creatinine ratio of 5 is thus consistent with 5 g/d per 1.73 m². Quantification of urine protein excretion on spot urines has largely supplanted formal 24-h urine collections, due to the greater ease and the need to verify a complete 24-h collection. The total protein:creatinine ratio does not detect microalbuminuria, a level of albumin excretion that is below the level of detection by tests for total protein; urine albumin:creatinine measurement is therefore preferred as a screening tool for lesser proteinuria.

In addition to edema, the complications of NS can include renal vein thrombosis and other thromboembolic events, infection, vitamin D deficiency, protein malnutrition, and drug toxicities due to decreased protein binding.

In adults, the most common cause of NS is diabetes. A minority of cases are secondary to SLE, amyloidosis, drugs, neoplasia, or other disorders

TABLE 152-3 CAUSES OF NEPHROTIC SYNDROME (NS)

Systemic Causes	Glomerular Disease
Diabetes mellitus, SLE, amyloidosis, HIV-associated nephropathy	Membranous
	Minimal change disease
Drugs: gold, penicillamine, probenecid, street heroin, NSAIDs, pamidronate, interferons	Focal glomerulosclerosis
Infections: bacterial endocarditis, hepatitis B, shunt infections, syphilis, malaria, hepatic schistosomiasis	Membranoproliferative GN
Malignancy: multiple myeloma, light chain deposition disease, Hodgkin's and other lymphomas, leukemia, carcinoma of breast and GI tract	Mesangioproliferative GN
	Immunotactoid and fibrillary GN

Abbreviations: GI, gastrointestinal; GN, glomerulonephritis; NSAIDs, nonsteroidal anti-inflammatory drugs; SLE, systemic lupus erythematosus.
Source: Modified from RJ Glassock, BM Brenner: HPIM-13.

(Table 152-3). By exclusion, the remainder are idiopathic. With the exception of diabetic nephropathy, a renal biopsy is required to make the diagnosis and determine therapy in NS.

Minimal Change Disease

Causes about 10–15% of idiopathic NS in adults, but 70–90% of NS in children. Blood pressure is normal; GFR is normal or slightly reduced; urinary sediment is benign or may show few RBCs. Protein selectivity is variable in adults. Recent upper respiratory infection, allergies, or immunizations are present in some cases; nonsteroidal anti-inflammatory drugs can cause minimal change disease with interstitial nephritis. Acute renal failure may rarely occur, particularly among elderly persons. Renal biopsy shows only foot process fusion on electron microscopy. Remission of proteinuria with glucocorticoids carries a good prognosis; cytotoxic therapy may be required for relapse. Progression to renal failure is uncommon. Focal sclerosis has been suspected in some cases refractory to steroid therapy.

Membranous GN

Characterized by subepithelial IgG deposits; accounts for ~30% of idiopathic adult NS. Pts present with edema and nephrotic proteinuria. Blood pressure, GFR, and urine sediment are usually normal at initial presentation. Hypertension, mild renal insufficiency, and abnormal urine sediment develop later. Renal vein thrombosis is relatively common, more so than with other forms of NS. Underlying diseases such as SLE, hepatitis B, and solid tumors and exposure to such drugs as high-dose captopril or penicillamine should be sought. The majority of pts with idiopathic membranous GN have detectable circulating autoantibodies to the M-type phospholipase

A$_2$ (PLA$_2$R), which is expressed in glomerular podocytes. Some pts progress to end-stage renal disease (ESRD); however, 20–33% may experience a spontaneous remission. Male gender, older age, hypertension, and persistence of significant proteinuria (>6 g/d) are associated with a higher risk of progressive disease. Optimal immunosuppressive therapy is controversial. Glucocorticoids alone are ineffective. Cytotoxic agents may promote complete or partial remission in some pts, as may cyclosporine. Anti-CD20 antibody therapy with rituximab has recently shown considerable promise, consistent with a role for B cells and anti-PLA$_2$R antibodies in the pathophysiology. Reduction of proteinuria with angiotensin-converting enzyme (ACE) inhibitors and/or angiotensin receptor blockers (ARBs) is also an important mainstay of therapy.

Focal Glomerulosclerosis (FGS)

Can be primary or secondary. Primary tends to be more acute, similar to minimal change disease in abruptness of NS, but with added features of hypertension, renal insufficiency, and hematuria. Involves fibrosis of portions of some (primarily juxtamedullary) glomeruli and is found in ~35% of pts with NS. There are several different pathologic subtypes of idiopathic FGS, with prognostic implications. In particular, the "collapsing glomerulopathy" variant has pathologic similarity to HIV-associated nephropathy (HIVAN); both nephropathies cause rapidly progressive disease.

African Americans are disproportionately affected by FGS, HIVAN, and other nondiabetic renal disease, with higher incidence, greater susceptibility (HIVAN), and a much higher risk of developing ESRD. "African-specific" variants in the *APOL1* gene, which encodes apolipoprotein L1 expressed in glomerular podocytes, have recently been implicated in this enhanced genetic risk.

Treatment of primary FGS typically begins with an extended course of steroids; fewer than half of pts undergo remission. Cyclosporine is an alternative therapy for maintenance of remission and for steroid-resistant pts. As in other glomerulopathies, reduction of proteinuria with ACE inhibitors and/or ARBs is also an important component of therapy. Finally, primary FGS may recur after renal transplant, when it may lead to loss of the allograft.

Secondary FGS can occur in the late stages of any form of kidney disease associated with nephron loss (e.g., remote GN, pyelonephritis, sickle cell disease, vesicoureteral reflux). Treatment includes anti-proteinuric therapy with ACE inhibition and blood pressure control. There is no benefit of glucocorticoids in secondary FGS. Clinical history, kidney size, biopsy findings, and associated conditions usually allow differentiation of primary versus secondary causes.

Membranoproliferative Glomerulonephritis (MPGN)

Mesangial expansion and proliferation extend into the capillary loop. Two ultrastructural variants exist. In MPGN I, subendothelial electron-dense deposits are present, C3 is deposited in a granular pattern indicative of immune-complex pathogenesis, and IgG and the early components of complement may or may not be present. In MPGN II, the lamina densa of the GBM is transformed into an electron-dense character, as is the basement membrane in Bowman's capsule and tubules. C3 is found irregularly in the GBM. Small amounts of Ig (usually IgM) are present, but early components of complement are absent. Serum complement levels are decreased. MPGN affects young adults. Blood pressure and GFR are abnormal, and the urine sediment is active. Some have acute nephritis or hematuria. Similar lesions occur in SLE and hemolytic-uremic syndrome. Infection with hepatitis C virus (HCV) has been linked to MPGN, often with associated cryoglobulinemia. Treatment with interferon α and ribavirin has resulted in remission of renal disease in some cases, depending on HCV serotype; however, renal insufficiency typically precludes ribavirin therapy. Glucocorticoids, cytotoxic agents, antiplatelet agents, and plasmapheresis have been used with limited success; rituximab is a newer therapy with greater evident efficacy. MPGN may recur in allografts.

Diabetic Nephropathy

The most common cause of NS. Although prior duration of diabetes mellitus (DM) is variable, in type 1 DM proteinuria may develop 10–15 years after onset of diabetes, progress to NS, and then lead to renal failure over 3–5 years. Retinopathy is nearly universal in type 1 diabetics with nephropathy, so much so that the absence of retinopathy should prompt consideration of another glomerular lesion (e.g., membranous nephropathy). In contrast, only ~60% of type 2 diabetics with diabetic nephropathy have retinopathy. Clinical features include proteinuria, progressive hypertension, and progressive renal insufficiency. Pathologic changes include mesangial sclerosis, diffuse, and/or nodular (Kimmelstiel-Wilson) glomerulosclerosis. However, pts rarely undergo renal biopsy; to the extent that yearly measurement of microalbuminuria is routine management for all diabetics, the natural history is an important component of the diagnosis. Pts typically demonstrate progression from microalbuminuria (30–300 mg/24 h) to dipstick-positive proteinuria (>300 mg albuminuria) and then progressively overt proteinuria and chronic kidney disease. However, proteinuria can be quite variable in diabetic nephropathy, with as much as 25 g/24 h in the absence of profound renal insufficiency or alternatively with progressive renal insufficiency and stable, modest proteinuria.

Treatment with ACE inhibitors delays the onset of nephropathy and of ESRD in type 1 diabetics with microalbuminuria and/or declining renal function and should be instituted in all pts tolerant to that class of drug. If a cough develops in a pt treated with an ACE inhibitor, an ARB is the next best choice. Type 2 diabetics with microalbuminuria or proteinuria can be treated with ACE inhibitors or ARBs. Although long-term studies are lacking, many authorities advocate combining inhibitors of the renin-angiotensin-aldosterone system (RAAS), i.e., ARBs, ACE inhibitors, mineralocorticoid receptor blockers, and/or renin inhibitors, in pts with persistent, significant proteinuria. Hyperkalemia, hypotension, and/or worsening GFR can limit single or combined therapy with RAAS inhibitors. If hyperkalemia develops and cannot be controlled with (1) optimizing glucose control, (2) loop diuretics (if otherwise appropriate), or (3) treatment

TABLE 152-4 EVALUATION OF NEPHROTIC SYNDROME

Random spot urine for protein and creatinine

Serum albumin, cholesterol, complement

Urine protein electrophoresis

Rule out SLE, diabetes mellitus

Review drug exposure

Renal biopsy

Consider malignancy (in elderly pt with membranous GN or minimal change disease)

Consider renal vein thrombosis (if membranous GN or symptoms of pulmonary embolism are present)

Abbreviations: GN, glomerulonephritis; SLE, systemic lupus erythematosus.

TABLE 152-5 GLOMERULAR CAUSES OF ASYMPTOMATIC URINARY ABNORMALITIES

I. Hematuria with or without proteinuria

  A. Primary glomerular diseases

    1. Berger's disease (IgA nephropathy)[a]

    2. Mesangiocapillary glomerulonephritis

    3. Other primary glomerular hematurias accompanied by "pure" mesangial proliferation, focal and segmental proliferative glomerulonephritis, or other lesions

    4. "Thin basement membrane" disease (? forme fruste of Alport's syndrome)

  B. Associated with multisystem or hereditary diseases

    1. Alport's syndrome and other "benign" familial hematurias

    2. Fabry's disease

    3. Sickle cell disease

  C. Associated with infections

    1. Resolving poststreptococcal glomerulonephritis

    2. Other postinfectious glomerulonephritides

II. Isolated nonnephrotic proteinuria

  A. Primary glomerular diseases

    1. "Orthostatic" proteinuria

    2. Focal and segmental glomerulosclerosis

    3. Membranous glomerulonephritis

  B. Associated with multisystem or heredofamilial diseases

    1. Diabetes mellitus

    2. Amyloidosis

    3. Nail-patella syndrome

[a]Most common.
Source: RJ Glassock, BM Brenner: HPIM-13.

TABLE 152-6 SEROLOGIC FINDINGS IN SELECTED MULTISYSTEM DISEASES CAUSING GLOMERULAR DISEASE

Disease	C3	Ig	FANA	Anti-dsDNA	Anti-GBM	Cryo-Ig	CIC	ANCA
SLE	↓	↑ IgG	+++	±	–	±	+++	±
Goodpasture's syndrome	–	–	–	–	+++	–	±	+ (10–15%)
Henoch-Schönlein purpura	–	↑ IgA	–	–	–	±	++	–
Polyarteritis	↓↑	IgG	+	±	–	+	+++	+++
Granulomatosis with polyangiitis (Wegener's)	↓↑	↑ IgA, IgE	–	–	–	±	++	+++
Cryoglobulinemia	↓	±	–	–	–	+++	+++	–
		↓↑ IgG						
		IgA, IgD						
Multiple myeloma	–	IgG	–	–	–	+	–	–
Waldenström's macroglobulinemia	–	↑ IgM	–	–	–	–	–	–
Amyloidosis	–	± Ig	–	–	–	–	–	–

Abbreviations: ANCA, antineutrophil cytoplasmic antibody; anti-dsDNA, antibody to double-stranded (native) DNA; anti-GBM, antibody to glomerular basement membrane antigens; CIC, circulating immune complexes; cryo-Ig, cryoimmunoglobulin; C3, complement component 3; FANA, fluorescent antinuclear antibody assay; Ig, immunoglobulin levels; SLE, systemic lupus erythematosus; –, normal; +, occasionally slightly abnormal; ++, often abnormal; +++, severely abnormal.

Source: RJ Glassock, BM Brenner: HPIM-13.

of metabolic acidosis (if present), then tight control of blood pressure with alternative agents is warranted.

Evaluation of NS is shown in Table 152-4.

ASYMPTOMATIC URINARY ABNORMALITIES

Proteinuria in the nonnephrotic range and/or hematuria unaccompanied by edema, reduced GFR, or hypertension can be due to multiple causes (Table 152-5).

Thin Basement Membrane Nephropathy

Also known as benign familial hematuria, may cause up to 25% of isolated, sustained hematuria without proteinuria. Diffuse thinning of the glomerular basement membrane on renal biopsy, with minimal other changes. May be hereditary, caused in some instances by defects in type IV collagen. Pts have persistent glomerular hematuria, with minimal proteinuria. The renal prognosis is controversial but appears to be relatively benign.

IgA Nephropathy

Another very common cause of recurrent hematuria of glomerular origin; is most frequent in young men. Episodes of macroscopic hematuria are present with flulike symptoms, without skin rash, abdominal pain, or arthritis. Renal biopsy shows diffuse mesangial deposition of IgA, often with lesser amounts of IgG, nearly always by C3 and properdin but not by C1q or C4. Prognosis is variable; 50% develop ESRD within 25 years; men with hypertension and heavy proteinuria are at highest risk. Glucocorticoids and other immunosuppressive agents have not proved successful, except in pts who present with rapidly progressive GN. A randomized clinical trial of fish oil supplementation suggested a modest therapeutic benefit. Rarely recurs in allografts.

Glomerulopathies Associated with Multisystem Disease (Table 152-6)

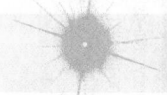

For a more detailed discussion, see Lewis JB, Neilson EG: Glomerular Diseases, Chap. 283, p. 2334, in HPIM-18.

CHAPTER **153**
Renal Tubular Disease

Tubulointerstitial diseases constitute a diverse group of acute and chronic, hereditary and acquired disorders involving the renal tubules and supporting structures (Table 153-1). Functionally, they may result in a wide variety of physiologic phenotypes, including nephrogenic diabetes insipidus (DI) with polyuria, non-anion-gap metabolic acidosis, salt wasting, and hypo- or hyperkalemia. Azotemia is common, owing to associated glomerular fibrosis and/or ischemia. Compared with glomerulopathies, proteinuria

TABLE 153-1 PRINCIPAL CAUSES OF TUBULOINTERSTITIAL DISEASE OF THE KIDNEY

Toxins

Exogenous toxins	Metabolic toxins
Analgesic nephropathy[a]	Acute uric acid nephropathy
Lead nephropathy	Gouty nephropathy[a]
Chinese herb nephropathy	Hypercalcemic nephropathy
Balkan endemic nephropathy	Hypokalemic nephropathy
Miscellaneous nephrotoxins (e.g., antibiotics, cyclosporine, radiographic contrast media, heavy metals)[a,b]	Miscellaneous metabolic toxins (e.g., hyperoxaluria, cystinosis, Fabry's disease)

Neoplasia

Lymphoma

Leukemia

Multiple myeloma (cast nephropathy, AL amyloidosis)

Immune disorders

Acute (allergic) interstitial nephritis[a,b]	Transplant rejection
Sjögren's syndrome	HIV-associated nephropathy
Amyloidosis	

Vascular disorders

Arteriolar nephrosclerosis[a]	Sickle cell nephropathy
Atheroembolic disease	Acute tubular necrosis[a,b]

Hereditary renal diseases

Disorders associated with renal failure	Hereditary tubular disorders
Autosomal dominant polycystic kidney disease	Bartter's syndrome (hereditary hypokalemic alkalosis)
Autosomal recessive polycystic kidney disease	Gitelman's syndrome (hereditary hypokalemic alkalosis)
Medullary cystic kidney disease	Pseudohypoaldosteronism type I (hypotension/salt wasting and hyperkalemia)
Hereditary nephritis (Alport's syndrome)	Pseudohypoaldosteronism type II (hereditary hypertension and hyperkalemia)
	Liddle's syndrome (hypertension and hypokalemia)
	Hereditary hypomagnesemia

(*continued*)

TABLE 153-1 PRINCIPAL CAUSES OF TUBULOINTERSTITIAL DISEASE OF THE KIDNEY (CONTINUED)

Hereditary renal diseases

Hereditary nephrogenic diabetes insipidus

X-linked (AVP receptor dysfunction)

Autosomal (aquaporin-2 dysfunction)

Infectious injury

Acute pyelonephritis[a,b]

Chronic pyelonephritis

Miscellaneous disorders

Chronic urinary tract obstruction[a]

Vesicoureteral reflux[a]

Radiation nephritis

[a]Common.
[b]Typically acute.

and hematuria are less dramatic, and hypertension is less common. The functional consequences of tubular dysfunction are outlined in Table 153-2.

ACUTE INTERSTITIAL NEPHRITIS (AIN)

Drugs are a leading cause of this type of renal failure, usually identified by a gradual rise in the serum creatinine at least several days after the institution of therapy, occasionally accompanied by fever, eosinophilia, rash, and arthralgias. The onset of renal dysfunction may be very rapid in pts who have previously been sensitized to the offending agent; this is particularly true for rifampin, for which intermittent or interrupted therapy appears to be associated with the development of AIN. In addition to azotemia, there may be evidence of tubular dysfunction (e.g., hyperkalemia, metabolic acidosis). Urinalysis may show hematuria, pyuria, white cell casts, and eosinophiluria on Hansel's or Wright's stain; notably, however, eosinophiluria is not specific for AIN, occurring in other causes of acute kidney injury (AKI), including atheroemboli.

Drugs that commonly cause AIN are listed in Table 153-3. Some drugs have a particular predilection for causing AIN, e.g., nafcillin; however, less frequent causes may be apparent only from case reports, such that a detailed history and literature review may be required to make the association with AIN. Many drugs, nonsteroidal anti-inflammatory drugs (NSAIDs) in particular, may elicit a glomerular lesion with similarity to minimal change disease, in addition to AIN; these pts typically have nephrotic-range proteinuria, versus the modest proteinuria typically associated with tubulointerstitial disease.

Renal dysfunction in drug-associated AIN usually improves after withdrawal of the offending drug, but complete recovery may be delayed and

TABLE 153-2 TRANSPORT DYSFUNCTION IN TUBULOINTERSTITIAL DISEASE

Defect	Cause(s)
Reduced GFR[a]	Obliteration of microvasculature and obstruction of tubules
Fanconi syndrome	Damage to proximal tubular reabsorption of solutes, primarily glucose, amino acids, and phosphate; may also exhibit hypouricemia, proximal tubular acidosis, low-molecular-weight proteinuria
Hyperchloremic acidosis[a]	1. Reduced ammonia production (CKD) or excretion (hyperkalemia) 2. Inability to acidify the collecting duct fluid (distal renal tubular acidosis) 3. Proximal bicarbonate wasting (proximal RTA)
Polyuria, isothenuria[a]	Damage to medullary tubules (thick ascending limb and/or collecting duct) and vasculature
Hypokalemic alkalosis	Damage or hereditary dysfunction of the thick ascending limb or distal convoluted tubule (Bartter's and Gitelman's syndromes)
Magnesium wasting	Damage or hereditary dysfunction of the thick ascending limb or distal convoluted tubules
Hyperkalemia[a]	Potassium secretory defects including aldosterone resistance
Salt wasting	Distal tubular damage with impaired sodium reabsorption

[a]Common.
Abbreviations: CKD, chronic kidney disease; GFR, glomerular filtration rate; RTA, renal tubular acidosis.

incomplete. In uncontrolled studies, glucocorticoids have been shown to promote earlier recovery of renal function and reduce fibrosis; this therapy is generally reserved to avoid or reduce the duration of dialytic therapy in pts who fail to respond to medication withdrawal.

AIN may also occur in the context of systemic infections, classically leptospirosis, *Legionella* infection, and streptococcal bacterial infection. Interstitial nephritis characterized by a dense infiltrate of IgG4-expressing plasma cells can occur as part of IgG4-related systemic disease; pancreatitis, retroperitoneal fibrosis, and a chronic sclerosing sialadenitis may variably be present. Finally, the tubulointerstitial nephritis and uveitis syndrome (TINU) is another increasingly recognized form of AIN. In addition to uveitis, which may precede or follow the AIN in pts with TINU, systemic symptoms and signs are common, e.g., weight loss, fever, malaise, arthralgias, and an elevated erythrocyte sedimentation rate. The renal disease is typically self-limited; those with progressive disease are often treated with prednisone.

TABLE 153-3 CAUSES OF ACUTE INTERSTITIAL NEPHRITIS

Drugs (70%, antibiotics in one-third)

  Antibiotics

    Methicillin, nafcillin, oxacillin

    Rifampin

    Penicillins, cephalosporins

    Ciprofloxacin

    Sulfamethoxazole and other sulfonamides

  Proton pump inhibitors, e.g., omeprazole

  H_2 blockers, e.g., cimetidine

  Allopurinol

  5-Aminosalicylates

  NSAIDs, including COX-2 inhibitors

Infections (16%)

  Leptospirosis, *Legionella*, streptococcal, tuberculosis

Tubulointerstitial nephritis and uveitis syndrome (TINU) (5%)

Idiopathic (8%)

Sarcoidosis (1%)

IgG4-related systemic disease

Abbreviations: COX-2, cyclooxygenase 2; NSAIDs, nonsteroidal anti-inflammatory drugs.

CHRONIC INTERSTITIAL NEPHRITIS (IN)

Analgesic nephropathy is an important cause of chronic kidney disease that results from the cumulative (in quantity and duration) effects of combination analgesic agents, usually phenacetin and aspirin. It is thought to be a more common cause of end-stage renal disease (ESRD) in Australia/New Zealand than elsewhere owing to the larger per capita ingestion of analgesic agents in that region of the world. Transitional cell carcinoma may develop. Analgesic nephropathy should be suspected in pts with a history of chronic headache or back pain with chronic kidney disease (CKD) that is otherwise unexplained. Manifestations include papillary necrosis, calculi, sterile pyuria, and azotemia.

A severe form of chronic tubulointerstitial fibrosis has been associated with the ingestion of Chinese herbal medicines, typically employed as part of a dieting regimen; Balkan endemic nephropathy (BEN), geographically restricted to pts from this region of southeastern Europe, shares many similarities with Chinese herbal nephropathy. These disorders are thought to be caused by exposure to aristolochic acid and/or other plant, endemic (in BEN), and medical toxins (the appetite suppressants fenfluramine and diethylpropion, in Chinese herbal nephropathy). Like analgesic nephropathies, these syndromes are both characterized by a high incidence of genitourinary malignancy.

Chronic therapy with lithium can also cause a chronic tubulointerstitial nephritis, often accompanied by nephrogenic DI that persists following discontinuation of the medication. If at all feasible, lithium-treated pts with evolving CKD should be transitioned to alternative medications for their psychiatric disease (e.g., valproic acid).

Metabolic causes of chronic IN include hypercalcemia (with nephrocalcinosis), oxalosis (primary or secondary, e.g., with intestinal disease and hyperabsorption of dietary oxalate), hypokalemia, and hyperuricemia or hyperuricosuria. The renal pathology associated with chronic hypokalemia includes a relatively specific proximal tubular vacuolization, interstitial nephritis, and renal cysts; both chronic and acute renal failure have been described. Chronic IN can occur in association with several systemic diseases, including sarcoidosis, Sjögren's syndrome, and following radiation or chemotherapy exposure (e.g., ifosfamide, cisplatin).

MONOCLONAL IMMUNOGLOBULINS AND RENAL DISEASE

Monoclonal immunoglobulins are associated with a wide variety of renal manifestations (Table 153-4), of which myeloma-associated cast nephropathy is the most common. The physiochemical characteristics of the monoclonal immunoglobulin light or heavy chains determine the clinical phenotype in individual pts, most commonly cast nephropathy, light chain deposition disease, and AL amyloidosis. In cast nephropathy, filtered light chains aggregate and cause tubular obstruction, tubular damage, and interstitial inflammation.

TABLE 153-4 RENAL DISEASES ASSOCIATED WITH MONOCLONAL IMMUNOGLOBULINS

Disease	Notes
Cast nephropathy	Most common cause of CKD in myeloma
	Tubular obstruction with light chains
	Interstitial inflammation
	Acute or chronic renal failure
Light chain deposition disease	Nephrotic syndrome, chronic renal failure, ~40% have associated myeloma
Heavy chain deposition disease	Nephrotic syndrome, chronic renal failure
AL amyloidosis	Nephrotic syndrome, cardiac/endocrine/ neuropathic involvement
	~10% have associated myeloma
	Renal tubular dysfunction (RTA, nephrogenic DI, etc.)
Hypercalcemia	With myeloma
Hyperviscosity syndrome	With Waldenström's macroglobulinemia
Fanconi syndrome	Glucosuria, aminoaciduria, phosphaturia, ± hypouricemia, proximal RTA, etc.

Abbreviations: CKD, chronic kidney disease; DI, diabetes insipidus; RTA, renal tubular acidosis.

Pts can present with CKD or with AKI; important predisposing factors in acute cast nephropathy include hypercalcemia and volume depletion.

Diagnosis of cast nephropathy relies on the detection of monoclonal light chains in serum and/or urine, typically by protein electrophoresis and immunofixation. Dipstick analysis of the urine for protein is classically negative in cast nephropathy, despite the excretion of up to several grams a day of light chain protein; light chains are not detected by this screening test, which tests only for albuminuria. In contrast, the glomerular deposition of light chains in light chain deposition disease or AL amyloidosis can result in nephrotic-range proteinuria (Table 153-4), with strongly *positive* urine dipstick for protein.

Management of cast nephropathy encompasses aggressive hydration, treatment of hypercalcemia if present, and chemotherapy for the associated multiple myeloma. Some experts advocate the use of plasmapheresis for pts with severe AKI, high levels of serum monoclonal light chains, and a renal biopsy demonstrating cast nephropathy.

Filtered light chains and multiple other low-molecular-weight proteins are also endocytosed and metabolized by the proximal tubule. Rarely, specific light chains generate crystalline depositions within proximal tubule cells, causing a Fanconi syndrome; again, this property appears to be caused by the specific physicochemical characteristics of the associated light chains. Fanconi syndrome or dysfunction of the distal nephron (hyperkalemic acidosis or nephrogenic DI) may also complicate renal amyloidosis.

POLYCYSTIC KIDNEY DISEASE

Autosomal dominant polycystic kidney disease (ADPKD) is the most common life-threatening monogenic genetic disorder, caused by autosomal dominant mutations in the *PKD1* and *PKD2* genes; it is a quantitatively important cause of ESRD. Autosomal recessive polycystic disease is a less much common cause of renal failure, typically presenting in infancy; hepatic involvement is much more prominent. The massive renal cysts in ADPKD can lead to progressive CKD, episodic flank pain, hematuria (often gross), hypertension, and/or urinary tract infection. The kidneys are often palpable and occasionally of very large size. Hepatic cysts and intracranial aneurysms may also be present; pts with ADPKD and a family history of ruptured intracranial aneurysms should undergo presymptomatic screening. Other common extrarenal features include diverticulosis and mitral valve prolapse.

The expression of ADPKD is highly variable, with the age of onset of ESRD ranging from childhood to old age. The renal phenotype is much milder in pts with mutations in *PKD1*, who on average develop ESRD approximately 15 years earlier than those with *PKD2* mutations. Indeed, some pts with ADPKD discover the disease incidentally in late adult life, having had mild to moderate hypertension earlier.

The diagnosis is usually made by ultrasonography. In a 15- to 29-year-old at-risk individual from a family with ADPKD, the presence of at least two renal cysts (unilateral or bilateral) is sufficient for diagnosis. Notably, however, renal cysts are a common ultrasound finding in older pts without ADPKD, particularly those with CKD. Therefore, in at-risk individuals 30–59 years of age, the presence of at least two cysts in each kidney is required for the diagnosis; this increases to four cysts in each kidney for those older than 60. Conversely, the absence of at least two cysts in each kidney excludes the diagnosis of ADPKD in at-risk individuals between the ages of 30 and 59.

Hypertension is common in ADPKD, often in the absence of an apparent reduction in glomerular filtration rate. Activation of the renin-angiotensin system appears to play a dominant role; angiotensin-converting enzyme inhibitors or angiotensin receptor blockers are the recommended antihypertensive agents, with a target blood pressure of 120/80 mmHg. Promising treatment modalities for halting progression of CKD in ADPKD include vasopressin antagonists, which dramatically reduce cyst enlargement and renal progression in animal models.

Urinary tract infections are also common in ADPKD. In particular, pts may develop cyst infections, often with negative urine cultures and an absence of pyuria. Pts with an infected cyst may have a discrete area of tenderness, as opposed to the more diffuse discomfort of pyelonephritis; however, clinical distinction between these two possibilities can be problematic. Many commonly used antibiotics, including penicillins and aminoglycosides, fail to penetrate cysts and are ineffective; therapy of kidney infections in ADPKD should use an antibiotic that is known to penetrate cysts (e.g., quinolones), guided initially by local antimicrobial susceptibility patterns.

RENAL TUBULAR ACIDOSIS (RTA)

This describes a number of pathophysiologically distinct entities of tubular function whose common feature is the presence of a non-anion-gap metabolic acidosis. Diarrhea, CKD, and RTA together constitute the vast majority of cases of non-anion-gap metabolic acidosis. Pts with earlier stages of CKD (Table 52-1) typically develop a non-anion-gap acidosis, with a superimposed increase in the anion gap at later stages (Chap. 2). Acidosis may develop at an earlier stage of CKD in those with prominent injury to the distal nephron, as for example in reflux nephropathy.

Distal Hypokalemic (Type I) RTA

Pts are unable to acidify the urine despite systemic acidosis; the urinary anion gap is positive, reflective of a decrease in ammonium excretion (Chap. 2). Distal hypokalemic RTA may be inherited (both autosomal dominant and autosomal recessive) or acquired due to autoimmune and inflammatory diseases (e.g., Sjögren's syndrome, sarcoidosis), urinary tract obstruction, or amphotericin B therapy. Chronic type I RTA is typically associated with hypercalciuria and osteomalacia, a consequence of the long-term buffering of acidosis by bone.

Proximal (Type II) RTA

There is a defect in bicarbonate reabsorption, usually associated with features of Fanconi syndrome, including glycosuria, aminoaciduria, phosphaturia, and uricosuria (indicating proximal tubular dysfunction). Isolated proximal RTA is caused by hereditary dysfunction of the basolateral sodium-bicarbonate cotransporter. Fanconi syndrome may be inherited or acquired due to myeloma, chronic IN (e.g., Chinese herbal nephropathy), or drugs (e.g., ifosfamide, tenofovir). Treatment requires large doses of bicarbonate (5–15 mmol/kg per day), which may aggravate hypokalemia.

Type IV RTA

This may be due to hyporeninemic hypoaldosteronism or to resistance of the distal nephron to aldosterone. Hyporeninemic hypoaldosteronism is typically associated with volume expansion and most commonly seen in elderly and/ or diabetic pts with CKD. The hyperkalemia associated with NSAIDs and cyclosporine is at least partially due to hyporeninemic hypoaldosteronism. Pts with hyporeninemic hypoaldosteronism are typically hyperkalemic; they may also exhibit a mild non-anion-gap acidosis, with urine pH <5.5 and a positive urinary anion gap. Acidosis often improves with reduction in serum [K$^+$]; hyperkalemia appears to interfere with medullary concentration of ammonium by the renal countercurrent mechanism. Should reduction in serum [K$^+$] not improve acidosis, pts should be treated with oral bicarbonate or citrate. Finally, various forms of distal tubular injury and tubulointerstitial disease, e.g., interstitial nephritis, are associated with distal insensitivity to aldosterone; urine pH is classically >5.5, again with a positive urinary anion gap.

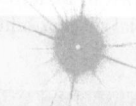

For a more detailed discussion, see Beck LH, Salant DJ: Tubulointerstitial Diseases of the Kidney, Chap. 285, p. 2367, in HPIM-18.

CHAPTER **154**
Urinary Tract Infections and Interstitial Cystitis

URINARY TRACT INFECTIONS

Definitions

The term *urinary tract infection* (UTI) encompasses a variety of clinical entities: *cystitis* (symptomatic disease of the bladder), *pyelonephritis* (symptomatic disease of the kidney), *prostatitis* (symptomatic disease of the prostate), and asymptomatic bacteriuria (ABU). *Uncomplicated UTI* refers to acute disease in nonpregnant outpatient women without anatomic abnormalities or instrumentation of the urinary tract; *complicated UTI* refers to all other types of UTI.

Epidemiology

UTI occurs far more commonly in females than in males, although obstruction from prostatic hypertrophy causes men >50 years old to have an incidence of UTI comparable to that among women of the same age.

- 50–80% of women have at least one UTI during their lifetime, and 20–30% of women have recurrent episodes.
- Risk factors for acute cystitis include recent use of a diaphragm with spermicide, frequent sexual intercourse, a history of UTI, diabetes mellitus, and incontinence; many of these factors also increase the risk of pyelonephritis.

Microbiology

In the United States, *Escherichia coli* accounts for 75–90% of cystitis isolates; *Staphylococcus saprophyticus* for 5–15%; and *Klebsiella* species, *Proteus* species, *Enterococcus* species, *Citrobacter* species, and other organisms for 5–10%.

- The spectrum of organisms causing uncomplicated pyelonephritis is similar, with *E. coli* predominating.
- Gram-positive bacteria (e.g., enterococci and *Staphylococcus aureus*) and yeasts are also important pathogens in complicated UTI.

Pathogenesis

In the majority of UTIs, bacteria establish infection by ascending from the urethra to the bladder. Continuing ascent up the ureter to the kidney is the pathway for most renal parenchymal infections.

- The pathogenesis of candiduria is distinct in that the hematogenous route is common.
- The presence of *Candida* in the urine of a noninstrumented immunocompetent pt implies either genital contamination or potentially widespread visceral dissemination.

Clinical Manifestations

When a UTI is suspected, the most important issue is to classify it as ABU; as uncomplicated cystitis, pyelonephritis, or prostatitis; or as complicated UTI.

- *Asymptomatic bacteriuria* is diagnosed when a screening urine culture performed for a reason unrelated to the genitourinary tract is incidentally found to contain bacteria, but the pt has no local or systemic symptoms referable to the urinary tract.
- *Cystitis* presents with dysuria, urinary frequency, and urgency; nocturia, hesitancy, suprapubic discomfort, and gross hematuria are often noted as well. Unilateral back or flank pain and fever are signs that the upper urinary tract is involved.
- *Pyelonephritis* presents with fever, lower-back or costovertebral-angle pain, nausea, and vomiting. Bacteremia develops in 20–30% of cases.
  - *Papillary necrosis* can occur in pts with obstruction, diabetes, sickle cell disease, or analgesic nephropathy.
  - *Emphysematous pyelonephritis* is particularly severe, is associated with the production of gas in renal and perinephric tissues, and occurs almost exclusively in diabetic pts.
  - *Xanthogranulomatous pyelonephritis* occurs when chronic urinary obstruction (often by staghorn calculi), together with chronic infection, leads to suppurative destruction of renal tissue.
- *Prostatitis* can be either infectious or noninfectious; noninfectious cases are far more common. Acute bacterial prostatitis presents with dysuria,

urinary frequency, fever, chills, symptoms of bladder outlet obstruction, and pain in the prostatic, pelvic, or perineal area.

- *Complicated UTI* presents as symptomatic disease in a man or woman with an anatomic predisposition to infection, with a foreign body in the urinary tract, or with factors predisposing to a delayed response to therapy.

Diagnosis

The clinical history itself has a high predictive value in diagnosing uncomplicated cystitis; in a pt presenting with both dysuria and urinary frequency in the absence of vaginal discharge, the likelihood of UTI is 96%.

- A urine dipstick test positive for nitrite or leukocyte esterase can confirm the diagnosis of uncomplicated cystitis in pts with a high pretest probability of disease.
- The detection of bacteria in a urine culture is the diagnostic gold standard for UTI. A colony count threshold of $>10^2$ bacteria/mL is more sensitive (95%) and specific (85%) than a threshold of 10^5/mL for the diagnosis of acute cystitis in women with symptoms of cystitis.

TREATMENT Urinary Tract Infections

- **Uncomplicated cystitis in women** See Table 154-1 for effective therapeutic regimens.
  - Trimethoprim-sulfamethoxazole (TMP-SMX) has been recommended as first-line treatment for acute cystitis, but should be avoided in regions with resistance rates >20%.
  - Nitrofurantoin is another first-line agent with low rates of resistance.
  - Fluoroquinolones should be used only when other antibiotics are not suitable because of increasing resistance or their role in prompting nosocomial outbreaks of *Clostridium difficile* infection.
  - Except for pivmecillinam, β-lactam agents are associated with lower rates of pathogen eradication and higher rates of relapse.
- **Pyelonephritis** Given high rates of TMP-SMX-resistant *E. coli*, fluoroquinolones (e.g., ciprofloxacin, 500 mg PO bid for 7 days) are first-line agents for the treatment of acute uncomplicated pyelonephritis. Oral TMP-SMX (one double-strength tablet bid for 14 days) is effective against susceptible uropathogens.
- **UTI in pregnant women** Nitrofurantoin, ampicillin, and the cephalosporins are considered relatively safe in early pregnancy.
- **UTI in men** In men with apparently uncomplicated UTI, a 7- to 14-day course of a fluoroquinolone or TMP-SMX is recommended.
  - If acute bacterial prostatitis is suspected, antibiotics should be initiated after urine and blood are obtained for cultures.
  - Therapy can be tailored to urine culture results and should be continued for 2–4 weeks; a 4- to 6-week course is often necessary for chronic bacterial prostatitis.
- **Asymptomatic bacteriuria** ABU should be treated only in pregnant women, in pts undergoing urologic surgery, and perhaps in neutropenic pts and renal transplant recipients; antibiotic choice is guided by culture results.

TABLE 154-1 TREATMENT STRATEGIES FOR ACUTE UNCOMPLICATED CYSTITIS

Drug and Dose	Estimated Clinical Efficacy (%)	Estimated Bacterial Efficacy (%)	Common Side Effects
Nitrofurantoin, 100 mg bid × 5–7 d	84–95	86–92	Nausea, headache
TMP-SMX, 1 DS tablet bid × 3 d	90–100	91–100	Rash, urticaria, nausea, vomiting, hematologic abnormalities
Fosfomycin, 3-g single-dose sachet	70–91	78–83	Diarrhea, nausea, headache
Pivmecillinam, 400 mg bid × 3–7 d	55–82	74–84	Nausea, vomiting, diarrhea
Fluoroquinolones, dose varies by agent; 3-d regimen	85–95	81–98	Nausea, vomiting, diarrhea, headache, drowsiness, insomnia
β-Lactams, dose varies by agent; 5- to 7-d regimen	79–98	74–98	Diarrhea, nausea, vomiting, rash, urticaria

Note: Efficacy rates are averages or ranges calculated from the data and studies included in the 2010 Infectious Diseases Society of America/European Society of Clinical Microbiology and Infectious Diseases guidelines for treatment of uncomplicated UTI.
Abbreviations: DS, double-strength; TMP-SMX, trimethoprim-sulfamethoxazole.

- **Catheter-associated UTI** Urine culture results are essential to guide therapy.
  - Replacing the catheter during treatment is generally necessary. Candiduria, a common complication of indwelling catheterization, resolves in ~1/3 of cases with catheter removal.
  - Treatment (fluconazole, 200–400 mg/d for 14 days) is recommended for pts who have symptomatic cystitis or pyelonephritis and for those who are at high risk for disseminated disease.

Prevention of Recurrent UTI

Women experiencing symptomatic UTIs ≥2 times a year are candidates for prophylaxis—either continuous or postcoital—or pt-initiated therapy. Continuous prophylaxis and postcoital prophylaxis usually entail low doses of TMP-SMX, a fluoroquinolone, or nitrofurantoin. Pt-initiated therapy involves supplying the pt with materials for urine culture and for self-medication with a course of antibiotics at the first symptoms of infection.

Prognosis

In the absence of anatomic abnormalities, recurrent infection in children and adults does not lead to chronic pyelonephritis or to renal failure.

INTERSTITIAL CYSTITIS

Interstitial cystitis (painful bladder syndrome) is a chronic condition characterized by pain perceived to be from the urinary bladder, urinary urgency and frequency, and nocturia.

Epidemiology

In the United States, 2–3% of women and 1–2% of men have interstitial cystitis. Among women, the average age at onset is the early forties, but the range is from childhood through the early sixties.

Etiology

The etiology remains unknown.

- Theoretical possibilities include chronic bladder infection, inflammatory factors such as mast cells, autoimmunity, increased permeability of the bladder mucosa, and abnormal pain sensitivity.
- However, few data support any of these factors as an inciting cause.

Clinical Manifestations

The cardinal symptoms of pain (often at ≥2 sites), urinary urgency and frequency, and nocturia occur in no consistent order. Symptoms can begin acutely or gradually.

- Unlike pelvic pain arising from other sources, pain caused by interstitial cystitis is exacerbated by bladder filling and relieved by bladder emptying.
- 85% of pts void >10 times per day; some do so as often as 60 times per day.
- Many pts with interstitial cystitis have comorbid functional somatic syndromes (e.g., fibromyalgia, chronic fatigue syndrome, irritable bowel syndrome, vulvodynia, migraine).

Diagnosis

The diagnosis is based on the presence of appropriate symptoms and the exclusion of diseases with a similar presentation (e.g., diseases that manifest with pelvic pain and/or urinary symptoms, functional somatic syndromes with urinary symptoms); physical exam and laboratory findings are insensitive and/or nonspecific. Cystoscopy may reveal an ulcer (10% of pts) or petechial hemorrhages after bladder distension, but neither of these findings is specific.

TREATMENT   Interstitial Cystitis

The goal of therapy is the relief of symptoms, which often requires a multifaceted approach (e.g., education, dietary changes, medications such as nonsteroidal anti-inflammatory drugs or amitriptyline, pelvic-floor physical therapy, and treatment of associated functional somatic syndromes).

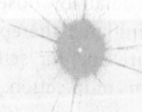

For a more detailed discussion, see Gupta K, Trautner BW: Urinary Tract Infections, Pyelonephritis, and Prostatitis, Chap. 288, p. 2387, in HPIM-18.

CHAPTER **155**
Renovascular Disease

Ischemic injury to the kidney depends on the rate, site, severity, and duration of vascular compromise. Manifestations range from painful infarction to acute kidney injury (AKI), impaired glomerular filtration rate (GFR), hematuria, or tubular dysfunction. Renal ischemia of any etiology may cause renin-mediated hypertension.

ACUTE OCCLUSION OF A RENAL ARTERY

Can be due to thrombosis or embolism (from valvular disease, endocarditis, mural thrombi, or atrial arrhythmias) or to intraoperative occlusion, e.g., during endovascular repair of abdominal aortic aneurysms.

Thrombosis of Renal Arteries

Large renal infarcts cause pain, vomiting, nausea, hypertension, fever, proteinuria, hematuria, and elevated lactate dehydrogenase (LDH) and aspartate aminotransferase. In unilateral lesion, renal functional loss depends on contralateral function. IV pyelogram or radionuclide scan shows unilateral hypofunction; ultrasound is typically normal until scarring develops. Renal arteriography establishes diagnosis. With occlusions of large arteries, surgery may be required; anticoagulation should be used for occlusions of small arteries. Pts should be evaluated for a thrombotic diathesis, e.g., antiphospholipid syndrome. Occlusion of one or both of the renal arteries can also rarely occur in pts treated with angiotensin-converting enzyme (ACE) inhibitors, typically in association with significant underlying renal artery stenosis.

Renal Atheroembolism

Usually arises when aortic or coronary angiography or surgery causes cholesterol embolization of small renal vessels in a pt with diffuse atherosclerosis. May also be spontaneous or associated with thrombolysis, or rarely may occur after the initiation of anticoagulation (e.g., with warfarin). Renal insufficiency may develop suddenly, a few days or weeks after a procedure or intervention, or gradually; the pace may alternatively be progressive or "stuttering," with punctuated drops in GFR. Associated findings can include retinal ischemia with cholesterol emboli visible on funduscopic examination, pancreatitis, neurologic deficits (especially confusion), livedo reticularis, peripheral embolic phenomena (e.g., gangrenous toes with palpable pedal pulses), abdominal pain from mesenteric emboli, and hypertension (sometimes malignant). Systemic symptoms may also occur, including fever, myalgias, headache, and weight loss. Peripheral eosinophilia, eosinophiluria, and hypocomplementemia may be observed, mimicking other forms of acute and subacute renal injury. Indeed, atheroembolic renal disease is the "great imitator" of clinical nephrology, presenting in rare instances with malignant hypertension, with nephrotic syndrome, or with what looks like rapidly progressive glomerulonephritis with an "active" urinary sediment; the diagnosis is made by history, clinical findings, and/or the renal biopsy.

Renal biopsy is usually successful in detecting the cholesterol emboli in the renal microvasculature, which are seen as needle-shaped clefts after solvent fixation of the biopsy specimen; these emboli are typically associated with an exuberant intravascular inflammatory response.

There is no specific therapy, and pts have a poor overall prognosis due to the associated burden of atherosclerotic vascular disease. However, there is often a partial improvement in renal function several months after the onset of renal impairment.

RENAL VEIN THROMBOSIS

This occurs in a variety of settings, including pregnancy, oral contraceptive use, trauma, nephrotic syndrome (especially membranous nephropathy; see Chap. 152), dehydration (in infants), extrinsic compression of the renal vein (lymph nodes, aortic aneurysm, tumor), and invasion of the renal vein by renal cell carcinoma. Definitive diagnosis is established by selective renal renography. Thrombolytic therapy may be effective. Oral anticoagulants (warfarin) are usually prescribed for longer-term therapy.

RENAL ARTERY STENOSIS AND ISCHEMIC NEPHROPATHY (SEE TABLE 155-1)

Main cause of renovascular hypertension. Due to (1) atherosclerosis (two-thirds of cases; usually men age >60 years, advanced retinopathy, history or findings of generalized atherosclerosis, e.g., femoral bruits) or (2) fibromuscular dysplasia (one-third of cases; usually white women age <45 years, brief history of hypertension). Renal hypoperfusion due to renal artery stenosis (RAS) activates the renin-angiotensin-aldosterone (RAA) axis. Suggestive clinical features include onset of hypertension <30 or >50 years of age, abdominal or femoral bruits, hypokalemic alkalosis, moderate to severe retinopathy, acute onset of hypertension or malignant hypertension, recurrent episodes of acute, otherwise unexplained pulmonary edema (typically with bilateral RAS or RAS in a solitary kidney), and hypertension resistant to medical therapy. Malignant hypertension (Chap. 126) may also be caused by renal vascular occlusion. Pts, particularly those with bilateral atherosclerotic disease, may develop chronic kidney disease (ischemic nephropathy). Although the incidence is difficult to assess, ischemic nephropathy is clearly a major cause of end-stage renal disease (ESRD) in those over 50.

Nitroprusside, labetalol, or calcium antagonists are generally effective in lowering blood pressure (bp) acutely; inhibitors of the RAA axis (e.g., ACE inhibitors, angiotensin II receptor blockers) are the most effective long-term treatment.

The "gold standard" in diagnosis of renal artery stenosis is conventional arteriography. Magnetic resonance angiography (MRA) has been used in many centers, given the risk of radiographic contrast nephropathy in pts with renal insufficiency; however, the newly appreciated risk of nephrogenic systemic fibrosis (NSF) in pts with renal insufficiency, attributed to gadolinium-containing MRI contrast agents, has dramatically restricted this practice in most institutions. Duplex ultrasonography is an alternative, but only if experienced operators are available. In pts with normal renal function and hypertension, the captopril (or enalaprilat) renogram may be

TABLE 155-1 CLINICAL FINDINGS ASSOCIATED WITH RENAL ARTERY STENOSIS

Hypertension

   Abrupt onset of hypertension before the age of 50 years (suggestive of fibromuscular dysplasia)

   Abrupt onset of hypertension at or after the age of 50 years (suggestive of atherosclerotic renal artery stenosis)

   Accelerated or malignant hypertension; can sometimes be associated with polydipsia and hyponatremia

   Refractory hypertension (not responsive to therapy with ≥3 drugs)

Renal abnormalities

   Unexplained azotemia (suggestive of atherosclerotic renal artery stenosis)

   Azotemia induced by treatment with an angiotensin-converting enzyme inhibitor

   Unilateral small kidney

   Unexplained hypokalemia

Other findings

   Abdominal bruit, flank bruit, or both

   Severe retinopathy

   Carotid, coronary, or peripheral vascular disease

   Unexplained congestive heart failure or acute pulmonary edema

Source: From RD Safian, SC Textor: New Engl J Med 344:431, 2001, reprinted with permission.

used as a screening test. Lateralization of renal function [accentuation of the difference between affected and unaffected (or "less affected") sides] is suggestive of significant vascular disease. Test results may be falsely negative in the presence of bilateral disease.

Medical therapy is advocated for most pts with renal artery stenosis, such that investigation of suspected RAS should be reserved for those in whom an intervention is anticipated. Medical management of atherosclerotic RAS should include lifestyle modification and management of dyslipidemia (Fig. 155-1). Intervention, i.e., revascularization, should be considered in the following scenarios: (1) progressive, otherwise-unexplained reduction in GFR during treatment of systemic hypertension; (2) poorly controlled hypertension despite multiple agents at maximally tolerated dosages; (3) rapid or recurrent decline in GFR in association with reduction in systemic pressure; and/or (4) recurrent episodes of acute, otherwise unexplained pulmonary edema. Notably, pts should always be re-evaluated frequently (every 3–6 months) for the progression of RAS and the development of an indication for revascularization (Fig. 155-1).

The choice of nonmedical management options depends on the type of lesion (atherosclerotic vs fibromuscular), the location of the lesion (ostial vs. nonostial), localized surgical and/or interventional expertise, and the presence of other localized comorbidities (i.e., aortic aneurysm or severe

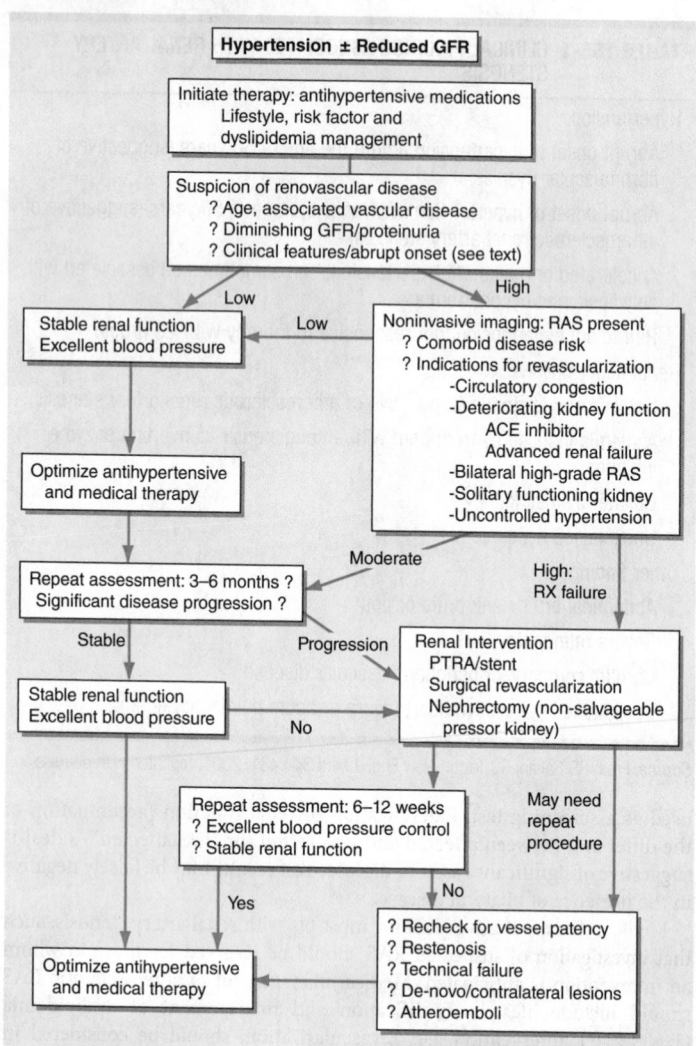

FIGURE 155-1 Management of pts with renal artery stenosis and/or ischemic nephropathy. ACE, angiotensin-converting enzyme; GFR, glomerular filtration rate; PTRA, percutaneous transluminal renal angioplasty; RAS, renal artery stenosis. *[From Textor SC: Renovascular hypertension and ischemic nephropathy, in Brenner BM (ed). The Kidney, 8th ed. Philadelphia, Saunders 2008; with permission.]*

aortoiliac disease). Thus fibromuscular lesions, typically located at a distance away from the renal artery ostium, are generally amenable to percutaneous angioplasty; ostial atherosclerotic lesions require stenting. Surgery is more commonly reserved for those who require aortic surgery, but it may be appropriate for those with severe bilateral disease. Again, periodic re-evaluation is needed to follow the response to intervention and, if necessary, investigate for restenosis (Fig. 155-1).

Pts who respond to vascularization will typically have a reduction in bp of 25–30 mmHg systolic, generally within the first 48 h or so after the procedure. For those with renal dysfunction, only ~25% are expected to demonstrate renal improvement, with deterioration in renal function in another 25% and stable function in ~50%. Small kidneys (<8 cm by ultrasound) are much less likely to respond favorably to revascularization.

SCLERODERMA

Scleroderma commonly affects the kidney; 52% of pts with widespread scleroderma have renal involvement. Scleroderma renal crisis can cause sudden oliguric renal failure and severe hypertension due to small-vessel occlusion in previously stable pts. Aggressive control of bp with ACE inhibitors and dialysis, if necessary, improve survival and may restore renal function.

ARTERIOLAR NEPHROSCLEROSIS

Persistent hypertension causes arteriosclerosis of the renal arterioles and loss of renal function (nephrosclerosis). "Benign" nephrosclerosis is associated with loss of cortical kidney mass and thickened afferent arterioles and mild to moderate impairment of renal function. Renal biopsy will also demonstrate glomerulosclerosis and interstitial nephritis; pts will typically exhibit moderate proteinuria, i.e., <1 g/d. Malignant nephrosclerosis is characterized by accelerated rise in bp and the clinical features of malignant hypertension, including renal failure (Chap. 126). Malignant nephrosclerosis may be seen in association with cocaine use, which also increases the risk of renal progression in pts with "benign" arteriolar nephrosclerosis.

Aggressive control of bp can usually but not always halt or reverse the deterioration of renal function, and some pts have a return of renal function to near normal. Risk factors for progressive renal injury include a history of severe, longstanding hypertension; however, African Americans are at particularly high risk of progressive renal injury (Chap. 152). The African American Study of Kidney Disease and Hypertension (AASK) established the superiority of ACE inhibitors over beta blockers or calcium channel blockers, with respect to progression of kidney disease.

THROMBOTIC MICROANGIOPATHIES

The thrombotic microangiopathies (TMAs) are classically subdivided into two general syndromes: thrombotic thrombocytopenic purpura (TTP) and hemolytic uremic syndrome (HUS). TMAs are thus broadly characterized by the presence of AKI, microangiopathic hemolytic anemia, thrombocytopenia, and neurologic dysfunction. Pts with TTP may suffer from the classic pentad of microangiopathic hemolytic anemia, fever, thrombocytopenia, neurologic symptoms and signs, and renal dysfunction. Extrarenal symptoms are in contrast less prominent or common, but not unheard of, in postdiarrheal HUS.

The major causes of TMA are listed in Table 155-2; the common pathogenic pathway is endothelial injury. In idiopathic and familial TTP, pts have

TABLE 155-2 CAUSES OF THROMBOTIC MICROANGIOPATHY

Genetic

    TTP: deficiency of ADAMTS13 (vWF protease)

    HUS: deficiency of complement regulatory proteins: factor H, complement factor I, complement factor B, complement factor H-related protein 1 (CHFR1, CHFR3, CHFR5, membrane cofactor protein

Idiopathic

    TTP: acquired antibodies to ADAMTS13 (vWF protease)

    HUS: acquired antibodies to complement factor H, typically in pts with genetic deficiency of this and other complement regulatory proteins

Infectious

    Bacterial: *Escherichia coli* O157:H7 and other strains, *Shigella*, *Salmonella*, *Campylobacter*, etc.

    Viral: HIV, CMV, EBV, etc.

Drug-related

    Calcineurin inhibitors: tacrolimus and cyclosporine

    Antiplatelet agents: ticlopidine, clopidogrel

    Quinine

    Chemotherapy: mitomycin C, gemcitabine, cisplatin

    OKT3 monoclonal antibody

    Angiogenesis/VEGF inhibitors: bevacizumab, sunitinib, sorafenib

Autoimmune

    Antiphospholipid antibody syndrome

    SLE, vasculitis

Miscellaneous

    Post–bone marrow transplantation

    Disseminated malignancy

    Pregnancy

Abbreviations: ADAMTS13, a disintegrin-like and metalloprotease with thrombospondin type I motif-13; CMV, cytomegalovirus; EBV, Epstein-Barr virus; HUS, hemolytic uremic syndrome; SLE, systemic lupus erythematosus; TTP, thrombotic thrombocytopenic purpura; VEGF, vascular endothelial growth factor; vWF, von Willebrand factor.

a marked deficiency in the ADAMTS13 protease, leading to accumulation of ultra-large, unprocessed von Willebrand factor (vWF) polymers, platelet aggregation, and TMA. In contrast, postdiarrheal HUS is associated with presence of a bacterial toxin (Shiga toxin or verotoxin) that causes endothelial injury; children and the elderly are particularly susceptible. Pts with atypical or nondiarrheal HUS may in turn have inherited or acquired deficiencies in membrane-associated regulatory proteins of the alternative complement pathway, enhancing endothelial sensitivity to complement.

Laboratory evaluation will usually reveal evidence of a microangiopathic hemolytic anemia, although this may be absent in certain causes, e.g., antiphospholipid antibody syndrome. The reticulocyte count should be elevated, along with an increase in the red cell distribution width. Hemolysis should increase levels of LDH and decrease circulating haptoglobin, with a negative Coombs' test. Examination of the peripheral smear is key, since the presence of schistocytes will help establish the diagnosis. Specific diagnostic tests—e.g., HIV testing, antiphospholipid antibody screens—may be useful in the differential diagnosis. Measurement of vWF protease activity promises considerable diagnostic and therapeutic utility; however, at this point, this is not routinely available in a time frame suitable for routine clinical use. Renal biopsy will classically demonstrate fibrin- and/or vWF-positive thrombi in arterioles and glomeruli, endothelial injury, and widening of the subendothelial space leading to a "double contour" appearance of the glomerular capillaries.

Treatment of TMA depends on the underlying pathogenesis. Idiopathic TTP is due to the presence of circulating antibody inhibitors of ADAMTS13 and thus responds to plasma exchange, combining plasmapheresis (removal of antibody) and infusion of fresh-frozen plasma (repletion with native ADAMTS13/vWF protease). Pts with atypical HUS due to deficiencies in complement regulatory proteins respond to therapy with eculizumab, a monoclonal antibody to C5 that prevents the production of the terminal complement components C5a and the membrane attack complex C5b-9.

TOXEMIAS OF PREGNANCY

Preeclampsia is characterized by hypertension, proteinuria, edema, consumptive coagulopathy, sodium retention, hyperuricemia, and hyperreflexia; eclampsia is the further development of seizures. Glomerular swelling and/or ischemia causes renal insufficiency. Coagulation abnormalities and AKI may occur. Treatment consists of bed rest, sedation, control of neurologic manifestations with magnesium sulfate, control of hypertension with vasodilators and other antihypertensive agents proven safe in pregnancy, and delivery of the infant.

VASCULITIS

Renal complications are frequent and severe in polyarteritis nodosa, hypersensitivity angiitis, granulomatosis with polyangiitis (Wegener's), and other forms of vasculitis (Chap. 170). Therapy is directed toward the underlying disease.

SICKLE CELL NEPHROPATHY

The hypertonic and relatively hypoxic renal medulla coupled with slow blood flow in the vasa recta favors sickling. Papillary necrosis, cortical infarcts, functional tubule abnormalities (nephrogenic diabetes insipidus), glomerulopathy, nephrotic syndrome, and, rarely, ESRD may be complications.

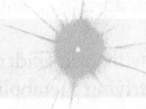

For a more detailed discussion, see Textor SC, Leung N: Vascular Injury to the Kidney, Chap. 286, p. 2375, in HPIM-18.

CHAPTER **156**
Nephrolithiasis

Renal calculi are common, affecting ~1% of the population, and recurrent in more than half of pts. Stone formation begins when urine becomes supersaturated with insoluble components due to (1) low urinary volume, (2) excessive or insufficient excretion of selected compounds, or (3) other factors (e.g., urinary pH) that diminish solubility. Approximately 75% of stones are Ca-based (the majority Ca oxalate; also Ca phosphate and other mixed stones), 15% struvite (magnesium-ammonium-phosphate), 5% uric acid, and 1% cystine, reflecting the metabolic disturbance(s) from which they arise.

SIGNS AND SYMPTOMS

Stones in the renal pelvis may be asymptomatic or cause hematuria alone; with passage, obstruction may occur at any site along the collecting system. Obstruction related to the passing of a stone leads to severe pain, often radiating to the groin, sometimes accompanied by intense visceral symptoms (i.e., nausea, vomiting, diaphoresis, light-headedness), hematuria, pyuria, urinary tract infection (UTI), and, rarely, hydronephrosis. In contrast, staghorn calculi, associated with recurrent UTI with urea-splitting organisms (*Proteus, Klebsiella, Providencia, Morganella,* and others), may be completely asymptomatic, presenting with loss of renal function.

STONE COMPOSITION

Most stones are composed of Ca oxalate. These may be associated with hypercalciuria and/or hyperoxaluria. Hypercalciuria can be seen in association with a very high-Na diet, loop diuretic therapy, distal (type I) renal tubular acidosis (RTA), sarcoidosis, Cushing's syndrome, aldosterone excess, or conditions associated with hypercalcemia (e.g., primary hyperparathyroidism, vitamin D excess, milk-alkali syndrome), or it may be idiopathic.

Hyperoxaluria may be seen with intestinal (especially ileal) malabsorption syndromes (e.g., inflammatory bowel disease, pancreatitis), due to reduced intestinal secretion of oxalate and/or the binding of intestinal Ca by fatty acids within the bowel lumen, with enhanced absorption of free oxalate and hyperoxaluria. Ca oxalate stones may also form due to (1) a deficiency of urinary citrate, an inhibitor of stone formation that is underexcreted with metabolic acidosis; and (2) hyperuricosuria (see below). Ca phosphate stones are much less common and tend to occur in the setting of an abnormally high urinary pH (7–8), usually in association with a complete or partial distal RTA.

Struvite stones form in the collecting system when infection with urea-splitting organisms is present. Struvite is the most common component of staghorn calculi and obstruction. Risk factors include previous UTI, nonstruvite stone disease, urinary catheters, neurogenic bladder (e.g., with diabetes or multiple sclerosis), and instrumentation.

Uric acid stones develop when the urine is saturated with uric acid in the presence of an acid urine pH; pts typically have underlying metabolic syndrome and insulin resistance, often with clinical gout, associated with a relative defect in ammoniagenesis and urine pH that is <5.4 and often <5.0. Pts with myeloproliferative disorders and other causes of secondary hyperuricemia and hyperuricosuria due to increased purine biosynthesis and/or urate production are at risk for stones if the urine volume diminishes. Hyperuricosuria without hyperuricemia may be seen in association with certain drugs (e.g., probenecid, high-dose salicylates).

Cystine stones are the result of a rare inherited defect in renal and intestinal transport of several dibasic amino acids; the overexcretion of cystine (cysteine disulfide), which is relatively insoluble, leads to nephrolithiasis. Stones begin in childhood and are a rare cause of staghorn calculi; they occasionally lead to end-stage renal disease. Cystine stones are more likely to form in acidic urinary pH.

WORKUP

Although some have advocated a complete workup after a first stone episode, others would defer that evaluation until there has been evidence of recurrence or if there is no obvious cause (e.g., low fluid intake during the summer months with obvious dehydration). Table 156-1 outlines a reasonable workup for an outpatient with an uncomplicated kidney stone. On occasion, a stone is recovered and can be analyzed for content, yielding important clues to pathogenesis and management. For example, a predominance of Ca phosphate suggests underlying distal RTA or hyperparathyroidism.

TREATMENT   Nephrolithiasis

Treatment of renal calculi is often empirical, based on odds (Ca oxalate stones most common), clinical history, and/or the metabolic workup. An increase in fluid intake to at least 2.5–3 L/d is perhaps the single most effective intervention, regardless of the type of stone. Conservative recommendations for pts with Ca oxalate stones (i.e., low-salt, low-fat,

---

TABLE 156-1 WORKUP FOR AN OUTPATIENT WITH A RENAL STONE

1. Dietary and fluid intake history
2. Careful medical history and physical examination, focusing on systemic diseases
3. Noncontrast helical CT, with 5-mm CT cuts
4. Routine UA; presence of crystals, hematuria, measurement of urine pH
5. Serum chemistries: BUN, Cr, uric acid, calcium, phosphate, chloride, bicarbonate, PTH
6. Timed urine collections (at least 1 day during week, 1 day on weekend): Cr, Na, K, urea nitrogen, uric acid, calcium, phosphate, oxalate, citrate, pH

Abbreviations: BUN, blood urea nitrogen; Cr, creatinine; PTH, parathyroid hormone; UA, urinalysis.

TABLE 156-2 SPECIFIC THERAPIES FOR NEPHROLITHIASIS

Stone Type	Dietary Modifications	Other
Calcium oxalate	Increase fluid intake	Citrate supplementation (calcium or potassium salts > sodium)
	Moderate sodium intake	
	Moderate oxalate intake	Cholestyramine or other therapy for fat malabsorption
	Moderate protein intake	
	Moderate fat intake	Thiazides if hypercalciuric
		Allopurinol if hyperuricosuric
Calcium phosphate	Increase fluid intake	Thiazides if hypercalciuric
	Moderate sodium intake	Treat hyperparathyroidism if present
		Alkali for distal renal tubular acidosis
Struvite	Increase fluid intake; same as calcium oxalate if evidence of calcium oxalate nidus for struvite	Methenamine and vitamin C or daily suppressive antibiotic therapy (e.g., trimethoprim-sulfamethoxazole)
Uric acid	Increase fluid intake	Allopurinol
	Moderate dietary protein intake	Alkali therapy (K^+ citrate) to raise urine pH to 6.0–6.5
Cystine	Increase fluid intake	Alkali therapy
		Penicillamine

Note: Sodium excretion correlates with calcium excretion.

moderate-protein diet) are thought to be healthful in general and therefore advisable in pts whose condition is otherwise uncomplicated. In contrast to prior assumptions, dietary calcium intake does not contribute to stone risk; rather, dietary calcium may help to reduce oxalate absorption and reduce stone risk. Table 156-2 outlines stone-specific therapies for pts with complex or recurrent nephrolithiasis.

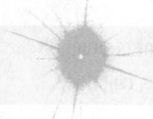

For a more detailed discussion, see Asplin JR, Coe FL, Favus MJ: Nephrolithiasis, Chap. 287, p. 2382, in HPIM-18.

CHAPTER **157**
Urinary Tract Obstruction

Urinary tract obstruction (UTO), a potentially reversible cause of renal failure (RF), should be considered in all cases of acute or abrupt worsening of chronic RF. Consequences depend on duration and severity and whether the obstruction is unilateral or bilateral. UTO may occur at any level from collecting tubule to urethra. It is preponderant in women (pelvic tumors), elderly men (prostatic disease), diabetic pts (papillary necrosis), pts with neurologic diseases (spinal cord injury or multiple sclerosis, with neurogenic bladder), and individuals with retroperitoneal lymphadenopathy or fibrosis, vesicoureteral reflux, nephrolithiasis, or other causes of functional urinary retention (e.g., anticholinergic drugs).

CLINICAL MANIFESTATIONS

Pain can occur in some settings (obstruction due to stones) but is not common. In men, there is frequently a history of prostatism. Physical exam may reveal an enlarged bladder by percussion over the lower abdominal wall; bedside ultrasound assessment ("bladder scan") can be helpful to assess the post-void bladder volume. Other findings depend on the clinical scenario. Prostatic hypertrophy can be determined by digital rectal examination. A bimanual examination in women may show a pelvic or rectal mass. The workup of pts with RF suspected of having UTO is shown in Fig. 157-1. Laboratory studies may show marked elevations of blood urea nitrogen and creatinine; if the obstruction has been of sufficient duration, there may be evidence of tubulointerstitial disease (e.g., hyperkalemia, non-anion-gap metabolic acidosis, mild hypernatremia). Urinalysis is most often benign or with a small number of cells; heavy proteinuria is rare. An obstructing stone may be visualized on abdominal radiography or helical noncontrast CT with 5-mm cuts.

Ultrasonography can be used to assess the degree of hydronephrosis and the integrity of the renal parenchyma; CT or IV urography may be required to localize the level of obstruction. Calyceal dilation is commonly seen; it may be absent with hyperacute obstruction, upper tract encasement by tumor or retroperitoneal fibrosis, or indwelling staghorn calculi. Imaging in retroperitoneal fibrosis with associated periaortitis classically reveals a periaortic, confluent mass encasing the anterior and lateral sides of the aorta. Kidney size may indicate the duration of obstruction. It should be noted that unilateral obstruction may be prolonged and severe (ultimately leading to loss of renal function in the obstructed kidney), with no hint of abnormality on physical exam and laboratory survey.

TREATMENT	Urinary Tract Obstruction

Management of acute RF associated with UTO is dictated by (1) the level of obstruction (upper vs. lower tract), and (2) the acuity of the obstruction and its clinical consequences, including renal dysfunction and

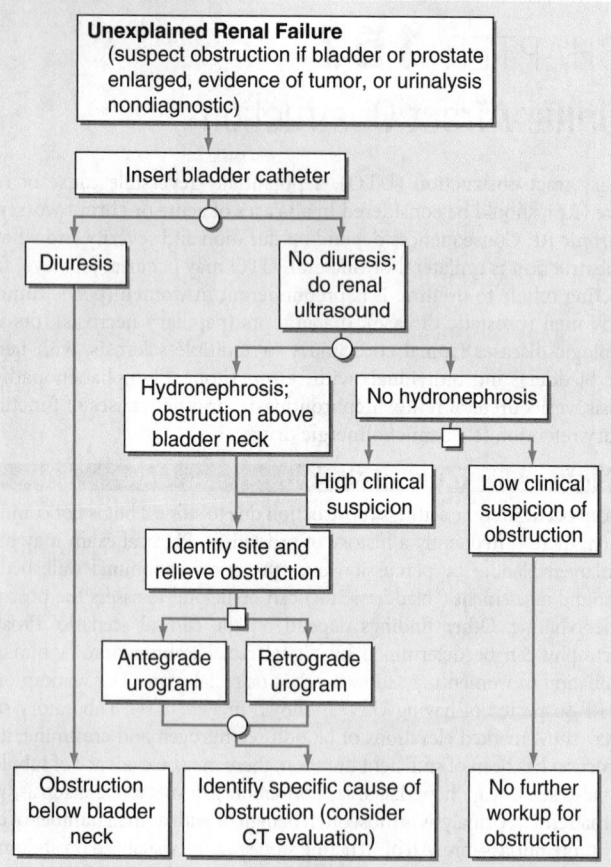

FIGURE 157-1 Diagnostic approach for urinary tract obstruction in unexplained renal failure. Circles represent diagnostic procedures and squares indicate clinical decisions based on available data.

infection. Benign causes of UTO, including bladder outlet obstruction and nephrolithiasis, should be ruled out because conservative management, including Foley catheter placement and IV fluids, respectively, will usually relieve the obstruction in most cases.

Among more seriously ill pts, ureteral obstruction due to tumor is the most common and concerning cause of UTO. If technically feasible, ureteral obstruction due to tumor is best managed by cystoscopic placement of a ureteral stent. Otherwise, the placement of nephrostomy tubes with external drainage may be required. IV antibiotics should also be given if there are signs of pyelonephritis or urosepsis. In addition to ureteral stenting, pts with idiopathic retroperitoneal fibrosis are typically treated with immunosuppression (prednisone, mycophenolate mofetil, and/or tamoxifen).

Fluid and electrolyte status should be carefully monitored after obstruction is relieved. There may be a physiologic natriuresis/diuresis related to volume overload. However, there may be an "inappropriate" natriuresis/diuresis related to (1) elevated urea nitrogen, leading to an osmotic diuresis; and (2) acquired nephrogenic diabetes insipidus. Hypernatremia, sometimes of a severe degree, may develop.

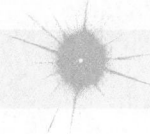

For a more detailed discussion, see Seifter JL: Urinary Tract Obstruction, Chap. 289, p. 2396, in HPIM-18.

CHAPTER **158**
Peptic Ulcer and Related Disorders

PEPTIC ULCER DISEASE (PUD)

PUD occurs most commonly in duodenal bulb (duodenal ulcer, DU) and stomach (gastric ulcer, GU). It may also occur in esophagus, pyloric channel, duodenal loop, jejunum, Meckel's diverticulum. PUD results when "aggressive" factors (gastric acid, pepsin) overwhelm "defensive" factors involved in mucosal resistance (gastric mucus, bicarbonate, microcirculation, prostaglandins, mucosal "barrier"), and from effects of *Helicobacter pylori*.

■ CAUSES AND RISK FACTORS

General

H. pylori is a spiral urease-producing organism that colonizes gastric antral mucosa in up to 100% of persons with DU and 80% with GU. It is also found in normals (increasing prevalence with age) and in those of low socioeconomic status. *H. pylori* is invariably associated with histologic evidence of active chronic gastritis, which over years can lead to atrophic gastritis and gastric cancer. The other major cause of ulcers (those not due to *H. pylori*) is nonsteroidal anti-inflammatory drugs (NSAIDs). Fewer than 1% are due to gastrinoma (Zollinger-Ellison syndrome). Other risk factors and associations: hereditary (? increased parietal cell number), smoking, hypercalcemia, mastocytosis, blood group O (antigens may bind *H. pylori*). Unproven: stress, coffee, alcohol.

Duodenal Ulcer

Mild gastric acid hypersecretion resulting from (1) increased release of gastrin, presumably due to (a) stimulation of antral G cells by cytokines released by inflammatory cells and (b) diminished production of somatostatin by D cells, both resulting from *H. pylori* infection; and (2) an exaggerated acid response to gastrin due to an increased parietal cell mass resulting from gastrin stimulation. These abnormalities reverse rapidly with eradication of *H. pylori*. However, a mildly elevated maximum gastric acid output in response to exogenous gastrin persists in some pts long after eradication of *H. pylori*, suggesting that gastric acid hypersecretion may be, in part, genetically determined. *H. pylori* may also result in elevated serum pepsinogen levels. Mucosal defense in duodenum is compromised by toxic effects of *H. pylori* infection on patches of gastric metaplasia that result from gastric acid hypersecretion or rapid gastric emptying. Other risk factors include glucocorticoids, NSAIDs, chronic renal failure, renal transplantation, cirrhosis, chronic lung disease.

Gastric Ulcer

H. pylori is also principal cause. Gastric acid secretory rates are usually normal or reduced, possibly reflecting earlier age of infection by *H. pylori* than in DU pts. Gastritis due to reflux of duodenal contents (including bile) may play a role. Chronic salicylate or NSAID use may account for 15–30% of GUs and increase risk of associated bleeding, perforation.

■ CLINICAL FEATURES

Duodenal Ulcer

Burning epigastric pain 90 min to 3 h after meals, often nocturnal, relieved by food.

Gastric Ulcer

Burning epigastric pain made worse by or unrelated to food; anorexia, food aversion, weight loss (in 40%). Great individual variation. Similar symptoms may occur in persons without demonstrated peptic ulcers ("nonulcer dyspepsia"); less responsive to standard therapy.

■ COMPLICATIONS

Bleeding, obstruction, penetration causing acute pancreatitis, perforation, intractability.

■ DIAGNOSIS

Duodenal Ulcer

Upper endoscopy or upper GI barium radiography.

Gastric Ulcer

Upper endoscopy preferable to exclude possibility that ulcer is malignant (brush cytology, ≥6 pinch biopsies of ulcer margin). Radiographic features suggesting malignancy: ulcer within a mass, folds that do not radiate from ulcer margin, a large ulcer (>2.5–3 cm).

■ DETECTION OF *H. PYLORI*

Detection of antibodies in serum (inexpensive, preferred when endoscopy is not required); rapid urease test of antral biopsy (when endoscopy is required). Urea breath test generally used to confirm eradication of *H. pylori*, if necessary. The fecal antigen test is sensitive, specific, and inexpensive (Table 158-1).

TREATMENT ▶ Peptic Ulcer Disease

MEDICAL Objectives: pain relief, healing, prevention of complications, prevention of recurrences. For GU, exclude malignancy (follow endoscopically to healing). Dietary restriction unnecessary with contemporary drugs; discontinue NSAIDs; smoking may prevent healing and should be stopped. Eradication of *H. pylori* markedly reduces rate of ulcer relapse and is indicated for all DUs and GUs associated with *H. pylori* (Table 158-2). Acid suppression is generally included in regimen. Reinfection rates are <1%/year. Standard drugs (H$_2$ receptor blockers,

TABLE 158-1 TESTS FOR DETECTION OF *H. PYLORI*

Test	Sensitivity/Specificity, %	Comments
Invasive (endoscopy/biopsy required)		
Rapid urease	80–95/95–100	Simple, false negative with recent use of PPIs, antibiotics, or bismuth compounds
Histology	80–90/>95	Requires pathology processing and staining; provides histologic information
Culture	—/—	Time-consuming, expensive, dependent on experience; allows determination of antibiotic susceptibility
Noninvasive		
Serology	>80/>90	Inexpensive, convenient; not useful for early follow-up
Urea breath test	>90/>90	Simple, rapid; useful for early follow-up; false negatives with recent therapy (see rapid urease test); exposure to low-dose radiation with ^{14}C test
Stool antigen	>90/>90	Inexpensive, convenient; not established for eradication but promising

Abbreviation: PPIs, proton pump inhibitors.

sucralfate, antacids) heal 80–90% of DUs and 60% of GUs in 6 weeks; healing is more rapid with omeprazole (20 mg/d).

SURGERY Used for complications (persistent or recurrent bleeding, obstruction, perforation) or, uncommonly, intractability (first screen for surreptitious NSAID use and gastrinoma). For DU, see Table 158-3. For GU, perform subtotal gastrectomy.

COMPLICATIONS OF SURGERY (1) Obstructed afferent loop (Billroth II), (2) bile reflux gastritis, (3) dumping syndrome (rapid gastric emptying with abdominal distress + postprandial vasomotor symptoms), (4) post-vagotomy diarrhea, (5) bezoar, (6) anemia (iron, B_{12}, folate malabsorption), (7) malabsorption (poor mixing of gastric contents, pancreatic juices, bile; bacterial overgrowth), (8) osteomalacia and osteoporosis (vitamin D and Ca malabsorption), (9) gastric remnant carcinoma.

APPROACH TO THE PATIENT | **Peptic Ulcer Disease**

Optimal approach is uncertain. Serologic testing for *H. pylori* and treating, if present, may be cost-effective. Other options include trial of acid-suppressive therapy, endoscopy only in treatment failures, or initial endoscopy in all cases.

**TABLE 158-2 REGIMENS RECOMMENDED FOR ERADICATION OF
H. PYLORI INFECTION**

Drug	Dose
Triple therapy	
1. Bismuth subsalicylate *plus*	2 tablets qid
Metronidazole *plus*	250 mg qid
Tetracycline[a]	500 mg qid
2. Ranitidine bismuth citrate *plus*	400 mg bid
Tetracycline *plus*	500 mg bid
Clarithromycin or metronidazole	500 mg bid
3. Omeprazole (lansoprazole) *plus*	20 mg bid (30 mg bid)
Clarithromycin *plus*	250 or 500 mg bid
Metronidazole[b] *or*	500 mg bid
Amoxicillin[c]	1 g bid
Quadruple therapy	
Omeprazole (lansoprazole)	20 mg (30 mg) daily
Bismuth subsalicylate	2 tablets qid
Metronidazole	250 mg qid
Tetracycline	500 mg qid

[a]Alternative: use prepacked Helidac.
[b]Alternative: use prepacked Prevpac.
[c]Use either metronidazole or amoxicillin, not both.

GASTROPATHIES

■ EROSIVE GASTROPATHIES

Hemorrhagic gastritis, multiple gastric erosions may be caused by aspirin and other NSAIDs (lower risk with newer agents, e.g., nabumetone and etodolac, which do not inhibit gastric mucosal prostaglandins) or severe stress (burns, sepsis, trauma, surgery, shock, or respiratory, renal, or liver failure). Pt may be asymptomatic or experience epigastric discomfort, nausea, hematemesis, or melena. Diagnosis is made by upper endoscopy.

TABLE 158-3 SURGICAL TREATMENT OF DUODENAL ULCER

Operation	Recurrence Rate	Complication Rate
Vagotomy + antrectomy (Billroth I or II)[a]	1%	Highest
Vagotomy and pyloroplasty	10%	Intermediate
Parietal cell (proximal gastric, superselective) vagotomy	≥10%	Lowest

[a]Billroth I, gastroduodenostomy; Billroth II, gastrojejunostomy.

| **TREATMENT** | Erosive Gastropathies |

Removal of offending agent and maintenance of O_2 and blood volume as required. For prevention of stress ulcers in critically ill pts, hourly oral administration of liquid antacids (e.g., Maalox 30 mL), IV H_2 receptor antagonist (e.g., cimetidine, 300-mg bolus + 37.5–50 mg/h IV), or both is recommended to maintain gastric pH > 4. Alternatively, sucralfate slurry, 1 g PO q6h, can be given; does not raise gastric pH and may thus avoid increased risk of aspiration pneumonia associated with liquid antacids. Pantoprazole can be administered IV to suppress gastric acid in the critically ill. Misoprostol, 200 µg PO qid, or profound acid suppression (e.g., famotidine, 40 mg PO bid) can be used with NSAIDs to prevent NSAID-induced ulcers.

■ CHRONIC GASTRITIS

Identified histologically by an inflammatory cell infiltrate dominated by lymphocytes and plasma cells with scant neutrophils. In its early stage, the changes are limited to the lamina propria (*superficial gastritis*). When the disease progresses to destroy glands, it becomes *atrophic gastritis*. The final stage is *gastric atrophy,* in which the mucosa is thin and the infiltrate sparse. Chronic gastritis can be classified based on predominant site of involvement.

Type A Gastritis

This is the body-predominant and less common form. Generally asymptomatic, common in elderly; autoimmune mechanism may be associated with achlorhydria, pernicious anemia, and increased risk of gastric cancer (value of screening endoscopy uncertain). Antibodies to parietal cells present in >90%.

Type B Gastritis

This is antral-predominant disease and caused by *H. pylori*. Often asymptomatic but may be associated with dyspepsia. Atrophic gastritis, gastric atrophy, gastric lymphoid follicles, and gastric B cell lymphomas may occur. Infection early in life or in setting of malnutrition or low gastric acid output is associated with gastritis of entire stomach (including body) and increased risk of gastric cancer. Eradication of *H. pylori* (Table 158-2) not routinely recommended unless PUD or gastric mucosa-associated lymphoid tissue (MALT) lymphoma is present.

■ SPECIFIC TYPES OF GASTROPATHY OR GASTRITIS

Alcoholic gastropathy (submucosal hemorrhages), Ménétrier's disease (hypertrophic gastropathy), eosinophilic gastritis, granulomatous gastritis, Crohn's disease, sarcoidosis, infections (tuberculosis, syphilis, fungi, viruses, parasites), pseudolymphoma, radiation, corrosive gastritis.

ZOLLINGER-ELLISON (Z-E) SYNDROME (GASTRINOMA)

Consider when ulcer disease is severe, refractory to therapy, associated with ulcers in atypical locations, or associated with diarrhea. Tumors are usually pancreatic or in duodenum (submucosal, often small), may be multiple,

TABLE 158-4 DIFFERENTIAL DIAGNOSTIC TESTS

Condition	Fasting Gastrin	Gastrin Response to	
		IV Secretin	Food
DU	N (≤150 ng/L)	NC	Slight ↑
Z-E	↑↑↑	↑↑↑	NC
Antral G (gastrin) cell hyperplasia	↑	↑, NC	↑↑↑

Abbreviations: DU, duodenal ulcer; N, normal; NC, no change; Z-E, Zollinger-Ellison syndrome.

slowly growing; >60% malignant; 25% associated with MEN 1, i.e., multiple endocrine neoplasia type 1 (gastrinoma, hyperparathyroidism, pituitary neoplasm), often duodenal, small, multicentric, less likely to metastasize to liver than pancreatic gastrinomas but often metastasize to local lymph nodes.

■ DIAGNOSIS

Suggestive

Basal acid output >15 mmol/h; basal/maximal acid output >60%; large mucosal folds on endoscopy or upper GI radiograph.

Confirmatory

Serum gastrin > 1000 ng/L or rise in gastrin of 200 ng/L following IV secretin and, if necessary, rise of 400 ng/L following IV calcium (Table 158-4).

■ DIFFERENTIAL DIAGNOSIS

Increased Gastric Acid Secretion

Z-E syndrome, antral G cell hyperplasia or hyperfunction (? due to *H. pylori*), postgastrectomy retained antrum, renal failure, massive small bowel resection, chronic gastric outlet obstruction.

Normal or Decreased Gastric Acid Secretion

Pernicious anemia, chronic gastritis, gastric cancer, vagotomy, pheochromocytoma.

TREATMENT	Zollinger-Ellison Syndrome

Omeprazole (or lansoprazole), beginning at 60 mg PO q A.M. and increasing until maximal gastric acid output is <10 mmol/h before next dose, is drug of choice during evaluation and in pts who are not surgical candidates; dose can often be reduced over time. Radiolabeled octreotide scanning has emerged as the most sensitive test for detecting primary tumors and metastases; may be supplemented by endoscopic ultrasonography. Exploratory laparotomy with resection of primary tumor and solitary metastases is done when possible. In pts with MEN 1, tumor is often multifocal and unresectable; treat hyperparathyroidism first (hypergastrinemia may improve). For unresectable tumors, parietal cell vagotomy may enhance control of ulcer disease by drugs. Chemotherapy is used for metastatic tumor to control symptoms (e.g., streptozocin, 5-fluorouracil, doxorubicin, or interferon α); 40% partial response rate. Newer agents effective in pancreatic neuroendocrine tumors have not been evaluated.

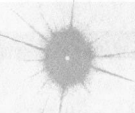

For a more detailed discussion, see Del Valle J: Peptic Ulcer Disease and Related Disorders, Chap. 293, p. 2438, in HPIM-18.

CHAPTER **159**
Inflammatory Bowel Diseases

Inflammatory bowel diseases (IBD) are chronic inflammatory disorders of unknown etiology involving the GI tract. Peak occurrence is between ages 15 and 30 and between ages 60 and 80, but onset may occur at any age. Epidemiologic features are shown in Table 159-1. Pathogenesis of IBD involves activation of immune cells by unknown inciting agent (? microorganism, dietary component, bacterial or self-antigen) leading to release of cytokines and inflammatory mediators. Genetic component suggested by increased risk in first-degree relatives of pts with IBD and concurrence of type of IBD, location of Crohn's disease (CD), and clinical course. Reported associations include HLA-DR2 in Japanese pts with ulcerative colitis and a CD-related gene called *CARD15* on chromosome 16p. *CARD15*

TABLE 159-1 EPIDEMIOLOGY OF IBD

	Ulcerative Colitis	Crohn's Disease
Incidence (North America) per person-years	2.2–14.3:100,000	3.1–14.6:100,000
Age of onset	15–30 and 60–80	15–30 and 60–80
Ethnicity	Jewish > non-Jewish white > African American > Hispanic > Asian	
Male/female ratio	1:1	1.1–1.8:1
Smoking	May prevent disease	May cause disease
Oral contraceptives	No increased risk	Odds ratio 1.4
Appendectomy	Protective	Not protective
Monozygotic twins	6% concordance	58% concordance
Dizygotic twins	0% concordance	4% concordance

mutations may account for 10% of CD risk. Other potential pathogenic factors include serum antineutrophil cytoplasmic antibodies (ANCA) in 70% of pts with ulcerative colitis (also in 5–10% of CD pts) and antibodies to *Saccharomyces cerevisiae* (ASCA) in 60–70% of CD pts (also in 10–15% of ulcerative colitis pts and 5% of normal controls). Granulomatous angiitis (vasculitis) may occur in CD. Acute flares may be precipitated by infections, nonsteroidal anti-inflammatory drugs (NSAIDs), stress. Onset of ulcerative colitis often follows cessation of smoking.

ULCERATIVE COLITIS (UC)

■ PATHOLOGY

Colonic mucosal inflammation; rectum almost always involved, with inflammation extending continuously (no skip areas) proximally for a variable extent; histologic features include epithelial damage, inflammation, crypt abscesses, loss of goblet cells.

■ CLINICAL MANIFESTATIONS

Bloody diarrhea, mucus, fever, abdominal pain, tenesmus, weight loss; spectrum of severity (majority of cases are mild, limited to rectosigmoid). In severe cases dehydration, anemia, hypokalemia, hypoalbuminemia.

■ COMPLICATIONS

Toxic megacolon, colonic perforation; cancer risk related to extent and duration of colitis; often preceded by or coincident with dysplasia, which may be detected on surveillance colonoscopic biopsies.

■ DIAGNOSIS

Sigmoidoscopy/colonoscopy: mucosal erythema, granularity, friability, exudate, hemorrhage, ulcers, inflammatory polyps (pseudopolyps). Barium enema: loss of haustrations, mucosal irregularity, ulcerations.

CROHN'S DISEASE (CD)

■ PATHOLOGY

Any part of GI tract, usually terminal ileum and/or colon; transmural inflammation, bowel wall thickening, linear ulcerations, and submucosal thickening leading to cobblestone pattern; discontinuous (skip areas); histologic features include transmural inflammation, granulomas (often absent), fissures, fistulas.

■ CLINICAL MANIFESTATIONS

Fever, abdominal pain, diarrhea (often without blood), fatigue, weight loss, growth retardation in children; acute ileitis mimicking appendicitis; anorectal fissures, fistulas, abscesses. Clinical course falls into three broad patterns: (1) inflammatory, (2) stricturing, and (3) fistulizing.

■ COMPLICATIONS

Intestinal obstruction (edema vs. fibrosis); rarely toxic megacolon or perforation; intestinal fistulas to bowel, bladder, vagina, skin, soft tissue, often with abscess formation; bile salt malabsorption leading to cholesterol gallstones and/or oxalate kidney stones; intestinal malignancy; amyloidosis.

■ DIAGNOSIS

Sigmoidoscopy/colonoscopy, barium enema, upper GI and small-bowel series: nodularity, rigidity, ulcers that may be deep or longitudinal, cobblestoning, skip areas, strictures, fistulas. CT may show thickened, matted bowel loops or an abscess.

DIFFERENTIAL DIAGNOSIS
■ INFECTIOUS ENTEROCOLITIS

Shigella, Salmonella, Campylobacter, Yersinia (acute ileitis), *Plesiomonas shigelloides, Aeromonas hydrophila, Escherichia coli* serotype O157:H7, *Gonorrhea, Lymphogranuloma venereum, Clostridium difficile* (pseudomembranous colitis), tuberculosis, amebiasis, cytomegalovirus, AIDS.

■ OTHERS

Ischemic bowel disease, appendicitis, diverticulitis, radiation enterocolitis, bile salt–induced diarrhea (ileal resection), drug-induced colitis (e.g., NSAIDs), bleeding colonic lesion (e.g., neoplasm), irritable bowel syndrome (no bleeding), microscopic (lymphocytic) or collagenous colitis (chronic watery diarrhea)—normal colonoscopy, but biopsies show superficial colonic epithelial inflammation and, in collagenous colitis, a thick subepithelial layer of collagen; response to aminosalicylates and glucocorticoids variable.

EXTRAINTESTINAL MANIFESTATIONS OF UC AND CD

1. *Joint:* Peripheral arthritis—parallels activity of bowel disease; ankylosing spondylitis and sacroiliitis (associated with HLA-B27)—activity independent of bowel disease.
2. *Skin:* Erythema nodosum, aphthous ulcers, pyoderma gangrenosum, cutaneous Crohn's disease.
3. *Eye:* Conjunctivitis, episcleritis, iritis, uveitis.
4. *Liver:* Fatty liver, "pericholangitis" (intrahepatic sclerosing cholangitis), primary sclerosing cholangitis, cholangiocarcinoma, chronic hepatitis.
5. *Others:* Autoimmune hemolytic anemia, phlebitis, pulmonary embolus (hypercoagulable state), kidney stones, metabolic bone disease.

> **TREATMENT** Inflammatory Bowel Diseases (See Fig. 159-1)
>
> **SUPPORTIVE** Antidiarrheal agents (diphenoxylate and atropine, loperamide) in mild disease; IV hydration and blood transfusions in severe disease; parenteral nutrition or defined enteral formulas—effective as primary therapy in CD, although high relapse rate when oral feeding is resumed; should not replace drug therapy; important role in preoperative preparation of malnourished pt; emotional support.
>
> **SULFASALAZINE AND AMINOSALICYLATES** Active component of sulfasalazine is 5-aminosalicylic acid (5-ASA) linked to sulfapyridine carrier; useful in colonic disease of mild to moderate severity (1–1.5 g PO qid); efficacy in maintaining remission demonstrated only for UC (500 mg PO qid). Toxicity (generally due to sulfapyridine component):

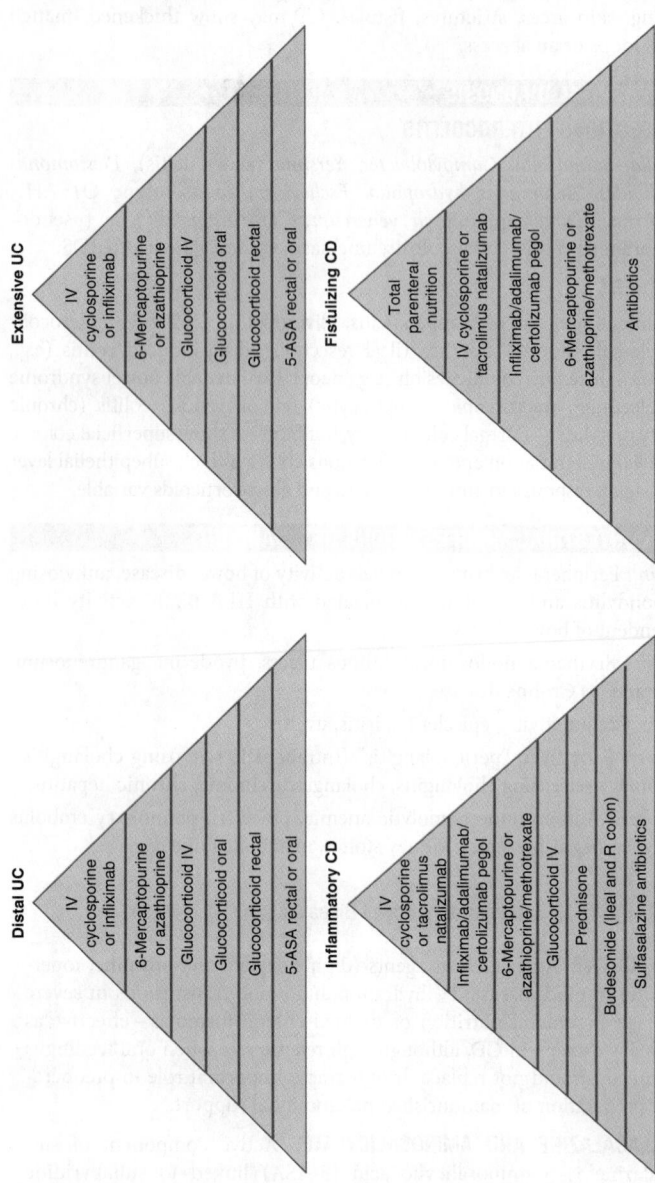

FIGURE 159-1 Medical management of IBD. 5-ASA, 5-aminosalicylic acid; CD, Crohn's disease; UC, ulcerative colitis.

Distal UC

- IV cyclosporine or infliximab
- 6-Mercaptopurine or azathioprine
- Glucocorticoid IV
- Glucocorticoid oral
- Glucocorticoid rectal
- 5-ASA rectal or oral

Extensive UC

- IV cyclosporine or infliximab
- 6-Mercaptopurine or azathioprine
- Glucocorticoid IV
- Glucocorticoid oral
- Glucocorticoid rectal
- 5-ASA rectal or oral

Inflammatory CD

- IV cyclosporine or tacrolimus natalizumab
- Infliximab/adalimumab/ certolizumab pegol
- 6-Mercaptopurine or azathioprine/methotrexate
- Glucocorticoid IV
- Prednisone
- Budesonide (Ileal and R colon)
- Sulfasalazine antibiotics

Fistulizing CD

- Total parenteral nutrition
- IV cyclosporine or tacrolimus natalizumab
- Infliximab/adalimumab/ certolizumab pegol
- 6-Mercaptopurine or azathioprine/methotrexate
- Antibiotics

dose-related—nausea, headache, rarely hemolytic anemia—may resolve when drug dose is lowered; idiosyncratic—fever, rash, neutropenia, pancreatitis, hepatitis, etc.; miscellaneous—oligospermia. Newer aminosalicylates are as effective as sulfasalazine but with fewer side effects. Enemas containing 4 g of 5-ASA (mesalamine) may be used in distal UC, 1 nightly retained qhs until remission, then q2hs or q3hs. Suppositories containing 500 mg of 5-ASA may be used in proctitis.

GLUCOCORTICOIDS Useful in severe disease and ileal or ileocolonic CD. Prednisone, 40–60 mg PO qd, then taper; IV hydrocortisone, 100 mg tid or equivalent, in hospitalized pts; IV adrenocorticotropic hormone drip (120 U qd) may be preferable in first attacks of UC. Nightly hydrocortisone retention enemas in proctosigmoiditis. Numerous side effects make long-term use problematic.

IMMUNOSUPPRESSIVE AGENTS Azathioprine, 6-mercaptopurine—50 mg PO qd up to 2.0 or 1.5 mg/kg qd, respectively. Useful as steroid-sparing agents and in intractable or fistulous CD (may require 2- to 6-month trial before efficacy seen). Toxicity—immunosuppression, pancreatitis, ?carcinogenicity. Avoid in pregnancy.

METRONIDAZOLE Appears effective in colonic CD (500 mg PO bid) and refractory perineal CD (10–20 mg/kg PO qd). Toxicity—peripheral neuropathy, metallic taste, ?carcinogenicity. Avoid in pregnancy. Other antibiotics (e.g., ciprofloxacin 500 mg PO bid) may be of value in terminal ileal and perianal CD, and broad-spectrum IV antibiotics are indicated for fulminant colitis and abscesses.

OTHERS Cyclosporine [potential value in a dose of 4 (mg/kg)/d IV for 7–14 days in severe UC and possibly intractable Crohn's fistulas]; experimental—tacrolimus, methotrexate, chloroquine, fish oil, nicotine, others. Infliximab [monoclonal antibody to tumor necrosis factor (TNF)] 5 mg/kg IV induces responses in 65% (complete in 33%) of CD pts refractory to 5-ASA, glucocorticoids, and 6-mercaptopurine. In UC, 27–49% of pts respond.

Adalimumab is a humanized version of the anti-TNF antibody that is less likely to elicit neutralizing antibodies in the pt. Pegylated versions of anti-TNF antibody may be used once monthly.

Natalizumab is an anti-integrin antibody with activity against Crohn's disease, but some pts develop progressive multifocal leukoencephalopathy.

SURGERY UC: Colectomy (curative) for intractability, toxic megacolon (if no improvement with aggressive medical therapy in 24–48 h), cancer, dysplasia. Ileal pouch—anal anastomosis is operation of choice in UC, but contraindicated in CD and in elderly. CD: Resection for fixed obstruction (or stricturoplasty), abscesses, persistent symptomatic fistulas, intractability.

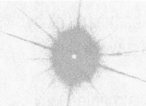

For a more detailed discussion, see Friedman S, Blumberg RS: Inflammatory Bowel Disease, Chap. 295, p. 2477, in HPIM-18.

CHAPTER **160**
Colonic and Anorectal Diseases

IRRITABLE BOWEL SYNDROME (IBS)

Characterized by altered bowel habits, abdominal pain, and absence of detectable organic pathology. Most common GI disease in clinical practice. Three types of clinical presentations: (1) spastic colon (chronic abdominal pain and constipation), (2) alternating constipation and diarrhea, or (3) chronic, painless diarrhea.

■ PATHOPHYSIOLOGY

Visceral hyperalgesia to mechanoreceptor stimuli is common. Reported abnormalities include altered colonic motility at rest and in response to stress, cholinergic drugs, cholecystokinin; altered small-intestinal motility; enhanced visceral sensation (lower pain threshold in response to gut distention); and abnormal extrinsic innervation of the gut. Pts presenting with IBS to a physician have an increased frequency of psychological disturbances—depression, hysteria, obsessive-compulsive disorder. Specific food intolerances and malabsorption of bile acids by the terminal ileum may account for a few cases.

■ CLINICAL MANIFESTATIONS

Onset often before age 30; females:males = 2:1. Abdominal pain and irregular bowel habits. Additional symptoms often include abdominal distention, relief of abdominal pain with bowel movement, increased frequency of stools with pain, loose stools with pain, mucus in stools, and sense of incomplete evacuation. Associated findings include pasty stools, ribbony

---

TABLE 160-1 DIAGNOSTIC CRITERIA FOR IRRITABLE BOWEL SYNDROME[a]

Recurrent abdominal pain or discomfort[b] at least 3 days per month in the last 3 months associated with *two or more* of the following:

1. Improvement with defecation
2. Onset associated with a change in frequency of stool
3. Onset associated with a change in form (appearance) of stool

[a]Criteria fulfilled for the last 3 months with symptom onset at least 6 months prior to diagnosis.

[b]Discomfort means an uncomfortable sensation not described as pain. In pathophysiology research and clinical trials, a pain/discomfort frequency of at least 2 days a week during screening evaluation is required for subject eligibility.

Source: Adapted from Longstreth GF et al: Functional bowel disorders. Gastroenterology 130:1480, 2006.

or pencil-thin stools, heartburn, bloating, back pain, weakness, faintness, palpitations, urinary frequency.

■ DIAGNOSIS

IBS is a diagnosis of exclusion. Rome criteria for diagnosis are shown in Table 160-1. Consider sigmoidoscopy and barium radiographs to exclude inflammatory bowel disease or malignancy; consider excluding giardiasis, intestinal lactase deficiency, hyperthyroidism.

| TREATMENT | Irritable Bowel Syndrome (Table 160-2) |

Reassurance and supportive physician-pt relationship, avoidance of stress or precipitating factors, dietary bulk (fiber, psyllium extract, e.g., Metamucil 1 tbsp daily or bid); for diarrhea, trials of loperamide (2-mg tabs PO q A.M. then 1 PO after each loose stool to a maximum of 8/d, then titrate), diphenoxylate (Lomotil) (up to 2-mg tabs PO qid), or cholestyramine (up to 1-g packet mixed in water PO qid); for pain, anticholinergics (e.g., dicyclomine HCl 10–40 mg PO qid) or

TABLE 160-2 POSSIBLE DRUGS FOR A DOMINANT SYMPTOM IN IBS

Symptom	Drug	Dose
Diarrhea	Loperamide	2–4 mg when necessary/maximum 12 g/d
	Cholestyramine resin	4 g with meals
	Alosetron[a]	0.5–1 mg bid (for severe IBS, women)
Constipation	Psyllium husk	3–4 g bid with meals, then adjust
	Methylcellulose	2 g bid with meals, then adjust
	Calcium polycarbophil	1 g qd to qid
	Lactulose syrup	10–20 g bid
	70% sorbitol	15 mL bid
	Polyethylene glycol 3350	17 g in 250 mL water qd
	Lubiprostone (Amitiza)	24 mg bid
	Magnesium hydroxide	30–60 mL qd
Abdominal pain	Smooth-muscle relaxant	qd to qid ac
	Tricyclic antidepressants	Start 25–50 mg hs, then adjust
	Selective serotonin reuptake inhibitors	Begin small dose, increase as needed

[a]Available only in the United States.
Source: Adapted from Longstreth GF et al:Functional bowel disorders. Gastroenterology 130:1480, 2006.

hyoscyamine as Levsin 1–2 PO q4h prn. Amitriptyline 25–50 mg PO qhs or other antidepressants in low doses may relieve pain. Selective serotonin reuptake inhibitors such as paroxetine are being evaluated in constipation-dominant pts, and serotonin receptor antagonists such as alosetron are being evaluated in diarrhea-dominant pts. Altering gut flora with probiotics (*Bifidobacterium infantis* 35624) or oral nonabsorbable antibiotics (rifaximin) is being evaluated with some promising early results. Psychotherapy, hypnotherapy of possible benefit in severe refractory cases.

DIVERTICULAR DISEASE

Herniations or saclike protrusions of the mucosa through the muscularis at points of nutrient artery penetration; possibly due to increased intraluminal pressure, low-fiber diet; most common in sigmoid colon.

■ CLINICAL PRESENTATION

1. *Asymptomatic* (detected by barium enema or colonoscopy).
2. *Pain*: Recurrent left lower quadrant pain relieved by defecation; alternating constipation and diarrhea. Diagnosis by barium enema.
3. *Diverticulitis*: Pain, fever, altered bowel habits, tender colon, leukocytosis. Best confirmed and staged by CT after opacification of bowel. (In pts who recover with medical therapy, perform elective barium enema or colonoscopy in 4–6 weeks to exclude cancer.) Complications: pericolic abscess, perforation, fistula (to bladder, vagina, skin, soft tissue), liver abscess, stricture. Frequently require surgery or, for abscesses, percutaneous drainage.
4. *Hemorrhage*: Usually in absence of diverticulitis, often from ascending colon and self-limited. If persistent, manage with mesenteric arteriography and intraarterial infusion of vasopressin, or surgery (Chap. 47).

TREATMENT   Diverticular Disease

PAIN High-fiber diet, psyllium extract (e.g., Metamucil 1 tbsp PO qd or bid), anticholinergics (e.g., dicyclomine HCl 10–40 mg PO qid).

DIVERTICULITIS NPO, IV fluids, antibiotics for 7–10 d (e.g., trimethoprim/sulfamethoxazole or ciprofloxacin and metronidazole; add ampicillin to cover enterococci in nonresponders); for ambulatory pts, ampicillin/clavulanate (clear liquid diet); surgical resection in refractory or frequently recurrent cases, young persons (<age 50), immunosuppressed pts, or when there is inability to exclude cancer.

Pts who have had at least two documented episodes and those who respond slowly to medical therapy should be offered surgical options to achieve removal of the diseased colonic segment, controlling sepsis, eliminating obstructions or fistulas, and restoring intestinal continuity.

INTESTINAL PSEUDOOBSTRUCTION

Recurrent attacks of nausea, vomiting, and abdominal pain and distention mimicking mechanical obstruction; may be complicated by steatorrhea due to bacterial overgrowth.

■ CAUSES

Primary: Familial visceral neuropathy, familial visceral myopathy, idiopathic. *Secondary*: Scleroderma, amyloidosis, diabetes, celiac disease, parkinsonism, muscular dystrophy, drugs, electrolyte imbalance, postsurgical.

> **TREATMENT** Intestinal Pseudoobstruction
>
> For acute attacks: intestinal decompression with long tube. Oral antibiotics for bacterial overgrowth (e.g., metronidazole 250 mg PO tid, tetracycline 500 mg PO qid, or ciprofloxacin 500 mg bid 1 week out of each month, usually in an alternating rotation of at least two antibiotics). Avoid surgery. In refractory cases, consider long-term parenteral hyperalimentation.

VASCULAR DISORDERS (SMALL AND LARGE INTESTINE)

■ MECHANISMS OF MESENTERIC ISCHEMIA

(1) Occlusive: embolus (atrial fibrillation, valvular heart disease); arterial thrombus (atherosclerosis); venous thrombosis (trauma, neoplasm, infection, cirrhosis, oral contraceptives, antithrombin-III deficiency, protein S or C deficiency, lupus anticoagulant, factor V Leiden mutation, idiopathic); vasculitis (systemic lupus erythematosus, polyarteritis, rheumatoid arthritis, Henoch-Schönlein purpura); (2) nonocclusive: hypotension, heart failure, arrhythmia, digitalis (vasoconstrictor).

■ ACUTE MESENTERIC ISCHEMIA

Periumbilical pain out of proportion to tenderness; nausea, vomiting, distention, GI bleeding, altered bowel habits. Abdominal x-ray shows bowel distention, air-fluid levels, thumbprinting (submucosal edema), but may be normal early in course. Peritoneal signs indicate infarcted bowel requiring surgical resection. Early celiac and mesenteric arteriography is recommended in all cases following hemodynamic resuscitation (avoid vasopressors, digitalis). Intraarterial vasodilators (e.g., papaverine) can be administered to reverse vasoconstriction. Laparotomy indicated to restore intestinal blood flow obstructed by embolus or thrombosis or to resect necrotic bowel. Postoperative anticoagulation indicated in mesenteric venous thrombosis, controversial in arterial occlusion.

■ CHRONIC MESENTERIC INSUFFICIENCY

"Abdominal angina": dull, crampy periumbilical pain 15–30 min after a meal and lasting for several hours; weight loss; occasionally diarrhea. Evaluate with mesenteric arteriography for possible bypass graft surgery.

■ ISCHEMIC COLITIS

Usually due to nonocclusive disease in pts with atherosclerosis. Severe lower abdominal pain, rectal bleeding, hypotension. Abdominal x-ray shows colonic dilatation, thumbprinting. Sigmoidoscopy shows submucosal hemorrhage, friability, ulcerations; rectum often spared. Conservative management (NPO, IV fluids); surgical resection for infarction or postischemic stricture.

COLONIC ANGIODYSPLASIA

In persons over age 60, vascular ectasias, usually in right colon, account for up to 40% of cases of chronic or recurrent lower GI bleeding. May be associated with aortic stenosis. Diagnosis is by arteriography (clusters of small vessels, early and prolonged opacification of draining vein) or colonoscopy (flat, bright red, fernlike lesions). For bleeding, treat by colonoscopic electro- or laser coagulation, band ligation, arteriographic embolization, or, if necessary, right hemicolectomy (Chap. 47).

ANORECTAL DISEASES

■ HEMORRHOIDS

Due to increased hydrostatic pressure in hemorrhoidal venous plexus (associated with straining at stool, pregnancy). May be external, internal, thrombosed, acute (prolapsed or strangulated), or bleeding. Treat pain with bulk laxative and stool softeners (psyllium extract, dioctyl sodium sulfosuccinate 100–200 mg/d), sitz baths 1–4 per day, witch hazel compresses, analgesics as needed. Bleeding may require rubber band ligation or injection sclerotherapy. Operative hemorrhoidectomy in severe or refractory cases.

■ ANAL FISSURES

Medical therapy as for hemorrhoids. Relaxation of the anal canal with nitroglycerin ointment (0.2%) applied tid or botulinum toxin type A up to 20 U injected into the internal sphincter on each side of the fissure. Internal anal sphincterotomy in refractory cases.

■ PRURITUS ANI

Often of unclear cause; may be due to poor hygiene, fungal or parasitic infection. Treat with thorough cleansing after bowel movement, topical glucocorticoid, antifungal agent if indicated.

■ ANAL CONDYLOMAS (GENITAL WARTS)

Wartlike papillomas due to sexually transmitted papillomavirus. Treat with cautious application of liquid nitrogen or podophyllotoxin or with intralesional interferon α. Tend to recur. May be prevented by vaccination with HPV vaccine.

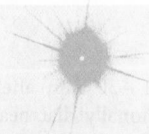

For a more detailed discussion, see Owyang C: Irritable Bowel Syndrome, Chap. 296, p. 2496; Gearhart SL: Diverticular Disease and Common Anorectal Disorders, Chap. 297, p. 2502; and Gearhart SL: Mesenteric Vascular Insufficiency, Chap. 298, p. 2510, in HPIM-18.

CHAPTER **161**
Cholelithiasis, Cholecystitis, and Cholangitis

CHOLELITHIASIS

There are two major types of gallstones: cholesterol and pigment stones. Cholesterol gallstones contain >50% cholesterol monohydrate. Pigment stones have <20% cholesterol and are composed primarily of calcium bilirubinate. In the United States, 80% of stones are cholesterol and 20% are pigment.

◼ EPIDEMIOLOGY

One million new cases of cholelithiasis per year in the United States. Predisposing factors include demographic/genetics (increased prevalence in North American Indians), obesity, weight loss, female sex hormones, age, ileal disease, pregnancy, type IV hyperlipidemia, and cirrhosis.

◼ SYMPTOMS AND SIGNS

Many gallstones are "silent," i.e., present in asymptomatic pts. Symptoms occur when stones trigger inflammation or cause obstruction of the cystic or common bile ducts. Major symptoms: (1) biliary colic—a severe steady ache in the RUQ or epigastrium that begins suddenly; often occurs 30–90 min after meals, lasts for several hours, and occasionally radiates to the right scapula or back; (2) nausea, vomiting. Physical exam may be normal or show epigastric or RUQ tenderness.

◼ LABORATORY

Occasionally, mild and transient elevations in bilirubin [<85 μmol/L (<5 mg/dL)] accompany biliary colic.

◼ IMAGING

Only 10% of cholesterol gallstones are radiopaque. Ultrasonography is best diagnostic test. The oral cholecystogram has been largely replaced by ultrasound, but may be used to assess the patency of the cystic duct and gallbladder emptying function (Table 161-1).

◼ DIFFERENTIAL DIAGNOSIS

Includes peptic ulcer disease (PUD), gastroesophageal reflux, irritable bowel syndrome, and hepatitis.

◼ COMPLICATIONS

Cholecystitis, pancreatitis, cholangitis.

TREATMENT Cholelithiasis

In asymptomatic pts, risk of developing complications requiring surgery is small. Elective cholecystectomy should be reserved for: (1) symptomatic

TABLE 161-1 DIAGNOSTIC EVALUATION OF THE BILE DUCTS

Diagnostic Advantages	Diagnostic Limitations
Hepatobiliary ultrasound	
Rapid	Bowel gas
Simultaneous scanning of GB, liver, bile ducts, pancreas	Massive obesity
	Ascites
Accurate identification of dilated bile ducts	Barium
Not limited by jaundice, pregnancy	Partial bile duct obstruction
Guidance for fine-needle biopsy	Poor visualization of distal CBD
Computed tomography	
Simultaneous scanning of GB, liver, bile ducts, pancreas	Extreme cachexia
	Movement artifact
Accurate identification of dilated bile ducts, masses	Ileus
	Partial bile duct obstruction
Not limited by jaundice, gas, obesity, ascites	
High-resolution image	
Guidance for fine-needle biopsy	
Magnetic resonance cholangiopancreatography	
Useful modality for visualizing pancreatic and biliary ducts	Cannot offer therapeutic intervention
Has excellent sensitivity for bile duct dilatation, biliary stricture, and intraductal abnormalities	High cost
Can identify pancreatic duct dilatation or stricture, pancreatic duct stenosis, and pancreas divisum	
Endoscopic retrograde cholangiopancreatography	
Simultaneous pancreatography	Gastroduodenal obstruction
Best visualization of distal biliary tract	?Roux-en-Y biliary-enteric anastomosis
Bile or pancreatic cytology	
Endoscopic sphincterotomy and stone removal	
Biliary manometry	
Percutaneous transhepatic cholangiogram	
Extremely successful when bile ducts dilated	Nondilated or sclerosed ducts
Best visualization of proximal biliary tract	
Bile cytology/culture	
Percutaneous transhepatic drainage	
Endoscopic ultrasound	
Most sensitive method to detect ampullary stones	

pts (i.e., biliary colic despite low-fat diet); (2) persons with previous complications of cholelithiasis (see below); and (3) presence of an underlying condition predisposing to an increased risk of complications (calcified or porcelain gallbladder). Pts with gallstones >3 cm or with an anomalous gallbladder containing stones should also be considered for surgery. Laparoscopic cholecystectomy is minimally invasive and is the procedure of choice for most pts undergoing elective cholecystectomy. Oral dissolution agents (ursodeoxycholic acid) partially or completely dissolve small radiolucent stones in 50% of selected pts within 6–24 months. Because of the frequency of stone recurrence and the effectiveness of laparoscopic surgery, the role of oral dissolution therapy has been largely confined to pts who are not candidates for elective cholecystectomy.

ACUTE CHOLECYSTITIS

Acute inflammation of the gallbladder is usually caused by cystic duct obstruction by an impacted stone. Inflammatory response is evoked by: (1) mechanical inflammation from increased intraluminal pressure; (2) chemical inflammation from release of lysolecithin; (3) bacterial inflammation, which plays a role in 50–85% of pts with acute cholecystitis.

■ ETIOLOGY

90% calculous; 10% acalculous. Acalculous cholecystitis is associated with higher complication rate and acute illness (i.e., burns, trauma, major surgery), fasting, hyperalimentation leading to gallbladder stasis, vasculitis, carcinoma of gallbladder or common bile duct, some gallbladder infections (*Leptospira, Streptococcus, Salmonella,* or *Vibrio cholerae*), but in >50% of cases an underlying explanation is not found.

■ SYMPTOMS AND SIGNS

(1) Biliary colic (RUQ or epigastric pain) that progressively worsens; (2) nausea, vomiting, anorexia; and (3) fever. Examination typically reveals RUQ tenderness; palpable RUQ mass found in 20% of pts. *Murphy's sign* is present when deep inspiration or cough during palpation of the RUQ produces increased pain or inspiratory arrest.

■ LABORATORY

Mild leukocytosis; serum bilirubin, alkaline phosphatase, and AST may be mildly elevated.

■ IMAGING

Ultrasonography is useful for demonstrating gallstones and occasionally a phlegmonous mass surrounding the gallbladder. Radionuclide scans (HIDA, DIDA, DISIDA, etc.) may identify cystic duct obstruction.

■ DIFFERENTIAL DIAGNOSIS

Includes acute pancreatitis, appendicitis, pyelonephritis, peptic ulcer disease, hepatitis, and hepatic abscess.

■ COMPLICATIONS

Empyema, hydrops, gangrene, perforation, fistulization, gallstone ileus, porcelain gallbladder.

> **TREATMENT** Acute Cholecystitis
>
> No oral intake, nasogastric suction, IV fluids and electrolytes, analgesia (meperidine or NSAIDs), and antibiotics (ureidopenicillins, ampicillin sulbactam, ciprofloxacin, third-generation cephalosporins; anaerobic coverage should be added if gangrenous or emphysematous cholecystitis is suspected; imipenem/meropenem cover the spectrum of bacteria causing ascending cholangitis but should be reserved for the most life-threatening infections when other antibiotics have failed). Acute symptoms will resolve in 70% of pts. Optimal timing of surgery depends on pt stabilization and should be performed as soon as feasible. Urgent cholecystectomy is appropriate in most pts with a suspected or confirmed complication. Delayed surgery is reserved for pts with high risk of emergent surgery and where the diagnosis is in doubt.

CHRONIC CHOLECYSTITIS

■ ETIOLOGY

Chronic inflammation of the gallbladder; almost always associated with gallstones. Results from repeated acute/subacute cholecystitis or prolonged mechanical irritation of gallbladder wall.

■ SYMPTOMS AND SIGNS

May be asymptomatic for years, may progress to symptomatic gallbladder disease or to acute cholecystitis, or present with complications.

■ LABORATORY

Tests are usually normal.

■ IMAGING

Ultrasonography preferred; usually shows gallstones within a contracted gallbladder (Table 161-1).

■ DIFFERENTIAL DIAGNOSIS

Peptic ulcer disease, esophagitis, irritable bowel syndrome.

> **TREATMENT** Chronic Cholecystitis
>
> Surgery indicated if pt is symptomatic.

CHOLEDOCHOLITHIASIS/CHOLANGITIS

■ ETIOLOGY

In pts with cholelithiasis, passage of gallstones into common bile duct (CBD) occurs in 10–15%; increases with age. At cholecystectomy, undetected stones are left behind in 1–5% of pts.

■ SYMPTOMS AND SIGNS

Choledocholithiasis may present as an incidental finding, biliary colic, obstructive jaundice, cholangitis, or pancreatitis. Cholangitis usually presents as fever, RUQ pain, and jaundice (*Charcot's triad*).

■ LABORATORY

Elevations in serum bilirubin, alkaline phosphatase, and aminotransferases. Leukocytosis usually accompanies cholangitis; blood cultures are frequently positive. Amylase is elevated in 15% of cases.

■ IMAGING

Diagnosis usually made by cholangiography either preoperatively by endoscopic retrograde cholangiopancreatography (ERCP) or intraoperatively at the time of cholecystectomy. Ultrasonography may reveal dilated bile ducts but is not sensitive for detecting CBD stones (Table 161-1).

■ DIFFERENTIAL DIAGNOSIS

Acute cholecystitis, renal colic, perforated viscus, pancreatitis.

■ COMPLICATIONS

Cholangitis, obstructive jaundice, gallstone-induced pancreatitis, and secondary biliary cirrhosis.

TREATMENT   Choledocholithiasis/Cholangitis

Laparoscopic cholecystectomy and ERCP have decreased the need for choledocholithotomy and T-tube drainage of the bile ducts. When CBD stones are suspected prior to laparoscopic cholecystectomy, preoperative ERCP with endoscopic papillotomy and stone extraction is the preferred approach. CBD stones should be suspected in gallstone pts with (1) history of jaundice or pancreatitis, (2) abnormal LFT, and (3) ultrasound evidence of a dilated common bile duct or stones in the duct. Cholangitis treated like acute cholecystitis; no oral intake, hydration, analgesia, and antibiotics are the mainstays; stones should be removed surgically or endoscopically.

PRIMARY SCLEROSING CHOLANGITIS (PSC)

PSC is a sclerosing, inflammatory, and obliterative process involving the biliary tree.

■ ETIOLOGY

Associations: inflammatory bowel disease (75% of cases of PSC—especially ulcerative colitis), AIDS, rarely retroperitoneal fibrosis.

■ SYMPTOMS AND SIGNS

Pruritus, RUQ pain, jaundice, fever, weight loss, and malaise. 44% may be asymptomatic at diagnosis. May progress to cirrhosis with portal hypertension.

■ LABORATORY

Evidence of cholestasis (elevated bilirubin and alkaline phosphatase) common.

■ RADIOLOGY/ENDOSCOPY

Transhepatic or endoscopic cholangiograms reveal stenosis and dilation of the intra- and extrahepatic bile ducts.

■ DIFFERENTIAL DIAGNOSIS

Cholangiocarcinoma, Caroli disease (cystic dilation of bile ducts), *Fasciola hepatica* infection, echinococcosis, and ascariasis.

TREATMENT	**Primary Sclerosing Cholangitis**

No satisfactory therapy. Cholangitis should be treated as outlined above. Cholestyramine may control pruritus. Supplemental vitamin D and calcium may retard bone loss. Glucocorticoids, methotrexate, and cyclosporine have not been shown to be effective. Ursodeoxycholic acid improves liver tests but has not been shown to affect survival. Surgical relief of biliary obstruction may be appropriate but has a high complication rate. Liver transplantation should be considered in pts with end-stage cirrhosis. Median survival: 9–12 years after diagnosis, with age, bilirubin level, histologic stage, and splenomegaly being predictors of survival.

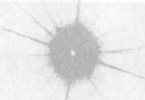

For a more detailed discussion, see Greenberger NJ, Paumgartner G: Diseases of the Gallbladder and Bile Ducts, Chap. 311, p. 2615, in HPIM-18.

CHAPTER 162
Pancreatitis

ACUTE PANCREATITIS

The pathologic spectrum of acute pancreatitis varies from *interstitial pancreatitis*, which is usually a mild and self-limited disorder, to *necrotizing pancreatitis*, in which the degree of pancreatic necrosis correlates with the severity of the attack and its systemic manifestations.

■ ETIOLOGY

Most common causes in the United States are cholelithiasis and alcohol. Others are listed in Table 162-1.

■ CLINICAL FEATURES

Can vary from mild abdominal pain to shock. *Common symptoms:* (1) steady, boring midepigastric pain radiating to the back that is frequently increased in the supine position; (2) nausea, vomiting.

Physical exam: (1) low-grade fever, tachycardia, hypotension; (2) erythematous skin nodules due to subcutaneous fat necrosis; (3) basilar rales, pleural effusion (often on the left); (4) abdominal tenderness and rigidity,

TABLE 162-1 CAUSES OF ACUTE PANCREATITIS

Common Causes
Gallstones (including microlithiasis)
Alcohol (acute and chronic alcoholism)
Hypertriglyceridemia
Complication of endoscopic retrograde cholangiopancreatography (ERCP), especially after biliary manometry
Trauma (especially blunt abdominal trauma)
Postoperative (abdominal and nonabdominal operations)
Drugs (azathioprine, 6-mercaptopurine, sulfonamides, estrogens, tetracycline, valproic acid, anti-HIV medications)
Sphincter of Oddi dysfunction
Uncommon Causes
Vascular causes and vasculitis (ischemic-hypoperfusion states after cardiac surgery)
Connective tissue disorders and thrombotic thrombocytopenic purpura (TTP)
Cancer of the pancreas
Hypercalcemia
Periampullary diverticulum
Pancreas divisum
Hereditary pancreatitis
Cystic fibrosis
Renal failure
Rare Causes
Infections (mumps, coxsackievirus, cytomegalovirus, echovirus, parasites) Autoimmune (e.g., Sjögren's syndrome)
Causes to Consider in Patients with Recurrent Bouts of Acute Pancreatitis without an Obvious Etiology
Occult disease of the biliary tree or pancreatic ducts, especially microlithiasis, sludge
Drugs
Hypertriglyceridemia
Pancreas divisum
Pancreatic cancer
Sphincter of Oddi dysfunction
Cystic fibrosis
Idiopathic

diminished bowel sounds, palpable upper abdominal mass; (5) Cullen's sign: blue discoloration in the periumbilical area due to hemoperitoneum; (6) Turner's sign: blue-red-purple or green-brown discoloration of the flanks due to tissue catabolism of hemoglobin.

■ LABORATORY

1. *Serum amylase*: Large elevations (>3 × normal) virtually assure the diagnosis if salivary gland disease and intestinal perforation/infarction are excluded. However, normal serum amylase does not exclude the diagnosis of acute pancreatitis, and the degree of elevation does not predict severity of pancreatitis. Amylase levels typically return to normal in 48–72 h.

2. *Urinary amylase–creatinine clearance ratio*: no more sensitive or specific than blood amylase levels.

3. *Serum lipase level*: increases in parallel with amylase level and measurement of both tests increases the diagnostic yield.

4. *Other tests*: Hypocalcemia occurs in ~25% of pts. *Leukocytosis* (15,000–20,000/μL) occurs frequently. *Hypertriglyceridemia* occurs in 15–20% of cases and can cause a spuriously normal serum amylase level. *Hyperglycemia* is common. *Serum bilirubin, alkaline phosphatase,* and *aspartame aminotransferase* can be transiently elevated. *Hypoalbuminemia* and marked elevations of *serum lactic dehydrogenase* (LDH) are associated with an increased mortality rate. *Hypoxemia* is present in 25% of pts. Arterial pH <7.32 may spuriously elevate serum amylase.

■ IMAGING

1. *Abdominal radiographs* are abnormal in 30–50% of pts but are not specific for pancreatitis. Common findings include total or partial ileus ("sentinel loop") and the "colon cut-off sign," which results from isolated distention of the transverse colon. Useful for excluding diagnoses such as intestinal perforation with free air.

2. *Ultrasound* often fails to visualize the pancreas because of overlying intestinal gas but may detect gallstones, pseudocysts, mass lesions, or edema or enlargement of the pancreas.

3. *CT* can confirm the clinical impression of acute pancreatitis. It can also be helpful in indicating the severity of acute pancreatitis via the CT severity index (CTSI—see Table 313-3, p. 2637, HPIM-18), assessing the risk of morbidity and mortality and in evaluating the complications of acute pancreatitis.

■ DIFFERENTIAL DIAGNOSIS

Intestinal perforation (especially peptic ulcer), cholecystitis, acute intestinal obstruction, mesenteric ischemia, renal colic, myocardial ischemia, aortic dissection, connective tissue disorders, pneumonia, and diabetic ketoacidosis.

TREATMENT Acute Pancreatitis

Most (90%) cases subside over a period of 3–7 days. Conventional measures: (1) analgesics, such as meperidine; (2) IV fluids and colloids; (3) no oral alimentation. The benefit of antibiotic prophylaxis in necrotizing acute pancreatitis remains controversial. Current recommendation is use of an antibiotic such as imipenem-cilastatin, 500 mg tid for 2 weeks. Not effective: cimetidine (or related agents), H_2 blockers, protease inhibitors, glucocorticoids, nasogastric suction, glucagon, peritoneal lavage, and anticholinergic medications. Precipitating factors (alcohol, medications) must be eliminated. In mild or moderate pancreatitis, a clear liquid diet can usually be started after 3–6 days. pts with severe gallstone-induced pancreatitis often benefit from early (<3 days) papillotomy.

■ **COMPLICATIONS**

It is important to identify pts who are at risk of poor outcome. Risk factors and markers of severe acute pancreatitis are listed in Table 162-2. Fulminant pancreatitis requires aggressive fluid support and meticulous management. Mortality is largely due to infection.

TABLE 162-2 SEVERE ACUTE PANCREATITIS

Risk Factors for Severity
• Age >60 years
• Obesity, BMI >30
• Comorbid disease
Markers of Severity within 24 Hours
• SIRS [temperature >38° or <36°C (>100.4° or 96.8°F), Pulse >90, Tachypnea >24, ↑ WBC >12,000]
• Hemoconcentration (Hct >44%)
• BISAP
– (B) Blood urea nitrogen (BUN) >22 mg%
– (I) Impaired mental status
– (S) SIRS: 2/4 present
– (A) Age >60 years
– (P) Pleural effusion
• Organ Failure
– Cardiovascular: systolic BP <90 mmHg, heart rate >130
– Pulmonary: Pao$_2$ <60 mmHg
– Renal serum creatinine >2.0 mg%
Markers of Severity during Hospitalization
• Persistent organ failure
• Pancreatic necrosis
• Hospital-acquired infection

Abbreviations: BISAP, bedside index of severity in acute pancreatitis.

Systemic

Shock, GI bleeding, common duct obstruction, ileus, splenic infarction or rupture, disseminated intravascular coagulation, subcutaneous fat necrosis, acute respiratory distress syndrome, pleural effusion, acute renal failure, sudden blindness.

Local

1. Sterile or infected *pancreatic necrosis*—necrosis may become secondarily infected in 40–60% of pts, typically within 1–2 weeks after the onset of pancreatitis. Most frequent organisms: gram-negative bacteria of alimentary origin, but intraabdominal *Candida* infection increasing in frequency. Necrosis can be visualized by contrast-enhanced dynamic CT, with infection diagnosed by CT-guided needle aspiration. Laparotomy with removal of necrotic material and adequate drainage should be considered for pts with sterile acute necrotic pancreatitis, if pt continues to deteriorate despite conventional therapy. Infected pancreatic necrosis requires aggressive surgical debridement and antibiotics.

2. *Pancreatic pseudocysts* develop over 1–4 weeks in 15% of pts. Abdominal pain is the usual complaint, and a tender upper abdominal mass may be present. Can be detected by abdominal ultrasound or CT. In pts who are stable and uncomplicated, treatment is supportive; pseudocysts that are >5 cm in diameter and persist for >6 weeks should be considered for drainage. In pts with an expanding pseudocyst or one complicated by hemorrhage, rupture, or abscess, surgery should be performed.

3. *Pancreatic abscess*—ill-defined liquid collection of pus that evolves over 4–6 weeks. Can be treated surgically or in selected cases by percutaneous drainage.

4. *Pancreatic ascites* and *pleural effusions* are usually due to disruption of the main pancreatic duct. Treatment involves nasogastric suction and parenteral alimentation for 2–3 weeks. If medical management fails, pancreatography followed by surgery should be performed.

CHRONIC PANCREATITIS

Chronic pancreatitis may occur as recurrent episodes of acute inflammation superimposed upon a previously injured pancreas or as chronic damage with pain and malabsorption.

■ ETIOLOGY

Chronic alcoholism is most frequent cause of pancreatic exocrine insufficiency in U.S. adults; in 25% of adults, etiology is unknown. Other causes are listed in Table 162-3.

■ SYMPTOMS AND SIGNS

Pain is cardinal symptom. Weight loss, steatorrhea, and other signs and symptoms of malabsorption common. Physical exam often unremarkable.

■ LABORATORY

No specific laboratory test for chronic pancreatitis. Serum amylase and lipase levels are often normal. Serum bilirubin and alkaline phosphatase

TABLE 162-3 CHRONIC PANCREATITIS AND PANCREATIC EXOCRINE INSUFFICIENCY: TIGAR-O CLASSIFICATION SYSTEM

Toxic-Metabolic	**Autoimmune**
Alcoholic	Isolated autoimmune CP
Tobacco smoking	Autoimmune CP associated with
Hypercalcemia	Sjögren's syndrome
Hyperlipidemia	Inflammatory bowel disease
Chronic renal failure	Primary biliary cirrhosis
Medications—phenacetin abuse	
Toxins—organotin compounds (e.g., DBTC)	**Recurrent and severe acute pancreatitis**
	Postnecrotic (severe acute pancreatitis)
	Recurrent acute pancreatitis
	Vascular diseases/ischemia
Idiopathic	Postirradiation
Early onset	
Late onset	**Obstructive**
Tropical	Pancreas divisum
	Sphincter of Oddi disorders (controversial)
Genetic	Duct obstruction (e.g., tumor)
Hereditary pancreatitis	Preampullary duodenal wall cysts
Cationic trypsinogen	Posttraumatic pancreatic duct scars
CFTR mutations	
SPINK1 mutations	

Abbreviations: CP, chronic pancreatitis; TIGAR-O, toxic-metabolic, idiopathic, genetic, autoimmune, recurrent and severe acute pancreatitis, obstructive.

may be elevated. Steatorrhea (fecal fat concentration ≥9.5%) late in the course. The bentiromide test, a simple, effective test of pancreatic exocrine function, may be helpful. D-Xylose urinary excretion test is usually normal. Impaired glucose tolerance is present in >50% of pts. Secretin stimulation test is a relatively sensitive test for pancreatic exocrine deficiency.

■ **IMAGING**

Plain films of the abdomen reveal pancreatic calcifications in 30–60%. *Ultrasound* and *CT scans* may show dilation of the pancreatic duct. *ERCP* and endoscopic ultrasound (*EUS*) provide information about the main pancreatic and smaller ducts.

■ **DIFFERENTIAL DIAGNOSIS**

Important to distinguish from pancreatic carcinoma; may require radiographically guided biopsy.

TREATMENT Chronic Pancreatitis

Aimed at controlling pain and malabsorption. Intermittent attacks treated like acute pancreatitis. Alcohol and large, fatty meals must be avoided. Narcotics for severe pain, but subsequent addiction is common. pts unable to maintain adequate hydration should be hospitalized, while those with milder symptoms can be managed on an ambulatory basis. Surgery may control pain if there is a ductal stricture. Subtotal pancreatectomy may also control pain but at the cost of exocrine insufficiency and diabetes. Malabsorption is managed with a low-fat diet and pancreatic enzyme replacement. Because pancreatic enzymes are inactivated by acid, agents that reduce acid production (e.g., omeprazole or sodium bicarbonate) may improve their efficacy (but should not be given with enteric-coated preparations). Insulin may be necessary to control serum glucose.

■ COMPLICATIONS

Vitamin B$_{12}$ malabsorption in 40% of alcohol-induced and all cystic fibrosis cases. Impaired glucose tolerance. Nondiabetic retinopathy due to vitamin A and/or zinc deficiency. GI bleeding, icterus, effusions, subcutaneous fat necrosis, and bone pain occasionally occur. Increased risk for pancreatic carcinoma. Narcotic addiction common.

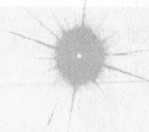

For a more detailed discussion, see Greenberger NJ, Conwell DL, Banks PA: Approach to the Patient With Pancreatic Disease, Chap. 312, p. 2629; Greenberger NJ, Conwell DL, Wu BU, Banks PA: Acute and Chronic Pancreatitis, Chap. 313, p. 2634, in HPIM-18.

CHAPTER **163**
Acute Hepatitis

VIRAL HEPATITIS

Acute viral hepatitis is a systemic infection predominantly affecting the liver. Clinically characterized by malaise, nausea, vomiting, diarrhea, and low-grade fever followed by dark urine, jaundice, and tender hepatomegaly; may be subclinical and detected on basis of elevated aspartate and alanine aminotransferase (AST and ALT) levels. Hepatitis B may be associated with immune-complex phenomena, including arthritis, serum sickness-like illness, glomerulonephritis, and a polyarteritis nodosa–like vasculitis. Hepatitis-like illnesses may be caused not only by hepatotropic viruses (A, B, C, D, E) but also by other viruses (Epstein-Barr, CMV, coxsackievirus, etc.), alcohol, drugs, hypotension and ischemia, and biliary tract disease (Table 163-1).

TABLE 163-1 THE HEPATITIS VIRUSES

	HAV	HBV	HCV	HDV	HEV
Viral Properties					
Size, nm	27	42	~55	~36	~32
Nucleic acid	RNA	DNA	RNA	RNA	RNA
Genome length, kb	7.5	3.2	9.4	1.7	7.5
Classification	Picornavirus	Hepadnavirus	Flavivirus-like	—	Calicivirus-like or alpha-virus-like
Incubation, days	15–45	30–180	15–160	21–140	14–63
Transmission					
Fecal-oral	+++	—	—	—	+++
Percutaneous	Rare	+++	+++	+++	—
Sexual	?	++	Uncommon	++	—
Perinatal	—	+++	Uncommon	+	—
Clinical Features					
Severity	Usually mild	Moderate	Mild	May be severe	Usually mild
Chronic infection	No	1–10%; up to 90% in neonates	80–90%	Common	No
Carrier state	No	Yes	Yes	Yes	No
Fulminant hepatitis	0.1%	1%	Rare	Up to 20% in superinfection	10–20% in pregnant women
Hepatocellular carcinoma	No	Yes	Yes	?	No
Prophylaxis	Ig; vaccine	HBIg; vaccine	None	None (HBV vaccine for susceptibles)	None

Note: HAV, hepatitis A virus; HBV, hepatitis B virus; HCV, hepatitis C virus; HDV, hepatitis D virus; HEV, hepatitis E virus; Ig, immune globulin; + +, sometimes; + + +, often; ?, possibly.

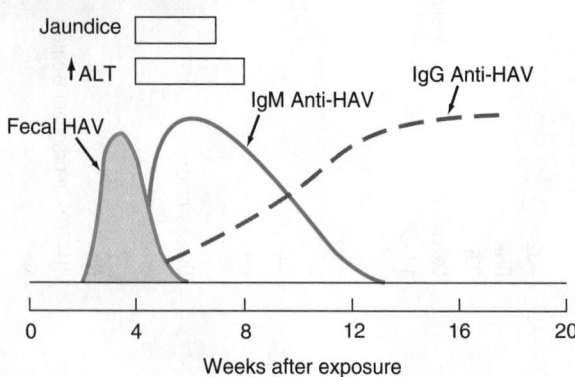

FIGURE 163-1 Scheme of typical clinical and laboratory features of HAV.

■ HEPATITIS A (HAV)

27-nm picornavirus (hepatovirus) with single-stranded RNA genome.

Clinical Course See Fig. 163-1.

Outcome

Recovery within 6–12 months, usually with no clinical sequelae; a small proportion will have one or two apparent clinical and serologic relapses; in some cases, pronounced cholestasis suggesting biliary obstruction may occur; rare fatalities (fulminant hepatitis), no chronic carrier state.

Diagnosis

IgM anti-HAV in acute or early convalescent serum sample.

Epidemiology

Fecal-oral transmission; endemic in underdeveloped countries; food-borne and waterborne epidemics; outbreaks in day-care centers, residential institutions.

Prevention

After exposure: immune globulin 0.02 mL/kg IM within 2 weeks to household and institutional contacts (not casual contacts at work). *Before exposure*: inactivated HAV vaccine 1 mL IM (unit dose depends on formulation); half dose to children; repeat at 6–12 months; target travelers, military recruits, animal handlers, day-care personnel, laboratory workers, and pts with chronic liver disease (especially hepatitis C).

■ HEPATITIS B (HBV)

42-nm hepadnavirus with outer surface coat (HBsAg), inner nucleocapsid core (HBcAg), DNA polymerase, and partially double-stranded DNA genome of 3200 nucleotides. Circulating form of HBcAg is HBeAg, a marker of viral replication and infectivity. Multiple serotypes and genetic heterogeneity.

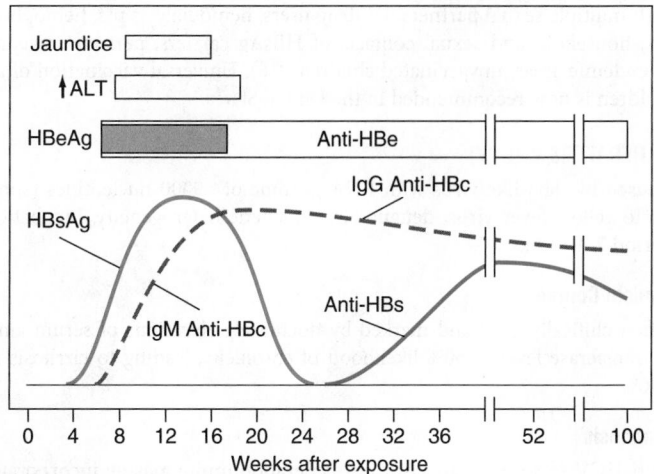

FIGURE 163-2 Scheme of typical clinical and laboratory features of HBV.

Clinical Course See Fig. 163-2.

Outcome

Recovery >90%, fulminant hepatitis (<1%), chronic hepatitis or carrier state (only 1–2% of immunocompetent adults; higher in neonates, elderly, immunocompromised), cirrhosis, and hepatocellular carcinoma (especially following chronic infection beginning in infancy or early childhood) (Chap. 165). Reactivation of HBV has been observed with immunosuppression, particularly with rituximab.

Diagnosis

HBsAg in serum (acute or chronic infection); IgM anti-HBc (early anti-HBc indicative of acute or recent infection). Most sensitive test is detection of HBV DNA in serum; not generally required for routine diagnosis.

Epidemiology

Percutaneous (needle stick), sexual, or perinatal transmission. Endemic in sub-Saharan Africa and Southeast Asia, where up to 20% of population acquire infection, usually early in life.

Prevention

After exposure in unvaccinated persons: hepatitis B immune globulin (HBIg) 0.06 mL/kg IM immediately after needle stick to within 14 days of sexual exposure in combination with vaccine series. For perinatal exposure (HbsAg+ mother) HBIg 0.05 mL in the thigh immediately after birth with the vaccine series started within the first 12 h of life. *Before exposure*: recombinant hepatitis B vaccine IM (dose depends on formulation as well as adult or pediatric and hemodialysis); at 0, 1, and 6 months; deltoid, not gluteal injection. Has been targeted to high-risk groups (e.g., health workers, persons with multiple sexual partners, IV drug users, hemodialysis pts, hemophiliacs, household and sexual contacts of HBsAg carriers, persons traveling in endemic areas, unvaccinated children <18). Universal vaccination of all children is now recommended in the United States.

◼ HEPATITIS C (HCV)

Caused by flavi-like virus with RNA genome of >9000 nucleotides (similar to yellow fever virus, dengue virus); genetic heterogeneity. Incubation period 7–8 weeks.

Clinical Course

Often clinically mild and marked by fluctuating elevations of serum aminotransferase levels; >50% likelihood of chronicity, leading to cirrhosis in >20%.

Diagnosis

Anti-HCV in serum. Current third-generation immunoassay incorporates proteins from the core, NS3, and NS5 regions. The most sensitive indicator of HCV infection is HCV RNA (Fig. 163-3).

Epidemiology

HCV accounts for >90% of transfusion-associated hepatitis cases. IV drug use accounts >50% of reported cases of hepatitis C. Little evidence for frequent sexual or perinatal transmission.

Prevention

Exclusion of paid blood donors, testing of donated blood for anti-HCV. Anti-HCV detected by enzyme immunoassay in blood donors with normal ALT is often falsely positive (30%); result should be confirmed by HCV RNA in serum.

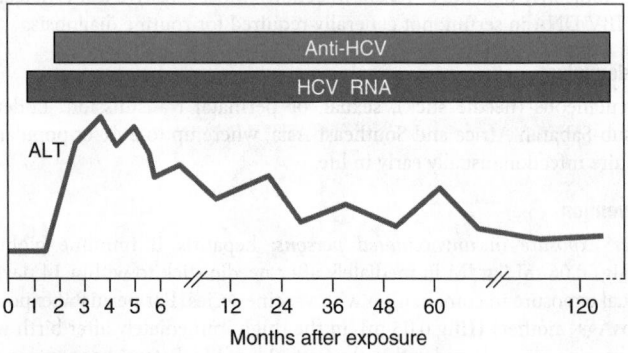

FIGURE 163-3 Scheme of typical laboratory features during acute hepatitis C progressing to chronicity. HCV RNA is the first detectable event, preceding alanine aminotransferase (ALT) elevation and the appearance of anti-HCV.

■ HEPATITIS D (HDV, DELTA AGENT)

Defective 37-nm RNA virus that requires HBV for its replication; either co-infects with HBV or superinfects a chronic HBV carrier. Enhances severity of HBV infection (acceleration of chronic hepatitis to cirrhosis, occasionally fulminant acute hepatitis).

Diagnosis

Anti-HDV in serum (acute hepatitis D—often in low titer, is transient; chronic hepatitis D—in higher titer, is sustained).

Epidemiology

Endemic among HBV carriers in Mediterranean Basin, where it is spread predominantly by nonpercutaneous means. In nonendemic areas (e.g., northern Europe, United States) HDV is spread percutaneously among HbsAg+ IV drug users or by transfusion in hemophiliacs and to a lesser extent among HbsAg+ men who have sex with men.

Prevention

Hepatitis B vaccine (noncarriers only).

■ HEPATITIS E (HEV)

Caused by 29- to 32-nm agent thought to be related to caliciviruses. Enterically transmitted and responsible for waterborne epidemics of hepatitis in India, parts of Asia and Africa, and Central America. Self-limited illness with high (10–20%) mortality rate in pregnant women.

TREATMENT   Viral Hepatitis

Activity as tolerated, high-calorie diet (often tolerated best in morning), IV hydration for severe vomiting, cholestyramine up to 4 g PO four times daily for severe pruritus, avoid hepatically metabolized drugs; no role for glucocorticoids. Liver transplantation for fulminant hepatic failure and grades III–IV encephalopathy. In rare instances of severe acute HBV, lamivudine has been used successfully. Most authorities would recommend antiviral therapy for severe acute HBV (Chap. 164). Meta-analyses and small clinical trials suggest that treatment of acute HCV infection with interferon α may be effective at reducing the rate of chronicity. Based on these data, many experts feel that acute HCV infection should be treated with a 24-week course of the best available regimens currently used to treat chronic HCV infection (Chap. 164).

TOXIC AND DRUG-INDUCED HEPATITIS

■ DOSE-DEPENDENT (DIRECT HEPATOTOXINS)

Onset is within 48 h, predictable, necrosis around terminal hepatic venule–e.g., carbon tetrachloride, benzene derivatives, mushroom poisoning, acetaminophen, or microvesicular steatosis (e.g., tetracyclines, valproic acid).

■ IDIOSYNCRATIC

Variable dose and time of onset; small number of exposed persons affected; may be associated with fever, rash, arthralgias, eosinophilia. In many cases, mechanism may actually involve toxic metabolite, possibly determined on genetic basis—e.g., isoniazid, halothane, phenytoin, methyldopa, carbamazepine, diclofenac, oxacillin, sulfonamides.

TREATMENT Toxic and Drug-Induced Hepatitis

Supportive as for viral hepatitis; withdraw suspected agent, and include use of gastric lavage and oral administration of charcoal or cholestyramine. Liver transplantation if necessary. In acetaminophen overdose, more specific therapy is available in the form of sulfhydryl compounds (e.g., N-acetylcysteine). These agents appear to act by providing a reservoir of sulfhydryl groups to bind the toxic metabolites or by stimulating synthesis of hepatic glutathione. Therapy should be begun within 8 h of ingestion but may be effective even if given as late as 24–36 h after overdose.

ACUTE HEPATIC FAILURE

Massive hepatic necrosis with impaired consciousness occurring within 8 weeks of the onset of illness.

■ CAUSES

Infections [viral, including HAV, HBV, HCV (rarely), HDV, HEV; bacterial, rickettsial, parasitic], drugs and toxins, ischemia (shock), Budd-Chiari syndrome, idiopathic chronic active hepatitis, acute Wilson's disease, microvesicular fat syndromes (Reye's syndrome, acute fatty liver of pregnancy).

■ CLINICAL MANIFESTATIONS

Neuropsychiatric changes—delirium, personality change, stupor, coma; cerebral edema—suggested by profuse sweating, hemodynamic instability, tachyarrhythmias, tachypnea, fever, papilledema, decerebrate rigidity (though all may be absent); deep jaundice, coagulopathy, bleeding, renal failure, acid-base disturbance, hypoglycemia, acute pancreatitis, cardiorespiratory failure, infections (bacterial, fungal).

■ ADVERSE PROGNOSTIC INDICATORS

Age <10 or >40, certain causes (e.g., halothane, hepatitis C), duration of jaundice >7 d before onset of encephalopathy, serum bilirubin > 300 μmol/L (>18 mg/dL), coma (survival <20%), rapid reduction in liver size, respiratory failure, marked prolongation of PT, factor V level < 20%. In acetaminophen overdose, adverse prognosis is suggested by blood pH <7.30, serum creatinine >266 μmol/L (>3 mg/dL), markedly prolonged PT.

TREATMENT Acute Hepatic Failure

Endotracheal intubation often required. Monitor serum glucose—IV D10 or D20 as necessary. Prevent GI bleeding with H_2 receptor antagonists and antacids (maintain gastric pH ≥3.5). In many centers intracranial pressure is monitored—more sensitive than CT in detecting cerebral edema. Value of dexamethasone for cerebral edema unclear; IV mannitol may be beneficial. Liver transplantation should be considered in pts with grades III–IV encephalopathy and other adverse prognostic indicators.

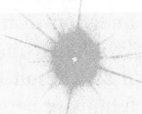

For a more detailed discussion, see Dienstag JL: Acute Viral Hepatitis, Chap. 304, p.2537, and Dienstag JL: Toxic and Drug-Induced Hepatitis, Chap. 305, p. 2558, in HPIM-18.

CHAPTER **164**
Chronic Hepatitis

A group of disorders characterized by a chronic inflammatory reaction in the liver for at least 6 months.

OVERVIEW

■ ETIOLOGY

Hepatitis B virus (HBV), hepatitis C virus (HCV), hepatitis D virus (HDV, delta agent), drugs (methyldopa, nitrofurantoin, isoniazid, dantrolene), autoimmune hepatitis, Wilson's disease, hemochromatosis, α_1-antitrypsin deficiency.

■ HISTOLOGIC CLASSIFICATION

Chronic hepatitis can be classified by *grade* and *stage*. The grade is a histologic assessment of necrosis and inflammatory activity and is based on examination of the liver biopsy. The stage of chronic hepatitis reflects the level of disease progression and is based on the degree of fibrosis (see Table 306-2, p. 2568, HPIM-18).

■ PRESENTATION

Wide clinical spectrum ranging from asymptomatic serum aminotransferase elevations to apparently acute, even fulminant, hepatitis. Common symptoms include fatigue, malaise, anorexia, low-grade fever; jaundice is frequent in severe disease. Some pts may present with complications of cirrhosis: ascites, variceal bleeding, encephalopathy, coagulopathy, and hypersplenism. In chronic HBV or HCV and autoimmune hepatitis, extrahepatic features may predominate.

CHRONIC HEPATITIS B

Follows up to 1–2% of cases of acute hepatitis B in immunocompetent hosts; more frequent in immunocompromised hosts. Spectrum of disease: asymptomatic antigenemia, chronic hepatitis, cirrhosis, hepatocellular cancer; early phase often associated with continued symptoms of hepatitis, elevated aminotransferase levels, presence in serum of HBeAg and HBV DNA, and presence in liver of replicative form of HBV; later phase in some pts may be associated with clinical and biochemical improvement, disappearance of HBeAg and HBV DNA and appearance of anti-HBeAg in serum, and integration of HBV DNA into host hepatocyte genome. In Mediterranean and European countries as well as in Asia, a frequent variant is characterized by readily detectable HBV DNA, but without HBeAg (anti-HBeAg-reactive). Most of these cases are due to a mutation in the pre-C region of the HBV genome that prevents HBeAg synthesis (may appear during course of chronic wild-type HBV infection as a result of immune pressure and may also account for some cases of fulminant hepatitis B). Chronic hepatitis B ultimately leads to cirrhosis in 25–40% of cases (particularly in pts with HDV superinfection or the pre-C mutation) and hepatocellular carcinoma in many of these pts (particularly when chronic infection is acquired early in life).

■ EXTRAHEPATIC MANIFESTATIONS (IMMUNE COMPLEX–MEDIATED)

Rash, urticaria, arthritis, polyarteritis nodosa–like vasculitis, polyneuropathy, glomerulonephritis.

TREATMENT Chronic Hepatitis B

There are currently seven approved drugs for the treatment of chronic HBV: interferon α (IFN-α), pegylated interferon (PEG IFN), lamivudine, adefovir dipivoxil, entecavir, telbivudine, and tenofovir (see Table 164-1). Use of IFN-α has been supplanted by PEG-IFN. Table 164-2 summarizes recommendations for treatment of chronic HBV.

CHRONIC HEPATITIS C

Follows 50–70% of cases of transfusion-associated and sporadic hepatitis C. Clinically mild, often waxing and waning aminotransferase elevations; mild chronic hepatitis on liver biopsy. Extrahepatic manifestations include cryoglobulinemia, porphyria cutanea tarda, membranoproliferative glomerulonephritis, and lymphocytic sialadenitis. Diagnosis confirmed by detecting anti-HCV in serum. May lead to cirrhosis in ≥20% of cases after 20 years.

TREATMENT Chronic Hepatitis C

Therapy should be considered in pts with detectable HCV RNA in serum and biopsy evidence of at least moderate chronic hepatitis (portal or bridging fibrosis). The current agents used in the treatment of chronic HCV, as well as their dosage and duration, depend on HCV genotype (see Tables 164-3 and Table 164-4). For pts with genotype 1, PEG IFN/ribavirin should be combined with a protease inhibitor (boceprevir, telaprevir) where available. Protease inhibitors should never be used alone due to development of resistance. Since the presently available HCV protease inhibitors have not been studied on pts with genotypes other than I, their use in these populations is not recommended (see Table 164-3).

TABLE 164-1 COMPARISON OF PEGYLATED INTERFERON (PEG IFN), LAMIVUDINE, ADEFOVIR, ENTECAVIR, TELBIVUDINE, AND TENOFOVIR THERAPY FOR CHRONIC HEPATITIS B[a]

Feature	PEG IFN[b]	Lamivudine	Adefovir	Entecavir	Telbivudine	Tenofovir
Route of administration	Subcutaneous injection	Oral	Oral	Oral	Oral	Oral
Duration of therapy[c]	48–52 weeks	≥52 weeks	≥48 weeks	≥48 weeks	≥52 weeks	≥48 weeks
Tolerability	Poorly tolerated	Well tolerated	Well tolerated; creatinine monitoring recommended	Well tolerated	Well tolerated	Well tolerated; creatinine monitoring recommended
HBeAg seroconversion						
1 yr Rx	18–20%	16–21%	12%	21%	22%	21%
>1 yr Rx	NA	up to 50% @ 5 yrs	43% @ 3 yrs[d]	31% @ 2 yrs 39% @ 3 yrs	30% @ 2 yrs	27% @ 2 yrs
Log₁₀ HBV DNA reduction (mean copies/mL)						
HBeAg-reactive	4.5	5.5	median 3.5–5	6.9	6.4	6.2
HBeAg-negative	4.1	4.4–4.7	median 3.5–3.9	5.0	5.2	4.6

(continued)

TABLE 164-1 COMPARISON OF PEGYLATED INTERFERON (PEG IFN), LAMIVUDINE, ADEFOVIR, ENTECAVIR, TELBIVUDINE, AND TENOFOVIR THERAPY FOR CHRONIC HEPATITIS B[a] (CONTINUED)

Feature	PEG IFN[b]	Lamivudine	Adefovir	Entecavir	Telbivudine	Tenofovir
HBV DNA PCR negative (<300–400 copies/mL; <1000 copies/mL for adefovir) end of yr 1						
HBeAg-reactive	10–25%	36–44%	13–21%	67% (91% @ 4 yrs)	60%	76%
HBeAg-negative	63%	60–73%	48–77%	90%	88%	93%
ALT normalization at end of yr 1						
HBeAg-reactive	39%	41–75%	48–61%	68%	77%	68%
HBeAg-negative	34–38%	62–79%	48–77%	78%	74%	76%
HBsAg loss yr 1	3–4%	≤1%	0%	2%	<1%	3%
yr 2	12% 5 yr after 1 yr of Rx	no data	5% at yr 5	5%	No data	6%
Histologic improvement (≥2-point reduction in HAI) at yr 1						
HBeAg-reactive	38% 6 months after	49–62%	53–68%	72%	65%	74%
HBeAg-negative	48% 6 months after	61–66%	64%	70%	67%	72%

Viral resistance	None	15-30% @ 1 yr 70% @ 5 yrs	None @ 1 yr 29% at 5 yrs	≤1% @ 1 yr[e] 1.2% @ 5 yr[e]	up to 5% @ yr 1 up to 22% @ yr 2	0% @ yr 1 0% through yr 3
Cost (US $) for 1 yr	~$18,000	~$2500	~$6500	~$8700[f]	~$6000	~$6000

[a]Generally, these comparisons are based on data on each drug tested individually versus placebo in registration clinical trials; because, with rare exception, these comparisons are not based on head-to-head testing of these drugs, relative advantages and disadvantages should be interpreted cautiously.

[b]Although standard IFN-α administered daily or three times a week is approved as therapy for chronic hepatitis B, it has been supplanted by PEG IFN, which is administered once a week and is more effective. Standard IFN has no advantages over PEG IFN.

[c]Duration of therapy in clinical efficacy trials; use in clinical practice may vary.

[d]Because of a computer-generated randomization error that resulted in misallocation of drug versus placebo during the second year of clinical-trial treatment, the frequency of HBeAg seroconversion beyond the first year is an estimate (Kaplan-Meier analysis) based on the small subset in whom adefovir was administered correctly.

[e]7% during a year of therapy (43% at year 4) in lamivudine-resistant pts.

[f]~17,400 for lamivudine-refractory pts.

Abbreviations: ALT, alanine aminotransferase; HAI, histologic activity index; HBeAg, hepatitis B e antigen; HBsAg, hepatitis B surface antigen; HBV, hepatitis B virus; NA, not applicable; PEG IFN, pegylated interferon; PCR, polymerase chain reaction; Rx, therapy; yr, year.

TABLE 164-2 RECOMMENDATIONS FOR TREATMENT OF CHRONIC HEPATITIS B[a]

HBeAg Status	Clinical	HBV DNA (IU/mL)	ALT	Recommendation
HBeAg-reactive [b]		>2 × 10⁴	≤2 × ULN[d]	No treatment; monitor. In pts >40, with family history of hepatocellular carcinoma, and/or ALT persistently at the high end of the twofold range, liver biopsy may help in decision to treat
	Chronic hepatitis	>2 × 10⁴ [d]	>2 × ULN[d]	Treat[e]
	Cirrhosis compensated	>2 × 10³	< or > ULN	Treat[e] with oral agents, not PEG IFN
		<2 × 10³	>ULN	Consider treatment[f]
	Cirrhosis decompensated	Detectable	< or > ULN	Treat[e] with oral agents[g], not PEG IFN; refer for liver transplantation
		Undetectable	< or > ULN	Observe; refer for liver transplantation
HBeAg-negative [b]		≤2 × 10³	≤ULN	Inactive carrier; treatment not necessary
	Chronic hepatitis	>10³	1–>2 × ULN[d]	Consider liver biopsy; treat[h] if biopsy shows moderate to severe inflammation or fibrosis
	Chronic hepatitis	>10⁴	>2 × ULN[d]	Treat[h,i]

Cirrhosis compensated	>2 × 10³	< or > ULN	Treat[e] with oral agents, not PEG IFN
	<2 × 10³	>ULN	Consider treatment[f]
Cirrhosis decompensated	Detectable	< or > ULN	Treat[h] with oral agents[g], not PEG IFN; refer for liver transplantation
	Undetectable	< or > ULN	Observe; refer for liver transplantation

[a]Based on practice guidelines of the American Association for the Study of Liver Diseases (AASLD). Except as indicated in footnotes, these guidelines are similar to those issued by the European Association for the Study of the Liver (EASL).

[b]Liver disease tends to be mild or inactive clinically; most pts do not undergo liver biopsy.

[c]This pattern is common during early decades of life in Asian pts infected at birth.

[d]According to the EASL guidelines, treat if HBV DNA is >2 × 10³ IU/mL and ALT >ULN.

[e]One of the potent oral drugs with a high barrier to resistance (entecavir or tenofovir) or PEG IFN can be used as first-line therapy (see text). These oral agents, but not PEG IFN, should be used for IFN-refractory/intolerant and immunocompromised pts. PEG IFN is administered weekly by SC injection for a year; the oral agents are administered daily for at least a year and continued indefinitely or until at least 6 months after HBeAg seroconversion.

[f]According to EASL guidelines, pts with compensated cirrhosis and detectable HBV DNA at any level, even with normal ALT, are candidates for therapy. Most authorities would treat indefinitely, even in HBeAg-positive disease after HBeAg seroconversion.

[g]Because the emergence of resistance can lead to loss of antiviral benefit and further deterioration in decompensated cirrhosis, a low-resistance regimen is recommended—entecavir or tenofovir monotherapy or combination therapy with the more resistance-prone lamivudine (or telbivudine) plus adefovir. Therapy should be instituted urgently.

[h]Because HBeAg seroconversion is not an option, the goal of therapy is to suppress HBV DNA and maintain a normal ALT. PEG IFN is administered by SC injection weekly for a year; caution is warranted in relying on a 6-month posttreatment interval to define a sustained response, because the majority of such responses are lost thereafter. Oral agents, entecavir or tenofovir, are administered daily, usually indefinitely or, until as very rarely occurs, virologic and biochemical responses are accompanied by HBsAg seroconversion.

[i]For older pts and those with advanced fibrosis, consider lowering the HBV DNA threshold to >2 × 10³ IU/mL.

Abbreviations: ALT, alanine aminotransferase; AASLD, American Association for the Study of Liver Diseases; EASL, European Association for the Study of the Liver; HBeAg, hepatitis B e antigen; HBV, hepatitis B virus; PEG IFN, pegylated interferon; ULN, upper limits of normal.

TABLE 164-3 PEGYLATED INTERFERON α-2A AND α-2B FOR CHRONIC HEPATITIS C

	PEG IFN α-2b	PEG IFN α-2a
PEG size	12 kDa linear	40 kDa branched
Elimination half-life	54 h	65 h
Clearance	725 mL/h	60 mL/h
Dose	1.5 μg/kg (weight-based)	180 μg
Storage	Room temperature	Refrigerated
Ribavirin dose		
Genotype 1	800–1400 mg[a]	1000–1200 mg[b]
Genotype 2/3	800 mg	800 mg
Duration of therapy		
Genotype 1[c]	48 weeks	48 weeks
Genotype 2/3	48 weeks[d]	24 weeks
Efficacy of combination Rx[e]	54%	56%
Genotype 1[c]	40–42%	41–51%
Genotype 2/3	82%	76–78%

[a]In the registration trial for PEG IFN α-2b plus ribavirin, the optimal regimen was 1.5 μg of PEG IFN plus 800 mg of ribavirin; however, a post-hoc analysis of this study suggested that higher ribavirin doses are better. In subsequent trials of PEG IFN α-2b with ribavirin in pts with genotype 1, the following daily ribavirin doses have been validated: 800 mg for pts weighing <65 kg, 1000 mg for pts weighing >65–85 kg, 1200 mg for pts weighing >85–105 kg, and 1400 mg for pts weighing >105 kg.
[b]1000 mg for pts weighing <75 kg; 1200 mg for pts weighing ≥75 kg.
[c]Based on PEG IFN/ribavirin-based regimens without protease inhibitors.
[d]In the registration trial for PEG IFN α-2b plus ribavirin, all pts were treated for 48 weeks; however, data from other trials of standard IFNs and the other PEG IFN demonstrated that 24 weeks suffices for pts with genotypes 2 and 3. For pts with genotype 3 who have advanced fibrosis/cirrhosis and/or high-level HCV RNA, a full 48 weeks is preferable.
[e]Attempts to compare the two PEG IFN preparations based on the results of registration clinical trials are confounded by differences between trials of the two agents in methodologic details (different ribavirin doses, different methods for recording depression, and other side effects) and study-population composition (different proportion with bridging fibrosis/cirrhosis, proportion from the United States versus international, mean weight, proportion with genotype 1, and proportion with high-level HCV RNA). In the head-to-head comparison of the two PEG IFN preparations in the IDEAL trial reported in 2009, the two drugs were comparable in tolerability and efficacy. PEG IFN α-2b was administered at a weekly weight-based dose of 1.0 μg/kg or 1.5 μg/kg, and PEG IFN α-2a was administered at a weekly fixed dose of 180 μg. For PEG IFN α-2b, daily ribavirin weight-based doses ranged between 800–1400 mg based on weight criteria,[a] while for PEG IFN α-2a, daily ribavirin weight-based doses ranged between 1000 and 1200 mg.[b] For the two PEG IFN α-2b study arms, ribavirin dose reductions for ribavirin-associated adverse effects were done in 200- to 400-mg decrements; for PEG IFN α-2a, the ribavirin dose was reduced to 600 mg for intolerability. Sustained virologic responses occurred in 38.0% of the low-dose PEG IFN α-2b group; 39.8% of the standard, full-dose PEG IFN α-2b group; and 40.9% of the PEG IFN α-2a group.

Abbreviations: PEG, polyethylene glycol; PEG IFN, pegylated interferon; HCV RNA, hepatitis C virus RNA.

TABLE 164-4 INDICATIONS AND RECOMMENDATIONS FOR ANTIVIRAL THERAPY OF CHRONIC HEPATITIS C

Standard Indications for Therapy

Detectable HCV RNA (with or without elevated ALT)

Portal/bridging fibrosis or moderate to severe hepatitis on liver biopsy

Re-Treatment Recommended

Genotype 1

Relapsers, partial responders, or nonresponders after a previous course of standard IFN monotherapy or combination standard IFN/ribavirin therapy or PEG IFN/ribavirin

    A course of PEG-IFN/ribavirin plus protease inhibitor as below

Genotype 2, 3, 4

Relapsers after a previous course of standard IFN monotherapy or combination standard IFN/ribavirin therapy

    A course of PEG IFN plus ribavirin

Nonresponders to a previous course of standard IFN monotherapy or combination standard IFN/ribavirin therapy

    A course of PEG IFN plus ribavirin—more likely to achieve a sustained virologic response in Caucasian pts without previous ribavirin therapy, with low baseline HCV RNA levels, with a 2-$\log_{10}$ reduction in HCV RNA during previous therapy, with genotypes 2 and 3, and without reduction in ribavirin dose.

Antiviral Therapy Management Decisions Made on an Individual Basis

Children (age <18 years)—protease inhibitors not recommended

Age >60

Mild hepatitis on liver biopsy

Persons with severe renal insufficiency

Long-Term Maintenance Therapy Recommended

Cryoglobulinemic vasculitis associated with chronic hepatitis C

Long-Term Maintenance Therapy in Nonresponders Not Recommended

Antiviral Therapy Not Recommended

Decompensated cirrhosis

Pregnancy (teratogenicity of ribavirin)

Contraindications to medications

Therapeutic Regimens

HCV genotype 1

    PEG IFN-α2a 180 μg weekly plus ribavirin 1000 mg/d (weight <75 kg) to 1200 mg/d (weight ≥75 kg) or

    PEG IFN-α2b 1.5 μg/kg weekly plus ribavirin 800 mg/d (the dose used in registration clinical trials, but the higher, weight-based ribavirin doses above are recommended for both types of PEG IFN)

(continued)

TABLE 164-4 INDICATIONS AND RECOMMENDATIONS FOR ANTIVIRAL THERAPY OF CHRONIC HEPATITIS C (CONTINUED)

Therapeutic Regimens

Plus a protease inhibitor consisting of one of the following two:

Boceprevir 800 mg three times daily started after a lead in treatment of 4 weeks with PEG IFN/ribavirin

- Pts with undetectable HCV RNA at 8 and 24 weeks should receive triple therapy (PEG-IFN/ribavirin, boceprevir) through week 28 (4 weeks of PEG IFN/ribavirin then 24 weeks of triple therapy). If there is detectable HCV RNA at 4 weeks, continuing therapy through 48 weeks (4 weeks of PEG IFN/ribavirin then 44 weeks of triple therapy) may increase the sustained response rate.

- Pts with detectable HCV RNA at 8 weeks and undetectable at 24 weeks should receive triple therapy (PEG-IFN/ribavirin, boceprevir) through week 36 (4 weeks of PEG IFN/ribavirin then 32 weeks of triple therapy) followed by a return to PEG IFN/ribavirin for 12 more weeks, making a total treatment duration of 48 weeks.

- Pts with cirrhosis who are treatment naïve and have undetectable HCV RNA at week 8 and 24 should continue triple therapy (PEG IFN/ribavirin, boceprevir) through 48 weeks (4 weeks of PEG IFN/ribavirin then 44 weeks of triple therapy).

Telaprevir 750 mg three times daily started at the beginning of therapy without a PEG IFN/ribavirin lead-in.

- Pts with undetectable HCV RNA at 4 and 12 weeks should receive triple therapy (PEG IFN/ribavirin, telaprevir) for 12 weeks then PEG-IFN and ribavirin for another 12 weeks for a total of 24 weeks.

- Pts with cirrhosis who are treatment naïve and have undetectable HCV RNA at 4 and 12 weeks should receive triple therapy for 12 weeks then PEG-FN, ribavirin for another 36 weeks to total 48 weeks.

HCV genotype 1 where protease inhibitors unavailable or contraindicated—48 weeks of therapy

PEG IFN-α2a 180 μg weekly plus ribavirin 1000 mg/d (weight <75 kg) to 1200 mg/d (weight ≥75 kg) or

PEG IFN-α2b 1.5 μg/kg weekly plus ribavirin 800 mg/d (the dose used in registration clinical trials, but the higher, weight-based ribavirin doses above are recommended for both types of PEG IFN)

HCV genotype 4—48 weeks of therapy

PEG IFN-α2a 180 μg weekly plus ribavirin 1000 mg/d (weight <75 kg) to 1200 mg/d (weight ≥75 kg) or

PEG IFN-α2b 1.5 μg/kg weekly plus ribavirin 800 mg/d (the dose used in registration clinical trials, but the higher, weight-based ribavirin doses above are recommended for both types of PEG IFN)

- Treatment should be discontinued in pts who do not achieve an early virologic response at week 12.

TABLE 164-4 INDICATIONS AND RECOMMENDATIONS FOR ANTIVIRAL THERAPY OF CHRONIC HEPATITIS C (CONTINUED)

Therapeutic Regimens

- Pts who do achieve an early virologic response should be retested at week 24 and treatment should be discontinued if HCV RNA remains positive.

HCV genotypes 2 and 3–24 weeks of therapy

　PEG IFN-α2a 180 μg weekly plus ribavirin 800 mg/d or

　PEG IFN-α2b 1.5 μg/kg weekly plus ribavirin 800 mg/d (for pts with genotype 3 who have advanced fibrosis and/or high-level HCV RNA, a full 48 weeks of therapy may be preferable)

For HCV-HIV co-infected pts: 48 weeks, regardless of genotype, of weekly PEG IFN-α2a (180 μg) or PEG IFN-α2b (1.5 μg/kg) plus a daily ribavirin dose of at least 600–800 mg, up to full weight-based 1000- to 1200-mg dosing if tolerated. Protease inhibitors for genotype I are not recommended in this population at the current time due to potential interaction with anti-HIV drugs.

Features Associated with Reduced Responsiveness

Single-nucleotide polymorphism (SNP) T allele (as opposed to C allele) at IL28B locus

Genotype 1

High-level HCV RNA (>2 million copies/mL or >800,000 IU/mL)

Advanced fibrosis (bridging fibrosis, cirrhosis)

Long-duration disease

Age >40

High HCV quasispecies diversity

Immunosuppression

African-American ethnicity

Latino ethnicity

Obesity

Hepatic steatosis

Insulin resistance, type 2 diabetes mellitus

Reduced adherence (lower drug doses and reduced duration of therapy)

Abbreviations: ALT, alanine aminotransferase; HCV, hepatitis C virus; IFN, interferon; PEG IFN, pegylated interferon; IU, international units (1 IU/mL is equivalent to ~2.5 copies/mL).

Monitoring of HCV plasma RNA is useful in assessing response to therapy. The goal of treatment is to eradicate HCV RNA, which is predicted by the absence of HCV RNA by polymerase chain reaction 6 months after stopping treatment ("sustained viral response"). The failure to achieve a 2-log drop in HCV RNA by week 12 of therapy ("early virologic response") makes it unlikely that further therapy will result in a sustained virologic response. Thus, it is recommended that HCV RNA be measured at baseline and at weeks 4, 12, and 24 to assess response to treatment and to aid in decisions regarding treatment duration as well as after 12 weeks of therapy. Pts with genotype I receiving boceprevir should additionally have HCV RNA measured at week 8, as this may influence the duration of therapy. The current consensus view is that therapy can be stopped if an early virologic response is not achieved.

HEPATITIS A

Although hepatitis A rarely causes fulminant hepatic failure, it may do so more frequently in pts with chronic liver disease—especially those with chronic hepatitis B or C. The hepatitis A vaccine is immunogenic and well tolerated in pts with chronic hepatitis. Thus, pts with chronic liver disease, especially those with chronic hepatitis B or C, should be vaccinated against hepatitis A.

AUTOIMMUNE HEPATITIS

■ CLASSIFICATION

Type I: classic autoimmune hepatitis, anti–smooth-muscle and/or anti-nuclear antibodies (ANA). *Type II*: associated with anti-liver/kidney microsomal (anti-LKM) antibodies, which are directed against cytochrome P450IID6 (seen primarily in southern Europe). *Type III* pts lack ANA and anti-LKM, have antibodies reactive with hepatocyte cytokeratins; clinically similar to type I. Criteria have been suggested by an international group for establishing a diagnosis of autoimmune hepatitis.

■ CLINICAL MANIFESTATIONS

Classic autoimmune hepatitis (type I): 80% women, third to fifth decades. Abrupt onset (acute hepatitis) in a third. Insidious onset in two-thirds: progressive jaundice, anorexia, hepatomegaly, abdominal pain, epistaxis, fever, fatigue, amenorrhea. Leads to cirrhosis; >50% 5-year mortality if untreated.

■ EXTRAHEPATIC MANIFESTATIONS

Rash, arthralgias, keratoconjunctivitis sicca, thyroiditis, hemolytic anemia, nephritis.

■ SEROLOGIC ABNORMALITIES

Hypergammaglobulinemia, positive rheumatoid factor, smooth-muscle antibody (40–80%), ANA (20–50%), antimitochondrial antibody (10–20%), false-positive anti-HCV enzyme immunoassay but usually not HCV RNA, atypical p-ANCA. Type II: anti-LKM antibody.

> **TREATMENT** Autoimmune Hepatitis
>
> Indicated for symptomatic disease with biopsy evidence of severe chronic hepatitis (bridging necrosis), marked aminotransferase elevations (5- to 10-fold), and hypergammaglobulinemia. Prednisone or prednisolone 30–60 mg/d PO tapered to 10–15 mg/d over several weeks; often azathioprine 50 mg/d PO is also administered to permit lower

glucocorticoid doses and avoid steroid side effects. Monitor liver function tests monthly. Symptoms may improve rapidly, but biochemical improvement may take weeks or months and subsequent histologic improvement (to lesion of mild chronic hepatitis or normal biopsy) up to 18–24 months. Therapy should be continued for at least 12–18 months. Relapse occurs in at least 50% of cases (re-treat). For frequent relapses, consider maintenance therapy with low-dose glucocorticoids or azathioprine 2 (mg/kg)/d.

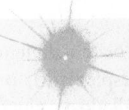

For a more detailed discussion, see Dienstag JL: Chronic Hepatitis, Chap. 306, p. 2567, in HPIM-18.

CHAPTER **165**
Cirrhosis and Alcoholic Liver Disease

CIRRHOSIS

Cirrhosis is defined histopathologically and has a variety of causes, clinical features, and complications. In cirrhosis, there is the development of liver fibrosis to the point that there is architectural distortion with the formation of regenerative nodules, which results in decreased liver function.

■ CAUSES (SEE TABLE 165-1)

■ CLINICAL MANIFESTATIONS
May be absent, with cirrhosis being incidentally found at surgery.

TABLE 165-1 CAUSES OF CIRRHOSIS

Alcoholism	Cardiac cirrhosis
Chronic viral hepatitis	Inherited metabolic liver disease
Hepatitis B	Hemochromatosis
Hepatitis C	Wilson's disease
Autoimmune hepatitis	α_1-Antitrypsin deficiency
Nonalcoholic steatohepatitis	Cystic fibrosis
Biliary cirrhosis	Cryptogenic cirrhosis
Primary biliary cirrhosis	
Primary sclerosing cholangitis	
Autoimmune cholangiopathy	

Symptoms

Anorexia, nausea, vomiting, diarrhea, vague RUQ pain, fatigue, weakness, fever, jaundice, amenorrhea, impotence, infertility.

Signs

Spider telangiectases, palmar erythema, jaundice, scleral icterus, parotid and lacrimal gland enlargement, clubbing, Dupuytren's contracture, gynecomastia, testicular atrophy, hepatosplenomegaly, ascites, gastrointestinal bleeding (e.g., varices), hepatic encephalopathy.

Laboratory Findings

Anemia (microcytic due to blood loss, macrocytic due to folate deficiency; hemolytic called *Zieve's syndrome*), pancytopenia (hypersplenism), prolonged PT, rarely overt DIC; hyponatremia, hypokalemic alkalosis, glucose disturbances, hypoalbuminemia.

■ DIAGNOSTIC STUDIES

Depend on clinical setting. Serum: HBsAg, anti-HBc, anti-HBs, anti-HCV, anti-HDV, Fe, total iron-binding capacity, ferritin, antimitochondrial antibody (AMA), smooth-muscle antibody (SMA), anti-liver/kidney microsomal (anti-LKM) antibody, ANA, ceruloplasmin, α_1 antitrypsin (and phenotyping); abdominal ultrasound with Doppler study, CT or MRI (may show cirrhotic liver, splenomegaly, collaterals, venous thrombosis). Definitive diagnosis often depends on liver biopsy (percutaneous, transjugular, or open).

■ COMPLICATIONS (SEE TABLE 165-2 AND CHAPS. 48, 49, AND 166)

The Child-Pugh scoring system has been used to predict the severity of cirrhosis and the risk of complications (Table 165-3).

TABLE 165-2 COMPLICATIONS OF CIRRHOSIS

Portal hypertension	Coagulopathy
Gastroesophageal varices	Factor deficiency
Portal hypertensive gastropathy	Fibrinolysis
Splenomegaly, hypersplenism	Thrombocytopenia
Ascites	Bone disease
Spontaneous bacterial peritonitis	Osteopenia
Hepatorenal syndrome	Osteoporosis
Type 1	Osteomalacia
Type 2	Hematologic abnormalities
Hepatic encephalopathy	Anemia
Hepatopulmonary syndrome	Hemolysis
Portopulmonary hypertension	Thrombocytopenia
Malnutrition	Neutropenia

TABLE 165-3 CHILD-PUGH CLASSIFICATION OF CIRRHOSIS

Factor	Units	1	2	3
Serum bilirubin	µmol/L	<34	34–51	>51
	mg/dL	<2.0	2.0–3.0	>3.0
Serum albumin	g/L	>35	30–35	<30
	g/dL	>3.5	3.0–3.5	<3.0
Prothrombin time	Seconds prolonged	0–4	4–6	>6
	INR	<1.7	1.7–2.3	>2.3
Ascites		None	Easily controlled	Poorly controlled
Hepatic encephalopathy		None	Minimal	Advanced

Note: The Child-Pugh score is calculated by adding the scores of the five factors and can range from 5–15. Child-Pugh class is either A (a score of 5–6), B (7–9), or C (10 or above). Decompensation indicates cirrhosis with a Child-Pugh score of 7 or more (class B). This level has been the accepted criterion for listing for liver transplantation.

ALCOHOLIC LIVER DISEASE

Excessive alcohol use can cause fatty liver, alcoholic hepatitis, cirrhosis. Alcoholic cirrhosis accounts for about 40% of the deaths due to cirrhosis. History of excessive alcohol use often denied. Severe forms (hepatitis, cirrhosis) associated with ingestion of 160 g/d for 10–20 years; women more susceptible than men and develop advanced liver disease with less alcohol intake. Hepatitis B and C may be cofactors in the development of liver disease. Malnutrition may contribute to development of cirrhosis.

■ FATTY LIVER

Often presents as asymptomatic hepatomegaly and mild elevations in biochemical liver tests. Reverses on withdrawal of ethanol; does not lead to cirrhosis.

■ ALCOHOLIC HEPATITIS

Clinical presentation ranges from asymptomatic to severe liver failure with jaundice, ascites, GI bleeding, and encephalopathy. Typically anorexia, nausea, vomiting, fever, jaundice, tender hepatomegaly. Occasional cholestatic picture mimicking biliary obstruction. Aspartate aminotransferase (AST) usually <400 U/L and more than twofold higher than alanine aminotransferase (ALT). Bilirubin and WBC may be elevated. Diagnosis defined by liver biopsy findings: hepatocyte swelling, alcoholic hyaline (Mallory bodies), infiltration of PMNs, necrosis of hepatocytes, pericentral venular fibrosis.

■ OTHER METABOLIC CONSEQUENCES OF ALCOHOLISM

Increased NADH/NAD ratio leads to lactic acidemia, ketoacidosis, hyperuricemia, hypoglycemia, hypomagnesemia, hypophosphatemia. Also mitochondrial dysfunction, induction of microsomal enzymes resulting in altered drug metabolism, lipid peroxidation leading to membrane damage, hypermetabolic state; many features of alcoholic hepatitis are attributable to toxic effects of acetaldehyde and cytokines (interleukins 1 and 6, and TNF, released because of impaired detoxification of endotoxin).

ADVERSE PROGNOSTIC FACTORS

Critically ill pts with alcoholic hepatitis have 30-day mortality rates >50%. Severe alcoholic hepatitis characterized by PT >5 × above control, bilirubin >137 μmol/L (>8 mg/dL), hypoalbuminemia, azotemia. A discriminant function can be calculated as 4.6 × (pt's PT in seconds) (control PT in seconds) + serum bilirubin (mg/dL). Values ≥32 are associated with poor prognosis. Ascites, variceal hemorrhage, encephalopathy, hepatorenal syndrome predict a poor prognosis.

TREATMENT   Alcoholic Liver Disease

Abstinence is essential; 8500- to 12,500-kJ (2000- to 3000-kcal) diet with 1 g/kg protein (less if encephalopathy). Daily multivitamin, thiamine 100 mg, folic acid 1 mg. Correct potassium, magnesium, and phosphate deficiencies. Transfusions of packed red cells, plasma as necessary. Monitor glucose (hypoglycemia in severe liver disease). Prednisone 40 mg/d or prednisolone 32 mg/d PO for 1 month may be beneficial in severe alcoholic hepatitis with encephalopathy (in absence of GI bleeding, renal failure, infection). Pentoxifylline demonstrated improved survival and led to the inclusion of this agent as an alternative to glucocorticoids in the treatment of severe alcoholic hepatitis. Liver transplantation may be an option in carefully selected cirrhotic pts who have been abstinent >6 months.

PRIMARY BILIARY CIRRHOSIS (PBC)

PBC is a progressive nonsuppurative destructive intrahepatic cholangitis. Strong female predominance, median age of 50 years. Presents as asymptomatic elevation in alkaline phosphatase (better prognosis) or with pruritus, progressive jaundice, consequences of impaired bile excretion, and ultimately cirrhosis and liver failure.

CLINICAL MANIFESTATIONS

Pruritus, fatigue, jaundice, xanthelasma, xanthomata, osteoporosis, steatorrhea, skin pigmentation, hepatosplenomegaly, portal hypertension; elevations in serum alkaline phosphatase, bilirubin, cholesterol, and IgM levels.

ASSOCIATED DISEASES

Sjögren's syndrome, collagen vascular diseases, thyroiditis, glomerulonephritis, pernicious anemia, renal tubular acidosis.

DIAGNOSIS

Antimitochondrial antibodies (AMA) in 90% (directed against enzymes of the pyruvate dehydrogenase complex and other 2-oxo-acid dehydrogenase mitochondrial enzymes). Liver biopsy most important in AMA-negative PBC. Biopsies identify 4 stages: stage 1—destruction of interlobular bile ducts, granulomas; stage 2—ductular proliferation; stage 3—fibrosis; stage 4—cirrhosis.

■ PROGNOSIS

Correlates with age, serum bilirubin, serum albumin, prothrombin time, edema.

TREATMENT ▶ Primary Biliary Cirrhosis

Ursodeoxycholic acid 13–15 mg/kg per day has been shown to improve the biochemical and histologic features of disease. Response is greatest when given early. Cholestyramine 4 g PO with meals for pruritus; in refractory cases consider rifampin, naltrexone, plasmapheresis. Calcium, vitamin D, and bisphosphonates are given for osteoporosis. Liver transplantation for end-stage disease.

LIVER TRANSPLANTATION

Consider in the absence of contraindications for chronic, irreversible, progressive liver disease or fulminant hepatic failure when no alternative therapy is available (Table 165-4).

■ CONTRAINDICATIONS (SEE TABLE 165-5)

TABLE 165-4 INDICATIONS FOR LIVER TRANSPLANTATION

Children	Adults
Biliary atresia	Primary biliary cirrhosis
Neonatal hepatitis	Secondary biliary cirrhosis
Congenital hepatic fibrosis	Primary sclerosing cholangitis
Alagille syndrome[a]	Autoimmune hepatitis
Byler disease[b]	Caroli disease[c]
α_1-Antitrypsin deficiency	Cryptogenic cirrhosis
Inherited disorders of metabolism	Chronic hepatitis with cirrhosis
Wilson's disease	Hepatic vein thrombosis
Tyrosinemia	Fulminant hepatitis
Glycogen storage diseases	Alcoholic cirrhosis
Lysosomal storage diseases	Chronic viral hepatitis
Protoporphyria	Primary hepatocellular malignancies
Crigler-Najjar disease type I	Hepatic adenomas
Familial hypercholesterolemia	Nonalcoholic steatohepatitis
Primary hyperoxaluria type I	Familial amyloid polyneuropathy
Hemophilia	

[a]Arteriohepatic dysplasia, with paucity of bile ducts, and congenital malformations, including pulmonary stenosis.
[b]Intrahepatic cholestasis, progressive liver failure, mental and growth retardation.
[c]Multiple cystic dilatations of the intrahepatic biliary tree.

TABLE 165-5 CONTRAINDICATIONS TO LIVER TRANSPLANTATION

Absolute	Relative
Uncontrolled extrahepatobiliary infection	Age >70
Active, untreated sepsis	Prior extensive hepatobiliary surgery
Uncorrectable, life-limiting congenital anomalies	Portal vein thrombosis
Active substance or alcohol abuse	Renal failure not attributable to liver disease
Advanced cardiopulmonary disease	Previous extrahepatic malignancy (not including nonmelanoma skin cancer)
Extrahepatobiliary malignancy (not including nonmelanoma skin cancer)	Severe obesity
Metastatic malignancy to the liver	Severe malnutrition/wasting
Cholangiocarcinoma	Medical noncompliance
AIDS	HIV seropositivity with failure to control HIV viremia or CD4 <100/µL
Life-threatening systemic diseases	Intrahepatic sepsis
	Severe hypoxemia secondary to right-to-left intrapulmonary shunts (Po_2<50 mmHg)
	Severe pulmonary hypertension (mean pulmonary artery pressure >35 mmHg)
	Uncontrolled psychiatric disorder

■ SELECTION OF DONOR

Matched for ABO blood group compatibility and liver size (reduced-size grafts may be used, esp. in children). Should be negative for HIV, HBV, and HCV. Living-donor transplant has gained increased popularity with transplantation of the right hepatic lobe from a healthy adult donor to an adult. Living-donor transplant of the left lobe accounts for one-third of all liver transplants in children.

■ IMMUNOSUPPRESSION

Various combinations of tacrolimus or cyclosporine and glucocorticoids, sirolimus, mycophenolate mofetil, or OKT3 (monoclonal antithymocyte globulin).

■ MEDICAL COMPLICATIONS AFTER TRANSPLANTATION

Liver graft dysfunction (primary nonfunction, acute or chronic rejection, ischemia, hepatic artery thrombosis, biliary obstruction or leak, recurrence of primary disease); infections (bacterial, viral, fungal, opportunistic); renal dysfunction; neuropsychiatric disorders, cardiovascular instability, pulmonary compromise.

■ SUCCESS RATE

Currently, 5-year survival rates exceed 60%; less for certain conditions (e.g., chronic hepatitis B, hepatocellular carcinoma).

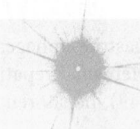

For a more detailed discussion, see Bacon BR: Cirrhosis and Its Complications, Chap. 308, p. 2592; Mailliard ME, Sorrell MF: Alcoholic Liver Disease, Chap. 307, p. 2589; Dienstag JL, Chung RT: Liver Transplantation, Chap. 310, p. 2606, in HPIM-18.

CHAPTER **166**
Portal Hypertension

Portal hypertension is defined as elevation of the hepatic venous pressure gradient to >5 mmHg, which occurs as a consequence of cirrhosis (Chap. 165). It is caused by increased intrahepatic resistance to the passage of blood flow through the liver due to cirrhosis together with increased splanchnic blood flow due to vasodilatation within the splanchnic vascular bed.

■ **CLASSIFICATION (SEE TABLE 166-1)**

TABLE 166-1 CLASSIFICATION OF PORTAL HYPERTENSION

Prehepatic
Portal vein thrombosis
Splenic vein thrombosis
Massive splenomegaly (Banti's syndrome)
Hepatic
Presinusoidal
Schistosomiasis
Congenital hepatic fibrosis
Sinusoidal
Cirrhosis—many causes
Alcoholic hepatitis
Postsinusoidal
Hepatic sinusoidal obstruction (venoocclusive syndrome)
Posthepatic
Budd-Chiari syndrome
Inferior vena caval webs
Cardiac causes
Restrictive cardiomyopathy
Constrictive pericarditis
Severe congestive heart failure

■ CONSEQUENCES

The primary complications of portal hypertension are gastroesophageal varices with hemorrhage, ascites (Chap. 49), hypersplenism, hepatic encephalopathy, spontaneous bacterial peritonitis (Chap. 49), hepatorenal syndrome (Chap. 49), hepatocellular carcinoma (Chap. 78).

ESOPHAGOGASTRIC VARICES

About one-third of pts with cirrhosis have varices, and one-third of pts with varices will develop bleeding. Bleeding is a life-threatening complication; risk of bleeding correlates with variceal size and location, the degree of portal hypertension (portal venous pressure >12 mmHg), and the severity of cirrhosis, e.g., Child-Pugh classification (see Table 165-3).

■ DIAGNOSIS

Esophagogastroscopy: procedure of choice for evaluation of upper GI hemorrhage in pts with known or suspected portal hypertension. *Celiac* and *mesenteric arteriography* are alternatives when massive bleeding prevents endoscopy and to evaluate portal vein patency (portal vein may also be studied by ultrasound with Doppler and MRI).

TREATMENT	Esophagogastric Varices

See Chap. 47 for general measures to treat GI bleeding.

CONTROL OF ACUTE BLEEDING

Choice of approach depends on clinical setting and availability.

1. Endoscopic intervention is employed as first-line treatment to control bleeding acutely. Endoscopic variceal ligation (EVL) is used to control acute bleeding in >90% of cases. EVL is less successful when varices extend into proximal stomach. Some endoscopists will use variceal injection (sclerotherapy) as initial therapy, particularly when bleeding is vigorous.

2. Vasoconstricting agents: somatostatin or octreotide (50–100 µg/h by continuous infusion).

3. Balloon tamponade (Blakemore-Sengstaken or Minnesota tube). Can be used when endoscopic therapy is not immediately available or in pts who need stabilization prior to endoscopic therapy. Complications—obstruction of pharynx, asphyxiation, aspiration, esophageal ulceration. Generally reserved for massive bleeding, failure of vasopressin and/or endoscopic therapy.

4. Transjugular intrahepatic portosystemic shunt (TIPS)—portacaval shunt placed by interventional radiologic technique, reserved for failure of other approaches; risk of hepatic encephalopathy (20–30%), shunt stenosis or occlusion (30–60%), infection.

PREVENTION OF RECURRENT BLEEDING

1. EVL should be repeated until obliteration of all varices is accomplished.

2. Propranolol or nadolol—nonselective beta blockers that act as portal venous antihypertensives; may decrease the risk of variceal hemorrhage and mortality due to hemorrhage.

3. TIPS—regarded as useful "bridge" to liver transplantation in pt who has failed pharmacologic therapy and is awaiting a donor liver.

4. Portosystemic shunt surgery used less commonly with the advent of TIPS; could be considered for pts with good hepatic synthetic function.

PREVENTION OF INITIAL BLEED

For pts at high risk of variceal bleeding, consider prophylaxis with EVL and/or nonselective beta blockers.

HEPATIC ENCEPHALOPATHY

An alteration in mental status and cognitive function occurring in the presence of liver failure; may be acute and reversible or chronic and progressive.

◼ CLINICAL FEATURES

Confusion, slurred speech, change in personality that can include being violent and hard to manage, being sleepy and difficult to arouse, asterixis (flapping tremor). Can progress to coma; initially responsive to noxious stimuli, later unresponsive.

◼ PATHOPHYSIOLOGY

Gut-derived neurotoxins that are not removed by the liver because of vascular shunting and decreased hepatic mass reach the brain and cause the symptoms of hepatic encephalopathy. Ammonia levels are typically elevated in encephalopathy, but the correlation between the severity of liver disease and height of ammonia levels is often poor. Other compounds that may contribute include false neurotransmitters and mercaptans.

◼ PRECIPITANTS

GI bleeding, azotemia, constipation, high-protein meal, hypokalemic alkalosis, CNS depressant drugs (e.g., benzodiazepines and barbiturates), hypoxia, hypercarbia, sepsis.

TREATMENT   Hepatic Encephalopathy

Remove precipitants; correct electrolyte imbalances. Lactulose (nonabsorbable disaccharide) results in colonic acidification and diarrhea and is the mainstay of treatment; goal is to produce 2–3 soft stools per day. Poorly absorbed antibiotics are often used in pts who do not tolerate lactulose, with alternating administration of neomycin and metronidazole being used to reduce the individual side effects of each. Rifaximin has recently also been used; zinc supplementation is sometimes helpful. Liver transplantation when otherwise indicated.

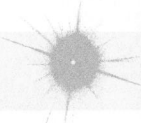

For a more detailed discussion, see Bacon BR: Cirrhosis and Its Complications, Chap. 308, p. 2592; in HPIM-18.

CHAPTER **167**
Diseases of Immediate-Type Hypersensitivity

■ DEFINITION

These diseases result from IgE-dependent release of mediators from sensitized basophils and mast cells upon contact with an offending antigen (allergen). Associated disorders include anaphylaxis, allergic rhinitis, urticaria, asthma, and eczematous (atopic) dermatitis. Atopic allergy implies a familial tendency to the development of these disorders singly or in combination.

■ PATHOPHYSIOLOGY

IgE binds to the surface of mast cells and basophils through a high-affinity receptor. Cross-linking of this IgE by antigen causes cellular activation with subsequent release of preformed and newly synthesized mediators including histamine, prostaglandins, leukotrienes (C_4, D_4, and E_4, collectively known as *slow-reacting substance of anaphylaxis*—SRS-A), acid hydrolases, neutral proteases, proteoglycans, and cytokines (Fig. 167-1). These mediators have been

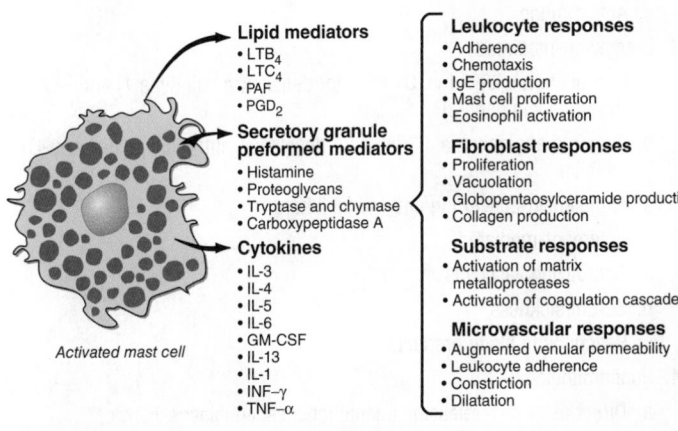

FIGURE 167-1 Bioactive mediators of three categories generated by IgE-dependent activation of murine mast cells can elicit common but sequential target cell effects leading to acute and sustained inflammatory responses. LT, leukotriene; PAF, platelet-activating factor; PGD_2, prostaglandin D_2; IL, interleukin; GM-CSF, granulocyte-macrophage colony-stimulating factor; INF, interferon; TNF, tumor necrosis factor.

implicated in many pathophysiologic events associated with immediate-type hypersensitivity, such as vasodilatation, increased vasopermeability, smooth-muscle contraction, and chemotaxis of neutrophils and other inflammatory cells. The clinical manifestations of each allergic reaction depend largely on the anatomic site(s) and time course of mediator release.

URTICARIA AND ANGIOEDEMA

■ DEFINITION

May occur together or separately. *Urticaria* involves only the superficial dermis and presents as circumscribed wheals with raised serpiginous borders and blanched centers; wheals may coalesce. *Angioedema* involves deeper layers of skin and may include subcutaneous tissue. The classification of urticaria-angioedema focuses on mechanisms that elicit clinical disease and can be useful for differential diagnosis (see Table 167-1).

■ PATHOPHYSIOLOGY

Characterized by massive edema formation in the dermis (and subcutaneous tissue in angioedema). Presumably the edema is due to increased vasopermeability caused by mediator release from mast cells or other cell populations.

TABLE 167-1 CLASSIFICATION OF URTICARIA AND/OR ANGIOEDEMA

1. IgE-dependent
    a. Specific antigen sensitivity (pollens, foods, drugs, fungi, molds, Hymenoptera venom, helminths)
    b. Physical: dermographism, cold, solar
    c. Autoimmune
2. Bradykinin-mediated
    a. Hereditary angioedema: C1 inhibitor deficiency: null (type 1) and dysfunctional (type 2)
    b. Acquired angioedema: C1 inhibitor deficiency: anti-idiotype and anti-C1 inhibitor
    c. Angiotensin-converting enzyme inhibitors
3. Complement-mediated
    a. Necrotizing vasculitis
    b. Serum sickness
    c. Reactions to blood products
4. Nonimmunologic
    a. Direct mast cell–releasing agents (opiates, antibiotics, curare, D-tubocurarine, radiocontrast media)
    b. Agents that alter arachidonic acid metabolism (aspirin and nonsteroidal anti-inflammatory agents, azo dyes, and benzoates)
5. Idiopathic

■ DIAGNOSIS

History, with special attention to possible offending exposures and/or ingestion as well as the duration of lesions. Vasculitic urticaria typically persists >72 h, whereas conventional urticaria often lasts <48 h.

- Skin testing to food and/or inhalant antigens.
- Physical provocation, e.g., challenge with vibratory or cold stimuli.
- Laboratory exam: complement levels, ESR (neither an elevated ESR nor hypocomplementemia is observed in IgE-mediated urticaria or angioedema); C1 inhibitor (C1INH) testing for deficiency of C1INH antigen (type 1) or a nonfunctional protein (type 2) if history suggests hereditary angioedema; cryoglobulins, hepatitis B antigen, and antibody studies; autoantibody screen.
- Skin biopsy may be necessary.

■ DIFFERENTIAL DIAGNOSIS

Atopic dermatitis, contact sensitivity, cutaneous mastocytosis (urticaria pigmentosa), systemic mastocytosis.

■ PREVENTION

Identification and avoidance of offending agent(s), if possible.

TREATMENT   Urticaria and Angioedema

- H_1 antihistamines may be helpful: e.g., chlorpheniramine up to 24 mg PO daily; diphenhydramine 25–50 mg PO qid; hydroxyzine 40–200 mg PO daily; cyproheptadine 8–32 mg PO daily; or the low or nonsedating class, e.g., loratidine 10 mg PO daily; desloratidine 5mg PO daily; fexofenadine up to 180 mg PO daily; cetirizine 5–10 mg PO daily; levocetirizine 5 mg PO daily.
- H_2 antihistamines: e.g., ranitidine 150 mg PO bid may add benefit.
- Leukotriene receptor antagonists can be add-on therapy: e.g., montelukast 10 mg daily or zafirlukast 20 mg bid.
- Topical glucocorticoids are of no value in the management of urticaria and/or angioedema. Systemic glucocorticoids should not be used in the treatment of idiopathic, allergen-induced, or physical urticaria because of their long-term toxicity.

ALLERGIC RHINITIS

■ DEFINITION

An inflammatory condition of the nose characterized by sneezing, rhinorrhea, and obstruction of nasal passages; may be associated with conjunctival and pharyngeal itching, lacrimation, and sinusitis. Seasonal allergic rhinitis is commonly caused by exposure to pollens, especially from grasses, trees, weeds, and molds. Perennial allergic rhinitis is frequently due to contact with house dust (containing dust mite antigens) and animal danders.

■ PATHOPHYSIOLOGY

Deposition of pollens and other allergens on nasal mucosa of sensitized individuals results in IgE-dependent triggering of mast cells with subsequent release of mediators that cause development of mucosal hyperemia, swelling, and fluid transudation. Inflammation of nasal mucosal surface probably allows penetration of allergens deeper into tissue, where they contact perivenular mast cells. Obstruction of sinus ostia may result in development of secondary sinusitis, with or without bacterial infection.

■ DIAGNOSIS

Accurate history of symptoms correlated with time of seasonal pollination of plants in a given locale; special attention must be paid to other potentially sensitizing antigens such as materials associated with pets, e.g., dander.

- Physical examination: nasal mucosa may be boggy or erythematous; nasal polyps may be present; conjunctivae may be inflamed or edematous; manifestations of other allergic conditions (e.g., asthma, eczema) may be present.
- Skin tests to inhalant and/or food antigens.
- Nasal smear may reveal large numbers of eosinophils; presence of neutrophils may suggest infection.
- Total and specific serum IgE (as assessed by immunoassay) may be elevated.

■ DIFFERENTIAL DIAGNOSIS

Vasomotor rhinitis, URI, irritant exposure, pregnancy with nasal mucosal edema, rhinitis medicamentosa, non-allergic rhinitis with eosinophilia, rhinitis due to α-adrenergic agents.

■ PREVENTION

Identification and avoidance of offending antigen(s).

TREATMENT	Allergic Rhinitis

- Older antihistamines (e.g., chlorpheniramine, diphenhydramine) are effective but cause sedation and psychomotor impairment including reduced hand-eye coordination and impaired automobile driving skills. Newer anti-histamines (e.g., fexofenadine, loratadine, desloratadine, cetirizine, levocetirizine, olopatadine, bilastine, and azelastine) are equally effective but are less sedating and more H1 specific.
- Oral sympathomimetics, e.g., pseudoephedrine 30–60 mg PO qid; may aggravate hypertension; combination antihistamine/decongestant preparations may balance side effects and provide improved pt convenience.
- Topical vasoconstrictors—should be used sparingly due to rebound congestion and chronic rhinitis associated with prolonged use.
- Topical nasal glucocorticoids, e.g., beclomethasone, 2 sprays in each nostril bid, or fluticasone, 2 sprays in each nostril once daily.
- Topical nasal cromolyn sodium, 1–2 sprays in each nostril qid.
- Montelukast 10 mg PO daily is approved for seasonal and perennial rhinitis.
- Hyposensitization therapy, if more conservative therapy is unsuccessful.

SYSTEMIC MASTOCYTOSIS

■ DEFINITION

A systemic disorder characterized by mast cell hyperplasia; generally involves bone marrow, skin, GI mucosa, liver, and spleen. Classified as (1) indolent, (2) associated with concomitant hematologic disorder, (3) aggressive, (4) mastocytic leukemia, and (5) mast cell sarcoma.

■ PATHOPHYSIOLOGY AND CLINICAL MANIFESTATIONS

The clinical manifestations of systemic mastocytosis are due to tissue occupancy by the mast cell mass, the tissue response to that mass (fibrosis), and the release of bioactive substances acting both locally (urticaria pigmentosa, crampy abdominal pain, gastritis, peptic ulcer) and at distal sites (headache, pruritus, flushing, vascular collapse). Clinical manifestations may be aggravated by alcohol, use of narcotics (e.g., codeine), ingestion of NSAIDs.

■ DIAGNOSIS

Although the diagnosis of mastocytosis may be suspected on the basis of clinical and laboratory findings, it can be established only by tissue biopsy (usually bone marrow biopsy). The diagnostic criteria for systemic mastocytosis are shown in Table 167-2. Laboratory studies that can help support a diagnosis of systemic mastocytosis include measurement of urinary or blood levels of mast cell products such as histamine, histamine metabolites, prostaglandin D_2 (PGD_2) metabolites, or mast cell tryptase. Other studies including bone scan, skeletal survey, GI contrast studies may be helpful. Other flushing disorders (e.g., carcinoid syndrome, pheochromocytoma) should be excluded.

TREATMENT Systemic Mastocystosis

- H_1 and H_2 antihistamines.
- Proton pump inhibitors for gastric hypersecretion.
- Oral cromolyn sodium for diarrhea and abdominal pain.
- NSAIDs (in nonsensitive pts) may help by blocking PGD_2 production.

TABLE 167-2 DIAGNOSTIC CRITERIA FOR SYSTEMIC MASTOCYTOSIS[a]

Major: Multifocal dense infiltrates of mast cells in bone marrow or other extracutaneous tissues with confirmation by immunodetection of tryptase or metachromasia
Minor: Abnormal mast cell morphology with a spindle shape and/or multilobed or eccentric nucleus
Aberrant mast cell surface phenotype with expression of CD25 and CD2 (IL-2 receptor) in addition to C117 (c-*kit*)
Detection of codon 816 mutation in peripheral blood cells, bone marrow cells, or lesional tissue
Total serum tryptase (mostly alpha) >20 ng/mL

[a]Diagnosis requires either major and one minor or three minor criteria.

- Systemic glucocorticoids may help, but frequently are associated with complications.
- Hydroxyurea to reduce mast cell lineage progenitors may have merit in aggressive systemic mastocytosis.
- Chemotherapy for frank leukemias.

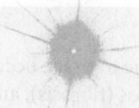

For a more detailed discussion, see Austen KF: Allergies, Anaphylaxis, and Systemic Mastocytosis, Chap. 317, p. 2707, in HPIM-18.

CHAPTER **168**
Primary Immune Deficiency Diseases

DEFINITION

Primary immunodeficiencies are genetic diseases that can involve all possible aspects of immune responses, from innate through adaptive, as well as cell differentiation, effector function, and immune regulation (Table 168-1). The consequences of primary immunodeficiencies vary widely as a function of the molecules that are defective and include vulnerability to infection by pathogenic and opportunistic infection, immunopathologic responses such as allergy, lymphoproliferations, and autoimmunity, and increased risk of cancers. The locations and sites of infection and the causal microorganisms often aid the physician in diagnosis.

DIAGNOSIS (SEE TABLE 168-2)

CLASSIFICATION (TABLE 168-1)

■ DEFICIENCIES OF THE INNATE IMMUNE SYSTEM
Account for ~10% of all primary immunodeficiencies (Table 168-1).

■ DEFICENCES OF THE ADAPTIVE IMMUNE SYSTEM

T Lymphocyte Deficiency Syndromes

Severe Combined Immunodeficiency (SCID) Group of rare primary immunodeficiencies characterized by a profound block in T cell development as a consequence of an intrinsic deficiency. Clinical consequences occur within 3–6 months following birth. The most frequent clinical manifestations are recurrent oral candidiasis, failure to thrive, protracted diarrhea, *Pneumocystis jiroveci* infections. Six distinct causative mechanisms have been identified:

TABLE 168-1 CLASSIFICATION OF PRIMARY IMMUNE DEFICIENCY DISEASES

Deficiencies of the Innate Immune System	
• Phagocytic cells	
– Impaired production: severe congenital neutropenia (SCN)	
– Asplenia	
– Impaired adhesion: leukocyte adhesion deficiency (LAD)	
– Impaired killing: chronic granulomatous disease (CGD)	
• Innate immunity receptors and signal transduction	
– Defects in Toll-like receptor signaling	
– Mendelian susceptibility to mycobacterial disease	
• Complement deficiencies	
– Classic, alternative, and lectin pathways	
– Lytic phase	

Deficiencies of the Adaptive Immune System	
• T lymphocytes	
– Impaired development	Severe combined immune deficiencies (SCIDs) DiGeorge syndrome
– Impaired survival, migration, function	Severe combined immunodeficiencies
	Hyper-IgE syndrome (autosomal dominant)
	CD40 ligand deficiency
	Wiskott-Aldrich syndrome
	Ataxia-telangiectasia and other DNA repair deficiencies
• B lymphocytes	
– Impaired development	XL and AR agammaglobulinemia
– Impaired function	Hyper-IgM syndrome
	Common variable immunodeficiency (CVID)
	IgA deficiency

Regulatory Defects	
• Innate immunity	Autoinflammatory syndromes (outside the scope of this chapter)
	Severe colitis
• Adaptive immunity	Hemophagocytic lymphohistiocytosis (HLH)
	Autoimmune lymphoproliferation syndrome (ALPS)
	Autoimmunity and inflammatory diseases (IPEX, APECED)

Abbreviations: APECED, autoimmune polyendocrinopathy candidiasis ectodermal dysplasia; AR, autosomal recessive; IPEX, immunodysregulation polyendocrinopathy enteropathy X-linked syndrome; XL, X-linked.

TABLE 168-2 TEST MOST FREQUENTLY USED TO DIAGNOSE A PRIMARY IMMUNE DEFICIENCY (PID)

Test	Information	PID Disease
Blood cell counts and cell morphology	Neutrophil counts	↓Severe congenital neutropenia, ↑↑ LAD
	Lymphocyte counts*	T cell ID
	Eosinophilia	WAS, Hyper-IgE syndrome
	Howell-Jolly bodies	Asplenia
Chest x-ray	Thymic shadow	SCID, DiGeorge syndrome
	Costochondral junctions	Adenosine deaminase deficiency
Bone x-ray	Metaphyseal ends	Cartilage hair hypoplasia
Immunoglobulin serum levels	IgG, IgA, IgM	B cell ID
	IgE	Hyper-IgE syndrome, WAS, T cell ID
Lymphocyte phenotype	T, B lymphocyte counts	T cell ID, agammaglobulinemia
Dihydrorhodamine fluorescence (DHR) assay	Reactive oxygen species production by PMN	Chronic granulomatous disease
Nitroblue tetrazolium (NBT) assay		
CH50, AP50	Classic and alternative complement pathways	Complement deficiencies
Ultrasonography of the abdomen	Spleen size	Asplenia

*Normal counts vary with age. For example, the lymphocyte count is between 3000 and 9000/μL of blood below the age of 3 months and between 1500 and 2500/μL in adults.
Abbreviations: ID, immunodeficiency; LAD, leukocyte adhesion deficiency; PMNs, polymorphonuclear leukocytes; SCID, severe combined immunodeficiency; WAS, Wiskott-Aldrich syndrome.

- *Cytokine signaling deficiency*: Most frequent SCID accounting for 40–50% of cases with the absence of T and NK cells. These pts have a deficiency in the gamma chain receptor shared by several cytokine receptors (interleukins 2, 4, 7, 9, 15, 21). The same phenotype seen in X-linked SCID can be inherited as an autosomal recessive disease due to mutations in the JAK3 protein kinase gene.
- *Purine metabolism deficiency*: About 20% of SCID pts are deficient in adenosine deaminase (ADA) due to mutations in the *ADA* gene.
- *Defective rearrangements of T and B cell receptors*: Account for ~20–30% of SCID cases. Main deficiencies involve recombinase activating genes

(RAG-1, RAG-2) DNA dependent protein kinase, DNA ligase 4, and Cernunnos deficiencies.
- *Defective (pre-) T cell receptor signaling in the thymus*: Rare deficiencies in CD3 subunits associated with the (pre) TCR and CD45.
- *Reticular dysgenesis*: Extremely rare. Results from adenylate kinase 2 deficiency.
- *Defective egress of lymphocytes*: Defective egress of T cells from the thymus resulting from deficiency in coronin-1A.

TREATMENT Severe Combined Immunodeficiency

Curative treatment relies on hematopoietic stem cell transplant (HSCT).

Other T cell–Related Primary Immunodeficiencies
- *DiGeorge syndrome*: Maldevelopment of the thymus.
- *Hyper-IgE syndrome*
- *CD40 ligand deficiency*
- *Wiskott-Aldrich syndrome*
- *Ataxia-telangiectasia and other DNA repair deficiencies*

TREATMENT Other T Cell Immunodeficiencies

Treatment is complex and largely investigational. HSCT plays a role in some diseases. Live vaccines and blood transfusions containing viable T cells should be strictly avoided. Prophylaxis for *Pneumocystis jiroveci* pneumonia should be considered in selected pts with severe T cell deficiency.

B Lymphocyte Deficiency Syndromes

Deficiencies that affect B cells are the most common primary immunodeficiencies and account for ~60–70% of all cases. Defective antibody production predisposes to invasive pyogenic bacterial infections as well as recurrent sinus and pulmonary infections. Complete lack of antibody production (agammaglobulinemia) predisposes to disseminated enteroviral infections causing meningoencephalitis, hepatitis, and a dermatomyositis-like disease. Diagnosis relies on the determination of serum Ig level.
- *Agammaglobulinemia*: Due to an X-linked mutation in the Bruton's tyrosine kinase (Btk) gene in 85% of cases.
- *Hyper IgM*: In most pts this syndrome results from an X linked defect in the gene encoding CD40 ligand. Pts exhibit normal or increased serum IgM with low or absent IgG and IgA.
- *Common variable immunodeficiency (CVID)*: Heterogeneous group of syndromes characterized by low serum levels of one or more Ig isotypes. Prevalence estimated to be 1 in 20,000. Besides infections, pts may develop lymphoproliferation, granulomatous lesions, colitis, antibody-mediated autoimmune diseases, and lymphomas.
- *Isolated IgA deficiency*: Most common immunodeficiency; affects 1 in 600 people. The majority of affected individuals do not have increased

infections; antibodies against IgA may lead to anaphylaxis during transfusion of blood or plasma; may progress to CVID.
- *Selective antibody deficiency to polysaccharide antigens.*

TREATMENT   **B Cell/Immunoglobulin Deficiency Syndromes**

IV immunoglobulin administration (only for pts who have recurrent
bacterial infections and are deficient in IgG):
- Starting dose 400–500 mg/kg given every 3–4 weeks
- Adjust dose to keep trough IgG level 800 mg/dL
- SC administration usually once a week can be considered in selected pts.

■ REGULATORY DEFECTS

Rare but increasingly described primary immunodeficiencies that cause
homeostatic dysregulation of the immune system either alone or in association with increased vulnerability to infection (Table 168-1).

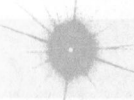

For a more detailed discussion, see Fischer A: Primary Immune
Deficiency Diseases, Chap. 316, p. 2695, in HPIM-18.

CHAPTER **169**
SLE, RA, and Other Connective Tissue Diseases

CONNECTIVE TISSUE DISEASE

■ DEFINITION

Heterogeneous disorders that share certain common features, including
inflammation of skin, joints, and other structures rich in connective tissue;
as well as altered patterns of immunoregulation, including production of
autoantibodies and abnormalities of cell-mediated immunity. While distinct clinical entities can be defined, manifestations may vary considerably
from one pt to the next, and overlap of clinical features between and among
specific diseases can occur.

SYSTEMIC LUPUS ERYTHEMATOSUS (SLE)

■ DEFINITION AND PATHOGENESIS

Disease of unknown etiology in which tissues and cells undergo damage
mediated by tissue-binding autoantibodies and immune complexes. Genetic,
environmental, and sex hormonal factors are likely of pathogenic importance.
T and B cell hyperactivity, production of autoantibodies with specificity for
nuclear antigenic determinants, and abnormalities of T cell function occur.

■ CLINICAL MANIFESTATIONS

90% of pts are women, usually of child-bearing age; more common in blacks than whites. Course of disease is often characterized by periods of exacerbation and relative quiescence. May involve virtually any organ system and have a wide range of disease severity. Common features include:

- *Constitutional*—fatigue, fever, malaise, weight loss
- *Cutaneous*—rashes (especially malar "butterfly" rash), photosensitivity, vasculitis, alopecia, oral ulcers
- *Arthritis*—inflammatory, symmetric, nonerosive
- *Hematologic*—anemia (may be hemolytic), neutropenia, thrombocytopenia, lymphadenopathy, splenomegaly, venous or arterial thrombosis
- *Cardiopulmonary*—pleuritis, pericarditis, myocarditis, endocarditis. Pts are also at increased risk of myocardial infarction usually due to accelerated atherosclerosis.
- *Nephritis*—classification is primarily histologic (Table 319-2, p. 2727, in HPIM-18)
- *GI*—peritonitis, vasculitis
- *Neurologic*—organic brain syndromes, seizures, psychosis, cerebritis

Drug-Induced Lupus

A clinical and immunologic picture similar to spontaneous SLE may be induced by drugs; in particular: procainamide, hydralazine, isoniazid, chlorpromazine, methyldopa, minocycline, anti-TNF agents. Features are predominantly constitutional, joint, and pleuropericardial; CNS and renal disease are rare. All pts have antinuclear antibodies (ANA); antihistone antibodies may be present, but antibodies to dsDNA and hypocomplementemia are uncommon. Most pts improve following withdrawal of offending drug.

■ EVALUATION

- Hx and physical exam
- Presence of ANA is a cardinal feature, but a (+) ANA is not specific for SLE. Laboratory assessment should include: CBC, ESR, ANA and ANA subtypes (antibodies to dsDNA, ssDNA, Sm, Ro, La, histone), complement levels (C3, C4, CH50), serum immunoglobulins, VDRL, PT, PTT, anticardiolipin antibody, lupus anticoagulant, urinalysis.
- Appropriate radiographic studies
- ECG
- Consideration of renal biopsy if evidence of glomerulonephritis

■ DIAGNOSIS

Made in the presence of four or more published criteria (Table 319-3, p. 2728, in HPIM-18).

TREATMENT	Systemic Lupus Erythematosus

Choice of therapy is based on type and severity of disease manifestations. Goals are to control acute, severe flares and to develop maintenance strategies whereby symptoms are suppressed to an acceptable level. Treatment choices depend on (1) whether disease is life-threatening or likely to cause organ damage; (2) whether manifestations are reversible; and (3) the best approach to prevent complications of disease and treatment (Fig. 319-2, p. 2729, and Table 319-5, p. 2732, in HPIM-18).

CONSERVATIVE THERAPIES FOR NON-LIFE-THREATENING DISEASE

- *NSAIDs* (e.g., ibuprofen 400–800 mg three to four times a day). Must consider renal, GI, and cardiovascular complications.
- *Antimalarials* (hydroxychloroquine 400 mg/d)—may improve constitutional, cutaneous, articular manifestations. Ophthalmologic evaluation required before and during Rx to rule out ocular toxicity.
- *Belimumab* (10 mg/kg IV at weeks 0, 2, 4 then monthly). B lymphocyte stimulator (BLyS)-specific inhibitor. Should not be used in severe SLE such as nephritis or CNS disease and limited to pts with mild to moderate active disease.

TREATMENTS FOR LIFE-THREATENING SLE

- *Systemic glucocorticoids.*
- *Cytotoxic/immunosuppressive agents*—added to glucocorticoids to treat serious SLE.
  1. Cyclophosphamide—administered as IV pulse 500–750 mg/M^2 IV × 6 months followed by maintenance with mycophenolate mofetil or azathioprine. European studies have found cyclophosphamide 500 mg every 2 weeks for 6 doses may be effective, but it remains unclear whether these data will apply to U.S. populations.
  2. Mycophenolate mofetil—2–3 g/d; efficacy data limited to nephritis. A higher proportion of black pts appear to respond to mycophenolate mofetil compared with cyclophosphamide.
  3. Azathioprine—may be effective but is slower in inducing therapeutic response.

RHEUMATOID ARTHRITIS (RA)

■ DEFINITION AND PATHOGENESIS

A chronic multisystem disease of unknown etiology characterized by persistent inflammatory synovitis, usually involving peripheral joints symmetrically. Although cartilaginous destruction, bony erosions, and joint deformity are hallmarks, the course of RA can be quite variable. An association with HLA-DR4 has been noted; both genetic and environmental factors may play a role in initiating disease. The propagation of RA is an immunologically mediated event in which joint injury occurs from synovial hyperplasia; lymphocytic infiltration of synovium; and local production of cytokines and chemokines by activated lymphocytes, macrophages, and fibroblasts.

■ CLINICAL MANIFESTATIONS

RA occurs in 0.5–1.0% of the population; women affected three times more often than men; prevalence increases with age, onset most frequent in fourth and fifth decades.

Articular Manifestations

Typically a symmetric polyarthritis of peripheral joints with pain, tenderness, and swelling of affected joints; morning stiffness is common; PIP and MCP joints frequently involved; joint deformities may develop after persistent inflammation.

Extraarticular Manifestations

Cutaneous—rheumatoid nodules, vasculitis

Pulmonary—nodules, interstitial disease, bronchiolitis obliterans–organizing pneumonia (BOOP), pleural disease, Caplan's syndrome [sero (+) RA associated with pneumoconiosis]

Ocular—keratoconjunctivitis sicca, episcleritis, scleritis

Hematologic—anemia, Felty's syndrome (splenomegaly and neutropenia)

Cardiac—pericarditis, myocarditis

Neurologic—myelopathies secondary to cervical spine disease, entrapment, vasculitis

■ EVALUATION

- Hx and physical exam with careful examination of all joints.
- Rheumatoid factor (RF) is present in >66% of pts; its presence correlates with severe disease, nodules, extraarticular features.
- Antibodies to cyclic citrullinated protein (anti-CCP) have similar sensitivity but higher specificity than RF; may be most useful in early RA; presence most common in pts with aggressive disease with a tendency for developing bone erosions.
- Other laboratory data: CBC, ESR.
- Synovial fluid analysis—useful to rule out crystalline disease, infection.
- Radiographs—juxta-articular osteopenia, joint space narrowing, marginal erosions. Chest x-ray should be obtained.

■ DIAGNOSIS

Not difficult in pts with typical established disease. May be confusing early. Classification criteria were updated in 2010 (Table 321-1, p. 2745, in HPIM-18).

■ DIFFERENTIAL DIAGNOSIS

Gout, SLE, psoriatic arthritis, infectious arthritis, osteoarthritis, sarcoid.

> **TREATMENT** Rheumatoid Arthritis
>
> Goals: lessen pain, reduce inflammation, improve/maintain function, prevent long-term joint damage, control of systemic involvement. Increasing trend to treat RA more aggressively earlier in disease course (Table 321-2, HPIM-18, pp. 2748–2749). All RA therapies have individual toxicities, with many requiring pretreatment screening and monitoring.
> - Pt education on disease, joint protection.
> - Physical and occupational therapy—strengthen periarticular muscles, consider assistive devices.

- Aspirin or NSAIDs.
- Intra-articular glucocorticoids.
- Systemic glucocorticoids.
- Disease-modifying antirheumatic drugs (DMARDs)—e.g., methotrexate, hydroxychloroquine, sulfasalazine, leflunomide.
- Biologic therapies.
- TNF modulatory agents (etanercept, infliximab, adalimumab, golimumab, certolizumab)—effective at controlling RA in many pts and can slow the rate of progression of radiographic joint damage and decrease disability; carry potential for serious infection and individual toxicities.
- Abatacept (CTLA4-Ig)—inhibits T cell activation, can be given with or without methotrexate.
- Rituximab—a chimeric antibody directed to CD20 that depletes mature B cells, is approved for refractory RA.
- Tocilizumab—humanized monoclonal antibody directed against the IL-6 receptor.
- Anakinra—an IL-1 receptor antagonist approved for RA but rarely used in RA due to only modest clinical efficacy.
- Surgery—may be considered for severe functional impairment due to deformity.

SYSTEMIC SCLEROSIS (SCLERODERMA, SSC)

■ DEFINITION AND PATHOGENESIS

Systemic sclerosis (SSc) is a multisystem disorder characterized by thickening of the skin (scleroderma) and distinctive involvement of multiple internal organs (chiefly GI tract, lungs, heart, and kidney). Pathogenesis unclear; involves immunologic mechanisms leading to vascular endothelial damage and activation of fibroblasts.

■ CLINICAL MANIFESTATIONS

- *Cutaneous*—edema followed by fibrosis of the skin (chiefly extremities, face, trunk); telangiectasis; calcinosis; Raynaud's phenomenon
- *Arthralgias and/or arthritis*
- *GI*—esophageal hypomotility; intestinal hypofunction
- *Pulmonary*—fibrosis, pulmonary hypertension, alveolitis
- *Cardiac*—pericarditis, cardiomyopathy, conduction abnormalities
- *Renal*—hypertension; renal crisis/failure

Two distinct subsets can be identified:

1. *Diffuse cutaneous SSc*—rapid development of symmetric skin thickening of proximal and distal extremity, face, and trunk. At high risk for development of visceral disease early in course.
2. *Limited cutaneous SSc*—often have long-standing Raynaud's phenomenon before other features appear; skin involvement limited to fingers (sclerodactyly), extremity distal to elbows, and face; associated with better prognosis; a subset of limited SSc has features of *CREST syndrome* (calcinosis, Raynaud's, esophageal dysmotility, sclerodactyly, telangiectasias).

■ EVALUATION

- Hx and physical exam with particular attention to blood pressure (heralding feature of renal disease).
- Laboratories: ESR, ANA (anticentromere pattern associated with limited SSc), specific antibodies may include antitopoisomerase I (Scl-70), UA. An increased range of autoantibodies correlating with specific clinical features have become recognized (Table 323-3, HPIM-18, p. 2760)
- Radiographs: CXR, barium swallow if indicated, hand x-rays may show distal tuft resorption and calcinosis.
- Additional studies: ECG, echo, PFT, consider skin biopsy.

TREATMENT   Systemic Sclerosis

- Education regarding warm clothing, smoking cessation, antireflux measures.
- Calcium channel blockers (e.g., nifedipine) useful for Raynaud's phenomenon. Other agents with potential benefit include sildenafil, losartan, nitroglycerin paste, fluoxetine, bosentan, digital sympathectomy.
- ACE inhibitors—particularly important for controlling hypertension and limiting progression of renal disease.
- Antacids, H2 antagonists, omeprazole, and metoclopramide may be useful for esophageal reflux.
- D-Penicillamine—controversial benefit to reduce skin thickening and prevent organ involvement; no advantages to using doses >125 mg every other day.
- Glucocorticoids—no efficacy in slowing progression of SSc; indicated for inflammatory myositis or pericarditis; high doses early in disease may be associated with development of renal crisis.
- Cyclophosphamide—improves lung function and survival in pts with alveolitis.
- Epoprostenol (prostacyclin) and bosentan (endothelin-1 receptor antagonist)—may improve cardiopulmonary hemodynamics in pts with pulmonary hypertension.

MIXED CONNECTIVE TISSUE DISEASE (MCTD)

■ DEFINITION

Syndrome characterized by a combination of clinical features similar to those of SLE, SSc, polymyositis, and RA; unusually high titers of circulating antibodies to a nuclear ribonucleoprotein (RNP) are found. It is controversial whether MCTD is a truly distinct entity or a subset of SLE or SSc.

■ CLINICAL MANIFESTATIONS

Raynaud's phenomenon, polyarthritis, swollen hands or sclerodactyly, esophageal dysfunction, pulmonary fibrosis, inflammatory myopathy. Renal involvement occurs in about 25%. Laboratory abnormalities include high-titer ANAs, very high titers of antibody to RNP, positive RF in 50% of pts.

■ EVALUATION

Similar to that for SLE and SSc.

> **TREATMENT** Mixed Connective Tissue Disease
>
> Few published data. Treat based on manifestations with similar approach to that used if feature occurred in SLE/SSc/polymyositis/RA.

SJÖGREN'S SYNDROME

■ DEFINITION

An immunologic disorder characterized by progressive lymphocytic destruction of exocrine glands most frequently resulting in symptomatic eye and mouth dryness; can be associated with extraglandular manifestations; predominantly affects middle-age females; may be primary or secondary when it occurs in association with other autoimmune diseases.

■ CLINICAL MANIFESTATIONS

- *Constitutional*—fatigue
- *Sicca symptoms*—keratoconjunctivitis sicca (KCS) and xerostomia
- *Dryness of other surfaces*—nose, vagina, trachea, skin
- *Extraglandular features*—arthralgia/arthritis, Raynaud's, lymphadenopathy, interstitial pneumonitis, vasculitis (usually cutaneous), nephritis, lymphoma

■ EVALUATION

- Hx and physical exam—with special attention to oral, ocular, lymphatic exam and presence of other autoimmune disorders.
- Presence of autoantibodies is a hallmark of disease (ANA, RF, anti-Ro, anti-La).
- Other laboratory tests—ESR; CBC; renal, liver, and thyroid function tests; serum protein electrophoresis (SPEP) (hypergammaglobulinemia or monoclonal gammopathy common); UA.
- Ocular studies—to diagnose and quantitate KCS; Schirmer's test, Rose bengal staining.
- Oral exam—unstimulated salivary flow, dental exam.
- Labial salivary gland biopsy—demonstrates lymphocytic infiltration and destruction of glandular tissue.

■ DIAGNOSIS

International classification criteria based on clinical and laboratory features have been established (Table 324-5, HPIM-18, p. 2772).

> **TREATMENT** Sjögren's Syndrome
>
> - Regular follow-up with dentist and ophthalmologist.
> - Dry eyes—artificial tears, ophthalmic lubricating ointments, local stimulation with cyclic adenosine monophosphate or cyclosporine drops.

- Xerostomia—frequent sips of water, sugarless candy.
- Pilocarpine or cevimeline—may help sicca manifestations.
- Hydroxychloroquine—may help arthralgias.
- Glucocorticoids—not effective for sicca Sx but may have role in treatment of extraglandular manifestations.

ANTIPHOSPHOLIPID ANTIBODY SYNDROME (APS)

■ DEFINITION

Autoantibody-mediated acquired thrombophilia characterized by recurrent arterial or venous thromboses and/or pregnancy morbidity in the presence of autoantibodies against phospholipid (PL)-binding plasma proteins. Can occur alone (primary) or in association with another autoimmune disease (secondary).

■ CLINICAL MANIFESTATIONS

Consist of vascular thrombotic features and pregnancy morbidity (Table 320-2 in HPIM-18, p. 2737). Catastrophic APS (CAPS) is rapidly progressive thromboembolic disease involving three or more organ systems that can be life-threatening.

■ EVALUATION

Laboratory examination of clotting parameters to include partial thrombo-plastin time, kaolin clotting time, dilute Russell viper venom test, antibodies directed against cardiolipin, β2 glycoprotein, prothrombin. Antibodies should be measured on two occasions 12 weeks apart.

■ DIAGNOSIS

Suggested by the presence of at least one clinical and one laboratory feature.

TREATMENT	Antiphospholipid Antibody Syndrome

- After first thrombotic event, warfarin for life to achieve an INR 2.5–3.5.
- Pregnancy morbidity prevented by heparin with aspirin 80 mg daily. IV immunoglobulins (IVIG) may also prevent pregnancy loss. Glucocorticoids are ineffective.
- For CAPS, consider IVIG, anti-CD20 and use of antithrombotics such as fondaparinux or rivaroxaban.

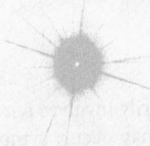

For a more detailed discussion, see Hahn BH: Systemic Lupus Erythematosus, Chap. 319, p. 2724; Shah A, St. Clair EW: Rheumatoid Arthritis, Chap. 321, p. 2738; Varga J: Systemic Sclerosis (Scleroderma) and Related Disorders, Chap. 323, p. 2757; Moutsopoulos HM, Tzioufas AG: Sjögren's Syndrome, Chap. 324, p. 2770; and Moutsopoulos HM, Vlachoyiannopoulos PG: Antiphospholipid Antibody Syndrome, Chap. 320, p. 2736, in HPIM-18.

CHAPTER **170**
Vasculitis

◾ DEFINITION AND PATHOGENESIS

A clinicopathologic process characterized by inflammation of and damage to blood vessels, compromise of vessel lumen, and resulting ischemia. Clinical manifestations depend on size and location of affected vessel. Most vasculitic syndromes appear to be mediated by immune mechanisms. May be primary or sole manifestation of a disease or secondary to another disease process. Unique vasculitic syndromes can differ greatly with regards to clinical features, disease severity, histology, and treatment.

◾ PRIMARY VASCULITIS SYNDROMES

Granulomatosis with Polyangiitis (Wegener's)

Granulomatous vasculitis of upper and lower respiratory tracts together with glomerulonephritis; upper airway lesions affecting the nose and sinuses can cause purulent or bloody nasal discharge, mucosal ulceration, septal perforation, and cartilaginous destruction (saddlenose deformity). Lung involvement may be asymptomatic or cause cough, hemoptysis, dyspnea; eye involvement may occur; glomerulonephritis can be rapidly progressive and asymptomatic and can lead to renal failure.

Churg-Strauss Syndrome

Granulomatous vasculitis of multiple organ systems, particularly the lung; characterized by asthma, peripheral eosinophilia, eosinophilic tissue infiltration; glomerulonephritis can occur.

Polyarteritis Nodosa (PAN)

Medium-sized muscular arteries involved; frequently associated with arteriographic aneurysms; commonly affects renal arteries, liver, GI tract, peripheral nerves, skin, heart; can be associated with hepatitis B.

Microscopic Polyangiitis

Small-vessel vasculitis that can affect the glomerulus and lungs; medium-sized vessels also may be affected.

Giant Cell Arteritis

Inflammation of medium- and large-sized arteries; primarily involves temporal artery but systemic and large vessel involvement may occur; symptoms include headache, jaw/tongue claudication, scalp tenderness, fever, musculoskeletal symptoms (*polymyalgia rheumatica*); sudden blindness from involvement of optic vessels is a dreaded complication.

Takayasu's Arteritis

Vasculitis of the large arteries with strong predilection for aortic arch and its branches; most common in young women; presents with inflammatory or ischemic symptoms in arms and neck, systemic inflammatory symptoms, aortic regurgitation.

Henoch-Schönlein Purpura

Characterized by involvement of skin, GI tract, kidneys; more common in children; may recur after initial remission.

Cryoglobulinemic Vasculitis

Majority of cases are associated with hepatitis C where an aberrant immune response leads to formation of cryoglobulin; characterized by cutaneous vasculitis, arthritis, peripheral neuropathy, and glomerulonephritis.

Idiopathic Cutaneous Vasculitis

Cutaneous vasculitis is defined broadly as inflammation of the blood vessels of the dermis; due to underlying disease in >70% of cases (see "Secondary Vasculitis Syndromes," below) with 30% occurring idiopathically.

Miscellaneous Vasculitic Syndromes

- Kawasaki disease (mucocutaneous lymph node syndrome)
- Isolated vasculitis of the central nervous system
- Behçet's syndrome
- Cogan's syndrome
- Polyangiitis overlap syndrome

■ SECONDARY VASCULITIS SYNDROMES

- Drug-induced vasculitis
- Serum sickness
- Vasculitis associated with infection, malignancy, rheumatic disease

■ EVALUATION (SEE FIG. 170-1)

- Thorough Hx and physical exam—special reference to ischemic manifestations and systemic inflammatory signs/symptoms.
- Laboratories—important in assessing organ involvement: CBC with differential, ESR, renal function tests, UA. Should also be obtained to rule out other diseases: ANA, rheumatoid factor, anti-GBM, hepatitis B/C serologies, HIV.
- Antineutrophil cytoplasmic autoantibodies (ANCA)—associated with granulomatosis with polyangiitis (Wegener's), microscopic polyangiitis, and some pts with Churg-Strauss syndrome; presence of ANCA is adjunctive and should not be used in place of biopsy as a means of diagnosis or to guide treatment decisions.
- Radiographs—CXR should be performed even in the absence of symptoms.
- Diagnosis—can usually be made only by arteriogram or biopsy of affected organ(s).

■ DIFFERENTIAL DIAGNOSIS

Guided by organ manifestations. In many instances includes infections and neoplasms, which must be ruled out prior to beginning immunosuppressive

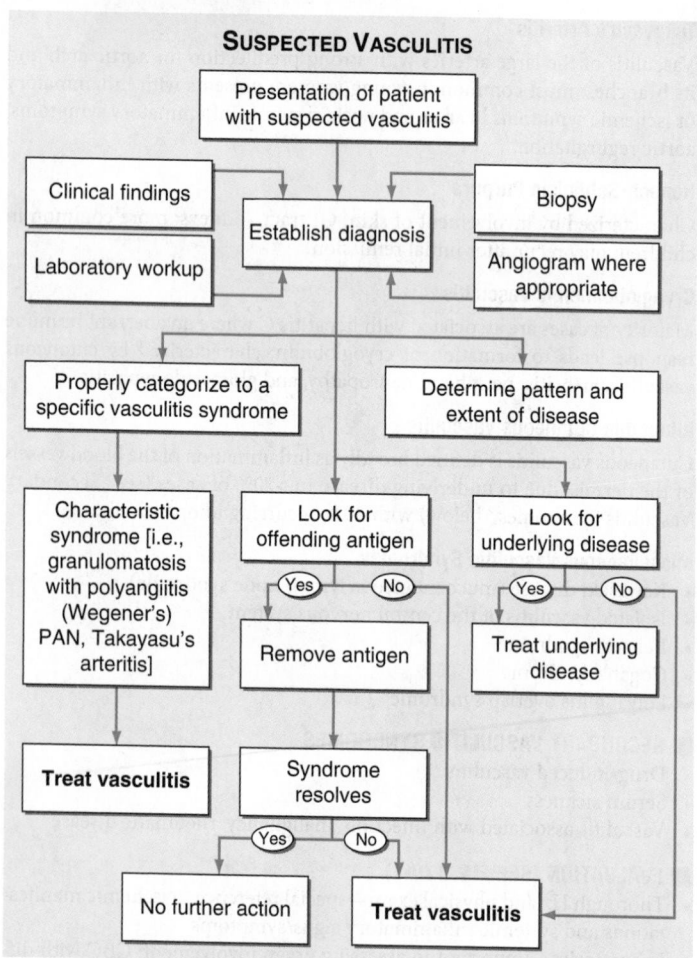

FIGURE 170-1 Algorithm for the approach to a pt with suspected diagnosis of vasculitis. PAN, polyarteritis nodosa.

therapy. Consideration must also be given for diseases that can mimic vasculitis (Table 170-1).

TREATMENT Vasculitis

Therapy is based on the specific vasculitic syndrome and the severity of its manifestations. Immunosuppressive therapy should be avoided in disease that rarely results in irreversible organ system dysfunction or that usually does not respond to such agents (e.g., isolated cutaneous vasculitis). Antiviral agents play an important role in treating vasculitis

TABLE 170-1 CONDITIONS THAT CAN MIMIC VASCULITIS

Infectious diseases
    Bacterial endocarditis
    Disseminated gonococcal infection
    Pulmonary histoplasmosis
    Coccidioidomycosis
    Syphilis
    Lyme disease
    Rocky Mountain spotted fever
    Whipple's disease

Coagulopathies/thrombotic microangiopathies
    Antiphospholipid antibody syndrome
    Thrombotic thrombocytopenic purpura

Neoplasms
    Atrial myxoma
    Lymphoma
    Carcinomatosis

Drug toxicity
    Cocaine
    Amphetamines
    Ergot alkaloids
    Methysergide
    Arsenic

Sarcoidosis

Atheroembolic disease

Anti–glomerular basement membrane antibody disease (Goodpasture's syndrome)

Amyloidosis

Migraine

occurring with hepatitis B or C. Glucocorticoids alone may control giant cell arteritis and Takayasu's arteritis. Therapy that combines glucocorticoids with another immunosuppressive agent is particularly important in syndromes with life-threatening organ system involvement, especially active glomerulonephritis. Frequently used agents:

- Prednisone 1 (mg/kg)/d initially, then tapered.
- Cyclophosphamide 2 (mg/kg)/d, adjusted to avoid severe leukopenia. Morning administration with a large amount of fluid is important in minimizing bladder toxicity. IV cyclophosphamide (15 mg/kg

every 2 weeks for 3 doses then every 3 weeks thereafter) can also induce remission but may be associated with a higher relapse rate. Treatment should be limited to 3–6 months followed by transition to maintenance therapy with methotrexate or azathioprine.

- Rituximab 375 (mg/m^2)/week for 4 weeks. As effective as cyclophosphamide to induce remission of granulomatosis with polyangiitis (Wegener's) or microscopic polyangiitis. Relapse rate, long-term safety, repeat dosing frequency are unclear.
- Methotrexate in weekly doses up to 25 mg/week may be used to induce remission in granulomatosis with polyangiitis (Wegener's) or microscopic polyangiitis pts who do not have immediately life-threatening disease or cannot tolerate cyclophosphamide. It may also be used for maintaining remission after induction with cyclophosphamide. Cannot be used in renal insufficiency or chronic liver disease.
- Azathioprine 2 (mg/kg)/d. Less effective in treating active disease but useful in maintaining remission after induction with cyclophosphamide.
- Mycophenolate mofetil 1000 mg bid. Less than azathioprine to maintain remission but an option in pts who cannot take or who have relapsed with methotrexate and azathioprine.
- Plasmapheresis may have an adjunctive role in rapidly progressive glomerulonephritis.

For a more detailed discussion, see Langford CA, Fauci AS: The Vasculitis Syndromes, Chap. 326, p. 2785; in HPIM-18.

CHAPTER **171**
Ankylosing Spondylitis

■ DEFINITION

Chronic and progressive inflammatory disease of the axial skeleton with sacroiliitis (usually bilateral) as its hallmark. Peripheral joints and extraarticular structures may also be affected. Most frequently presents in young men in second or third decade; strong association with histocompatibility antigen HLA-B27.

■ CLINICAL MANIFESTATIONS

- *Back pain and stiffness*—not relieved by lying down, often present at night forcing pt to leave bed, worse in the morning, improves with activity, insidious onset, duration >3 months (often called symptoms of "inflammatory" back pain).

- *Extraaxial arthritis*—hip and shoulders 25–35%, other peripheral joint involvement up to 30%, usually asymmetric.
- *Chest pain*—from involvement of thoracic skeleton and muscular insertions.
- *Extra/juxtaarticular pain*—due to "enthesitis": inflammation at insertion of tendons and ligaments into bone; frequently affects greater trochanter, iliac crests, ischial tuberosities, tibial tubercles, heels.
- *Extraarticular findings*—include acute anterior uveitis in about 20% of pts, aortitis, aortic insufficiency, GI inflammation, cardiac conduction defects, amyloidosis, bilateral upper lobe pulmonary fibrosis.
- *Constitutional symptoms*—fever, fatigue, weight loss may occur.
- *Neurologic complications*—related to spinal fracture/dislocation (can occur with even minor trauma), atlantoaxial subluxation (can lead to spinal cord compression), cauda equina syndrome.

■ PHYSICAL EXAMINATION

- Tenderness over involved joints
- Diminished chest expansion
- Diminished anterior flexion of lumbar spine (Schober test)

■ EVALUATION

- Erythrocyte sedimentation rate (ESR) and C-reactive protein elevated in majority.
- Mild anemia.
- Rheumatoid factor and ANA negative.
- HLA-B27 may be helpful in pts with inflammatory back Sx but negative x-rays.
- Radiographs: early may be normal. Sacroiliac joints: usually symmetric; bony erosions with "pseudowidening" followed by fibrosis and ankylosis. Spine: squaring of vertebrae; syndesmophytes; ossification of annulus fibrosis and anterior longitudinal ligament causing "bamboo spine." Sites of enthesitis may ossify and be visible on x-ray. MRI is procedure of choice when plain radiographs do not reveal sacroiliac abnormalities and can show early intraarticular inflammation, cartilage changes, and bone marrow edema.

■ DIAGNOSIS (TABLE 171-1)

Differential Diagnosis

Spondyloarthropathy associated with reactive arthritis, psoriatic arthritis, enteropathic arthritis (Table 171-2). Diffuse idiopathic skeletal hyperostosis.

TREATMENT	Ankylosing Spondylitis

- Exercise program to maintain posture and mobility is important.
- TNF modulatory agents (etanercept, infliximab, adalimumab, golimumab) have been found to suppress disease activity and improve function.
- NSAIDs (e.g., indomethacin 75 mg slow-release daily or bid) useful in most pts.

TABLE 171-1 ASAS CRITERIA FOR CLASSIFICATION OF AXIAL SPONDYLOARTHRITIS (TO BE APPLIED FOR PATIENTS WITH BACK PAIN ≥3 MONTHS AND AGE OF ONSET <45 YEARS)[a]

Sacroiliitis on Imaging Plus ≥1 SpA Feature	or	HLA-B27 Plus ≥ 2 Other SpA Features
Sacroiliitis on imaging		SpA features
• Active (acute) inflammation on MRI highly suggestive of SpA-associated sacroiliitis[b]		• Inflammatory back pain[d]
		• Arthritis[e]
		• Enthesitis (heel)[f]
and/or		• Anterior uveitis[g]
		• Dactylitis[e]
• Definite radiographic sacroiliitis according to modified New York criteria[c]		• Psoriasis[e]
		• Crohn's disease or ulcerative colitis[e]
		• Good response to NSAIDs[h]
		• Family history of SpA[i]
		• HLA-B27
		• Elevated CRP[j]

[a]Sensitivity 83%, specificity 84%. The imaging arm (sacroiliitis) alone has a sensitivity of 66% and a specificity of 97%.
[b]Bone marrow edema and/or osteitis on short tau inversion recovery (STIR) or gadolinium-enhanced T1 image.
[c]Bilateral grade ≥2 or unilateral grade 3 or 4.
[d]See text for criteria.
[e]Past or present, diagnosed by a physician.
[f]Past or present pain or tenderness on examination at calcaneus insertion of Achilles tendon or plantar fascia.
[g]Past or present, confirmed by an ophthalmologist.
[h]Substantial relief of back pain at 24–48 h after a full dose of NSAID.
[i]First- or second-degree relatives with ankylosing spondylitis (AS), psoriasis, uveitis, reactive arthritis (ReA), or inflammatory bowel disease (IBD).
[j]After exclusion of other causes of elevated CRP.
Abbreviations: ASAS, Assessment of Spondyloarthritis International Society; CRP, C-reactive protein; NSAIDs, nonsteroidal anti-inflammatory drugs; SpA, spondyloarthritis.
Source: From M Rudwaleit et al: Ann Rheum Dis 68:777, 2009. Copyright 2009, with permission from BMJ Publishing Group Ltd.

- Sulfasalazine 2–3 g/d is of modest benefit, primarily for peripheral arthritis.
- Methotrexate, widely used but has not been of proven benefit.
- No documented therapeutic role for systemic glucocorticoids.
- Intraarticular glucocorticoids for persistent enthesitis or peripheral synovitis; ocular glucocorticoids for uveitis with systemic immunosuppression required in some cases; surgery for severely affected or deformed joints.

TABLE 171-2 EUROPEAN SPONDYLOARTHROPATHY STUDY GROUP (ESSG) CRITERIA FOR SPONDYLOARTHRITIS[a]

Inflammatory Back Pain[b]	*or* / *and*	Synovitis • Asymmetric *or* • Predominantly in Lower Extremities

One or more of the following:

- Family history of SpA[b]
- Psoriasis[b]
- Crohn's disease or ulcerative colitis[c]
- Nongonococcal urethritis, cervicitis, or acute diarrhea within 1 month before arthritis
- Alternating buttock pain[d]
- Enthesitis[b]
- Radiographic sacroiliitis[b]

[a]Sensitivity >85%, specificity >85%.
[b]See definition in Table 171-1.
[c]Past or present, diagnosed by a physician and confirmed by endoscopy or radiography.
[d]Past or present pain alternating between the right and left gluteal regions. SpA, spondyloarthritis.
Sources: From M Dougados et al; J Sieper J et al. Copyright 2009, with permission from BMJ Publishing Group Ltd.

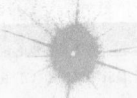

For a more detailed discussion, see Taurog JD: The Spondyloarthritides, Chap. 325, p. 2774, in HPIM-18.

CHAPTER **172**
Psoriatic Arthritis

DEFINITION

Psoriatic arthritis is a chronic inflammatory arthritis that affects 5–30% of persons with psoriasis. Some pts, especially those with spondylitis, will carry the HLA-B27 histocompatibility antigen. Onset of psoriasis usually precedes development of joint disease; approximately 15–20% of pts develop arthritis prior to onset of skin disease. Nail changes are seen in 90% of pts with psoriatic arthritis.

PATTERNS OF JOINT INVOLVEMENT

There are 5 patterns of joint involvement in psoriatic arthritis.

- Asymmetric oligoarthritis: often involves distal interphalangeal/ proximal interphalangeal (DIP/PIP) joints of hands and feet, knees, wrists, ankles; "sausage digits" may be present, reflecting tendon sheath inflammation.

- Symmetric polyarthritis (40%): resembles rheumatoid arthritis except rheumatoid factor is negative, absence of rheumatoid nodules.
- Predominantly DIP joint involvement (15%): high frequency of association with psoriatic nail changes.
- "Arthritis mutilans" (3–5%): aggressive, destructive form of arthritis with severe joint deformities and bony dissolution.
- Spondylitis and/or sacroiliitis: axial involvement is present in 20–40% of pts with psoriatic arthritis; may occur in absence of peripheral arthritis.

■ EVALUATION

- Negative tests for rheumatoid factor.
- Hypoproliferative anemia, elevated erythrocyte sedimentation rate (ESR).
- Hyperuricemia may be present.
- HIV infection should be suspected in fulminant disease.
- Inflammatory synovial fluid and biopsy without specific findings.
- Radiographic features include erosion at joint margin, bony ankylosis, tuft resorption of terminal phalanges, "pencil-in-cup" deformity (bone proliferation at base of distal phalanx with tapering of proximal phalanx), axial skeleton with asymmetric sacroiliitis, asymmetric nonmarginal syndesmophytes.

TABLE 172-1 THE CASPAR (CLASSIFICATION CRITERIA FOR PSORIATIC ARTHRITIS) CRITERIA[a]

To meet the CASPAR criteria, a pt must have inflammatory articular disease (joint, spine, or entheseal) with ≥3 points from any of the following five categories:

1. Evidence of current psoriasis,[b, c] a personal history of psoriasis, or a family history of psoriasis[d]
2. Typical psoriatic nail dystrophy[e] observed on current physical examination
3. A negative test result for rheumatoid factor.
4. Either current dactylitis[f] or a history of dactylitis recorded by a rheumatologist
5. Radiographic evidence of juxtaarticular new bone formation[g] in the hand or foot

[a]Specificity of 99% and sensitivity of 91%.
[b]Current psoriasis is assigned 2 points; all other features are assigned 1 point.
[c]Psoriatic skin or scalp disease present at the time of examination, as judged by a rheumatologist or dermatologist.
[d]History of psoriasis in a first- or second-degree relative.
[e]Onycholysis, pitting, or hyperkeratosis.
[f]Swelling of an entire digit.
[g]Ill-defined ossification near joint margins, excluding osteophyte formation.
Source: From Taylor W et al: Classification criteria for psoriatic arthritis. Development of new criteria from a large international study. Arthritis Rheum, 54:2665, 2006.

■ **DIAGNOSIS** (TABLE 172-1)

> **TREATMENT** Psoriatic Arthritis
>
> - Coordinated therapy is directed at the skin and joints.
> - Pt education, physical and occupational therapy.
> - TNF modulatory agents (etanercept, infliximab, adalimumab, golimumab) can improve skin and joint disease and delay radiographic progression.
> - Alefacept in combination with methotrexate can benefit skin and joint disease.
> - NSAIDs.
> - Intraarticular steroid injections—useful in some settings. Systemic glucocorticoids should rarely be used as may induce rebound flare of skin disease upon tapering.
> - Efficacy of gold salts and antimalarials controversial.
> - Methotrexate 15–25 mg/week and sulfasalazine 2–3 g/d have clinical efficacy but do not halt joint erosion.
> - Leflunomide may be of benefit for skin and joint disease.

> For a more detailed discussion, see Taurog JD: The Spondyloarthritides, Chap. 325, p. 2774, in HPIM-18.

CHAPTER **173**
Reactive Arthritis

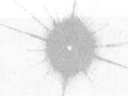

■ **DEFINITION**

Reactive arthritis refers to acute nonpurulent arthritis complicating an infection elsewhere in the body. The term has been used primarily to refer to spondyloarthritides following enteric or urogenital infections occurring predominantly in HLA-B27-positive individuals.

■ **PATHOGENESIS**

Up to 85% of pts possess the HLA-B27 alloantigen. It is thought that in individuals with appropriate genetic background, reactive arthritis may be triggered by an enteric infection with any of several *Shigella, Salmonella, Yersinia,* and *Campylobacter* species; by genitourinary infection with *Chlamydia* trachomatis; and possibly by other agents.

■ **CLINICAL MANIFESTATIONS**

The male:female ratio following enteric infection is 1:1; however, genitourinary-acquired reactive arthritis is predominantly seen in young males.

In a majority of cases, Hx will elicit Sx of genitourinary or enteric infection 1–4 weeks prior to onset of other features.

Constitutional—fatigue, malaise, fever, weight loss.

Arthritis—usually acute, asymmetric, oligoarticular, involving predominantly lower extremities; sacroiliitis may occur.

Enthesitis—inflammation at insertion of tendons and ligaments into bone; dactylitis or "sausage digit," plantar fasciitis, and Achilles tendinitis are common.

Ocular features—conjunctivitis, usually minimal; uveitis, keratitis, and optic neuritis rarely present.

Urethritis—discharge intermittent and may be asymptomatic.

Other urogenital manifestations—prostatitis, cervicitis, salpingitis.

Mucocutaneous lesions—painless lesions on glans penis (circinate balanitis) and oral mucosa in approximately a third of pts; *keratoderma blennorrhagica*: cutaneous vesicles that become hyperkeratotic, most common on soles and palms.

Uncommon manifestations—pleuropericarditis, aortic regurgitation, neurologic manifestations, secondary amyloidosis.

Reactive arthritis is associated with and may be the presenting sign and Sx of HIV.

■ EVALUATION

- Pursuit of triggering infection by culture, serology, or molecular methods as clinically suggested.
- Rheumatoid factor and ANA negative.
- Mild anemia, leukocytosis, elevated ESR may be seen.
- HLA-B27 may be helpful in atypical cases.
- HIV screening should be performed in all pts.
- Synovial fluid analysis—often very inflammatory; negative for crystals or infection.
- Radiographs—erosions may be seen with new periosteal bone formation, ossification of entheses, sacroiliitis (often unilateral).

■ DIFFERENTIAL DIAGNOSIS

Includes septic arthritis (gram +/−), gonococcal arthritis, crystalline arthritis, psoriatic arthritis.

TREATMENT Reactive Arthritis

- Controlled trials have failed to demonstrate any benefit of antibiotics in reactive arthritis. Prompt antibiotic treatment of acute chlamydial urethritis may prevent subsequent reactive arthritis.
- NSAIDs (e.g., indomethacin 25–50 mg PO tid) benefit most pts.
- Intra-articular glucocorticoids.
- Sulfasalazine up to 3 g/d in divided doses may help some pts with persistent arthritis.
- Cytotoxic therapy, such as azathioprine [1–2 (mg/kg)/d] or methotrexate (7.5–15 mg/week) may be considered for debilitating disease refractory to other modalities; contraindicated in HIV disease.

- Anti-TNF agents can be considered in severe chronic cases.
- Uveitis may require therapy with ocular or systemic glucocorticoids.

◼ OUTCOME

Prognosis is variable; 30–60% will have recurrent or sustained disease, with 15–25% developing permanent disability.

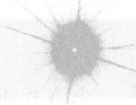

For a more detailed discussion, see Taurog JD: The Spondyloarthritides, Chap. 325, p. 2774, in HPIM-18.

CHAPTER **174**
Osteoarthritis

◼ DEFINITION

Osteoarthritis (OA) is a disorder characterized by progressive joint failure in which all structures of the joint have undergone pathologic change. The pathologic sine qua non of OA is hyaline articular cartilage loss accompanied by increasing thickness and sclerosis of the subchondral bone plate, outgrowth of osteophytes at the joint margin, stretching of the articular capsule, and weakness of the muscles bridging the joint. There are numerous pathways that lead to OA, but the initial step is often joint injury in the setting of a failure of protective mechanisms.

◼ EPIDEMIOLOGY

OA is the most common type of arthritis. The prevalence of OA correlates strikingly with age, and it is much more common in women than in men. Joint vulnerability and joint loading are the two major risk factors contributing to OA. These are influenced by factors that include age, female sex, race, genetic factors, nutritional factors, joint trauma, previous damage, malalignment, proprioceptive deficiencies, and obesity.

◼ PATHOGENESIS

The earliest changes of OA may begin in cartilage. The two major components of cartilage are type 2 collagen, which provides tensile strength, and aggrecan, a proteoglycan. OA cartilage is characterized by gradual depletion of aggrecan, unfurling of the collagen matrix, and loss of type 2 collagen, which leads to increased vulnerability.

◼ CLINICAL MANIFESTATIONS

OA can affect almost any joint but usually occurs in weight-bearing and frequently used joints such as the knee, hip, spine, and hands. The hand joints that are typically affected are the DIP, PIP, or first carpometacarpal (thumb base); metacarpophalangeal joint involvement is rare.

Symptoms

- Use-related pain affecting one or a few joints (rest and nocturnal pain less common)
- Stiffness after rest or in morning may occur but is usually brief (<30 min)
- Loss of joint movement or functional limitation
- Joint instability
- Joint deformity
- Joint crepitation ("crackling")

Physical Examination

- Chronic monarthritis or asymmetric oligo/polyarthritis
- Firm or "bony" swellings of the joint margins, e.g., Heberden's nodes (hand DIP) or Bouchard's nodes (hand PIP)
- Mild synovitis with a cool effusion can occur but is uncommon
- Crepitance—audible creaking or crackling of joint on passive or active movement
- Deformity, e.g., OA of knee may involve medial, lateral, or patellofemoral compartments resulting in varus or valgus deformities
- Restriction of movement, e.g., limitation of internal rotation of hip
- Objective neurologic abnormalities may be seen with spine involvement (may affect intervertebral disks, apophyseal joints, and paraspinal ligaments)

■ EVALUATION

- Routine lab work usually normal.
- ESR usually normal but may be elevated in pts who have synovitis.
- Rheumatoid factor, ANA studies negative.
- Joint fluid is straw-colored with good viscosity; fluid WBCs <1000/μL; of value in ruling out crystal-induced arthritis, inflammatory arthritis, or infection.
- Radiographs may be normal at first but as disease progresses may show joint space narrowing, subchondral bone sclerosis, subchondral cysts, and osteophytes. Erosions are distinct from those of rheumatoid and psoriatic arthritis as they occur subchondrally along the central portion of the joint surface.

■ DIAGNOSIS

Usually established on basis of pattern of joint involvement. Radiographic features, normal laboratory tests, and synovial fluid findings can be helpful if signs suggest an inflammatory arthritis.

Differential Diagnosis

Osteonecrosis, Charcot joint, rheumatoid arthritis, psoriatic arthritis, crystal-induced arthritides.

TREATMENT	Osteoarthritis

- Treatment goal—alleviate pain and minimize loss of physical function.
- Nonpharmacotherapy strategies aimed at altering loading across the painful joint—include pt education, weight reduction, appropriate use of cane and other supports, isometric exercises to strengthen muscles around affected joints, bracing/orthotics to correct malalignment.
- Topical capsaicin cream may help relieve hand or knee pain.

- Acetaminophen, salicylates, NSAIDs, COX-2 inhibitors—must weigh individual risks and benefits.
- Tramadol—may be considered in pts whose symptoms are inadequately controlled with NSAIDs; as it is a synthetic opioid agonist, habituation is a potential concern.
- Intraarticular glucocorticoids—may provide symptomatic relief but typically short-lived.
- Intraarticular hyaluronan—can be given for symptomatic knee and hip OA, but it is controversial whether it has efficacy beyond placebo.
- Glucosamine and chondroitin—although widely sold, is not FDA approved for use in OA. Proof of efficacy has not been established.
- Systemic glucocorticoids have no place in the treatment of OA.
- Arthroscopic debridement and lavage—can be helpful in the subgroup of pts with knee OA in whom disruption of the meniscus causes mechanical symptoms such as locking or buckling. In pts who do not have mechanical symptoms, this modality appears to be of no greater benefit than placebo.
- Joint replacement surgery may be considered in pts with advanced OA who have intractable pain and loss of function in whom aggressive medical management has failed.

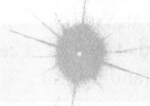

For a more detailed discussion, see Felson DT: Osteoarthritis, Chap. 332, p. 2828, in HPIM-18.

CHAPTER **175**
Gout, Pseudogout, and Related Diseases

GOUT

■ DEFINITION

Gout is a metabolic disease most often affecting middle-aged to elderly men and postmenopausal women. Hyperuricemia is the biologic hallmark of gout. When present, plasma and extracellular fluids become supersaturated with uric acid, which, under the right conditions, may crystallize and result in a spectrum of clinical manifestations that may occur singly or in combination.

■ PATHOGENESIS

Uric acid is the end product of purine nucleotide degradation; its production is closely linked to pathways of purine metabolism, with the intracellular concentration of 5-phosphoribosyl-1-pyrophosphate (PRPP) being the major determinant of the rate of uric acid biosynthesis. Uric acid is excreted primarily by the kidney through mechanisms of glomerular filtration, tubular secretion, and reabsorption. Hyperuricemia may thus arise in a wide range of settings that cause overproduction or reduced excretion of uric acid or a combination of the two (Table 359-2, p. 3183, HPIM-18).

Acute Gouty Arthritis

Monosodium urate (MSU) crystals present in the joint are phagocytosed by leukocytes; release of inflammatory mediators and lysosomal enzymes leads to recruitment of additional phagocytes into the joint and to synovial inflammation.

■ CLINICAL MANIFESTATIONS

Acute arthritis—most frequent early clinical manifestation of gout. Usually initially affects one joint, but may be polyarticular in later episodes. The first metatarsophalangeal joint (*podagra*) is often involved. Acute gout frequently begins at night with dramatic pain, swelling, warmth, and tenderness. Attack will generally subside spontaneously after 3–10 days. Although some pts may have a single attack, most pts have recurrent episodes with intervals of varying length with no symptoms between attacks. Acute gout may be precipitated by dietary excess, trauma, surgery, excessive ethanol ingestion, hypouricemic therapy, and serious medical illnesses such as myocardial infarction and stroke.

Chronic arthritis—a proportion of gout pts may have a chronic nonsymmetric synovitis; may rarely be the only manifestation. Can also present with periarticular *tophi* (aggregates of MSU crystals surrounded by a giant cell inflammatory reaction). Occurs in the setting of long-standing gout.

Extraarticular tophi—often occur in olecranon bursa, helix and anthelix of ears, ulnar surface of forearm, Achilles tendon.

Tenosynovitis

Urate nephropathy—deposition of MSU crystals in renal interstitium and pyramids. Can cause chronic renal insufficiency.

Acute uric acid nephropathy—reversible cause of acute renal failure due to precipitation of urate in the tubules; pts receiving cytotoxic treatment for neoplastic disease are at risk.

Uric acid nephrolithiasis—responsible for 10% of renal stones in the United States.

■ DIAGNOSIS

- Synovial fluid analysis—should be performed to confirm gout even when clinical appearance is strongly suggestive; joint aspiration and demonstration of both intracellular and extracellular needle-shaped negatively birefringent MSU crystals by polarizing microscopy. Gram stain and culture should be performed on all fluid to rule out infection. MSU crystals can also be demonstrated in chronically involved joints or tophaceous deposits.
- Serum uric acid—normal levels do not rule out gout.
- Urine uric acid—excretion of >800 mg/d on regular diet in the absence of drugs suggests overproduction.
- Screening for risk factors or sequelae—urinalysis; serum creatinine, liver function tests, glucose and lipids; complete blood counts.

- If overproduction is suspected, measurement of erythrocyte hypoxanthine guanine phosphoribosyl transferase (HGPRT) and PRPP levels may be indicated.
- Joint x-rays—may demonstrate cystic changes, erosions with sclerotic margins in advanced chronic arthritis.
- If renal stones suspected, abdominal flat plate (stones often radiolucent), possibly IVP.
- Chemical analysis of renal stones.

Differential Diagnosis

Septic arthritis, reactive arthritis, calcium pyrophosphate dihydrate (CPPD) deposition disease, rheumatoid arthritis.

TREATMENT   Gout

ASYMPTOMATIC HYPERURICEMIA As only ~5% of hyperuricemic pts develop gout, treatment of asymptomatic hyperuricemia is not indicated. Exceptions are pts about to receive cytotoxic therapy for neoplasms.

ACUTE GOUTY ARTHRITIS Treatment is given for symptomatic relief only since attacks are self-limited and will resolve spontaneously. Toxicity of therapy must be considered in each pt.

- Analgesia
- NSAIDs—Rx of choice when not contraindicated.
- Colchicine—generally only effective within first 24 h of attack; overdose has potentially life-threatening side effects; use is contraindicated in pts with renal insufficiency, cytopenias, LFTs >2 × normal, sepsis. PO—0.6 mg qh until pt improves, has GI side effects, or maximal dose of 4 mg is reached.
- Intraarticular glucocorticoids—septic arthritis must be ruled out prior to injection.
- Systemic glucocorticoids—brief taper may be considered in pts with a polyarticular gouty attack for whom other modalities are contraindicated and where articular or systemic infection has been ruled out.

URIC ACID–LOWERING AGENTS Indications for initiating uric acid–lowering therapy include recurrent frequent acute gouty arthritis, polyarticular gouty arthritis, tophaceous gout, renal stones, prophylaxis during cytotoxic therapy. Should not start during an acute attack. Initiation of such therapy can precipitate an acute flare; consider concomitant PO colchicine 0.6 mg qd until uric acid <5.0 mg/dL, then discontinue.

1. *Xanthine oxidase inhibitors* (allopurinol, febuxostat): Decrease uric acid synthesis. Allopurinol must be dose-reduced in renal insufficiency. Both have side effects and drug interactions.
2. *Uricosuric drugs* (probenecid, sulfinpyrazone): Increases uric acid excretion by inhibiting its tubular reabsorption; ineffective in renal insufficiency; should not be used in these settings: age >60, renal stones, tophi, increased urinary uric acid excretion, prophylaxis during cytotoxic therapy.

3. *Pegloticase*: Recombinant uricase that lowers uric acid by oxidizing urate to allantoin. Risk of severe infusion reactions. Should be used only in selected pts with chronic tophaceous gout refractory to conventional therapy.

CALCIUM PYROPHOSPHATE DIHYDRATE (CPPD) DEPOSITION DISEASE (PSEUDOGOUT)

■ DEFINITION AND PATHOGENESIS

CPPD disease is characterized by acute and chronic inflammatory joint disease, usually affecting older individuals. The knee and other large joints are most commonly affected. Calcium deposits in articular cartilage (*chondrocalcinosis*) may be seen radiographically; these are not always associated with symptoms.

CPPD is most often idiopathic but can be associated with other conditions (Table 175-1).

Crystals are thought not to form in synovial fluid but are probably shed from articular cartilage into joint space, where they are phagocytosed by neutrophils and incite an inflammatory response.

■ CLINICAL MANIFESTATIONS

- *Acute CPPD arthritis ("pseudogout")*—knee is most frequently involved, but polyarticular in two-thirds of cases; involved joint is erythematous, swollen, warm, and painful. Most pts have evidence of chondrocalcinosis.
- *Chronic arthropathy*—progressive degenerative changes in multiple joints; can resemble osteoarthritis (OA). Joint distribution may suggest CPPD with common sites including knee, wrist, MCP, hips, and shoulders.
- *Symmetric proliferative synovitis*—seen in familial forms with early onset; clinically similar to RA.

TABLE 175-1   CONDITIONS ASSOCIATED WITH CPPD DEPOSITION DISEASE

Aging
Disease-associated
Primary hyperparathyroidism
Hemochromatosis
Hypophosphatasia
Hypomagnesemia
Chronic gout
Postmeniscectomy
Epiphyseal dysplasias
Hereditary: Slovakian-Hungarian, Spanish, Spanish-American (Argentinian,[a] Colombian, and Chilean), French,[a] Swedish, Dutch, Canadian, Mexican-American, Italian-American,[a] German-American, Japanese, Tunisian, Jewish, English[a]

[a]Mutations in the *ANKH* gene.

- *Intervertebral disk and ligament calcification*
- *Spinal stenosis*

■ DIAGNOSIS

- Synovial fluid analysis—demonstration of CPPD crystals that appear as short blunt rods, rhomboids, and cuboids with weak positive birefringence by polarizing microscopy
- Radiographs may demonstrate chondrocalcinosis and degenerative changes (joint space narrowing, subchondral sclerosis/cysts).
- Secondary causes of CPPD deposition disease should be considered in pts <50 years old.

Differential Diagnosis

OA, RA, gout, septic arthritis.

TREATMENT	Pseudogout

- NSAIDs
- Intraarticular injection of glucocorticoids
- Colchicine (variably effective)

CALCIUM APATITE DEPOSITION DISEASE

Apatite is the primary mineral of normal bone and teeth. Abnormal accumulation can occur in a wide range of clinical settings (Table 175-2). Apatite

TABLE 175-2 CONDITIONS ASSOCIATED WITH CALCIUM APATITE DEPOSITION DISEASE

Aging
Osteoarthritis
Hemorrhagic shoulder effusions in the elderly (Milwaukee shoulder)
Destructive arthropathy
Tendinitis, bursitis
Tumoral calcinosis (sporadic cases)
Disease-associated
Hyperparathyroidism
Milk-alkali syndrome
Renal failure/long-term dialysis
Connective tissue diseases (e.g., systemic sclerosis, idiopathic myositis, SLE)
Heterotopic calcification following neurologic catastrophes (e.g., stroke, spinal cord injury)
Heredity
Bursitis, arthritis
Tumoral calcinosis
Fibrodysplasia ossificans progressiva

Abbreviation: SLE, systemic lupus erythematosus.

is an important factor in *Milwaukee shoulder*, a destructive arthropathy of the elderly that occurs in the shoulders and knees. Apatite crystals are small; clumps may stain purplish on Wright's stain and bright red with alizarin red S. Definitive identification requires electron microscopy or x-ray diffraction studies. Radiographic appearance resembles CPPD disease. *Treatment*: NSAIDs, repeated aspiration, and rest of affected joint.

CALCIUM OXALATE DEPOSITION DISEASE

CaOx crystals may be deposited in joints in primary oxalosis (rare) or secondary oxalosis (a complication of end-stage renal disease). Clinical syndrome similar to gout and CPPD disease. *Treatment*: marginally effective.

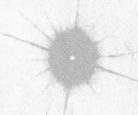

For a more detailed discussion, see Burns CM, Wortmann RL: Disorders of Purine and Pyrimidine Metabolism, Chap. 359, p. 3181; and Schumacher HR, Chen LX: Gout and Other Crystal-Associated Arthropathies, Chap. 333, p. 2837, in HPIM-18.

CHAPTER **176**
Other Musculoskeletal Disorders

ENTEROPATHIC ARTHRITIS

Both peripheral and axial arthritis may be associated with the inflammatory bowel diseases (IBD) of ulcerative colitis or Crohn's disease. The arthritis can occur after or before the onset of intestinal symptoms. Peripheral arthritis is episodic and asymmetric; it most frequently affects knee and ankle. Attacks usually subside within several weeks and characteristically resolve completely without residual joint damage. Enthesitis (inflammation at insertion of tendons and ligaments into bone) can occur with manifestations of "sausage digit," Achilles tendinitis, plantar fasciitis. Axial involvement can manifest as spondylitis and/or sacroiliitis (often symmetric). Laboratory findings are nonspecific; rheumatoid factor (RF) absent; only 30–70% HLA-B27 positive; radiographs of peripheral joints usually normal; axial involvement is often indistinguishable from ankylosing spondylitis.

TREATMENT Enteropathic Arthritis

Directed at underlying IBD; NSAIDs may alleviate joint symptoms but can precipitate flares of IBD; sulfasalazine may benefit peripheral arthritis; treatment of Crohn's disease with infliximab or adalimumab has improved arthritis.

■ WHIPPLE'S DISEASE

Characterized by arthritis in up to 75% of pts that usually precedes appearance of other symptoms. Usually oligo- or polyarticular, symmetric, transient but may become chronic. Joint manifestations respond to antibiotic therapy.

NEUROPATHIC JOINT DISEASE

Also known as *Charcot's joint*, this is a severe destructive arthropathy that occurs in joints deprived of pain and position sense; may occur in diabetic neuropathy, tabes dorsalis, syringomyelia, amyloidosis, spinal cord or peripheral nerve injury. Distribution depends on the underlying joint disease. Joint effusions are usually noninflammatory but can be hemorrhagic. Radiographs can reveal either bone resorption or new bone formation with bone dislocation and fragmentation.

> **TREATMENT** Neuropathic Joint Disease
>
> Stabilization of joint; surgical fusion may improve function.

RELAPSING POLYCHONDRITIS

An idiopathic disorder characterized by recurrent inflammation of cartilaginous structures. Cardinal manifestations include ear and nose involvement with floppy ear and saddlenose deformities, inflammation and collapse of tracheal and bronchial cartilaginous rings, asymmetric episodic nondeforming polyarthritis. Other features can include scleritis, conjunctivitis, iritis, keratitis, aortic regurgitation, glomerulonephritis, and other features of systemic vasculitis. Onset is frequently abrupt, with the appearance of 1–2 sites of cartilaginous inflammation. Diagnosis is made clinically and may be confirmed by biopsy of affected cartilage.

> **TREATMENT** Relapsing Polychondritis
>
> Glucocorticoids (prednisone 40–60 mg/d with subsequent taper) may suppress acute features and reduce the severity/frequency of recurrences. Cytotoxic agents should be reserved for unresponsive disease or for pts who require high glucocorticoid doses. When airway obstruction is severe, tracheostomy is required.

HYPERTROPHIC OSTEOARTHROPATHY

Syndrome consisting of periosteal new bone formation, digital clubbing, and arthritis. Most commonly seen in association with lung carcinoma but, also occurs with chronic lung or liver disease; congenital heart, lung, or liver disease in children; and idiopathic and familial forms. Symptoms include burning and aching pain most pronounced in distal extremities. Radiographs show periosteal thickening with new bone formation of distal ends of long bones.

> **TREATMENT** Hypertrophic Osteoarthropathy
>
> Identify and treat associated disorder; aspirin, NSAIDs, other analgesics, vagotomy, or percutaneous nerve block may help to relieve symptoms.

FIBROMYALGIA

A common disorder characterized by chronic widespread musculo-skeletal pain, aching, stiffness, paresthesia, disturbed sleep, and easy fatigability along with multiple tender points. More common in women than in men. Diagnosis is made clinically; evaluation reveals soft tissue tender points but no objective joint abnormalities by exam, laboratory, or radiograph.

TREATMENT Fibromyalgia

Pregabalin, duloxetine, and milnacipran have shown benefit for fibro-myalgia. Benzodiazepines or tricyclics for sleep disorder, local mea-sures (heat, massage, injection of tender points), NSAIDs.

POLYMYALGIA RHEUMATICA (PMR)

Clinical syndrome characterized by aching and morning stiffness in the shoulder girdle, hip girdle, or neck for >1 month, elevated ESR, and rapid response to low-dose prednisone (15 mg qd). Rarely occurs before age 50; more common in women. PMR can occur in association with giant cell (temporal) arteritis, which requires treatment with higher doses of predni-sone. Evaluation should include a careful history to elicit Sx suggestive of giant cell arteritis (Chap. 170); ESR; labs to rule out other processes usually include RF, ANA, CBC, CPK, serum protein electrophoresis; and renal, hepatic, and thyroid function tests.

TREATMENT PMR

Pts rapidly improve on prednisone, 10–20 mg qd, but may require treatment over months to years.

OSTEONECROSIS (AVASCULAR NECROSIS)

Caused by death of cellular elements of bone, believed to be due to impair-ment in blood supply. Frequent associations include glucocorticoid treat-ment, connective tissue disease, trauma, sickle cell disease, embolization, alcohol use, and HIV disease. Commonly involved sites include femoral and humeral heads, femoral condyles, proximal tibia. Hip disease is bilateral in >50% of cases. Clinical presentation is usually the abrupt onset of articular pain. Early changes are not visible on plain radiograph and are best seen by MRI; later stages demonstrate bone collapse ("crescent sign"), flattening of articular surface with joint space loss.

TREATMENT Osteonecrosis

Limited weight-bearing of unclear benefit; NSAIDs for Sx. Surgical procedures to enhance blood flow may be considered in early-stage disease but are of controversial efficacy; joint replacement may be nec-essary in late-stage disease for pain unresponsive to other measures.

PERIARTICULAR DISORDERS

■ BURSITIS

Inflammation of the thin-walled bursal sac surrounding tendons and muscles over bony prominences. The subacromial and greater trochanteric bursae are most commonly involved.

> **TREATMENT** Bursitis
>
> Prevention of aggravating conditions, rest, NSAIDs, and local glucocorticoid injections.

■ TENDINITIS

May involve virtually any tendon but frequently affects tendons of the rotator cuff around shoulder, especially the supraspinatus. Pain is dull and aching but becomes acute and sharp when tendon is squeezed below acromion.

> **TREATMENT** Tendinitis
>
> NSAIDs, glucocorticoid injection, and physical therapy may be beneficial. The rotator cuff tendons or biceps tendon may rupture acutely, frequently requiring surgical repair.

■ CALCIFIC TENDINITIS

Results from deposition of calcium salts in tendon, usually supraspinatus. The resulting pain may be sudden and severe.

■ ADHESIVE CAPSULITIS ("FROZEN SHOULDER")

Results from conditions that enforce prolonged immobility of shoulder joint. Shoulder is painful and tender to palpation, and both active and passive range of motion is restricted.

> **TREATMENT** Adhesive Capsulitis
>
> Spontaneous improvement may occur; NSAIDs, local injections of glucocorticoids, and physical therapy may be helpful.

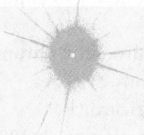

For a more detailed discussion, see Taurog JD: The Spondyloarthritides, Chap. 325, p. 2774; Crofford LJ: Fibromyalgia, Chap. 335, p. 2849; Langford CA, Mandell BF: Arthritis Associated With Systemic Disease, and Other Arthritides, Chap. 336, p. 2852; Langford CA, Gilliland BC: Periarticular Disorders of the Extremities, Chap. 337, p. 2860; and Langford CA: Relapsing Polychondritis, Chap. 328, p. 2802, in HPIM-18.

CHAPTER **177**
Sarcoidosis

■ **DEFINITION**

An inflammatory multisystem disease characterized by the presence of noncaseating granulomas of unknown etiology.

■ **PATHOPHYSIOLOGY**

The cause of sarcoid is unknown, and current evidence suggests that the triggering of an inflammatory response by an unidentified antigen in a genetically susceptible host is involved. The granuloma is the pathologic hallmark of sarcoidosis. The initial inflammatory response is an influx of CD4+ (helper) T cells and an accumulation of activated monocytes. This leads to an increased release of cytokines and the formation of a granuloma. The granuloma may resolve or lead to chronic disease, including fibrosis.

■ **CLINICAL MANIFESTATIONS**

In 10–20% of cases, sarcoidosis may first be detected as asymptomatic hilar adenopathy. Sarcoid manifests clinically in organs where it affects function or where it is readily observed. *Löfgren's syndrome* consists of hilar adenopathy, erythema nodosum, acute arthritis presenting in one or both ankles spreading to involve other joints, and uveitis.

Disease manifestations of sarcoid include:

- *Lung*—most commonly involved organ; >90% of pts with sarcoidosis will have abnormal CXR sometime during course. Features include hilar adenopathy, alveolitis, interstitial pneumonitis; airways may be involved and cause obstruction to airflow; pleural disease and hemoptysis are uncommon.
- *Lymph nodes*—intrathoracic nodes enlarged in 75–90% of pts. Extrathoracic lymph nodes affected in 15%.
- *Skin*—25% will have skin involvement; lesions include erythema nodosum, plaques, maculopapular eruptions, subcutaneous nodules, and *lupus pernio* (indurated blue-purple shiny lesions on face, fingers, and knees).
- *Eye*—uveitis in 30%; may progress to blindness.
- *Upper respiratory tract*—nasal mucosa involved in up to 20%, larynx 5%.
- *Bone marrow and spleen*—mild anemia and thrombocytopenia may occur.
- *Liver*—involved on biopsy in 60–90%; rarely important clinically.
- *Kidney*—parenchymal disease <5%, nephrolithiasis secondary to abnormalities of calcium metabolism.
- *Nervous system*—occurs in 5–10%; cranial/peripheral neuropathy, chronic meningitis, pituitary involvement, space-occupying lesions, seizures.
- *Heart*—disturbances of rhythm and/or contractility, pericarditis.
- *Musculoskeletal*—bone lesions involving cortical bone seen in 3–13%, consisting of cysts in areas of expanded bone or lattice-like changes; dactylitis; joint involvement occurs in 25–50% with chronic mono- or oligoarthritis of knee, ankle, proximal interphalangeal joints.
- *Constitutional symptoms*—fever, weight loss, anorexia, fatigue.
- *Other organ systems*—endocrine/reproductive, exocrine glands, GI.

▮ EVALUATION

- Hx and physical exam to rule out exposures and other causes of interstitial lung disease.
- CBC, Ca^{2+}, LFTs, ACE, PPD, and control skin tests.
- CXR and/or chest CT, ECG, PFTs.
- Biopsy of lung or other affected organ.
- Bronchoalveolar lavage and gallium scan of lungs may help decide when treatment is indicated and may help to follow therapy; however, these are not uniformly accepted.

▮ DIAGNOSIS

Made on basis of clinical, radiographic, and histologic findings. Biopsy of lung or other affected organs is mandatory to establish diagnosis before starting therapy. Transbronchial lung biopsy usually adequate to make the diagnosis. No blood findings are diagnostic. Differential diagnosis includes neoplasms, infections including HIV, other granulomatous processes.

TREATMENT Sarcoidosis

As sarcoidosis may remit spontaneously, treatment is based largely on the level of symptoms and extent of organ involvement (Figs. 177-1 and 177-2). When systemic therapy is indicated, glucocorticoids are the mainstay of therapy. Other immunomodulatory agents have been used in refractory or severe cases or when prednisone cannot be tapered.

▮ OUTCOME

Sarcoidosis is usually a self-limited, non-life-threatening disease. Overall, 50% of pts with sarcoidosis have some permanent organ dysfunction; death directly due to disease occurs in 5% of cases usually related to lung, cardiac, neurologic, or liver involvement. Respiratory tract abnormalities cause most of the morbidity and mortality related to sarcoid.

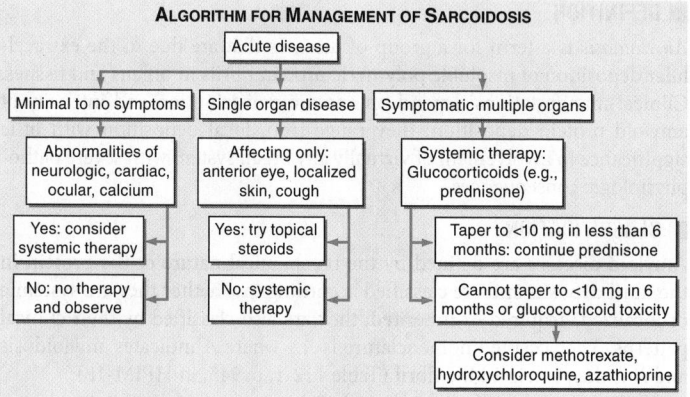

FIGURE 177-1 The management of acute sarcoidosis is based on level of symptoms and extent of organ involvement. In pts with mild symptoms, no therapy may be needed unless specified manifestations are noted.

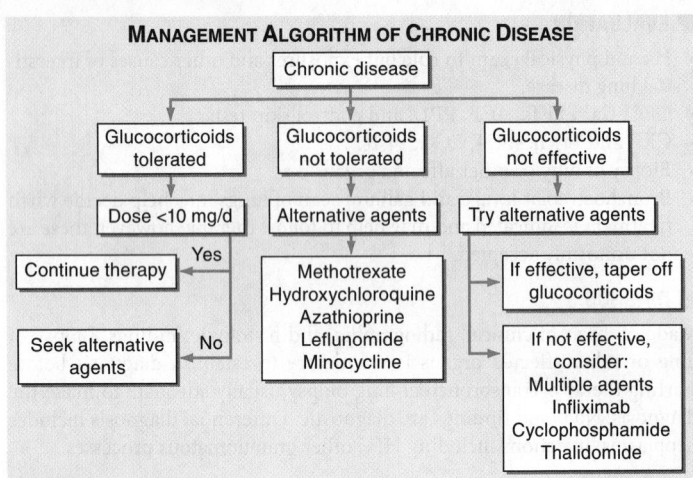

MANAGEMENT ALGORITHM OF CHRONIC DISEASE

FIGURE 177-2 Approach to chronic disease is based on whether glucocorticoid therapy is tolerated.

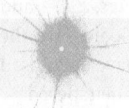

For a more detailed discussion, see Baughman RP, Lower EE: Sarcoidosis, Chap. 329, p. 2805, in HPIM-18.

CHAPTER 178
Amyloidosis

■ DEFINITION

Amyloidosis is a term for a group of diseases that are due to the extracellular deposition of insoluble polymeric protein fibrils in organs and tissues. Clinical manifestations depend on anatomic distribution and intensity of amyloid protein deposition; they range from local deposition with little significance to involvement of virtually any organ system with severe pathophysiologic consequences.

■ CLASSIFICATION

Amyloid diseases are defined by the biochemical nature of the protein in the fibril deposits and are classified according to whether they are systemic or localized, acquired or inherited; they are also classified by their clinical patterns. The accepted nomenclature is *AX* where *A* indicates amyloidosis and *X* is the protein in the fibril (Table 112-1, p. 945, in HPIM-18).

- AL (immunoglobulin light chains): *Primary amyloidosis*; most common form of systemic amyloidosis; arises from a clonal B cell disorder, usually multiple myeloma.

- AA (serum amyloid A): *Secondary amyloidosis;* can occur in association with almost any chronic inflammatory state [e.g., RA, SLE, familial Mediterranean fever (FMF), Crohn's disease] or chronic infections.
- AF (familial amyloidoses): number of different types that are dominantly transmitted in association with a mutation that enhances protein misfolding and fibril formation; most commonly due to transthyretin.
- $A\beta_2M$: composed of β_2 microglobulin; occurs in end-stage renal disease of long duration.
- Localized or organ-limited amyloidoses: most common form is $A\beta$ found in Alzheimer's disease derived from abnormal proteolytic processing of the amyloid precursor protein.

■ CLINICAL MANIFESTATIONS

Clinical features are varied and depend entirely on biochemical nature of the fibril protein. Frequent sites of involvement:

- *Kidney*—seen with AA and AL; proteinuria, nephrosis, azotemia.
- *Liver*—occurs in AA, AL, and AF; hepatomegaly.
- *Skin*—characteristic of AL but can be seen in AA; raised waxy papules.
- *Heart*—common in AL and AF; CHF, cardiomegaly, arrhythmias.
- *GI*—common in all types; GI obstruction or ulceration, hemorrhage, protein loss, diarrhea, macroglossia, disordered esophageal motility.
- *Joints*—usually AL, frequently with myeloma; periarticular amyloid deposits, "shoulder pad sign": firm amyloid deposits in soft tissue around the shoulder, symmetric arthritis of shoulders, wrists, knees, hands.
- *Nervous system*—prominent in AF; peripheral neuropathy, postural hypotension, dementia. Carpal tunnel syndrome may occur in AL and $A\beta_2M$.
- *Respiratory*—lower airways can be affected in AL; localized amyloid can cause obstruction along upper airways.

■ DIAGNOSIS

Diagnosis relies on the identification of fibrillar deposits in tissues and typing of the amyloid (Fig. 178-1). Congo red staining of abdominal fat will demonstrate amyloid deposits in >80% of pts with systemic amyloid.

■ PROGNOSIS

Outcome is variable and depends on type of amyloidosis and organ involvement. Average survival of AL amyloid is ~12 months; prognosis is poor when associated with myeloma. Cardiac dysfunction associated with death in 75% of pts.

TREATMENT   Amyloidosis

For AL most effective treatment is high-dose IV melphalan followed by autologous stem-cell transplantation. Only 50% are eligible for such aggressive treatment, and peritransplant mortality is higher than for other hematologic diseases because of impaired organ function. In pts who are not candidates for hematopoietic cell transplant, cyclic melphalan and glucocorticoids can decrease the plasma cell burden but produce remission

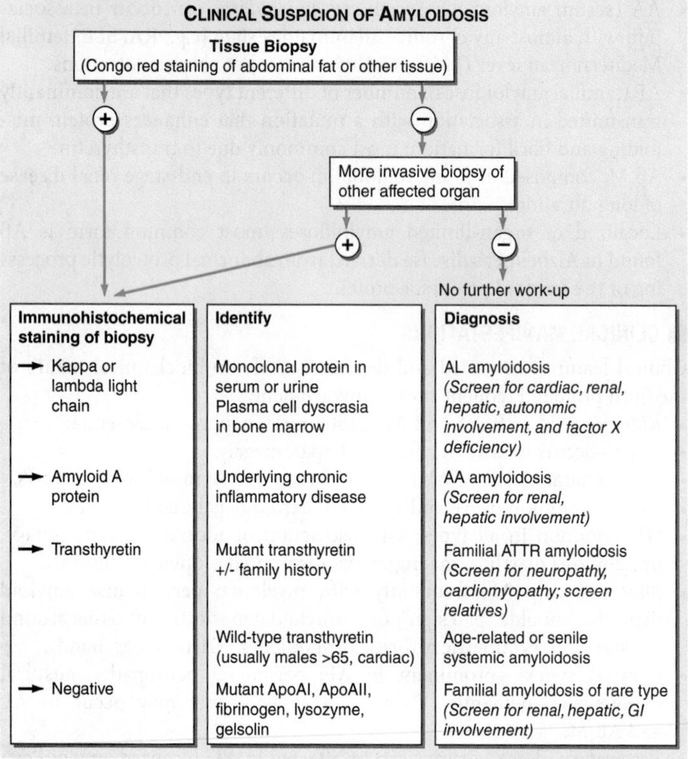

CLINICAL SUSPICION OF AMYLOIDOSIS

Tissue Biopsy
(Congo red staining of abdominal fat or other tissue)

⊕ ⊖

More invasive biopsy of other affected organ

⊕ ⊖

No further work-up

Immunohistochemical staining of biopsy	Identify	Diagnosis
→ Kappa or lambda light chain	Monoclonal protein in serum or urine Plasma cell dyscrasia in bone marrow	AL amyloidosis *(Screen for cardiac, renal, hepatic, autonomic involvement, and factor X deficiency)*
→ Amyloid A protein	Underlying chronic inflammatory disease	AA amyloidosis *(Screen for renal, hepatic involvement)*
→ Transthyretin	Mutant transthyretin +/- family history	Familial ATTR amyloidosis *(Screen for neuropathy, cardiomyopathy; screen relatives)*
	Wild-type transthyretin (usually males >65, cardiac)	Age-related or senile systemic amyloidosis
→ Negative	Mutant ApoAI, ApoAII, fibrinogen, lysozyme, gelsolin	Familial amyloidosis of rare type *(Screen for renal, hepatic, GI involvement)*

FIGURE 178-1 Algorithm for the diagnosis of amyloidosis and determination of type: Clinical suspicion: unexplained nephropathy, cardiomyopathy, neuropathy, enteropathy, arthropathy, and macroglossia. ApoAI, apolipoprotein AI, ApoAII, apolipoprotein AII, GI, gastrointestinal.

in only a few percent of pts with a minimal improvement in survival (median, 2 years). Treatment of AA is directed toward controlling the underlying inflammatory condition. Colchicine (1–2 mg/d) may prevent acute attacks in FMF and thus may block amyloid deposition. Eprodisate slowed the decline of renal function in AA, but had no significant effect on progression to end-stage renal disease or risk of death. In certain forms of AF, genetic counseling is important and liver transplantation is a successful form of therapy.

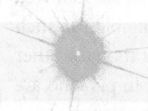

For a more detailed discussion, see Seldin DC, Skinner M: Amyloidosis, Chap. 112, p. 945, in HPIM-18.

CHAPTER **179**
Disorders of the Anterior Pituitary and Hypothalamus

The anterior pituitary is often referred to as the "master gland" because, together with the hypothalamus, it orchestrates the complex regulatory functions of multiple other glands (Fig. 179-1). The anterior pituitary produces six major hormones: (1) prolactin (PRL); (2) growth hormone (GH); (3) adrenocorticotropin hormone (ACTH); (4) luteinizing hormone (LH); (5) follicle-stimulating hormone (FSH); and (6) thyroid-stimulating hormone (TSH). Pituitary hormones are secreted in a pulsatile manner, reflecting intermittent stimulation by specific hypothalamic-releasing factors. Each of these pituitary hormones elicits specific responses in peripheral target glands. The hormonal products of these peripheral glands, in turn, exert feedback control at the level of the hypothalamus and pituitary to modulate pituitary function. Disorders of the pituitary include neoplasms or other lesions (granulomas, hemorrhage) that lead to mass effects and clinical syndromes due to excess or deficiency of one or more pituitary hormones.

PITUITARY TUMORS

Pituitary adenomas are benign monoclonal tumors that arise from one of the five anterior pituitary cell types and may cause clinical effects from either overproduction of a pituitary hormone or compressive/destructive effects on surrounding structures, including the hypothalamus, pituitary, optic chiasm, and cavernous sinus. About one-third of all adenomas are clinically nonfunctioning and produce no distinct clinical hypersecretory syndrome. Among hormonally functioning neoplasms, tumors secreting prolactin are most common (~50%); they have a greater prevalence in women than in men. GH- and ACTH-secreting tumors each account for about 10–15% of functioning pituitary tumors. Adenomas are classified as microadenomas (<10 mm) or macroadenomas (≥10 mm). Pituitary adenomas (especially PRL- and GH-producing tumors) may be part of genetic familial syndromes such as MEN 1, Carney syndrome, or mutant aryl hydrocarbon receptor inhibitor protein (AIP) syndrome. Other entities that can present as a sellar mass include craniopharyngiomas, Rathke's cleft cysts, sella chordomas, meningiomas, pituitary metastases, gliomas, and granulomatous disease (e.g., histiocytosis X, sarcoidosis).

Clinical Features

Symptoms from mass effects include headache; visual loss through compression of the optic chiasm superiorly (classically a bitemporal hemianopia); and diplopia, ptosis, ophthalmoplegia, and decreased facial sensation from

1105

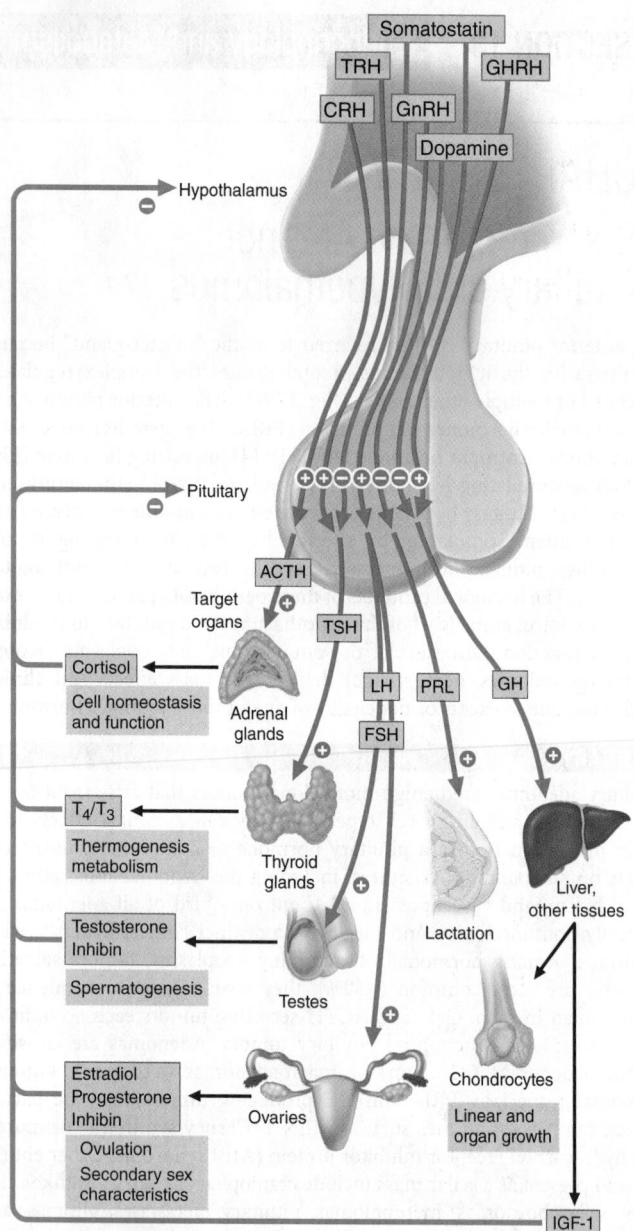

FIGURE 179-1 Diagram of pituitary axes. Hypothalamic hormones regulate anterior pituitary tropic hormones that, in turn, determine target gland secretion. Peripheral hormones feed back to regulate hypothalamic and pituitary hormones. GHRH, growth hormone-releasing hormone; SRIF, Somatostatin, somatotropin release-inhibiting factor; TRH, thyrotropin-releasing hormone; for other abbreviations, see text.

cranial nerve compression laterally. Pituitary stalk compression from the tumor may also result in mild hyperprolactinemia. Symptoms of hypopituitarism or hormonal excess may be present as well (see below).

Pituitary apoplexy, typically resulting from hemorrhage into a pre-existing adenoma or post-partum as Sheehan's syndrome, is an endocrine emergency that typically presents with features that include severe headache, bilateral visual changes, ophthalmoplegia, and, in severe cases, cardiovascular collapse and loss of consciousness. It may result in hypotension, severe hypoglycemia, CNS hemorrhage, and death. Pts with no evident visual loss or impaired consciousness can usually be observed and managed conservatively with high-dose glucocorticoids; surgical decompression should be considered when visual or neurologic symptoms/signs are present.

Diagnosis

Sagittal and coronal T1-weighted MRI images with specific pituitary cuts should be obtained before and after administration of gadolinium. In pts with lesions close to the optic chiasm, visual field assessment that uses perimetry techniques should be performed. Initial hormonal evaluation is listed in Table 179-1.

In pituitary apoplexy, CT or MRI of the pituitary may reveal signs of sellar hemorrhage, with deviation of the pituitary stalk and compression of pituitary tissue.

TREATMENT   Pituitary Tumors

Pituitary surgery is indicated for mass lesions that impinge on surrounding structures or to correct hormonal hypersecretion, except in the case of prolactinoma, where medical treatment is usually effective (see below). Transsphenoidal surgery, rather than transfrontal resection,

---

TABLE 179-1 INITIAL HORMONAL EVALUATION OF PITUITARY ADENOMAS

Pituitary Hormone	Test for Hyperfunction	Test for Deficiency
Prolactin	Prolactin	
Growth hormone	Insulin-like growth factor I (IGF-I)	IGF-I, GH stimulation tests
ACTH	24-h urinary free cortisol *or* 1-mg overnight dexamethasone suppression test	8 A.M. serum cortisol *or* ACTH stimulation test
Gonadotropins	FSH, LH	Testosterone in men
		Menstrual history in women
TSH	TSH, free T$_4$	TSH, free T$_4$
Other	α-subunit	

is the desired surgical approach for most pts. The goal is selective resection of the pituitary mass lesion without damage to the normal pituitary tissue, to decrease the likelihood of hypopituitarism. Transient or permanent diabetes insipidus, hypopituitarism, CSF rhinorrhea, visual loss, and oculomotor palsy may occur postoperatively. Tumor invasion outside of the sella is rarely amenable to surgical cure, but debulking procedures may relieve tumor mass effects and reduce hormonal hypersecretion. Radiation may be used as an adjunct to surgery, but efficacy is delayed and >50% of pts develop hormonal deficiencies within 10 years, usually due to hypothalamic damage. GH-, and TSH-secreting tumors may also be amenable to medical therapy; in PRL-secreting tumors medical therapy is the initial treatment of choice.

PITUITARY HORMONE HYPERSECRETION SYNDROMES

■ HYPERPROLACTINEMIA

Prolactin is unique among the pituitary hormones in that the predominant central control mechanism is inhibitory, reflecting dopamine-mediated suppression of prolactin release. Prolactin acts to induce and maintain lactation and decrease reproductive function and drive [via suppression of gonadotropin-releasing hormone (GnRH), gonadotropins, and gonadal steroidogenesis].

Etiology

Physiologic elevation of prolactin occurs in pregnancy and lactation. Otherwise, prolactin-secreting pituitary adenomas (prolactinomas) are the most common cause of prolactin levels >100 μg/L. Less pronounced hyperprolactinemia is commonly caused by medications [risperidone, chlorpromazine, perphenazine, haloperidol, metoclopramide, opiates, H$_2$ antagonists, amitriptyline, selective serotonin reuptake inhibitors (SSRIs), verapamil, estrogens], pituitary stalk damage (tumors, lymphocytic hypophysitis, granulomas, trauma, irradiation), primary hypothyroidism, or renal failure. Nipple stimulation may also cause acute prolactin increases.

Clinical Features

In women, amenorrhea, galactorrhea, and infertility are the hallmarks of hyperprolactinemia. In men, symptoms of hypogonadism (Chap. 185) or mass effects are the usual presenting symptoms, and galactorrhea is rare.

Diagnosis

Fasting, morning prolactin levels should be measured; when clinical suspicion is high, measurement of levels on several different occasions may be required. If hyperprolactinemia is present, nonneoplastic causes should be excluded (e.g., pregnancy test, hypothyroidism, medications).

TREATMENT Hyperprolactinemia

If the pt is taking a medication that is known to cause hyperprolactinemia, the drug should be withdrawn, if possible. A pituitary MRI should be performed if the underlying cause of prolactin elevation is unknown. Resection of hypothalamic or sellar mass lesions can reverse hyperprolactinemia due to stalk compression. Medical therapy with a dopamine agonist is indicated in microprolactinomas for control of symptomatic galactorrhea, for restoration of gonadal function, or when fertility is desired. Alternatively, estrogen replacement may be indicated if fertility is not desired, but tumor size should be carefully monitored. Dopamine agonist therapy for macroprolactinomas generally results in both adenoma shrinkage and reduction of prolactin levels. Cabergoline (initial dose 0.5 mg a week, usual dose 0.5–1 mg twice a week) or bromocriptine (initial dose 0.625–1.25 mg qhs, usual dose 2.5 PO three times a day) are the two most frequently used dopamine agonists. Cabergoline is the more effective and better-tolerated drug. These medications should initially be taken at bedtime with food, followed by gradual dose increases, to reduce the side effects of nausea and postural hypotension. Other side effects include constipation, nasal stuffiness, dry mouth, nightmares, insomnia, or vertigo; decreasing the dose usually alleviates these symptoms. Dopamine agonists may also precipitate or worsen underlying psychiatric conditions. Cabergoline in high doses can cause cardiac valvular disease. At doses typically used for prolactinoma treatment the risk for valvulopathy is small. Nevertheless, cardiac echocardiography should be performed before and 6–12 months after starting cabergoline therapy. In pts with microadenomas successfully treated (normal PRL, full tumors shrinkage), therapy may be withdrawn after 2 years, followed by careful monitoring for tumor recurrence. Spontaneous remission of microadenomas, presumably caused by infarction, occurs in some pts. Surgical debulking may be required for macroprolactinomas that do not adequately respond to medical therapy.

Women with microprolactinomas who become pregnant should discontinue dopaminergic therapy, as the risk for significant tumor growth during pregnancy is low. In those with macroprolactinomas, visual field testing should be performed at each trimester. A pituitary MRI should be performed if severe headache and/or visual defects occur.

■ ACROMEGALY

Etiology

GH hypersecretion is primarily the result of pituitary somatotrope adenomas, mostly sporadic, but also in conjunction with MEN 1, Carney syndrome, McCune-Albright syndrome, and familial AIP mutations. Extrapituitary causes of acromegaly (ectopic GHRH production) are very rare.

Clinical Features

The peak occurrence of acromegaly is at age 40–45. In children, GH hypersecretion prior to long bone epiphyseal closure results in gigantism.

The presentation of acromegaly in adults is usually indolent, and diagnosis is typically delayed by up to a decade. Pts may note a change in facial features, widened teeth spacing, deepening of the voice, snoring, increased shoe or glove size, ring tightening, hyperhidrosis, oily skin, arthropathy, and carpal tunnel syndrome. Frontal bossing, mandibular enlargement with prognathism, macroglossia, an enlarged thyroid, skin tags, thick heel pads, and hypertension may be present on examination. Associated conditions include cardiomyopathy, left ventricular hypertrophy, diastolic dysfunction, sleep apnea, glucose intolerance, diabetes mellitus, colon polyps, and colonic malignancy. Overall mortality is increased approximately threefold.

Diagnosis

Insulin-like growth factor type I (IGF-I) levels are a useful screening measure, with elevation suggesting acromegaly. Due to the pulsatility of GH, measurement of a single random GH level is not useful for screening. The diagnosis of acromegaly is confirmed by demonstrating the failure of GH suppression to <1 μg/L within 1–2 h of a 75-g oral glucose load. MRI of the pituitary usually reveals a macroadenoma.

TREATMENT Acromegaly

The primary treatment modality for acromegaly is transsphenoidal surgery. GH levels are not normalized by surgery alone in many pts with macroadenomas; in those, somatostatin analogues provide adjunctive medical therapy that suppresses GH secretion with modest to no effect on tumor size. Octreotide (50 μg SC three times a day) is used for initial therapy to determine response. Once a positive response and tolerance of side effects (nausea, abdominal discomfort, diarrhea, flatulence) is established, pts are changed to long-acting depot formulations (octreotide LAR 20–30 mg IM every 2–4 weeks or lanreotide autogel 90–120 mg IM once a month). Dopamine agonists (bromocriptine, cabergoline) can be used as adjunctive therapy but are generally not very effective. The GH receptor antagonist pegvisomant (10–30 mg SC daily) can be added in pts who do not respond to somatostatin analogues. Pegvisomant is highly effective in lowering IGF-I levels but does not lower GH levels or decrease tumor size. Pituitary irradiation may also be required as adjuvant therapy but has a slow therapeutic onset and a high rate of late hypopituitarism.

■ **CUSHING'S DISEASE (SEE CHAP. 182)**

■ **NONFUNCTIONING AND GONADOTROPIN-PRODUCING ADENOMAS**

These tumors are the most common type of pituitary neoplasm and usually present with symptoms of one or more hormonal deficiencies or mass effect. They typically produce small amounts of intact gonadotropins (usually FSH) as well as uncombined α-subunit and LHβ and FSHβ subunits. Surgery is indicated for mass effects or hypopituitarism; asymptomatic small adenomas may be followed with regular MRI and visual field testing. Diagnosis is based on immunohistochemical analysis of resected tumor tissue. Medical therapy is usually ineffective in shrinking these tumors.

■ TSH-SECRETING ADENOMAS

TSH-producing adenomas are rare but often large and locally invasive when they occur. Pts present with goiter and hyperthyroidism, and/or sella mass effects. Diagnosis is based on elevated serum free T_4 levels in the setting of inappropriately normal or high TSH secretion and MRI evidence of a pituitary adenoma. Surgery is indicated and is usually followed by somatostatin analogue therapy to treat residual tumor. Somatostatin analogue therapy leads to normalization of TSH and euthyroidism in most and tumor shrinkage in 50–75% of pts. If necessary, thyroid ablation or antithyroid drugs can be used to reduce thyroid hormone levels.

HYPOPITUITARISM

Etiology

A variety of disorders may cause deficiencies of one or more pituitary hormones. These disorders may be genetic, congenital, traumatic (pituitary surgery, cranial irradiation, head injury), neoplastic (large pituitary adenoma, parasellar mass, craniopharyngioma, metastases, meningioma), infiltrative (hemochromatosis, lymphocytic hypophysitis, sarcoidosis, histiocytosis X), vascular (pituitary apoplexy, postpartum necrosis, sickle cell disease), or infectious (tuberculous, fungal, parasitic). The most common cause of hypopituitarism is neoplastic in origin (macroadenomatous destruction, or following hypophysectomy or radiation therapy). Pituitary hormone failure due to compression, destruction, or radiation therapy typically follows a sequential pattern: GH>FSH>LH>TSH>ACTH. Genetic causes of hypopituitarism may affect several hormones (e.g., pituitary dysplasia, PROP-1 and PIT-1 mutations) or be restricted to single pituitary hormones or axes (e.g., isolated GH deficiency, Kallmann syndrome, isolated ACTH deficiency). Hypopituitarism following cranial irradiation develops over 5–15 years. Varying degrees of partial to complete hormone deficiencies occur during evolution of pituitary destruction.

Clinical Features

Each hormone deficiency is associated with specific findings:

- GH: growth disorders in children; increased intraabdominal fat, reduced lean body mass, hyperlipidemia, reduced bone mineral density, decreased stamina, and social isolation in adults
- FSH/LH: menstrual disorders and infertility in women (Chap. 186); hypogonadism in men (Chap. 185)
- ACTH: features of hypocortisolism (Chap. 182) without mineralocorticoid deficiency
- TSH: growth retardation in children, features of hypothyroidism in children and adults (Chap. 181)
- PRL: failure to lactate post-partum

Diagnosis

Biochemical diagnosis of pituitary insufficiency is made by demonstrating low or inappropriately normal levels of pituitary hormones in the setting of low target hormone levels. Initial testing should include an 8 A.M. cortisol level, TSH and free T_4, IGF-I, testosterone in men, assessment of menstrual cycles in women, and prolactin level. Provocative tests are required for definitive diagnosis of GH and ACTH deficiency. Adult GH deficiency is diagnosed by demonstrating a subnormal GH response to a standard provocative test (insulin tolerance test, L-arginine + GHRH). Acute ACTH deficiency may be diagnosed by a subnormal response in an insulin tolerance test, metyrapone test, or corticotropin-releasing hormone (CRH) stimulation test. Standard ACTH (cosyntropin) stimulation tests may be normal in acute ACTH deficiency; with adrenal atrophy, the cortisol response to cosyntropin is blunted.

TABLE 179-2 HORMONE REPLACEMENT THERAPY FOR ADULT HYPOPITUITARISM[a]

Trophic Hormone Deficit	Hormone Replacement
ACTH	Hydrocortisone (10–20 mg A.M.; 5–10 mg P.M.)
	Cortisone acetate (25 mg A.M.; 12.5 mg P.M.)
	Prednisone (5 mg A.M.)
TSH	L-Thyroxine (0.075–0.15 mg daily)
FSH/LH	Males
	Testosterone enanthate (200 mg IM every 2 weeks)
	Testosterone gel (5–10 g/d applied to skin)
	Females
	Conjugated estrogen (0.625–1.25 mg qd for 25 days)
	Progesterone (5–10 mg qd) on days 16–25
	Estradiol skin patch (0.5 mg, every other day)
	For fertility: Menopausal or biosynthetic gonadotropins, human chorionic gonadotropins
GH	Adults: Somatotropin (0.1–1.25 mg SC qd)
	Children: Somatotropin [0.02–0.05 (mg/kg per day)]
Vasopressin	Intranasal desmopressin (5–20 μg twice daily)
	Oral desmopressin (300–600 μg qd)

[a]All doses shown should be individualized for specific pts and should be reassessed during stress, surgery, or pregnancy. Male and female fertility requirements should be managed as discussed in Chaps. 185 and 186.
Note: For abbreviations, see text.

TREATMENT Hypopituitarism

Hormonal replacement should aim to mimic physiologic hormone production. Effective dose schedules are outlined in Table 179-2. Doses should be individualized, particularly for GH, glucocorticoids and L-thyroxine. GH therapy, particularly when excessive, may be associated with fluid retention, joint pain, and carpal tunnel syndrome. Glucocorticoid replacement should always precede L-thyroxine therapy to avoid precipitation of adrenal crisis. Pts requiring glucocorticoid replacement should wear a medical alert bracelet and should be instructed to take additional doses during stressful events such as acute illness, dental procedures, trauma, and acute hospitalization.

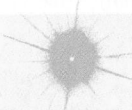

For a more detailed discussion, see Melmed S, Jameson JL: Disorders of the Anterior Pituitary and Hypothalamus, Chap. 339, p. 2876, in HPIM-18.

CHAPTER **180**
Diabetes Insipidus and SIADH

The neurohypophysis, or posterior pituitary gland, produces two hormones: (1) arginine vasopressin (AVP), also known as antidiuretic hormone (ADH), and (2) oxytocin. AVP acts on the renal tubules to induce water retention, leading to concentration of the urine. Oxytocin stimulates postpartum milk letdown in response to suckling. Its physiologic role in parturition is not established. Clinical syndromes may result from deficiency or excess of AVP.

◼ DIABETES INSIPIDUS

Etiology

Diabetes insipidus (DI) results from insufficient AVP production by the hypothalamus or from impaired AVP action in the kidney. AVP deficiency is characterized by production of large amounts of dilute urine. In *central DI*, insufficient AVP is released in response to physiologic stimuli. Causes include acquired (head trauma; neoplastic or inflammatory conditions affecting the hypothalamus/posterior pituitary), congenital, and genetic disorders, but almost half of cases are idiopathic. In *gestational DI*, increased metabolism of plasma AVP by an aminopeptidase (vasopressinase) produced by the placenta leads to a relative deficiency of AVP during pregnancy. *Primary polydipsia* results in secondary insufficiency of AVP due to physiologic inhibition of AVP secretion by excessive fluid intake. *Nephrogenic DI* is caused by AVP resistance in the kidney; it can be genetic or acquired from drug exposure (lithium, demeclocycline, amphotericin B), metabolic conditions (hypercalcemia, hypokalemia), or renal damage.

Clinical Features

Symptoms include polyuria, excessive thirst, and polydipsia, with a 24-h urine output of >50 mL/kg/day and a urine osmolality that is less than that of serum (<300 mosmol/kg; specific gravity <1.010). DI can be partial or complete; in the latter case the urine is maximally diluted (<100 mosmol/kg) and the daily urine output can reach 10–20 L. Clinical or laboratory signs of dehydration, including hypernatremia, occur only if the pt simultaneously has a thirst defect (not uncommon in pts with CNS disease) or does not have access to water. Other etiologies of hypernatremia are described in Chap. 2.

Diagnosis

DI must be differentiated from other etiologies of polyuria (Chap. 52). Unless an inappropriately dilute urine is present in the setting of serum hyperosmolality, a fluid deprivation test is used to make the diagnosis of DI. This test should be started in the morning, and body weight, plasma osmolality, serum sodium, and urine volume and osmolality should be measured hourly. The test should be stopped when body weight decreases by 5% or plasma osmolality/sodium exceed the upper limit of normal. If the urine osmolality is <300 mosmol/kg with serum hyperosmolality, desmopressin (0.03 µg/kg SC) should be administered with repeat measurement of urine osmolality 1–2 h later. An increase of >50% indicates severe pituitary DI, whereas a smaller or absent response suggests nephrogenic DI. Measurement of AVP levels before and after fluid deprivation may be required to diagnose partial DI. Occasionally, hypertonic saline infusion may be required if fluid deprivation does not achieve the requisite level of hypertonic dehydration, but this should be administered with caution.

TREATMENT   **Diabetes Insipidus**

Pituitary DI can be treated with desmopressin (DDAVP) subcutaneously (1–2 µg once or twice per day), via nasal spray (10–20 µg two or three times a day), or orally (100–400 µg two or three times a day), with recommendations to drink to thirst. Symptoms of nephrogenic DI may be ameliorated by treatment with a thiazide diuretic and/or amiloride in conjunction with a low-sodium diet, or with prostaglandin synthesis inhibitors (e.g., indomethacin).

■ SYNDROME OF INAPPROPRIATE ANTIDIURETIC HORMONE (SIADH)

Etiology

Excessive or inappropriate production of AVP predisposes to hyponatremia, reflecting water retention. The evaluation of hyponatremia is described in Chap. 2. Etiologies of SIADH include neoplasms, lung infections, CNS disorders, and drugs (Table 180-1).

Clinical Features

If hyponatremia develops gradually, it may be asymptomatic until it reaches a severe stage. However, if it develops acutely, symptoms of water intoxication

TABLE 180-1 CAUSES OF SYNDROME OF INAPPROPRIATE ANTIDIURETIC HORMONE (SIADH)

Neoplasms	Neurologic
Carcinomas	Guillain-Barré syndrome
Lung	Multiple sclerosis
Duodenum	Delirium tremens
Pancreas	Amyotrophic lateral sclerosis
Ovary	Hydrocephalus
Bladder, ureter	Psychosis
Other neoplasms	Peripheral neuropathy
Thymoma	Congenital malformations
Mesothelioma	Agenesis corpus callosum
Bronchial adenoma	Cleft lip/palate
Carcinoid	Other midline defects
Gangliocytoma	Metabolic
Ewing's sarcoma	Acute intermittent porphyria
Head trauma	Pulmonary
Infections	Asthma
Pneumonia, bacterial or viral	Pneumothorax
Abscess, lung or brain	Positive-pressure respiration
Cavitation (aspergillosis)	Drugs
Tuberculosis, lung or brain	Vasopressin or desmopressin
Meningitis, bacterial or viral	Chlorpropamide
Encephalitis	Oxytocin, high dose
AIDS	Vincristine
Vascular	Carbamazepine
Cerebrovascular occlusions, hemorrhage	Nicotine
	Phenothiazines
Cavernous sinus thrombosis	Cyclophosphamide
Genetic	Tricyclic antidepressants
X-linked recessive	Monoamine oxidase inhibitors
(V_2 receptor gene)	Serotonin reuptake inhibitors

may include mild headache, confusion, anorexia, nausea, vomiting, coma, and convulsions. Laboratory findings include low BUN, creatinine, uric acid, and albumin; serum Na <130 meq/L and plasma osmolality <270 mosmol/kg; urine is not maximally diluted and frequently hypertonic to plasma, and urinary Na$^+$ is usually >20 mmol/L.

TREATMENT ▸ SIADH

Fluid intake should be restricted to 500 mL less than urinary output. In pts with severe symptoms or signs, hypertonic (3%) saline can be infused at ≤0.05 mL/kg body weight IV per minute, with hourly sodium levels measured until Na increases by 12 meq/L or to 130 meq/L, whichever occurs first. However, if the hyponatremia has been present for >24–48 h and is corrected too rapidly, saline infusion has the potential to produce central pontine myelinolysis, a serious, potentially fatal neurologic complication caused by osmotic fluid shifts. Demeclocycline (150–300 mg PO three or four times a day) or fludrocortisone (0.05–0.2 mg PO twice a day) may be required to manage chronic SIADH. Vasopressin antagonists (conivaptan, tolvaptan) are available, but experience with these agents in SIADH treatment is limited.

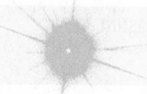

For a more detailed discussion, see Robertson GL: Disorders of the Neurohypophysis, Chap. 340, p. 2902, in HPIM-18.

CHAPTER **181**
Thyroid Gland Disorders

Disorders of the thyroid gland result primarily from autoimmune processes that stimulate the overproduction of thyroid hormones (*thyrotoxicosis*) or cause glandular destruction and underproduction of thyroid hormones (*hypothyroidism*). *Neoplastic processes* in the thyroid gland can lead to benign nodules or thyroid cancer.

Thyroidal production of the hormones thyroxine (T$_4$) and triiodothyronine (T$_3$) is controlled via a classic endocrine feedback loop (see Fig. 179-1). Some T$_3$ is secreted by the thyroid, but most is produced by deiodination of T$_4$ in peripheral tissues. Both T$_4$ and T$_3$ are bound to carrier proteins [thyroid-binding globulin (TBG), transthyretin (binds T$_4$ only), and albumin] in the circulation. Increased levels of total T$_4$ and T$_3$ with normal free levels are seen in states of increased carrier proteins (pregnancy, estrogens, cirrhosis, hepatitis, and inherited disorders). Conversely, decreased total T$_4$ and T$_3$ levels with normal free levels are seen in severe systemic illness, chronic liver disease, and nephrosis.

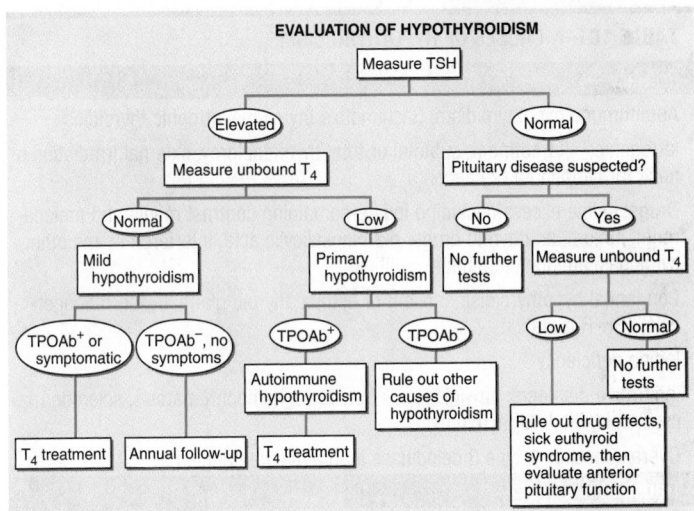

EVALUATION OF HYPOTHYROIDISM

FIGURE 181-1 Evaluation of hypothyroidism. TPOAb⁺, thyroid peroxidase antibodies present; TPOAb⁻, thyroid peroxidase antibodies not present; TSH, thyroid-stimulating hormone.

HYPOTHYROIDISM

Etiology

Deficient thyroid hormone secretion can be due to thyroid failure (primary hypothyroidism) or, less commonly, pituitary or hypothalamic disease (secondary hypothyroidism) (Table 181-1). Transient hypothyroidism may occur in silent or subacute thyroiditis. *Subclinical* (or *mild*) *hypothyroidism* is a state of normal free thyroid hormone levels and mild elevation of TSH; despite the name, some pts may have minor symptoms. With higher TSH levels and low free T_4 levels, symptoms become more readily apparent in *clinical* (or *overt*) *hypothyroidism*. In areas of iodine sufficiency, autoimmune disease and iatrogenic causes are the most common causes of hypothyroidism. The peak age of occurrence is around 60 years, and prevalence increases with age. Congenital hypothyroidism is present in 1 of 4000 newborns; the importance of its recognition and prompt treatment for child development has led to the adoption of neonatal screening programs.

Clinical Features

Symptoms of hypothyroidism include lethargy, dry hair and skin, cold intolerance, hair loss, difficulty concentrating, poor memory, constipation, mild weight gain with poor appetite, dyspnea, hoarse voice, muscle cramping, and menorrhagia. Cardinal features on examination include bradycardia, mild diastolic hypertension, prolongation of the relaxation phase of deep tendon reflexes, and cool peripheral extremities. Goiter may be palpated, or the thyroid may be atrophic and nonpalpable. Carpal tunnel syndrome may be present. Cardiomegaly may be present due to pericardial

TABLE 181-1   CAUSES OF HYPOTHYROIDISM

Primary
Autoimmune hypothyroidism: Hashimoto's thyroiditis, atrophic thyroiditis
Iatrogenic: [131]I treatment, subtotal or total thyroidectomy, external irradiation of neck for lymphoma or cancer
Drugs: iodine excess (including iodine-containing contrast media and amiodarone), lithium, antithyroid drugs, *p*-aminosalicylic acid, interferon α and other cytokines, aminoglutethimide, sunitinib
Congenital hypothyroidism: absent or ectopic thyroid gland, dyshormonogenesis, TSH-R mutation
Iodine deficiency
Infiltrative disorders: amyloidosis, sarcoidosis, hemochromatosis, scleroderma, cystinosis, Riedel's thyroiditis
Overexpression of type 3 deiodinase in infantile hemangioma
Transient
Silent thyroiditis, including postpartum thyroiditis
Subacute thyroiditis
Withdrawal of thyroxine treatment in individuals with an intact thyroid
After ^{131}I treatment or subtotal thyroidectomy for Graves' disease
Secondary
Hypopituitarism: tumors, pituitary surgery or irradiation, infiltrative disorders, Sheehan's syndrome, trauma, genetic forms of combined pituitary hormone deficiencies
Isolated TSH deficiency or inactivity
Bexarotene treatment
Hypothalamic disease: tumors, trauma, infiltrative disorders, idiopathic

Abbreviations: TSH, thyroid-stimulating hormone; TSH-R, TSH receptor.

effusion. The most extreme presentation is a dull, expressionless face, sparse hair, periorbital puffiness, large tongue, and pale, doughy, cool skin. The condition may progress into a hypothermic, stuporous state (*myxedema coma*) with respiratory depression. Factors that predispose to myxedema coma include cold exposure, trauma, infection, and administration of narcotics. In mild hypothyroidism, the classic findings of overt hypothyroidism may not be present, and the clinical picture may be dominated by fatigue and ill-defined symptoms.

Diagnosis

Decreased serum free T_4 is common to all varieties of hypothyroidism. An elevated serum TSH is a sensitive marker of primary hypothyroidism but is not found in secondary hypothyroidism. A summary of the investigations used to determine the existence and cause of hypothyroidism is provided in Fig. 181-1. Thyroid peroxidase (TPO) antibodies are increased in >90%

of pts with autoimmune-mediated hypothyroidism. Elevated cholesterol, increased creatine phosphokinase, and anemia may be present; bradycardia, low-amplitude QRS complexes, and flattened or inverted T waves may be present on ECG.

TREATMENT Hypothyroidism

Adult pts <60 years without evidence of heart disease may be started on 50–100 μg of levothyroxine (T_4) daily. In the elderly or in pts with known coronary artery disease, the starting dose of levothyroxine is 12.5–25 μg/d. The dose should be adjusted in 12.5- to 25-μg increments every 6–8 weeks on the basis of TSH levels, until a normal TSH level is achieved. The average daily replacement dose is 1.6 μg/kg/d, but dosing should be individualized and guided by TSH measurement. In *secondary* hypothyroidism, TSH levels cannot be used, and therapy needs to be guided by free T_4 measurement. Women on levothyroxine replacement should have a TSH level checked as soon as pregnancy is diagnosed, as the replacement dose typically increases by 30–50% during pregnancy. Failure to recognize and treat maternal hypothyroidism may adversely affect fetal neural development. Therapy for myxedema coma should include levothyroxine (500 μg) as a single IV bolus followed by daily treatment with levothyroxine (50–100 μg/d), along with hydrocortisone (50 mg every 6 h) for impaired adrenal reserve, ventilatory support, space blankets, and treatment of precipitating factors.

THYROTOXICOSIS

Etiology

Causes of thyroid hormone excess include primary hyperthyroidism (Graves' disease, toxic multinodular goiter, toxic adenoma, iodine excess); thyroid destruction (subacute thyroiditis, silent thyroiditis, amiodarone, radiation); extrathyroidal sources of thyroid hormone (thyrotoxicosis factitia, struma ovarii, functioning follicular carcinoma); and secondary hyperthyroidism [TSH-secreting pituitary adenoma, thyroid hormone resistance syndrome, human chorionic gonadotropin (hCG)-secreting tumors, gestational thyrotoxicosis]. Graves' disease, caused by activating TSH-receptor antibodies, is the most common cause of thyrotoxicosis and accounts for 60–80% of cases. Its prevalence in women is 10-fold higher than in men; its peak occurrence is at age 20–50 years.

Clinical Features

Symptoms include nervousness, irritability, heat intolerance, excessive sweating, palpitations, fatigue and weakness, weight loss with increased appetite, frequent bowel movements, and oligomenorrhea. Pts are anxious, restless, and fidgety. Skin is warm and moist, and fingernails may separate from the nail bed (Plummer's nails). Eyelid retraction and lid lag may be present. Cardiovascular findings include tachycardia, systolic hypertension, systolic murmur, and atrial fibrillation. A fine tremor, hyperreflexia, and proximal muscle weakness also may be present. Long-standing thyrotoxicosis may lead to osteopenia. In the elderly, the classic signs of thyrotoxicosis may not be apparent, the main manifestations being weight loss and fatigue ("apathetic thyrotoxicosis").

In Graves' disease, the thyroid is usually diffusely enlarged to two to three times its normal size, and a bruit or thrill may be present. Infiltrative ophthalmopathy (with variable degrees of proptosis, periorbital swelling, and ophthalmoplegia) and dermopathy (pretibial myxedema) also may be found; these are extrathyroidal manifestations of the autoimmune process. In subacute thyroiditis, the thyroid is exquisitely tender and enlarged with referred pain to the jaw or ear, and sometimes accompanied by fever and preceded by an upper respiratory tract infection. Solitary or multiple nodules may be present in toxic adenoma or toxic multinodular goiter.

Thyrotoxic crisis, or thyroid storm, is rare, presents as a life-threatening exacerbation of hyperthyroidism, and can be accompanied by fever, delirium, seizures, arrhythmias, coma, vomiting, diarrhea, and jaundice.

Diagnosis

Investigations used to determine the existence and causes of thyrotoxicosis are summarized in Fig. 181-2. Serum TSH is a sensitive marker of thyrotoxicosis caused by Graves' disease, autonomous thyroid nodules, thyroiditis, and exogenous levothyroxine treatment. Associated laboratory abnormalities include elevation of bilirubin, liver enzymes, and ferritin. Thyroid radioiodine uptake may be required to distinguish the various etiologies: high uptake in Graves' disease and nodular disease vs. low uptake in thyroid destruction, iodine excess, and extrathyroidal sources of thyroid hormone. (*Note:* Radioiodine is the nuclide required for quantitative thyroid uptake, whereas technetium is sufficient for imaging purposes.) The ESR is elevated in subacute thyroiditis.

TREATMENT Thyrotoxicosis

Graves' disease may be treated with antithyroid drugs or radioiodine; subtotal thyroidectomy is rarely indicated. The main antithyroid drugs are methimazole or carbimazole (10–20 mg two to three times a day initially, titrated to 2.5–10 mg/d) and propylthiouracil (100–200 mg every 8 h initially, titrated to 50 mg once or twice a day). Methimazole is preferred in most pts because of easier dosing. Thyroid function tests should be checked 3–4 weeks after initiation of treatment, with adjustments to maintain a normal free T_4 level. Since TSH recovery from suppression is delayed, serum TSH levels should not be used for dose adjustment in the first few months. The common side effects are rash, urticaria, fever, and arthralgia (1–5% of pts). Uncommon but major side effects include hepatitis, an SLE-like syndrome, and, rarely, agranulocytosis (<1%). All pts should be given written instructions regarding the symptoms of possible agranulocytosis (sore throat, fever, mouth ulcers) and the need to stop treatment pending a complete blood count to confirm that agranulocytosis is not present. Propranolol (20–40 mg

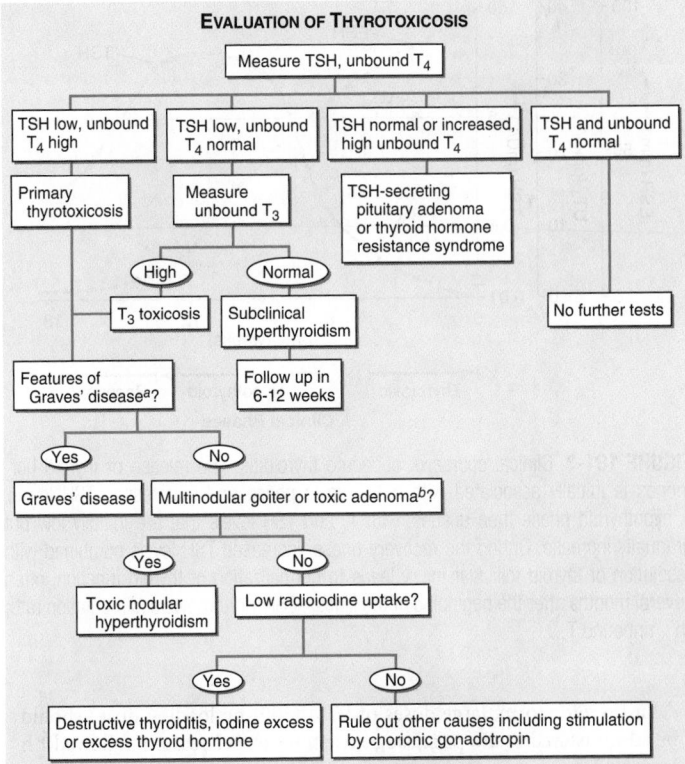

EVALUATION OF THYROTOXICOSIS

FIGURE 181-2 Evaluation of thyrotoxicosis. [a]Diffuse goiter, positive TPO antibodies, ophthalmopathy, dermopathy; [b]can be confirmed by radionuclide scan. TSH, thyroid-stimulating hormone.

every 6 h) or longer-acting beta blockers such as atenolol (50 mg/d) may be useful at the start of treatment to control adrenergic symptoms until euthyroidism is reached. Anticoagulation with warfarin should be considered in all pts with atrial fibrillation. Radioiodine can also be used as initial treatment or in pts who do not undergo remission after a 1- to 2-year trial of antithyroid drugs. Antecedent treatment with antithyroid drugs should be considered in elderly pts and those with cardiac problems, with cessation of antithyroid drugs 3–5 days prior to radioiodine administration. Radioiodine treatment is contraindicated in pregnancy; instead, symptoms should be controlled with the lowest effective dose of propylthiouracil (PTU). (Methimazole is not recommended in pregnancy because of reports of fetal agenesis cutis.) Corneal drying may be relieved with artificial tears and taping the eyelids shut during sleep. Progressive exophthalmos with chemosis, ophthalmoplegia, or vision loss is treated with large doses of prednisone (40–80 mg/d) and ophthalmologic referral; orbital decompression may be required.

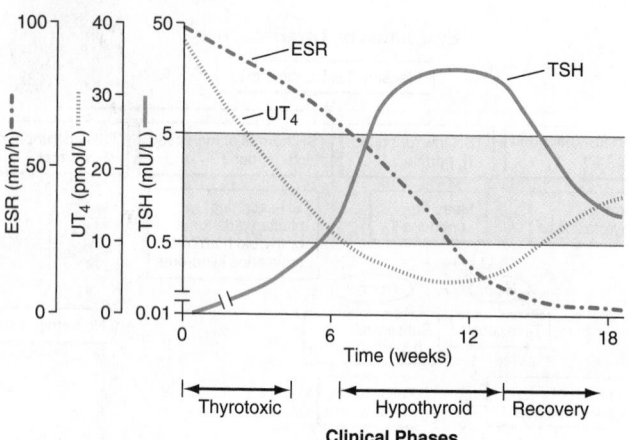

FIGURE 181-3 Clinical course of subacute thyroiditis. The release of thyroid hormones is initially associated with a thyrotoxic phase and suppressed TSH levels. A hypothyroid phase then ensues, with T_4 and TSH levels that are initially low but gradually increase. During the recovery phase, increased TSH levels combined with resolution of thyroid follicular injury leads to normalization of thyroid function, often several months after the beginning of the illness. ESR, erythrocyte sedimentation rate; UT_4, unbound T_4.

In thyroid storm, large doses of PTU (600-mg loading dose) should be administered orally, per nasogastric tube, or per rectum, followed 1 h later by 5 drops saturated solution of KI (SSKI) q6h. PTU (200–300 mg every 6 h) should be continued, along with propranolol (40–60 mg PO q4h or 2 mg IV every 4 h) and dexamethasone (2 mg every 6 h). Any underlying precipitating cause should be identified and treated.

Radioiodine is the treatment of choice for toxic nodules. Subacute thyroiditis in its thyrotoxic phase should be treated with NSAIDs and beta blockade to control symptoms, with monitoring of the TSH and free T_4 levels every 4 weeks. Antithyroid drugs are not effective in thyroiditis. The clinical course of subacute thyroiditis is summarized in Fig. 181-3. Transient levothyroxine replacement (50–100 μg/d) may be required if the hypothyroid phase is prolonged. Silent thyroiditis (or postpartum thyroiditis if within 3–6 months of delivery) should be treated with beta blockade during the thyrotoxic phase and levothyroxine in the hypothyroid phase, with withdrawal after 6–9 months to assess recovery.

SICK EUTHYROID SYNDROME

Any acute, severe illness can cause abnormalities of circulating thyroid hormone levels or TSH, even in the absence of underlying thyroid disease. Therefore, the routine testing of thyroid function should be avoided in acutely ill pts unless a thyroid disorder is strongly suspected. The most common pattern in sick euthyroid syndrome is a decrease in total and free T_3 levels, with normal levels of TSH and T_4. This is considered an adaptive response to a catabolic state. More ill pts may additionally have a fall in total T_4 levels, with normal free T_4 levels. TSH levels may range from <0.1 to >20 mU/L, with normalization after recovery from illness. The pathogenesis of this condition is not fully understood but may involve altered binding of T_4 to TBG and effects of high glucocorticoid and cytokine levels. Unless there is historic or unequivocal clinical evidence of hypothyroidism, thyroid hormone should not be administered and thyroid function tests should be repeated after recovery.

AMIODARONE

Amiodarone is a type III antiarrhythmic agent that has some structural similarity to thyroid hormone and has a high iodine content. Amiodarone treatment leads to substantial iodine overload and is associated with (1) acute, transient suppression of thyroid function, (2) hypothyroidism, or (3) thyrotoxicosis. These effects are only partially attributable to iodine overload. Hypothyroidism can occur in pts with preexisting thyroid disease, with an inability to escape from the suppressive effect of excess iodine. Pts with hypothyroidism can be easily managed with levothyroxine replacement therapy, without a need to stop amiodarone. There are two major forms of amiodarone-induced thyrotoxicosis (AIT). Type 1 AIT is associated with an underlying thyroid abnormality (preclinical Graves' disease or nodular goiter). Thyroid hormone synthesis becomes excessive as a result of increased iodine exposure. Type 2 AIT occurs in pts with no intrinsic thyroid abnormalities and is the result of destructive thyroiditis. Differentiation between type 1 and type 2 AIT may be difficult as the high iodine load interferes with thyroid scans. The drug should be stopped, if possible, although this is often difficult to achieve without compromising the arrhythmia management. Amiodarone has a long biologic half-life, and its effects persist for weeks following discontinuation. Therapy of type 1 AIT consists of high-dose antithyroid drugs, but efficacy may be limited. In type 2 AIT, sodium ipodate (500 mg/d) or sodium tyropanoate (500 mg, 1–2 doses/d) can be used to rapidly lower thyroid hormone levels. Potassium perchlorate (200 mg every 6 h) can be used to deplete the thyroid of iodine, but long-term use carries a risk of agranulocytosis. Glucocorticoids in high doses are partially effective. Lithium can be used to block thyroid hormone release. In some cases, subacute thyroidectomy may be necessary to control thyrotoxicosis.

NONTOXIC GOITER

Goiter refers to an enlarged thyroid gland (>20–25 g), which can be diffuse or nodular. Goiter is more common in women than men. Biosynthetic defects, iodine deficiency, autoimmune disease, dietary goitrogens (cabbage, cassava root), and nodular diseases can lead to goiter. Worldwide, iodine deficiency is the most common etiology of goiter. Nontoxic multinodular goiter is common in both iodine-deficient and iodine-replete populations, with a prevalence of up to 12%. The etiology, other than iodine deficiency, is usually not known and may be multifactorial. If thyroid function is preserved, most goiters are asymptomatic. Substernal goiter may obstruct the thoracic inlet and should be evaluated with respiratory flow measurements and CT or MRI in pts with obstructive signs or symptoms (difficulty swallowing, tracheal compression, or plethora). Thyroid function tests should be performed in all pts with goiter to exclude thyrotoxicosis or hypothyroidism. Ultrasound is not generally indicated in the evaluation of diffuse goiter, unless a nodule is palpable on physical exam.

Iodine or thyroid hormone replacement induces variable regression of goiter in iodine deficiency. Thyroid hormone replacement is rarely effective in significantly shrinking a nontoxic goiter that is not due to iodine deficiency or a biosynthetic defect. Radioiodine reduces goiter size by about 50% in the majority of pts. Surgery is rarely indicated for diffuse goiter but may be required to alleviate compression in pts with nontoxic multinodular goiter.

TOXIC MULTINODULAR GOITER AND TOXIC ADENOMA

■ TOXIC MULTINODULAR GOITER (MNG)

In addition to features of goiter, the clinical presentation of toxic MNG includes subclinical hyperthyroidism or mild thyrotoxicosis. The pt is usually elderly and may present with atrial fibrillation or palpitations, tachycardia, nervousness, tremor, or weight loss. Recent exposure to iodine, from contrast dyes or other sources, may precipitate or exacerbate thyrotoxicosis; this may be prevented by prior administration of an antithyroid drug. The TSH level is low. T_4 may be normal or minimally increased; T_3 is often elevated to a greater degree than T_4. Thyroid scan shows heterogeneous uptake with multiple regions of increased and decreased uptake; 24-h uptake of radioiodine may not be increased. Cold nodules in a multinodular goiter should be evaluated in the same way as solitary nodules (see below). Antithyroid drugs, often in combination with beta blockers, can normalize thyroid function and improve clinical features of thyrotoxicosis but do not induce remission. A trial of radioiodine should be considered before subjecting pts, many of whom are elderly, to surgery. Subtotal thyroidectomy provides definitive treatment of goiter and thyrotoxicosis. Pts should be rendered euthyroid with antithyroid drugs before surgical intervention.

■ TOXIC ADENOMA

A solitary, autonomously functioning thyroid nodule is referred to as *toxic adenoma*. Most cases are cause by somatic activating mutations of the TSH receptor. Thyrotoxicosis is typically mild. A thyroid scan provides a definitive diagnostic test, demonstrating focal uptake in the hyperfunctioning nodule and diminished uptake in the remainder of the gland, as activity of the normal thyroid is suppressed. Radioiodine ablation with relatively large doses (e.g., 10–29.9 mCi ^{131}I) is usually the treatment of choice.

THYROID NEOPLASMS

Etiology

Thyroid neoplasms may be benign (adenomas) or malignant (carcinomas). Carcinomas of the follicular epithelium include papillary, follicular, and anaplastic thyroid cancer. Thyroid cancer incidence is ~9/100,000 per year.

Papillary thyroid cancer is the most common type of thyroid cancer (70–90%). It tends to be multifocal and to invade locally. Follicular thyroid cancer is difficult to diagnose via fine-needle aspiration (FNA) because the distinction between benign and malignant follicular neoplasms rests largely on evidence of invasion into vessels, nerves, or adjacent structures. It tends to spread hematogenously, leading to bone, lung, and CNS metastases. Anaplastic carcinoma is rare, highly malignant, and rapidly fatal. Thyroid lymphoma often arises in the background of Hashimoto's thyroiditis and occurs in the setting of a rapidly expanding thyroid mass. Medullary thyroid carcinoma arises from parafollicular (C) cells producing calcitonin and may occur sporadically or as a familial disorder, sometimes in association with multiple endocrine neoplasia type 2.

Clinical Features

Features suggesting carcinoma include recent or rapid growth of a nodule or mass, history of neck irradiation, lymph node involvement, hoarseness, and fixation to surrounding tissues. Glandular enlargement may result in compression and displacement of the trachea or esophagus and obstructive symptoms. Age <20 or >45, male sex, and larger nodule size are associated with a worse prognosis.

Diagnosis

An approach to the evaluation of a solitary nodule is outlined in Fig. 181-4.

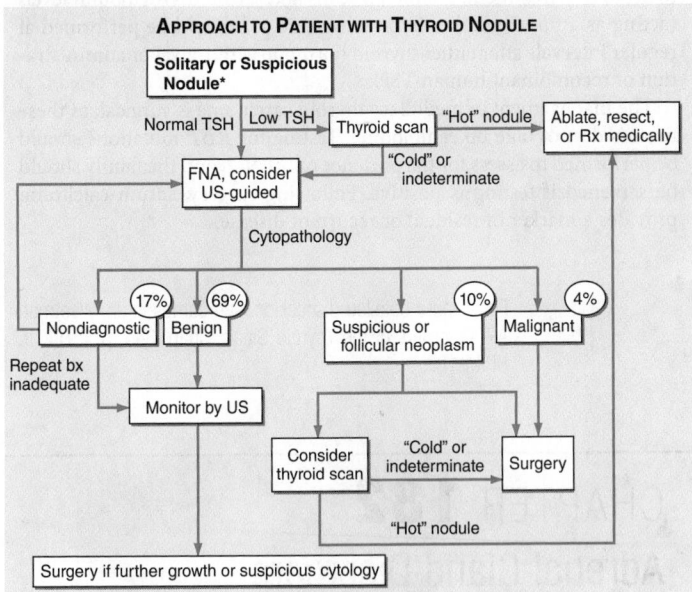

FIGURE 181-4 Approach to the pt with a thyroid nodule. *About one-third of nodules are cystic or mixed solid-cystic. FNA, fine-needle aspiration; TSH, thyroid-stimulating hormone; US, ultrasound.

TREATMENT Thyroid Neoplasms

Benign nodules should be monitored via serial examination. TSH suppression with levothyroxine results in decreased nodule size in about 30% of pts. Suppressive therapy should not exceed 6–12 months if unsuccessful.

Follicular adenomas cannot be distinguished from follicular carcinomas on the basis of cytologic analysis of FNA specimens. The extent of surgical resection (lobectomy vs. near-total thyroidectomy) should be discussed prior to surgery.

Near-total thyroidectomy is required for papillary and follicular carcinoma and should be performed by a surgeon who is highly experienced in the procedure. If risk factors and pathologic features indicate the need for radioiodine treatment, the pt should be treated for several weeks postoperatively with liothyronine (T_3, 25 µg two to three times a day), followed by withdrawal for an additional 2 weeks, in preparation for postsurgical radioablation of remnant tissue. A therapeutic dose of ^{131}I is administered when the TSH level is >50 IU/L. Alternatively, recombinant TSH can be used to raise the preablation TSH level. This appears to be equally effective as thyroid hormone withdrawal for radioablation therapy. Subsequent levothyroxine suppression of TSH to a low, but detectable, level (0.1–0.5 IU/L) should be attempted in pts with a low risk of recurrence, and to a completely suppressed level in those with a high risk of recurrence. In the latter case, free T_4 should be monitored to avoid overtreatment. Follow-up scans and serum thyroglobulin levels (acting as a tumor marker in an athyreotic pt) should be performed at regular intervals after either thyroid hormone withdrawal or administration of recombinant human TSH.

The management of medullary thyroid carcinoma is surgical, as these tumors do not take up radioiodine. Testing for *RET* mutations should be performed to assess for the presence of MEN-2, and the family should be screened if testing is positive. Following surgery, serum calcitonin provides a marker of residual or recurrent disease.

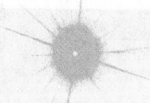

For a more detailed discussion, see Jameson JL, Weetman AP: Disorders of the Thyroid Gland, Chap. 341, p. 2911, in HPIM-18.

CHAPTER **182**
Adrenal Gland Disorders

The adrenal cortex produces three major classes of steroids: (1) glucocorticoids, (2) mineralocorticoids, and (3) adrenal androgens. Clinical syndromes may result from deficiencies or excesses of these hormones.

The adrenal medulla produces catecholamines, with excess leading to pheochromocytoma (Chap. 126).

HYPERFUNCTION OF THE ADRENAL GLAND

■ CUSHING'S SYNDROME

Etiology

The most common cause of Cushing's syndrome is iatrogenic, due to administration of glucocorticoids for therapeutic reasons. Endogenous Cushing's syndrome results from production of excess cortisol (and other steroid hormones) by the adrenal cortex. The major cause is bilateral adrenal hyperplasia secondary to hypersecretion of adrenocorticotropic hormone (ACTH) by the pituitary (Cushing's disease) or from ectopic sources such as small cell carcinoma of the lung; carcinoids of the bronchus, thymus, gut and ovary, medullary carcinoma of the thyroid; or pheochromocytoma. Adenomas or carcinoma of the adrenal gland account for about 15–20% of endogenous Cushing's syndrome cases. There is a female preponderance in endogenous Cushing's syndrome except for the ectopic ACTH syndrome.

Clinical Features

Some common manifestations (central obesity, hypertension, osteoporosis, psychological disturbances, acne, hirsutism, amenorrhea, and diabetes mellitus) are relatively nonspecific. More specific findings include easy bruising, purple striae, proximal myopathy, fat deposition in the face and nuchal areas (moon facies and buffalo hump), and rarely virilization. Thin, fragile skin and plethoric moon facies also may be found. Hypokalemia and metabolic alkalosis are prominent, particularly with ectopic production of ACTH.

Diagnosis

The diagnosis of Cushing's syndrome requires demonstration of increased cortisol production and abnormal cortisol suppression in response to dexamethasone. For initial screening, measurement of 24-h urinary free cortisol, the 1-mg overnight dexamethasone test [8 A.M. plasma cortisol <1.8 μg/dL (50 nmol/L)], or late-night salivary cortisol measurement is appropriate. Repeat testing or performance of more than one screening test may be required. Definitive diagnosis is established in equivocal cases by inadequate suppression of urinary cortisol [<10 μg/d (25 nmol/d)] or plasma cortisol [<5 μg/dL (140 nmol/L)] after 0.5 mg dexamethasone every 6 h for 48 h. Once the diagnosis of Cushing's syndrome is established, further biochemical testing is required to localize the source. This evaluation is best performed by an experienced endocrinologist. Low levels of plasma ACTH levels suggest an adrenal adenoma or carcinoma; inappropriately normal or high plasma ACTH levels suggest a pituitary or ectopic source. In 95% of ACTH-producing pituitary microadenomas, cortisol production is suppressed by high-dose dexamethasone (2 mg every 6 h for 48 h). MRI of the pituitary should be obtained but may not reveal a microadenoma because these tumors are typically very small. Furthermore, because up to 10% of ectopic sources of ACTH may also suppress after high-dose dexamethasone testing, inferior petrosal sinus sampling may be required to distinguish pituitary from peripheral sources of ACTH. Testing with corticotropin-releasing hormone (CRH) also may be helpful in determining the source of ACTH. Imaging of the chest and abdomen is required to localize the source of ectopic ACTH production; small bronchial carcinoids may escape detection by conventional CT. Pts with chronic alcoholism, depression, or obesity may have false-positive results in testing for Cushing's syndrome—a condition named pseudo-Cushing's syndrome. Similarly, pts with acute illness may have abnormal laboratory test results, since major stress alters the normal regulation of ACTH secretion.

TREATMENT Cushing's Syndrome

Uncontrolled hypercorticism carries a poor prognosis, and treatment of Cushing's syndrome is therefore necessary. Transsphenoidal surgery for pituitary ACTH-secreting microadenomas is curative in 70–80% when performed by a highly experienced surgeon, but long-term follow-up is required because these tumors may recur. Radiation therapy may be used when a surgical cure is not achieved (Chap. 179). Therapy of adrenal adenoma or carcinoma requires surgical excision; stress doses of glucocorticoids must be given pre- and postoperatively. Metastatic and unresectable adrenal carcinomas are treated with mitotane in doses gradually increased to 6 g/d in three or four divided doses. On occasion, debulking of lung carcinoma or resection of carcinoid tumors can result in remission of ectopic Cushing's syndrome. If the source of ACTH cannot be resected, medical management with ketoconazole (600–1200 mg/d), metyrapone (2–3 g/d), or mitotane (2–3 mg/d) may relieve manifestations of cortisol excess. In some cases, bilateral total adrenalectomy is required to control hypercorticism. Pts with unresectable pituitary adenomas who have had bilateral adrenalectomy are at risk for Nelson's syndrome (aggressive pituitary adenoma enlargement).

■ HYPERALDOSTERONISM

Etiology

Aldosteronism is caused by hypersecretion of the adrenal mineralocorticoid aldosterone. *Primary hyperaldosteronism* refers to an adrenal cause and can be due to either an adrenal adenoma or bilateral adrenal hyperplasia. Rare causes include glucocorticoid-remediable hyperaldosteronism, some forms of congenital adrenal hyperplasia, and other disorders of true or apparent mineralocorticoid excess (see Table 342-3, HPIM-18). The term *secondary hyperaldosteronism* is used when an extraadrenal stimulus for renin secretion is present, as in renal artery stenosis, decompensated liver cirrhosis, or diuretic therapy.

Clinical Features

Most pts with primary hyperaldosteronism have difficult to control hypertension (especially diastolic) and hypokalemia. Headaches are common. Edema is characteristically absent, unless congestive heart failure or renal disease is present. Hypokalemia, caused by urinary potassium losses, may cause muscle weakness, fatigue, and polyuria, although potassium levels may be normal in mild primary hyperaldosteronism. Metabolic alkalosis is a typical feature.

Diagnosis

The diagnosis is suggested by treatment-resistant hypertension that is associated with persistent hypokalemia in a nonedematous pt who is not receiving potassium-wasting diuretics. In pts receiving potassium-wasting diuretics, the diuretic should be discontinued and potassium supplements should be administered for 1–2 weeks. If hypokalemia persists after supplementation, screening using a serum aldosterone and plasma renin activity should be performed. Ideally, antihypertensives should be stopped before testing, but that is often impractical. Aldosterone receptor antagonists, beta-adrenergic blockers, ACE inhibitors, and angiotensin receptor blockers interfere with testing and should be substituted for other antihypertensives if possible. A ratio of serum aldosterone (in ng/dL) to plasma renin activity (in ng/mL per hour) >30 and an absolute level of aldosterone >15 ng/dL suggest primary aldosteronism. Failure to suppress plasma aldosterone (to <5 ng/dL after 500 mL/h of normal saline × 4 h) or urinary aldosterone after saline or sodium loading (to <10 μg/d on day 3 of 200 mmol/d oral NaCl + fludrocortisone 0.2 mg twice daily × 3 days) confirms primary hyperaldosteronism. Caution should be used with sodium loading in a hypertensive pt. Localization should then be undertaken with a high-resolution CT scan of the adrenal glands. If the CT scan is negative, bilateral adrenal vein sampling may be required to diagnose a unilateral aldosterone-producing adenoma. Secondary hyperaldosteronism is associated with elevated plasma renin activity.

TREATMENT ▶ Hyperaldosteronism

Surgery can be curative in pts with adrenal adenoma but is not effective for adrenal hyperplasia, which is managed with sodium restriction and spironolactone (25–100 mg twice daily) or eplerenone (25–50 mg twice daily). The sodium channel blocker amiloride (5–10 mg twice a day) also can be used. Secondary hyperaldosteronism is treated with salt restriction and correction of the underlying cause.

■ SYNDROMES OF ADRENAL ANDROGEN EXCESS

See Chap. 186 for discussion of hirsutism and virilization.

HYPOFUNCTION OF THE ADRENAL GLAND

Primary adrenal insufficiency is due to failure of the adrenal gland, whereas *secondary adrenal insufficiency* is due to failure of ACTH production or release.

■ ADDISON'S DISEASE

Etiology

Addison's disease occurs when >90% of adrenal tissue is destroyed. The most common cause is autoimmune destruction (alone, or as part of type I or type II polyglandular autoimmune syndromes). Tuberculosis used to be the leading etiology. Other granulomatous diseases (histoplasmosis, coccidioidomycosis, cryptococcosis, sarcoidosis), bilateral adrenalectomy, bilateral tumor metastases, bilateral hemorrhage, CMV, HIV, amyloidosis, and congenital diseases (some types of congenital adrenal hypoplasia, adrenal hypoplasia congenita, and adrenoleukodystrophy) are additional etiologies.

Clinical Features

Manifestations include fatigue, weakness, anorexia, nausea and vomiting, weight loss, abdominal pain, cutaneous and mucosal pigmentation, salt craving, hypotension (especially orthostatic), and, occasionally, hypoglycemia. Routine laboratory parameters may be normal, but typically serum Na is reduced and serum K increased. Extracellular fluid depletion accentuates hypotension. In secondary adrenal insufficiency, pigmentation is diminished and serum potassium is not elevated. Serum Na tends to be low because of hemodilution stemming from excess vasopressin secreted in the setting of cortisol deficiency.

Diagnosis

The best screening test is the cortisol response 60 min after 250 μg ACTH (cosyntropin) IV or IM. Cortisol levels should exceed 18 μg/dL 30–60 min after the ACTH. If the response is abnormal, then primary and secondary deficiency may be distinguished by measurement of aldosterone from the same blood samples. In secondary, but not primary, adrenal insufficiency, the aldosterone increment from baseline will be normal (≥5 ng/dL). Furthermore, in primary adrenal insufficiency, plasma ACTH is elevated, whereas in secondary adrenal insufficiency, plasma ACTH values are low or inappropriately normal. Pts with recent onset or partial pituitary insufficiency may have a normal response to the rapid ACTH stimulation test. In these pts, alternative testing (metyrapone test or insulin tolerance testing) can be used for diagnosis.

TREATMENT   Addison's Disease

Hydrocortisone, at 15–25 mg/d divided into ⅔ in the morning and ⅓ in the afternoon, is the mainstay of glucocorticoid replacement. Some pts benefit from doses administered three times daily, and other glucocorticoids may be given at equivalent doses. Mineralocorticoid supplementation is usually needed for primary adrenal insufficiency, with administration of 0.05–0.1 mg fludrocortisone PO qd and maintenance of adequate Na intake. Doses should be titrated to normalize Na and K levels and to maintain normal blood pressure without postural changes. Measurement of plasma renin levels may also be useful in titrating the dose. Mineralocorticoid replacement is not needed in pts with secondary adrenal insufficiency. All pts with adrenal insufficiency should be instructed in the parenteral self-administration of steroids and should be registered with a medical alert system. During periods of intercurrent illness, the dose of hydrocortisone should be doubled. During adrenal crisis, high-dose hydrocortisone (10 mg/h continuous IV or 100-mg bolus IV three times a day) should be administered along with normal saline. Thereafter, if the pt is improving and is afebrile, the dose can be tapered by 20–30% daily to usual replacement doses.

■ HYPOALDOSTERONISM

Isolated aldosterone deficiency accompanied by normal cortisol production occurs with hyporeninism, as an inherited aldosterone synthase deficiency, postoperatively following removal of aldosterone-secreting adenomas (transient), and during protracted heparin therapy. Hyporeninemic hypoaldosteronism is seen most commonly in adults with diabetes mellitus and mild renal failure; it is characterized by mild to moderate hyperkalemia. This is usually a benign condition that can be managed by observation. If needed, oral fludrocortisone (0.05–0.15 mg/d PO) restores electrolyte balance if salt intake is adequate. In pts with hypertension, mild renal insufficiency, or congestive heart failure, an alternative approach is to reduce salt intake and to administer furosemide.

INCIDENTAL ADRENAL MASSES

Adrenal masses are common findings on abdominal CT or MRI scans (1–7% prevalence with increasing age). The majority (70–80%) of such "incidentalomas" are clinically nonfunctional, and the probability of an adrenal carcinoma is low (<0.01%). Genetic syndromes such as MEN 1, MEN 2, Carney syndrome, and McCune-Albright syndrome are all associated with adrenal masses. The first step in evaluation is to determine the functional status by measurement of plasma free metanephrines to screen for pheochromocytoma (Fig. 182-1). In a pt with a known extraadrenal malignancy, there is a 30–50% chance that the incidentaloma is a metastasis. Additional hormonal evaluation should include overnight 1-mg dexamethasone suppression testing in all pts, plasma renin activity/aldosterone ratio in hypertensives, DHEAS in women with signs of androgen excess, and estradiol in males with feminization. Fine-needle aspiration is rarely indicated and absolutely contraindicated if a pheochromocytoma is suspected. Adrenocortical cancer is suggested by large size (>4–6 cm), irregular margins, tumor inhomogeneity, soft tissue calcifications, and high unenhanced CT attenuation values (>10 HU).

CLINICAL USES OF GLUCOCORTICOIDS

Glucocorticoids are pharmacologic agents used for a variety of disorders such as asthma, rheumatoid arthritis, and psoriasis. The almost certain development of complications (weight gain, hypertension, Cushingoid facies, diabetes mellitus, osteoporosis, myopathy, increased intraocular pressure, ischemic bone necrosis, infection, and hyperlipidemia) must be weighed against the potential therapeutic benefits of glucocorticoid therapy. These side effects can be minimized by a careful choice of steroid preparations (Table 182-1), dose minimization, and alternate-day or interrupted therapy; the use of topical steroids, i.e., inhaled, intranasal, or dermal, whenever possible; the judicious use of nonsteroid therapies; monitoring of

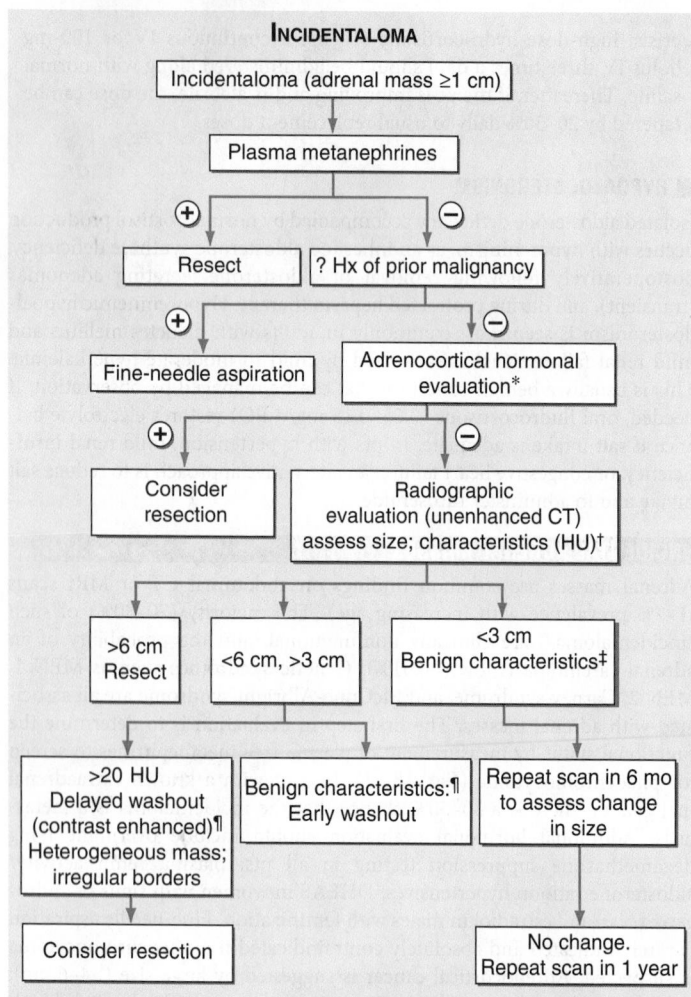

FIGURE 182-1 Incidentaloma. *Adrenocortical hormonal evaluation: Dexamethasone suppression test in all pts; plasma renin activity/aldosterone ratio for hypertensives; sex steroid (DHEA sulfate, estradiol) for clinical signs in females and males, respectively. †Hounsfield units (HU): a measurement of x-ray attenuation or lipid content of neoplasms. A lipid-rich mass (<10 HU) is diagnostic of a benign cortical adenoma. ‡Benign characteristics: homogeneous mass, smooth borders, HU <10. ¶Benign adrenal adenomas are also characterized by earlier washout of contrast enhancement than other neoplasms.

TABLE 182-1 GLUCOCORTICOID PREPARATIONS

Generic Name	Relative Potency		Dose Equivalent
	Glucocorticoid	Mineralocorticoid	
Short-acting			
Hydrocortisone	1.0	1.0	20.0
Cortisone	0.8	0.8	25.0
Intermediate-acting			
Prednisone	4.0	0.25	5.0
Methylprednisolone	5.0	0	4.0
Triamcinolone	5.0	0	4.0
Long-acting			
Dexamethasone	30.0	0	0.75
Betamethasone	25.0	0	0.8

TABLE 182-2 A CHECKLIST FOR USE PRIOR TO THE ADMINISTRATION OF GLUCOCORTICOIDS IN PHARMACOLOGIC DOSES

Presence of tuberculosis or other chronic infection (chest x-ray, tuberculin test)

Evidence of glucose intolerance, history of gestational diabetes mellitus, or high risk for type 2 diabetes mellitus

Evidence of preexisting osteoporosis (bone density assessment in organ transplant recipients or postmenopausal pts)

History of peptic ulcer, gastritis, or esophagitis (stool guaiac test)

Evidence of hypertension, cardiovascular disease, or hypertriglyceridemia

History of psychological disorders

caloric intake; and instituting measures to minimize bone loss. Pts should be evaluated for the risk of complications before the initiation of glucocorticoid therapy (Table 182-2). Higher doses of glucocorticoids may be required during periods of stress, since the hypothalamo-pituitary-adrenal axis is suppressed and the adrenal gland may atrophy in the setting of exogenous glucocorticoids. In addition, following long-term use, glucocorticoids should be tapered with the dual goals of allowing the pituitary-adrenal axis to recover and the avoidance of underlying disease flare.

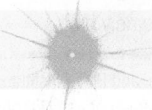

For a more detailed discussion, see Arlt W: Disorders of the Adrenal Cortex, Chap. 342, p. 2940, in HPIM-18.

CHAPTER **183**
Obesity

Obesity is a state of excess adipose tissue mass. Obesity should not be defined by body weight alone, as muscular individuals may be overweight by arbitrary standards without having increased adiposity. The most widely used method to classify weight status and risk of disease is the *body mass index* (BMI), which is equal to weight/height^2 in kg/m^2 (Table 183-1). At a similar BMI, women have more body fat than men. Furthermore, regional fat distribution may influence the risks associated with obesity. Central (primarily visceral) obesity [high ratio of the circumference of the waist to the circumference of the hips (waist-to-hip ratio), >0.9 in women and 1.0 in men] is independently associated with a higher risk for metabolic syndrome, diabetes mellitus, hyperandrogenism in women, and cardiovascular disease. The prevalence of obesity has increased dramatically over the past 3 decades. In the United States in 2008, 34% of adults age >20 were obese (BMI >30), and another 34% were overweight (BMI 25–30). Most alarming is the same trend among children, where 17% between ages 2 and 19 were obese, and another 18% were overweight. This has led to an epidemic of type 2 diabetes in children, a condition almost never seen until recently. These trends to increased obesity are not limited to Western societies but are occurring worldwide.

◾ ETIOLOGY

Obesity can result from increased energy intake, decreased energy expenditure, or a combination of the two. Excess accumulation of body fat is the consequence of environmental and genetic factors; social factors and economic conditions also represent important influences. The recent increase in obesity can be attributed to a combination of excess caloric intake and decreasing physical activity. Poorly understood reasons for increased food

TABLE 183-1 CLASSIFICATION OF WEIGHT STATUS AND RISK OF DISEASE

	BMI (kg/m^2)	Obesity Class	Risk of Disease
Underweight	<18.5		
Healthy weight	18.5–24.9		
Overweight	25.0–29.9		Increased
Obesity	30.0–34.9	I	High
Obesity	35.0–39.9	II	Very high
Extreme obesity	≥40	III	Extremely high

Source: Adapted from National Institutes of Health, National Heart, Lung, and Blood Institute: *Clinical Guidelines on the Identification, Evaluation, and Treatment of Overweight and Obesity in Adults.* U.S. Department of Health and Human Services, Public Health Service, 1998.

assimilation due to dietary composition have also been postulated, as have sleep deprivation and an unfavorable gut flora. The susceptibility to obesity is polygenic in nature, and 30–50% of the variability in total fat stores is believed to be genetically determined. Among monogenic causes, mutations in the melanocortin receptor 4 are most common and account for ~1% of obesity in the general population and ~6% in severe, early-onset obesity. Syndromic obesity forms include Prader-Willi syndrome and Laurence-Moon-Biedl syndrome. Other monogenetic or syndromic causes are extremely rare. Secondary causes of obesity include hypothalamic injury, hypothyroidism, Cushing's syndrome, and hypogonadism. Drug-induced weight gain is also common in those who use antidiabetes agents (insulin, sulfonylureas, thiazolidinediones), glucocorticoids, psychotropic agents, mood stabilizers (lithium), antidepressants (tricyclics, monoamine oxidase inhibitors, paroxetine, mirtazapine), or antiepileptic drugs (valproate, gabapentin, carbamazepine). Insulin-secreting tumors can cause overeating and weight gain.

■ CLINICAL FEATURES

Obesity has major adverse effects on health. Increased mortality from obesity is primarily due to cardiovascular disease, hypertension, gall bladder disease, diabetes mellitus, and several types of cancer, such as cancer of the esophagus, colon, rectum, pancreas, liver, and prostate, and gallbladder, bile ducts, breasts, endometrium, cervix, and ovaries in women. Sleep apnea in severely obese individuals poses serious health risks. Obesity is also associated with an increased incidence of steatohepatitis, gastroesophageal reflux, osteoarthritis, gout, back pain, skin infections, and depression. Hypogonadism in men and infertility in both sexes are prevalent in obesity; in women this may be associated with hyperandrogenism (polycystic ovarian syndrome).

TREATMENT	Obesity

Obesity is a chronic medical condition that requires ongoing treatment and lifestyle modifications. Treatment is important because of the associated health risks, but is made difficult by a limited repertoire of effective therapeutic options. Weight regain after weight loss is common with all forms of therapy. The urgency and selection of treatment modalities should be based on BMI and a risk assessment.

Diet, exercise, and behavior therapy are recommended for all pts with a BMI ≥25 kg/m². Behavior modification including group counseling, diet diaries, and changes in eating patterns should be initiated. Food-related behaviors should be monitored carefully (avoid cafeteria-style settings, eat small and frequent meals, eat breakfast). A deficit of 7500 kcal will produce a weight loss of approximately 1 kg. Therefore, eating 100 kcal/d less for a year should cause a 5-kg weight loss, and a deficit of 1000 kcal/d should cause a loss of ~1 kg per week. Physical activity should be increased to a minimum of 150 min of moderate intensity physical activity per week.

Pharmacotherapy may be added to a lifestyle program for pts with a BMI ≥30 kg/m² or ≥27 kg/m² with concomitant obesity-related diseases. Orlistat is the only pharmacologic agent currently approved by the U.S. Food and Drug Administration for treatment of obesity; several others have been withdrawn from the market because of significant adverse effects. Orlistat, an inhibitor of intestinal lipase, causes modest weight loss (9–10% at 12 months with lifestyle measures) due to drug-induced fat malabsorption. Metformin, exenatide, and liraglutide tend to decrease body weight in pts with obesity and type 2 diabetes mellitus, but they are not indicated for pts without diabetes.

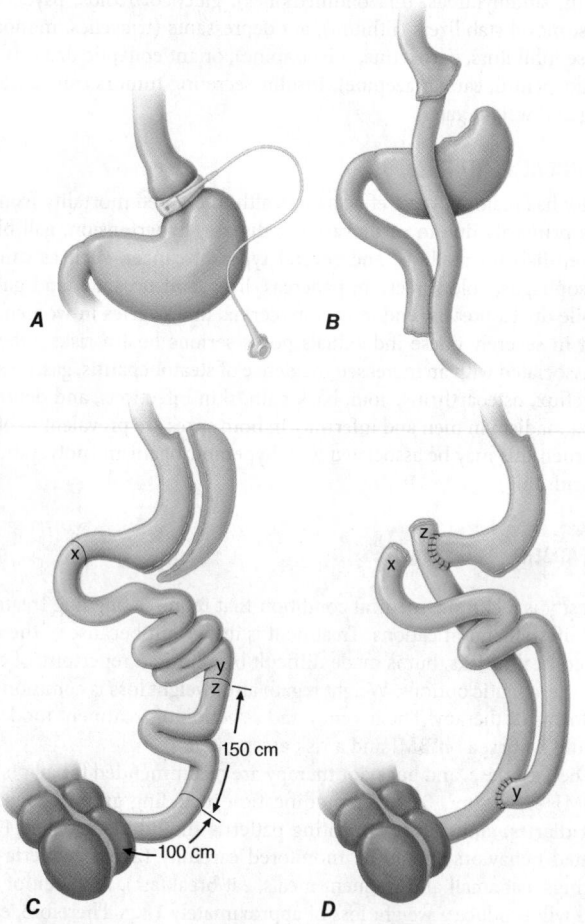

FIGURE 183-1 Bariatric surgical procedures. Examples of operative interventions used for surgical manipulation of the gastrointestinal tract. **A.** Laparoscopic gastric band (LAGB). **B.** The Roux-en-Y gastric bypass. **C.** Biliopancreatic diversion with duodenal switch. **D.** Biliopancreatic diversion. (*From ML Kendrick, GF Dakin, Surgical approaches to obesity. Mayo Clinic Proc 815:518, 2006; with permission.*)

Bariatric surgery should be considered for pts with severe obesity (BMI ≥40 kg/m²) or moderate obesity (BMI ≥35 kg/m²) associated with a serious medical condition, with repeated failures of other therapeutic approaches, at eligible weight for >3 years, capable of tolerating surgery, and without addictions or major psychopathology. Weight-loss surgeries are either restrictive (limiting the amount of food the stomach can hold and slowing gastric emptying), such as laparoscopic adjustable silicone gastric banding, or restrictive-malabsorptive, such as Roux-en-Y gastric bypass (Fig. 183-1). These procedures generally produce a 30–35% weight loss that is maintained in about 40% of pts at 4 years. Complications include stomal stenosis, marginal ulcers, and dumping syndrome. Procedures with a malabsorptive component require lifelong supplementation of micronutrients (iron, folate, calcium, vitamins B$_{12}$ and D) and are associated with a risk of islet cell hyperplasia and hypoglycemia.

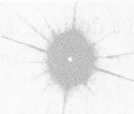

For a more detailed discussion, see Flier JS, Maratos-Flier E: Biology of Obesity, Chap. 77, p. 622 and Kushner RF: Evaluation and Management of Obesity, Chap. 78, p. 629, in HPIM-18.

CHAPTER **184**
Diabetes Mellitus

■ ETIOLOGY AND PREVALENCE

Diabetes mellitus (DM) comprises a group of metabolic disorders that share the common phenotype of hyperglycemia. DM is currently classified on the basis of the pathogenic process that leads to hyperglycemia. Type 1 DM is characterized by insulin deficiency and a tendency to develop ketosis, whereas type 2 DM is a heterogeneous group of disorders characterized by variable degrees of insulin resistance, impaired insulin secretion, and excessive hepatic glucose production. Other specific types include DM caused by genetic defects [maturity-onset diabetes of the young (MODY) and other rare monogenic disorders], diseases of the exocrine pancreas (chronic pancreatitis, cystic fibrosis, hemochromatosis), endocrinopathies (acromegaly, Cushing's syndrome, glucagonoma, pheochromocytoma, hyperthyroidism), drugs (nicotinic acid, glucocorticoids, thiazides, protease inhibitors), and pregnancy (gestational DM). The phenotype of these monogenetic and secondary types of DM typically resembles type 2 DM; its severity depends on the degree of beta cell dysfunction and prevailing insulin resistance. Type 1 DM usually results from autoimmune destruction of pancreatic beta cells; it is also known as juvenile-onset diabetes because its peak incidence is in children and adolescents.

The prevalence of DM is increasing rapidly; type 2 DM frequency in particular is rising in parallel with the epidemic of obesity (Chap. 183).

Between 1985 and 2010, the worldwide prevalence of DM has risen almost 10-fold, from 30 million to 285 million cases. In the United States, DM prevalence in 2010 is estimated at 26 million, or 8.4% of the population. A significant portion of persons with DM are undiagnosed.

DM is attended by serious morbidity and significant mortality; it is the fifth leading cause of death worldwide.

■ DIAGNOSIS

Criteria for the diagnosis of DM include one of the following:

- Fasting plasma glucose ≥7.0 mmol/L (≥126 mg/dL)
- Symptoms of diabetes plus a random blood glucose concentration ≥11.1 mmol/L (≥200 mg/dL)
- 2-h plasma glucose ≥11.1 mmol/L (≥200 mg/dL) during a 75-g oral glucose tolerance test.
- Hemoglobin A_{1c} >6.5%

These criteria should be confirmed by repeat testing on a different day, unless unequivocal hyperglycemia is present.

Two intermediate categories also have been designated:

- Impaired fasting glucose (IFG) for a fasting plasma glucose level of 5.6–6.9 mmol/L (100–125 mg/dL)
- Impaired glucose tolerance (IGT) for plasma glucose levels of 7.8–11.1 mmol/L (140–199 mg/dL) 2 h after a 75-g oral glucose load

Individuals with IFG or IGT do not have DM but are at substantial risk for developing type 2 DM and cardiovascular disease in the future.

Screening with a fasting plasma glucose level is recommended every 3 years for individuals over the age of 45, as well as for younger individuals who are overweight (body mass index ≥25 kg/m²) and have one or more additional risk factors (Table 184-1).

The *metabolic syndrome* (also known as *insulin resistance syndrome* or *syndrome X*) is a term used to describe a commonly found constellation of metabolic derangements that includes insulin resistance (with or without diabetes), hypertension, dyslipidemia, central or visceral obesity, and endothelial dysfunction and is associated with accelerated cardiovascular disease (Chap. 127).

■ CLINICAL FEATURES

Common presenting symptoms of DM include polyuria, polydipsia, weight loss, fatigue, weakness, blurred vision, frequent superficial infections, and poor wound healing. In early type 2 DM, symptoms may be more subtle and consist of fatigue, poor wound healing, and paresthesias. The lack of symptoms is the main reason for the delayed diagnosis of type 2 DM. A complete medical history should be obtained with special emphasis on weight, exercise, smoking, ethanol use, family history of DM, and risk factors for cardiovascular disease. In a pt with established DM, assessment of prior diabetes care, HbA_{1c} levels, self-monitoring blood glucose results, frequency of hypoglycemia, and pt's knowledge about DM

TABLE 184-1 CRITERIA FOR TESTING FOR PRE-DIABETES AND DIABETES IN ASYMPTOMATIC INDIVIDUALS[a]

Risk Factors
• First-degree relative with diabetes
• Physical inactivity
• Race/ethnicity (e.g., African American, Latino, Native American, Asian American, Pacific Islander)
• Previously identified IFG, IGT, or a hemoglobin A_{1c} of 5.7–6.4%
• History of GDM or delivery of baby >4 kg (>9 lb)
• Hypertension (blood pressure ≥140/90 mmHg)
• HDL cholesterol level ≤0.90 mmol/L (35 mg/dL) and/or a triglyceride level ≥2.82 mmol/L (250 mg/dL)
• Polycystic ovary syndrome or acanthosis nigricans
• History of vascular disease

[a]Testing should be considered in all adults at age 45 and adults <45 y with BMI ≥25 kg/m^2 and one or more of the following risk factors for diabetes.
Abbreviations: BMI, body mass index; GDM, gestational diabetes mellitus; HDL, high-density lipoprotein; IFG, impaired fasting glucose; IGT, impaired glucose tolerance.
Source: Adapted from American Diabetes Association, 2011.

should be obtained. Special attention should be given on physical exam to retinal exam, orthostatic bp, foot exam (including vibratory sensation and monofilament testing), peripheral pulses, and insulin injection sites. Acute complications of DM that may be seen on presentation include diabetic ketoacidosis (DKA) (type 1 DM) and hyperglycemic hyperosmolar state (type 2 DM) (Chap. 24).

The chronic complications of DM are listed below:

- Ophthalmologic: nonproliferative or proliferative diabetic retinopathy, macular edema, rubeosis of iris, glaucoma, cataracts
- Renal: proteinuria, end-stage renal disease (ESRD), type IV renal tubular acidosis
- Neurologic: distal symmetric polyneuropathy, polyradiculopathy, mononeuropathy, autonomic neuropathy
- Gastrointestinal: gastroparesis, diarrhea, constipation
- Genitourinary: cystopathy, erectile dysfunction, female sexual dysfunction, vaginal candidiasis
- Cardiovascular: coronary artery disease, congestive heart failure, peripheral vascular disease, stroke
- Lower extremity: foot deformity (hammer toe, claw toe, Charcot foot), ulceration, amputation
- Dermatologic: Infections (folliculitis, furunculosis, cellulitis), necrobiosis, poor healing, ulcers, gangrene
- Dental: Periodontal disease

TREATMENT Diabetes Mellitus

Optimal treatment of DM requires more than plasma glucose management. Comprehensive diabetes care should also detect and manage DM-specific complications and modify risk factors for DM-associated diseases. The pt with type 1 or type 2 DM should receive education about nutrition, exercise, care of diabetes during illness, and medications to lower the plasma glucose. In general, the target HbA_{1c} level should be <7.0%, although individual considerations (age, ability to implement a complex treatment regimen, and presence of other medical conditions) should also be taken into account. Intensive therapy reduces long-term complications but is associated with more frequent and more severe hypoglycemic episodes. Goal preprandial capillary plasma glucose levels should be 3.9–7.2 mmol/L (70–130 mg/dL) and postprandial levels should be <10.0 mmol/L (<180 mg/dL) 1–2 h after a meal.

In general, pts with type 1 DM require 0.5–1.0 U/kg per day of insulin divided into multiple doses. Combinations of insulin preparations with different times of onset and duration of action should be used (Table 184-2). Preferred regimens include injection of glargine at bedtime with preprandial lispro, glulisine, or insulin aspart or continuous SC insulin using an infusion device. Pramlintide, an injectable amylin analogue, can be used as adjunct therapy to control postprandial glucose excursions.

Pts with type 2 DM may be managed with diet and exercise alone or in conjunction with oral glucose-lowering agents, insulin, or a combination of oral agents and insulin. The classes of oral glucose-lowering agents and dosing regimens are listed in Table 184-3. In addition, exenatide and liraglutide are injectable glucagon-like peptide 1 (GLP-1, an incretin) analogues that may be used in combination with metformin or sulfonylureas. A reasonable treatment algorithm for initial therapy proposes metformin as initial therapy because of its efficacy (1–2% decrease in HbA_{1c}), known side-effect profile, and relatively low cost (Fig. 184-1). Metformin has the advantage that it promotes mild weight loss, lowers insulin levels, improves the lipid profile slightly, lowers cancer risk, and does not cause hypoglycemia when used as monotherapy, although it is contraindicated in renal insufficiency, congestive heart failure, any form of acidosis, liver disease, or severe hypoxia, and should be temporarily discontinued in pts who are seriously ill or receiving radiographic contrast material. Metformin therapy can be followed by addition of a second oral agent (insulin secretagogue, DPP-IV inhibitor, thiazolidinedione, or α-glucosidase inhibitor). Combinations of two oral agents may be used with additive effects, with stepwise addition of bedtime insulin or a third oral agent if adequate control is not achieved. As endogenous insulin production falls, multiple injections of long-acting and short-acting insulin may be required, as in type 1 DM. Individuals who require >1 U/kg per day of long-acting insulin should be considered for combination therapy with an insulin-sensitizing agent such as metformin or a thiazolidinedione. Insulin-requiring type 2 DM pts may also benefit from addition of pramlintide.

TABLE 184-2 PROPERTIES OF INSULIN PREPARATIONS

Preparation	Onset, h	Peak, h	Effective Duration, h
		Time of Action	
Short-acting			
Aspart	<0.25	0.5–1.5	3–4
Glulisine	<0.25	0.5–1.5	3–4
Lispro	<0.25	0.5–1.5	3–4
Regular	0.5–1.0	2–3	4–6
Long-acting			
Detemir	1–4	—[a]	Up to 24
Glargine	1–4	—[a]	Up to 24
NPH	1–4	6–10	10–16
Insulin combinations			
75/25–75% protamine lispro, 25% lispro	<0.25	1.5 h	Up to 10–16
70/30–70% protamine aspart, 30% aspart	<0.25	1.5 h	Up to 10–16
50/50–50% protamine lispro, 50% lispro	<0.25	1.5 h	Up to 10–16
70/30–70% NPH, 30% regular	0.5–1	Dual[b]	10–16

[a]Glargine and detemir have minimal peak activity.
[b]Dual: two peaks—one at 2–3 h and the second one several hours later.
Source: Adapted from JS Skyler: *Therapy for Diabetes Mellitus and Related Disorders,* American Diabetes Association, Alexandria, VA, 2004.

The morbidity and mortality of DM-related complications can be greatly reduced by timely and consistent surveillance procedures (Table 184-4). A routine urinalysis may be performed as an initial screen for diabetic nephropathy. If it is positive for protein, quantification of protein on a 24-h urine collection should be performed. If the urinalysis is negative for protein, a spot collection for microalbuminuria should be performed (present if 30–300 μg/mg creatinine on two of three tests within a 3- to 6-month period). A resting ECG should be performed in adults, with more extensive cardiac testing for high-risk pts. Therapeutic goals to prevent complications of DM include management of protein-uria with ACE inhibitor or angiotensin receptor blocker therapy, bp control (<130/80 mmHg if no proteinuria, <125/75 if proteinuria), and dyslipidemia management [LDL <2.6 mmol/L (<100 mg/dL), HDL >1.1 mmol/L (>40 mg/dL) in men and >1.38 mmol/L (50 mg/dL) in women, triglycerides <1.7 mmol/L (<150 mg/dL)]. In addition, any diabetic pt >40 years should take a statin, regardless of the LDL cholesterol, and in

TABLE 184-3 ORAL GLUCOSE-LOWERING AGENTS

Agent	Daily Dose, mg	Doses/d	Contraindications
Biguanide			Creatinine >133 μmol/L (1.5 mg/dL) (men); >124 μmol/L (1.4 mg/dL) (women); CHF; liver disease
Metformin	500–2500	1–3	
Sulfonylureas			Renal/liver disease
Glimepiride	1–8	1	
Glipizide	2.5–40	1–2	
Glipizide (ext. release)	5–10	1	
Glyburide	1.25–20	1–2	
Glyburide (micronized)	0.75–12	1–2	
Non-sulfonylurea secretagogue			Renal/liver disease
Repaglinide	0.5–16	1–4	
Nateglinide	180–360	1–3	
α-Glucosidase inhibitor			IBD, liver disease, or Cr >177 μmol/L (2.0 mg/dL)
Acarbose	25–300	1–3	
Miglitol	25–300	1–3	
Thiazolidinedione			Liver disease, CHF
Pioglitazone	15–45	1	
DPP-IV inhibitor			↓ Dose with renal failure
Sitagliptin	100	1	
Saxagliptin	2.5–5	1	
Linagliptin	5	1	
Vildagliptin	50–100	1	

those with existing cardiovascular disease, the LDL target should be <1.8 mmol/L (70 mg/dL).

MANAGEMENT OF THE HOSPITALIZED PATIENT

The goals of diabetes management during hospitalization are near-normal glycemic control, avoidance of hypoglycemia, and transition back to the outpatient diabetes treatment regimen. Pts with type 1 DM undergoing general anesthesia and surgery, or with serious illness, should receive continuous insulin, either through an IV insulin infusion or by

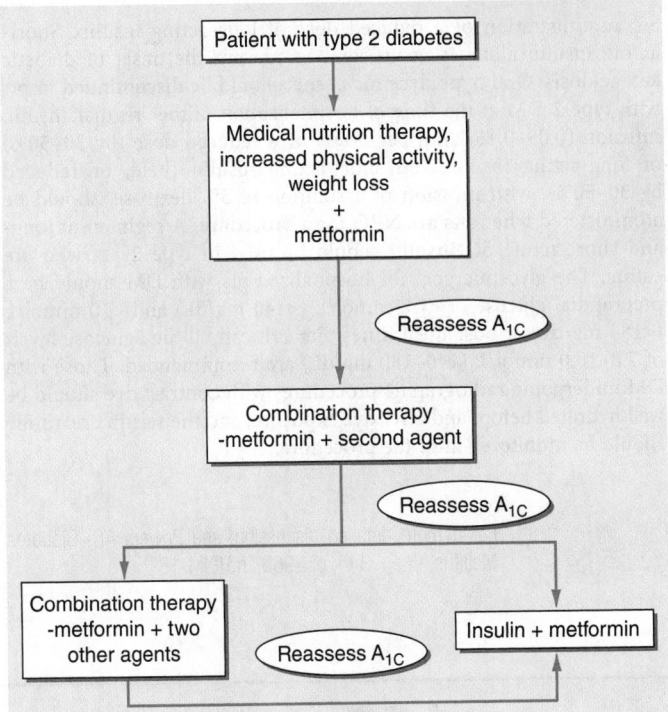

FIGURE 184-1 Glycemic management of type 2 diabetes. Agents that can be combined with metformin include insulin secretagogues, thiazolidinediones, α-glucosidase inhibitors, DPP-IV inhibitors, and GLP-1 receptor agonists. A_{1c}, hemoglobin A_{1c}.

TABLE 184-4 GUIDELINES FOR ONGOING MEDICAL CARE FOR PATIENTS WITH DIABETES

- Self-monitoring of blood glucose (individualized frequency)
- A_{1c} testing (2–4 times/year)
- Pt education in diabetes management (annual)
- Medical nutrition therapy and education (annual)
- Eye examination (annual)
- Foot examination (1–2 times/year by physician; daily by pt)
- Screening for diabetic nephropathy (annual; see Fig. 344-11)
- Blood pressure measurement (quarterly)
- Lipid profile and serum creatinine (estimate GFR) (annual)
- Influenza/pneumococcal immunizations
- Consider antiplatelet therapy (see text)

Abbreviation: A_{1c}, hemoglobin A_{1c}.

SC administration of a reduced dose of long-acting insulin. Short-acting insulin alone is insufficient to prevent the onset of diabetic ketoacidosis. Oral hypoglycemic agents should be discontinued in pts with type 2 DM at the time of hospitalization. Either regular insulin infusion (0.05–0.15 U/kg per hour) or a reduced dose (by 30–50%) of long-acting insulin and short-acting insulin (held, or reduced by 30–50%), with infusion of a solution of 5% dextrose, should be administered when pts are NPO for a procedure. A regimen of long- and short-acting SC insulin should be used in type 2 pts who are eating. The glycemic goal for hospitalized pts with DM should be a preprandial glucose of <7.8 mmol/L (<140 mg/dL) and <10 mmol/L (<180 mg/dL) at post-meal times. For critically ill pts, glucose levels of 7.8–10.0 mmol/L (140–180 mg/dL) are recommended. Those with DM undergoing radiographic procedures with contrast dye should be well hydrated before and after dye exposure, and the serum creatinine should be monitored after the procedure.

For a more detailed discussion, see Powers AC: Diabetes Mellitus, Chap. 344, p. 2968, in HPIM-18.

CHAPTER **185**
Disorders of the Male Reproductive System

The testes produce sperm and testosterone. Inadequate production of sperm can occur in isolation or in the presence of androgen deficiency, which impairs spermatogenesis secondarily.

◼ ANDROGEN DEFICIENCY

Etiology

Androgen deficiency can be due to either testicular failure (*primary hypogonadism*) or hypothalamic-pituitary defects (*secondary hypogonadism*).

Primary hypogonadism is diagnosed when testosterone levels are low and gonadotropin levels [luteinizing hormone (LH) and follicle-stimulating hormone (FSH)] are high. Klinefelter's syndrome is the most common cause (~1 in 1000 male births) and is due to the presence of one or more extra X chromosomes, usually a 47,XXY karyotype. Other genetic causes of testicular development, androgen biosynthesis, or androgen action are uncommon. Acquired primary testicular failure usually results from viral orchitis but may be due to trauma, testicular torsion, cryptorchidism, radiation damage, or systemic diseases such as amyloidosis, Hodgkin's disease, sickle cell disease, or granulomatous diseases. Testicular failure can occur as a part of polyglandular autoimmune failure syndrome. Malnutrition, AIDS, renal failure, liver cirrhosis, myotonic dystrophy, paraplegia, and toxins such as alcohol, marijuana, heroin, methadone, lead, and antineoplastic and chemotherapeutic agents also can cause testicular failure. Testosterone synthesis may be blocked by ketoconazole, and testosterone action may be blocked at the androgen receptor level by spironolactone or cimetidine.

Secondary hypogonadism is diagnosed when levels of both testosterone and gonadotropins are low (*hypogonadotropic hypogonadism*). Kallmann syndrome is due to maldevelopment of neurons producing gonadotropin-releasing hormone (GnRH) and is characterized by GnRH deficiency, low levels of LH and FSH, and anosmia. Several other types of GnRH deficiency or gonadotropin deficiency present without anosmia. Acquired causes of isolated hypogonadotropic hypogonadism include critical illness, excessive stress, obesity, Cushing's syndrome, opioid and marijuana use, hemochromatosis, and hyperprolactinemia (due to pituitary adenomas or drugs such as phenothiazines). Destruction of the pituitary gland by tumors, infection, trauma, or metastatic disease causes hypogonadism in conjunction with deficiency of other pituitary hormones (see Chap. 179). Normal aging is associated with a progressive decline of testosterone production, which is due to downregulation of the entire hypothalamo-pituitary-testicular axis.

Clinical Features

The history should focus on developmental stages such as puberty and growth spurts, as well as androgen-dependent events such as early morning erections, frequency and intensity of sexual thoughts, and frequency of masturbation or intercourse. The physical examination should focus on secondary sex characteristics such as hair growth in the face, axilla, chest, and pubic regions; gynecomastia; testicular volume; prostate; and height and body proportions. Eunuchoidal proportions are defined as an arm span >2 cm greater than height and suggest that androgen deficiency occurred prior to epiphyseal fusion. Normal testicular size ranges from 3.5–5.5 cm in length, which corresponds to a volume of 12–25 mL. The presence of varicocele should be sought by palpation of the testicular veins with the pt standing. Pts with Klinefelter's syndrome have small (1–2 mL), firm testes.

A morning total testosterone level <10.4 nmol/L (<300 ng/dL), in association with symptoms, suggests testosterone deficiency. A level of >12.1 nmol/L (>350 ng/dL) makes the diagnosis of androgen deficiency unlikely. In men with testosterone levels between 6.9 and 12.1 nmol/L (200 and 350 ng/dL), the total testosterone level should be repeated and a free testosterone level should be measured by a reliable method. In older men and in pts with other clinical states that are associated with alterations in sex hormone–binding globulin levels, a direct measurement of free testosterone by equilibrium dialysis can be useful in unmasking testosterone deficiency. When androgen deficiency has been confirmed by low testosterone concentrations, LH should be measured to classify the pt as having primary (high LH) or secondary (low or inappropriately normal LH) hypogonadism. In men with primary hypogonadism of unknown cause, a karyotype should be performed to exclude Klinefelter's syndrome. Measurement of a prolactin level and MRI of the hypothalamic-pituitary region should be considered in men with secondary hypogonadism. Gynecomastia in the absence of androgen deficiency should be further evaluated (Fig. 185-1).

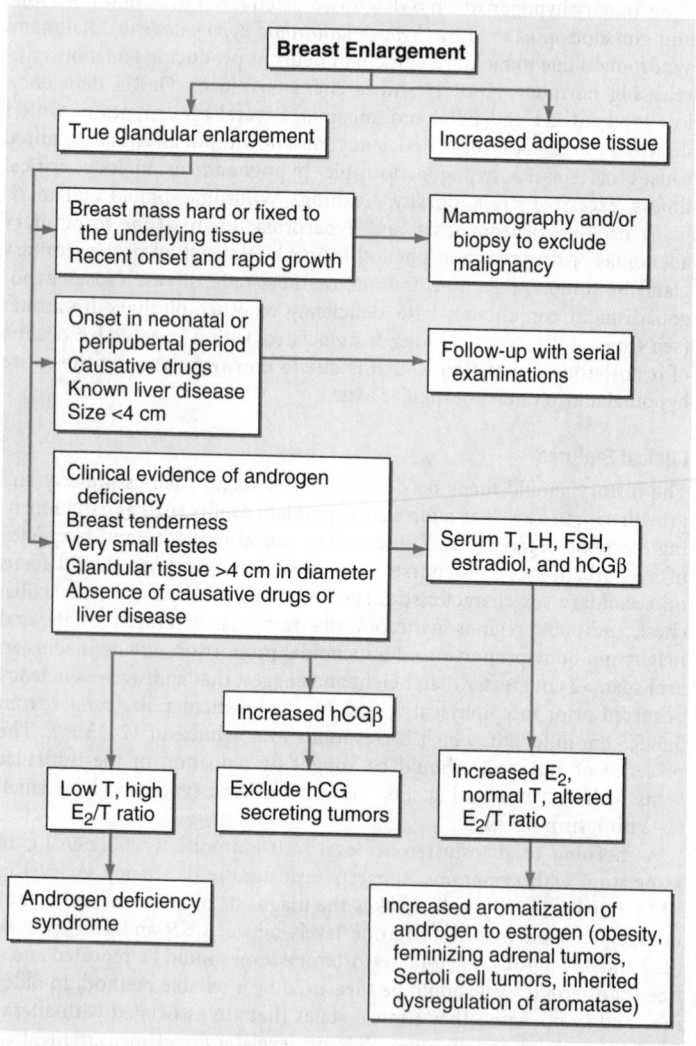

FIGURE 185-1 Evaluation of gynecomastia. T, testosterone; LH, luteinizing hormone; FSH, follicle-stimulating hormone; hCGβ, human chorionic gonadotropin β; E2, 17β-estradiol.

> **TREATMENT** Androgen Deficiency
>
> Treatment of hypogonadal men with androgens restores normal male secondary sexual characteristics (beard, body hair, external genitalia), male sexual drive, and masculine somatic development (hemoglobin, muscle mass), but not fertility. Administration of gradually increasing doses of testosterone is recommended for disorders in which hypogonadism occurred prior to puberty. Testosterone levels in the normal range may be achieved through daily application of transdermal testosterone patches (5–10 mg/d) or gel (50–100 mg/d), parenteral administration of a long-acting testosterone ester (e.g., 100–200 mg testosterone enanthate at 1- to 3-week intervals) or buccal testosterone tablets (30 mg/d). Hematocrit should be monitored initially during testosterone therapy and the dose lowered if Hct is >54%. Prostate cancer, severe symptoms of lower urinary tract obstruction, baseline hematocrit >50%, severe sleep apnea, and class IV congestive heart failure are contraindications for androgen replacement. Gonadotropin therapy for secondary hypogonadism should be reserved for fertility induction.

■ MALE INFERTILITY

Etiology

Male infertility plays a role in 25% of infertile couples (couples who fail to conceive after 1 year of unprotected intercourse). Known causes of male infertility include primary hypogonadism (30–40%), disorders of sperm transport (10–20%), and secondary hypogonadism (2%), with an unknown etiology in up to half of men with suspected male factor infertility (see Fig. 186-3). Impaired spermatogenesis occurs with testosterone deficiency but may also be present without testosterone deficiency. Y chromosome microdeletions and substitutions, viral orchitis, tuberculosis, STDs, radiation, chemotherapeutic agents, and environmental toxins have all been associated with isolated impaired spermatogenesis. Prolonged elevations of testicular temperature, as in varicocele, in cryptorchidism, or after an acute febrile illness, may impair spermatogenesis. Ejaculatory obstruction can be a congenital (cystic fibrosis, in utero diethylstilbestrol exposure, or idiopathic) or acquired (vasectomy, accidental ligation of the vas deferens, or obstruction of the epididymis) etiology of male infertility. Androgen abuse by male athletes can lead to testicular atrophy and a low sperm count.

Clinical Features

Evidence of hypogonadism may or may not be present. Testicular size and consistency may be abnormal, and a varicocele may be apparent on palpation. When the seminiferous tubules are damaged prior to puberty, the testes are small (usually <12 mL) and firm, whereas postpubertal damage causes the testes to be soft (the capsule, once enlarged, does not contract to its previous size). The key diagnostic test is a *semen analysis*. Sperm counts of <13 million/mL, motility of <32%, and <9% normal morphology are associated with subfertility. Testosterone levels should be measured if the sperm count is low on repeated exam or if there is clinical evidence of hypogonadism.

TREATMENT   Male Infertility

Men with primary hypogonadism occasionally respond to androgen therapy if there is minimal damage to the seminiferous tubules, whereas those with secondary hypogonadism require gonadotropin therapy to achieve fertility. Fertility occurs in about half of men with varicocele who undergo surgical repair. In vitro fertilization is an option for men with mild to moderate defects in sperm quality; intracytoplasmic sperm injection (ICSI) has been a major advance for men with severe defects in sperm quality.

■ ERECTILE DYSFUNCTION

Etiology

Erectile dysfunction (ED) is the failure to achieve erection, ejaculation, or both. It affects 10–25% of middle-aged and elderly men. ED may result from three basic mechanisms: (1) failure to initiate (psychogenic, endocrinologic, or neurogenic); (2) failure to fill (arteriogenic); or (3) failure to store adequate blood volume within the lacunar network (venooclusive dysfunction). Diabetic, atherosclerotic, and drug-related causes account for >80% of cases of ED in older men. The most common organic cause of ED is vasculogenic; 35–75% of men with diabetes have ED due to a combination of vascular and neurologic complications. Psychogenic causes of ED include performance anxiety, depression, relationship conflict, sexual inhibition, history of sexual abuse in childhood, and fear of pregnancy or sexually transmitted disease. Among the antihypertensive agents, the thiazide diuretics and beta blockers have been implicated most frequently. Estrogens, GnRH agonists and antagonists, H_2 antagonists, and spironolactone suppress gonadotropin production or block androgen action. Antidepressant and antipsychotic agents—particularly neuroleptics, tricyclics, and selective serotonin reuptake inhibitors—are associated with erectile, ejaculatory, orgasmic, and sexual desire difficulties. Recreational drugs, including ethanol, cocaine, and marijuana, also may cause ED. Any disorder that affects the sacral spinal cord or the sensory nerves or autonomic fibers innervating the penis may lead to ED.

Clinical Features

Men with sexual dysfunction may complain of loss of libido, inability to initiate or maintain an erection, ejaculatory failure, premature ejaculation, or inability to achieve orgasm, but frequently are too embarrassed to bring up the subject unless specifically asked by the physician. Initial questions should focus on the onset of symptoms, the presence and duration of partial erections, the progression of ED, and ejaculation. Psychosocial history, libido, relationship issues, sexual orientation and sexual practices should be part of the clinical assessment. A history of nocturnal or early morning erections is useful for distinguishing physiologic from psychogenic ED. Relevant risk factors should be identified, such as diabetes mellitus, coronary artery disease, lipid disorders, hypertension, peripheral vascular disease, smoking, alcoholism, and endocrine or neurologic disorders. The pt's surgical history should be explored, with an emphasis on bowel, bladder, prostate, or vascular procedures. Evaluation includes a detailed general as well as genital physical exam. Penile abnormalities (Peyronie's disease), testicular size, and gynecomastia should be noted. Peripheral pulses should be palpated, and bruits should be sought. Neurologic exam should assess anal sphincter tone, perineal sensation, and bulbocavernosus reflex. Serum testosterone and prolactin should be measured. Penile arteriography, electromyography, or penile Doppler ultrasound is occasionally performed.

TREATMENT   Erectile Dysfunction

An approach to the evaluation and treatment of ED is summarized in Fig. 185-2. Correction of the underlying disorders or discontinuation of responsible medications should be attempted. Oral inhibitors of phosphodiesterase-5 (sildenafil, tadalafil, and vardenafil) enhance erections after sexual stimulation, with an onset of approximately 60–120 min. They are contraindicated in men receiving any form of nitrate therapy and should be avoided in those with congestive heart failure. Vacuum

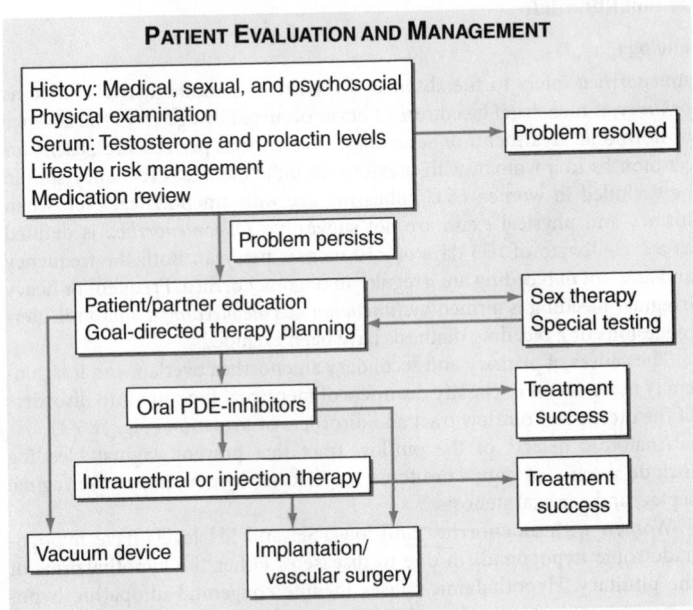

PATIENT EVALUATION AND MANAGEMENT

FIGURE 185-2 Algorithm for the evaluation and management of pts with ED. PDE, phosphodiesterase.

constriction devices or injection of alprostadil into the urethra or corpora cavernosa may also be effective. The insertion of a penile prosthesis is reserved for pts with refractory ED.

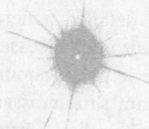

For a more detailed discussion, see Bhasin S, Jameson JL: Disorders of the Testes and Male Reproductive System, Chap. 346, p. 3010; Hall JE: The Female Reproductive System, Infertility, and Contraception, Chap. 347, p. 3028; and McVary KT: Sexual Dysfunction, Chap. 48, p. 374, in HPIM-18.

CHAPTER **186**
Disorders of the Female Reproductive System

The pituitary hormones, luteinizing hormone (LH) and follicle-stimulating hormone (FSH), stimulate ovarian follicular development and result in ovulation at about day 14 of the 28-day menstrual cycle.

■ AMENORRHEA

Etiology

Amenorrhea refers to the absence of menstrual periods. It is classified as *primary*, if menstrual bleeding has never occurred by age 15 in the absence of hormonal treatment, or *secondary*, if menstrual periods are absent for >3 months in a woman with previous periodic menses. Pregnancy should be excluded in women of childbearing age with amenorrhea, even when history and physical exam are not suggestive. *Oligomenorrhea* is defined as a cycle length of >35 days or <10 menses per year. Both the frequency and amount of bleeding are irregular in oligomenorrhea. Frequent or heavy irregular bleeding is termed *dysfunctional uterine bleeding* if anatomic uterine lesions or a bleeding diathesis have been excluded.

The causes of primary and secondary amenorrhea overlap, and it is generally more useful to classify disorders of menstrual function into disorders of the uterus and outflow tract and disorders of ovulation (Fig. 186-1).

Anatomic defects of the outflow tract that prevent vaginal bleeding include absence of vagina or uterus, imperforate hymen, transverse vaginal septae, and cervical stenosis.

Women with amenorrhea and low FSH and LH levels have hypogonadotropic hypogonadism due to disease of either the hypothalamus or the pituitary. Hypothalamic causes include congenital idiopathic hypogonadotropic hypogonadism, hypothalamic lesions (craniopharyngiomas and other tumors, tuberculosis, sarcoidosis, metastatic tumors), hypothalamic trauma or irradiation, vigorous exercise, eating disorders, stress,

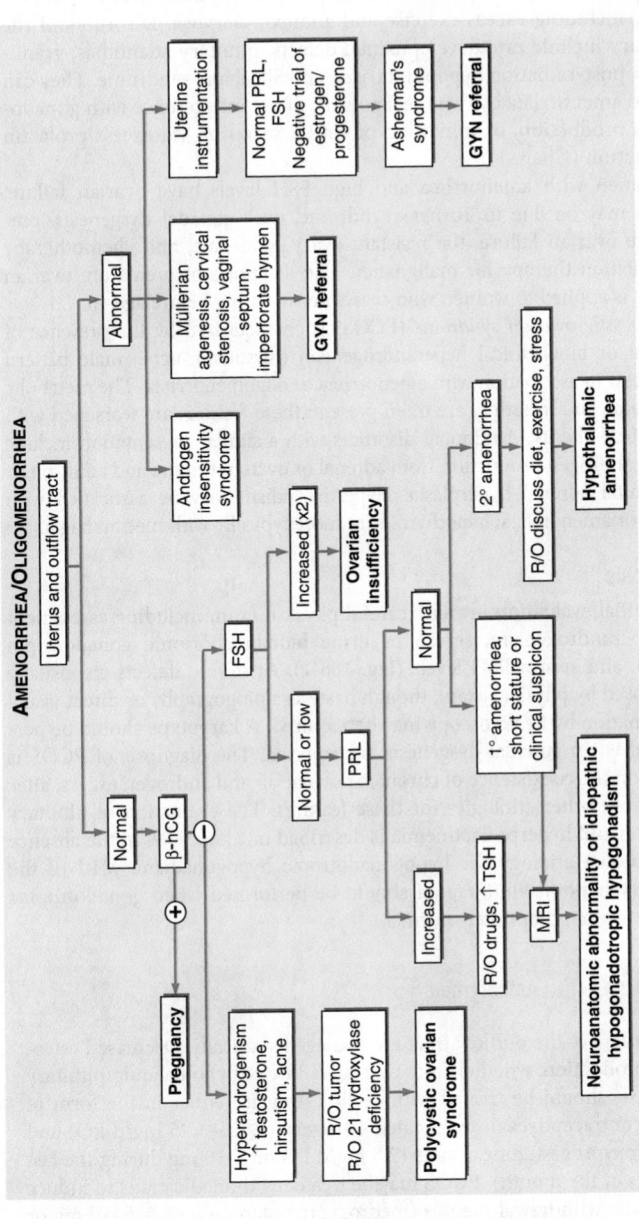

FIGURE 186-1 Algorithm for evaluation of amenorrhea. β-hCG, human chorionic gonadotropin; FSH, follicle-stimulating hormone; PRL, prolactin; TSH, thyroid-stimulating hormone.

and chronic debilitating diseases (end-stage renal disease, malignancy, malabsorption). The most common form of hypothalamic amenorrhea is functional, reversible GnRH deficiency due to psychological or physical stress, including excess exercise and anorexia nervosa. Disorders of the pituitary include rare developmental defects, pituitary adenomas, granulomas, post-radiation hypopituitarism, and Sheehan's syndrome. They can lead to amenorrhea by two mechanisms: direct interference with gonadotropin production, or inhibition of GnRH secretion via excess prolactin production (Chap. 179).

Women with amenorrhea and high FSH levels have ovarian failure, which may be due to Turner's syndrome, pure gonadal dysgenesis, premature ovarian failure, the resistant-ovary syndrome, and chemotherapy or radiation therapy for malignancy. The diagnosis of premature ovarian failure is applied to women who cease menstruating before age 40.

Polycystic ovarian syndrome (PCOS) is characterized by the presence of clinical or biochemical hyperandrogenism (hirsutism, acne, male pattern baldness) in association with amenorrhea or oligomenorrhea. The metabolic syndrome and infertility are often present; these features are worsened with coexistent obesity. Additional disorders with a similar presentation include excess androgen production from adrenal or ovarian tumors and adult-onset congenital adrenal hyperplasia. Hyperthyroidism may be associated with oligo- or amenorrhea; hypothyroidism more typically with metrorrhagia.

Diagnosis

The initial evaluation involves careful physical exam including assessment of hyperandrogenism, serum or urine human chorionic gonadotropin (hCG), and serum FSH levels (Fig. 186-1). Anatomic defects are usually diagnosed by physical exam, though hysterosalpingography or direct visual examination by hysteroscopy may be required. A karyotype should be performed when gonadal dysgenesis is suspected. The diagnosis of PCOS is based on the coexistence of chronic anovulation and androgen excess, after ruling out other etiologies for these features. The evaluation of pituitary function and hyperprolactinemia is described in Chap. 179. In the absence of a known etiology for hypogonadotropic hypogonadism, MRI of the pituitary-hypothalamic region should be performed when gonadotropins are low or inappropriately normal.

TREATMENT Amenorrhea

Disorders of the outflow tract are managed surgically. Decreased estrogen production, whether from ovarian failure or hypothalamic/pituitary disease, should be treated with cyclic estrogens, either in the form of oral contraceptives or conjugated estrogens (0.625–1.25 mg/d PO) and medroxyprogesterone acetate (2.5 mg/d PO or 5–10 mg during the last 5 days of the month). PCOS may be treated with medications to induce periodic withdrawal menses (medroxyprogesterone acetate 5–10 mg or progesterone 200 mg daily for 10–14 days of each month, or oral contraceptive agents) and weight reduction, along with treatment of hirsutism and, if desired, ovulation induction (see below). Individuals with PCOS may benefit from insulin-sensitizing drugs, such as metformin, and should be screened for diabetes mellitus.

■ PELVIC PAIN

Etiology

Pelvic pain may be associated with normal or abnormal menstrual cycles and may originate in the pelvis or be referred from another region of the body. A high index of suspicion must be entertained for extrapelvic disorders that refer to the pelvis, such as appendicitis, diverticulitis, cholecystitis, intestinal obstruction, and urinary tract infections. A thorough history including the type, location, radiation, and status with respect to increasing or decreasing severity can help to identify the cause of acute pelvic pain. Associations with vaginal bleeding, sexual activity, defecation, urination, movement, or eating should be sought. Determination of whether the pain is acute versus chronic, constant versus spasmodic, and cyclic versus noncyclic will direct further investigation (Table 186-1).

Acute Pelvic Pain

Pelvic inflammatory disease most commonly presents with bilateral lower abdominal pain. Unilateral pain suggests adnexal pathology from rupture, bleeding, or torsion of ovarian cysts, or, less commonly, neoplasms of the ovary, fallopian tubes, or paraovarian areas. Ectopic pregnancy is associated with right- or left-sided lower abdominal pain, vaginal bleeding, and menstrual cycle abnormalities, with clinical signs appearing 6–8 weeks after the last normal menstrual period. Orthostatic signs and fever may be present. Uterine pathology includes endometritis and degenerating leiomyomas.

TABLE 186-1 CAUSES OF PELVIC PAIN

	Acute	Chronic
Cyclic pelvic pain		Premenstrual symptoms
		Mittelschmerz
		Dysmenorrhea
		Endometriosis
Noncyclic pelvic pain	Pelvic inflammatory disease	Pelvic congestion syndrome
	Ruptured or hemorrhagic ovarian cyst or ovarian torsion	Adhesions and retroversion of the uterus
	Ectopic pregnancy	Pelvic malignancy
	Endometritis	Vulvodynia
	Acute growth or degeneration of uterine myoma	History of sexual abuse

Chronic Pelvic Pain

Many women experience lower abdominal discomfort with ovulation (*mittelschmerz*), characterized as a dull, aching pain at midcycle that lasts minutes to hours. In addition, ovulatory women may experience somatic symptoms during the few days prior to menses, including edema, breast engorgement, and abdominal bloating or discomfort. A symptom complex of cyclic irritability, depression, and lethargy is known as *premenstrual syndrome* (PMS). Severe or incapacitating cramping with ovulatory menses in the absence of demonstrable disorders of the pelvis is termed *primary dysmenorrhea*. *Secondary dysmenorrhea* is caused by underlying pelvic pathology such as endometriosis, adenomyosis, or cervical stenosis.

Diagnosis

Evaluation includes a history, pelvic exam, hCG measurement, tests for chlamydial and gonococcal infections, and pelvic ultrasound. Laparoscopy or laparotomy is indicated in some cases of pelvic pain of undetermined cause.

TREATMENT   Pelvic Pain

Primary dysmenorrhea is best treated with NSAIDs or oral contraceptive agents. Secondary dysmenorrhea not responding to NSAIDs suggests pelvic pathology, such as endometriosis. Infections should be treated with the appropriate antibiotics. Symptoms from PMS may improve with selective serotonin reuptake inhibitor (SSRI) therapy. The majority of unruptured ectopic pregnancies are treated with methotrexate, which has an 85–95% success rate. Surgery may be required for structural abnormalities.

◼ HIRSUTISM

Etiology

Hirsutism, defined as excessive male-pattern hair growth, affects ~10% of women. It may be familial or caused by PCOS, ovarian or adrenal neoplasms, congenital adrenal hyperplasia, Cushing's syndrome, pregnancy, and drugs (androgens, oral contraceptives containing androgenic progestins). Other drugs, such as minoxidil, phenytoin, diazoxide, and cyclosporine, can cause excessive growth of non-androgen-dependent vellus hair, leading to hypertrichosis.

Clinical Features

An objective clinical assessment of hair distribution and quantity is central to the evaluation. A commonly used method to grade hair growth is the Ferriman-Gallwey score (see Fig. 49-1, p. 382, in HPIM-18). Associated manifestations of androgen excess include acne and male-pattern balding (androgenic alopecia). *Virilization*, on the other hand, refers to the state in which androgen levels are sufficiently high to cause deepening of the voice, breast atrophy, increased muscle bulk, clitoromegaly, and increased libido. Historic elements include menstrual history and the age of onset, rate of progression, and distribution of hair growth. Sudden development of hirsutism, rapid progression, and virilization suggest an ovarian or adrenal neoplasm.

Diagnosis

An approach to testing for androgen excess is depicted in Fig. 186-2. PCOS is a relatively common cause of hirsutism. The dexamethasone androgen-suppression test (0.5 mg PO every 6 h × 4 days, with free testosterone levels obtained before and after administration of dexamethasone) may distinguish ovarian from adrenal overproduction. Incomplete suppression suggests ovarian androgen excess. Congenital adrenal hyperplasia due to 21-hydroxylase deficiency can be excluded by a 17-hydroxyprogesterone level that is <6 nmol/L (<2 μg/L) either in the morning during the follicular phase or 1 h after administration of 250 μg of cosyntropin. CT may localize an adrenal mass, and ultrasound may identify an ovarian mass, if evaluation suggests these possibilities.

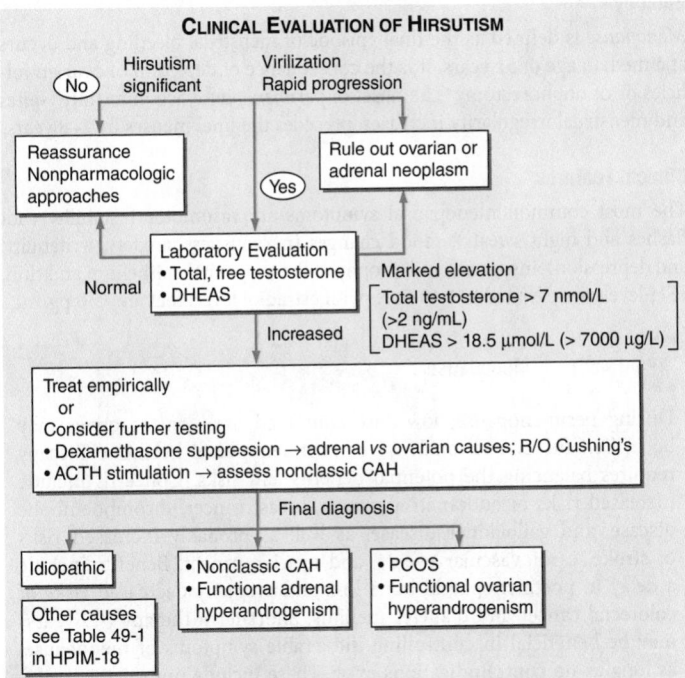

FIGURE 186-2 Algorithm for the evaluation and differential diagnosis of hirsutism. ACTH, adrenocorticotropic hormone; CAH, congenital adrenal hyperplasia; DHEAS, sulfated form of dehydroepiandrosterone; PCOS, polycystic ovarian syndrome.

TREATMENT Hirsutism

Treatment of a remediable underlying cause (e.g., Cushing's syndrome, adrenal or ovarian tumor) also improves hirsutism. In idiopathic hirsutism or PCOS, symptomatic physical or pharmacologic treatment is indicated. Nonpharmacologic treatments include (1) bleaching; (2) depilatory such as shaving and chemical treatments; and (3) epilatory such as plucking, waxing, electrolysis, and laser therapy. Pharmacologic therapy includes oral contraceptives with a low androgenic progestin and spironolactone (100–200 mg/d PO), often in combination. Flutamide is also effective as an antiandrogen, but its use is limited by hepatotoxicity. Glucocorticoids (dexamethasone, 0.25–0.5 mg at bedtime, or prednisone, 5–10 mg at bedtime) are the mainstay of treatment in pts with congenital adrenal hyperplasia. Attenuation of hair growth with pharmacologic therapy is typically not evident until 6 months after initiation of medical treatment and therefore should be used in conjunction with nonpharmacologic treatments.

■ MENOPAUSE

Etiology

Menopause is defined as the final episode of menstrual bleeding and occurs at a median age of 51 years. It is the consequence of depletion of ovarian follicles or of oophorectomy. The onset of *perimenopause*, when fertility wanes and menstrual irregularity increases, precedes the final menses by 2–8 years.

Clinical Features

The most common menopausal symptoms are vasomotor instability (hot flashes and night sweats), mood changes (nervousness, anxiety, irritability, and depression), insomnia, and atrophy of the urogenital epithelium and skin. FSH levels are elevated to ≥40 IU/L with estradiol levels that are <30 pg/mL.

TREATMENT Menopause

During perimenopause, low-dose combined oral contraceptives may be of benefit. The rational use of postmenopausal hormone therapy requires balancing the potential benefits and risks. Concerns include increased risks of endometrial cancer, breast cancer, thromboembolic disease, and gallbladder disease, as well as probably increased risks of stroke, cardiovascular events, and ovarian cancer. Benefits include a delay in postmenopausal bone loss and probably decreased risks of colorectal cancer and diabetes mellitus. Short-term therapy (<5 years) may be beneficial in controlling intolerable symptoms of menopause, as long as no contraindications exist. These include unexplained vaginal bleeding, active liver disease, venous thromboembolism, history of endometrial cancer (except stage I without deep invasion), breast cancer, preexisting cardiovascular disease, and diabetes. Hypertriglyceridemia

(>400 mg/dL) and active gallbladder disease are relative contrain-dications. Alternative therapies for symptoms include venlafaxine, fluoxetine, paroxetine, gabapentin, clonidine, vitamin E, or soy-based products. Vaginal estradiol tablets may be used for genitourinary symptoms. Long-term therapy (≥5 years) should be undertaken only after careful consideration , particularly in light of alternative therapies for osteoporosis (bisphosphonates, raloxifene) and of the risks of venous thromboembolism and breast cancer. Estrogens should be given in the minimal effective doses (conjugated estrogen, 0.625 mg/d PO; micronized estradiol, 1.0 mg/d PO; or transdermal estradiol, 0.05–1.0 mg once or twice a week). Women with an intact uterus should be given estrogen in combination with a progestin (medroxyprogesterone either cyclically, 5–10 mg/d PO for days 15–25 each month, or continuously, 2.5 mg/d PO) to avoid the increased risk of endometrial carcinoma seen with unopposed estrogen use.

■ CONTRACEPTION

The most widely used methods for fertility control include (1) barrier methods, (2) oral contraceptives, (3) intrauterine devices, (4) long-acting progestins, (5) sterilization, and (6) abortion.

Oral contraceptive agents are widely used for both prevention of pregnancy and control of dysmenorrhea and anovulatory bleeding. Combination oral contraceptive agents contain synthetic estrogen (ethinyl estradiol or mestranol) and synthetic progestins. Some progestins possess an inherent androgenic action. Low-dose norgestimate and third-generation progestins (desogestrel, gestodene, drospirenone) have a less androgenic profile; levonorgestrel appears to be the most androgenic of the progestins and should be avoided in pts with hyperandrogenic symptoms. The three major formulation types include fixed-dose estrogen-progestin, phasic estrogen-progestin, and progestin only.

Despite overall safety, oral contraceptive users are at risk for venous thromboembolism, hypertension, and cholelithiasis. Risks for myocardial infarction and stroke are increased with smoking and aging. Side effects, including breakthrough bleeding, amenorrhea, breast tenderness, and weight gain, are often responsive to a change in formulation.

Absolute contraindications to the use of oral contraceptives include previous thromboembolic disorders, cerebrovascular or coronary artery disease, carcinoma of the breasts or other estrogen-dependent neoplasia, liver disease, hypertriglyceridemia, heavy smoking with age over 35, undiagnosed uterine bleeding, or known or suspected pregnancy. Relative contraindications include hypertension and anticonvulsant drug therapy.

New methods include a weekly contraceptive patch, a monthly contraceptive injection, and a monthly vaginal ring. Long-term progestins may be administered in the form of Depo-Provera or a subdermal progestin implant.

Emergency contraceptive pills, containing progestin only or estrogen and progestin, can be used within 72 h of unprotected intercourse for prevention of pregnancy. Both Plan B and Preven are emergency contraceptive kits specifically designed for postcoital contraception. In addition, certain oral contraceptive pills may be dosed within 72 h for emergency contraception (Ovral, 2 tabs, 12 h apart; Lo/Ovral, 4 tabs, 12 h apart). Side effects include nausea, vomiting, and breast soreness. Mifepristone (RU486) also may be used, with fewer side effects.

■ INFERTILITY

Etiology

Infertility is defined as the inability to conceive after 12 months of unprotected sexual intercourse. The causes of infertility are outlined in Fig. 186-3. Male infertility is discussed in Chap. 185.

Clinical Features

The initial evaluation includes discussion of the appropriate timing of intercourse, semen analysis in the male, confirmation of ovulation in the female, and, in the majority of situations, documentation of tubal patency in the female. Abnormalities in menstrual function constitute the most common cause of female infertility (Fig. 186-1). A history of regular, cyclic, predictable, spontaneous menses usually indicates ovulatory cycles, which may be confirmed by urinary ovulation predictor kits, basal body temperature graphs, or plasma progesterone measurements during the luteal phase of

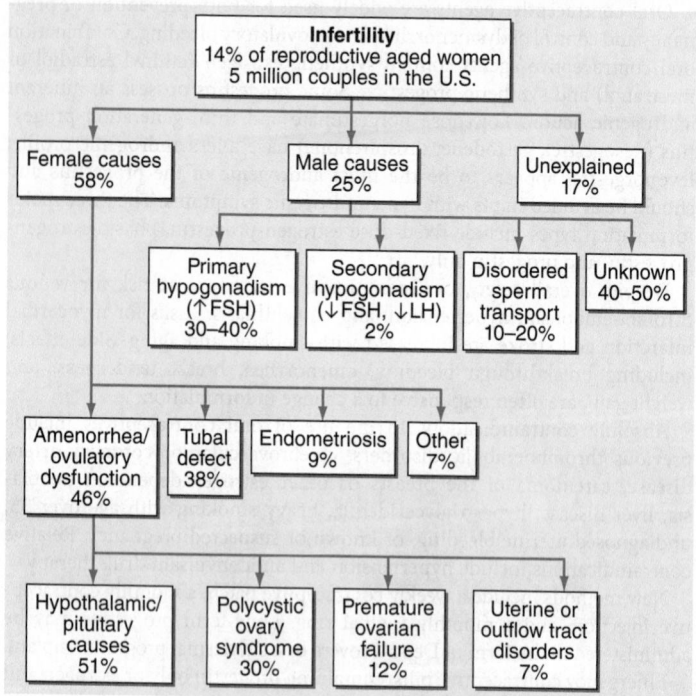

FIGURE 186-3 Causes of infertility. FSH, follicle-stimulating hormone; LH, luteinizing hormone.

the cycle. An FSH level <10 IU/mL on day 3 of the cycle predicts adequate ovarian oocyte reserve. Tubal disease can be evaluated by obtaining a hysterosalpingogram or by diagnostic laparoscopy. Endometriosis may be suggested by history and exam, but is often clinically silent and can only be excluded definitively by laparoscopy.

TREATMENT Infertility

The treatment of infertility should be tailored to the problems unique to each couple. Treatment options include expectant management, clomiphene citrate with or without intrauterine insemination (IUI), gonadotropins with or without IUI, and in vitro fertilization (IVF). In specific situations, surgery, pulsatile GnRH therapy, intracytoplasmic sperm injection (ICSI), or assisted reproductive technologies with donor egg or sperm may be required.

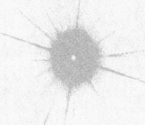

For a more detailed discussion, see Ehrmann DA: Hirsutism and Virilization, Chap. 49, p. 380; Hall JE: Menstrual Disorders and Pelvic Pain, Chap. 50, p. 384; Hall JE: The Female Reproductive System: Infertility and Contraception, Chap. 347, p. 3028; and Manson JE, Bassuk SS: The Menopause Transition and Postmenopausal Hormone Therapy, Chap. 348, p. 3040, in HPIM-18.

CHAPTER **187**
Hypercalcemia and Hypocalcemia

■ HYPERCALCEMIA

Hypercalcemia from any cause can result in fatigue, depression, mental confusion, anorexia, nausea, constipation, renal tubular defects, polyuria, a short QT interval, and arrhythmias. CNS and GI symptoms can occur at levels of serum calcium >2.9 mmol/L (>11.5 mg/dL), and nephrocalcinosis and impairment of renal function occur when serum calcium is >3.2 mmol/L (>13 mg/dL). Severe hypercalcemia, usually defined as >3.7 mmol/L (>15 mg/dL), can be a medical emergency, leading to coma and cardiac arrest.

Etiology

The regulation of the calcium homeostasis is depicted in Fig. 187-1. The causes of hypercalcemia are listed in Table 187-1. Hyperparathyroidism and malignancy account for 90% of cases.

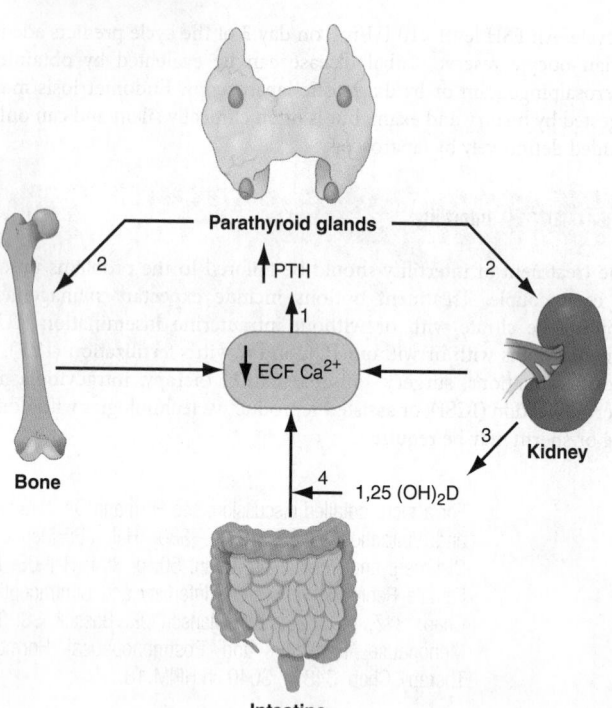

FIGURE 187-1 Feedback mechanisms maintaining extracellular calcium concentrations within a narrow, physiologic range [8.9–10.1 mg/dL (2.2–2.5 m*M*)]. A decrease in extracellular (ECF) ionized calcium (Ca²⁺) triggers an increase in parathyroid hormone (PTH) secretion **(1)** via activation of the calcium sensor receptor on parathyroid cells. PTH, in turn, results in increased tubular reabsorption of calcium by the kidney **(2)** and resorption of calcium from bone (2) and also stimulates renal 1,25(OH)₂D production **(3)**. 1,25(OH)₂D, in turn, acts principally on the intestine to increase calcium absorption **(4)**. Collectively, these homeostatic mechanisms serve to restore serum calcium levels to normal.

Primary hyperparathyroidism is a generalized disorder of bone metabolism due to increased secretion of parathyroid hormone (PTH) by an adenoma (81%) or rarely a carcinoma in a single gland, or by parathyroid hyperplasia (15%). Familial hyperparathyroidism may be part of multiple endocrine neoplasia type 1 (MEN 1), which also includes pituitary and pancreatic islet tumors, or of MEN 2A, in which hyperparathyroidism occurs with pheochromocytoma and medullary carcinoma of the thyroid.

Hypercalcemia associated with malignancy is often severe and difficult to manage. Mechanisms for this include excess production and release of PTH-related protein (PTHrP) in lung, kidney, and squamous cell carcinoma (humoral hypercalcemia of malignancy); local bone destruction in

---

TABLE 187-1 CLASSIFICATION OF CAUSES OF HYPERCALCEMIA

I. Parathyroid-related

    A. Primary hyperparathyroidism

        1. Solitary adenomas or rarely carcinoma

        2. Multiple endocrine neoplasia

    B. Lithium therapy

    C. Familial hypocalciuric hypercalcemia

II. Malignancy-related

    A. Solid tumor with humoral mediation of hypercalcemia (lung, kidney, squamous cell carcinoma)

    B. Solid tumor with metastases (breast)

    C. Hematologic malignancies (multiple myeloma, lymphoma, leukemia)

III. Vitamin D–related

    A. Vitamin D intoxication

    B. ↑ $1,25(OH)_2D$; sarcoidosis and other granulomatous diseases

    C. Idiopathic hypercalcemia of infancy

IV. Associated with high bone turnover

    A. Hyperthyroidism

    B. Immobilization

    C. Thiazides

    D. Vitamin A intoxication

V. Associated with renal failure

    A. Severe secondary or tertiary hyperparathyroidism

    B. Aluminum intoxication

    C. Milk-alkali syndrome

---

myeloma and breast carcinoma; activation of lymphocytes leading to release of IL-1 and TNF in myeloma and lymphoma; or an increased synthesis of $1,25(OH)_2D$ in lymphoma.

Several other conditions have been associated with hypercalcemia. These include sarcoidosis and other granulomatous diseases, which lead to increased synthesis of $1,25(OH)_2D$; vitamin D intoxication from chronic ingestion of large vitamin doses (50–100 × physiologic requirements); lithium therapy, which results in hyperfunctioning of the parathyroid glands; and familial hypocalciuric hypercalcemia (FHH) due autosomal dominant inheritance of an inactivating mutation in the calcium-sensing receptor, which results in inappropriately normal or even high secretion of PTH, despite hypercalcemia and enhanced renal calcium resorption. Severe secondary hyperparathyroidism associated with end-stage renal disease may progress to tertiary hyperthyroidism, in which PTH hypersecretion becomes autonomous, causes hypercalcemia, and is no longer responsive to medical therapy.

Clinical Features

Most pts with mild to moderate hyperparathyroidism are asymptomatic, even when the disease involves the kidneys and the skeletal system. Pts frequently have hypercalciuria and polyuria, and calcium can be deposited in the renal parenchyma (nephrocalcinosis) or form calcium oxalate stones. The characteristic skeletal lesion is osteopenia or osteoporosis; rarely, the more severe disorder osteitis fibrosa cystica occurs as a manifestation of long-standing, more severe hyperparathyroidism. Increased bone resorption primarily involves cortical rather than trabecular bone. Hypercalcemia may be intermittent or sustained, and serum phosphate is usually low but may be normal.

Diagnosis

Primary hyperparathyroidism is confirmed by demonstration of an inappropriately high PTH level for the degree of hypercalcemia. Hypercalciuria helps to distinguish this disorder from FHH, in which PTH levels are usually in the normal range and the urine calcium level is low. Differentiation between primary hyperparathyroidism and FHH is important because the latter does not respond to parathyroid surgery. Levels of PTH are low in hypercalcemia of malignancy (Table 187-2).

Total serum calcium should be corrected when serum albumin is abnormal [addition of 0.2 mM (0.8 mg/dL) to calcium value for every 1.0-g/dL decrement in albumin below 4.1 g/dL, or the converse for an increase in albumin]. Alternatively, ionized calcium can be measured. Third-generation PTH assays should be used for PTH measurement, especially in pts with renal impairment.

TABLE 187-2 DIFFERENTIAL DIAGNOSIS OF HYPERCALCEMIA: LABORATORY CRITERIA

	Blood[a]			
	Ca	P_i	1,25(OH)$_2$D	iPTH
Primary hyperparathyroidism	↑	↓	↑↔	↑(↔)
Malignancy-associated hypercalcemia:				
Humoral hypercalcemia	↑↑	↓	↓↔	↓
Local destruction (osteolytic metastases)	↑	↔	↓↔	↓

[a]Symbols in parentheses refer to values rarely seen in the particular disease.
Abbreviations: P_i, inorganic phosphate; iPTH, immunoreactive parathyroid hormone.
Source: JT Potts Jr: HPIM-12, p. 1911.

TREATMENT Hypercalcemia

The type of treatment is based on the severity of the hypercalcemia and the nature of the associated symptoms. Table 187-3 shows general recommendations that apply to therapy of severe hypercalcemia [levels of >3.2 mmol/L (>13 mg/dL)] from any cause.

In pts with severe primary hyperparathyroidism, surgical parathyroidectomy should be performed promptly. Asymptomatic disease may not require surgery; usual surgical indications include age <50, nephrolithiasis, creatinine clearance <60 mL/min, reduction in bone mass (T score <−2.5), or serum calcium >0.25 mmol/L (>1 mg/dL) above the normal range. A minimally invasive approach may be used if preoperative localization via sestamibi scans with SPECT or neck ultrasound demonstrates a solitary adenoma and intraoperative PTH assays are

TABLE 187-3 THERAPIES FOR SEVERE HYPERCALCEMIA

Treatment	Onset of Action	Duration of Action	Advantages	Disadvantages
Hydration with saline (≤6 L/d)	Hours	During infusion	Rehydrates; rapid action	Volume overload; electrolyte disturbance
Forced diuresis (furosemide along with aggressive hydration)	Hours	During treatment	Rapid action	Monitoring required to avoid dehydration
Pamidronate 30–90 mg IV over 4 h	1–2 days	10–14 days	High potency; intermediate onset of action	Fever in 20%, ↓ Ca, ↓ phosphate, ↓ Mg, rarely jaw necrosis
Zoledronate 4–8 mg IV over 15 min	1–2 days	>3 weeks	High potency; prolonged action; rapid infusion	Minor: Fever; rare ↓ Ca, ↓ phosphate, jaw necrosis
Calcitonin (2–8 U/kg SC q6-12h)	Hours	1–2 days	Rapid onset	Limited effect; rapid tachyphylaxis
Glucocorticoids (prednisone 10–25 mg PO qid)	Days	Days-weeks	Useful in myeloma, lymphoma, breast CA, sarcoid, vitamin D intox	Effects limited to certain disorders; glucocorticoid side effects
Dialysis	Hours	During use–2 days	Useful in renal failure; immediate effect	Complex procedure

available. Otherwise, neck exploration is required. Surgery in a center experienced in parathyroid interventions is recommended. Postoperative management requires close monitoring of calcium and phosphorus, as transient hypocalcemia is common. Calcium supplementation is given for symptomatic hypocalcemia.

Hypercalcemia of malignancy is managed by treating the underlying tumor. Adequate hydration and parenteral bisphosphonates can be used to reduce calcium levels. Long-term control of hypercalcemia is difficult unless the underlying cause can be eliminated.

No therapy is recommended for FHH. Secondary hyperparathyroidism should be treated with phosphate restriction, the use of nonabsorbable antacids or sevelamer, and calcitriol. Tertiary hyperparathyroidism requires parathyroidectomy.

■ HYPOCALCEMIA

Chronic hypocalcemia is less common than hypercalcemia, but is usually symptomatic and requires treatment. Symptoms include peripheral and perioral paresthesia, muscle spasms, carpopedal spasm, tetany, laryngeal spasm, seizure, and respiratory arrest. Increased intracranial pressure and papilledema may occur with long-standing hypocalcemia, and other manifestations may include irritability, depression, psychosis, intestinal cramps, and chronic malabsorption. Chvostek's and Trousseau's signs are frequently positive, and the QT interval is prolonged. Both hypomagnesemia and alkalosis lower the threshold for tetany.

Etiology

Transient hypocalcemia often occurs in critically ill pts with burns, sepsis, and acute renal failure; following transfusion with citrated blood; or with medications such as protamine and heparin. Hypoalbuminemia can reduce serum calcium below normal, although ionized calcium levels remain normal. The above-mentioned correction (see "Hypercalcemia") can be used to assess whether the serum calcium concentration is abnormal when serum proteins are low. Alkalosis increases calcium binding to proteins, and in this setting direct measurements of ionized calcium should be used.

The causes of hypocalcemia can be divided into those in which PTH is absent (hereditary or acquired hypoparathyroidism, hypomagnesemia), PTH is ineffective (chronic renal failure, vitamin D deficiency, anticonvulsant therapy, intestinal malabsorption, pseudohypoparathyroidism), or PTH is overwhelmed (severe, acute hyperphosphatemia in tumor lysis, acute renal failure, or rhabdomyolysis; hungry bone syndrome following parathyroidectomy). The most common forms of chronic severe hypocalcemia are autoimmune hypoparathyroidism and postoperative hypoparathyroidism following neck surgery. Chronic renal insufficiency is associated with mild hypocalcemia compensated for by secondary hyperparathyroidism. The cause of hypocalcemia associated with acute pancreatitis is unclear.

| TREATMENT | Hypocalcemia |

Symptomatic hypocalcemia may be treated with IV calcium gluconate (bolus of 1–2 g IV over 10–20 min followed by infusion of 10 ampoules of 10% calcium gluconate diluted in 1 L D_5W infused at 30–100 mL/h). Management of chronic hypocalcemia requires a high oral calcium intake, usually with vitamin D supplementation (Chap. 188). Hypoparathyroidism requires administration of calcium (1–3 g/d) and calcitriol (0.25–1 μg/d), adjusted according to serum calcium levels and urinary excretion. Restoration of magnesium stores may be required to reverse hypocalcemia in the setting of severe hypomagnesemia.

◼ HYPOPHOSPHATEMIA

Mild hypophosphatemia is not usually associated with clinical symptoms. In severe hypophosphatemia, pts may have muscle weakness, numbness, paresthesia, and confusion. Rhabdomyolysis may develop during rapidly progressive hypophosphatemia. Respiratory insufficiency can result from diaphragm muscle weakness.

Etiology

The causes of hypophosphatemia include: decreased intestinal absorption (vitamin D deficiency, phosphorus-binding antacids, malabsorption); urinary losses (hyperparathyroidism, hyperglycemic states, X-linked hypophosphatemic rickets, oncogenic osteomalacia, alcoholism, or certain toxins); and shifts of phosphorus from extracellular to intracellular compartments (administration of insulin in diabetic ketoacidosis or by hyperalimentation or refeeding in a malnourished pt). In syndromes of severe primary renal phosphate wasting (X-linked hypophosphatemic rickets, autosomal dominant hypophosphatemic rickets, oncogenic osteomalacia), the phosphatonin hormone FGF23 (fibroblast growth factor 23) plays a key pathogenetic role.

| TREATMENT | Hypophosphatemia |

Mild hypophosphatemia can be replaced orally with milk, carbonated beverages, or Neutra-Phos or K-Phos (up to 2 g/d in divided doses). For severe hypophosphatemia [0.75 mmol/L; (<2.0 mg/dL)], IV phosphate may be administered at initial doses of 0.2–0.8 mmol/kg of elemental phosphorus over 6 h. The total body phosphate depletion cannot be predicted from the serum phosphate level; careful monitoring of therapy is therefore required. Hypocalcemia should be corrected first, and the dose reduced 50% in hypercalcemia. Serum calcium and phosphate levels should be measured every 6–12 h; a serum calcium × phosphate product of >50 must be avoided.

◼ HYPERPHOSPHATEMIA

In adults, hyperphosphatemia is defined as a level >1.8 mmol/L (>5.5 mg/dL). The most common causes are acute and chronic renal failure, but it may also be seen in hypoparathyroidism, vitamin D intoxication, acromegaly, acidosis, rhabdomyolysis, and hemolysis. The clinical consequences of severe hyperphosphatemia are hypocalcemia and calcium phosphate deposition in tissues. Depending on the location of tissue calcifications, serious chronic or acute complications may ensue (e.g., nephrocalcinosis, cardiac arrhythmias). Therapy consists of treating the underlying disorder and limiting dietary phosphorus intake and absorption. Oral aluminum phosphate binders or sevelamer may be used, and hemodialysis should be considered in severe cases.

■ HYPOMAGNESEMIA

Hypomagnesemia usually indicates significant whole body magnesium depletion. Muscle weakness, prolonged PR and QT intervals, and cardiac arrhythmias are the most common manifestations of hypomagnesemia. Magnesium is important for effective PTH secretion as well as the renal and skeletal responsiveness to PTH. Therefore, hypomagnesemia is often associated with hypocalcemia.

Etiology

Hypomagnesemia generally results from a derangement in renal or intestinal handling of magnesium and is classified as primary (hereditary) or secondary (acquired). Hereditary causes include both disorders of absorption (rare) and those of renal loss (e.g., Bartter's and Gitelman syndromes). Secondary causes are much more common, with renal losses being due to volume expansion, hypercalcemia, osmotic diuresis, loop diuretics, alcohol, aminoglycosides, cisplatin, cyclosporine, and amphotericin B, and gastrointestinal losses most commonly resulting from vomiting and diarrhea.

TREATMENT Hypomagnesemia

For mild deficiency, oral replacement in divided doses totaling 20–30 mmol/d (40–60 meq/d) is effective, although diarrhea may result. Parenteral magnesium administration is usually needed for serum levels <0.5 mmol/L (<1.2 mg/dL), with a continuous infusion of magnesium chloride IV to deliver 50 mmol/d over a 24-h period (dose reduced by 50–75% in renal failure). Therapy may be required for several days in order to replete tissue magnesium stores; serum Mg should be monitored every 12–24 h during treatment. Other electrolyte disturbances should be treated simultaneously. Pts with associated seizures or acute arrhythmias can be given 1–2 g of magnesium sulfate IV over 5–10 min.

■ HYPERMAGNESEMIA

Hypermagnesemia is rare but can be seen in renal failure when pts are taking magnesium-containing antacids, laxatives, enemas, or infusions, or in acute rhabdomyolysis. The most readily detectable clinical sign of hypermagnesemia is the disappearance of deep tendon reflexes, but hypocalcemia, hypotension, paralysis of respiratory muscles, complete heart block, and cardiac arrest can occur. Treatment includes stopping the preparation, clearing the intestines of residual offending laxatives or antacids with magnesium-free enemas or cathartics, dialysis against a low magnesium bath, or, if associated with life-threatening complications, 100–200 mg of elemental calcium IV over 1–2 h.

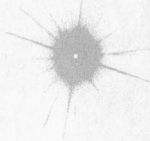

For a more detailed discussion, see Bringhurst FR, Demay MB, Krane SM, Kronenberg HM: Bone and Mineral Metabolism in Health and Disease, Chap. 352, p. 3082; Khosla S: Hypercalcemia and Hypocalcemia, Chap. 46, p. 360; and Potts JT Jr, Jüppner H: Disorders of the Parathyroid Gland and Calcium Homeostasis, Chap. 353, p. 3096, in HPIM-18.

CHAPTER **188**
Osteoporosis and Osteomalacia

■ OSTEOPOROSIS

Osteoporosis is defined as a reduction in bone mass [or bone mineral density (BMD)] or the presence of fragility fracture. It is defined operationally as a bone density that falls 2.5 SD below the mean for a young normal individual (a T-score of <-2.5). Those with a T-score of <1.0 (osteopenia) have low bone density and are at increased risk for osteoporosis. The most common sites for osteoporosis-related fractures are the vertebrae, hip, and distal radius.

Osteoporosis is a common condition in the elderly; women are at particularly high risk. In the United States, 8 million women and 2 million men have osteoporosis; an additional 18 million have osteopenia. The annual incidence of osteoporosis-related fractures is at least 1.5 million; almost half of them are vertebral crush fractures, followed in frequency by hip and wrist fractures. Hip fractures are associated with significant morbidity (thromboembolism) and a 5–20% mortality within a year.

Etiology

Low bone density may result from low peak bone mass or increased bone loss. Risk factors for an osteoporotic fracture are listed in Table 188-1, and diseases associated with osteoporosis are listed in Table 188-2. Certain drugs, primarily glucocorticoids, cyclosporine, cytotoxic drugs, thiazolidinediones, anticonvulsants, aluminum, heparin, excessive levothyroxine, GnRH agonists, and aromatase inhibitors also have detrimental effects on the skeleton.

Clinical Features

Pts with multiple vertebral crush fractures may have height loss, kyphosis, and secondary pain from altered biomechanics of the back. Thoracic

TABLE 188-1 RISK FACTORS FOR OSTEOPOROSIS FRACTURE

Nonmodifiable	Estrogen deficiency
Personal history of fracture as an adult	Early menopause (<45 years) or bilateral ovariectomy
History of fracture in first-degree relative	Prolonged premenopausal amenorrhea (>1 year)
Female sex	Low calcium intake
Advanced age	Alcoholism
White race	Impaired eyesight despite adequate correction
Dementia	
Potentially modifiable	Recurrent falls
Current cigarette smoking	Inadequate physical activity
Low body weight [<58 kg (127 lb)]	Poor health/frailty

fractures can be associated with restrictive lung disease, whereas lumbar fractures are sometimes associated with abdominal symptoms or nerve compression leading to sciatica. Dual-energy x-ray absorptiometry (DEXA) has become the standard for measuring bone density. The U.S. Preventive Health Services Task Force recommends that women age 65 and older be screened routinely for osteoporosis, and screening should begin at age 60 for women with increased risk. Criteria approved for Medicare reimbursement of bone mass measurement are summarized in Table 188-3. A general laboratory evaluation includes complete blood count, serum and 24-h urine calcium, 25(OH)D level, and renal and hepatic function tests. Further testing is based on clinical suspicion and may include thyroid-stimulating hormone (TSH), urinary free cortisol, parathyroid hormone (PTH), serum and urine electrophoresis, and testosterone levels (in men). Tissue transglutaminase Ab testing may identify asymptomatic celiac disease. Markers of bone resorption (e.g., urine cross-linked N-telopeptide) may be helpful in detecting an early response to antiresorptive therapy if measured prior to and 4–6 months after initiating therapy.

TREATMENT Osteoporosis

Treatment involves the management of acute fractures, modifying risk factors, and treating any underlying disorders that lead to reduced bone mass. Treatment decisions are based on an individual's risk factors, but active treatment is generally recommended if the T-score is ≤2.5. Risk factor reduction is a key part of management; smoking cessation and reduced alcohol intake should be encouraged; offending drugs should be discontinued or doses minimized (e.g., glucocorticoids), an exercise program should be instituted, and fall prevention strategies should be put in place. Oral calcium (1–1.5 g/d of elemental calcium in divided

TABLE 188-2 DISEASES ASSOCIATED WITH AN INCREASED RISK OF GENERALIZED OSTEOPOROSIS IN ADULTS

Hypogonadal states	Hematologic disorders/malignancy
Turner's syndrome	Multiple myeloma
Klinefelter's syndrome	Lymphoma and leukemia
Anorexia nervosa	Malignancy-associated parathyroid hormone–related (PTHrP) production
Hypothalamic amenorrhea	Mastocytosis
Hyperprolactinemia	Hemophilia
Other primary or secondary hypogonadal states	Thalassemia
Endocrine disorders	Selected inherited disorders
Cushing's syndrome	Osteogenesis imperfecta
Hyperparathyroidism	Marfan syndrome
Thyrotoxicosis	Hemochromatosis
Type 1 diabetes mellitus	Hypophosphatasia
Acromegaly	Glycogen storage diseases
Adrenal insufficiency	Homocystinuria
Nutritional and gastrointestinal disorders	Ehlers-Danlos syndrome
	Porphyria
Malnutrition	Menkes' syndrome
Parenteral nutrition	Epidermolysis bullosa
Malabsorption syndromes	Other disorders
Gastrectomy	Immobilization
Severe liver disease, especially biliary cirrhosis	Chronic obstructive pulmonary disease
	Pregnancy and lactation
Pernicious anemia	Scoliosis
Rheumatologic disorders	Multiple sclerosis
Rheumatoid arthritis	Sarcoidosis
Ankylosing spondylitis	Amyloidosis

doses) and vitamin D (400–800 IU/d) should be initiated in all pts with osteoporosis. Adequate vitamin D status should be verified by measuring serum 25(OH)D, the value of which should be at least 75 nmol/L (30 ng/mL). Some pts may require higher vitamin D supplements than those recommended above. Moderate sun exposure also generates vitamin D, although recommending outdoor exposure is controversial because of concerns about skin cancer. Bisphosphonates (alendronate, 70 mg PO weekly; risedronate, 35 mg PO weekly; ibandronate, 150 mg PO monthly or 3 mg IV every 3 mo; zoledronic acid, 5 mg IV annually)

TABLE 188-3 FDA-APPROVED INDICATIONS FOR BMD TESTS[a]

Estrogen-deficient women at clinical risk of osteoporosis

    Vertebral abnormalities on x-ray suggestive of osteoporosis (osteopenia, vertebral fracture)

    Glucocorticoid treatment equivalent to ≥7.5 mg of prednisone, or duration of therapy >3 months

Primary hyperparathyroidism

Monitoring response to an FDA-approved medication for osteoporosis

    Repeat BMD evaluations at >23-month intervals, or more frequently, if medically justified

[a]Criteria adapted from the 1998 Bone Mass Measurement Act.
Abbreviations: BMD, bone mineral density; FDA, U.S. Food and Drug Administration

inhibit bone resorption, augment bone density, and decrease fracture rates. Oral bisphosphonates are poorly absorbed and should be taken in the morning on an empty stomach with 0.25 L (8 oz) of tap water. Long-term bisphosphonate treatment may be associated with atypical femur fractures; a tentative recommendation is to limit therapy to 5 years. Osteonecrosis of the jaw is a rare complication of bisphosphonate treatment mainly seen with high-dose IV zoledronic acid or pamidronate administered in cancer pts. Estrogen decreases the rate of bone reabsorption, but therapy should be carefully weighed in the context of increased risks of cardiovascular disease and breast cancer. Raloxifene (60 mg/d PO), a selective estrogen receptor modulator (SERM), is an alternative antiresorptive agent that can be used in lieu of estrogen. It increases bone density and decreases total and LDL cholesterol without stimulating endometrial hyperplasia, although it may precipitate hot flashes. A new antiresorptive agent is denosumab, a monoclonal antibody against RANKL, an osteoclast differentiation factor. It is approved for pts at high risk for fracture and is given as an injection twice a year (60 mg SC every 6 months). Clinical experience with denosumab is still limited.

The only available drug that induces bone *formation* is teriparatide [PTH(1-34)]. It is indicated for treatment of severe osteoporosis and is administered as a daily injection for a maximum of 2 years. Teriparatide therapy must be followed by antiresorptive agent therapy to prevent rapid loss of the newly formed bone.

◼ OSTEOMALACIA

Etiology

Defective mineralization of the organic matrix of bone results in *osteomalacia*. The childhood form of osteomalacia is called rickets. Osteomalacia is caused by inadequate intake or malabsorption of vitamin D (chronic pancreatic insufficiency, gastrectomy, malabsorption) and disorders of vitamin D metabolism (anticonvulsant therapy, chronic renal failure, genetic disorders of vitamin D activation or action). Osteomalacia can also be caused by long-standing hypophosphatemia, which can be due to renal phosphate wasting (e.g., X-linked hypophosphatemic rickets or oncogenic osteomalacia) or excessive use of phosphate binders.

Clinical Features

Skeletal deformities may be overlooked until fractures occur after minimal trauma. Symptoms include diffuse skeletal pain and bony tenderness and may be subtle. Proximal muscle weakness is a feature of vitamin D deficiency and may mimic primary muscle disorders. A decrease in bone density is usually associated with loss of trabeculae and thinning of the cortices. Characteristic x-ray findings are radiolucent bands (Looser's zones or pseudofractures) ranging from a few millimeters to several centimeters in length, usually perpendicular to the surface of the femur, pelvis, and scapula. Changes in serum calcium, phosphorus, 25(OH)D, and 1,25(OH)$_2$D levels vary depending on the cause. The most specific test for vitamin D deficiency in an otherwise healthy individual is a low serum 25(OH)D level. Even modest vitamin D deficiency leads to compensatory secondary hyperparathyroidism characterized by increased levels of PTH and alkaline phosphatase, hyperphosphaturia, and low serum phosphate. With advancing osteomalacia, hypocalcemia may develop due to impaired calcium mobilization from undermineralized bone. 1,25-Dihydroxyvitamin D levels may be preserved, reflecting upregulation of 1α-hydroxylase activity.

TREATMENT   Osteomalacia

In osteomalacia due to vitamin D deficiency [serum 25(OH)D <50 nmol/L (<20 ng/mL)], vitamin D$_2$ (ergocalciferol) is given orally in doses of 50,000 IU weekly for 8 weeks, followed by maintenance therapy with 800 IU daily. Osteomalacia due to malabsorption requires larger doses of vitamin D (up to 50,000 IU/d orally or 250,000 IU IM biannually). In pts taking anticonvulsants or those with disorders of abnormal vitamin D activation, vitamin D should be administered in doses that maintain the serum calcium and 25(OH)D levels in the normal range. Calcitriol (0.25–0.5 μg/d PO) is effective in treating hypocalcemia or osteodystrophy caused by chronic renal failure. Vitamin D deficiency should always be repleted in conjunction with calcium supplementation (1.5–2.0 g of elemental calcium daily). Serum and urinary calcium measurements are efficacious for monitoring resolution of vitamin D deficiency, with a goal 24-h urinary calcium excretion of 100–250 mg/24 h.

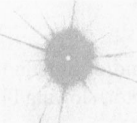

For a more detailed discussion, see Bringhurst FR, Demay MB, Krane SM, Kronenberg HM: Bone and Mineral Metabolism in Health and Disease, Chap. 352, p. 3082; and Lindsay R, Cosman F: Osteoporosis, Chap. 354, p. 3120, in HPIM-18.

CHAPTER **189**

Hypercholesterolemia and Hypertriglyceridemia

Hyperlipoproteinemia may be characterized by hypercholesterolemia, isolated hypertriglyceridemia, or both (Table 189-1). Diabetes mellitus, obesity, ethanol consumption, oral contraceptives, glucocorticoids, renal disease, hepatic disease, and hypothyroidism can cause secondary hyperlipoproteinemias or worsen underlying hyperlipoproteinemic states.

Standard lipoprotein analysis assesses total cholesterol, HDL cholesterol, and triglycerides with a calculation of LDL cholesterol levels using the following equation: LDL cholesterol = total cholesterol − HDL cholesterol − (triglycerides/5). The LDL cholesterol concentration can be estimated using this method only if triglycerides are <4.0 mmol/L (<350 mg/dL). Both LDL and HDL cholesterol levels are temporarily decreased for several weeks after myocardial infarction or acute inflammatory states, but can be accurately measured if blood is obtained within 8 h of the event.

ISOLATED HYPERCHOLESTEROLEMIA

Elevated levels of fasting plasma total cholesterol [>5.2 mmol/L (>200 mg/dL)] in the presence of normal levels of triglycerides are almost always associated with increased concentrations of plasma LDL cholesterol. A rare individual with markedly elevated HDL cholesterol may also have increased plasma total cholesterol levels. Elevations of LDL cholesterol can result from single-gene defects, from polygenic disorders, or from the secondary effects of other disease states.

■ FAMILIAL HYPERCHOLESTEROLEMIA (FH)

FH is a codominant genetic disorder due to mutations in the gene for the LDL receptor. Plasma LDL levels are elevated at birth and remain so throughout life. In untreated heterozygous adults, total cholesterol levels range from 7.1 to 12.9 mmol/L (275–500 mg/dL). Plasma triglyceride levels are typically normal, and HDL cholesterol levels are normal or reduced. Heterozygotes, especially men, are prone to accelerated atherosclerosis and premature coronary artery disease (CAD). *Tendon xanthomas* (most commonly of the Achilles tendons and the extensor tendons of the knuckles), *tuberous xanthomas* (softer, painless nodules on the ankles and buttocks), and *xanthelasmas* (deposits on the eyelids) are common. In its homozygous form, FH leads to severe atherosclerosis during childhood.

■ FAMILIAL DEFECTIVE APO B-100

This autosomal dominant disorder impairs the synthesis and/or function of apo B-100, thereby reducing the affinity for the LDL receptor, slowing LDL catabolism, and causing a phenocopy of FH.

TABLE 189-1 CHARACTERISTICS OF CLASSIC HYPERLIPIDEMIAS

Lipid Phenotype	Plasma Lipid Levels, mmol/L (mg/dL)	Lipoproteins Elevated	Phenotype	Clinical Signs
Isolated Hypercholesterolemia				
Familial hypercholesterolemia	Heterozygotes: total chol = 7–13 (275–500)	LDL	IIa	Usually develop xanthomas in adulthood and vascular disease at 30–50 years
	Homozygotes: total chol >13 (>500)	LDL	IIa	Usually develop xanthomas and vascular disease in childhood
Familial defective apo B-100	Heterozygotes: total chol = 7–13 (275–500)	LDL	IIa	
Polygenic hypercholesterolemia	Total chol = 6.5–9.0 (250–350)	LDL	IIa	Usually asymptomatic until vascular disease develops; no xanthomas
Isolated Hypertriglyceridemia				
Familial hypertriglyceridemia	TG = 2.8–8.5 (250–750) (plasma may be cloudy)	VLDL	IV	Asymptomatic; may be associated with increased risk of vascular disease
Familial lipoprotein lipase deficiency	TG >8.5 (>750) (plasma may be milky postprandially)	Chylomicrons	I, V	May be asymptomatic; may be associated with pancreatitis, abdominal pain, hepatosplenomegaly
Familial apo CII deficiency	TG >8.5 (>750) (plasma may be milky postprandially)	Chylomicrons	I, V	As above

(continued)

1173

TABLE 189-1 CHARACTERISTICS OF CLASSIC HYPERLIPIDEMIAS (CONTINUED)

Lipid Phenotype	Plasma Lipid Levels, mmol/L (mg/dL)	Lipoproteins Elevated	Phenotype	Clinical Signs
Hypertriglyceridemia and Hypercholesterolemia				
Combined hyperlipidemia	TG = 2.8–8.5 (250–750) Total chol = 6.5–13.0 (250–500)	VLDL, LDL	IIb	Usually asymptomatic until vascular disease develops; familial form may also present as isolated high TG or an isolated high LDL cholesterol
Dysbetalipoproteinemia	TG = 2.8–5.6 (250–500) Total chol = 6.5–13.0 (250–500)	VLDL, IDL; LDL normal	III	Usually asymptomatic until vascular disease develops; may have palmar or tuberoeruptive xanthomas

Note: Total chol, the sum of free and esterified cholesterol. The lipoprotein phenotype is designated according to the Fredrickson classification.
Abbreviations: IDL, intermediate-density lipoprotein; LDL, low-density lipoprotein; TG, triglycerides; VLDL, very low-density lipoprotein.
Source: From HN Ginsberg, IJ Goldberg: HPIM-15, p. 2250.

■ POLYGENIC HYPERCHOLESTEROLEMIA

Most moderate hypercholesterolemia [<9.1 mmol/L (<350 mg/dL)] arises from an interaction of multiple genetic defects and environmental factors such as diet, age, and exercise. Plasma HDL and triglyceride levels are normal, and xanthomas are not present.

TREATMENT Isolated Hypercholesterolemia

An algorithm for the evaluation and treatment of hypercholesterolemia is displayed in Fig. 189-1. Therapy for all of these disorders includes restriction of dietary cholesterol and HMG-CoA reductase inhibitors (statins). Cholesterol absorption inhibitors and bile acid sequestrants or nicotinic acid may also be required (Table 189-2).

ISOLATED HYPERTRIGLYCERIDEMIA

The diagnosis of hypertriglyceridemia is made by measuring plasma lipid levels after an overnight fast (≥12 h). Hypertriglyceridemia in adults is defined as a triglyceride level >2.3 mmol/L (>200 mg/dL). An isolated increase in plasma triglycerides indicates that chylomicrons and/or very low-density lipoprotein (VLDL) are increased. Plasma is usually clear when triglyceride levels are <4.5 mmol/L (<400 mg/dL) and cloudy when levels are higher due to VLDL (and/or chylomicron) particles becoming large enough to scatter light. When chylomicrons are present, a creamy layer floats to the top of plasma after refrigeration for several hours. Tendon xanthomas and xanthelasmas do not occur with isolated hypertriglyceridemia, but *eruptive xanthomas* (small orange-red papules) can appear on the trunk and extremities and *lipemia retinalis* (orange-yellow retinal vessels) may be seen when the triglyceride levels are >11.3 mmol/L (>1000 mg/dL). Pancreatitis is associated with these high concentrations.

■ FAMILIAL HYPERTRIGLYCERIDEMIA

In this relatively common (~1 in 500) autosomal dominant disorder, increased plasma VLDL causes elevated plasma triglyceride concentrations. Obesity, hyperglycemia, and hyperinsulinemia are characteristic, and diabetes mellitus, ethanol consumption, oral contraceptives, and hypothyroidism may exacerbate the condition. The diagnosis is suggested by the triad of elevated plasma triglycerides [2.8–11.3 mmol/L (250–1000 mg/dL)], normal or only mildly increased cholesterol levels [<6.5 mmol/L (<250 mg/dL)], and reduced plasma HDL. Secondary forms of hypertriglyceridemia due to the conditions listed above should be ruled out before making the diagnosis of familial hypertriglyceridemia. The identification of other first-degree relatives with hypertriglyceridemia is useful in making the diagnosis. Familial dysbetalipoproteinemia and familial combined hyperlipidemia should be ruled out, as these two conditions are associated with accelerated atherosclerosis.

■ LIPOPROTEIN LIPASE DEFICIENCY

This rare autosomal recessive disorder results from the absence or deficiency of lipoprotein lipase, which in turn impairs the metabolism of

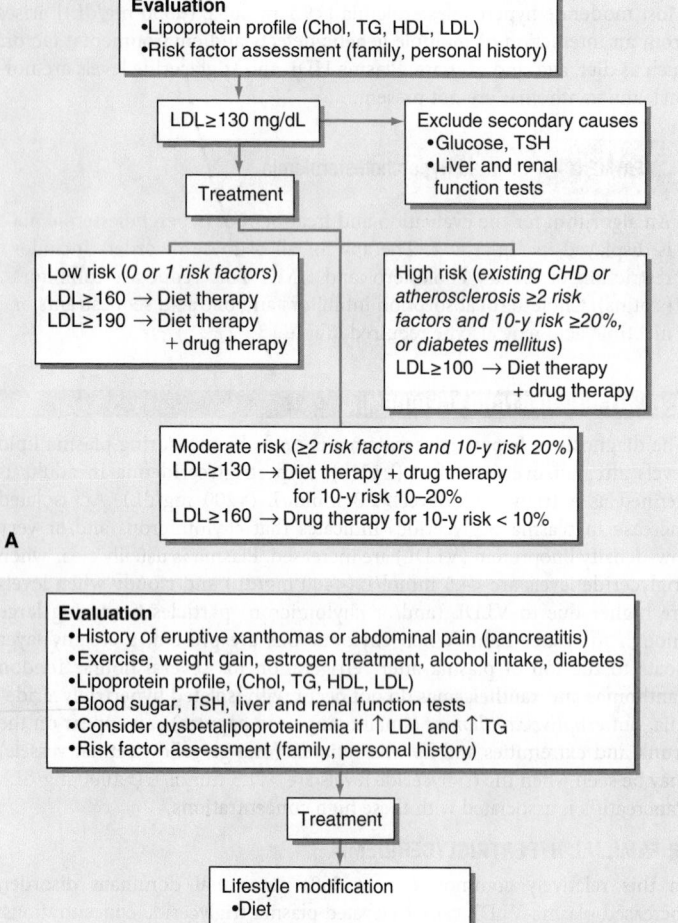

FIGURE 189-1 Algorithms for the evaluation and treatment of hypercholesterolemia **A** and hypertriglyceridemia **B**. Statin, HMG-CoA reductase inhibitor; Chol, cholesterol; HDL, high-density lipoprotein; LDL, low-density lipoprotein; TG, triglyceride; TSH, thyroid-stimulating hormone; CHD, coronary heart disease.

TABLE 189-2 HYPOLIPIDEMIC DRUGS

Drugs and dosing	Lipoprotein Class Affected	Common Side Effects	Contraindications
HMG-CoA reductase inhibitors	↓ LDL 18–55%	Myalgias, arthralgias, ↑ transaminases, dyspepsia	Acute or chronic liver disease; risk of myositis increased by impaired renal function and in combination with a fibrate
Lovastatin 20–80 mg/d	↓ TG 7–30%		
Pravastatin 40–80 mg qhs	↑ HDL 5–15%		
Simvastatin 20–80 mg qhs			
Fluvastatin 20–80 mg/d			
Atorvastatin 10–80 mg qhs			
Rosuvastatin 10–40 mg qhs			
Cholesterol absorption inhibitors	↓ LDL 18%	↑ Transaminases	
Ezetimibe 10 mg qd	↓ TG 8%		
Bile acid sequestrant	↓ LDL 15–30%	Constipation, gastric discomfort, nausea	Biliary tract obstruction, gastric outlet obstruction
Cholestyramine 4–32 g/d	↑ TG 10%		
Colestipol 5–40 g/d	↑ HDL 3–5%		
Colesevelam 3750–4375 mg/d			
Nicotinic acid	↓ LDL 5–25% ↓ TG 20–50% ↑ HDL 15–35%	Flushing (may be relieved by aspirin), hepatic dysfunction, nausea, diarrhea, glucose intolerance, hyperuricemia	Peptic ulcer disease, hepatic disease, gout
Immediate release 100 mg tid, gradual increase to 1 g tid			
Sustained release 250 mg–1.5 g bid			

(continued)

TABLE 189-2 HYPOLIPIDEMIC DRUGS (CONTINUED)

Drugs and dosing	Lipoprotein Class Affected	Common Side Effects	Contraindications
Extended release 500 mg–2 g qhs			
Fibric acid derivatives	↑ or ↓ LDL	↓ Absorption of other drugs	Hepatic or biliary disease, renal insufficiency associated with ↑ risk of myositis
Gemfibrozil 600 mg bid	↓ TG 20–50%	↑ Gallstones, dyspepsia, hepatic dysfunction, myalgia	
Fenofibrate 145 mg qd	↑ HDL 10–20%		
Fish oils 3–6 g qd	↓ TG 5–10%	Dyspepsia, diarrhea, fishy odor to breath	

Abbreviations: HDL, high-density lipoprotein; LDL, low-density lipoprotein; LPL, lipoprotein lipase; TG, triglycerides; VLDL, very low density lipoprotein.

chylomicrons. Accumulation of chylomicrons in plasma causes recurrent bouts of pancreatitis, usually beginning in childhood, and hepatosplenomegaly is present. Accelerated atherosclerosis is not a feature.

APO CII DEFICIENCY

This rare autosomal recessive disorder is due to the absence of apo CII, an essential cofactor for lipoprotein lipase. As a result, chylomicrons and triglycerides accumulate and cause manifestations similar to those in lipoprotein lipase deficiency.

TREATMENT Isolated Hypertriglyceridemia

An algorithm for the evaluation and treatment of hypertriglyceridemia is displayed in Fig. 189-1. Pts with severe hypertriglyceridemia should be placed on a fat-free diet with fat-soluble vitamin supplementation. Pts with moderate hypertriglyceridemia should restrict fat, carbohydrate, and alcohol intake. In those with familial hypertriglyceridemia, fibric acid derivatives should be administered if dietary measures fail (Table 189-2).

HYPERCHOLESTEROLEMIA AND HYPERTRIGLYCERIDEMIA

Elevations of both triglycerides and cholesterol are caused by elevations in both VLDL and LDL or in VLDL remnant particles.

FAMILIAL COMBINED HYPERLIPIDEMIA (FCHL)

This inherited disorder, present in 1/200 persons, can cause different lipoprotein abnormalities in affected individuals, including hypercholesterolemia (elevated LDL), hypertriglyceridemia (elevated triglycerides and VLDL), or both. Atherosclerosis is accelerated. A mixed dyslipidemia [plasma triglycerides 2.3–9.0 mmol/L (200–800 mg/dL), cholesterol levels 5.2–10.3 mmol/L (200–400 mg/dL), and HDL levels <10.3 mmol/L (<40 mg/dL) in men and <12.9 mmol/L (<50 mg/dL) in women] and a family history of hyperlipidemia and/or premature cardiovascular disease suggest the diagnosis of FCHL. Many of these pts also have the metabolic syndrome (Chap. 127), and it may be difficult to differentiate familial from secondary causes of hyperlipidemia. All pts should restrict dietary cholesterol and fat and avoid alcohol and oral contraceptives; pts with diabetes should be treated aggressively. An HMG-CoA reductase inhibitor is usually required, and many pts will require a second drug (cholesterol absorption inhibitor, niacin, or fibrate) for optimal control.

■ DYSBETALIPOPROTEINEMIA

This rare genetic disorder is associated with homozygosity for an apoprotein variant (apoE2) that has reduced affinity for the LDL receptor. Development of disease requires additional environmental and/or genetic factors. Plasma cholesterol [6.5–13.0 mmol/L (250–500 mg/dL)] and triglycerides [2.8–5.6 mmol/L (250–500 mg/dL)] are increased due to accumulation of VLDL and chylomicron remnant particles. Pts usually present in adulthood with xanthomas and premature coronary and peripheral vascular disease. Cutaneous xanthomas are distinctive, in the form of *palmar* and *tuberoeruptive xanthomas*. Triglycerides and cholesterol are both elevated. Diagnosis is established by lipoprotein electrophoresis (showing a broad beta band) or a ratio of VLDL (by ultracentrifugation) to total plasma triglycerides of >0.3. The disorder is associated with accelerated atherosclerosis. Dietary modifications should be instituted, and HMG-CoA reductase inhibitors, fibrates, and/or niacin may be necessary. Comorbidities, such as diabetes mellitus, obesity, or hypothyroidism, should be optimally managed.

PREVENTION OF THE COMPLICATIONS OF ATHEROSCLEROSIS

The National Cholesterol Education Program guidelines (Fig. 189-1) are based on plasma LDL levels and estimations of other risk factors. The goal in pts with the highest risk (known coronary heart or other atherosclerotic disease, 10-year Framingham Study risk for coronary heart disease >20%, or diabetes mellitus) is to lower LDL cholesterol to <2.6 mmol/L (<100 mg/dL). In pts with very high risk, clinical trials suggest additional benefit by reducing LDL cholesterol to <1.8 mmol/L (<70 mg/dL). The goal is an LDL cholesterol <3.4 mmol/L (<130 mg/dL) in pts with two or more risk factors for atherosclerotic heart disease and a 10-year absolute risk of 10–20%, although a treatment goal of <2.6 mmol/L (<100 mg/dL) can be considered. The intensity of LDL-lowering drug treatment in high- and moderately high-risk pts should achieve at least a 30% reduction in LDL levels. Risk factors include (1) men age >45, women age >55 or after menopause; (2) family history of early CAD (<55 years in a male parent or sibling and <65 years in a female parent or sibling); (3) hypertension (even if it is controlled with medications); (4) cigarette smoking

(>10 cigarettes/day); and (5) HDL cholesterol <1.0 mmol/L (<40 mg/dL). Therapy begins with a low-fat diet and lifestyle modification, but pharmacologic intervention is often required (Table 189-2).

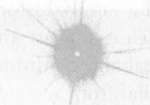

For a more detailed discussion, see Rader DJ, Hobbs HH: Disorders of Lipoprotein Metabolism, Chap. 356, p. 3145; in HPIM-18.

CHAPTER **190**
Hemochromatosis, Porphyrias, and Wilson's Disease

HEMOCHROMATOSIS

Hemochromatosis is a disorder of iron storage that results in increased intestinal iron absorption with Fe deposition and damage to many tissues. The classic clinical constellation of hemochromatosis is a pt presenting with bronze skin, liver disease, diabetes, arthropathy, cardiac conduction abnormalities, and hypogonadism. Two major causes of hemochromatosis exist: hereditary (due to inheritance of mutant *HFE* genes) and secondary iron overload (usually the result of ineffective erythropoiesis, such as thalassemia or sideroblastic anemia). *HFE* encodes a protein that is involved in cellular iron sensing and in regulating intestinal iron absorption. *HFE* mutations are very common in populations of Northern European origin (1 in 10 is a carrier). Heterozygotes are asymptomatic; homozygotes show a disease penetrance of ~30%. There is progressive iron overload, with clinical manifestations appearing after age 30–40, typically earlier in men than in women. Alcoholic liver disease and chronic excessive Fe ingestion may also be associated with a moderate increase in hepatic Fe and elevated body Fe stores.

Clinical Features

Early symptoms include weakness, lassitude, weight loss, a bronze pigmentation or darkening of skin, abdominal pain, and loss of libido. Hepatomegaly occurs in 95% of pts, sometimes in the presence of normal LFTs. If untreated, liver disease progresses to cirrhosis, and further to hepatocellular carcinoma in ~30% of pts with cirrhosis. Other manifestations include skin pigmentation (bronzing), diabetes mellitus (65% of pts), arthropathy (25–59%), cardiac arrhythmias and CHF (15%), and hypogonadotropic hypogonadism. Diabetes mellitus is more common in pts with a family history of diabetes, and hypogonadism may be an isolated early manifestation. Typical signs of portal hypertension and decompensated hepatic cirrhosis may appear late in the clinical course. Adrenal insufficiency, hypothyroidism, and hypoparathyroidism rarely occur.

Diagnosis

Serum Fe, percent transferrin saturation, and serum ferritin levels are increased. In an otherwise-healthy person, a fasting serum transferrin saturation >50% is abnormal and suggests homozygosity for hemochromatosis. In most untreated pts with hemochromatosis, the serum ferritin level is also greatly increased. If either the percent transferrin saturation or the serum ferritin level is abnormal, genetic testing for hemochromatosis should be performed. All first-degree relatives of pts with hemochromatosis should be tested for the C282Y and H63D mutations in *HFE*. Liver biopsy may be required in affected individuals to evaluate possible cirrhosis and to quantify tissue iron. An algorithm for evaluating pts with possible hemochromatosis is shown in Fig. 190-1. Death in untreated pts results from cardiac failure (30%), cirrhosis (25%), and hepatocellular carcinoma (30%); the latter may develop despite adequate Fe removal.

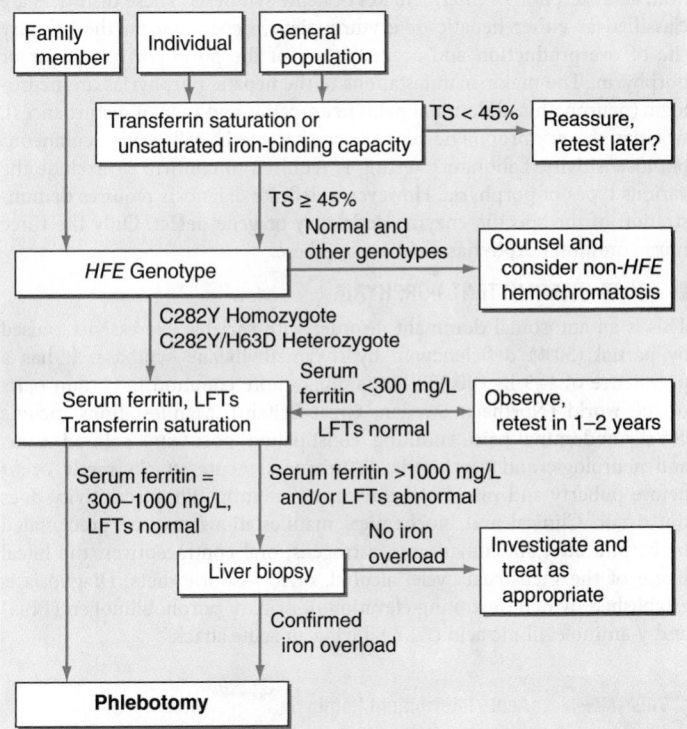

FIGURE 190-1 Algorithm for screening for *HFE*-associated hemochromatosis. LFT, liver function tests; TS, transferrin saturation. (*From EJ Eijkelkamp et al: Can J Gastroenterol 14:2, 2000; with permission.*)

TREATMENT Hemochromatosis

Therapy involves removal of excess body Fe, usually by intermittent phlebotomy, and supportive treatment of damaged organs. Since 1 unit of blood contains ~250 mg Fe, and since up to 25 g of Fe must be removed, phlebotomy is performed weekly for 1–2 years. Less frequent phlebotomy is then used to maintain serum Fe at 9–18 μmol/L (50–100 μg/dL). Chelating agents such as deferoxamine (infused subcutaneously using a portable pump) remove 10–20 mg iron per day, a fraction of that mobilized by weekly phlebotomy. Chelation therapy is indicated, however, when phlebotomy is inappropriate, such as with anemia or hypoproteinemia. Alcohol consumption should be eliminated. End-stage liver disease may require liver transplantation.

PORPHYRIAS

The porphyrias are inherited disturbances in heme biosynthesis. Each of the nine disorders causes a unique pattern of overproduction, accumulation, and excretion of intermediates of heme synthesis. These disorders are classified as either hepatic or erythropoietic, depending on the primary site of overproduction and accumulation of the porphyrin precursor or porphyrin. The major manifestations of the hepatic porphyrias are neurologic (neuropathic abdominal pain, neuropathy, and mental disturbances), whereas the erythropoietic porphyrias characteristically cause cutaneous photosensitivity. Laboratory testing is required to confirm or exclude the various types of porphyria. However, a definite diagnosis requires demonstration of the specific enzyme deficiency or gene defect. Only the three most common porphyrias are discussed here.

■ ACUTE INTERMITTENT PORPHYRIA

This is an autosomal dominant disorder with variable expressivity caused by partial (50%) deficiency in hydroxymethylbilane synthase. It has a prevalence of 1–3 in 100,000 but is much more common in certain parts of the world (Northern Sweden, Great Britain). Manifestations include colicky abdominal pain, vomiting, constipation, port wine–colored urine, and neurologic and psychiatric disturbances. Acute attacks rarely occur before puberty and may last from days to months. Photosensitivity does not occur. Clinical and biochemical manifestations may be precipitated by barbiturates, anticonvulsants, estrogens, oral contraceptives, the luteal phase of the menstrual cycle, alcohol, or low-calorie diets. Diagnosis is established by demonstrating elevation of urinary porphobilinogen (PBG) and γ-aminolevulinic acid (ALA) during an acute attack.

TREATMENT Acute Intermittent Porphyria

As soon as possible after the onset of an attack, 3–4 mg of heme, in the form of heme arginate, heme albumin, or hematin, should be infused daily for 4 days. Heme acts by inhibiting ALA synthase, thereby restraining

ALA and PBG production. Administration of IV glucose at rates up to 20 g/h or parenteral nutrition, if oral feeding is not possible for long periods, can be effective in acute attacks. Narcotic analgesics may be required during acute attacks for abdominal pain, and phenothiazines are useful for nausea, vomiting, anxiety, and restlessness. Treatment between attacks involves adequate nutritional intake, avoidance of drugs known to exacerbate the disease, and prompt treatment of other intercurrent diseases or infections.

■ PORPHYRIA CUTANEA TARDA

This is the most common porphyria (2–4 in 100,000) and is characterized by cutaneous photosensitivity and, usually, hepatic disease. It is due to partial deficiency (familial, sporadic, or acquired) of hepatic uroporphyrinogen decarboxylase. Photosensitivity causes facial pigmentation, increased fragility of skin, erythema, and vesicular and ulcerative lesions, typically involving face, forehead, and forearms. Neurologic manifestations are not observed. Contributing factors include excess alcohol, iron, and estrogens. Pts with liver disease are at risk for cirrhosis and hepatocellular carcinoma. Plasma and urine uroporphyrin and 7-carboxylate porphyrin are increased.

> **TREATMENT** Porphyria Cutanea Tarda
>
> Avoidance of precipitating factors, including abstinence from alcohol, estrogens, iron supplements, and other exacerbating drugs, is the first line of therapy. A complete response can almost always be achieved by repeated phlebotomy (every 1–2 weeks) until hepatic iron is reduced. Chloroquine or hydroxychloroquine may be used in low doses (e.g., 125 mg chloroquine phosphate twice weekly) to promote porphyrin excretion in pts unable to undergo or unresponsive to phlebotomy.

■ ERYTHROPOIETIC PROTOPORPHYRIA

Erythropoietic protoporphyria is an autosomal dominant disorder due to partial deficiency of ferrochelatase, the last enzyme in the heme biosynthetic pathway. Its prevalence is 1 in 100,000. Porphyrins (primarily protoporphyrin IX) from bone marrow erythrocytes and plasma are deposited in the skin and lead to cutaneous photosensitivity. Skin photosensitivity usually begins in childhood. The skin manifestations differ from those of other porphyrias, in that vesicular lesions are uncommon. Redness, swelling, burning, and itching can develop within minutes of sun exposure and resemble angioedema. Symptoms may seem out of proportion to the visible skin lesions. Chronic skin changes may include lichenification, leathery pseudovesicles, labial grooving, and nail changes. Liver function is usually normal, but liver disease and gallstones may occur. Protoporphyrin levels are increased in bone marrow, circulating erythrocytes, plasma, bile, and feces; protoporphyrin in erythrocytes is free rather than zinc-complexed as it is in other types of porphyria or hematologic disorders. Urinary porphyrin levels are normal. Diagnosis is confirmed by identifying a mutation in the ferrochelatase gene.

> **TREATMENT** Erythropoietic Protoporphyria
>
> Avoidance of sun exposure is essential. Oral β-carotene (120–180 mg/d) improves tolerance to sunlight in many pts. The dosage may be adjusted to maintain serum carotene levels between 10 and 15 μmol/L (600–800 μg/dL). Cholestyramine or activated charcoal may promote fecal excretion of protoporphyrin. Plasmapheresis or IV heme therapy may be beneficial.

WILSON'S DISEASE

Wilson's disease is a rare inherited disorder of copper metabolism, resulting in the toxic accumulation of copper in the liver, brain, and other organs. Individuals with Wilson's disease have mutations in the *ATP7B* gene, which encodes a membrane-bound copper-transporting ATPase. Deficiency of this protein impairs copper excretion into the bile and copper incorporation into ceruloplasmin, leading to its rapid degradation.

Clinical Features

Clinical manifestations typically appear in the mid- to late-teen years but may occur later. Hepatic disease may present as hepatitis, cirrhosis, or hepatic decompensation. In other pts, neurologic or psychiatric disturbances are the first clinical sign and are always accompanied by Kayser-Fleischer rings (corneal deposits of copper). Dystonia, incoordination, or tremor may be present, and dysarthria and dysphagia are common. Autonomic disturbances also may be present. Microscopic hematuria is common. In about 5% of pts, the first manifestation may be primary or secondary amenorrhea or repeated spontaneous abortions.

Diagnosis

Serum ceruloplasmin levels are often low but may be normal in up to 10% of pts. Urine copper levels are elevated. The "gold standard" for diagnosis is an elevated copper level on liver biopsy. Genetic testing is not currently practical because of the large number of mutations that can be responsible.

> **TREATMENT** Wilson's Disease
>
> Hepatitis or cirrhosis without decompensation should be treated with zinc acetate (50 mg elemental Zn PO three times a day). Zinc is effective by blocking intestinal copper absorption and inducing metallothionein, which sequesters copper in an nontoxic complex. For pts with hepatic decompensation, the chelator trientene (500 mg PO twice a day) plus zinc (separated by at least 1 h to avoid zinc chelation in the intestinal lumen) is recommended, although liver transplantation should be considered

for severe hepatic decompensation. For initial neurologic therapy, trientine and zinc are recommended for 8 weeks, followed by therapy with zinc alone. Tetrathiomolybdate is an alternative therapeutic option available in the future. Penicillamine is no longer first-line therapy. Zinc treatment does not require monitoring for toxicity, and 24-h urine copper can be followed for a therapeutic response. Trientine may induce bone marrow suppression and proteinuria. With chelation therapy, measuring free serum copper levels (adjusting total serum copper for ceruloplasmin copper) rather than urine copper is used to monitor therapeutic response. Anticopper therapy must be lifelong.

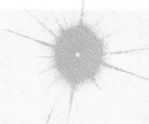

For a more detailed discussion, see Powell LW: Hemochromatosis, Chap. 357, p. 3162; Desnick RJ, Balwani M: The Porphyrias, Chap. 358, p. 3167; and Brewer GJ: Wilson's Disease, Chap. 360, p. 3188, in HPIM-18.

CHAPTER **191**
The Neurologic Examination

MENTAL STATUS EXAM

- *The bare minimum: During the interview, look for difficulties with communication and determine whether the pt has recall and insight into recent and past events.*

The mental status examination is underway as soon as the physician begins observing and talking with the pt. The goal of the mental status exam is to evaluate attention, orientation, memory, insight, judgment, and grasp of general information. Attention is tested by asking the pt to respond every time a specific item recurs in a list. Orientation is evaluated by asking about the day, date, and location. Memory can be tested by asking pt to immediately recall a sequence of numbers and by testing recall of a series of objects after defined times (e.g., 5 and 15 min). More remote memory is evaluated by assessing pt's ability to provide a cogent chronologic history of the illness or personal life events. Recall of historic events or dates of current events can be used to assess knowledge. Evaluation of language function should include assessment of spontaneous speech, naming, repetition, reading, writing, and comprehension. Additional tests such as ability to draw and copy, perform calculations, interpret proverbs or logic problems, identify right vs. left, name and identify body parts, etc., are also important.

A useful screening examination of cognitive function is the mini-mental status examination (MMSE) (Table 191-1).

CRANIAL NERVE (CN) EXAM

- *The bare minimum: Check the fundi, visual fields, pupil size and reactivity, extraocular movements, and facial movements.*

CN I

Occlude each nostril sequentially and ask pt to gently sniff and identify a mild test stimulus, such as soap, toothpaste, coffee, or lemon oil.

CN II

Check visual acuity with eyeglasses or contact lens correction using a Snellen chart or similar tool. Map visual fields (VFs) by confrontation testing in each quadrant of visual field for each eye individually. The best method is to sit facing pt (2–3 ft apart) and then have pt cover one eye gently and fix uncovered eye on examiner's nose. A small white object (e.g., a cotton-tipped applicator) is then moved slowly from periphery of field toward center until seen. Pt's VF should be mapped against examiner's for

TABLE 191-1 THE MINI-MENTAL STATUS EXAMINATION

	Points
Orientation	
Name: season/date/day/month/year	5 (1 for each name)
Name: hospital floor/town/state/country	5 (1 for each name)
Registration	
Identify three objects by name and ask pt to repeat	3 (1 for each object)
Attention and calculation	
Serial 7s; subtract from 100 (e.g., 93–86–79–72–65)	5 (1 for each subtraction)
Recall	
Recall the three objects presented earlier	3 (1 for each object)
Language	
Name pencil and watch	2 (1 for each object)
Repeat "No ifs, ands, or buts"	1
Follow a 3-step command (e.g., "Take this paper, fold it in half, and place it on the table")	3 (1 for each command)
Write "close your eyes" and ask pt to obey written command	1
Ask pt to write a sentence	1
Ask pt to copy a design (e.g., intersecting pentagons)	1
TOTAL	30

comparison. Formal perimetry and tangent screen exam are essential to identify and delineate small defects. Optic fundi should be examined with an ophthalmoscope, and the color, size, and degree of swelling or elevation of the optic disc recorded. The retinal vessels should be checked for size, regularity, AV nicking at crossing points, hemorrhage, exudates, and aneurysms. The retina, including the macula, should be examined for abnormal pigmentation and other lesions.

CN III, IV, VI

Describe size, regularity, and shape of pupils; reaction (direct and consensual) to light; and convergence (pt follows an object as it moves closer). Check for lid drooping, lag, or retraction. Ask pt to follow your finger as you move it horizontally to left and right and vertically with each eye first fully adducted then fully abducted. Check for failure to move fully in particular directions and for presence of regular, rhythmic, involuntary oscillations of eyes (nystagmus). Test quick voluntary eye movements (saccades) as well as pursuit (e.g., follow the finger).

CN V

Feel the masseter and temporalis muscles as pt bites down and test jaw opening, protrusion, and lateral motion against resistance. Examine sensation over entire face. Testing of the corneal reflex is indicated when suggested by the history.

CN VII

Look for asymmetry of face at rest and with spontaneous movements. Test eyebrow elevation, forehead wrinkling, eye closure, smiling, frowning; check puff, whistle, lip pursing, and chin muscle contraction. Observe for differences in strength of lower and upper facial muscles. Taste on the anterior two-thirds of tongue can be affected by lesions of the seventh CN proximal to the chorda tympani.

CN VIII

Check ability to hear tuning fork, finger rub, watch tick, and whispered voice at specified distances with each ear. Check for air vs. mastoid bone conduction (Rinne) and lateralization of a tuning fork placed on center of forehead (Weber). Accurate, quantitative testing of hearing requires formal audiometry. Remember to examine tympanic membranes.

CN IX, X

Check for symmetric elevation of palate-uvula with phonation ("ahh"), as well as position of uvula and palatal arch at rest. Sensation in region of tonsils, posterior pharynx, and tongue may also require testing. Pharyngeal ("gag") reflex is evaluated by stimulating posterior pharyngeal wall on each side with a blunt object (e.g., tongue blade). Direct examination of vocal cords by laryngoscopy is necessary in some situations.

CN XI

Check shoulder shrug (trapezius muscle) and head rotation to each side (sternocleidomastoid muscle) against resistance.

CN XII

Examine bulk and power of tongue. Look for atrophy, deviation from midline with protrusion, tremor, and small flickering or twitching movements (fibrillations, fasciculations).

MOTOR EXAM

- *The bare minimum: Look for muscle atrophy and check limb tone. Assess upper limb strength by checking for pronator drift and strength of wrist or finger reflexes. Test for lower limb strength by asking pt to walk normally and on heels and toes.*

Power should be systematically tested for major movements at each joint (Table 191-2). Strength should be recorded using a reproducible scale (e.g., 0 = no movement, 1 = flicker or trace of contraction with no associated movement at a joint, 2 = movement present but cannot be sustained against gravity, 3 = movement against gravity but not against applied resistance,

TABLE 191-2 MUSCLES THAT MOVE JOINTS

	Muscle	Nerve	Segmental Innervation	Function
Shoulder	Supraspinatus	Suprascapular n.	C5,6	Abduction of upper arm
	Deltoid	Axillary n.	C5,6	Abduction of upper arm
Forearm	Biceps	Musculocutaneous n.	C5,6	Flexion of the supinated forearm
	Brachioradialis	Radial n.	C5,6	Forearm flexion with arm between pronation and supination
	Triceps	Radial n.	C6,7,8	Extension of forearm
	Ext. carpi radialis	Radial n.	C5,6	Extension and abduction of hand at the wrist
	Ext. carpi ulnaris	P. interosseous n.	C7,8	Extension and adduction of hand at the wrist
	Ext. digitorum	P. interosseous n.	C7,8	Extension of fingers at the MCP joints
	Supinator	P. interosseous n.	C6,7	Supination of the extended forearm
	Flex. carpi radialis	Median n.	C6,7	Flexion and abduction of hand at the wrist
	Flex. carpi ulnaris	Ulnar n.	C7,8,T1	Flexion and adduction of hand at the wrist
	Pronator teres	Median n.	C6,7	Pronation of the forearm
Wrist	Ext. carpi ulnaris	Ulnar n.	C7,8,T1	Extension/adduction at the wrist
	Flex. carpi radialis	Median n.	C6,7	Flexion/abduction at the wrist

Hand	Lumbricals	Median + ulnar n.	C8,T1	Extension of fingers at PIP joint with the MCP joint extended and fixed
	Interossei	Ulnar n.	C8,T1	Abduction/adduction of the fingers
	Flex. digitorum	Median + A. interosseous n.	C7,C8,T1	Flexion of the fingers
Thumb	Opponens pollicis	Median n.	C8,T1	Touching the base of the 5th finger with thumb
	Ext. pollicis	P. interosseous n.	C7,8	Extension of the thumb
	Add. pollicis	Median n.	C8,T1	Adduction of the thumb
	Abd. pollicis	Ulnar n.	C8,T1	Abduction of the thumb
	Flex. pollicis br.	Ulnar n.	C8,T1	Flexion of the thumb
Thigh	Iliopsoas	Femoral n.	L1,2,3	Flexion of the thigh
	Glutei	Sup. + inf. gluteal n.	L4,L5,S1,S2	Abduction, extension, and internal rotation of the leg
	Quadriceps	Femoral n.	L2,3,4	Extension of the leg at the knee
	Adductors	Obturator n.	L2,3,4	Adduction of the leg
	Hamstrings	Sciatic n.	L5,S1,S2	Flexion of the leg at the knee
Foot	Gastrocnemius	Tibial n.	S1,S2	Plantar flexion of the foot
	Tibialis ant.	Deep peroneal n.	L4,5	Dorsiflexion of the foot
	Peronei	Deep peroneal n.	L5,S1	Eversion of the foot
	Tibialis post.	Tibial n.	L4,5	Inversion of the foot
Toes	Ext. hallucis l.	Deep peroneal n.	L5,S1	Dorsiflexion of the great toe

4 = movement against some degree of resistance, and 5 = full power; 4 values can be supplemented with + and − signs to provide additional gradations). Speed of movement, ability to relax contractions promptly, and fatigue with repetition should all be noted. Loss in bulk and size of muscle (atrophy) should be noted, as well as the presence of irregular involuntary contraction (twitching) of groups of muscle fibers (fasciculations). Any involuntary movements should be noted at rest, during maintained posture, and with voluntary action.

REFLEXES

- *The bare minimum: Tap the biceps, patellar, and Achilles reflexes.*

Important muscle-stretch reflexes to test routinely and the spinal cord segments involved in their reflex arcs include biceps (C5, 6); brachioradialis (C5, 6); triceps (C7, 8); patellar (L3, 4); and Achilles (S1, 2). A common grading scale is 0 = absent, 1 = present but diminished, 2 = normal, 3 = hyperactive, and 4 = hyperactive with clonus (repetitive rhythmic contractions with maintained stretch). The plantar reflex should be tested by using a blunt-ended object such as the point of a key to stroke the outer border of the sole of the foot from the heel toward the base of the great toe. An abnormal response (Babinski sign) is extension (dorsiflexion) of the great toe at the metatarsophalangeal joint. In some cases this may be associated with abduction (fanning) of other toes and variable degrees of flexion at ankle, knee, and hip. Normal response is plantar flexion of the toes. Superficial abdominal and anal reflexes are important in certain situations; unlike muscle stretch reflexes, these cutaneous reflexes disappear with CNS lesions.

SENSORY EXAM

- *The bare minimum: Ask whether the pt can feel light touch and the temperature of a cool object in each distal extremity. Check double simultaneous stimulation using light touch on the hands.*

For most purposes it is sufficient to test sensation to pinprick, touch, position, and vibration in each of the four extremities (Figs. 191-1 and 191-2). Specific problems often require more thorough evaluation. Pts with cerebral lesions may have abnormalities in "discriminative sensation" such as the ability to perceive double simultaneous stimuli, to localize stimuli accurately, to identify closely approximated stimuli as separate (two-point discrimination), to identify objects by touch alone (stereognosis), or to judge weights, evaluate texture, or identify letters or numbers written on the skin surface (graphesthesia).

COORDINATION AND GAIT

- *The bare minimum: Test rapid alternating movements of the fingers and feet, and the finger-to-nose maneuver. Observe the pt while he or she is walking along a straight line.*

The ability to move the index finger accurately from the nose to the examiner's outstretched finger and the ability to slide the heel of each foot from the knee down the shin are tests of coordination. Additional tests (drawing objects in the air, following a moving finger, tapping with index finger against thumb or alternately against each individual finger) may also be useful. The ability to stand with feet together and eyes closed (Romberg test), to walk a straight line (tandem walk), and to turn should all be observed.

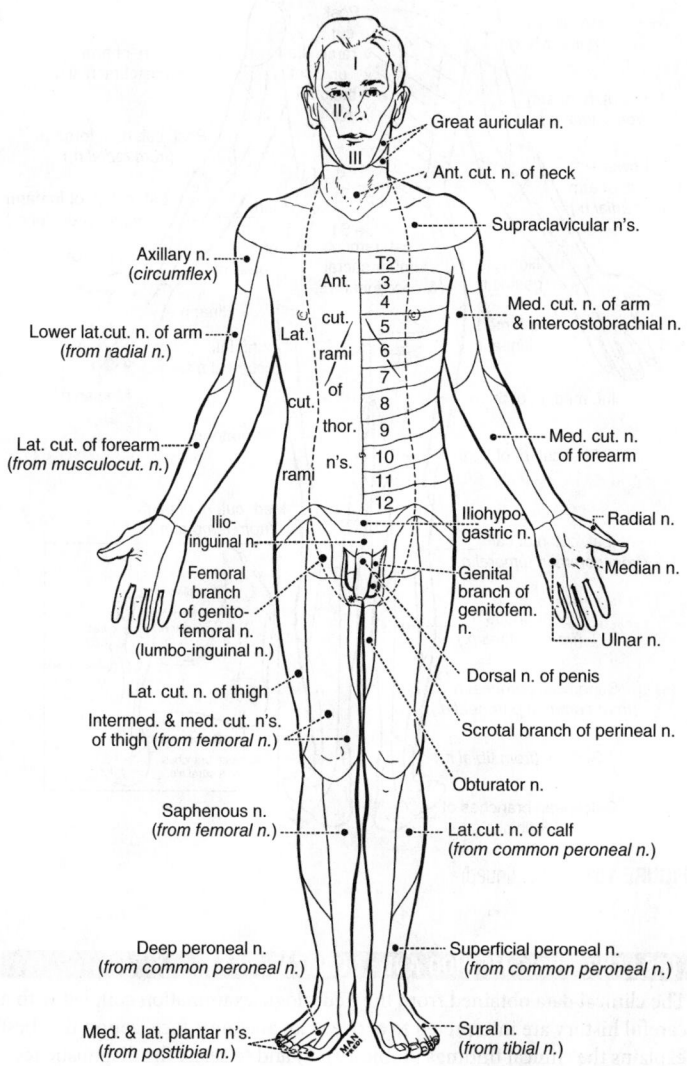

FIGURE 191-1 The cutaneous fields of peripheral nerves. *(Reproduced by permission from W Haymaker, B Woodhall:* Peripheral Nerve Injuries, *2nd ed. Philadelphia, Saunders, 1953.)*

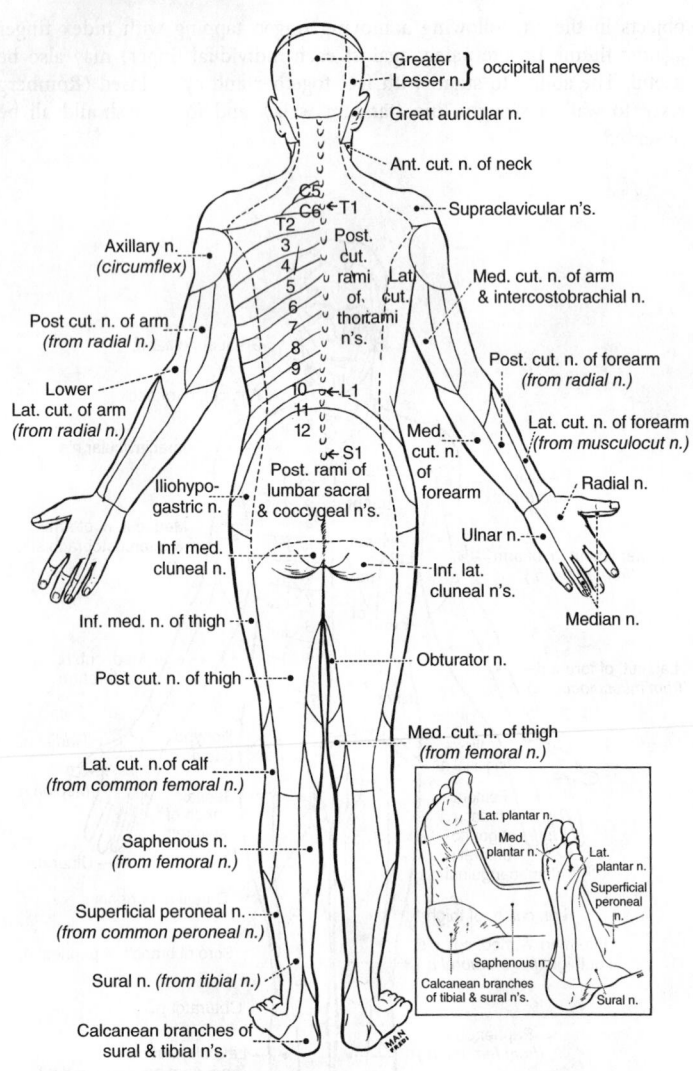

FIGURE 191-1 (Continued)

THE NEUROLOGIC METHOD AND LOCALIZATION

The clinical data obtained from the neurologic examination coupled with a careful history are interpreted to arrive at an anatomic localization that best explains the clinical findings (Table 191-3) and to select the diagnostic tests most likely to be informative in order to define the pathophysiology of the anatomic lesion.

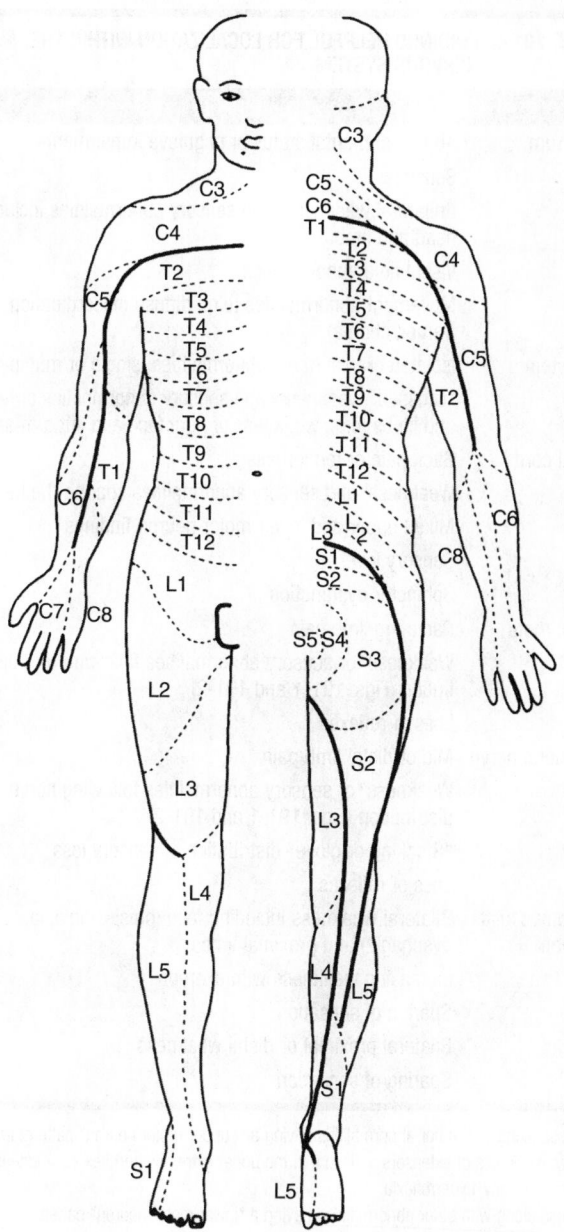

FIGURE 191-2 Distribution of the sensory spinal roots on the surface of the body (dermatomes). *(From D Sinclair:* Mechanisms of Cutaneous Sensation. *Oxford, UK, Oxford University Press, 1981; with permission from Dr. David Sinclair.)*

TABLE 191-3 FINDINGS HELPFUL FOR LOCALIZATION WITHIN THE NERVOUS SYSTEM

	Signs
Cerebrum	Abnormal mental status or cognitive impairment
	Seizures
	Unilateral weakness[a] and sensory abnormalities including head and limbs
	Visual field abnormalities
	Movement abnormalities (e.g., diffuse incoordination, tremor, chorea)
Brainstem	Isolated cranial nerve abnormalities (single or multiple)
	"Crossed" weakness[a] and sensory abnormalities of head and limbs (e.g., weakness of right face and left arm and leg)
Spinal cord	Back pain or tenderness
	Weakness[a] and sensory abnormalities sparing the head
	Mixed upper and lower motor neuron findings
	Sensory level
	Sphincter dysfunction
Spinal roots	Radiating limb pain
	Weakness[b] or sensory abnormalities following root distribution (Figs. 191-1 and 191-2)
	Loss of reflexes
Peripheral nerve	Mid or distal limb pain
	Weakness[b] or sensory abnormalities following nerve distribution (Figs. 191-1 and 191-2)
	"Stocking or glove" distribution of sensory loss
	Loss of reflexes
Neuromuscular junction	Bilateral weakness including face (ptosis, diplopia, dysphagia) and proximal limbs
	Increasing weakness with exertion
	Sparing of sensation
Muscle	Bilateral proximal or distal weakness
	Sparing of sensation

[a]Weakness along with other abnormalities having an "upper motor neuron" pattern, i.e., spasticity, weakness of extensors > flexors in the upper extremity and flexors > extensors in the lower extremity, hyperreflexia.
[b]Weakness along with other abnormalities having a "lower motor neuron" pattern, i.e., flaccidity and hyporeflexia.

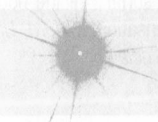

For a more detailed discussion, see Lowenstein DH, Martin JB, Hauser SL: Approach to the Patient With Neurologic Disease, Chap. 367, p. 3233, in HPIM-18

CHAPTER **192**
Neuroimaging

The clinician caring for pts with neurologic symptoms is faced with an expanding number of imaging options. MRI is more sensitive than CT for detection of many lesions affecting the nervous system, particularly those of the spinal cord, cranial nerves, and posterior fossa structures. Diffusion MR, a sequence that detects reduction of microscopic motion of water, is the most sensitive technique for detecting acute ischemic stroke and is useful in the detection of encephalitis, abscesses, and prion diseases. CT, however, can be quickly obtained and is widely available, making it a pragmatic choice for initial evaluation of pts with suspected acute stroke (especially when coupled with CT angiography and perfusion CT), hemorrhage, and intracranial or spinal trauma. CT is also more sensitive than MRI for visualizing fine osseous detail and is indicated in the initial evaluation of conductive hearing loss as well as lesions affecting the skull base and calvarium. MRI and CT-myelography have replaced conventional myelography for evaluation of disease of the spinal cord and canal. An increasing number of interventional neuroradiologic techniques are available including embolization, coiling, and stenting of vascular structures as well as spine interventions such as discography, selective nerve root injection, and epidural injection. Conventional angiography is now reserved for pts in whom small-vessel detail is essential for diagnosis or for whom interventional therapies are planned. Guidelines for initial selection of neuroimaging studies are shown in Table 192-1.

TABLE 192-1 GUIDELINES FOR THE USE OF CT, ULTRASOUND, AND MRI

Condition	Recommended Technique
Hemorrhage	
Acute parenchymal	CT, MR
Subacute/chronic	MRI
Subarachnoid hemorrhage	CT, CTA, lumbar puncture $\rightarrow$ angiography
Aneurysm	Angiography > CTA, MRA
Ischemic infarction	
Hemorrhagic infarction	CT or MRI
Bland infarction	MRI > CT, CTA, angiography
Carotid or vertebral dissection	MRI/MRA
Vertebral basilar insufficiency	CTA, MRI/MRA
Carotid stenosis	CTA > Doppler ultrasound, MRA

(*continued*)

TABLE 192-1 GUIDELINES FOR THE USE OF CT, ULTRASOUND, AND MRI (CONTINUED)

Condition	Recommended Technique
Suspected mass lesion	
Neoplasm, primary or metastatic	MRI + contrast
Infection/abscess	MRI + contrast
Immunosuppressed with focal findings	MRI + contrast
Vascular malformation	MRI ± angiography
White matter disorders	MRI
Demyelinating disease	MRI ± contrast
Dementia	MRI > CT
Trauma	
Acute trauma	CT (noncontrast)
Shear injury/chronic hemorrhage	MRI + gradient echo imaging
Headache/migraine	CT (noncontrast)/MRI
Seizure	
First time, no focal neurologic deficits	?CT as screen ± contrast
Partial complex/refractory	MRI with coronal T2W imaging
Cranial neuropathy	MRI with contrast
Meningeal disease	MRI with contrast
Spine	
Low back pain	
No neurologic deficits	MRI or CT after 4 weeks
With focal deficits	MRI > CT
Spinal stenosis	MRI or CT
Cervical spondylosis	MRI or CT myelography
Infection	MRI + contrast, CT
Myelopathy	MRI + contrast
Arteriovenous malformation	MRI, angiography

Abbreviations: CT, computed tomography; CTA, CT angiography; MRA, MR angiography; MRI, magnetic resonance imaging; T2W, T2-weighted.

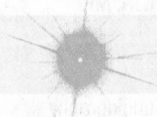

For a more detailed discussion, see Dillon WP: Neuroimaging in Neurologic Disorders, Chap. 368, p. 3240, in HPIM-18.

CHAPTER **193**
Seizures and Epilepsy

A *seizure* is a paroxysmal event due to abnormal excessive or synchronous neuronal activity in the brain. *Epilepsy* is diagnosed when there are recurrent seizures due to a chronic, underlying process.

> **APPROACH TO THE PATIENT** | **Seizure**

Seizure classification: This is essential for diagnosis, therapy, and prognosis (Table 193-1). Seizures are focal or generalized: *focal seizures* originate in networks limited to one cerebral hemisphere, and *generalized seizures* involve networks distributed across both hemispheres. *Focal seizures* can be described as with or without dyscognitive features depending on the presence of cognitive impairment.

Generalized seizures may occur as a primary disorder or result from secondary generalization of a focal seizure. *Tonic-clonic seizures* (grand mal) cause sudden loss of consciousness, loss of postural control, and tonic muscular contraction producing teeth-clenching and rigidity in extension (tonic phase), followed by rhythmic muscular jerking (clonic phase). Tongue-biting and incontinence may occur during the seizure. Recovery of consciousness is typically gradual over many minutes to hours. Headache and confusion are common postictal phenomena. In *absence seizures* (petit mal) there is sudden, brief impairment of consciousness without loss of postural control. Events rarely last longer than 5–10 s but can recur many times per day. Minor motor symptoms are common, while complex automatisms and clonic activity are not. Other types of generalized seizures include tonic, atonic, and myoclonic seizures.

Etiology: Seizure type and age of pt provide important clues to etiology (Table 193-2).

■ CLINICAL EVALUATION

Careful history is essential since diagnosis of seizures and epilepsy is often based solely on clinical grounds. Differential diagnosis (Table 193-3) includes syncope or psychogenic seizures ("pseudoseizures"). General exam includes search for infection, trauma, toxins, systemic illness, neurocutaneous abnormalities, and vascular disease. A number of drugs lower the seizure threshold (Table 193-4). Asymmetries in neurologic exam suggest brain tumor, stroke, trauma, or other focal lesions. An algorithmic approach is shown in Fig. 193-1.

■ LABORATORY EVALUATION

Routine blood studies are indicated to identify the more common metabolic causes of seizures such as abnormalities in electrolytes, glucose, calcium, or magnesium, and hepatic or renal disease. A screen for toxins in blood and

TABLE 193-1   CLASSIFICATION OF SEIZURES

1. Focal seizures

(Can be further described as having motor, sensory, autonomic, cognitive, or other features)

2. Generalized seizures

   a. Absence

     Typical

     Atypical

   b. Tonic clonic

   c. Clonic

   d. Tonic

   e. Atonic

   f. Myoclonic

3. May be focal, generalized, or unclear

   Epileptic spasms

urine should be obtained especially when no clear precipitating factor has been identified. A lumbar puncture is indicated if there is any suspicion of CNS infection such as meningitis or encephalitis; it is mandatory in HIV-infected pts even in the absence of symptoms or signs suggesting infection.

Electroencephalography (EEG)

All pts should be evaluated as soon as possible with an EEG, which measures electrical activity of the brain by recording from electrodes placed on the scalp. The presence of *electrographic seizure activity* during the clinically evident event, i.e., abnormal, repetitive, rhythmic activity having an abrupt onset and termination, clearly establishes the diagnosis. The absence of electrographic seizure activity does not exclude a seizure disorder, however. The EEG is always abnormal during generalized tonic-clonic seizures. Continuous monitoring for prolonged periods may be required to capture the EEG abnormalities. The EEG can show abnormal discharges during the interictal period that support the diagnosis of epilepsy and is useful for classifying seizure disorders, selecting anticonvulsant medications, and determining prognosis.

Brain Imaging

All pts with unexplained new-onset seizures should have a brain imaging study (MRI or CT) to search for an underlying structural abnormality; the only exception may be children who have an unambiguous history and examination suggestive of a benign, generalized seizure disorder such as absence epilepsy. Newer MRI methods have increased the sensitivity for detection of abnormalities of cortical architecture, including hippocampal atrophy associated with mesial temporal sclerosis, and abnormalities of cortical neuronal migration.

TABLE 193-2 CAUSES OF SEIZURES

Neonates (<1 month)	Perinatal hypoxia and ischemia
	Intracranial hemorrhage and trauma
	Acute CNS infection
	Metabolic disturbances (hypoglycemia, hypocalcemia, hypomagnesemia, pyridoxine deficiency)
	Drug withdrawal
	Developmental disorders
	Genetic disorders
Infants and children (>1 month and <12 years)	Febrile seizures
	Genetic disorders (metabolic, degenerative, primary epilepsy syndromes)
	CNS infection
	Developmental disorders
	Trauma
	Idiopathic
Adolescents (12–18 years)	Trauma
	Genetic disorders
	Infection
	Brain tumor
	Illicit drug use
	Idiopathic
Young adults (18–35 years)	Trauma
	Alcohol withdrawal
	Illicit drug use
	Brain tumor
	Idiopathic
Older adults (>35 years)	Cerebrovascular disease
	Brain tumor
	Alcohol withdrawal
	Metabolic disorders (uremia, hepatic failure, electrolyte abnormalities, hypoglycemia, hyperglycemia)
	Alzheimer's disease and other degenerative CNS diseases
	Idiopathic

Abbreviation: CNS, central nervous system.

TABLE 193-3 DIFFERENTIAL DIAGNOSIS OF SEIZURES

Syncope	Transient ischemic attack (TIA)
Vasovagal syncope	Basilar artery TIA
Cardiac arrhythmia	Sleep disorders
Valvular heart disease	Narcolepsy/cataplexy
Cardiac failure	Benign sleep myoclonus
Orthostatic hypotension	Movement disorders
Psychological disorders	Tics
Psychogenic seizure	Nonepileptic myoclonus
Hyperventilation	Paroxysmal choreoathetosis
Panic attack	Special considerations in children
Metabolic disturbances	Breath-holding spells
Alcoholic blackouts	Migraine with recurrent abdominal
Delirium tremens	pain and cyclic vomiting
Hypoglycemia	Benign paroxysmal vertigo
Hypoxia	Apnea
Psychoactive drugs	Night terrors
(e.g., hallucinogens)	Sleepwalking
Migraine	
Confusional migraine	
Basilar migraine	

TREATMENT   Seizures and Epilepsy

- Acute management of seizures
  - Pt should be placed in semiprone position with head to the side to avoid aspiration.
  - Tongue blades or other objects should not be forced between clenched teeth.
  - Oxygen should be given via face mask.
  - Reversible metabolic disorders (e.g., hypoglycemia, hyponatremia, hypocalcemia, drug or alcohol withdrawal) should be promptly corrected.
  - Treatment of status epilepticus is discussed in Chap. 23.
- Longer-term therapy includes treatment of underlying conditions, avoidance of precipitating factors, prophylactic therapy with anti-epileptic medications or surgery, and addressing various psychological and social issues.
- Choice of antiepileptic drug therapy depends on a variety of factors including seizure type, dosing schedule, and potential side effects (Tables 193-5 and 193-6).

TABLE 193-4 DRUGS AND OTHER SUBSTANCES THAT CAN CAUSE SEIZURES

Alkylating agents (e.g., busulfan, chlorambucil)	Psychotropics
	Antidepressants
Antimalarials (chloroquine, mefloquine)	Antipsychotics
Antimicrobials/antivirals	Lithium
β-Lactam and related compounds	Radiographic contrast agents
Quinolones	Theophylline
Acyclovir	Sedative-hypnotic drug withdrawal
Isoniazid	Alcohol
Ganciclovir	Barbiturates (short-acting)
Anesthetics and analgesics	Benzodiazepines (short-acting)
Meperidine	Drugs of abuse
Tramadol	Amphetamine
Local anesthetics	Cocaine
Dietary supplements	Phencyclidine
Ephedra (ma huang)	Methylphenidate
Gingko	Flumazenil[a]
Immunomodulatory drugs	
Cyclosporine	
Muromonab-(CD3)	
Tacrolimus	
Interferons	

[a]In benzodiazepine-dependent pts.

- Therapeutic goal is complete cessation of seizures without side effects using a single drug (monotherapy) and a dosing schedule that is easy for the pt to follow.
    - If ineffective, medication should be increased to maximal tolerated dose based primarily on clinical response rather than serum levels.
    - If still unsuccessful, a second drug should be added, and when control is obtained, the first drug can be slowly tapered. Some pts will require polytherapy with two or more drugs, although monotherapy should be the goal.
    - Pts with certain epilepsy syndromes (e.g., temporal lobe epilepsy) are often refractory to medical therapy and benefit from surgical excision of the seizure focus.

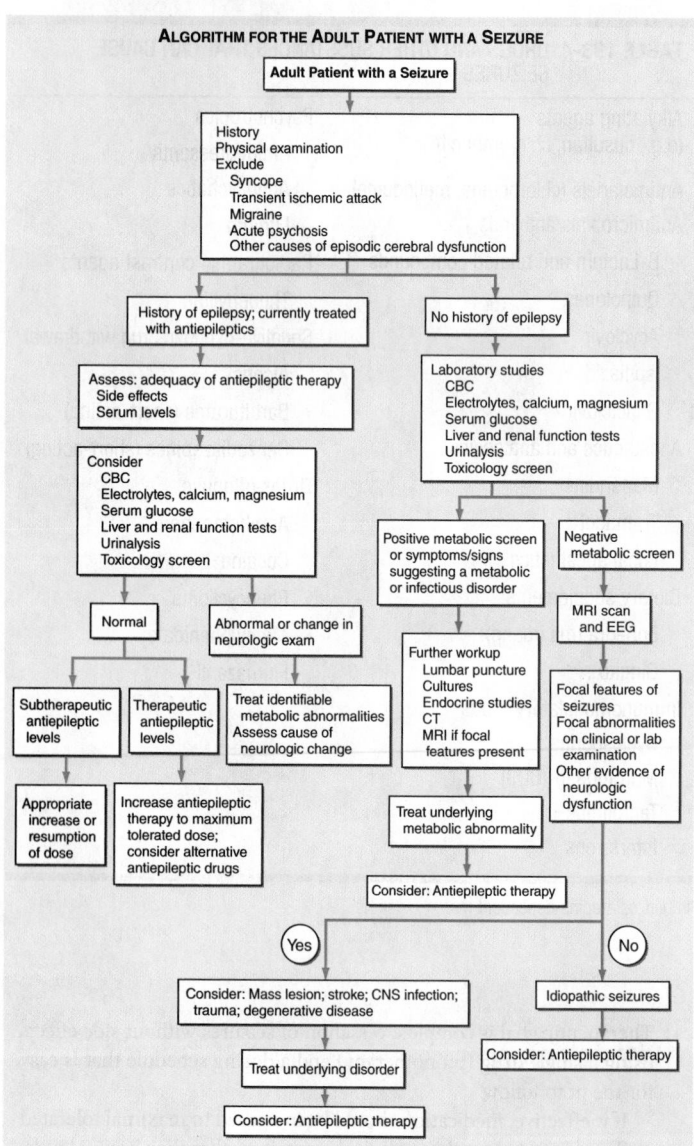

FIGURE 193-1 Evaluation of the adult pt with a seizure. CBC, complete blood count; CNS, central nervous system; CT, computed tomography; EEG, electroencephalogram; MRI, magnetic resonance imaging.

TABLE 193-5 DOSAGE AND ADVERSE EFFECTS OF COMMONLY USED ANTIEPILEPTIC DRUGS

Generic Name	Trade Name	Principal Uses	Typical Dose; Dose Interval	Half-Life	Therapeutic Range	Adverse Effects — Neurologic	Adverse Effects — Systemic	Drug Interactions
Phenytoin (diphenylhydantoin)	Dilantin	Tonic-clonic Focal-onset	300–400 mg/d (3–6 mg/kg, adult; 4–8 mg/kg, child); qd-bid	24 h (wide variation, dose-dependent)	10–20 μg/mL	Dizziness Diplopia Ataxia Incoordination Confusion	Gum hyperplasia Lymphadenopathy Hirsutism Osteomalacia Facial coarsening Skin rash	Level increased by isoniazid, sulfonamides, fluoxetine Level decreased by enzyme-inducing drugs[a] Altered folate metabolism
Carbamazepine	Tegretol[b] Carbatrol	Tonic-clonic Focal-onset	600–1800 mg/d (15–35 mg/kg, child); bid-qid	10–17 h	6–12 μg/mL	Ataxia Dizziness Diplopia Vertigo	Aplastic anemia Leukopenia Gastrointestinal irritation Hepatotoxicity Hyponatremia	Level decreased by enzyme-inducing drugs[a] Level increased by erythromycin, propoxyphene, isoniazid, cimetidine, fluoxetine

(continued)

TABLE 193-5 DOSAGE AND ADVERSE EFFECTS OF COMMONLY USED ANTIEPILEPTIC DRUGS (CONTINUED)

Generic Name	Trade Name	Principal Uses	Typical Dose; Dose Interval	Half-Life	Therapeutic Range	Adverse Effects		Drug Interactions
						Neurologic	Systemic	
Valproic acid	Depakene	Tonic-clonic	750–2000 mg/d (20–60 mg/kg); bid-qid	15 h	50–125 µg/mL	Ataxia	Hepatotoxicity	Level decreased by enzyme-inducing drugs[a]
	Depakote[b]	Absence				Sedation	Thrombocytopenia	
		Atypical absence				Tremor	Gastrointestinal irritation	
		Myoclonic					Weight gain	
		Focal-onset					Transient alopecia	
		Atonic					Hyperammonemia	
Lamotrigine	Lamictal[b]	Focal-onset	150–500 mg/d; bid	25 h	Not established	Dizziness	Skin rash	Level decreased by enzyme-inducing drugs[a] and oral contraceptives
		Tonic-clonic		14 h (with enzyme-inducers) 59 h (with valproic acid)		Diplopia	Stevens-Johnson syndrome	
		Atypical absence				Sedation		Level increased by valproic acid
		Myoclonic				Ataxia		
		Lennox-Gastaut syndrome				Headache		

Drug	Trade name	Seizure type	Dose	Half-life	Therapeutic level	Neurologic side effects	Systemic side effects	Drug interactions
Ethosuximide	Zarontin	Absence	750–1250 mg/d (20–40 mg/kg); qd-bid	60 h, adult; 30 h, child	40–100 µg/mL	Ataxia; Lethargy; Headache	Gastrointestinal irritation; Skin rash; Bone marrow suppression	Level decreased by enzyme-inducing drugs[a]; Level increased by valproic acid
Gabapentin	Neurontin	Focal-onset	900–2400 mg/d; tid-qid	5–9 h	Not established	Sedation; Dizziness; Ataxia; Fatigue	Gastrointestinal irritation; Weight gain; Edema	No known significant interactions
Topiramate	Topamax	Focal-onset; Tonic-clonic; Lennox-Gastaut syndrome	200–400 mg/d; bid	20–30 h	Not established	Psychomotor slowing; Sedation; Speech or language problems; Fatigue; Paresthesias	Renal stones (avoid use with other carbonic anhydrase inhibitors); Glaucoma; Weight loss; Hypohidrosis	Level decreased by enzyme-inducing drugs[a]

(continued)

TABLE 193-5 DOSAGE AND ADVERSE EFFECTS OF COMMONLY USED ANTIEPILEPTIC DRUGS (CONTINUED)

Generic Name	Trade Name	Principal Uses	Typical Dose; Dose Interval	Half-Life	Therapeutic Range	Adverse Effects Neurologic	Adverse Effects Systemic	Drug Interactions
Tiagabine	Gabitril	Focal-onset	32–56 mg/d; bid-qid	7–9 h	Not established	Confusion Sedation Depression Dizziness Speech or language problems Paresthesias Psychosis	Gastrointestinal irritation	Level decreased by enzyme-inducing drugs[a]
Phenobarbital	Luminal	Tonic-clonic Focal-onset	60–180 mg/d; qd	90 h	10–40 μg/mL	Sedation Ataxia Confusion Dizziness Decreased libido Depression	Skin rash	Level increased by valproic acid, phenytoin

Drug	Brand	Seizure type	Dosage	Half-life	Therapeutic level	Side effects		Drug interactions
Primidone	Mysoline	Tonic-clonic Focal-onset	750–1000 mg/d; bid-tid	Primidone, 8–15 h Phenobarbital, 90 h	Primidone, 4–12 µg/mL Phenobarbital, 10–40 µg/mL	Same as phenobarbital		Level increased by valproic acid, phenytoin
Clonazepam	Klonopin	Absence Atypical absence Myoclonic	1–12 mg/d; qd-tid	24–48 h	10–70 ng/mL	Ataxia Sedation Lethargy	Anorexia	Level decreased by enzyme-inducing drugs[a]
Felbamate	Felbatol	Focal-onset Lennox-Gastaut syndrome Tonic-clonic	2400–3600 mg/d, tid-qid	16–22 h	Not established	Insomnia Dizziness Sedation Headache	Aplastic anemia Hepatic failure Weight loss Gastrointestinal irritation	Increases phenytoin, valproic acid, active carbamazepine metabolite
Levetiracetam	Keppra[b]	Focal-onset	1000–3000 mg/d; qd-bid	6–8 h	Not established	Sedation Fatigue Incoordination Mood changes	Anemia Leukopenia	No known significant interactions

(continued)

1209

TABLE 193-5 DOSAGE AND ADVERSE EFFECTS OF COMMONLY USED ANTIEPILEPTIC DRUGS (CONTINUED)

Generic Name	Trade Name	Principal Uses	Typical Dose; Dose Interval	Half-Life	Therapeutic Range	Adverse Effects		Drug Interactions
						Neurologic	Systemic	
Zonisamide	Zonegran	Focal-onset	200–400 mg/d; qd-bid	50–68 h	Not established	Sedation	Anorexia	Level decreased by enzyme-inducing drugs[a]
		Tonic-clonic				Dizziness	Renal stones	
						Confusion	Hypohidrosis	
						Headache		
						Psychosis		
Oxcarbazepine	Trileptal	Focal-onset	900–2400 mg/d (30–45 mg/kg, child); bid	10–17 h (for active metabolite)	Not established	Fatigue	See carbamazepine	Level decreased by enzyme-inducing drugs[a]
		Tonic-clonic				Ataxia		May increase phenytoin
						Dizziness		
						Diplopia		
						Vertigo		
						Headache		

						Dizziness	GI irritation	Level decreased by enzyme-inducing drugs[a]
Lacosamide	Vimpat	Focal-onset	200–400 mg/d; bid	13 h	Not established	Ataxia Diplopia Vertigo	Cardiac conduction (PR interval prolongation)	
						Sedation	GI irritation	Level decreased by enzyme-inducing drugs[a]
Rufinamide	Banzel	Lennox-Gastaut syndrome	3200 mg/d (45 mg/kg, child); bid	6–10 h	Not established	Fatigue Dizziness Ataxia Headache Diplopia	Leukopenia Cardiac conduction (QT interval prolongation)	Level increased by valproic acid May increase phenytoin

[a]Phenytoin, carbamazepine, phenobarbital.
[b]Extended-release product available.

1211

TABLE 193-6 SELECTION OF ANTIEPILEPTIC DRUGS

Generalized-onset Tonic-Clonic	Focal	Typical Absence	Atypical Absence, Myoclonic, Atonic
First-line			
Valproic acid	Lamotrigine	Valproic acid	Valproic acid
Lamotrigine	Carbamazepine	Ethosuximide	Lamotrigine
Topiramate	Oxcarbazepine		Topiramate
	Phenytoin		
	Levetiracetam		
Alternatives			
Zonisamide[a]	Topiramate	Lamotrigine	Clonazepam
Phenytoin	Zonisamide[a]	Clonazepam	Felbamate
Carbamazepine	Valproic acid		
Oxcarbazepine	Tiagabine[a]		
Phenobarbital	Gabapentin[a]		
Primidone	Lacosamide[a]		
Felbamate	Phenobarbital		
	Primidone		
	Felbamate		

[a]As adjunctive therapy.

For a more detailed discussion, see Lowenstein DH: Seizures and Epilepsy, Chap. 369, p. 3251, in HPIM-18.

CHAPTER **194**
Dementia

Dementia

Dementia is an acquired deterioration in cognitive ability that impairs the successful performance of activities of daily living. Memory is the most common cognitive ability lost with dementia; 10% of persons over age 70 and 20–40% of individuals over age 85 have clinically identifiable memory loss. Other mental faculties are also affected in dementia, such as language, visuospatial ability, calculation, judgment, and problem solving. Neuropsychiatric and social deficits develop in many dementia syndromes, resulting in depression, withdrawal, hallucinations, delusions, agitation, insomnia, and disinhibition. Dementia is usually chronic and progressive.

Diagnosis

The mini-mental status examination (MMSE) is a useful screening test for dementia (Table 191-1). A score of <24 points (out of 30) indicates a need for more detailed cognitive and physical assessment. In some pts with early cognitive disorders, the MMSE may be normal and more detailed neuropsychological testing will be required.

| APPROACH TO THE PATIENT | Dementia |

Differential Diagnosis: Dementia has many causes (Table 194-1). It is essential to exclude treatable etiologies; the most common potentially reversible diagnoses are depression, hydrocephalus, and alcohol dependence. The major degenerative dementias can usually be distinguished by distinctive symptoms, signs, and neuroimaging features (Table 194-2).

History: A subacute onset of confusion may represent delirium and should trigger the search for intoxication, infection, or metabolic derangement (Chap. 17). An elderly person with slowly progressive memory loss over several years is likely to have Alzheimer's disease (AD). A change in personality, disinhibition, gain of weight, or compulsive eating suggests frontotemporal dementia (FTD), not AD; apathy, loss of executive function, progressive abnormalities in speech, or relative sparing of memory or visuospatial abilities also suggests FTD. Dementia with Lewy bodies (DLB) is suggested by the early presence of visual hallucinations, parkinsonism, tendency to delirium, sensitivity to psychoactive medications, or an REM behavior disorder (RBD, the loss of skeletal muscle paralysis during dreaming).

A history of stroke suggests vascular dementia, which may also occur with hypertension, atrial fibrillation, peripheral vascular disease, and diabetes. Rapid progression of dementia with myoclonus suggests a prion disease such as Creutzfeldt-Jakob disease (CJD). Gait disturbance is prominent with vascular dementia, Parkinson's disease, DLB, or normal-pressure hydrocephalus. Multiple sex partners or IV drug use should trigger search for an infection, especially HIV or syphilis. A history of head trauma could indicate chronic subdural hematoma, dementia pugilistica, or normal-pressure hydrocephalus. Alcoholism may suggest malnutrition and thiamine deficiency. A history of gastric surgery may result in loss of intrinsic factor and vitamin B$_{12}$ deficiency. A careful review of medications, especially of sedatives and tranquilizers, may raise the issue of drug intoxication. A family history of dementia is found in Huntington's disease and in familial forms of AD, FTD, DLB, or prion disorders. Insomnia or weight loss is often seen with depression-related cognitive impairments, which can also be caused by the recent death of a loved one.

Examination: It is essential to document the dementia, look for other signs of nervous system involvement, and search for clues of a systemic disease that might be responsible for the cognitive disorder. AD does not affect motor systems until late in the course. In contrast, FTD pts often develop axial rigidity, supranuclear gaze palsy, or features of

TABLE 194-1 DIFFERENTIAL DIAGNOSIS OF DEMENTIA

Most Common Causes of Dementia	
Alzheimer's disease	Alcoholism[a]
Vascular dementia	Parkinson's disease
Multi-infarct	Drug/medication intoxication[a]
Diffuse white matter disease (Binswanger's)	

Less Common Causes of Dementia	
Vitamin deficiencies	Toxic disorders
Thiamine (B$_1$): Wernicke's encephalopathy[a]	Drug, medication, and narcotic poisoning[a]
B$_{12}$ (subacute combined degeneration)[a]	Heavy metal intoxication[a]
Nicotinic acid (pellagra)[a]	Dialysis dementia (aluminum)
Endocrine and other organ failure	Organic toxins
Hypothyroidism[a]	Psychiatric
Adrenal insufficiency and Cushing's syndrome[a]	Depression (pseudodementia)[a]
Hypo- and hyperparathyroidism[a]	Schizophrenia[a]
Renal failure[a]	Conversion reaction[a]
Liver failure[a]	Degenerative disorders
Pulmonary failure[a]	Huntington's disease
Chronic infections	Dementia with Lewy bodies
HIV	Progressive supranuclear palsy
Neurosyphilis[a]	Multisystem atrophy
Papovavirus (JC virus) (progressive multifocal leukoencephalopathy)	Hereditary ataxias (some forms)
	Motor neuron disease [amyotrophic lateral sclerosis (ALS); some forms]
Tuberculosis, fungal, and protozoal[a]	Frontotemporal dementia
Whipple's disease[a]	Corticobasal degeneration
Head trauma and diffuse brain damage	Multiple sclerosis
Dementia pugilistica	Adult Down syndrome with Alzheimer's disease
Chronic subdural hematoma[a]	ALS–Parkinson's–dementia complex of Guam
Postanoxia	
Postencephalitis	Prion (Creutzfeldt-Jakob and Gerstmann-Sträussler-Scheinker diseases)
Normal-pressure hydrocephalus[a]	Miscellaneous
Neoplastic	Sarcoidosis[a]
Primary brain tumor[a]	Vasculitis[a]
	CADASIL, etc.
	Acute intermittent porphyria[a]

TABLE 194-1 DIFFERENTIAL DIAGNOSIS OF DEMENTIA (CONTINUED)

Less Common Causes of Dementia	
Metastatic brain tumor[a]	Recurrent nonconvulsive seizures[a]
Paraneoplastic limbic encephalitis	Additional conditions in children or adolescents
	Pantothenate kinase–associated neurodegeneration
	Subacute sclerosing panencephalitis
	Metabolic disorders (e.g., Wilson's and Leigh's diseases, leukodystrophies, lipid storage diseases, mitochondrial mutations)

[a]Potentially reversible dementia.
Abbreviation: CADASIL, Cerebral autosomal dominant arteriopathy with subcortical infarcts and leukoencephalopathy.

amyotrophic lateral sclerosis. In DLB, initial symptoms may be the new onset of a parkinsonian syndrome (resting tremor, cogwheel rigidity, bradykinesia, and festinating gait). Unexplained falls, axial rigidity, dysphagia, and gaze deficits suggest progressive supranuclear palsy (PSP).

Focal neurologic deficits may occur in vascular dementia or brain tumor. Dementia with a myelopathy and peripheral neuropathy suggests vitamin B_{12} deficiency. A peripheral neuropathy could also indicate an underlying vitamin deficiency or heavy metal intoxication. Dry cool skin, hair loss, and bradycardia suggest hypothyroidism. Confusion associated with repetitive stereotyped movements may indicate ongoing seizure activity. Hearing impairment or visual loss may produce confusion and disorientation misinterpreted as dementia. Such sensory deficits are common in the elderly.

Choice of Diagnostic Studies: A reversible or treatable cause must not be missed, yet no single etiology is common; thus a screen must employ multiple tests, each of which has a low yield. Table 194-3 lists most screening tests for dementia. Guidelines recommend the routine measurement of thyroid function, a vitamin B_{12} level, and a neuroimaging study (CT or MRI). Lumbar puncture need not be done routinely but is indicated if infection is a consideration; CSF levels of tau protein and amyloid β_{42} show differing patterns with the various dementias although their sensitivity and specificity are not yet sufficiently high to warrant routine use. An EEG is rarely helpful except to suggest a prion disease or an underlying nonconvulsive seizure disorder. The role of functional-metabolic imaging in the diagnosis of dementia is still under study; amyloid imaging has recently shown promise for the diagnosis of AD. Brain biopsy is not advised except to diagnose vasculitis, potentially treatable neoplasms, unusual infections, or systemic disorders such as sarcoid.

TABLE 194-2 CLINICAL DIFFERENTIATION OF THE MAJOR DEMENTIAS

Disease	First Symptom	Mental Status	Neuropsychiatry	Neurology	Imaging
AD	Memory loss	Episodic memory loss	Initially normal	Initially normal	Entorhinal cortex and hippocampal atrophy
FTD	Apathy; poor judgment/insight, speech/language; hyperorality	Frontal/executive, language; spares drawing	Apathy, disinhibition, hyperorality, euphoria, depression	May have vertical gaze palsy, axial rigidity, dystonia, alien hand, or MND	Frontal, insular, and/or temporal atrophy; spares posterior parietal lobe
DLB	Visual hallucinations, REM sleep disorder, delirium, Capgras syndrome, parkinsonism	Drawing and frontal/executive; spares memory; delirium prone	Visual hallucinations, depression, sleep disorder, delusions	Parkinsonism	Posterior parietal atrophy; hippocampi larger than in AD
CJD	Dementia, mood, anxiety, movement disorders	Variable, frontal/executive, focal cortical, memory	Depression, anxiety	Myoclonus, rigidity, parkinsonism	Cortical ribboning and basal ganglia or thalamus hyperintensity on diffusion/FLAIR MRI
Vascular	Often but not always sudden; variable; apathy, falls, focal weakness	Frontal/executive, cognitive slowing; can spare memory	Apathy, delusions, anxiety	Usually motor slowing, spasticity; can be normal	Cortical and/or subcortical infarctions, confluent white matter disease

Abbreviations: AD, Alzheimer's disease; CBD, cortical basal degeneration; CJD, Creutzfeldt-Jakob disease; DLB, dementia with Lewy bodies; FTD, frontotemporal dementia; MND, motor neuron disease; PSP, progressive supranuclear palsy.

ALZHEIMER'S DISEASE

Most common cause of dementia; 10% of all persons over age 70 have significant memory loss, and in more than half the cause is AD. Cost is >$50 billion/year.

TABLE 194-3 EVALUATION OF THE PATIENT WITH DEMENTIA

Routine Evaluation	Optional Focused Tests	Occasionally Helpful Tests
History	Psychometric testing	EEG
Physical examination	Chest x-ray	Parathyroid function
Laboratory tests	Lumbar puncture	Adrenal function
Thyroid function (TSH)	Liver function	Urine heavy metals
	Renal function	RBC sedimentation rate
Vitamin B_{12}	Urine toxin screen	Angiogram
Complete blood count	HIV	Brain biopsy
Electrolytes	Apolipoprotein E	SPECT
CT/MRI	RPR or VDRL	PET

Diagnostic Categories		

Reversible causes	Irreversible/ degenerative dementias	Psychiatric disorders
Examples	Examples	Depression
Hypothyroidism	Alzheimer's	Schizophrenia
Thiamine deficiency	Frontotemporal dementia	Conversion reaction
Vitamin B_{12} deficiency	Huntington's	
Normal-pressure hydrocephalus	Dementia with Lewy bodies	
Subdural hematoma	Vascular	
Chronic infection	Leukoencephalopathies	
Brain tumor	Parkinson's	
Drug intoxication		

Associated Treatable Conditions	
Depression	Agitation
Seizures	Caregiver "burnout"
Insomnia	Drug side effects

Abbreviations: PET, positron emission tomography; RPR, rapid plasma reagin (test); SPECT, single-photon emission CT; VDRL, Venereal Disease Research Laboratory (test for syphilis).

Clinical Manifestations

Cognitive changes follow a characteristic pattern beginning with memory impairment and spreading to language and visuospatial deficits. Memory loss is often not recognized initially, in part due to preservation of social graces until later phases; impaired activities of daily living (keeping track of finances, appointments) draw attention of friends/family. Once the memory loss becomes noticeable to the pt and spouse and falls 1.5 standard deviations below normal on standardized memory tests, the term *mild cognitive impairment* (MCI) is applied; Roughly 12% per year will progress to AD over 4 years. Disorientation, poor judgment, poor concentration, aphasia, and apraxia are increasingly evident as the disease progresses. Pts may be frustrated or unaware of deficit. In end-stage AD, pts become rigid, mute, incontinent, and bedridden. Help may be needed with the simplest tasks, such as eating, dressing, and toilet function. Often, death results from malnutrition, secondary infections, pulmonary emboli, heart disease, or, most commonly, aspiration. Typical duration is 8–10 years, but the course can range from 1 to 25 years.

Pathogenesis

Risk factors for AD are old age, positive family history. Pathology: neuritic plaques composed in part of Aβ amyloid, derived from amyloid precursor protein (APP); neurofibrillary tangles composed of abnormally phosphorylated tau protein. The apolipoprotein E (apo E) ε4 allele accelerates age of onset of AD and is associated with sporadic and late-onset familial cases. Apo E testing is not indicated as a predictive test. Rare genetic causes of AD are Down syndrome and mutations in APP, presenilin I, and presenilin II genes; all appear to increase production of Aβ amyloid. Genetic testing available for presenilin mutations; likely to be revealing only in early-age-of-onset familial AD.

TREATMENT **Alzheimer's Disease**

- AD cannot be cured, and no highly effective drug exists. The focus is on judicious use of cholinesterase inhibitor drugs; symptomatic management of behavioral problems; and building rapport with the pt, family members, and other caregivers.
- Donepezil, rivastigmine, galantamine, tacrine (tetrahydroaminoacridine), and memantine are approved by the FDA for treatment of AD. Due to hepatotoxicity, tacrine is no longer used. With the exception of memantine, their action is inhibition of cholinesterase, with a resulting increase in cerebral levels of acetylcholine. Memantine appears to act by blocking overexcited *N*-methyl-D-aspartate (NMDA) channels.
  - These compounds are only modestly efficacious and offer little or no benefit in the late stages of AD; they are associated with improved caregiver ratings of pts' functioning and with an apparent decreased rate of decline in cognitive test scores over periods of up to 3 years.
  - Donepezil (Aricept), 5–10 mg/d PO, has the advantages of few side effects and single daily dosage.
  - Dosing of memantine begins at 5 mg/d with gradual increases (over 1 month) to 10 mg twice a day.

- There is no role for hormone replacement therapy in prevention of AD in women, and no benefit has been found in the treatment of established AD with estrogen.
- Randomized trials of *Ginkgo biloba* have found it to be ineffective. Prospective studies are examining the role of NSAIDs and statin medications as well as lowering of serum homocysteine in order to slow the progression to dementia.
- Other experimental approaches target amyloid either through diminishing its production or promoting clearance by passive immunization with monoclonal antibodies.
- Depression, common in early stages of AD, may respond to antidepressants or cholinesterase inhibitors. Selective serotonin reuptake inhibitors (SSRIs) are often used due to their low anticholinergic side effects. Management of behavioral problems in conjunction with family and caregivers is essential. Mild sedation may help insomnia.
- Control of agitation usually involves low doses of atypical antipsychotic medications, but recent trials have questioned the efficacy of this approach; in addition, all of the antipsychotics carry a black box warning in the elderly, increasing the risk of cardiovascular complications and death, and therefore should be used with caution.
- Notebooks and posted daily reminders can function as memory aids in early stages. Kitchens, bathrooms, and bedrooms need evaluation for safety. Pts must eventually stop driving. Caregiver burnout is common; nursing home placement may be necessary. Local and national support groups (Alzheimer's Disease and Related Disorders Association) are valuable resources.

OTHER CAUSES OF DEMENTIA

Vascular Dementia

Typically follows a pattern of either multiple strokelike episodes (multi-infarct dementia) or diffuse white matter disease (leukoaraiosis, subcortical arteriosclerotic encephalopathy, Binswanger's disease) (Fig. 194-1). Unlike AD, focal neurologic signs (e.g., hemiparesis) may be apparent at presentation. Treatment focuses on underlying causes of atherosclerosis.

Frontotemporal Dementia

Often begins in the fifth to seventh decades; in this age group it is nearly as prevalent as AD. Unlike in AD, behavioral symptoms predominate in the early stages of FTD. Extremely heterogeneous; presents with combinations of disinhibition, dementia, apraxia, parkinsonism, and motor neuron disease. May be sporadic or inherited; some familial cases due to mutations of tau or progranulin genes. Treatment is symptomatic; no therapies known to slow progression or improve cognitive symptoms. Many of the behaviors that accompany FTD such as depression, hyperorality, compulsions, and irritability may be helped with SSRIs.

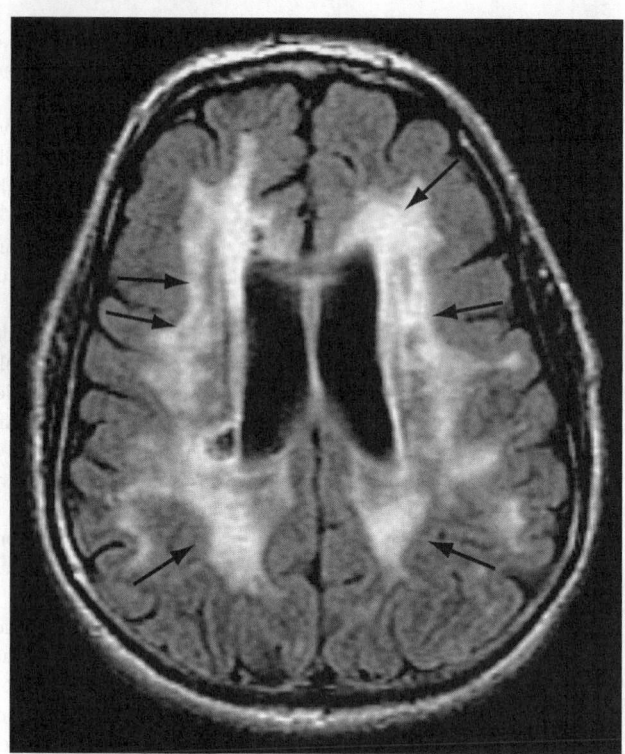

FIGURE 194-1 Diffuse white matter disease (Binswanger's disease). Axial T2-weighted MR image through the lateral ventricles reveals multiple areas of abnormal high signal intensity involving the periventricular white matter as well as the corona radiata and lentiform nuclei (arrows). While seen in some individuals with normal cognition, this appearance is more pronounced in pts with dementia of a vascular etiology.

Dementia with Lewy Bodies

Characterized by visual hallucinations, parkinsonism, fluctuating alertness, and falls. Dementia can precede or follow the appearance of parkinsonism; when it occurs after an established diagnosis of Parkinson's disease, many use the term Parkinson's disease dementia (PDD). Lewy bodies are intraneuronal cytoplasmic inclusions. Anticholinesterase compounds often provide significant benefit due to a severe cholinergic deficit in DLB. Exercise programs to maximize motor function, antidepressants to treat depressive syndromes, and possibly antipsychotics in low doses to alleviate psychosis may also be helpful.

Normal-Pressure Hydrocephalus (NPH)

Uncommon; presents as a gait disorder (ataxic or apractic), dementia, and urinary incontinence. Gait improves in some pts following ventricular shunting; dementia and incontinence do not improve. The diagnosis is difficult to make, and the clinical picture may overlap with several other causes of dementia including AD; historically many individuals treated for NPH have suffered from other dementias.

Huntington's Disease

Chorea, behavioral disturbance, and a frontal/executive disorder (Chap. 59). Typical onset fourth to fifth decade but can present at almost any age. Autosomal dominant inheritance due to expanded trinucleotide repeat in gene encoding the protein huntingtin. Diagnosis confirmed with genetic testing coupled with genetic counseling. Symptomatic treatment of movements and behaviors; SSRIs may help depression.

Creutzfeldt-Jakob Disease (CJD)

Prion disorders such as CJD are rare (~1 per million). CJD is a rapidly progressive disorder with dementia, focal cortical signs, rigidity, and myoclonus; death in <1 year from first symptom. The markedly abnormal periodic discharges on EEG and cortical and basal ganglia abnormalities on diffusion-weighted MR are unique diagnostic features. No proven treatments exist.

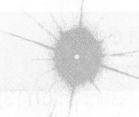

For a more detailed discussion, see Seeley WW, Miller BL: Dementia, Chap. 371, p. 3300, in HPIM-18.

CHAPTER **195**
Parkinson's Disease

■ CLINICAL FEATURES

Parkinsonism is a general term used to define a symptom complex manifest by bradykinesia (slowness of voluntary movements) with rigidity and/or tremor; it has a wide differential diagnosis (Table 195-1). *Parkinson's disease* (PD) is idiopathic parkinsonism without evidence of more widespread neurologic involvement. PD afflicts >1 million individuals in the United States. Peak age of onset in the 60s; course progressive over 10–25 years. Tremor ("pill rolling" of hands) at rest (4–6 Hz). Presentation with tremor confined to one limb or one side of body is common. Other findings: rigidity ("cogwheeling"—increased ratchet-like resistance to passive limb movements), bradykinesia, fixed expressionless face (facial masking) with reduced frequency of blinking, hypophonic voice, drooling, impaired rapid alternating movements, micrographia (small handwriting), reduced arm swing, and flexed "stooped" posture with walking, shuffling gait, difficulty initiating or stopping walking, en-bloc turning (multiple small steps required to turn), retropulsion

TABLE 195-1 DIFFERENTIAL DIAGNOSIS OF PARKINSONISM

Parkinson's Disease	Atypical Parkinsonisms	Secondary Parkinsonism	Other Neurodegenerative Disorders
Genetic	Multiple-system atrophy	Drug-induced	Wilson's disease
Sporadic	Cerebellar type (MSA-c)	Tumor	Huntington's disease
Dementia with Lewy bodies	Parkinson type (MSA-p)	Infection	Neurodegeneration with brain iron accumulation
	Progressive supra-nuclear palsy	Vascular	
	Corticobasal ganglionic degeneration	Normal-pressure hydrocephalus	SCA 3 (spinocerebellar ataxia)
		Trauma	Fragile X–associated ataxia-tremor-parkinsonism
	Frontotemporal dementia	Liver failure	
		Toxins (e.g., carbon monoxide, manganese, MPTP, cyanide, hexane, methanol, carbon disulfide)	Prion disease
			Dystonia-parkinsonism (DYT3)
			Alzheimer's disease with parkinsonism

Abbreviation: MPTP, 1-methyl-4-phenyl-1,2,3,6-tetrahydropyridine.

(tendency to fall backwards). Nonmotor aspects of PD include depression and anxiety, cognitive impairment, sleep disturbances, sensation of inner restlessness, loss of smell (*anosmia*), and disturbances of autonomic function. Normal muscular strength, deep tendon reflexes, and sensory exam. Diagnosis based on history and examination; neuroimaging, EEG, and CSF studies usually normal for age.

■ **PATHOPHYSIOLOGY**

Most PD cases occur sporadically and are of unknown cause. Degeneration of pigmented pars compacta neurons of the substantia nigra in the midbrain resulting in lack of dopaminergic input to striatum; accumulation of cytoplasmic intraneural inclusion granules (Lewy bodies). Cause of cell death is unknown, but it may result from generation of free radicals and oxidative stress; no environmental factor has yet been conclusively determined to cause PD. Rare genetic forms of parkinsonism exist (~5% of cases); most common are mutations in α-synuclein or parkin genes. Early age of onset suggests a possible genetic cause of PD, although one genetic form (*LLRK2*) causes PD in the same age range as sporadic PD and may be responsible for as much as 1% of all sporadic cases. Mutations in the glucocerebrosidase (GBA) gene are also associated with an increased risk of idiopathic PD.

■ DIFFERENTIAL DIAGNOSIS

Atypical parkinsonism refers to a group of neurodegenerative conditions that usually are associated with more widespread neurodegeneration than is found in PD including multiple-system atrophy (MSA), progressive supranuclear palsy (PSP), and corticobasal ganglionic degeneration (CBGD). Secondary parkinsonism can be associated with drugs (neuroleptics as well as GI medications such as metoclopramide, all of which block dopamine), infection, or exposure to toxins such as carbon monoxide or manganese. Some features to suggest that parkinsonism might be due to a condition other than PD are shown in Table 195-2.

TABLE 195-2 FEATURES SUGGESTING DIAGNOSIS OTHER THAN PD

Symptoms/Signs	Alternate Diagnosis to Consider
History	
Early speech and gait impairment	Atypical parkinsonism
Exposure to neuroleptics	Drug-induced parkinsonism
Onset prior to age 40	Genetic form of PD
Liver disease	Wilson's disease, non-Wilsonian hepatolenticular degeneration
Early hallucinations	Dementia with Lewy bodies
Diplopia	PSP
Poor or no response to an adequate trial of levodopa	Atypical or secondary parkinsonism
Physical Exam	
Dementia as first symptom	Dementia with Lewy bodies
Prominent orthostatic hypotension	MSA-p
Prominent cerebellar signs	MSA-c
Impairment of down gaze	PSP
High-frequency (8–10 Hz) symmetric postural tremor with a prominent kinetic component	Essential tremor

Abbreviations: MSA-c, multiple-system atrophy–cerebellar type; MSA-p, multiple-system atrophy–Parkinson type; PSP, progressive supranuclear palsy.

TREATMENT   Parkinson's Disease (see Fig. 195-1, Table 195-3**)**

Goals are to maintain function and avoid drug-induced complications; start therapy when symptoms interfere with quality of life. Bradykinesia, tremor, rigidity, and abnormal posture respond early in illness; cognitive symptoms, hypophonia, autonomic dysfunction, and balance difficulties respond poorly.

LEVODOPA

- Routinely administered in combination with a decarboxylase inhibitor to prevent its peripheral metabolism to dopamine and the development of nausea and vomiting. In the United States, levodopa is combined with carbidopa (Sinemet).
- Levodopa is also available in controlled-release formulations and in combination (e.g., as Stalevo) with a COMT inhibitor (see below).
- Levodopa remains the most effective symptomatic treatment for PD, and lack of response to the medication despite an adequate trial should cause the diagnosis to be questioned.
- Side effects include nausea, vomiting, and orthostatic hypotension that can be avoided by gradual titration.
- Levodopa-induced motor complications consist of fluctuations in motor response and involuntary movements known as dyskinesias.
- When pts initially take the drug, the benefits are long-lasting; with continued treatment, the duration of benefit following an individual dose becomes progressively shorter ("wearing-off effect").

DOPAMINE AGONISTS

- A diverse group of drugs that act directly on dopamine receptors. Second-generation non-ergot dopamine agonists are commonly used (e.g., pramipexole, ropinirole, rotigotine).
- Compared with levodopa, dopamine agonists are longer acting and thus provide a more uniform stimulation of dopamine receptors; less prone to induce dyskinesias compared with levodopa.
- They are effective as monotherapeutic agents and as adjuncts to carbidopa/levodopa therapy.
- Side effects include nausea, vomiting, and postural hypotension. Hallucinations and cognitive impairment are more common than with levodopa, so caution is urged in those older than 70.
- Recently, it has become recognized that dopamine agonists are associated with impulse-control disorders including pathologic gambling, hypersexuality, and compulsive eating and shopping.

MAO-B INHIBITORS

- Block central dopamine metabolism and increase synaptic concentrations of the neurotransmitter; generally safe and well tolerated.
- Provide modest antiparkinson benefits when used as monotherapy in early disease.
- Recent work has examined whether these drugs could have a disease-modifying effect; however, long-term significance is uncertain.

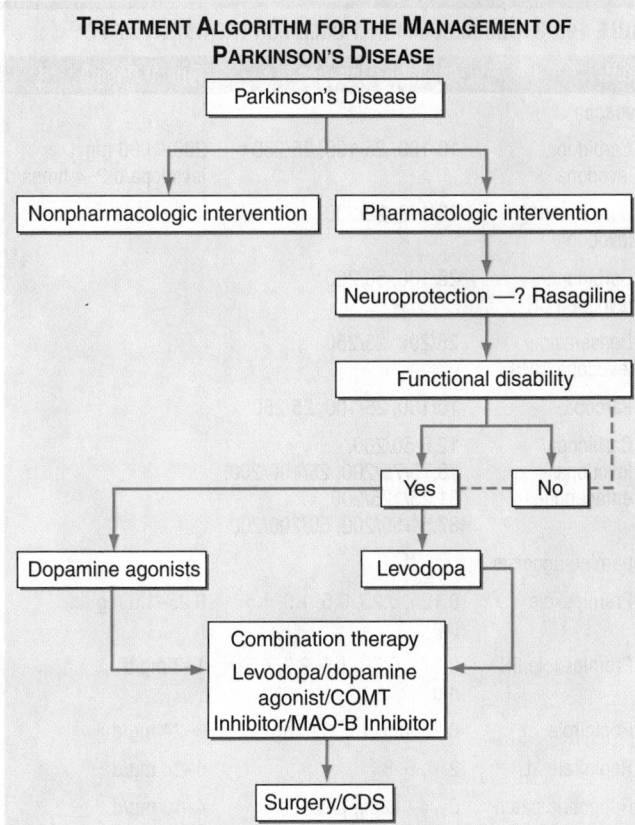

TREATMENT ALGORITHM FOR THE MANAGEMENT OF PARKINSON'S DISEASE

FIGURE 195-1 Treatment options for the management of PD. Decision points include:

a. Introduction of a neuroprotective therapy: No drug has been established to have or is currently approved for neuroprotection or disease modification, but there are several agents that have this potential based on laboratory and preliminary clinical studies (e.g., rasagiline 1 mg/d, coenzyme Q10 1200 mg/d, the dopamine agonists ropinirole and pramipexole).

b. When to initiate symptomatic therapy: There is a trend toward initiating therapy at the time of diagnosis or early in the course of the disease because pts may have some disability even at an early stage, and there is the possibility that early treatment may preserve beneficial compensatory mechanisms; however, some experts recommend waiting until there is functional disability before initiating therapy.

c. What therapy to initiate: Many experts favor starting with an MAO-B inhibitor in mildly affected pts because of the potential for a disease-modifying effect; dopamine agonists for younger pts with functionally significant disability to reduce the risk of motor complications; and levodopa for pts with more advanced disease, the elderly, or those with cognitive impairment.

d. Management of motor complications: Motor complications are typically approached with combination therapy to try and reduce dyskinesia and enhance the "on" time. When medical therapies cannot provide satisfactory control, surgical therapies can be considered.

e. Nonpharmacologic approaches: Interventions such as exercise, education, and support should be considered throughout the course of the disease. (*Adapted from CW Olanow et al: Neurology 72:S1, 2009.*)

TABLE 195-3 DRUGS COMMONLY USED FOR TREATMENT OF PD*

Agent	Available Dosages	Typical Dosing
Levodopa*		
Carbidopa/ levodopa	10/100, 25/100, 25/250	200–1000 mg levodopa/d 2–4 times/d
Benserazide/ levodopa	25/100, 50/200	
Carbidopa/ levodopa CR	25/100, 50/200	
Benserazide/ levodopa MDS	25/200, 25/250	
Parcopa	10/100, 25/100, 25/250	
Carbidopa/ levodopa/ entacapone	12.5/50/200, 18.75/75/200, 25/100/200, 31.25/125/200, 37.5/150/200, 50/200/200	
Dopamine agonists		
Pramipexole	0.125, 0.25, 0.5, 1.0, 1.5 mg	0.25–1.0 mg tid
Pramipexole ER	0.375, 0.75, 1.5. 3.0, 4.5 mg	1–3 mg/d
Ropinirole	0.25, 0.5, 1.0, 3.0 mg	6–24 mg/d
Ropinirole XL	2, 4, 6, 8	6–24 mg/d
Rotigotine patch	2-, 4-, 6-mg patches	4–10 mg/d
Apomorphine SC		2–8 mg
COMT Inhibitors		
Entacapone	200 mg	200 mg with each levodopa dose
Tolcapone	100, 200 mg	100–200 mg tid
MAO-B Inhibitors		
Selegiline	5 mg	5 mg bid
Rasagiline	0.5, 1.0 mg	1.0 mg QAM

*Treatment should be individualized. Generally, drugs should be started in low doses and titrated to optimal dose.
Note: Drugs should not be withdrawn abruptly but should be gradually lowered or removed as appropriate.
Abbreviations: COMT, catechol-*O*-methyltransferase; MAO-B, monoamine oxidase type B.

COMT INHIBITORS

- When levodopa is administered with a decarboxylase inhibitor, it is primarily metabolized by COMT; inhibitors of COMT increase the elimination half-life of levodopa and enhance its brain availability.
- Combining levodopa with a COMT inhibitor reduces wearing-off time.

OTHER MEDICAL THERAPIES

- Anticholinergics (trihexyphenidyl, benztropine) have their major clinical effect on tremor. Use in the elderly is limited due to propensity for inducing urinary dysfunction, glaucoma, and particularly cognitive impairment.
- The mechanism of action of amantadine is unknown; it has NMDA antagonist properties; it is most commonly used as an antidyskinesia agent in pts with advanced PD. Side effects include livedo reticularis, weight gain, and impaired cognitive function; discontinue slowly as pts can experience withdrawal symptoms.

SURGICAL TREATMENTS

- In refractory cases, surgical treatment of PD should be considered.
- The use of ablation (e.g., pallidotomy or thalamotomy) has decreased greatly since the introduction of deep-brain stimulation (DBS) of the subthalamic nucleus (STN) or globus pallidus interna (GPi).
- DBS is primarily indicated for pts who suffer disability resulting from levodopa-induced motor complications; the procedure is profoundly beneficial to many pts.
- Contraindications to surgery include atypical PD, cognitive impairment, major psychiatric illness, substantial medical comorbidities, and advanced age (a relative factor).
- Experimental surgical procedures including cell-based therapies, gene therapies, and trophic factors are under investigation.

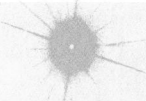

For a more detailed discussion, see Olanow CW, Schapira AHV: Parkinson's Disease and Other Extrapyramidal Movement Disorders, Chap. 372, p. 3317, in HPIM-18.

CHAPTER **196**
Ataxic Disorders

■ CLINICAL PRESENTATION

Symptoms and signs may include gait impairment, visual blurring due to nystagmus, unclear ("scanning") speech, hand incoordination, intention tremor (i.e., with movement). *Differential diagnosis:* Unsteady gait associated with vertigo from vestibular nerve or labyrinthine disease can resemble gait instability of cerebellar disease but produces a sensation of movement, dizziness, or light-headedness. Sensory disturbances also can simulate cerebellar disease; with sensory ataxia, imbalance dramatically worsens when visual input is removed (Romberg sign). Bilateral proximal leg weakness also can rarely mimic cerebellar ataxia.

APPROACH TO THE PATIENT	Ataxia

Causes are best grouped by determining whether ataxia is symmetric or focal and by the time course (Table 196-1). Also important to distinguish whether ataxia is present in isolation or is part of a multisystem neurologic disorder. Acute symmetric ataxia is usually due to medications, toxins, viral infection, or a postinfectious syndrome (especially varicella). Subacute or chronic symmetric ataxia can result from hypothyroidism, vitamin deficiencies, infections (Lyme disease, tabes dorsalis, prions), alcohol, other toxins, or an inherited condition (see below). An immune-mediated progressive ataxia is associated with antigliadin antibodies; biopsy of the small intestine may reveal villous atrophy of gluten enteropathy. Elevated serum anti–glutamic acid decarboxylase (GAD) antibodies have been associated with a progressive ataxic syndrome affecting speech and gait. Progressive nonfamilial cerebellar ataxia after age 45 suggests a paraneoplastic syndrome, either subacute cortical cerebellar degeneration (ovarian, breast, lung, Hodgkin's) or opsoclonus-myoclonus (neuroblastoma, breast, lung).

Unilateral ataxia suggests a focal lesion in the ipsilateral cerebellar hemisphere or its connections. An important cause of acute unilateral ataxia is stroke. Mass effect from cerebellar hemorrhage or swelling from cerebellar infarction can compress brainstem structures, producing altered consciousness and ipsilateral pontine signs (small pupils, sixth or seventh nerve palsies); limb ataxia may not be prominent. Other diseases producing asymmetric or unilateral ataxia include tumors, multiple sclerosis, progressive multifocal leukoencephalopathy (immunodeficiency states), and congenital malformations.

■ INHERITED ATAXIAS

May be autosomal dominant, autosomal recessive, or mitochondrial (maternal inheritance); more than 30 disorders recognized (see Table 373-2, pp. 3337–3340, in HPIM-18). Friedreich's ataxia is most common; autosomal recessive, onset before age 25; ataxia with areflexia, upgoing toes, vibration and position sense deficits, cardiomyopathy, hammer toes, scoliosis; linked to expanded trinucleotide repeat in the intron of gene encoding frataxin; a second form is associated with genetically determined vitamin E deficiency syndrome. Common dominantly inherited ataxias are spinocerebellar ataxia (SCA)1 (olivopontocerebellar atrophy; "ataxin-1" gene) (Fig. 196-1), SCA2 (ataxin-2; pts from Cuba and India) and SCA3 (Machado-Joseph disease); all may manifest as ataxia with brainstem and/or extrapyramidal signs; SCA3 may also have dystonia and amyotrophy; genes for each disorder contain unstable trinucleotide repeats in coding region.

TABLE 196-1 ETIOLOGY OF CEREBELLAR ATAXIA

Symmetric and Progressive Signs			Focal and Ipsilateral Cerebellar Signs		
Acute (Hours to Days)	Subacute (Days to Weeks)	Chronic (Months to Years)	Acute (Hours to Days)	Subacute (Days to Weeks)	Chronic (Months to Years)
Intoxication: alcohol, phenytoin, lithium, barbiturates (positive history and toxicology screen)	Intoxication: mercury, solvents, gasoline, glue; cytotoxic chemotherapeutic, hemotherapeutic drugs	Paraneoplastic syndrome	Vascular: cerebellar infarction, hemorrhage, or subdural hematoma	Neoplastic: cerebellar glioma or metastatic tumor (positive for neoplasm on MRI/CT)	Stable gliosis secondary to vascular lesion or demyelinating plaque (stable lesion on MRI/CT older than several months)
Acute viral cerebellitis (CSF supportive of acute viral infection)	Alcoholic-nutritional (vitamin B_1 and B_{12} deficiency)	Antigliadin antibody syndrome	Infectious: cerebellar abscess (mass lesion on MRI/CT, history in support of lesion)	Demyelinating: multiple sclerosis (history, CSF, and MRI are consistent)	Congenital lesion: Chiari or Dandy-Walker malformations (malformation noted on MRI/CT)
Postinfection syndrome	Lyme disease	Hypothyroidism		AIDS-related multifocal leukoencephalopathy (positive HIV test and CD4+ cell count for AIDS)	
		Inherited diseases			
		Tabes dorsalis (tertiary syphilis)			
		Phenytoin toxicity			
		Amiodarone			

Abbreviations: CSF, cerebrospinal fluid; CT, computed tomography; MRI, magnetic resonance imaging.

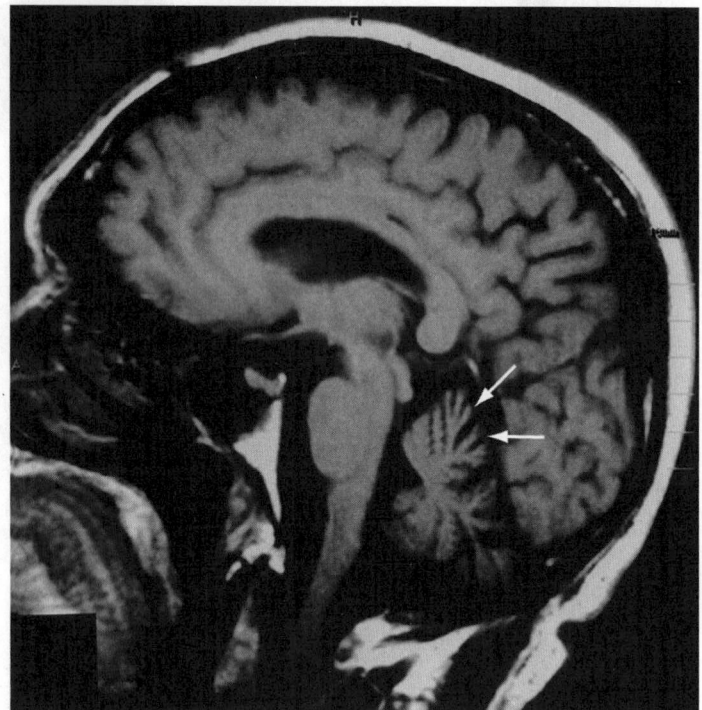

FIGURE 196-1 Sagittal MRI of the brain of a 60-year-old-man with gait ataxia and dysarthria due to SCA1, illustrating cerebellar atrophy (*arrows*). MRI, magnetic resonance imaging; SCA1, spinocerebellar ataxia type 1.

■ EVALUATION

Diagnostic approach is determined by the nature of the ataxia (Table 196-1). For symmetric ataxias, drug and toxicology screens; vitamin B_1, B_{12}, and E levels; thyroid function tests; antibody tests for syphilis and Lyme infection; antigliadin and anti-GAD antibodies; paraneoplastic antibodies (Chap. 84); and CSF studies often indicated. Genetic testing is available for many inherited ataxias. For unilateral or asymmetric ataxias, brain MRI or CT scan is the initial test of choice; CT is insensitive for nonhemorrhagic lesions of the cerebellum.

TREATMENT Ataxia

- The most important goal is to identify treatable entities including hypothyroidism, vitamin deficiency, and infectious causes.
- Parainfectious ataxia can be treated with glucocorticoids.
- Ataxia with antigliadin antibodies and gluten enteropathy may improve with a gluten-free diet.
- Paraneoplastic disorders are often refractory to therapy, but some pts improve following removal of the tumor or immunotherapy (Chap. 84).

- Vitamins B$_1$, B$_{12}$, and E should be administered to pts with deficient levels.
- The deleterious effects of phenytoin and alcohol on the cerebellum are well known, and these exposures should be avoided in pts with ataxia of any cause.
- There is no proven therapy for any of the autosomal dominant ataxias; family and genetic counseling are important.
- There is preliminary evidence that idebenone, a free-radical scavenger, can improve myocardial hypertrophy in Friedreich's ataxia; there is no evidence that it improves neurologic function.
- Cerebellar hemorrhage and other mass lesions of the posterior fossa may require emergent surgical treatment to prevent fatal brainstem compression.

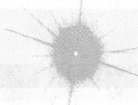

For a more detailed discussion, see Rosenberg RN: Ataxic Disorders, Chap. 373, p. 3335, in HPIM-18.

CHAPTER **197**
ALS and Other Motor Neuron Diseases

Amyotrophic lateral sclerosis (ALS) is the most common form of progressive motor neuron disease (Table 197-1). ALS is caused by degeneration of motor neurons at all levels of the CNS, including anterior horns of the spinal cord, brainstem motor nuclei, and motor cortex. Familial ALS (FALS) represents 5–10% of the total and is inherited usually as an autosomal dominant disorder.

◼ CLINICAL FEATURES

Onset is usually midlife, with most cases progressing to death in 3–5 years. In most societies there is an incidence of 1–3 per 100,000 and a prevalence of 3–5 per 100,000. Presentation is variable depending on whether upper motor or lower motor neurons are more prominently involved initially.

Common initial symptoms are weakness, muscle wasting, stiffness and cramping, and twitching in muscles of hands and arms, often first in the intrinsic hand muscles. Legs are less severely involved than arms, with complaints of leg stiffness, cramping, and weakness common. Symptoms of brainstem involvement include dysphagia, which may lead to aspiration pneumonia and compromised energy intake; there may be prominent wasting of the tongue leading to difficulty in articulation (dysarthria), phonation, and deglutition. Weakness of ventilatory muscles leads to respiratory insufficiency. Additional features that characterize ALS are lack of sensory

TABLE 197-1 SPORADIC MOTOR NEURON DISEASES

Chronic	Entity
Upper and lower motor neuron	Amyotrophic lateral sclerosis
Predominantly upper motor neuron	Primary lateral sclerosis
Predominantly lower motor neuron	Multifocal motor neuropathy with conduction block
	Motor neuropathy with paraproteinemia or cancer
	Motor predominant peripheral neuropathies
Other	
Associated with other neurodegenerative disorders	
Secondary motor neuron disorders (see Table 197-2)	
Acute	
Poliomyelitis	
Herpes zoster	
Coxsackie virus	

abnormalities, pseudobulbar palsy (e.g., involuntary laughter, crying), and absence of bowel or bladder dysfunction. Dementia is not a component of sporadic ALS; in some families ALS is co-inherited with frontotemporal dementia characterized by behavioral abnormalities due to frontal lobe dysfunction.

■ PATHOPHYSIOLOGY

Pathologic hallmark is death of lower motor neurons (consisting of anterior horn cells in the spinal cord and their brainstem homologues innervating bulbar muscles) and upper, or corticospinal, motor neurons (originating in layer five of the motor cortex and descending via the pyramidal tract to synapse with lower motor neurons). Although at onset ALS may involve selective loss of function of only upper or lower motor neurons, it ultimately causes progressive loss of both; the absence of clear involvement of both motor neuron types should call into question the diagnosis of ALS.

■ LABORATORY EVALUATION

EMG provides objective evidence of extensive muscle denervation not confined to the territory of individual peripheral nerves and nerve roots. CSF is usually normal. Muscle enzymes (e.g., CK) may be elevated.

Several types of secondary motor neuron disorders that resemble ALS are treatable (Table 197-2); therefore all pts should have a careful search for these disorders.

MRI or CT myelography is often required to exclude compressive lesions of the foramen magnum or cervical spine. When involvement is

TABLE 197-2 ETIOLOGY OF MOTOR NEURON DISORDERS

Diagnostic Category	Investigation
Structural lesions	MRI scan of head (including foramen magnum and cervical spine)
Parasagittal or foramen magnum tumors	
Cervical spondylosis	
Chiari malformation of syrinx	
Spinal cord arteriovenous malformation	
Infections	CSF exam, culture
Bacterial—tetanus, Lyme	Lyme titer
Viral—poliomyelitis, herpes zoster	Antiviral antibody
Retroviral—myelopathy	HTLV-1 titers
Intoxications, physical agents	24-h urine for heavy metals
Toxins—lead, aluminum, others	Serum lead level
Drugs—strychnine, phenytoin	
Electric shock, x-irradiation	
Immunologic mechanisms	Complete blood count[a]
Plasma cell dyscrasias	Sedimentation rate[a]
Autoimmune polyradiculopathy	Total protein[a]
Motor neuropathy with conduction block	Anti-GM1 antibodies[a]
Paraneoplastic	Anti-Hu antibody
Paracarcinomatous	MRI scan, bone marrow biopsy
Metabolic	Fasting blood sugar[a]
Hypoglycemia	Routine chemistries including calcium[a]
Hyperparathyroidism	PTH
Hyperthyroidism	Thyroid function[a]
Deficiency of folate, vitamin B$_{12}$, vitamin E	Vitamin B$_{12}$, vitamin E, folate[a]
Deficiency of copper, zinc	Serum zinc, copper[a]
Malabsorption	24-h stool fat, carotene, prothrombin time
Mitochondrial dysfunction	Fasting lactate, pyruvate, ammonia
	Consider mtDNA
Hyperlipidemia	Lipid electrophoresis
Hyperglycinuria	Urine and serum amino acids
	CSF amino acids
Hereditary disorders	WBC DNA for mutational analysis

(*continued*)

TABLE 197-2 ETIOLOGY OF MOTOR NEURON DISORDERS (CONTINUED)

Diagnostic Category	Investigation
Superoxide dismutase	
TDP43	
FUS/TLS	
Androgen receptor defect (Kennedy's disease)	
Hexosaminidase deficiency	
Infantile α-glucosidase deficiency (Pompe's disease)	

*a*Denotes studies that should be obtained in all cases.
Abbreviations: CSF, cerebrospinal fluid; FUS/TLS, fused in sarcoma/translocated in liposarcoma; HTLV-1, human T cell lymphotropic virus; PTH, parathyroid; WBC, white blood cell.

restricted to lower motor neurons only, another important entity is multi-focal motor neuropathy with conduction block (MMCB). A diffuse, lower motor axonal neuropathy mimicking ALS sometimes evolves in association with hematopoietic disorders such as lymphoma or multiple myeloma; an M-component in serum should prompt consideration of a bone marrow biopsy. Lyme disease may also cause an axonal, lower motor neuropathy, typically with intense proximal limb pain and a CSF pleocytosis. Other treatable disorders that occasionally mimic ALS are chronic lead poisoning and thyrotoxicosis.

Pulmonary function studies may aid in management of ventilation. Swallowing evaluation identifies those at risk for aspiration. Genetic testing is available for superoxide dismutase 1 (SOD1) (20% of FALS) and for rare mutations in other genes.

TREATMENT Amyotrophic Lateral Sclerosis

- There is no treatment that arrests the underlying pathologic process in ALS.
- The drug riluzole produces modest lengthening of survival; in one trial the survival rate at 18 months with riluzole (100 mg/d) was similar to placebo at 15 months. It may act by diminishing glutamate release and thereby decreasing excitotoxic neuronal cell death. Side effects of riluzole include nausea, dizziness, weight loss, and elevation of liver enzymes.
- Multiple therapies are presently in clinical trials for ALS including ceftriaxone, pramipexole, and tamoxifen; interventions such as antisense oligonucleotides that diminish expression of mutant SOD1 protein are in trial for SOD1-mediated ALS.
- A variety of rehabilitative aids may substantially assist ALS pts. Foot-drop splints facilitate ambulation, and finger extension splints can potentiate grip.

- Respiratory support may be life-sustaining. For pts electing against long-term ventilation by tracheostomy, positive-pressure ventilation by mouth or nose provides transient (several weeks) relief from hypercarbia and hypoxia. Also beneficial are respiratory devices that produce an artificial cough; these help to clear airways and prevent aspiration pneumonia.
- When bulbar disease prevents normal chewing and swallowing, gastrostomy is helpful in restoring normal nutrition and hydration.
- Speech synthesizers can augment speech when there is advanced bulbar palsy.
- Web-based information on ALS is offered by the Muscular Dystrophy Association (*www.mdausa.org*) and the Amyotrophic Lateral Sclerosis Association (*www.alsa.org*).

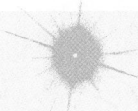

For a more detailed discussion, see Brown RH Jr: Amyotrophic Lateral Sclerosis and Other Motor Neuron Diseases, Chap. 374, p. 3345, in HPIM-18.

CHAPTER **198**
Autonomic Nervous System Disorders

The autonomic nervous system (ANS) (Fig. 198-1) innervates the entire neuraxis and permeates all organ systems. It regulates blood pressure (bp), heart rate, sleep, and bladder and bowel function. It operates automatically, so that its full importance becomes recognized only when ANS function is compromised, resulting in dysautonomia.

Key features of the ANS are summarized in Table 198-1. Responses to sympathetic or parasympathetic activation often have opposite effects; partial activation of both systems allows for simultaneous integration of multiple body functions.

Consider disorders of autonomic function in the differential diagnosis of pts with unexplained orthostatic hypotension, sleep dysfunction, impotence, bladder dysfunction (urinary frequency, hesitancy, or incontinence), diarrhea, constipation, upper gastrointestinal symptoms (bloating, nausea, vomiting of old food), impaired lacrimation, or altered sweating (hyperhidrosis or hypohidrosis).

Orthostatic hypotension (OH) is perhaps the most disabling feature of autonomic dysfunction. Syncope results when the drop in bp impairs cerebral perfusion (Chap. 56). Other manifestations of impaired baroreflexes are supine hypertension, a heart rate that is fixed regardless of posture, postprandial hypotension, and an excessively high nocturnal bp. Many pts

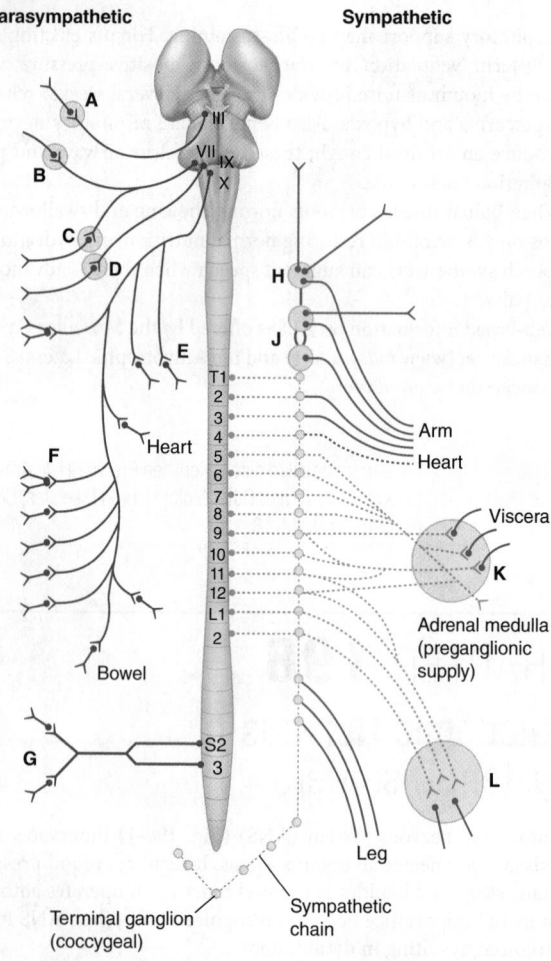

FIGURE 198-1 Schematic representation of the autonomic nervous system. (*From M. Moskowitz: Clin Endocrinol Metab 6:745, 1977.*)

TABLE 198-1 FUNCTIONAL CONSEQUENCES OF NORMAL ANS ACTIVATION

	Sympathetic	Parasympathetic
Heart rate	Increased	Decreased
Blood pressure	Increased	Mildly decreased
Bladder	Increased sphincter tone	Voiding (decreased tone)
Bowel motility	Decreased motility	Increased
Lung	Bronchodilation	Bronchoconstriction
Sweat glands	Sweating	—
Pupils	Dilation	Constriction
Adrenal glands	Catecholamine release	—
Sexual function	Ejaculation, orgasm	Erection
Lacrimal glands	—	Tearing
Parotid glands	—	Salivation

with OH have a preceding diagnosis of hypertension. The most common causes of OH are not neurologic in origin; these must be distinguished from the neurogenic causes.

APPROACH TO THE PATIENT Autonomic Nervous System Disorders

The first step in the evaluation of symptomatic OH is the exclusion of treatable causes. The history should include a review of medications that may cause OH (e.g., diuretics, antihypertensives, antidepressants, phenothiazines, ethanol, narcotics, insulin, dopamine agonists, barbiturates, and calcium channel blocking agents); the precipitation of OH by medications may also be the first sign of an underlying autonomic disorder. The history may reveal an underlying cause for symptoms (e.g., diabetes, Parkinson's disease) or specific underlying mechanisms (e.g., cardiac pump failure, reduced intravascular volume). The relationship of symptoms to meals (splanchnic pooling), standing on awakening in the morning (intravascular volume depletion), ambient warming (vasodilatation), or exercise (muscle arteriolar vasodilatation) should be sought.

Physical exam includes measurement of supine and standing pulse and bp. OH is defined as a sustained drop in systolic ($\geq$20 mmHg) or diastolic ($\geq$10 mmHg) bp within 3 min of standing. In nonneurogenic causes of OH (such as hypovolemia), the bp drop is accompanied by a compensatory increase in heart rate of >15 beats/min. A clue to neurogenic OH is aggravation or precipitation of OH by autonomic stressors (such as a meal, hot tub/hot bath, and exercise). Neurologic evaluation should include a mental status exam (to exclude neurodegenerative disorders), cranial nerve exam (impaired downgaze in progressive supranuclear palsy), pupils (Horner's or Adie's pupils), motor tone (Parkinson's), and sensory exam (polyneuropathies). In pts without a clear initial diagnosis, follow-up exams and laboratory evaluations over 1 to 2 years may reveal the underlying cause.

Autonomic Testing: Autonomic function tests are helpful when the history and physical exam findings are inconclusive; to detect subclinical involvement; or to follow the course of an autonomic disorder. Heart rate variation with deep breathing is a measure of vagal function. The Valsalva maneuver measures changes in heart rate and bp while a constant expiratory pressure of 40 mmHg is maintained for 15 s. The Valsalva ratio is the maximum heart rate during the maneuver divided by the minimum heart rate following the maneuver; the ratio reflects cardiovagal function. Tilt-table beat-to-beat bp measurements in the supine, 70° tilt, and tilt-back positions can be used to evaluate orthostatic failure in bp control in pts with unexplained syncope. Most pts with syncope do not have autonomic failure; the tilt-table test can be used to diagnose vasovagal syncope with high sensitivity, specificity, and reproducibility.

Other tests of autonomic function include the quantitative sudomotor axon reflex test (QSART) and the thermoregulatory sweat test (TST). The QSART provides quantitative measure of regional autonomic function mediated by ACh-induced sweating. The TST provides a qualitative measure of sweating in response to a standardized elevation of body temperature. For a more complete discussion of autonomic function tests, see Chap. 375, HPIM-18.

■ DISORDERS OF THE AUTONOMIC NERVOUS SYSTEM

Autonomic disorders may occur with a large number of disorders of the central and/or peripheral nervous systems (Table 198-2). Diseases of the CNS may cause ANS dysfunction at many levels, including hypothalamus, brainstem, or spinal cord.

Multiple system atrophy (MSA) is a progressive neurodegenerative disorder comprising autonomic failure (OH and/or a neurogenic bladder) combined with either parkinsonism (MSA-p) or cerebellar signs (MSA-c), often along with progressive cognitive dysfunction. Dysautonomia is also common in advanced Parkinson's disease and dementia with Lewy bodies.

Spinal cord injury may be accompanied by autonomic hyperreflexia affecting bowel, bladder, sexual, temperature-regulation, or cardiovascular functions. Markedly increased autonomic discharge (autonomic dysreflexia) can be elicited by stimulation of the bladder, skin, or muscles with spinal cord lesions above the C6 level. Bladder distention from palpation, catheter insertion, catheter obstruction, or urinary infection is a common and correctable trigger of autonomic dysreflexia. Dangerous increases or decreases in body temperature may result from the inability to experience the sensory accompaniments of heat or cold exposure below the level of the injury.

Peripheral neuropathies affecting the small myelinated and unmyelinated fibers of the sympathetic and parasympathetic nerves are the most common cause of chronic autonomic insufficiency (Chap. 205). Autonomic involvement in *diabetes mellitus* typically begins ~10 years after the onset of diabetes and slowly progresses. Diabetic enteric neuropathy may result in

TABLE 198-2 CLASSIFICATION OF CLINICAL AUTONOMIC DISORDERS

I. Autonomic disorders with brain involvement

  A. Associated with multisystem degeneration

    1. Multisystem degeneration: autonomic failure clinically prominent

      a. Multiple system atrophy (MSA)

      b. Parkinson's disease with autonomic failure

      c. Diffuse Lewy body disease (some cases)

    2. Multisystem degeneration: autonomic failure clinically not usually prominent

      a. Parkinson's disease

      b. Other extrapyramidal disorders [inherited spinocerebellar atrophies, progressive supranuclear palsy, corticobasal degeneration, Machado-Joseph disease, fragile X–associated tremor/ataxia syndrome (FXTAS)]

  B. Unassociated with multisystem degeneration (focal CNS disorders)

    1. Disorders mainly due to cerebral cortex involvement

      a. Frontal cortex lesions causing urinary/bowel incontinence

      b. Partial complex seizures (temporal lobe or anterior cingulate)

      c. Cerebral infarction of the insula

    2. Disorders of the limbic and paralimbic circuits

      a. Shapiro's syndrome (agenesis of corpus callosum, hyperhidrosis, hypothermia)

      b. Autonomic seizures

      c. Limbic encephalitis

    3. Disorders of the hypothalamus

      a. Wernicke-Korsakoff syndrome

      b. Diencephalic syndrome

      c. Neuroleptic malignant syndrome

      d. Serotonin syndrome

      e. Fatal familial insomnia

      f. Antidiuretic hormone syndromes (diabetes insipidus, inappropriate ADH secretion)

      g. Disturbances of temperature regulation (hyperthermia, hypothermia)

      h. Disturbances of sexual function

      i. Disturbances of appetite

      j. Disturbances of BP/HR and gastric function

      k. Horner's syndrome

    4. Disorders of the brainstem and cerebellum

      a. Posterior fossa tumors

      b. Syringobulbia and Arnold-Chiari malformation

(*continued*)

TABLE 198-2 CLASSIFICATION OF CLINICAL AUTONOMIC DISORDERS (CONTINUED)

    c. Disorders of BP control (hypertension, hypotension)

    d. Cardiac arrhythmias

    e. Central sleep apnea

    f. Baroreflex failure

    g. Horner's syndrome

    h. Vertebrobasilar and Wallenberg syndromes

    i. Brainstem encephalitis

II. Autonomic disorders with spinal cord involvement

  A. Traumatic quadriplegia

  B. Syringomyelia

  C. Subacute combined degeneration

  D. Multiple sclerosis and Devic disease

  E. Amyotrophic lateral sclerosis

  F. Tetanus

  G. Stiff-man syndrome

  H. Spinal cord tumors

III. Autonomic neuropathies

  A. Acute/subacute autonomic neuropathies

    1. Subacute autoimmune autonomic ganglionopathy (AAG)

      a. Subacute paraneoplastic autonomic neuropathy

      b. Guillain-Barré syndrome

      c. Botulism

      d. Porphyria

      e. Drug-induced autonomic neuropathies—stimulants, drug withdrawal, vasoconstrictors, vasodilators, beta receptor antagonists, beta agonists

      f. Toxic autonomic neuropathies

      g. Subacute cholinergic neuropathy

  B. Chronic peripheral autonomic neuropathies

    1. Distal small fiber neuropathy

    2. Combined sympathetic and parasympathetic failure

      a. Amyloid

      b. Diabetic autonomic neuropathy

      c. Autoimmune autonomic ganglionopathy (paraneoplastic and idiopathic)

      d. Sensory neuronopathy with autonomic failure

      e. Familial dysautonomia (Riley-Day syndrome)

TABLE 198-2 CLASSIFICATION OF CLINICAL AUTONOMIC DISORDERS (CONTINUED)

    f. Diabetic, uremic, or nutritional deficiency

    g. Dysautonomia of old age

  3. Disorders of reduced orthostatic intolerance—reflex syncope, POTS, associated with prolonged bed rest, associated with space flight, chronic fatigue

---

Abbreviations: BP, blood pressure; HR, heart rate; POTS, postural orthostatic tachycardia syndrome.

gastroparesis, nausea and vomiting, malnutrition, achlorhydria, and bowel incontinence. Impotence, urinary incontinence, pupillary abnormalities, and OH may occur as well. Prolongation of the QT interval increases the risk of sudden death. Autonomic neuropathy occurs in both sporadic and familial forms of *amyloidosis*. Pts typically present with distal, painful polyneuropathy. *Alcoholic polyneuropathy* produces symptoms of autonomic failure only when the neuropathy is severe. Attacks of *acute intermittent porphyria* (AIP) are associated with tachycardia, sweating, urinary retention, and hypertension; other prominent symptoms include anxiety, abdominal pain, nausea, and vomiting. Blood pressure fluctuation and cardiac arrhythmias can be severe in *Guillain-Barré syndrome. Autoimmune autonomic neuropathy* presents as the subacute development of autonomic failure featuring OH, enteric neuropathy (gastroparesis, ileus, constipation/diarrhea), loss of sweating, sicca complex, and a tonic pupil. Onset may follow a viral infection; serum antibodies to the ganglionic ACh receptor (A_3 AChR) are diagnostic, and some pts appear to respond to immunotherapy. Rare pts develop *dysautonomia* as a paraneoplastic disorder (Chap. 84). There are five known hereditary sensory and autonomic neuropathies (*HSAN I–V*).

Botulism is associated with blurred vision, dry mouth, nausea, unreactive or sluggishly reactive pupils, urinary retention, and constipation. *Postural orthostatic tachycardia syndrome* (POTS) presents with symptoms of orthostatic intolerance (not OH), including shortness of breath, light-headedness, and exercise intolerance accompanied by an increase in heart rate but no drop in bp. *Primary hyperhidrosis* affects 0.6–1.0% of the population; the usual symptoms are excessive sweating of the palms and soles. Onset is in adolescence, and symptoms tend to improve with age. Although not dangerous, this condition is socially embarrassing; treatment with either sympathectomy or local injection of botulinum toxin is often effective.

■ COMPLEX REGIONAL PAIN SYNDROME (REFLEX SYMPATHETIC DYSTROPHY AND CAUSALGIA)

Complex regional pain syndrome (CRPS) type I is a regional pain syndrome that usually develops after tissue trauma. *Allodynia* (the perception of a nonpainful stimulus as painful), *hyperpathia* (an exaggerated pain response to a painful stimulus), and *spontaneous pain* occur. The symptoms are unrelated to the severity of the initial trauma and are not confined to the distribution of a single peripheral nerve. CRPS type II is a regional pain syndrome that develops after injury to a peripheral nerve, usually a major nerve trunk. Spontaneous pain initially develops within the territory of the affected nerve but eventually may spread outside the nerve distribution.

- Early mobilization with physical therapy or a brief course of glucocorticoids may be helpful for CRPS type I.
- Other treatments include the use of adrenergic blockers, NSAIDs, calcium channel blockers, phenytoin, opioids, and calcitonin.
- Stellate ganglion blockade is a commonly used invasive therapeutic technique that often provides temporary pain relief, but the efficacy of repetitive blocks is uncertain.

TREATMENT Autonomic Nervous System Disorders

- Of particular importance is the removal of drugs or amelioration of underlying conditions that cause or aggravate the autonomic symptom. For instance, OH can be related to angiotensin-converting enzyme inhibitors, calcium channel blocking agents, tricyclic antidepressants, levodopa, alcohol, or insulin.
- Nonpharmacologic approaches are summarized in Table 198-3. Adequate intake of salt and fluids to produce a voiding volume between 1.5 and 2.5 L of urine (containing >170 meq of Na^+) each 24 h is essential. Sleeping with the head of the bed elevated will minimize the effects of supine nocturnal hypertension.
- Prolonged recumbency should be avoided. Pts are advised to sit with legs dangling over the edge of the bed for several minutes before attempting to stand in the morning. Compressive garments such as compression stockings and abdominal binders may be helpful if they can be tolerated. Anemia should be corrected, if necessary, with erythropoietin; the increased intravascular volume that accompanies the rise in hematocrit can exacerbate supine hypertension. Postprandial OH may respond to frequent, small, low-carbohydrate meals.
- If these measures are not sufficient, drug treatment might be necessary.
- Midodrine is a directly acting α_1 agonist that does not cross the blood-brain barrier. The dose is 5–10 mg orally three times a day, but some pts respond best to a decremental dose (e.g., 15 mg on awakening, 10 mg at noon, and 5 mg in the afternoon). Midodrine should not be taken after 6 P.M. Side effects include pruritus, uncomfortable piloerection, and supine hypertension.
- Pyridostigmine appears to improve OH without aggravating supine hypertension by enhancing ganglionic transmission (maximal when orthostatic, minimal supine).
- Fludrocortisone (0.1–0.3 mg PO twice daily) will reduce OH, but it aggravates supine hypertension. Susceptible pts may develop fluid overload, congestive heart failure, supine hypertension, or hypokalemia.

TABLE 198-3 INITIAL TREATMENT OF ORTHOSTATIC HYPOTENSION (OH)

Educate pt: mechanisms and stressors of OH

Implement high-salt diet (10–20 g/d)

Implement high fluid intake (2 L/d)

Elevate head of bed 10 cm (4 in.)

Maintain postural stimuli

Learn physical countermaneuvers

Wear compression garments

Correct anemia

For a more detailed discussion, see Low PA, Engstrom JW: Disorders of the Autonomic Nervous System, Chap. 375, p. 3351, in HPIM-18.

CHAPTER **199**
Trigeminal Neuralgia, Bell's Palsy, and Other Cranial Nerve Disorders

Disorders of vision and ocular movement are discussed in Chaps. 58 and 63, dizziness and vertigo in Chap. 57, and disorders of hearing in Chap. 63.

■ FACIAL PAIN OR NUMBNESS [TRIGEMINAL NERVE (V)]

(See Fig. 199-1)

Trigeminal Neuralgia (Tic Douloureux)

Frequent, excruciating paroxysms of pain in lips, gums, cheek, or chin (rarely in ophthalmic division of fifth nerve) lasting seconds to minutes. Typically presents in middle or old age. Pain is often stimulated at trigger points. Sensory deficit cannot be demonstrated. Must be distinguished from other forms of facial pain arising from diseases of jaw, teeth, or sinuses. Rare causes are herpes zoster or a tumor. Onset in young adulthood or if bilateral raises the possibility of multiple sclerosis (Chap. 202).

TREATMENT Trigeminal Neuralgia

- Carbamazepine is effective in 50–75% of cases. Begin at 100-mg single daily dose taken with food and advance by 100 mg every 1–2 days until substantial (50%) pain relief occurs. Most pts require 200 mg four times a day; doses >1200 mg daily usually provide no additional benefit.

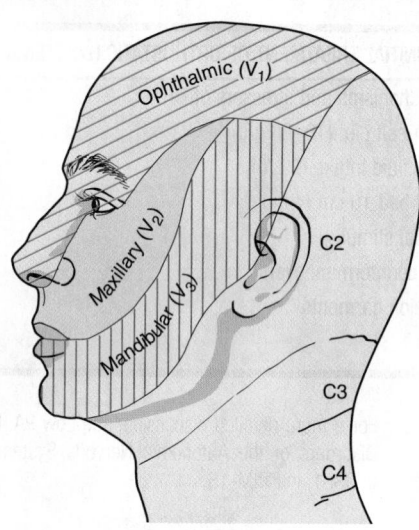

FIGURE 199-1 The three major sensory divisions of the trigeminal nerve consist of the ophthalmic, maxillary, and mandibular nerves.

- Oxcarbazepine (300–1200 mg bid) is an alternative with less bone marrow toxicity and probably similar efficacy.
- For nonresponders, lamotrigine (400 mg daily) or phenytoin (300–400 mg/d) can be tried.
- When medications fail, surgical microvascular decompression to relieve pressure on the trigeminal nerve can be offered.
- Other options include gamma knife radiosurgery and radiofrequency thermal rhizotomy.

Trigeminal Neuropathy

Usually presents as facial sensory loss or weakness of jaw muscles. Causes are varied (Table 199-1), including tumors of middle cranial fossa or trigeminal nerve, metastases to base of skull, or lesions in cavernous sinus (affecting first and second divisions of fifth nerve) or superior orbital fissure (affecting first division of fifth nerve).

■ FACIAL WEAKNESS [FACIAL NERVE (VII)] (SEE FIG. 199-2)

Look for hemifacial weakness that includes muscles of forehead and orbicularis oculi. If lesion is in middle ear portion, taste is lost over the anterior two-thirds of tongue and there may be hyperacusis; if lesion is at internal auditory meatus, there may be involvement of auditory and vestibular nerves; pontine lesions usually affect abducens nerve and often corticospinal tract. Peripheral nerve lesions with incomplete recovery may produce continuous contractions of affected musculature (*facial myokymia*); contraction of all facial muscles on attempts to move one group selectively (*synkinesis*); hemifacial spasms; or anomalous tears when facial muscles activated as in eating (*crocodile tears*).

TABLE 199-1 TRIGEMINAL NERVE DISORDERS

Nuclear (brainstem) lesions	Peripheral nerve lesions
Multiple sclerosis	Nasopharyngeal carcinoma
Stroke	Trauma
Syringobulbia	Guillain-Barré syndrome
Glioma	Sjögren's syndrome
Lymphoma	Collagen-vascular diseases
Preganglionic lesions	Sarcoidosis
Acoustic neuroma	Leprosy
Meningioma	Drugs (stilbamidine, trichloroethylene)
Metastasis	Idiopathic trigeminal neuropathy
Chronic meningitis	
Cavernous carotid aneurysm	
Gasserian ganglion lesions	
Trigeminal neuroma	
Herpes zoster	
Infection (spread from otitis media or mastoiditis)	

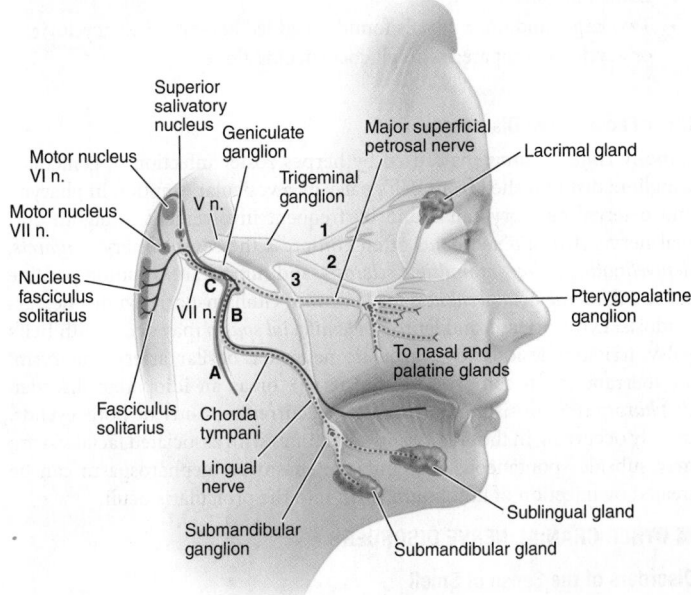

FIGURE 199-2 The facial nerve. A, B, and C denote lesions of the facial nerve at the stylomastoid foramen, distal and proximal to the geniculate ganglion, respectively. Green lines indicate the parasympathetic fibers, red lines indicate motor fibers, and purple lines indicate visceral afferent fibers (taste). *(Adapted from MB Carpenter: Core Text of Neuroanatomy, 2nd ed. Baltimore, Williams & Wilkins, 1978.)*

Bell's Palsy

Most common form of idiopathic facial paralysis; affects 1 in 60 persons over a lifetime. Association with herpes simplex virus type 1. Weakness evolves with maximal weakness by 48 h, sometimes preceded by retroaural pain. Hyperacusis may be present. Full recovery within several weeks or months in 80%; incomplete paralysis in first week is the most favorable prognostic sign.

Diagnosis can be made clinically in pts with (1) a typical presentation, (2) no risk factors or preexisting symptoms for other causes of facial paralysis, (3) no lesions of herpes zoster in the external ear canal, and (4) a normal neurologic examination with the exception of the facial nerve. In uncertain cases, an ESR, testing for diabetes mellitus, a Lyme titer, angiotensin-converting enzyme level and chest imaging study for possible sarcoidosis, a lumbar puncture for possible Guillain-Barré syndrome, or MRI scanning may be indicated.

TREATMENT   Bell's Palsy

- Protect the eye with paper tape to depress the upper eyelid during sleep and prevent corneal drying.
- Massage of the weakened muscle may help symptomatically as well
- Prednisone (60–80 mg/d over 5 days, tapered off over the next 5 days) modestly shortens the recovery period and improves functional outcome.
- Two large randomized trials found no added benefit for valacyclovir or acyclovir compared with glucocorticoids alone

---

Other Facial Nerve Disorders

Ramsay Hunt syndrome is caused by herpes zoster infection of geniculate ganglion; distinguished from Bell's palsy by a vesicular eruption in pharynx and external auditory canal, and by frequent involvement of eighth cranial nerve. *Acoustic neuromas* often compress the seventh nerve. *Infarcts, demyelinating lesions of multiple sclerosis,* and *tumors* are common pontine causes. *Bilateral facial weakness* may occur in Guillain-Barré syndrome, sarcoidosis, Lyme disease, and leprosy. *Hemifacial spasm* may occur with Bell's palsy, irritative lesions (e.g., acoustic neuroma, basilar artery aneurysm, an aberrant vessel compressing the nerve), or as an idiopathic disorder. *Blepharospasm* consists of involuntary recurrent spasms of both eyelids, usually occurring in the elderly and sometimes with associated facial spasm; may subside spontaneously. Hemifacial spasm or blepharospasm can be treated by injection of botulinum toxin into the orbicularis oculi.

■ OTHER CRANIAL NERVE DISORDERS

Disorders of the Sense of Smell

Olfactory nerve (I) disorders are due to interference with access of the odorant to the olfactory neuroepithelium (transport loss), injury to receptor region (sensory loss), or damage to central olfactory pathways (neural loss). The causes of olfactory disorders are summarized in Table 199-2); most common other than aging are severe upper respiratory infections,

TABLE 199-2 DISORDERS AND CONDITIONS ASSOCIATED WITH COMPROMISED OLFACTORY FUNCTION AS MEASURED BY OLFACTORY TESTING

22q11 deletion syndrome	Liver disease
AIDS/HIV infection	Lubag disease
Adenoid hypertrophy	Medications
Adrenal cortical insufficiency	Migraine
Age	Multiple sclerosis
Alcoholism	Multi-infarct dementia
Allergies	Narcolepsy with cataplexy
Alzheimer's disease	Neoplasms, cranial/nasal
Amyotrophic lateral sclerosis	Nutritional deficiencies
Anorexia nervosa	Obesity
Asperger's syndrome	Obsessive-compulsive disorder
Ataxias	Obstructive pulmonary disease
Attention deficit/hyperactivity disorder	Orthostatic tremor
Bardet-Biedl syndrome	Panic disorder
Chemical exposure	Parkinson's disease
Chronic obstructive pulmonary disease	Pick's disease
Congenital	Posttraumatic stress disorder
Cushing's syndrome	Pregnancy
Cystic fibrosis	Pseudohypoparathyroidism
Degenerative ataxias	Psychopathy
Diabetes	Radiation (therapeutic, cranial)
Down syndrome	Refsum disease
Epilepsy	REM behavior disorder
Facial paralysis	Renal failure/end-stage kidney disease
Frontotemporal lobe degeneration	Restless leg syndrome
Gonadal dysgenesis (Turner syndrome)	Rhinosinusitis/polyposis
Guamanian ALS/PD/dementia syndrome	Schizophrenia
Head trauma	Seasonal affective disorder
Herpes simplex encephalitis	Sjögren's syndrome
Huntington's disease	Stroke
Hypothyroidism	Tobacco smoking
Iatrogenesis	Toxic chemical exposure
Kallmann syndrome	Upper respiratory infections
Korsakoff's psychosis	Usher syndrome
Leprosy	Vitamin B_{12} deficiency

head trauma, and chronic rhinosinusitis. More than half of people between 65 and 80 years of age suffer from olfactory dysfunction that is idiopathic (*presbyosmia*). Pts often present with a complaint of loss of the sense of taste even though their taste thresholds may be within normal limits.

TREATMENT Disorders of the Sense of Smell

- Therapy for allergic rhinitis, bacterial rhinitis and sinusitis, polyps, neoplasms, and structural abnormalities of the nasal cavities is usually successful in restoring the sense of smell.
- There is no proven treatment for sensorineural olfactory losses; fortunately, spontaneous recovery can occur.
- Cases due to exposure to cigarette smoke and other airborne toxic chemicals can recover if the insult is discontinued.
- A nonblinded study reported that pts with hyposmia may benefit from smelling strong odors before going to bed and upon awakening over the course of several months

---

Glossopharyngeal Neuralgia

This form of neuralgia involves the ninth (glossopharyngeal) and sometimes portions of the tenth (vagus) cranial nerves. Paroxysmal, intense pain in tonsillar fossa of throat that may be precipitated by swallowing. There is no demonstrable sensory and motor deficit. Other diseases affecting this nerve include herpes zoster or compressive neuropathy due to tumor or aneurysm in region of jugular foramen (when associated with vagus and accessory nerve palsies).

TREATMENT Glossopharyngeal Neuralgia

- Medical therapy is similar to that for trigeminal neuralgia, and carbamazepine is generally the first choice.
- If drug therapy is unsuccessful, surgical procedures (including microvascular decompression, if vascular compression is evident, or rhizotomy of glossopharyngeal and vagal fibers in the jugular bulb) are frequently successful.

Dysphagia and Dysphonia

Lesions of the vagus nerve (X) may be responsible. Unilateral lesions produce drooping of soft palate, loss of gag reflex, and "curtain movement" of lateral wall of pharynx with hoarse, nasal voice. Etiologies include neoplastic and infectious processes of the meninges, tumors and vascular lesions in the medulla, motor neuron disease (e.g., ALS), or compression of the recurrent laryngeal nerve by intrathoracic processes. Aneurysm of the aortic arch, an enlarged left atrium, and tumors of the mediastinum and bronchi are much more frequent causes of an isolated vocal cord palsy than are intracranial disorders. A substantial number of cases of recurrent laryngeal palsy remain idiopathic.

With laryngeal palsy, first determine the site of the lesion. If intramedullary, there are usually other brainstem or cerebellar signs. If extramedullary, the glossopharyngeal (IX) and spinal accessory (XI) nerves are frequently involved (jugular foramen syndrome). If extracranial in the posterior laterocondylar or retroparotid space, there may be combinations of ninth, tenth, eleventh, and twelfth cranial nerve palsies and a Horner syndrome. If there is no sensory loss over the palate and pharynx and no palatal weakness or dysphagia, lesion is below the origin of the pharyngeal branches, which leave the vagus nerve high in the cervical region; the usual site of disease is then the mediastinum.

Neck Weakness

Isolated involvement of the accessory (XI) nerve can occur anywhere along its route, resulting in paralysis of the sternocleidomastoid and trapezius muscles. More commonly, involvement occurs in combination with deficits of the ninth and tenth cranial nerves in the jugular foramen or after exit from the skull. An idiopathic form of accessory neuropathy, akin to Bell's palsy, has been described; most pts recover but it may be recurrent in some cases.

Tongue Paralysis

The hypoglossal (XII) nerve supplies the ipsilateral muscles of the tongue. The nucleus of the nerve or its fibers of exit may be involved by intramedullary lesions such as tumor, poliomyelitis, or most often motor neuron disease. Lesions of the basal meninges and the occipital bones (platybasia, invagination of occipital condyles, Paget's disease) may compress the nerve in its extramedullary course or in the hypoglossal canal. Isolated lesions of unknown cause can occur. Atrophy and fasciculation of the tongue develop weeks to months after interruption of the nerve.

■ MULTIPLE CRANIAL NERVE PALSIES

APPROACH TO THE PATIENT Multiple Cranial Nerve Palsies

First determine whether the process is within the brainstem or outside it. Lesions on the surface of the brainstem tend to involve adjacent cranial nerves in succession with only late and slight involvement of long sensory and motor pathways. The opposite is true of processes within the brainstem. Involvement of multiple cranial nerves outside of the brainstem may be due to trauma, localized infections including varicella zoster virus, infectious and noninfectious (especially carcinomatous) causes of meningitis; granulomatous diseases such as Wagener's, Behçet's disease, vascular disorders including those associated with diabetes, enlarging saccular aneurysms, or locally infiltrating tumors. A purely motor disorder without atrophy raises the question of myasthenia gravis. *Facial diplegia* is common in Guillain-Barré syndrome. *Ophthalmoplegia* may occur with Guillain-Barré syndrome (Fisher variant) or Wernicke's encephalopathy.

The *cavernous sinus syndrome* (Fig. 199-3) is frequently life-threatening. It often presents as orbital or facial pain; orbital swelling and chemosis; fever; oculomotor neuropathy; and trigeminal neuropathy affecting the ophthalmic (V_1) and occasionally maxillary (V_2) divisions. Cavernous sinus thrombosis, often secondary to infection from orbital cellulitis, a cutaneous source on the face, or sinusitis, is the most frequent cause; other etiologies include aneurysm of the carotid artery, a carotid-cavernous fistula (orbital bruit may be present), meningioma, nasopharyngeal carcinoma, other tumors, or an idiopathic granulomatous disorder (Tolosa-Hunt syndrome). In infectious cases, prompt administration of broad-spectrum antibiotics, drainage of any abscess cavities, and identification of the offending organism are essential. Anticoagulant therapy may benefit cases of primary thrombosis. Repair or occlusion of the carotid artery may be required for treatment of fistulas or aneurysms. Tolosa-Hunt syndrome generally responds to glucocorticoids.

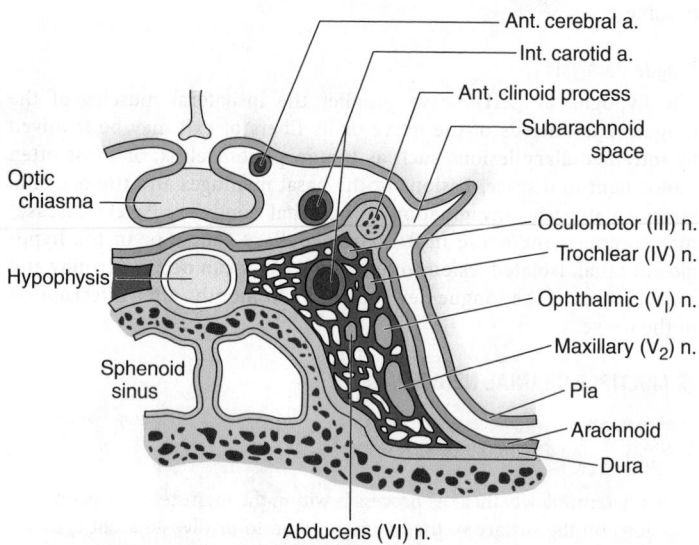

FIGURE 199-3 Anatomy of the cavernous sinus in coronal section, illustrating the location of the cranial nerves in relation to the vascular sinus, internal carotid artery (which loops anteriorly to the section), and surrounding structures.

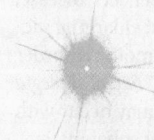

For a more detailed discussion, see Beal MF, Hauser SL: Trigeminal Neuralgia, Bell's Palsy, and Other Cranial Nerve Disorders, Chap. 376, p. 3360; and Doty RL, Bromley SM: Disorders of Smell and Taste, Chap. 29, p. 241, in HPIM-18.

CHAPTER **200**
Spinal Cord Diseases

Spinal cord disorders can be devastating, but many are treatable if recognized early (Table 200-1). Knowledge of relevant spinal cord anatomy is often the key to correct diagnosis (Fig. 200-1).

■ SYMPTOMS AND SIGNS

Sensory symptoms often include paresthesias; may begin in one or both feet and ascend. Sensory level to pin sensation or vibration often correlates well with location of transverse lesions. May have isolated pain/temperature sensation loss over the shoulders ("cape" or "syringomyelic" pattern) or loss of sensation to vibration/position on one side of the body and pain/temperature loss on the other (Brown-Séquard hemicord syndrome).

Motor symptoms are caused by disruption of corticospinal tracts that leads to quadriplegia or paraplegia with increased muscle tone, hyperactive deep tendon reflexes, and extensor plantar responses. With acute severe lesions there may be initial flaccidity and areflexia (spinal shock).

Autonomic dysfunction includes primarily urinary retention; should raise suspicion of spinal cord disease when associated with back or neck pain, weakness, and/or a sensory level.

Pain may be present. Midline back pain is of localizing value; interscapular pain may be first sign of midthoracic cord compression; radicular pain may mark site of more laterally placed spinal lesion; pain from lower cord (conus medullaris) lesion may be referred to low back.

■ SPECIFIC SIGNS BY SPINAL CORD LEVEL

Approximate indicators of level of lesion include the location of a sensory level, a band of hyperalgesia/hyperpathia at the upper end of the sensory disturbance, identification of isolated atrophy or fasciculations, or lost tendon reflex at a specific spinal cord segment.

Lesions Near the Foramen Magnum

Weakness of the ipsilateral shoulder and arm, followed by weakness of ipsilateral leg, then contralateral leg, then contralateral arm, with respiratory paralysis.

Cervical Cord

Best localized by noting pattern of motor weakness and areflexia; shoulder (C5), biceps (C5–6), brachioradialis (C6), triceps/finger and wrist extensors (C7), finger and wrist flexors (C8).

Thoracic Cord

Localized by identification of a sensory level on the trunk. Useful markers are the nipples (T4) and umbilicus (T10).

TABLE 200-1 TREATABLE SPINAL CORD DISORDERS

Compressive
Epidural, intradural, or intramedullary neoplasm
Epidural abscess
Epidural hemorrhage
Cervical spondylosis
Herniated disk
Posttraumatic compression by fractured or displaced vertebra or hemorrhage
Vascular
Arteriovenous malformation
Antiphospholipid syndrome and other hypercoagulable states
Inflammatory
Multiple sclerosis
Neuromyelitis optica
Transverse myelitis
Sarcoidosis
Sjögren's syndrome myelopathy
Systemic lupus erythematosus
Vasculitis
Infectious
Viral: VZV, HSV-1 and -2, CMV, HIV, HTLV-I, others
Bacterial and mycobacterial: *Borrelia, Listeria*, syphilis, others
Mycoplasma pneumoniae
Parasitic: schistosomiasis, toxoplasmosis
Developmental
Syringomyelia
Meningomyelocele
Tethered cord syndrome
Metabolic
Vitamin B_{12} deficiency (subacute combined degeneration)
Copper deficiency

Abbreviations: CMV, cytomegalovirus; HSV, herpes simplex virus; HTLV, human T cell lymphotropic virus; VZV, varicella-zoster virus.

Lumbar Cord

Upper lumbar cord lesions paralyze hip flexion and knee extension and abolish the patella reflex, whereas lower lumbar lesions affect foot and ankle movements, knee flexion, and thigh extension, and abolish the ankle jerks.

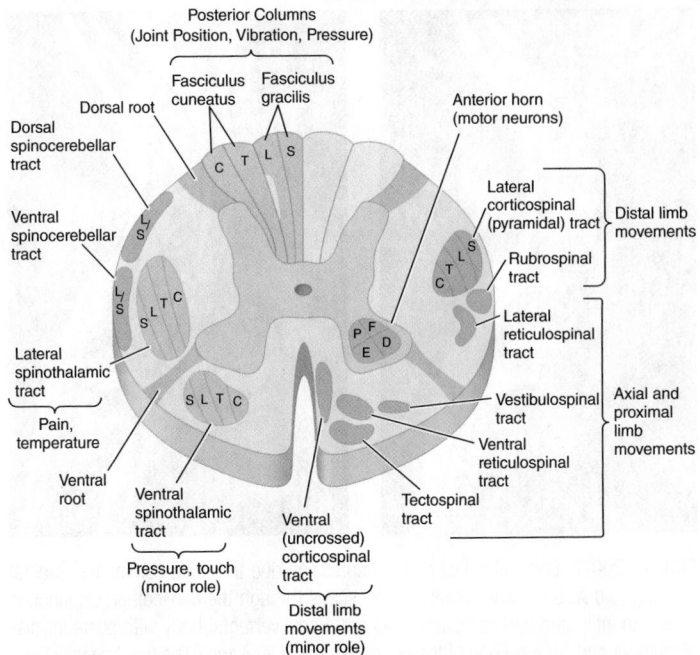

FIGURE 200-1 Transverse section through the spinal cord, composite representation, illustrating the principal ascending (*left*) and descending (*right*) pathways. The lateral and ventral spinothalamic tracts ascend contralateral to the side of the body that is innervated. C, cervical; D, distal; E, extensors; F, flexors; L, lumbar; P, proximal; S, sacral; T, thoracic.

Sacral Cord (Conus Medullaris)

Saddle anesthesia, early bladder/bowel dysfunction, impotence; muscle strength is largely preserved.

Cauda Equina (Cluster of Nerve Roots Derived from Lower Cord)

Lesions below spinal cord termination at the L1 vertebral level produce a flaccid, areflexic, asymmetric paraparesis with bladder/bowel dysfunction and sensory loss below L1; pain is common and projected to perineum or thighs.

■ INTRAMEDULLARY AND EXTRAMEDULLARY SYNDROMES

Spinal cord disorders may be intramedullary (arising from within the substance of the cord) or extramedullary (compressing the cord or its blood supply). Extramedullary lesions often produce radicular pain, early corticospinal signs, and sacral sensory loss. Intramedullary lesions produce poorly localized burning pain, less prominent corticospinal signs, and often spare perineal/sacral sensation.

■ ACUTE AND SUBACUTE SPINAL CORD DISEASES (SEE CHAP. 21)

Neoplastic spinal cord compression (Chap. 21): Most are epidural in origin, resulting from metastases to the adjacent spinal bones (Fig. 200-2). Almost any tumor can be responsible: breast, lung, prostate, lymphoma, and plasma

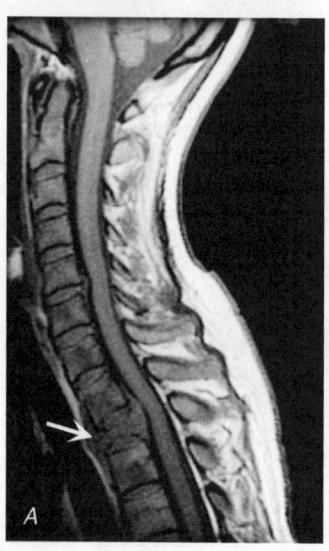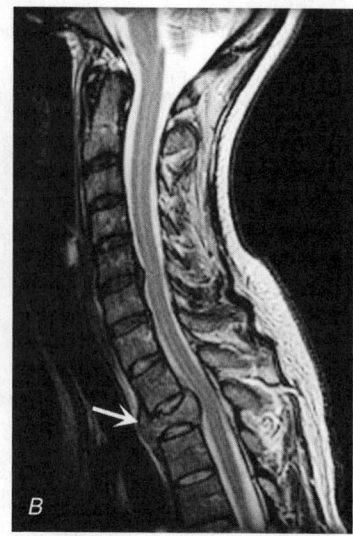

FIGURE 200-2 Epidural spinal cord compression due to breast carcinoma. Sagittal T1-weighted **A.** and T2-weighted **B.** MRI scans through the cervicothoracic junction reveal an infiltrated and collapsed second thoracic vertebral body with posterior displacement and compression of the upper thoracic spinal cord. The low-intensity bone marrow signal in (*A*) signifies replacement by tumor.

cell dyscrasias most frequent. Thoracic cord most commonly involved. Initial symptom is usually back pain, worse when recumbent, with local tenderness preceding other symptoms by many weeks. Spinal cord compression due to metastases is a medical emergency; in general, therapy will not reverse paralysis of >48 h duration.

Spinal epidural abscess: Triad of fever, localized midline dorsal spinal pain, and progressive limb weakness; once neurologic signs appear, cord compression rapidly progresses.

Spinal epidural hematoma: Presents as focal or radicular pain followed by variable signs of a spinal cord or conus medullaris disorder.

Acute disk herniation: Cervical and thoracic disk herniations are less common than lumbar.

Spinal cord infarction: Anterior spinal artery infarction produces paraplegia or quadriplegia, sensory loss affecting pain/temperature but sparing vibration/position sensation (supplied by posterior spinal arteries), and loss of sphincter control. Onset sudden or evolving over minutes or a few hours. Associated conditions: aortic atherosclerosis, dissecting aortic aneurysm, vertebral artery occlusion or dissection in the neck, aortic surgery, or profound hypotension. Therapy is directed at the predisposing condition.

Immune-mediated myelopathies: Acute transverse myelopathy (ATM) occurs in 1% of pts with SLE; associated with antiphospholipid antibodies. Sjögren's and Behçet's syndromes, mixed connective tissue disease, and p-ANCA vasculitis are other causes. Sarcoid can produce ATM with large edematous swelling of the spinal cord. Demyelinating diseases, either neuromyelitis optica (NMO) or multiple sclerosis, also can present as ATM; glucocorticoids, consisting of IV methylprednisolone followed by oral prednisone, are indicated for moderate to severe symptoms and refractory cases may respond to plasma exchange (Chap. 202). Treatment with mycophenolate mofetil (250 mg bid gradually increasing to 1000 mg bid) or anti-CD20 monoclonal antibody may protect against relapses in NMO. Other cases of ATM are idiopathic.

Infectious myelopathies: Herpes zoster is the most common viral agent, but herpes simplex virus types 1 and 2, EBV, CMV, and rabies virus are also well described; in cases of suspected viral myelitis, antivirals may be appropriately started pending laboratory confirmation. Bacterial and mycobacterial causes are less common. Schistosomiasis is an important cause worldwide.

◼ CHRONIC MYELOPATHIES

Spondylitic myelopathies: One of the most common causes of gait difficulty in the elderly. Presents as neck and shoulder pain with stiffness, radicular arm pain, and progressive spastic paraparesis with paresthesias and loss of vibration sense; in advanced cases, urinary incontinence may occur. A tendon reflex in the arms is often diminished at some level. Diagnosis is best made by MRI. Treatment is surgical (Chap. 54).

Vascular malformations: An important treatable cause of progressive or episodic myelopathy. May occur at any level; diagnosis is often suggested by contrast-enhanced MRI (Fig. 200-3), but is confirmed by selective spinal angiography. Treatment is embolization with occlusion of the major feeding vessels.

Retrovirus-associated myelopathies: Infection with HTLV-I may produce a slowly progressive spastic paraparesis with variable pain, sensory loss, and bladder disturbance; diagnosis is made by demonstration of specific serum antibody. Treatment is symptomatic. A progressive vacuolar myelopathy may also result from HIV infection.

Syringomyelia: Cavitary expansion of the spinal cord resulting in progressive myelopathy; may be an isolated finding or associated with protrusion of cerebellar tonsils into cervical spinal canal (Chiari type 1). Classic presentation is loss of pain/temperature sensation in the neck, shoulders, forearms, or hands with areflexic weakness in the upper limbs and progressive spastic paraparesis; cough headache, facial numbness, or thoracic kyphoscoliosis may occur. Diagnosis is made by MRI; treatment is surgical and often unsatisfactory.

Multiple sclerosis: Spinal cord involvement is common and is a major cause of disability in progressive forms of MS (Chap. 202).

Subacute combined degeneration (vitamin B_{12} deficiency): Paresthesias in hands and feet, early loss of vibration/position sense, progressive spastic/ataxic weakness, and areflexia due to associated peripheral neuropathy; mental changes ("megaloblastic madness") and optic atrophy may be present along with a serum macrocytic anemia. Diagnosis is confirmed by a low serum B_{12} level, elevated levels of homocysteine and methylmalonic acid. Treatment is vitamin replacement beginning with 1 mg of IM vitamin B_{12} repeated at regular intervals or by subsequent oral treatment.

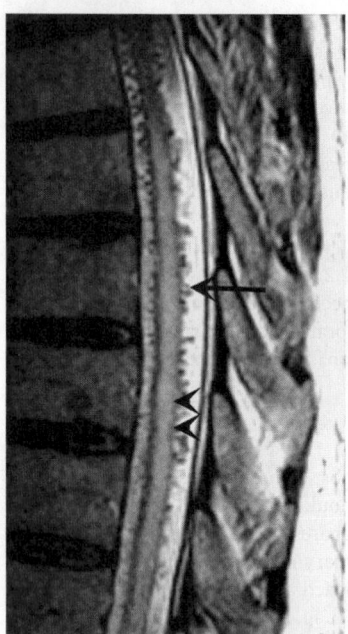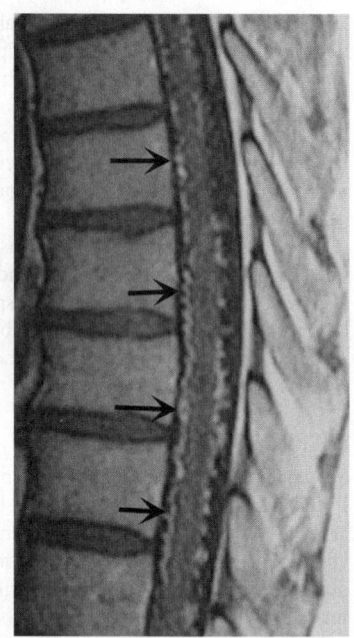

FIGURE 200-3 Arteriovenous malformation. Sagittal MR scans of the thoracic spinal cord: T2 fast spin-echo technique (*left*) and T1 post-contrast image (*right*). On the T2-weighted image (*left*), abnormally high signal intensity is noted in the central aspect of the spinal cord (*arrowheads*). Numerous punctate flow voids indent the dorsal and ventral spinal cord (*arrow*). These represent the abnormally dilated venous plexus supplied by the dural arteriovenous fistula. After contrast administration (*right*), multiple, serpentine, enhancing veins (*arrows*) on the ventral and dorsal aspect of the thoracic spinal cord are visualized, diagnostic of arteriovenous malformation. This pt was a 54-year-old man with a 4-year history of progressive paraparesis.

Hypocupric myelopathy: Clinically nearly identical to subacute combined degeneration (above). Low levels of serum copper and usually ceruloplasmin make the diagnosis. Some cases idiopathic and others follow GI procedures that hinder absorption. Treatment is oral copper supplementation.

Tabes dorsalis (tertiary syphilis): May present as lancinating pains, gait ataxia, bladder disturbances, and visceral crises. Cardinal signs are areflexia in the legs, impaired vibration/position sense, Romberg sign, and Argyll Robertson pupils, which fail to constrict to light but accommodate.

Familial spastic paraplegia: Progressive spasticity and weakness in the legs occurring on a familial basis; may be autosomal dominant, recessive, or X-linked. More than 20 different loci identified.

Adrenomyeloneuropathy: X-linked disorder that is a variant of adrenoleukodystrophy. Usually affected males have a history of adrenal insufficiency and then develop a progressive spastic paraparesis. Female heterozygotes may develop a slower progressive myelopathy without adrenal insufficiency. Diagnosis made by elevated very long chain fatty acids in serum.

No therapy is clearly effective although bone marrow transplantation and nutritional supplements have been tried.

■ **COMPLICATIONS**

Bladder dysfunction with risk of urinary tract infection; bowel dysmotility; pressure sores; in high cervical cord lesions, mechanical respiratory failure; paroxysmal hypertension or hypotension with volume changes; severe hypertension and bradycardia in response to noxious stimuli or bladder or bowel distention; venous thrombosis and pulmonary embolism.

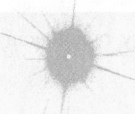

For a more detailed discussion, see Hauser SL, Ropper AH: Diseases of the Spinal Cord, Chap. 377, p. 3366, in HPIM-18.

CHAPTER **201**
Tumors of the Nervous System

APPROACH TO THE PATIENT | **Tumor of the Nervous System**

Clinical Presentation: Brain tumors of any type can present with general and/or focal symptoms and signs. General nonspecific symptoms include headache, cognitive difficulties, personality change, and gait disorder. The classic headache associated with a brain tumor is most evident in the morning and improves during the day, but this pattern is actually seen in only a minority of pts. Papilledema may suggest elevated intracranial pressure. Focal symptoms and signs include hemiparesis, aphasia, or visual field deficit that are typically subacute and progressive. Seizures are a common presentation, occurring in about 25% of pts with brain metastases or malignant glioma.

Evaluation: Primary brain tumors have no serologic features of malignancy such as an elevated ESR or tumor-specific antigens, unlike metastases. Cranial MRI with contrast is the preferred diagnostic test for any pt suspected of having a brain tumor; CT should be reserved for those pts unable to undergo MRI. Malignant brain tumors typically enhance with contrast and may have central areas of necrosis; they are characteristically surrounded by edema of the neighboring white matter. Low-grade gliomas typically do not enhance. Additional testing such as cerebral angiogram, EEG, or lumbar puncture is rarely indicated or helpful.

| TREATMENT | Tumors of the Nervous System |

SYMPTOMATIC TREATMENT
- Glucocorticoids (dexamethasone 12–16 mg/d in divided doses PO or IV) to temporarily reduce edema
- Anticonvulsants (levetiracetam, topiramate, lamotrigine, valproic acid, or lacosamide) for pts who present with seizures; there is no role for prophylactic anticonvulsant drugs
- Low-dose SC heparin for immobile pts

DEFINITIVE TREATMENT
- Based on the specific tumor types and includes surgery, radiotherapy (RT), and chemotherapy

■ PRIMARY INTRACRANIAL TUMORS

Astrocytomas

Infiltrative tumors with a presumptive glial cell of origin. Most common primary intracranial neoplasm. Only known risk factors are ionizing radiation and uncommon hereditary syndromes (neurofibromatosis, tuberous sclerosis). Infiltration along white matter pathways often prevents total resection. Imaging studies (Fig. 201-1) fail to indicate full tumor extent. Grade I tumors (pilocytic astrocytomas) are the most common tumor of childhood, typically in the cerebellum; can be cured if completely resected. Grade II astrocytomas usually present with seizures in young adults; if feasible should be surgically resected. RT and chemotherapeutic agents such as temozolomide are increasingly used and may be helpful. Grade III (anaplastic astrocytoma) and grade IV (glioblastoma) astrocytomas are treated similarly with maximal safe surgical resection followed by RT with concurrent and adjuvant temozolomide or with RT and adjuvant temozolomide alone. Median survival in glioblastoma is 12–15 months. Glioblastomas invariably recur and treatment options include reoperation, carmustine wafer implantation, and chemotherapeutic regimens including bevacizumab. The most important adverse prognostic factors in high-grade astrocytomas are older age, histologic features of glioblastoma, poor performance status, and unresectable tumor.

Oligodendrogliomas

Generally more responsive to therapy and have a better prognosis than pure astrocytic tumors. Usually nonenhancing; often partially calcified. Treated with surgery and, if necessary, RT and chemotherapy. Median survival in excess of 10 years. Chemotherapy response improved when deletions of chromosomes 1p and 19q present.

Ependymomas

Derived from ependymal cells; highly cellular. Location—spinal canal more than intracranial in adults. If total excision possible, may be curable. Partially resected tumors will recur and require irradiation.

Primary CNS Lymphomas

B cell malignancy; most occur in immunosuppressed pts (organ transplantation, AIDS). May present as a single mass lesion or as multiple mass

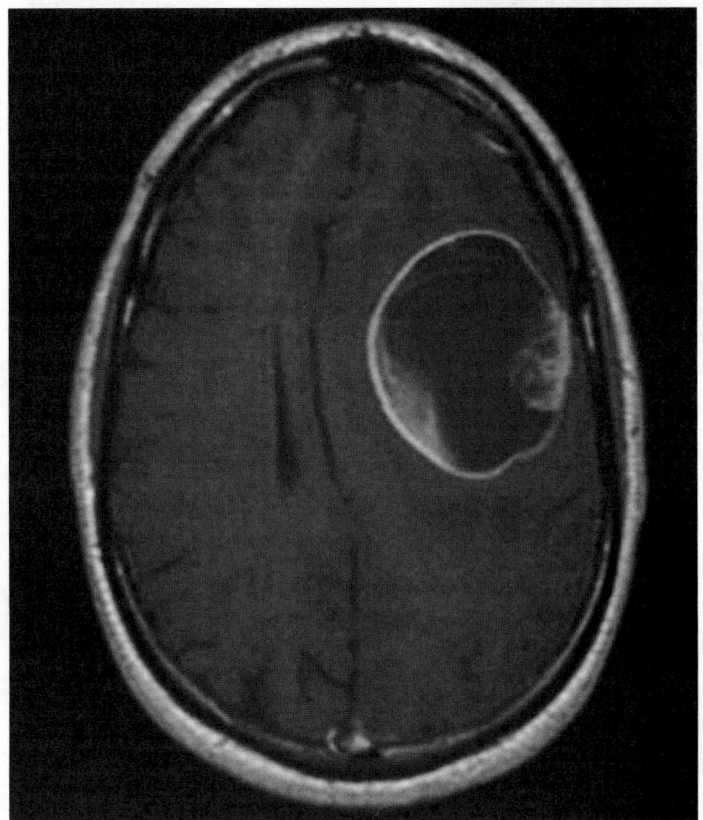

FIGURE 201-1 Postgadolinium T1 MRI of a large cystic left frontal glioblastoma.

lesions or meningeal disease. Dramatic, transient responses occur with glucocorticoids; therefore whenever possible steroids should be withheld until after biopsy has been obtained. Pts should be tested for HIV and the extent of disease assessed by performing PET or CT of the body, MRI of the spine, CSF analysis, and slit-lamp examination of the eye. In immuno-competent pts, high-dose methotrexate therapy produces median survival up to 50 months, which may be increased with concurrent whole-brain RT and additional combinations of other chemotherapeutic agents such as cytarabine or rituximab. In immunocompromised pts, prognosis is worse and treatment is with high-dose methotrexate, whole-brain RT, and, in HIV, antiretroviral therapy.

Medulloblastomas

Most common malignant brain tumor of childhood. Half in posterior fossa; highly cellular; derived from neural precursor cells. Treat with surgery, RT, and chemotherapy. Approximately 70% of pts have long-term survival but usually at the cost of significant neurocognitive impairment.

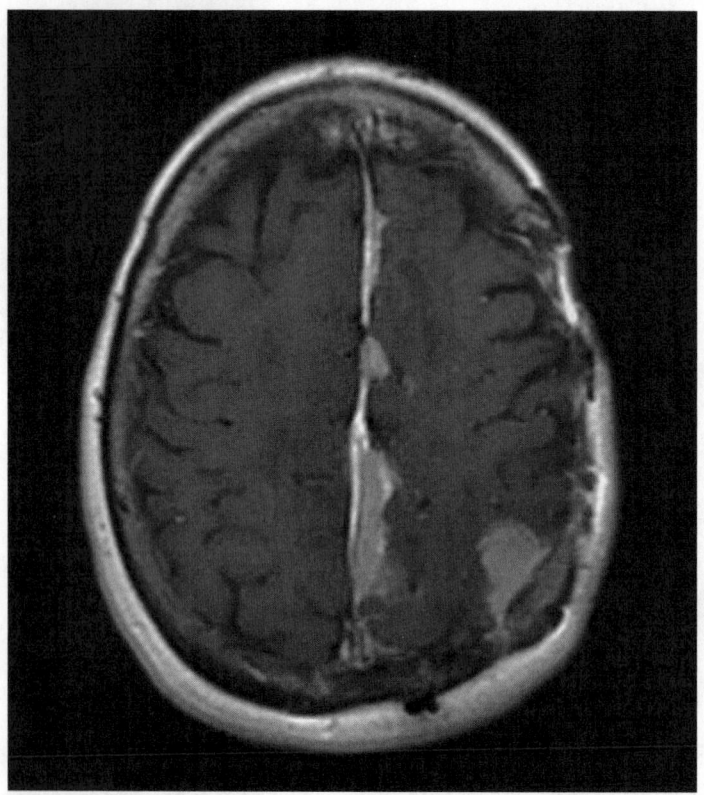

FIGURE 201-2 Postgadolinium T1 MRI demonstrating multiple meningiomas along the falx and left parietal cortex.

Meningiomas

The most common primary brain tumor. Extraaxial mass attached to dura; dense and uniform contrast enhancement is diagnostic (Fig. 201-2). Total surgical resection of large, symptomatic benign meningiomas is curative. With subtotal resection, local RT reduces recurrence. Small, asymptomatic meningiomas may be followed radiologically without surgery. Treat rare aggressive meningiomas with excision and RT.

Schwannomas

Vestibular schwannomas present as progressive, unexplained unilateral hearing loss. MRI reveals dense, uniformly enhancing tumor at the cerebellopontine angle. Surgical excision may preserve hearing.

■ TUMORS METASTATIC TO THE NERVOUS SYSTEM

Hematogenous spread most common. Skull metastases rarely invade CNS; may compress adjacent brain or cranial nerves or obstruct intracranial venous sinuses. Primary tumors that commonly metastasize to the nervous system are listed in Table 201-1. Brain metastases are well demarcated

TABLE 201-1 FREQUENCY OF NERVOUS SYSTEM METASTASES BY COMMON PRIMARY TUMORS

	Brain %	LM %	ESCC %
Lung	41	17	15
Breast	19	57	22
Melanoma	10	12	4
Prostate	1	1	10
GIT	7	—	5
Renal	3	2	7
Lymphoma	<1	10	10
Sarcoma	7	1	9
Other	11	—	18

Abbreviations: ESCC, epidural spinal cord compression; GIT, gastrointestinal tract; LM, leptomeningeal metastases.

by MRI and enhance with gadolinium. Ring enhancement is nonspecific; differential diagnosis includes brain abscess, radiation necrosis, toxoplasmosis, granulomas, tuberculosis, sarcoidosis, demyelinating lesions, primary brain tumors, CNS lymphoma, stroke, hemorrhage, and trauma. Screen for occult cancer: examine skin and thyroid gland; blood carcinoembryonic antigen (CEA) and liver function tests; CT of chest, abdomen, and pelvis. In approximately 10% of pts, a systemic cancer may present with brain metastases; biopsy of primary tumor or accessible brain metastasis is needed to plan treatment. Treatment with glucocorticoids, anticonvulsants, RT, or surgery. Whole-brain RT is often given because multiple microscopic tumor deposits are likely throughout the brain; stereotaxic radiosurgery is of benefit in pts with three or fewer metastases demonstrated by MRI. If a single metastasis is found, it may be surgically excised followed by whole-brain RT. Systemic chemotherapy may produce dramatic responses in rare cases of a highly chemosensitive tumor type such as germ cell tumors.

Leptomeningeal Metastases

Presents as headache, encephalopathy, cranial nerve or polyradicular symptoms. Diagnosis by CSF cytology, MRI (nodular meningeal tumor deposits or diffuse meningeal enhancement), or meningeal biopsy. Associated with hydrocephalus due to CSF pathway obstruction. Treatment is palliative, often with RT or chemotherapy.

Spinal Cord Compression from Metastases

(See Chap. 21) Expansion of vertebral body metastasis posteriorly into epidural space compresses cord. Most common primary tumors are lung, breast, or prostate primary. Back pain (>90%) precedes development of weakness, sensory level, or incontinence. Medical emergency; early recognition of impending spinal cord compression essential to avoid devastating sequelae. Diagnosis is by spine MRI.

■ COMPLICATIONS OF RADIATION THERAPY

Three patterns of radiation injury after CNS RT:

1. Acute—headache, sleepiness, worse neurologic deficits during or immediately after RT. Rarely seen with current protocols. Can be both prevented and treated with glucocorticoids.
2. Early delayed—somnolence (children), Lhermitte's sign; within weeks to months of RT. Increased T2 signal and sometimes enhancement on MRI. Self-limited and improves with glucocorticoids.
3. Late delayed—dementia or other progressive neurologic deficits; typically months to years after RT. White matter abnormalities on MRI (leukoencephalopathy) or ring-enhancing mass (radiation necrosis). PET can distinguish delayed necrosis from tumor recurrence. Progressive radiation necrosis is best treated palliatively with surgical resection unless it can be managed with glucocorticoids. Radiation injury of large arteries accelerates the development of atherosclerosis, increasing the risk of stroke years after RT. Endocrine dysfunction due to hypothalamus or pituitary gland injury can be due to delayed effects of RT. Development of a second neoplasm after RT also is a risk years after exposure.

> For a more detailed discussion, see DeAngelis LM, Wen PY: Primary and Metastatic Tumors of the Nervous System, Chap. 379, p. 3382, in HPIM-18.

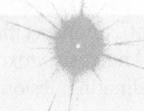

CHAPTER **202**
Multiple Sclerosis (MS)

Characterized by chronic inflammation and selective destruction of CNS myelin; peripheral nervous system is spared. Pathologically, the multifocal scarred lesions of MS are termed *plaques*. Etiology is thought to be autoimmune, with susceptibility determined by genetic and environmental factors. MS affects 350,000 Americans; onset is most often in early to middle adulthood, and women are affected approximately three times as often as men.

■ CLINICAL FEATURES

Onset may be abrupt or insidious. Some pts have symptoms that are so trivial that they may not seek medical attention for months or years. Most common are recurrent attacks of focal neurologic dysfunction, typically lasting weeks or months, and followed by variable recovery; some pts initially present with slowly progressive neurologic deterioration. Symptoms often transiently worsen with fatigue, stress, exercise, or heat. Manifestations of MS are protean but commonly include weakness and/or sensory symptoms involving a limb, visual difficulties, abnormalities of gait and coordination, urinary urgency or frequency, and abnormal fatigue. Motor involvement can present as a heavy, stiff, weak, or clumsy limb. Localized tingling, "pins and needles," and "dead" sensations are common. Optic neuritis can result in blurring of vision, especially in the central visual field, often with associated retroorbital pain accentuated by eye movement. Involvement of the brainstem may result in diplopia, nystagmus, vertigo, or facial pain, numbness, weakness, hemispasm, or myokymia (rippling muscular contractions). Ataxia, tremor, and dysarthria may reflect disease of cerebellar pathways. Lhermitte's symptom, a momentary electric shock–like sensation evoked by neck flexion, indicates disease in the cervical spinal cord. Diagnostic criteria are listed in Table 202-1; MS mimics are summarized in Table 202-2.

■ PHYSICAL EXAMINATION

Abnormal signs usually more widespread than expected from the history. Check for abnormalities in visual fields, loss of visual acuity, disturbed color perception, optic pallor or papillitis, afferent pupillary defect (paradoxical dilation to direct light following constriction to consensual light), nystagmus, internuclear ophthalmoplegia (slowness or loss of adduction in one eye with nystagmus in the abducting eye on lateral gaze), facial numbness or weakness, dysarthria, weakness and spasticity, hyperreflexia, ankle clonus, upgoing toes, ataxia, sensory abnormalities.

■ DISEASE COURSE

Four general categories:

- *Relapsing-remitting MS* (RRMS) is characterized by recurrent attacks of neurologic dysfunction with or without recovery; between attacks, no progression of neurologic impairment is noted. Accounts for 85% of new-onset MS cases.
- *Secondary progressive MS* (SPMS) always initially presents as RRMS but evolves to be gradually progressive. The majority of RRMS eventually evolves into SPMS (~2% each year).
- *Primary progressive MS* (PPMS) is characterized by gradual progression of disability from onset without discrete attacks; 15% of new-onset MS cases.
- *Progressive-relapsing MS* (PRMS) is a rare form that begins with a primary progressive course, but later superimposed relapses occur.

MS is a chronic illness; 15 years after diagnosis, only 20% of pts have no functional limitation; one-third to one-half will have progressed to SPMS and will require assistance with ambulation.

■ LABORATORY EVALUATION

MRI reveals multifocal bright areas on T2-weighted sequences in >95% of pts, often in periventricular location; gadolinium enhancement indicates acute lesions with disruption of blood-brain barrier (Fig. 202-1). MRI also useful to exclude MS mimics, although findings in MS are not completely specific for the disorder. CSF findings include mild lymphocytic pleocytosis (5–75 cells in 25%), oligoclonal bands (75–90%), elevated IgG (80%), and normal total protein level. Visual, auditory, and somatosensory evoked response tests can identify lesions that are clinically silent; one or more evoked response tests abnormal in 80–90% of pts. Urodynamic studies aid in management of bladder symptoms.

TABLE 202-1 DIAGNOSTIC CRITERIA FOR MS

Clinical Presentation	Additional Data Needed for MS Diagnosis
2 or more attacks; objective clinical evidence of 2 or more lesions or objective clinical evidence of 1 lesion with reasonable historical evidence of a prior attack	None
2 or more attacks; objective clinical evidence of 1 lesion	Dissemination in space, demonstrated by • ≥1 T2 lesion on MRI in at least two out of four MS-typical regions of the CNS (periventricular, juxtacortical, infratentorial, or spinal cord) *or* • Await a further clinical attack implicating a different CNS site
1 attack; objective clinical evidence of 2 or more lesions	Dissemination in time, demonstrated by • Simultaneous presence of asymptomatic gadolinium-enhancing and -nonenhancing lesions at any time *or* • A new T2 and/or gadolinium-enhancing lesion(s) on follow-up MRI, irrespective of its timing with reference to a baseline scan *or* • Await a second clinical attack
1 attack; objective clinical evidence of 1 lesion (clinically isolated syndrome)	Dissemination in space and time, demonstrated by: For dissemination in space • ≥1 T2 lesion in at least two out of four MS-typical regions of the CNS (periventricular, juxtacortical, infratentorial, or spinal cord) *or* • Await a second clinical attack implicating a different CNS site *and* For dissemination in time • Simultaneous presence of asymptomatic gadolinium-enhancing and -nonenhancing lesions at any time *or* • A new T2 and/or gadolinium-enhancing lesion(s) on follow-up MRI, irrespective of its timing with reference to a baseline scan *or* • Await a second clinical attack

(continued)

TABLE 202-1 DIAGNOSTIC CRITERIA FOR MS (CONTINUED)

Clinical Presentation	Additional Data Needed for MS Diagnosis
Insidious neurologic progression suggestive of MS (PPMS)	1 year of disease progression (retrospectively or prospectively determined)
	plus
	2 out of the 3 following criteria
	Evidence for dissemination in space in the *brain* based on ≥1 T2⁺ lesions in the MS-characteristic periventricular, juxtacortical, or infratentorial regions
	Evidence for dissemination in space in the *spinal cord* based on ≥2 T2⁺ lesions in the cord
	Positive CSF (isoelectric focusing evidence of oligoclonal bands and/or elevated IgG index)

Source: From Polman CH et al: Diagnostic criteria for multiple sclerosis: 2010 revisions to the "McDonald Criteria." Ann Neurol 69:292, 2011

TABLE 202-2 DISORDERS THAT CAN MIMIC MS

Acute disseminated encephalomyelitis (ADEM)

Antiphospholipid antibody syndrome

Behçet's disease

Cerebral autosomal dominant arteriopathy, subcortical infarcts, and leukoencephalopathy (CADASIL)

Congenital leukodystrophies (e.g., adrenoleukodystrophy, metachromatic leukodystrophy)

Human immunodeficiency virus (HIV) infection

Ischemic optic neuropathy (arteritic and nonarteritic)

Lyme disease

Mitochondrial encephalopathy with lactic acidosis and stroke (MELAS)

Neoplasms (e.g., lymphoma, glioma, meningioma)

Sarcoid

Sjögren's syndrome

Stroke and ischemic cerebrovascular disease

Syphilis

Systemic lupus erythematosus and related collagen vascular disorders

Tropical spastic paraparesis (HTLV I/II infection)

Vascular malformations (especially spinal dural AV fistulas)

Vasculitis (primary CNS or other)

Vitamin B_{12} deficiency

Abbreviations: AV, arteriovenous; CNS, central nervous system; HTLV, human T cell lymphotropic virus.

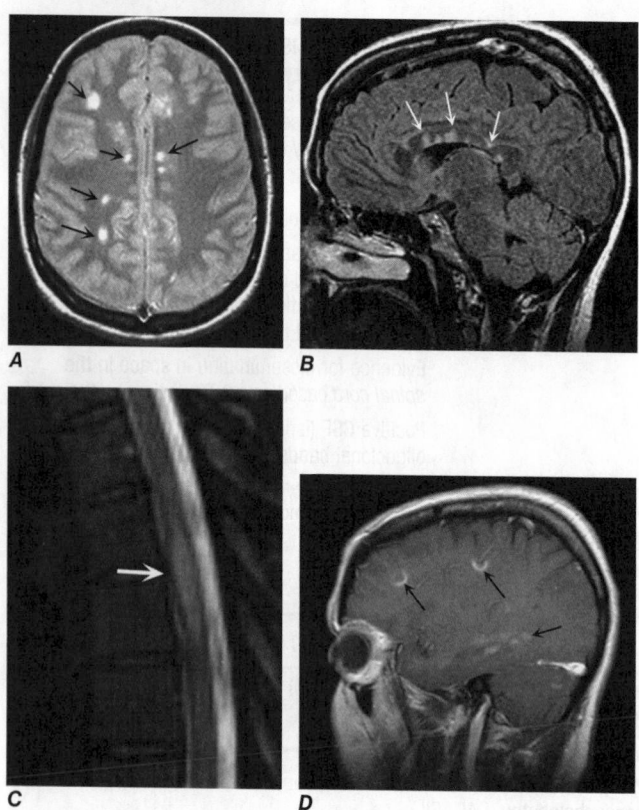

C *D*

FIGURE 202-1 MRI findings in MS. **A.** Axial first-echo image from T2-weighted sequence demonstrates multiple bright signal abnormalities in white matter, typical for MS. **B.** Sagittal T2-weighted FLAIR (fluid attenuated inversion recovery) image in which the high signal of CSF has been suppressed. CSF appears dark, while areas of brain edema or demyelination appear high in signal as shown here in the corpus callosum (*arrows*). Lesions in the anterior corpus callosum are frequent in MS and rare in vascular disease. **C.** Sagittal T2-weighted fast spin echo image of the thoracic spine demonstrates a fusiform high-signal-intensity lesion in the midthoracic spinal cord. **D.** Sagittal T1-weighted image obtained after the IV administration of gadolinium DPTA reveals focal areas of blood-brain barrier disruption, identified as high-signal-intensity regions (*arrows*).

TREATMENT Multiple Sclerosis (See Fig. 202-2)

DISEASE-MODIFYING THERAPIES FOR RELAPSING FORMS OF MS (RRMS, SPMS WITH EXACERBATIONS)

- Seven treatments are available in the U.S.: interferon (IFN)-β1a (Avonex; 30 μg IM once a week), IFN-β1a (Rebif; 44 μg SC thrice weekly), IFN-β1b (Betaseron; 250 μg SC every other day), glatiramer acetate (Copaxone;

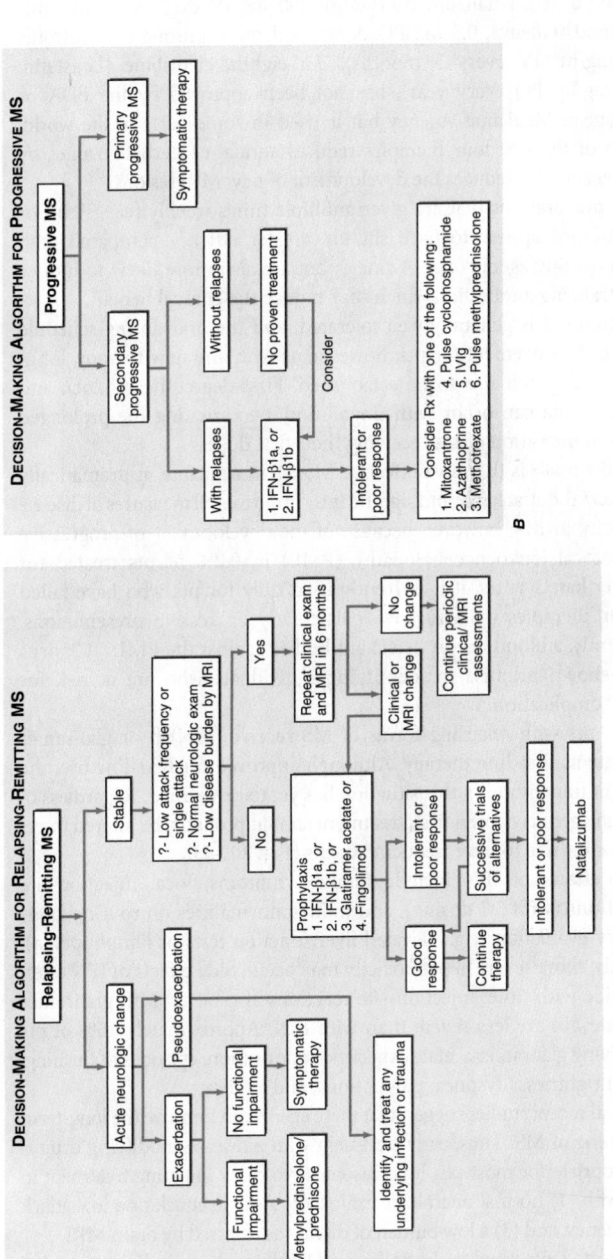

FIGURE 202-2 Therapeutic decision-making for MS.

12 mg/d SC), natalizumab (Tysabri; 300 mg IV every 4 weeks), fingolimod (Gilenya; 0.5 mg PO daily), and mitoxantrone (Novantrone; 12 mg/m² IV every 3 months). An eighth, cladribine (Leustatin; 3.5 mg/kg PO every year), has not been approved by the FDA or European Medicines Agency but is used in some parts of the world. Each of the first four therapies reduces annual exacerbation rates by ~30% and also reduces the development of new MRI lesions.

- IFN preparations that are given multiple times weekly (e.g., Rebif or Betaseron) appear to have slightly greater efficacy compared with once-weekly agents (e.g., Avonex), but are also more likely to induce neutralizing antibodies, which may reduce the clinical benefit.

- Fingolimod is generally well tolerated, and the oral dosing schedule makes it convenient for pts; however, as with any new therapy, long-term safety remains to be established. First-degree heart block and bradycardia can occur with fingolimod, necessitating the prolonged (6-h) observation of pts receiving their first dose.

- Natalizumab is the most effective MS agent available. It dramatically reduces the attack rate and significantly improves all measures of disease severity in MS; however, because of the development of progressive multifocal leukoencephalopathy (PML) in 0.2% of pts treated for more than 2 years, it is currently used only for pts who have failed other therapies or who have particularly aggressive presentations. Recently, a blood test to detect antibodies against the PML (JC) virus has shown promise in identifying individuals who are at risk for this complication.

- Most pts with relapsing forms of MS receive (IFN)-β or glatiramer acetate as first-line therapy. Although approved for first-line use, the role of fingolimod in this situation has yet to be defined. Regardless of which agent is chosen first, treatment should probably be altered in pts who continue to have frequent attacks (Fig. 202-2).

- Side effects of IFN include flulike symptoms, local injection-site reactions (with SC dosing), and mild abnormalities on routine laboratory evaluation (e.g., elevated liver function tests or lymphopenia). Rarely, more severe hepatotoxicity may occur. Side effects of IFN often subside with time. Injection-site reactions also occur with glatiramer acetate but are less severe than with IFN. Approximately 15% of pts receiving glatiramer acetate experience one or more episodes of flushing, chest tightness, dyspnea, palpitations, and anxiety.

- Several recent studies suggest that these agents can improve the long-term outcome of MS. Thus, early treatment with a disease-modifying drug is appropriate for most pts. It is reasonable to delay initiating treatment in pts with (1) normal neurologic exams, (2) a single attack or a low attack frequency, and (3) a low burden of disease as assessed by brain MRI.

- Untreated pts need to be followed closely with periodic brain MRI scans; the need for therapy is reassessed if the scans reveal evidence of ongoing disease.

ACUTE RELAPSES

- Acute relapses that produce functional impairment may be treated with a short course of IV methylprednisolone (1 g IV q A.M. × 3–5 days) followed by oral prednisone (60 mg q A.M. × 4; 40 mg q A.M. × 4; 20 mg q A.M. × 3). This regimen modestly reduces the severity and shortens the duration of attacks.
- Plasma exchange (7 exchanges: 40–60 mL/kg, every other day for 14 days) may benefit pts with fulminant attacks of demyelination (not only MS) that are unresponsive to glucocorticoids; cost is high and conclusive evidence of efficacy is lacking.

PROGRESSIVE SYMPTOMS

- For pts with secondary progressive MS who continue to experience relapses, treatment with one of the IFNs is reasonable; however, the IFNs are ineffective against purely progressive MS symptoms.
- The immunosuppressant/immunomodulatory drug mitoxantrone is approved in the U.S. for treatment of secondary progressive MS; however, the evidence for efficacy is relatively weak, and dose-related cardiac toxicity is an important concern.
- Methotrexate (7.5–20 mg PO once each week) or azathioprine (2–3 mg/kg per day PO) is sometimes tried, but efficacy is modest.
- Pulse therapy with cyclophosphamide is employed in some centers for young adults with aggressive forms of MS.
- Other smaller studies have examined monthly pulses of IV immunoglobulin (IVIg) or IV methylprednisolone.
- For pts with PPMS, symptomatic therapy only is recommended, although a preplanned secondary analysis of a negative rituximab trial was promising and a follow-up trial with a related agent is ongoing.

SYMPTOMATIC THERAPY

- Spasticity may respond to physical therapy, baclofen (20–120 mg/d), diazepam (2–40 mg/d), tizanidine (8–32 mg/d), dantrolene (25–400 mg/d), and cyclobenzaprine hydrochloride (10–60 mg/d).
- Dysesthesia may respond to carbamazepine (100–1000 mg/d in divided doses), phenytoin (300–600 mg/d), gabapentin (300–3600 mg/d), pregabalin (50–300 mg/d), or amitriptyline (25–150 mg/d).
- Treatment of bladder symptoms is based on the underlying pathophysiology investigated with urodynamic testing: bladder hyperreflexia is treated with evening fluid restriction and frequent voiding; if this fails, anticholinergics such as oxybutynin (5–15 mg/d) may be tried; hyporeflexia is treated with the cholinergic drug bethanechol (30–150 mg a day), and dyssynergia due to loss of coordination between bladder wall and sphincter muscles is treated with anticholinergics and intermittent catheterization.
- Depression should be treated aggressively.

■ CLINICAL VARIANTS OF MS

Neuromyelitis optica (NMO), or Devic's syndrome, consists of separate attacks of acute optic neuritis (bilateral or unilateral) and myelitis. In contrast to MS, the brain MRI is typically, but not always, normal. A focal enhancing region of swelling and cavitation, extending over three or more spinal cord segments, is typically seen on spinal MRI. A highly specific autoantibody directed against the water channel aquaporin-4 is present in the sera of more than half of pts with a clinical diagnosis of NMO. Acute attacks are usually treated with high-dose glucocorticoids as for MS exacerbations. Plasma exchange has also been used empirically for acute episodes that fail to respond to glucocorticoids. Prophylaxis against relapses can be achieved with mycophenolate mofetil, rituximab, or a combination of glucocorticoids plus azathioprine. *Acute MS* (Marburg's variant) is a fulminant demyelinating process that progresses to death within 1–2 years. No controlled trials of therapy exist; high-dose glucocorticoids, plasma exchange, and cyclophosphamide have been tried, with uncertain benefit.

■ ACUTE DISSEMINATED ENCEPHALOMYELITIS (ADEM)

A fulminant, often devastating, demyelinating disease that has a monophasic course and may be associated with antecedent immunization or infection. Signs of disseminated neurologic disease are consistently present (e.g., hemiparesis or quadriparesis, extensor plantar responses, lost or hyperactive tendon reflexes, sensory loss, and brainstem involvement). Fever, headache, meningismus, lethargy progressing to coma, and seizures may occur. CSF pleocytosis, generally 200 cells/µL, is common. MRI may reveal extensive gadolinium enhancement of white matter in brain and spinal cord. Initial treatment is with high-dose glucocorticoids. Pts who fail to respond may benefit from a course of plasma exchange or IVIg.

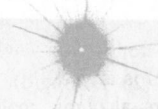

For a more detailed discussion, see Hauser SL, Goodin DS: Multiple Sclerosis and Other Demyelinating Diseases, Chap. 380, p. 3395, in HPIM-18.

CHAPTER **203**
Acute Meningitis and Encephalitis

Acute infections of the nervous system include bacterial meningitis, viral meningitis, encephalitis, focal infections such as brain abscess and subdural empyema, and infectious thrombophlebitis. Key goals: emergently distinguish between these conditions, identify the pathogen, and initiate appropriate antimicrobial therapy.

Acute Infection of the Nervous System

(Fig. 203-1) First identify whether infection predominantly involves the subarachnoid space (*meningitis*) or brain tissue (termed *encephalitis* when viral, *cerebritis* or *abscess* if bacterial, fungal, or parasitic). Nuchal rigidity is the pathognomonic sign of meningeal irritation and is present when the neck resists passive flexion.

Principles of management:

- Initiate empirical therapy whenever bacterial meningitis is considered.
- All pts with head trauma, immunocompromised states, known malignancies, or focal neurologic findings (including papilledema or stupor/coma) should undergo a neuroimaging study of the brain prior to LP. If bacterial meningitis is suspected, begin empirical antibiotic therapy prior to neuroimaging and LP.
- Stupor/coma, seizures, or focal neurologic deficits do not occur in viral meningitis; pts with these symptoms should be hospitalized and treated empirically for bacterial and viral meningoencephalitis.
- Immunocompetent pts with a normal level of consciousness, no prior antimicrobial treatment, and a CSF profile consistent with viral meningitis (lymphocytic pleocytosis and a normal glucose concentration) can often be treated as outpatients. Failure of a pt with suspected viral meningitis to improve within 48 h should prompt a reevaluation including follow-up exam, repeat imaging, and laboratory studies, often including a second LP.

ACUTE BACTERIAL MENINGITIS

Pathogens most frequently involved in immunocompetent adults are *Streptococcus pneumoniae* ("pneumococcus," ~50%) and *Neisseria meningitidis* ("meningococcus," ~25%). Predisposing factors for pneumococcal meningitis include infection (pneumonia, otitis, sinusitis), asplenia, hypogammaglobulinemia, complement deficiency, alcoholism, diabetes, and head trauma with CSF leak. *Listeria monocytogenes* is an important consideration in pregnant women, individuals >60 years, alcoholics, and immunocompromised individuals of all ages. Enteric gram-negative bacilli and group B streptococcus are increasingly common causes of meningitis in individuals with chronic medical conditions. *Staphylococcus aureus* and coagulase-negative staphylococci are important causes following invasive neurosurgical procedures, especially shunting procedures for hydrocephalus.

Clinical Features

Presents as an acute fulminant illness that progresses rapidly in a few hours or as a subacute infection that progressively worsens over several days. The classic clinical triad of meningitis is fever, headache, and nuchal rigidity ("stiff neck"). Alteration in mental status occurs in >75% of pts and can vary from lethargy to coma. Nausea, vomiting, and photophobia are also common. Seizures occur in 20–40% of pts. Raised intracranial pressure (ICP) is the major cause of obtundation and coma. The rash of

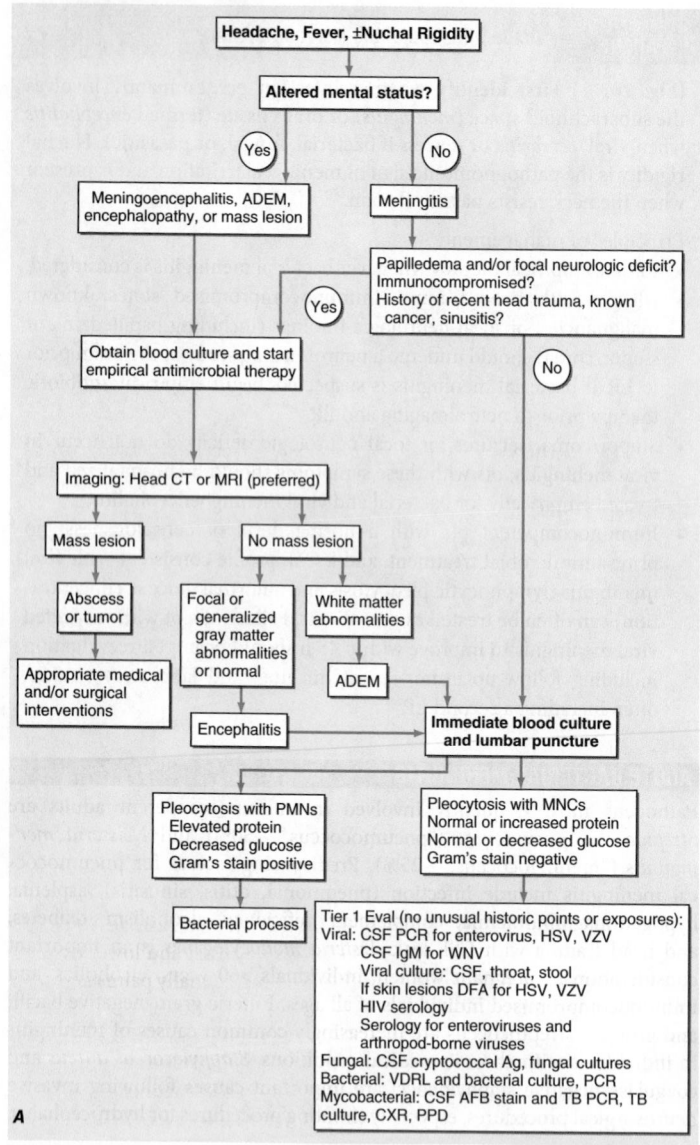

FIGURE 203-1 The management of pts with suspected CNS infection. ADEM, acute disseminated encephalomyelitis; AFB, acid-fast bacillus; Ag, antigen; CSF, cerebrospinal fluid; CT, computed tomography; CTFV, Colorado tick fever virus; CXR, chest x-ray; DFA, direct fluorescent antibody; EBV, Epstein-Barr virus; HHV, human herpesvirus; HSV, herpes simplex virus; LCMV, lymphocytic choriomeningitis virus; MNCs, mononuclear cells; MRI, magnetic resonance imaging; PCR, polymerase chain reaction; PMNs, polymorphonuclear leukocytes; PPD, purified protein derivative; TB, tuberculosis; VDRL, Venereal Disease Research Laboratory; VZV, varicella-zoster virus; WNV, West Nile virus.

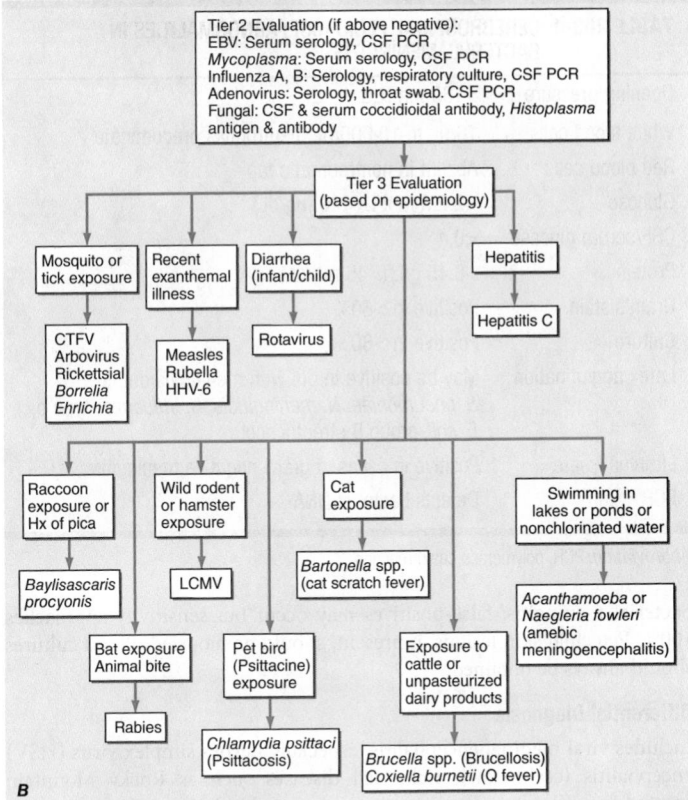

FIGURE 203-1 *(Continued)*

meningococcemia begins as a diffuse maculopapular rash resembling a viral exanthem but rapidly becomes petechial on trunk and lower extremities, mucous membranes and conjunctiva, and occasionally palms and soles.

Laboratory Evaluation

The CSF profile is shown in Table 203-1. CSF bacterial cultures are positive in >80% of pts, and CSF Gram's stain demonstrates organisms in >60%. A 16S rRNA conserved sequence broad-based bacterial PCR can detect small numbers of viable and nonviable organisms in the CSF and is useful for making a diagnosis in pts who have been pretreated with antibiotics and in whom Gram's stain and CSF cultures are negative. When positive, more specific PCR tests for individual organisms can be obtained. The latex agglutination (LA) test for detection of bacterial antigens of *S. pneumoniae*, *N. meningitidis*, *Haemophilus influenzae* type b, group B streptococcus, and *Escherichia coli* K1 strains in the CSF is being replaced by the CSF bacterial PCR assay. The Limulus amebocyte lysate assay rapidly detects gram-negative endotoxin in CSF and thus is useful in diagnosis of gram-negative

TABLE 203-1 CEREBROSPINAL FLUID (CSF) ABNORMALITIES IN BACTERIAL MENINGITIS

Opening pressure	>180 mmH$_2$O
White blood cells	10/μL to 10,000/μL; neutrophils predominate
Red blood cells	Absent in nontraumatic tap
Glucose	<2.2 mmol/L (<40 mg/dL)
CSF/serum glucose	<0.4
Protein	>0.45 g/L (>45 mg/dL)
Gram's stain	Positive in >60%
Culture	Positive in >80%
Latex agglutination	May be positive in pts with meningitis due to *S. pneumoniae, N. meningitidis, H. influenzae* type b, *E. coli,* group B streptococci
Limulus lysate	Positive in cases of gram-negative meningitis
PCR	Detects bacterial DNA

Abbreviation: PCR, polymerase chain reaction

bacterial meningitis; false-positives may occur but sensitivity approaches 100%. Petechial skin lesions, if present, should be biopsied. Blood cultures should always be obtained.

Differential Diagnosis

Includes viral meningoencephalitis, especially herpes simplex virus (HSV) encephalitis (see below); rickettsial diseases such as Rocky Mountain spotted fever (immunofluorescent staining of skin lesions); focal suppurative CNS infections including subdural and epidural empyema and brain abscess (see below); subarachnoid hemorrhage (Chap. 19); and the demyelinating disease acute disseminated encephalomyelitis (ADEM, Chap. 202).

TREATMENT   Acute Bacterial Meningitis

- Recommendations for empirical therapy are summarized in Table 203-2. Therapy is then modified based on results of CSF culture (Table 203-3).
- In general, the treatment course is 7 days for meningococcus, 14 days for pneumococcus, 21 days for gram-negative meningitis, and at least 21 days for *L. monocytogenes.*
- Adjunctive therapy with dexamethasone (10 mg IV), administered 15–20 min before the first dose of an antimicrobial agent and repeated every 6 h for 4 days, improves outcome from bacterial meningitis; benefits most striking in pneumococcal meningitis. Dexamethasone may decrease the penetration of vancomycin into CSF, and thus its potential benefit should be carefully weighed when vancomycin is the antibiotic of choice.

TABLE 203-2 ANTIBIOTICS USED IN EMPIRICAL THERAPY OF BACTERIAL MENINGITIS AND FOCAL CNS INFECTIONS[a]

Indication	Antibiotic
Preterm infants to infants <1 month	Ampicillin + cefotaxime
Infants 1–3 months	Ampicillin + cefotaxime or ceftriaxone
Immunocompetent children >3 months and adults <55	Cefotaxime, ceftriaxone or cefepime + vancomycin
Adults >55 and adults of any age with alcoholism or other debilitating illnesses	Ampicillin + cefotaxime, ceftriaxone or cefepime + vancomycin
Hospital-acquired meningitis, posttraumatic or postneurosurgery meningitis, neutropenic pts, or pts with impaired cell-mediated immunity	Ampicillin + ceftazidime or meropenem + vancomycin

Antimicrobial Agent	Total Daily Dose and Dosing Interval	
	Child (>1 month)	Adult
Ampicillin	200 (mg/kg)/d, q4h	12 g/d, q4h
Cefepime	150 (mg/kg)/d, q8h	6 g/d, q8h
Cefotaxime	200 (mg/kg)/d, q6h	12 g/d, q4h
Ceftriaxone	100 (mg/kg)/d, q12h	4 g/d, q12h
Ceftazidime	150 (mg/kg)/d, q8h	6 g/d, q8h
Gentamicin	7.5 (mg/kg)/d, q8h[b]	7.5 (mg/kg)/d, q8h
Meropenem	120 (mg/kg)/d, q8h	3 g/d, q8h
Metronidazole	30 (mg/kg)/d, q6h	1500–2000 mg/d, q6h
Nafcillin	100–200 (mg/kg)/d, q6h	9–12 g/d, q4h
Penicillin G	400,000 (U/kg)/d, q4h	20–24 million U/d, q4h
Vancomycin	60 (mg/kg)/d, q6h	2 g/d, q12h[b]

[a]All antibiotics are administered intravenously; doses indicated assume normal renal and hepatic function.
[b]Doses should be adjusted based on serum peak and trough levels: gentamicin therapeutic level: peak: 5–8 µg/mL; trough: <2 µg/mL; vancomycin therapeutic level: peak: 25–40 µg/mL; trough: 5–15 µg/mL.

- In meningococcal meningitis, all close contacts should receive prophylaxis with rifampin [600 mg in adults (10 mg/kg in children > 1 year)] every 12 h for 2 days; rifampin is not recommended in pregnant women. Alternatively, adults can be treated with one dose of azithromycin (500 mg), or one IM dose of ceftriaxone (250 mg).

TABLE 203-3 ANTIMICROBIAL THERAPY OF CNS BACTERIAL INFECTIONS BASED ON PATHOGEN[a]

Organism	Antibiotic
Neisseria meningitides	
Penicillin-sensitive	Penicillin G or ampicillin
Penicillin-resistant	Ceftriaxone or cefotaxime
Streptococcus pneumoniae	
Penicillin-sensitive	Penicillin G
Penicillin-intermediate	Ceftriaxone or cefotaxime or cefepime
Penicillin-resistant	(Ceftriaxone or cefotaxime or cefepime) + vancomycin
Gram-negative bacilli (except *Pseudomonas* spp.)	Ceftriaxone or cefotaxime
Pseudomonas aeruginosa	Ceftazidime or cefepime or meropenem
Staphylococci spp.	
Methicillin-sensitive	Nafcillin
Methicillin-resistant	Vancomycin
Listeria monocytogenes	Ampicillin + gentamicin
Haemophilus influenzae	Ceftriaxone or cefotaxime or cefepime
Streptococcus agalactiae	Penicillin G or ampicillin
Bacteroides fragilis	Metronidazole
Fusobacterium spp.	Metronidazole

[a]Doses are as indicated in Table 203-2.

Prognosis

Moderate or severe sequelae occur in ~25% of survivors; outcome varies with the infecting organism. Common sequelae include decreased intellectual function, memory impairment, seizures, hearing loss and dizziness, and gait disturbances.

VIRAL MENINGITIS

Presents as fever, headache, and meningeal irritation associated with a CSF lymphocytic pleocytosis. Fever may be accompanied by malaise, myalgia, anorexia, nausea and vomiting, abdominal pain, and/or diarrhea. A mild degree of lethargy or drowsiness may occur; however, a more profound alteration in consciousness should prompt consideration of alternative diagnoses, including encephalitis.

Etiology

Using a variety of diagnostic techniques, including CSF PCR, culture, and serology, a specific viral cause can be found in 75–90% of cases. The most important agents are enteroviruses, HSV type 2, HIV, and arboviruses (Table 203-4). The incidence of enteroviral and arboviral infections is greatly increased during the summer.

TABLE 203-4 VIRUSES CAUSING ACUTE MENINGITIS AND ENCEPHALITIS IN NORTH AMERICA

Acute Meningitis	
Common	**Less common**
Enteroviruses (coxsackieviruses, echoviruses, and human enteroviruses 68–71)	Varicella zoster virus
	Epstein-Barr virus
Herpes simplex virus 2	Lymphocytic choriomeningitis virus
Arthropod-borne viruses	
HIV	

Acute Encephalitis	
Common	**Less common**
Herpesviruses	Rabies
Herpes simplex virus 1	Eastern equine encephalitis virus
Varicella zoster virus	Western equine encephalitis virus
Epstein-Barr virus	Powassan virus
Arthropod-borne viruses	Cytomegalovirus[a]
La Crosse virus	Enteroviruses[a]
West Nile virus	Colorado tick fever
St. Louis encephalitis virus	Mumps

[a]Immunocompromised host.

Diagnosis

Most important test is examination of the CSF. The typical profile is a lymphocytic pleocytosis (25–500 cells/μL), a normal or slightly elevated protein concentration [0.2–0.8 g/L (20–80 mg/dL)], a normal glucose concentration, and a normal or mildly elevated opening pressure (100–350 mmH$_2$O). Organisms are *not* seen on Gram or acid-fast stained smears or india ink preparations of CSF. Rarely, polymorphonuclear leukocytes (PMN) predominate in the first 48 h of illness, especially with echovirus 9, West Nile virus (WNV), eastern equine encephalitis virus, or mumps. The total CSF cell count in viral meningitis is typically 25–500/μL. As a general rule, a lymphocytic pleocytosis with a low glucose concentration should suggest fungal, listerial, or tuberculous meningitis or noninfectious disorders (e.g., sarcoid, neoplastic meningitis).

CSF PCR testing is the procedure of choice for rapid, sensitive, and specific identification of enteroviruses, HSV, EBV, varicella zoster virus (VZV), human herpes virus 6 (HHV-6), and CMV. Attempts should also be made to culture virus from CSF and other sites and body fluids including blood, throat swabs, stool, and urine, although sensitivity of cultures is generally poor. Serologic studies, including those utilizing paired CSF and serum specimens, may be helpful for retrospective diagnosis; they are particularly important for diagnosis of WNV and other arbovirus etiologies.

Differential Diagnosis

Consider bacterial, fungal, tuberculous, spirochetal, and other infectious causes of meningitis; parameningeal infections; partially treated bacterial meningitis; neoplastic meningitis; noninfectious inflammatory diseases including sarcoid and Behçet's disease.

TREATMENT	Viral Meningitis

- Supportive or symptomatic therapy is usually sufficient, and hospitalization is not required.
- The elderly and immunocompromised pts should be hospitalized, as should individuals in whom the diagnosis is uncertain or those with significant alterations in consciousness, seizures, or focal neurologic signs or symptoms.
- Severe cases of meningitis due to HSV, EBV, and VZV can be treated with IV acyclovir (5–10 mg/kg every 8 h), followed by an oral drug (acyclovir (800 mg, five times daily; famciclovir 500 mg tid; or valacyclovir 1000 mg tid) for a total course of 7–14 days; for mildly affected pts, a 7–14 day course of oral antivirals may be appropriate.
- Additional supportive or symptomatic therapy can include analgesics and antipyretics.
- Prognosis for full recovery is excellent.
- Vaccination is an effective method of preventing the development of meningitis and other neurologic complications associated with poliovirus, mumps, measles, and VZV infection.

VIRAL ENCEPHALITIS

An infection of the brain parenchyma commonly associated with meningitis ("meningoencephalitis"). Clinical features are those of viral meningitis plus evidence of brain tissue involvement, commonly including altered consciousness such as behavioral changes and hallucinations; seizures; and focal neurologic findings such as aphasia, hemiparesis, involuntary movements, and cranial nerve deficits.

Etiology

The same organisms responsible for aseptic meningitis are also responsible for encephalitis, although relative frequencies differ. The most common causes of sporadic encephalitis in immunocompetent adults are herpesviruses (HSV, VZV, EBV) (Table 203-4). HSV encephalitis should be considered when focal findings are present and when involvement of the inferomedial frontotemporal regions of the brain is likely (olfactory hallucinations, anosmia, bizarre behavior, or memory disturbance). Epidemics of encephalitis are usually caused by arboviruses. WNV has been responsible for the majority of arbovirus meningitis and encephalitis cases in the United States. Since 2002, prominent motor manifestations, including acute poliomyelitis-like paralysis, may occur with WNV.

Diagnosis

CSF studies are essential; typical CSF profile is similar to viral meningitis. CSF PCR tests allow for rapid and reliable diagnosis of HSV, EBV, VZV, CMV, HHV-6, and enteroviruses. CSF virus cultures are generally negative. Serologic studies also have a role for some viruses. Demonstration of WNV IgM antibodies is diagnostic of WNV encephalitis.

MRI is the neuroimaging procedure of choice and demonstrates areas of increased T2 signal. Bitemporal and orbitofrontal areas of increased signal are seen in HSV encephalitis, but are not diagnostic (Fig. 203-2). The EEG may suggest seizures or show temporally predominant periodic spikes on a slow, low-amplitude background suggestive of HSV encephalitis.

Brain biopsy is now used only when CSF PCR studies fail to identify the cause, focal abnormalities on MRI are present, and progressive clinical deterioration occurs despite treatment with acyclovir and supportive therapy.

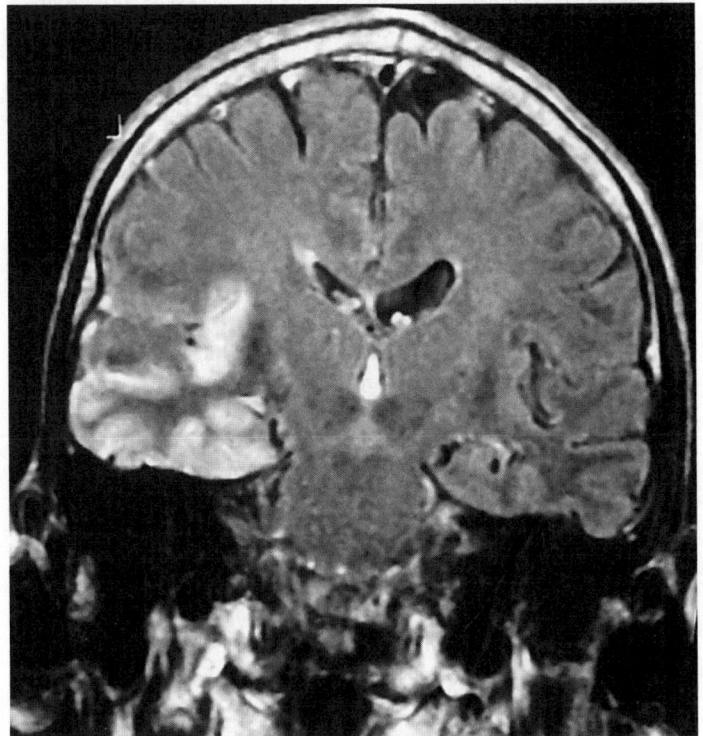

FIGURE 203-2 Coronal FLAIR magnetic resonance image from a pt with herpes simplex encephalitis. Note the area of increased signal in the right temporal lobe (left side of image) confined predominantly to the gray matter. This pt had predominantly unilateral disease; bilateral lesions are more common, but may be quite asymmetric in their intensity.

Differential Diagnosis

Includes both infectious and noninfectious causes of encephalitis, including vascular diseases; abscess and empyema; fungal (*Cryptococcus* and *Mucor*), spirochetal (*Leptospira*), rickettsial, bacterial (*Listeria*), tuberculous, and mycoplasmal infections; tumors; toxic encephalopathy; SLE; and acute disseminated encephalomyelitis.

TREATMENT   Viral Encephalitis

- All pts with suspected HSV encephalitis should be treated with IV acyclovir (10 mg/kg every 8 h) while awaiting diagnostic studies.
- Pts with a PCR-confirmed diagnosis of HSV encephalitis should receive a 14- to 21-day course of therapy. Consider repeat CSF PCR after completion of acyclovir therapy; pts with a persistently positive CSF PCR for HSV after completing a standard course of acyclovir therapy should receive additional treatment, followed by a repeat CSF PCR test.
- Acyclovir treatment may also be of benefit in severe encephalitis due to EBV and VZV. No therapy currently available for enteroviral, mumps, or measles encephalitis.
- IV ribavirin (15–25 mg/kg per day given in 3 divided doses) may benefit severe encephalitis due to California encephalitis (LaCrosse) virus.
- CMV encephalitis should be treated with ganciclovir (5 mg/kg every 12 h IV over 1 h, followed by maintenance therapy of 5 mg/kg every day), foscarnet (60 mg/kg every 8 h IV over 1 h, followed by maintenance therapy (60–120 mg/kg per day), or a combination of the two drugs; cidofovir (5 mg/kg IV once weekly for 2 weeks, then biweekly for two or more additional doses, depending on response; prehydrate with normal saline and pretreat with probenecid) may provide an alternative for nonresponders.
- No proven therapy is available for WNV encephalitis; small groups of pts have been treated with interferon, ribavirin, WNV-specific antisense oligonucleotides, IV immunoglobulin preparations of Israeli origin containing high-titer anti-WNV antibody, and humanized monoclonal antibodies directed against the viral envelope glycoprotein.

Prognosis

In HSV encephalitis treated with acyclovir, 81% survival in one series; neurologic sequelae were mild or absent in 46%, moderate in 12%, and severe in 42%.

BRAIN ABSCESS

A focal, suppurative infection within the brain parenchyma, typically surrounded by a vascularized capsule. The term *cerebritis* is used to describe a nonencapsulated brain abscess. Predisposing conditions include otitis media and mastoiditis, paranasal sinusitis, pyogenic infections in the chest or other body sites, head trauma, neurosurgical procedures, and dental infections. Many brain abscesses occur in immunocompromised hosts and are caused less often by bacteria than by fungi and parasites including *Toxoplasma gondii*, *Aspergillus* spp., *Nocardia* spp., *Candida* spp., and *Cryptococcus* neoformans. In Latin America and in immigrants from Latin America, the most common cause of brain abscess is *Taenia solium* (neurocysticercosis). In India and the Far East, mycobacterial infection (tuberculoma) remains a major cause of focal CNS mass lesions.

Clinical Features

Brain abscess typically presents as an expanding intracranial mass lesion, rather than as an infectious process. The classic triad of headache, fever, and a focal neurologic deficit is present in <50% of cases.

Diagnosis

MRI is better than CT for demonstrating abscesses in the early (cerebritis) stages and is superior to CT for identifying abscesses in the posterior fossa. A mature brain abscess appears on CT as a focal area of hypodensity surrounded by ring enhancement. The CT and MRI appearance, particularly of the capsule, may be altered by treatment with glucocorticoids. The distinction between a brain abscess and other focal lesions such as tumors may be facilitated with diffusion-weighted imaging (DWI) sequences in which brain abscesses typically show increased signal due to restricted diffusion.

Microbiologic diagnosis best determined by Gram's stain and culture of abscess material obtained by stereotactic needle aspiration. Up to 10% of pts will also have positive blood cultures. CSF analysis contributes nothing to diagnosis or therapy, and LP increases the risk of herniation.

TREATMENT   Brain Abscess

- Optimal therapy involves a combination of high-dose parenteral antibiotics and neurosurgical drainage.
- Empirical therapy of community-acquired brain abscess in an immunocompetent pt typically includes a third or fourth-generation cephalosporin (e.g., cefotaxime, ceftriaxone, or cefepime) and metronidazole (see Table 203-2 for antibiotic dosages).
- In pts with penetrating head trauma or recent neurosurgical procedures, treatment should include ceftazidime as the third-generation cephalosporin to enhance coverage of *Pseudomonas* spp. and vancomycin for coverage of resistant staphylococci. Meropenem plus vancomycin also provides good coverage in this setting.
- Aspiration and drainage essential in most cases. Empirical antibiotic coverage is modified based on the results of Gram's stain and culture of the abscess contents.
- Medical therapy alone is reserved for pts whose abscesses are neurosurgically inaccessible and for pts with small (<2–3 cm) or nonencapsulated abscesses (cerebritis).
- All pts should receive a minimum of 6–8 weeks of parenteral antibiotic therapy.
- Pts should receive prophylactic anticonvulsant therapy.
- Glucocorticoids should not be given routinely.

Prognosis

In modern series the mortality is typically <15%. Significant sequelae including seizures, persisting weakness, aphasia, or mental impairment occur in ≥20% of survivors.

PROGRESSIVE MULTIFOCAL LEUKOENCEPHALOPATHY (PML)

Clinical Features

A progressive disorder due to infection with the JC virus, a human polyoma virus; characterized pathologically by multifocal areas of demyelination of varying size distributed throughout the CNS but sparing the spinal cord and optic nerves. In addition, there are characteristic cytologic alterations in both astrocytes and oligodendrocytes. Pts often present with visual deficits (45%), typically a homonymous hemianopia, and mental impairment (38%) (dementia, confusion, personality change), weakness, and ataxia. Almost all pts have an underlying immunosuppressive disorder. More than 80% of currently diagnosed PML cases occur in pts with AIDS; it has been estimated that nearly 5% of AIDS pts will develop PML. Immunosuppressant drugs such as natalizumab have also been associated with PML.

Diagnostic Studies

MRI reveals multifocal asymmetric, coalescing white matter lesions located periventricularly, in the centrum semiovale, in the parietal-occipital region, and in the cerebellum. These lesions have increased T2 and decreased T1 signal, are generally nonenhancing (rarely they may show ring enhancement), and are not associated with edema or mass effect. CT scans, which are less sensitive than MRI for the diagnosis of PML, often show hypodense nonenhancing white matter lesions.

The CSF is typically normal, although mild elevation in protein and/or IgG may be found. Pleocytosis occurs in <25% of cases, is predominantly mononuclear, and rarely exceeds 25 cells/μL. PCR amplification of JC virus DNA from CSF has become an important diagnostic tool. A positive CSF PCR for JC virus DNA in association with typical MRI lesions in the appropriate clinical setting is diagnostic of PML. Pts with negative CSF PCR studies may require brain biopsy for definitive diagnosis as sensitivity of this test is variable; JC virus antigen and nucleic acid can be detected by immunocytochemistry, in situ hybridization, or PCR amplification on tissue. Detection of JC virus antigen or genomic material should be considered diagnostic of PML only if accompanied by characteristic pathologic changes, since both antigen and genomic material have been found in the brains of normal pts. Serologic studies are of no utility given high basal seroprevalence level (>80%).

TREATMENT   Progressive Multifocal Leukoencephalopathy

- No effective therapy is available.
- Some pts with HIV-associated PML have shown dramatic clinical gains associated with improvement in immune status following institution of highly active antiretroviral therapy (HAART).

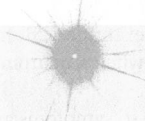

For a more detailed discussion, see Roos KL, Tyler KL: Meningitis, Encephalitis, Brain Abscess, and Empyema, Chap. 381, p. 3410, in HPIM-18; and HPIM-18 chapters covering specific organisms or infections.

CHAPTER **204**
Chronic Meningitis

Chronic inflammation of the meninges (pia, arachnoid, and dura) can produce profound neurologic disability and may be fatal if not successfully treated. The causes are varied. Five categories of disease account for most cases of chronic meningitis:

- Meningeal infections
- Malignancy
- Noninfectious inflammatory disorders
- Chemical meningitis
- Parameningeal infections

■ CLINICAL FEATURES

Neurologic manifestations consist of persistent headache with or without stiff neck and hydrocephalus; cranial neuropathies; radiculopathies; and/or cognitive or personality changes (Table 204-1). The diagnosis is usually

TABLE 204-1 SYMPTOMS AND SIGNS OF CHRONIC MENINGITIS

Symptom	Sign
Chronic headache	+/– Papilledema
Neck or back pain	Brudzinski's or Kernig's sign of meningeal irritation
Change in personality	Altered mental status—drowsiness, inattention, disorientation, memory loss, frontal release signs (grasp, suck, snout), perseveration
Facial weakness	Peripheral seventh CN palsy
Double vision	Palsy of CNs III, IV, VI
Visual loss	Papilledema, optic atrophy
Hearing loss	Eighth CN palsy
Arm or leg weakness	Myelopathy or radiculopathy
Numbness in arms or legs	Myelopathy or radiculopathy
Sphincter dysfunction	Myelopathy or radiculopathy Frontal lobe dysfunction (hydrocephalus)
Clumsiness	Ataxia

Abbreviation: CN, cranial nerve.

made when clinical presentation leads the physician to examine CSF for signs of inflammation; on occasion the diagnosis is made when a neuroimaging study shows contrast enhancement of the meninges.

Two clinical forms of chronic meningitis exist. In the first, symptoms are chronic and persistent, whereas in the second there are recurrent, discrete episodes with complete resolution of meningeal inflammation between episodes without specific therapy. In the latter group, likely etiologies are herpes simplex virus type 2, chemical meningitis due to leakage from a tumor, a primary inflammatory condition, or drug hypersensitivity.

APPROACH TO THE PATIENT | **Chronic Meningitis**

Once chronic meningitis is confirmed by CSF examination, effort is focused on identifying the cause (Tables 204-2 and 204-3) by (1) further analysis of the CSF, (2) diagnosis of an underlying systemic infection or noninfectious inflammatory condition, or (3) examination of meningeal biopsy tissue.

Proper analysis of the CSF is essential; if the possibility of raised intracranial pressure (ICP) exists, a brain imaging study should be performed before LP. In pts with communicating hydrocephalus caused by impaired resorption of CSF, LP is safe and may lead to temporary improvement. However, if ICP is elevated because of a mass lesion, brain swelling, or a block in ventricular CSF outflow (obstructive hydrocephalus), then LP carries the potential risk of brain herniation. Obstructive hydrocephalus usually requires direct ventricular drainage of CSF.

Contrast-enhanced MRI or CT studies of the brain and spinal cord can identify meningeal enhancement, parameningeal infections (including brain abscess), encasement of the spinal cord (malignancy or inflammation and infection), or nodular deposits on the meninges or nerve roots (malignancy or sarcoidosis). Imaging studies are also useful to localize areas of meningeal disease prior to meningeal biopsy. Cerebral angiography may identify arteritis.

A meningeal biopsy should be considered in pts who are disabled, who need chronic ventricular decompression, or whose illness is progressing rapidly. The diagnostic yield of meningeal biopsy can be increased by targeting regions that enhance with contrast on MRI or CT; in one series, diagnostic biopsies most often identified sarcoid (31%) or metastatic adenocarcinoma (25%). Tuberculosis is the most common condition identified in many reports outside of the United States.

In approximately one-third of cases, the diagnosis is not known despite careful evaluation. A number of the organisms that cause chronic meningitis may take weeks to be identified by culture. It is reasonable to wait until cultures are finalized if symptoms are mild and not progressive. However, in many cases progressive neurologic deterioration occurs, and rapid treatment is required. Empirical therapy in the United States consists of antimycobacterial agents, amphotericin for fungal infection, or glucocorticoids for noninfectious inflammatory causes (most common). It is important to direct empirical therapy of

TABLE 204-2 INFECTIOUS CAUSES OF CHRONIC MENINGITIS

Causative Agent	CSF Formula	Helpful Diagnostic Tests	Risk Factors and Systemic Manifestations
Common bacterial causes			
Partially treated suppurative meningitis	Mononuclear or mixed mononuclear-polymorphonuclear cells	CSF culture and Gram's stain	History consistent with acute bacterial meningitis and incomplete treatment
Parameningeal infection	Mononuclear or mixed polymorphonuclear-mononuclear cells	Contrast-enhanced CT or MRI to detect parenchymal, subdural, epidural, or sinus infection	Otitis media, pleuropulmonary infection, right-to-left cardiopulmonary shunt for brain abscess; focal neurologic signs; neck, back, ear, or sinus tenderness
Mycobacterium tuberculosis	Mononuclear cells except polymorphonuclear cells in early infection (commonly <500 WBC/µL; low CSF glucose, high protein	Tuberculin skin test may be negative; AFB culture of CSF (sputum, urine, gastric contents if indicated); tuberculostearic acid detection in CSF; identify tubercle bacillus on acid-fast stain of CSF or protein pellicle; PCR	Exposure history; previous tuberculous illness; immunosuppressed or AIDS; young children; fever, meningismus, night sweats, miliary TB on x-ray or liver biopsy; stroke due to arteritis
Lyme disease (Bannwarth's syndrome) *Borrelia burgdorferi*	Mononuclear cells; elevated protein	Serum Lyme antibody titer; Western blot confirmation; (pts with syphilis may have false-positive Lyme titer)	History of tick bite or appropriate exposure history; erythema chronicum migrans skin rash; arthritis, radiculopathy, Bell's palsy, meningoencephalitis–multiple sclerosis-like syndrome
Syphilis (secondary, tertiary) *Treponema pallidum*	Mononuclear cells; elevated protein	CSF VDRL; serum VDRL (or RPR); fluorescent treponemal antibody-absorbed (FTA) or MHA-TP; serum VDRL may be negative in tertiary syphilis	Appropriate exposure history; HIV- seropositive individuals at increased risk of aggressive infection; "dementia"; cerebral infarction due to endarteritis

(continued)

TABLE 204-2 INFECTIOUS CAUSES OF CHRONIC MENINGITIS (CONTINUED)

Causative Agent	CSF Formula	Helpful Diagnostic Tests	Risk Factors and Systemic Manifestations
Uncommon bacterial causes			
Actinomyces	Polymorphonuclear cells	Anaerobic culture	Parameningeal abscess or sinus tract (oral or dental focus); pneumonitis
Nocardia	Polymorphonuclear; occasionally mononuclear cells; weakly acid fast	Isolation may require weeks; weakly acid fast	Associated brain abscess may be present
Brucella	Mononuclear cells (rarely polymorphonuclear); elevated protein; often low glucose	CSF antibody detection; serum antibody detection	Intake of unpasteurized dairy products; exposure to goats, sheep, cows; fever, arthralgia, myalgia, vertebral osteomyelitis
Whipple's disease *Tropheryma whipplei*	Mononuclear cells	Biopsy of small bowel or lymph node; CSF PCR for *T. whipplei*; brain and meningeal biopsy (with PAS stain and EM examination)	Diarrhea, weight loss, arthralgias, fever; dementia, ataxia, paresis, ophthalmoplegia, oculomasticatory myoclonus
Rare bacterial causes			
Leptospirosis (occasionally if left untreated may last 3–4 weeks)			
Fungal causes			
Cryptococcus neoformans	Mononuclear cells; count not elevated in some pts with AIDS	India ink or fungal wet mount of CSF (budding yeast); blood and urine cultures; antigen detection in CSF	AIDS and immune suppression; pigeon exposure; skin and other organ involvement due to disseminated infection

Etiologic agent	CSF findings	Diagnostic tests	Comments
Coccidioides immitis	Mononuclear cells (sometimes 10–20% eosinophils); often low glucose	Antibody detection in CSF and serum	Exposure history—southwestern U.S.; increased virulence in dark-skinned races
Candida sp.	Polymorphonuclear or mononuclear	Fungal stain and culture of CSF	IV drug abuse; post surgery; prolonged IV therapy; disseminated candidiasis
Histoplasma capsulatum	Mononuclear cells; low glucose	Fungal stain and culture of large volumes of CSF; antigen detection in CSF, serum, and urine; antibody detection in serum, CSF	Exposure history—Ohio and central Mississippi River Valley; AIDS; mucosal lesions
Blastomyces dermatitidis	Mononuclear cells	Fungal stain and culture of CSF; biopsy and culture of skin, lung lesions; antibody detection in serum	Midwestern and southeastern U.S.; usually systemic infection; abscesses, draining sinus, ulcers
Aspergillus sp.	Mononuclear or polymorpho-nuclear	CSF culture	Sinusitis; granulocytopenia or immunosuppression
Sporothrix schenckii	Mononuclear cells	Antibody detection in CSF and serum; CSF culture	Traumatic inoculation; IV drug use; ulcerated skin lesion
Rare fungal causes			
Xylohypha (formerly *Cladosporium*) *trichoides* and other dark-walled (dematiaceous) fungi such as *Curvularia, Drechslera; Mucor,* and, after water aspiration, *Pseudallescheria boydii*			
Protozoal causes			
Toxoplasma gondii	Mononuclear cells	Biopsy or response to empirical therapy in clinically appropriate context (including presence of antibody in serum)	Usually with intracerebral abscesses; common in HIV-seropositive pts

(continued)

12

TABLE 204-2 INFECTIOUS CAUSES OF CHRONIC MENINGITIS (CONTINUED)

Causative Agent	CSF Formula	Helpful Diagnostic Tests	Risk Factors and Systemic Manifestations
Protozoal causes			
Trypanosomiasis *Trypanosoma gambiense, T. rhodesiense*	Mononuclear cells, elevated protein	Elevated CSF IgM; identification of trypanosomes in CSF and blood smear	Endemic in Africa; chancre, lymphadenopathy; prominent sleep disorder
Rare protozoal causes			
Acanthamoeba sp. causing granulomatous amebic encephalitis and meningoencephalitis in immunocompromised and debilitated individuals. *Balamuthia mandrillaris* causing chronic meningoencephalitis in immunocompetent hosts.			
Helminthic causes			
Cysticercosis (infection with cysts of *Taenia solium*)	Mononuclear cells; may have eosinophils; glucose level may be low	Indirect hemagglutination assay in CSF; ELISA immunoblotting in serum	Usually with multiple cysts in basal meninges and hydrocephalus; cerebral cysts, muscle calcification
Gnathostoma spinigerum	Eosinophils, mononuclear cells	Peripheral eosinophilia	History of eating raw fish; common in Thailand and Japan; subarachnoid hemorrhage; painful radiculopathy
Angiostrongylus cantonensis	Eosinophils, mononuclear cells	Recovery of worms from CSF	History of eating raw shellfish; common in tropical Pacific regions; often benign
Baylisascaris procyonis (raccoon ascarid)	Eosinophils, mononuclear cells		Infection follows accidental ingestion of *B. procyonis* eggs from raccoon feces; fatal meningoencephalitis

Rare helminthic causes

Trichinella spiralis (trichinosis); *Fasciola hepatica* (liver fluke), *Echinococcus* cysts; *Schistosoma* sp. The former may produce a lymphocytic pleocytosis whereas the latter two may produce an eosinophilic response in CSF associated with cerebral cysts (*Echinococcus*) or granulomatous lesions of brain or spinal cord

Viral causes

Mumps	Mononuclear cells	Antibody in serum	No prior mumps or immunization; may produce meningoencephalitis; may persist for 3–4 weeks
Lymphocytic choriomeningitis	Mononuclear cells	Antibody in serum	Contact with rodents or their excreta; may persist for 3–4 weeks
Echovirus	Mononuclear cells; may have low glucose	Virus isolation from CSF	Congenital hypogammaglobulinemia; history of recurrent meningitis
HIV (acute retroviral syndrome)	Mononuclear cells	p24 antigen in serum and CSF; high level of HIV viremia	HIV risk factors; rash, fever, lymphadenopathy; lymphopenia in peripheral blood; syndrome may persist long enough to be considered as "chronic meningitis"; or chronic meningitis may develop in later stages (AIDS) due to HIV
Herpes simplex (HSV)	Mononuclear cells	PCR for HSV, CMV DNA; CSF antibody for HSV, EBV	Recurrent meningitis due to HSV-2 (rarely HSV-1) often associated with genital recurrences; EBV associated with myeloradiculopathy, CMV with polyradiculopathy

Abbreviations: AFB, acid-fast bacillus; CMV, cytomegalovirus; CSF, cerebrospinal fluid; CT, computed tomography; EBV, Epstein-Barr virus; ELISA, enzyme-linked immunosorbent assay; EM, electron microscopy; FTA, fluorescent treponemal antibody absorption test; HSV, herpes simplex virus; MHA-TP, microhemagglutination assay–*T. pallidum*; MRI, magnetic resonance imaging; PAS, periodic acid–Schiff; PCR, polymerase chain reaction; RPR, rapid plasma reagin test; TB, tuberculosis; VDRL, Venereal Disease Research Laboratories test.

TABLE 204-3 NONINFECTIOUS CAUSES OF CHRONIC MENINGITIS

Causative Agents	CSF Formula	Helpful Diagnostic Tests	Risk Factors and Systemic Manifestations
Malignancy	Mononuclear cells, elevated protein, low glucose	Repeated cytologic examination of large volumes of CSF; CSF exam by polarizing microscopy; clonal lymphocyte markers; deposits on nerve roots or meninges seen on myelogram or contrast-enhanced MRI; meningeal biopsy	Metastatic cancer of breast, lung, stomach, or pancreas; melanoma, lymphoma, leukemia; meningeal gliomatosis; meningeal sarcoma; cerebral dysgerminoma; meningeal melanoma or B cell lymphoma
Chemical compounds (may cause recurrent meningitis)	Mononuclear or PMNs, low glucose, elevated protein; xanthochromia from sub-arachnoid hemorrhage in week prior to presentation with "meningitis"	Contrast-enhanced CT scan or MRI Cerebral angiogram to detect aneurysm	History of recent injection into the subarachnoid space; history of sudden onset of headache; recent resection of acoustic neuroma or craniopharyngioma; epidermoid tumor of brain or spine, sometimes with dermoid sinus tract; pituitary apoplexy
Primary Inflammation			
CNS sarcoidosis	Mononuclear cells; elevated protein; often low glucose	Serum and CSF angiotensin-converting enzyme levels; biopsy of extraneural affected tissues or brain lesion/meningeal biopsy	CN palsy, especially of CN VII; hypothalamic dysfunction, especially diabetes insipidus; abnormal chest radiograph; peripheral neuropathy or myopathy
Vogt-Koyanagi-Harada syndrome (recurrent meningitis)	Mononuclear cells		Recurrent meningoencephalitis with uveitis; retinal detachment, alopecia, lightening of eyebrows and lashes, dysacousia, cataracts, glaucoma

Condition	CSF findings	Diagnostic tests	Clinical features
Isolated granulomatous angiitis of the nervous system	Mononuclear cells, elevated protein	Angiography or meningeal biopsy	Subacute dementia; multiple cerebral infarctions; recent zoster ophthalmicus
Systemic lupus erythematosus	Mononuclear or PMNs	Anti-DNA antibody, antinuclear antibodies	Encephalopathy; seizures; stroke; transverse myelopathy; rash; arthritis
Behçet's syndrome (recurrent meningitis)	Mononuclear or PMNs, elevated protein		Oral and genital aphthous ulcers; iridocyclitis; retinal hemorrhages; pathergic lesions at site of skin puncture
Chronic benign lymphocytic meningitis	Mononuclear cells		Recovery in 2–6 months, diagnosis by exclusion
Mollaret's meningitis (recurrent meningitis)	Large endothelial cells and PMNs in first hours, followed by mononuclear cells	PCR for herpes; MRI/CT to rule out epidermoid tumor or dural cyst	Recurrent meningitis; exclude HSV-2; rare cases due to HSV-1; occasional case associated with dural cyst
Drug hypersensitivity	PMNs; occasionally mononuclear cells or eosinophils	Complete blood count (eosinophilia)	Exposure to non steroidal anti-inflammatory agents, sulfonamides, isoniazid, tolmetin, ciprofloxacin, penicillin, carbamazepine, lamotrigine, IV immunoglobulin, OKT3 antibodies, phenazopyridine; improvement after discontinuation of drug; recurrence with repeat exposure
Granulomatosis with polyangiitis (Wegener's)	Mononuclear cells	Chest and sinus radiographs; urinalysis; ANCA antibodies in serum	Associated sinus, pulmonary, or renal lesions; CN palsies; skin lesions; peripheral neuropathy

Other: multiple sclerosis, Sjögren's syndrome, neonatal-onset multisystemic inflammatory disease (NOMID), and rarer forms of vasculitis (e.g., Cogan's syndrome)

Abbreviations: ANCA, anti-neutrophil cytoplasmic antibodies; CN, cranial nerve; CSF, cerebrospinal fluid; CT, computed tomography; HSV, herpes simplex virus; MRI, magnetic resonance imaging; PCR, polymerase chain reaction; PMNs, polymorphonuclear cells.

lymphocytic meningitis at tuberculosis, particularly if the condition is associated with hypoglycorrhachia and sixth and other cranial nerve palsies, since untreated disease can be fatal in 4–8 weeks. Carcinomatous or lymphomatous meningitis may be difficult to diagnose initially, but the diagnosis becomes evident with time. Important causes of chronic meningitis in AIDS pts include infection with *Toxoplasma* (usually presents as intracranial abscesses), *Cryptococcus*, *Nocardia*, *Candida*, or other fungi; syphilis; and lymphoma.

For a more detailed discussion, see Koroshetz WJ, Swartz MN: Chronic and Recurrent Meningitis, Chap. 382, p. 3435, in HPIM-18.

CHAPTER **205**

Peripheral Neuropathies Including Guillain-Barré Syndrome (GBS)

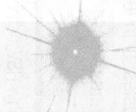

APPROACH TO THE PATIENT Peripheral Neuropathy

Peripheral neuropathy (PN) refers to a peripheral nerve disorder of any cause. Nerve involvement may be single (mononeuropathy) or multiple (polyneuropathy); pathology may be axonal or demyelinating. An approach to pts with suspected neuropathy appears in Fig. 205-1.

Address the following seven initial questions:

1. *What systems are involved?* It is important to determine if the pt's symptoms and signs are motor, sensory, autonomic, or a combination of these. If only weakness is present without any evidence of sensory or autonomic dysfunction, consider a motor neuropathy, neuromuscular junction disorder, or myopathy; myopathies usually have a proximal, symmetric pattern of weakness.

2. *What is the distribution of weakness?* Polyneuropathy involves widespread and symmetric dysfunction of the peripheral nerves that is usually distal more than proximal; mononeuropathy involves a single nerve usually due to trauma or compression; multiple mononeuropathies (mononeuropathy multiplex) can be a result of multiple entrapments, vasculitis, or infiltration.

3. *What is the nature of the sensory involvement?* Temperature loss or burning/stabbing pain suggests small fiber involvement. Vibratory or proprioceptive loss implicates large fibers.

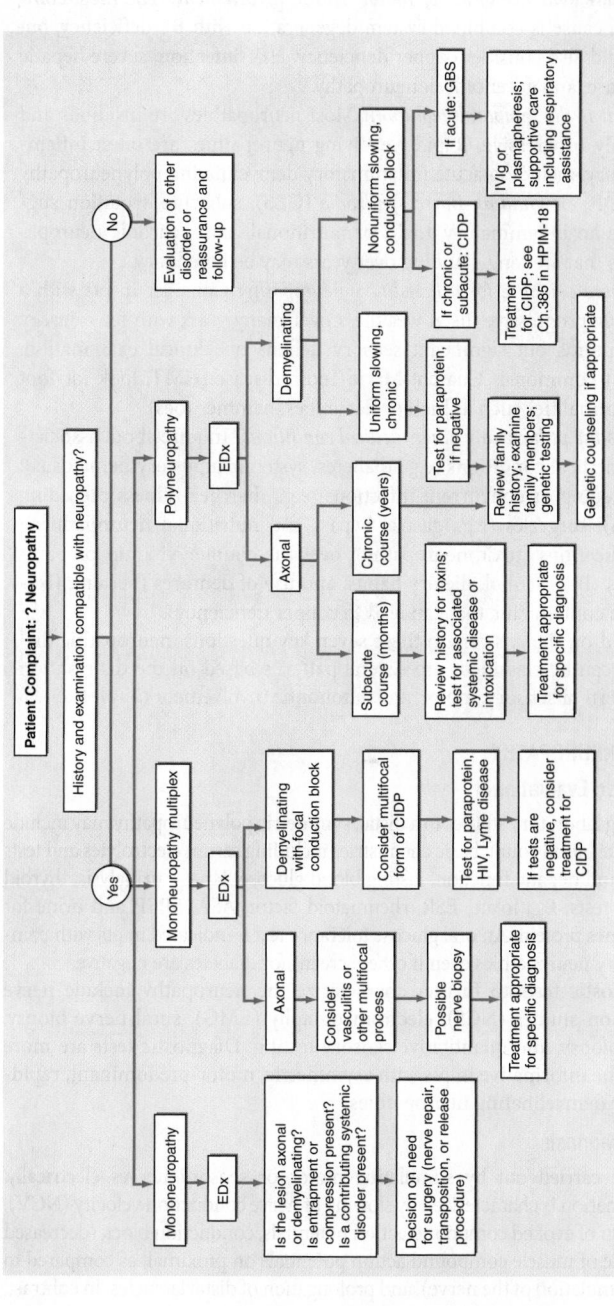

FIGURE 205-1 Approach to evaluation of peripheral neuropathies. CIDP, chronic inflammatory demyelinating polyradiculoneuropathy; EDX, electrodiagnostic studies; GBS, Guillain-Barré syndrome; IVIg, intravenous immunoglobulin.

4. *Is there evidence of upper motor neuron involvement?* The most common cause is combined system degeneration with B$_{12}$ deficiency, but should also consider copper deficiency, HIV infection, severe hepatic disease, and adrenomyeloneuropathy.

5. *What is the temporal evolution?* Most neuropathies are insidious and slowly progressive. Rapidly evolving neuropathies are often inflammatory, including acute inflammatory demyelinating polyneuropathy (AIDP) or *Guillain-Barré syndrome* (GBS); subacute evolution suggests an inflammatory, toxic, or nutritional cause; chronic neuropathies that are long-standing over years may be hereditary.

6. *Is there evidence for a hereditary neuropathy?* Consider in pts with a slowly progressive distal weakness over many years with few sensory symptoms but significant sensory deficits on clinical examination. Most common is Charcot-Marie-Tooth disease (CMT; look for foot abnormalities such as high or flat arches, hammer toes).

7. *Does the pt have any other medical conditions?* Inquire about associated medical conditions (e.g., diabetes, systemic lupus erythematosus); preceding or concurrent infections (e.g., diarrheal illness preceding GBS); surgeries (e.g., gastric bypass and nutritional neuropathies); medications (toxic neuropathy); over-the-counter vitamin preparations (B$_6$); alcohol, dietary habits; and use of dentures (because fixatives contain zinc that can lead to copper deficiency).

Based on the answers to these seven key questions, neuropathic disorders can be classified into several patterns based on the distribution or pattern of sensory, motor, and autonomic involvement (Table 205-1).

▪ POLYNEUROPATHY

Diagnostic Evaluation

Screening laboratory studies in a distal, symmetric polyneuropathy may include a complete blood count, basic chemistries including serum electrolytes and tests of renal and hepatic function, fasting blood glucose, HbA$_{1c}$, urinalysis, thyroid function tests, B$_{12}$, folate, ESR, rheumatoid factor, ASA, SPEP, and urine for Bence Jones protein. An oral glucose tolerance test is indicated in pts with painful sensory neuropathies even if other screens for diabetes are negative.

Diagnostic tests to further characterize the neuropathy include nerve conduction studies (NCS), electromyography (EMG), sural nerve biopsy, muscle biopsy, and quantitative sensory testing. Diagnostic tests are more likely to be informative in pts with asymmetric, motor-predominant, rapid-onset, or demyelinating neuropathies.

Electrodiagnosis

NCS are carried out by stimulating motor or sensory nerves electrically. Demyelination is characterized by slowing of nerve conduction velocity (NCV), dispersion of evoked compound action potentials, conduction block (decreased amplitude of muscle compound action potentials on proximal, as compared to distal, stimulation of the nerve), and prolongation of distal latencies. In contrast, axonal neuropathies exhibit reduced amplitude of evoked compound action potentials with relative preservation of NCV. EMG records electrical potentials

TABLE 205-1 PATTERNS OF NEUROPATHIC DISORDERS

Pattern 1: Symmetric proximal and distal weakness with sensory loss

Consider: inflammatory demyelinating polyneuropathy (GBS and CIDP)

Pattern 2: Symmetric distal sensory loss with or without distal weakness

Consider: cryptogenic or idiopathic sensory polyneuropathy (CSPN), diabetes mellitus and other metabolic disorders, drugs, toxins, hereditary (Charcot-Marie-Tooth, amyloidosis, and others)

Pattern 3: Asymmetric distal weakness with sensory loss

With involvement of multiple nerves

Consider: multifocal CIDP, vasculitis, cryoglobulinemia, amyloidosis, sarcoid, infectious (leprosy, Lyme, hepatitis B or C, HIV, CMV), hereditary neuropathy with liability to pressure palsies (HNPP), tumor infiltration

With involvement of single nerves/regions

Consider: may be any of the above but also could be compressive mononeuropathy, plexopathy, or radiculopathy

Pattern 4: Asymmetric proximal and distal weakness with sensory loss

Consider: polyradiculopathy or plexopathy due to diabetes mellitus, meningeal carcinomatosis or lymphomatosis, hereditary plexopathy (HNPP, HNA), idiopathic

Pattern 5: Asymmetric distal weakness without sensory loss

With upper motor neuron findings

Consider: motor neuron disease

Without upper motor neuron findings

Consider: progressive muscular atrophy, juvenile monomelic amyotrophy (Hirayama disease), multifocal motor neuropathy, multifocal acquired motor axonopathy

Pattern 6: Symmetric sensory loss and distal areflexia with upper motor neuron findings

Consider: Vitamin B_{12}, vitamin E, and copper deficiency with combined system degeneration with peripheral neuropathy, hereditary leukodystrophies (e.g., adrenomyeloneuropathy)

Pattern 7: Symmetric weakness without sensory loss

With proximal and distal weakness

Consider: spinal muscular atrophy

With distal weakness

Consider: hereditary motor neuropathy ("distal" SMA) or atypical CMT

Pattern 8: Asymmetric proprioceptive sensory loss without weakness

Consider causes of a sensory neuronopathy (ganglionopathy):

Cancer (paraneoplastic)

Sjögren's syndrome

Idiopathic sensory neuronopathy (possible GBS variant)

(*continued*)

TABLE 205-1 PATTERNS OF NEUROPATHIC DISORDERS (CONTINUED)

Pattern 8: Asymmetric proprioceptive sensory loss without weakness
Cisplatin and other chemotherapeutic agents
Vitamin B_6 toxicity
HIV-related sensory neuronopathy

Pattern 9: Autonomic symptoms and signs
Consider neuropathies associated with prominent autonomic dysfunction:
Hereditary sensory and autonomic neuropathy
Amyloidosis (familial and acquired)
Diabetes mellitus
Idiopathic pandysautonomia (may be a variant of Guillain-Barré syndrome)
Porphyria
HIV-related autonomic neuropathy
Vincristine and other chemotherapeutic agents

Abbreviations: CIDP, chronic inflammatory demyelinating polyneuropathy; CMT, Charcot-Marie-Tooth disease; CMV, cytomegalovirus; GBS, Guillain-Barré syndrome; HIV, human immunodeficiency virus; HNA, hereditary neuralgic amyotrophy; SMA, spinal muscular atrophy.

from a needle electrode in muscle, at rest and during voluntary contraction; it is most useful for distinguishing myopathic from neuropathic disorders. Myopathic disorders are marked by small, short-duration, polyphasic muscle action potentials; by contrast, neuropathic disorders are characterized by muscle denervation. Denervation decreases the number of motor units (e.g., an anterior horn cell, its axon, and the motor end plates and muscle fibers it innervates). In long-standing denervation, motor unit potentials become large and polyphasic due to collateral reinnervation of denervated muscle fibers by axonal sprouts from surviving motor axons. Other EMG features of denervation include fibrillations (random, unregulated firing of individual muscle fibers) and fasciculations (random, spontaneous firing of motor units).

TREATMENT   Polyneuropathy

- Treatment of the underlying disorder, pain management, and supportive care to protect and rehabilitate damaged tissue all need to be considered.
- Examples of specific therapies include tight glycemic control in diabetic neuropathy, vitamin replacement for B_{12} deficiency, IV immune globulin (IVIg) or plasmapheresis for GBS, and immunosuppression for vasculitis.
- Painful sensory neuropathies can be difficult to treat. Pain management usually begins with tricyclic antidepressants (TCAs), duloxetine hydrochloride, lidocaine patches, or anticonvulsants such as gabapentin (Table 205-2). Topical anesthetic agents including EMLA (lidocaine/prilocaine) and capsaicin cream can provide additional relief.

TABLE 205-2 TREATMENT OF PAINFUL SENSORY NEUROPATHIES

Therapy	Route	Dose	Side Effects
First-line			
Lidocaine 5% patch	Apply to painful area	Up to 3 patches qd	Skin irritation
Tricyclic antidepressants (e.g., amitriptyline, nortriptyline)	PO	10–100 mg qhs	Cognitive changes, sedation, dry eyes and mouth, urinary retention, constipation
Gabapentin	PO	300–1200 mg tid	Cognitive changes, sedation, peripheral edema
Pregabalin	PO	50–100 mg tid	Cognitive changes, sedation, peripheral edema
Duloxetine	PO	30–60 mg qd	Cognitive changes, sedation, dry eyes, diaphoresis, nausea, diarrhea, constipation
Second-line			
Carbamazepine	PO	200–400 mg q 6–8 h	Cognitive changes, dizziness, leukopenia, liver dysfunction
Phenytoin	PO	200–400 mg qhs	Cognitive changes, dizziness, liver dysfunction
Venlafaxine	PO	37.5–150 mg/d	Asthenia, sweating, nausea, constipation, anorexia, vomiting, somnolence, dry mouth, dizziness, nervousness, anxiety, tremor, and blurred vision as well as abnormal ejaculation/orgasm and impotence
Tramadol	PO	50 mg qid	Cognitive changes, GI upset
Third-line			
Mexiletine	PO	200–300 mg tid	Arrhythmias
Other agents			
EMLA cream 2.5% lidocaine 2.5% prilocaine	Cutaneous	qid	Local erythema
Capsaicin 0.025%–0.075% cream	Cutaneous	qid	Painful burning skin

Source: Modified from Amato AA, Russell J: *Neuromuscular Disease.* New York, McGraw-Hill, 2008.

- Physical and occupational therapy is important. Proper care of dener-vated areas prevents skin ulceration, which can lead to poor wound healing, tissue resorption, arthropathy, and ultimately amputation.

Specific Polyneuropathies

AIDP or *GBS*: an ascending, usually demyelinating, motor > sensory polyneu-ropathy accompanied by areflexia, motor paralysis, and elevated CSF **total** protein without pleocytosis. Over two-thirds are preceded by an acute respiratory or gastrointestinal infection. Maximum weakness is usually reached within 2 weeks; demyelination by EMG. Most pts are hospitalized; one-third require ventilatory assistance. 85% make a complete or near-complete recovery with supportive care. Variants of GBS include Fisher syndrome (ophthalmo-paresis, facial diplegia, ataxia, areflexia; associated with serum antibodies to ganglioside GQ1b) and acute motor axonal neuropathy (more severe course than demyelinating GBS; antibodies to GM_1 in some cases).

- IVIg (2 g/kg divided over 5 days) or plasmapheresis (40–50 mL/kg daily for 4–5 days) significantly shortens the course.
- Glucocorticoids are ineffective.

Chronic inflammatory demyelinating polyneuropathy (CIDP): a slowly pro-gressive or relapsing polyneuropathy characterized by diffuse hyporeflexia or areflexia, diffuse weakness, elevated CSF protein without pleocytosis, and demyelination by EMG.

- Begin treatment when progression is rapid or walking is compromised.
- Initial treatment is usually IVIg; most pts require periodic re-treatment at 4- to 6-week intervals.
- Other first-line treatment options include plasmapheresis or glucocorticoids
- Immunosuppressants (azathioprine, methotrexate, cyclosporine, cyclo-phosphamide) used in refractory cases.

Diabetic neuropathy: typically a distal symmetric, sensorimotor, axonal poly-neuropathy. A mixture of demyelination and axonal loss is frequent. Other variants include: isolated sixth or third cranial nerve palsies, asymmetric proximal motor neuropathy in the legs, truncal neuropathy, autonomic neu-ropathy, and an increased frequency of entrapment neuropathy (see below).

Mononeuropathy multiplex (MM): defined as involvement of multiple individual peripheral nerves. When an inflammatory disorder is the cause, *mononeuritis multiplex* is the term used. Both systemic (67%) and nonsys-temic (33%) vasculitis may present as MM. Immunosuppressive treatment of the underlying disease (usually with glucocorticoids and cyclophos-phamide) is indicated. A tissue diagnosis of vasculitis should be obtained before initiating treatment; a positive biopsy helps to justify the necessary long-term treatment with immunosuppressive medications, and pathologic confirmation is difficult after treatment has commenced.

■ MONONEUROPATHY

Clinical Features

Mononeuropathies are usually caused by trauma, compression, or entrap-ment. Sensory and motor symptoms are in the distribution of a single

TABLE 205-3   MONONEUROPATHIES

	Symptoms	Precipitating Activities	Examination	Electro-Diagnosis	Differential Diagnosis	Treatment
Carpal tunnel syndrome	Numbness, pain or paresthesias in fingers	Sleep or repetitive hand activity	Sensory loss in thumb, second, and third fingers Weakness in thenar muscles; inability to make a circle with thumb and index finger Tinel sign, Phalen maneuver	Slowing of sensory and motor conduction across carpal tunnel	C6 radiculopathy	Splint Surgery definitive treatment
Ulnar nerve entrapment at the elbow (UNE)	Numbness or paresthesias in ulnar aspect of hand	Elbow flexion during sleep; elbow resting on desk	Sensory loss in the little finger and ulnar half of ring finger Weakness of the interossei and thumb adductor; claw-hand	Focal slowing of nerve conduction velocity at the elbow	Thoracic outlet syndrome C8-T1 radiculopathy	Elbow pads Avoid further injury Surgery when conservative treatment fails
Ulnar nerve entrapment at the wrist	Numbness or weakness in the ulnar distribution in the hand	Unusual hand activities with tools, bicycling	Like UNE but sensory examination spares dorsum of the hand, and selected hand muscles affected	Prolongation of distal motor latency in the hand	UNE	Avoid precipitating activities

(continued)

TABLE 205-3 MONONEUROPATHIES (CONTINUED)

	Symptoms	Precipitating Activities	Examination	Electro-Diagnosis	Differential Diagnosis	Treatment
Radial neuropathy at the spiral groove	Wrist drop	Sleeping on arm after inebriation with alcohol—"Saturday night palsy"	Wrist drop with sparing of elbow extension (triceps spared); finger and thumb extensors paralyzed; sensory loss in radial region of wrist	Early—conduction block along the spiral groove Late—denervation in radial muscles; reduced radial SNAP	Posterior cord lesion; deltoid also weak Posterior interosseous nerve (PIN); isolated finger drop C7 radiculopathy	Splint Spontaneous recovery provided no ongoing injury
Thoracic outlet syndrome	Numbness, paresthesias in medial arm, forearm, hand, and fingers	Lifting heavy objects with the hand	Sensory loss resembles ulnar nerve and motor loss resembles median nerve	Absent ulnar sensory response and reduced median motor response	UNE	Surgery if correctable lesion present
Femoral neuropathy	Buckling of knee, numbness or tingling in thigh/medial leg	Abdominal hysterectomy; lithotomy position; hematoma, diabetes	Wasting and weakness of quadriceps; absent knee jerk; sensory loss in medial thigh and lower leg	EMG of quadriceps, iliopsoas, paraspinal muscles, adductor muscles	L2-4 radiculopathy Lumbar plexopathy	Physiotherapy to strengthen quadriceps and mobilize hip joint Surgery if needed
Obturator neuropathy	Weakness of the leg, thigh numbness	Stretch during hip surgery; pelvic fracture; childbirth	Weakness of hip adductors; sensory loss in upper medial thigh	EMG—denervation limited to hip adductors sparing the quadriceps	L3-4 radiculopathy Lumbar plexopathy	Conservative management Surgery if needed

Meralgia paresthetica	Pain or numbness in the anterior lateral thigh	Standing or walking; Recent weight gain	Sensory loss in the pant pocket distribution	Sometimes slowing of sensory response can be demonstrated across the inguinal ligament	L2 radiculopathy	Usually resolves spontaneously
Peroneal nerve entrapment at the fibular head	Footdrop	Usually an acute compressive episode identifiable; weight loss	Weak dorsiflexion, eversion of the foot; Sensory loss in the anterolateral leg and dorsum of the foot	Focal slowing of nerve conduction across fibular head; Denervation in tibialis anterior and peroneus longus muscles	L5 radiculopathy	Foot brace; remove external source of compression
Sciatic neuropathy	Flail foot and numbness in foot	Injection injury; fracture/dislocation of hip; prolonged pressure on hip (comatose pt)	Weakness of hamstring, plantar and dorsiflexion of foot; sensory loss in tibial and peroneal nerve distribution	NCS—abnormal sural, peroneal, and tibial amplitudes; EMG—denervation in sciatic nerve distribution sparing glutei and paraspinal	L5-S1 radiculopathies; Common peroneal neuropathy (partial sciatic nerve injury); LS plexopathies	Conservative follow up for partial sciatic nerve injuries; Brace and physiotherapy; Surgical exploration if needed
Tarsal tunnel syndrome	Pain and paresthesias in the sole of the foot but not in the heel	At the end of the day after standing or walking; nocturnal	Sensory loss in the sole of the foot; Tinel sign at tarsal tunnel	Reduced amplitude in sensory or motor components of medial and planter nerves	Polyneuropathy, foot deformity, poor circulation	Surgery if no external cause identified

nerve—most commonly the ulnar or median nerve in the arm or peroneal nerve in the leg. Intrinsic factors making pts more susceptible to entrapment include arthritis, fluid retention (pregnancy), amyloid, tumors, and diabetes mellitus. Clinical features favoring conservative management of median neuropathy at the wrist (carpal tunnel syndrome) or ulnar neuropathy at the elbow include sudden onset, no motor deficit, few or no sensory findings (pain or paresthesias may be present), and no evidence of axonal loss by EMG. Surgical decompression is considered for chronic mononeuropathies that are unresponsive to conservative treatment, if the site of entrapment is clearly defined. The most frequently encountered mononeuropathies are summarized in Table 205-3.

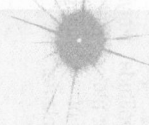

For a more detailed discussion, see Amato AA, Barohn RJ: Peripheral Neuropathy, Chap. 384, p. 3448; and Hauser SL, Amato AA: Guillain-Barré Syndrome and Other Immune-Mediated Neuropathies, Chap. 385, p. 3473, in HPIM-18.

CHAPTER **206**
Myasthenia Gravis (MG)

An autoimmune neuromuscular disorder resulting in weakness and fatigability of skeletal muscles, due to autoantibodies directed against acetylcholine receptors (AChRs) at neuromuscular junctions (NMJs).

■ CLINICAL FEATURES

May present at any age. Symptoms fluctuate throughout the day and are provoked by exertion. Characteristic distribution: cranial muscles (eyelids, extraocular muscles, facial weakness, "nasal" or slurred speech, dysphagia); in 85%, limb muscles (often proximal and asymmetric) become involved. Reflexes and sensation normal. May be limited to extraocular muscles only. Complications: aspiration pneumonia (weak bulbar muscles), respiratory failure (weak chest wall muscles), exacerbation of myasthenia due to administration of drugs with neuromuscular junction blocking effects (quinolones, macrolides, aminoglycosides, procainamide, propranolol, nondepolarizing muscle relaxants).

■ PATHOPHYSIOLOGY

Anti-AChR antibodies reduce the number of available AChRs at the NMJ. Postsynaptic folds are flattened or "simplified," with resulting inefficient neuromuscular transmission. During repeated or sustained muscle contraction, decrease in amount of ACh released per nerve impulse ("presynaptic rundown," a normal occurrence), combined with disease-specific decrease in postsynaptic AChRs, results in pathologic fatigue. Thymus is abnormal in 75% of pts (65% hyperplasia, 10% thymoma). Other autoimmune diseases may coexist: Hashimoto's thyroiditis, Graves' disease, rheumatoid arthritis, systemic lupus erythematosus.

■ DIFFERENTIAL DIAGNOSIS

Lambert-Eaton syndrome (autoantibodies to calcium channels in presynaptic motor nerve terminals)—reduced ACh release; may be associated with malignancy

Neurasthenia—weakness/fatigue without underlying organic disorder

Drug-induced myasthenia—penicillamine may cause MG; resolves weeks to months after discontinuing drug

Botulism—toxin inhibits presynaptic ACh release; most common form is food-borne.

Diplopia from an intracranial mass lesion—compression of nerves to extra-ocular muscles or brainstem lesions affecting cranial nerve nuclei

Hyperthyroidism

Progressive external ophthalmoplegia—seen in rare mitochondrial disorders that can be detected with muscle biopsy

■ LABORATORY EVALUATION

- AChR antibodies—levels do not correlate with disease severity; 85% of all MG pts are positive; only 50% with pure ocular findings are positive; positive antibodies are diagnostic. Muscle-specific kinase (MuSK) antibodies present in 40% of AChR antibody–negative pts with generalized MG.
- Tensilon (edrophonium) test—a short-acting anticholinesterase—look for rapid and transient improvement of strength; false-positive (placebo response, motor neuron disease) and false-negative tests occur. Atropine IV should be on hand if symptoms such as bradycardia occur.
- EMG—low-frequency (2–4 Hz) repetitive stimulation produces rapid decrement in amplitude (>10–15%) of evoked motor responses.
- Chest CT/MRI—search for thymoma.
- Consider thyroid and other studies (e.g., ANA) for associated autoimmune disease.
- Measurements of baseline respiratory function are useful.

TREATMENT	Myasthenia Gravis (See Fig. 206-1)

- The anticholinesterase drug pyridostigmine (Mestinon) titrated to assist pt with functional activities (chewing, swallowing, strength during exertion); usual initial dose of 30–60 mg 3–4 times daily; long-acting tablets help at night but have variable absorption so are not reliable during the day. Muscarinic side effects (diarrhea, abdominal cramps, salivation, nausea) blocked with atropine/diphenoxylate or loperamide if required.
- Plasmapheresis or IV immune globulin (IVIg; 400 mg/kg per day for 5 days) provides temporary boost for seriously ill pts; used to improve condition prior to surgery or during myasthenic crisis (see below).
- Thymectomy improves likelihood of long-term remission in adult pts (~85% improve; of these, ~35% achieve drug-free remission); benefit is usually delayed by months to years; whether it helps those with pure ocular disease, children, or those age >55 remains unclear.

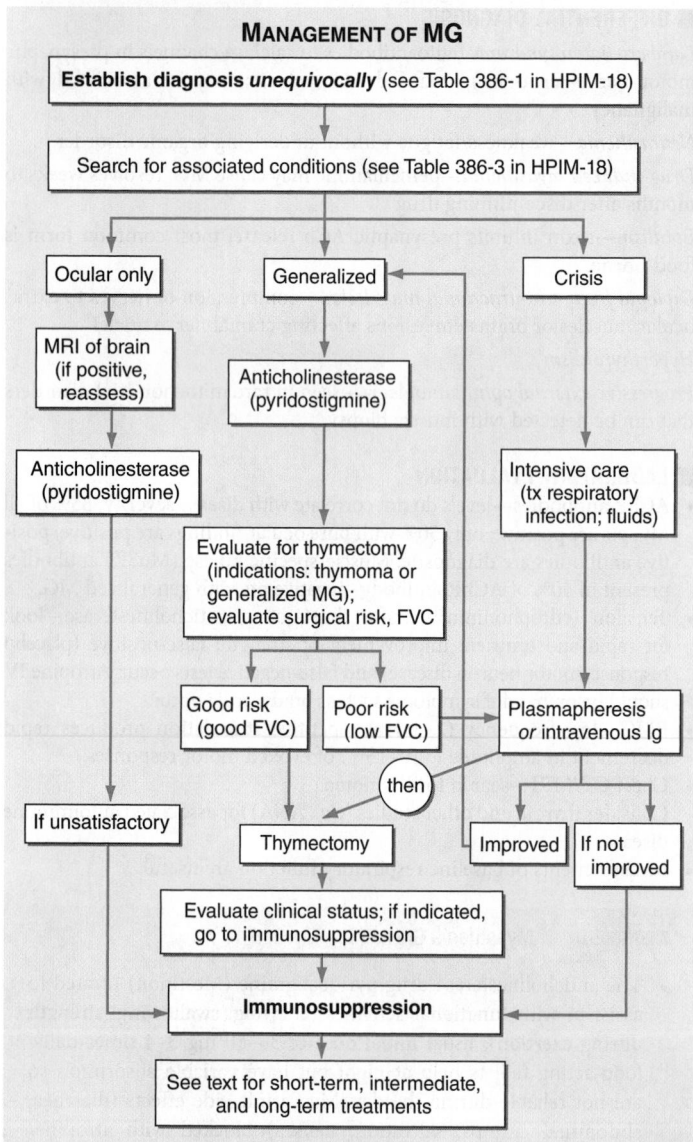

FIGURE 206-1 Algorithm for the management of myasthenia gravis. FVC, forced vital capacity.

- Glucocorticoids are a mainstay of chronic immunosuppressive treatment; begin prednisone at low dose (15–25 mg/d), increase by 5 mg/d every 2–3 days until marked clinical improvement or dose of 50–60 mg/d is reached. Maintain high dose for 1–3 months, then decrease to alternate-day regimen. Immunosuppressive drugs (mycophenolate mofetil, azathioprine, cyclosporine, tacrolimus, cyclophosphamide) may spare dose of prednisone required long-term to control symptoms.
- Myasthenic crisis is defined as an exacerbation of weakness, usually with respiratory failure, sufficient to endanger life; expert management in an intensive care setting essential as is prompt treatment with IVIg or plasmapheresis to hasten recovery.
- A number of drugs may exacerbate MG, potentially leading to crisis, and therefore should be avoided (Table 206-1).

TABLE 206-1 DRUGS WITH INTERACTIONS IN MYASTHENIA GRAVIS (MG)

Drugs That May Exacerbate MG
Antibiotics
Aminoglycosides: e.g., streptomycin, tobramycin, kanamycin
Quinolones: e.g., ciprofloxacin, levofloxacin, ofloxacin, gatifloxacin
Macrolides: e.g., erythromycin, azithromycin
Nondepolarizing muscle relaxants for surgery
D-Tubocurarine (curare), pancuronium, vecuronium, atracurium
Beta-blocking agents
Propranolol, atenolol, metoprolol
Local anesthetics and related agents
Procaine, lidocaine in large amounts
Procainamide (for arrhythmias)
Botulinum toxin
Botulinum toxin exacerbates weakness
Quinine derivatives
Quinine, quinidine, chloroquine, mefloquine (Lariam)
Magnesium
Decreases ACh release
Penicillamine
May cause MG

Drugs with Important Interactions in MG
Cyclosporine
Broad range of drug interactions, which may raise or lower cyclosporine levels
Azathioprine
Avoid allopurinol—combination may result in myelosuppression

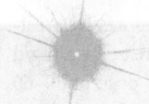

For a more detailed discussion, see Drachman DB: Myasthenia Gravis and Other Diseases of the Neuromuscular Junction, Chap. 386, p. 3480, in HPIM-18.

CHAPTER **207**
Muscle Diseases

APPROACH TO THE PATIENT | **Muscle Disease**

Muscle diseases (*myopathies*) may be intermittent or persistent and usually present with proximal, symmetric weakness with preserved reflexes and sensation. An associated sensory loss suggests injury to peripheral nerve or the central nervous system rather than myopathy; on occasion, disorders affecting the anterior horn cells, the neuromuscular junction, or peripheral nerves can mimic myopathy. Any disorder causing muscle weakness may be accompanied by *fatigue*, referring to an inability to maintain or sustain a force; this must be distinguished from asthenia, a type of fatigue caused by excess tiredness or lack of energy. Fatigue without abnormal clinical or laboratory findings almost never indicates a true myopathy.

Muscle disorders are usually painless; however, *myalgias*, or muscle pains, may occur. Myalgias must be distinguished from *muscle cramps*, i.e., painful, involuntary muscle contractions, usually due to neurogenic disorders. A *muscle contracture* due to an inability to relax after an active muscle contraction is associated with energy failure in glycolytic disorders. *Myotonia* is a condition of prolonged muscle contraction followed by slow muscle relaxation.

A limited battery of tests can be used to evaluate a suspected myopathy. CK is the preferred muscle enzyme to measure in the evaluation of myopathies. Electrodiagnostic studies (nerve conduction studies and electromyography, NCS-EMG) are usually necessary to distinguish myopathies from neuropathies and neuromuscular junction disorders. An approach to muscle weakness is presented in Figs. 207-1 and 207-2.

MUSCULAR DYSTROPHIES

A varied group of inherited, progressive degenerations of muscle, each with unique features.

■ DUCHENNE'S MUSCULAR DYSTROPHY

X-linked recessive mutation of the dystrophin gene that affects males almost exclusively. Progressive weakness in hip and shoulder girdle muscles beginning by age 5; by age 12, the majority are nonambulatory. Survival beyond age 25 is rare. Associated problems include tendon and muscle

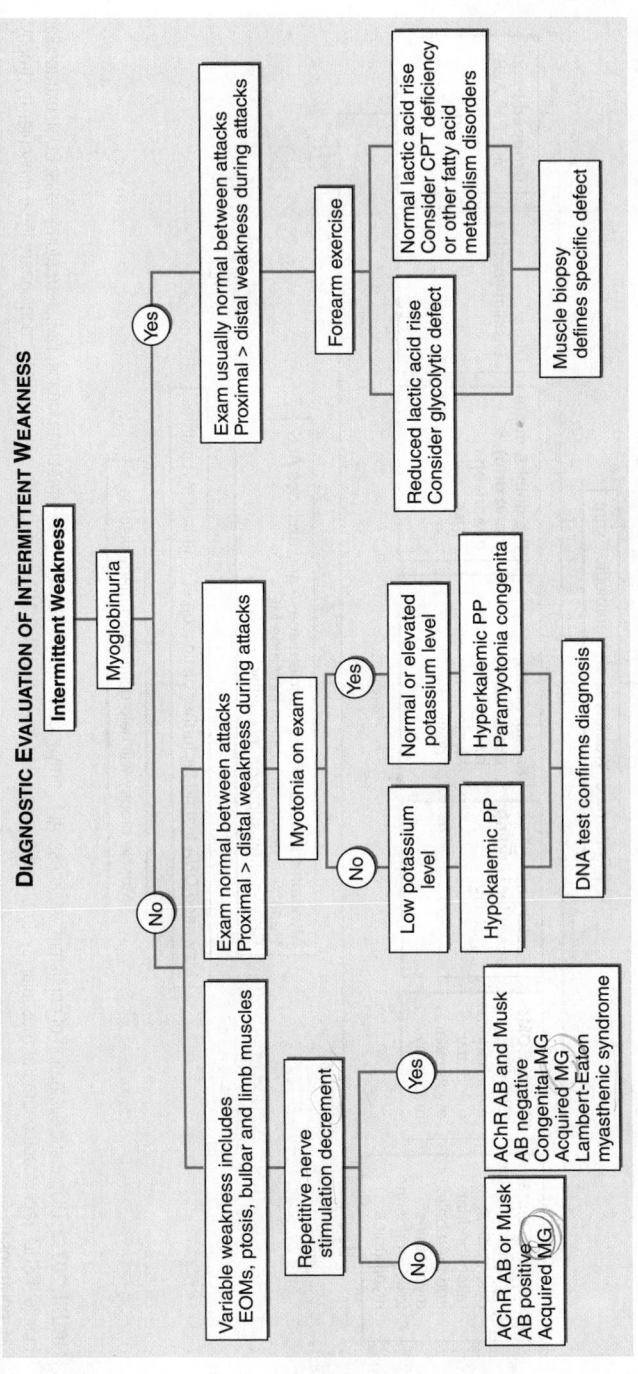

FIGURE 207-1 Diagnostic evaluation of intermittent weakness. AChR AB, acetylcholine receptor antibody; CPT, carnitine palmityl transferase; EOMs, extraocular muscles; MG, myasthenia gravis; PP, periodic paralysis.

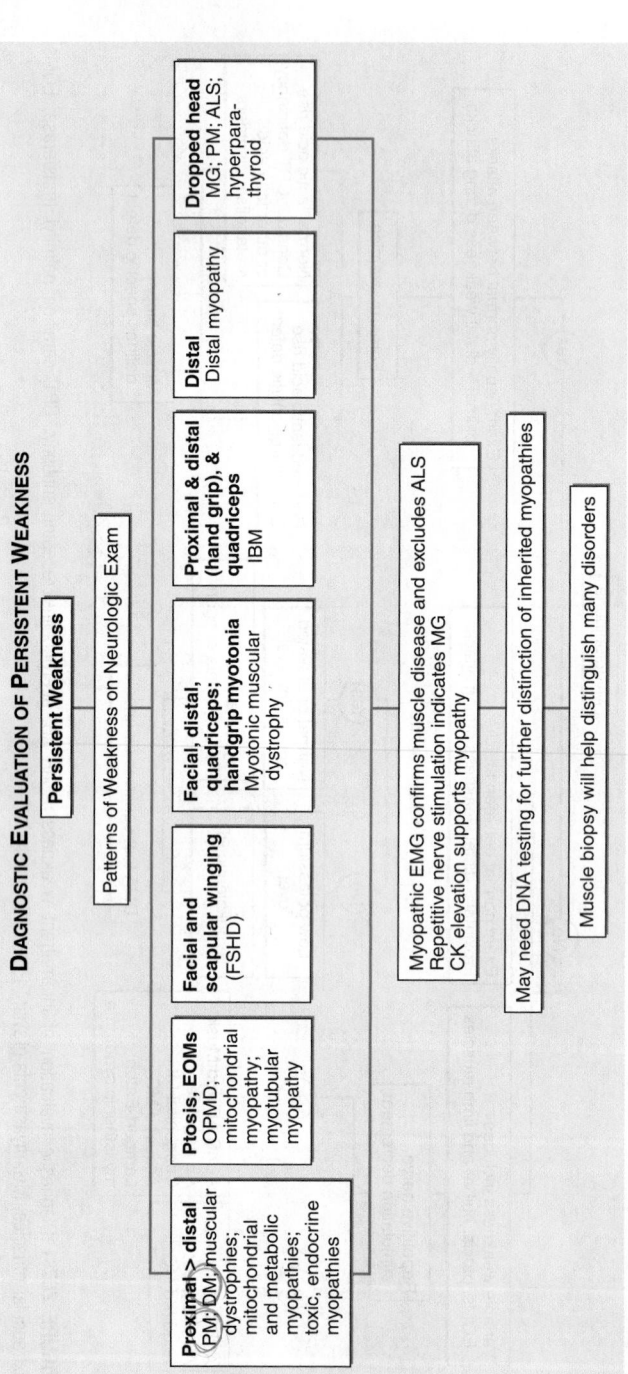

FIGURE 207-2 Diagnostic evaluation of persistent weakness. ALS, amyotrophic lateral sclerosis; CK, creatinine kinase; DM, dermatomyositis; EOM, extraocular muscle; FSHD, facioscapulohumeral muscular dystrophy; IBM, inclusion body myositis; MG, myasthenia gravis; OPMD, oculopharyngeal muscular dystrophy; PM, polymyositis.

contractures, progressive kyphoscoliosis, impaired pulmonary function, cardiomyopathy, and intellectual impairment. Palpable enlargement and firmness of some muscles. Becker dystrophy is a less severe form, with a slower course and later age of onset (5–15 yrs) but similar clinical, laboratory, and genetic features.

Laboratory findings include massive elevations (20–100 × normal) of serum CK, a myopathic pattern on EMG testing, and evidence of groups of necrotic muscle fibers with regeneration, phagocytosis, and fatty replacement of muscle on biopsy. Diagnosis is established by determination of dystrophin deficiency in muscle tissue or mutation analysis on peripheral blood leukocytes. Testing is available for detecting carriers and prenatal diagnosis.

TREATMENT Duchenne's Muscular Dystrophy

- Treatment is with glucocorticoids [prednisone (0.75 mg/kg)/d]. These slow progression of disease for up to 3 years; some pts cannot tolerate this therapy due to weight gain and increased risk of fractures.

■ LIMB-GIRDLE DYSTROPHY

A constellation of diseases with proximal weakness involving the pelvic and shoulder girdle musculature. Age of onset, rate of progression, severity of manifestations, inheritance pattern (autosomal dominant or autosomal recessive), and associated complications (e.g., cardiac, respiratory) vary with the specific subtype of disease.

■ MYOTONIC DYSTROPHY

Type 1 is an autosomal dominant disorder with genetic anticipation. Weakness typically becomes obvious in the second to third decade and initially involves the muscles of the face, neck, and distal extremities. This results in a distinctive facial appearance ("hatchet face") characterized by ptosis, temporal wasting, drooping of the lower lip, and sagging of the jaw. Myotonia manifests as a peculiar inability to relax muscles rapidly following a strong exertion (e.g., after tight hand grip) usually by the age of 5, as well as by sustained contraction of muscles following percussion (e.g., of tongue or thenar eminence).

Associated problems can include frontal baldness, posterior subcapsular cataracts, gonadal atrophy, respiratory and cardiac problems, endocrine abnormalities, intellectual impairment, and hypersomnia. Cardiac disturbances, including complete heart block, may be life-threatening. Respiratory function should be carefully followed, as chronic hypoxia may lead to cor pulmonale.

Laboratory studies show normal or mildly elevated CK, characteristic myotonia and myopathic features on EMG, and a typical pattern of muscle fiber injury on biopsy, including selective type I fiber atrophy in 50% of cases. Pts with myotonic dystrophy type 1 have an unstable region of DNA with an increased number of trinucleotide CTG repeats on chromosome 19q13.3 in a protein kinase gene. Genetic testing for early detection and prenatal diagnosis is possible.

TREATMENT   Myotonic Dystrophy

- Phenytoin or mexiletine may help alleviate myotonia, although pts are rarely bothered by this symptom.
- Pacemaker insertion may be required for syncope or heart block.
- Orthoses may control foot drop, stabilize the ankle, and decrease falling.
- Excessive daytime somnolence with or without sleep apnea is not uncommon; sleep studies, noninvasive respiratory support (BiPAP), and treatment with modafinil may be beneficial.

■ FACIOSCAPULOHUMERAL (FSH) DYSTROPHY

An autosomal dominant, slowly progressive disorder with onset in childhood or young adulthood. Weakness involves facial (usually the initial manifestation), shoulder girdle, and proximal arm muscles and can result in atrophy of biceps, triceps, and scapular winging. Facial weakness results in inability to smile, whistle, or fully close the eyes with loss of facial expressivity. Foot drop and leg weakness may cause falls and progressive difficulty with ambulation.

Laboratory studies reveal normal or slightly elevated CK and usually myopathic features on EMG and muscle biopsy. Pts have deletions at chromosome 4q35. Genetic testing is available for carrier detection and prenatal diagnosis.

TREATMENT   Facioscapulohumeral Dystrophy

- Ankle-foot orthoses are helpful for foot drop.
- Scapular stabilization procedures may help scapular winging but may not improve function.

■ OCULOPHARYNGEAL DYSTROPHY

Onset in the fourth to sixth decade of ptosis, limitation of extraocular movements, and facial and cricopharyngeal weakness. One of several disorders characterized by progressive external ophthalmoplegia. Dysphagia may be life-threatening. Most pts are of French-Canadian or Spanish-American descent. Mutation in a poly-RNA binding protein responsible.

INFLAMMATORY MYOPATHIES

The most common group of acquired and potentially treatable skeletal muscle disorders. Three major forms: polymyositis (PM), dermatomyositis (DM), and inclusion body myositis (IBM). Usually present as progressive and symmetric muscle weakness; extraocular muscles spared but pharyngeal weakness (dysphagia) and head drop from neck muscle weakness common. Respiratory muscles may be affected in advanced cases. IBM is characterized by early involvement of quadriceps (leading to falls) and

TABLE 207-1 FEATURES ASSOCIATED WITH INFLAMMATORY MYOPATHIES

Characteristic	Polymyositis	Dermatomyositis	Inclusion Body Myositis
Age at onset	>18 years	Adulthood and childhood	>50 years
Familial association	No	No	Yes, in some cases
Extramuscular manifestations	Yes	Yes	Yes
Associated conditions			
Connective tissue diseases	Yes[a]	Scleroderma and mixed connective tissue disease (overlap syndromes)	Yes, in up to 20% of cases[a]
Systemic autoimmune diseases[b]	Frequent	Infrequent	Infrequent
Malignancy	No	Yes, in up to 15% of cases	No
Viruses	Yes[c]	Unproven	Yes[c]
Drugs[d]	Yes	Yes, rarely	No
Parasites and bacteria[e]	Yes	No	No

[a]Systemic lupus erythematosus, rheumatoid arthritis, Sjögren's syndrome, systemic sclerosis, mixed connective tissue disease.

[b]Crohn's disease, vasculitis, sarcoidosis, primary biliary cirrhosis, adult celiac disease, chronic graft-versus-host disease, discoid lupus, ankylosing spondylitis, Behçet's syndrome, myasthenia gravis, acne fulminans, dermatitis herpetiformis, psoriasis, Hashimoto's disease, granulomatous diseases, agammaglobulinemia, monoclonal gammopathy, hypereosinophilic syndrome, Lyme disease, Kawasaki disease, autoimmune thrombocytopenia, hypergamma-globulinemic purpura, hereditary complement deficiency, IgA deficiency.

[c]HIV and HTLV-I (human T cell lymphotropic virus type I).

[d]Drugs include penicillamine (dermatomyositis and polymyositis), zidovudine (polymyositis), and contaminated tryptophan (dermatomyositis-like illness). Other myotoxic drugs may cause myopathy but not an inflammatory myopathy (see text for details).

[e]Parasites (protozoa, cestodes, nematodes), tropical and bacterial myositis (pyomyositis).

distal muscles; IBM may have an asymmetric pattern. Progression is over weeks or months in PM and DM, but typically over years in IBM. Skin involvement in DM may consist of a heliotrope rash (blue-purple discoloration) on the upper eyelids with edema, a flat red rash on the face and upper trunk, or erythema over knuckles (*Gottron's sign*). A variety of cancers are associated with DM. Features of each disorder are summarized in Table 207-1.

| TREATMENT | Inflammatory Myopathies |

Often effective for PM and DM but not for IBM.

- Step 1: Glucocorticoids (prednisone, 1 mg/kg per day for 3–4 weeks, then tapered very gradually)
- Step 2: Approximately 75% of pts require additional therapy with other immunosuppressive drugs. Azathioprine (up to 3 mg/kg per day), mycophenolate mofetil (up to 2.5–3 g/day in 2 divided doses), or methotrexate (7.5 mg/week gradually increasing to 25 mg/week), commonly used.
- Step 3: IV immunoglobulin (2 g/kg divided over 2–5 days)
- Step 4: A trial of one of the following agents: rituximab, cyclosporine, cyclophosphamide, or tacrolimus.

DISORDERS OF MUSCLE ENERGY METABOLISM

There are two principal sources of energy for skeletal muscle: fatty acids and glucose. Abnormalities in either glucose or lipid utilization can be associated with distinct clinical presentations that can range from an acute, painful syndrome that mimics polymyositis to a chronic, progressive muscle weakness simulating muscular dystrophy. Definitive diagnosis usually requires biochemical-enzymatic studies of biopsied muscle. However, muscle enzymes, EMG, and muscle biopsy all might be abnormal and may suggest specific disorders.

Progressive muscle weakness beginning usually in the third or fourth decade can be due to the adult form of *acid maltase deficiency (Pompe's disease)*. Respiratory failure is often the initial manifestation; treatment with enzyme replacement may be of benefit. Progressive weakness beginning after puberty occurs with *debranching enzyme deficiency*. *Glycolytic defects*, including *myophosphorylase deficiency* (McArdle's disease) or *phosphofructokinase deficiency*, present as exercise intolerance with myalgias. Disorders of fatty acid metabolism present with a similar picture. In adults, the most common cause is *carnitine palmitoyltransferase deficiency*. Exercise-induced cramps and myoglobinuria are common; strength is normal between the attacks. Dietary approaches (frequent meals and a low-fat high-carbohydrate diet, or a diet rich in medium-chain triglycerides) are of uncertain value.

MITOCHONDRIAL MYOPATHIES

More accurately referred to as *mitochondrial cytopathies* because multiple tissues are usually affected, these disorders result from defects in mitochondrial DNA. The clinical presentations vary greatly: muscle symptoms may include weakness, ophthalmoparesis, pain, or stiffness, or they may even be absent; age of onset ranges from infancy to adulthood; associated clinical presentations include ataxia, encephalopathy, seizures, strokelike episodes, and recurrent vomiting. Three groups: chronic progressive external ophthalmoplegia (CPEO), skeletal muscle–central nervous system syndromes, and pure myopathy syndromes simulating muscular dystrophy. The characteristic finding on muscle biopsy is "ragged red fibers," which are muscle fibers with accumulations of abnormal mitochondria. Genetics often show a maternal pattern of inheritance because mitochondrial genes are inherited almost exclusively from the oocyte.

Muscle membrane excitability is affected in a group of disorders referred to as *channelopathies*. Onset is usually in childhood or adolescence. Episodes typically occur after rest or sleep, often following earlier exercise. May be

TABLE 207-2 DRUG-INDUCED MYOPATHIES

Drugs	Major Toxic Reaction
Lipid-lowering agents Fibric acid derivatives HMG-CoA reductase inhibitors Niacin (nicotinic acid)	Drugs belonging to all three of the major classes of lipid-lowering agents can produce a spectrum of toxicity: asymptomatic serum creatine kinase elevation, myalgias, exercise-induced pain, rhabdomyolysis, and myoglobinuria.
Glucocorticoids	Acute, high-dose glucocorticoid treatment can cause acute quadriplegic myopathy. These high doses of steroids are often combined with nondepolarizing neuromuscular blocking agents but the weakness can occur without their use. Chronic steroid administration produces predominantly proximal weakness.
Nondepolarizing neuromuscular blocking agents	Acute quadriplegic myopathy can occur with or without concomitant glucocorticoids.
Zidovudine	Mitochondrial myopathy with ragged red fibers.
Drugs of abuse Alcohol Amphetamines	All drugs in this group can lead to widespread muscle breakdown, rhabdomyolysis, and myoglobinuria.
Cocaine Heroin Phencyclidine Meperidine	Local injections cause muscle necrosis, skin induration, and limb contractures.
Autoimmune toxic myopathy D-Penicillamine	Use of this drug may cause polymyositis and myasthenia gravis.
Amphophilic cationic drugs Amiodarone Chloroquine Hydroxychloroquine	All amphophilic drugs have the potential to produce painless, proximal weakness associated with autophagic vacuoles in the muscle biopsy.
Antimicrotubular drugs Colchicine	This drug produces painless, proximal weakness especially in the setting of renal failure. Muscle biopsy shows autophagic vacuoles.

due to genetic disorders of calcium [hypokalemic periodic paralysis (hypoKPP)], sodium (hyperkalemic periodic paralysis), chloride, or potassium channels.

- Attacks of hypoKPP are treated with potassium chloride (usually oral), and prophylaxis with acetazolamide (125–1000 mg/d in divided doses) is usually effective in hypoKPP type 1.
- Attacks of thyrotoxic periodic paralysis (usually in Asian men) resemble those of hypoKPP; attacks abate with treatment of the underlying thyroid condition.

ENDOCRINE AND METABOLIC MYOPATHIES

Abnormalities of thyroid function can cause a wide array of muscle disorders. Hypothyroidism is associated with muscle cramps, pain, and stiffness, and proximal muscle weakness occurs in one-third of pts; the relaxation phase of muscle stretch reflexes is characteristically prolonged, and serum CK is often elevated (up to 10 times normal).

Hyperthyroidism can produce proximal muscle weakness and atrophy; bulbar, respiratory, and even esophageal muscles are occasionally involved, causing dysphagia, dysphonia, and aspiration. Other neuromuscular disorders associated with hyperthyroidism include hypoKPP, myasthenia gravis, and a progressive ocular myopathy associated with proptosis (*Graves' ophthalmopathy*). Other endocrine conditions, including parathyroid, adrenal, and pituitary disorders, as well as diabetes mellitus, can also produce myopathy. Deficiencies of vitamins D and E are additional causes of muscle weakness.

DRUG-INDUCED MYOPATHIES

Drugs (including glucocorticoids and lipid-lowering agents) and toxins (e.g., alcohol) are associated with myopathies (Table 207-2). In most cases, weakness is symmetric and involves proximal limb girdle muscles. Weakness, myalgia, and cramps are common symptoms. An elevated CK is often an important indication of toxicity. Diagnosis often depends on resolution of signs and symptoms with removal of offending agent.

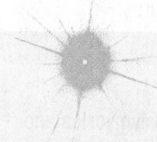

For a more detailed discussion, see Amato AA, Brown RH Jr.,: Muscular Dystrophies and Other Muscle Diseases, Chap. 387, p. 3487; Dalakas MC: Polymyositis, Dermatomyositis, and Inclusion Body Myositis, Chap. 388, p. 3509, in HPIM-18.

CHAPTER **208**
Psychiatric Disorders

Mental disorders are common in medical practice and may present either as a primary disorder or as a comorbid condition. The prevalence of mental or substance use disorders in the United States is ~30%, but only one-third of those individuals are currently receiving treatment.

Disorders of mood, thinking, and behavior may be due to a primary psychiatric diagnosis [DSM-IV *(Diagnostic and Statistical Manual,* 4th edition, American Psychiatric Association) Axis I major psychiatric disorders] or a personality disorder (DSM-IV Axis II disorders) or may be secondary to metabolic abnormalities, drug toxicities, focal cerebral lesions, seizure disorders, or degenerative neurologic disease (DSM-IV Axis III disorders). Any pt presenting with new onset of psychiatric symptoms must be evaluated for underlying psychoactive substance abuse and/or medical or neurologic illness. Psychiatric medications are discussed in Chap. 209. *The DSM-IV-PC (Primary Care) Manual* provides a synopsis of mental disorders commonly seen in medical practice.

MAJOR PSYCHIATRIC DISORDERS (AXIS I DIAGNOSES)

■ MOOD DISORDERS (MAJOR AFFECTIVE DISORDERS)

Mood disorders are characterized by a disturbance in the regulation of mood, behavior, and affect; subdivided into (1) depressive disorders, (2) bipolar disorders (depression plus manic or hypomanic episodes), and (3) depression in association with medical illness or alcohol and substance abuse (see Chaps. 211 and 212).

Major Depression

Clinical Features Affects 15% of the general population at some point in life; 6–8% of all outpatients in primary care settings satisfy diagnostic criteria. Diagnosis is made when five (or more) of the following symptoms have been present for 2 weeks (at least one of the symptoms must be #1 or #2 below):

1. Depressed mood
2. Loss of interest or pleasure
3. Change in appetite or weight
4. Insomnia or hypersomnia
5. Fatigue or loss of energy
6. Psychomotor agitation or retardation
7. Feelings of worthlessness or inappropriate guilt
8. Decreased ability to concentrate and make decisions
9. Recurrent thoughts of death or suicide.

A small number of pts with major depression will have psychotic symptoms (hallucinations and delusions) with their depressed mood. Negative life events can precipitate depression, but genetic factors influence the sensitivity to these events.

Onset of a first depressive episode is typically in early adulthood, although major depression can occur at any age. Untreated episodes generally resolve spontaneously in a few months to a year; however, a sizable number of pts suffer from chronic, unremitting depression or from partial treatment response. Half of all pts experiencing a first depressive episode will go on to a recurrent course. Untreated or partially treated episodes put the pt at risk for future problems with mood disorders. Within an individual, the nature of episodes may be similar over time. A family history of mood disorder is common and tends to predict a recurrent course. Major depression can also be the initial presentation of bipolar disorder (manic depressive illness).

Suicide Approximately 4–5% of all depressed pts will commit suicide, and most will have sought help from a physician within 1 month of their death. Physicians must always inquire about suicide when evaluating a pt with depression.

Depression with Medical Illness Virtually every class of medication can potentially induce or worsen depression. Antihypertensive drugs, anticholesterolemic agents, and antiarrhythmic agents are common triggers of depressive symptoms. Among the antihypertensive agents, β-adrenergic blockers and, to a lesser extent, calcium channel blockers are the most likely to cause depressed mood. Iatrogenic depression should also be considered in pts receiving glucocorticoids, antimicrobials, systemic analgesics, antiparkinsonian medications, and anticonvulsants.

Between 20–30% of cardiac pts manifest a depressive disorder. Tricyclic antidepressants (TCAs) are contraindicated in pts with bundle branch block, and TCA-induced tachycardia is an additional concern in pts with congestive heart failure. Selective serotonin reuptake inhibitors (SSRIs) appear not to induce ECG changes or adverse cardiac events, and thus, are reasonable first-line drugs for pts at risk for TCA-related complications. SSRIs may interfere with hepatic metabolism of anticoagulants, however, causing increased anticoagulation.

In *cancer*, the prevalence of depression is 25%, but it occurs in 40–50% of pts with cancers of the pancreas or oropharynx. Extreme cachexia from cancer may be misinterpreted as depression. Antidepressant medications in cancer pts improve quality of life as well as mood.

Diabetes mellitus is another consideration; the severity of the mood state correlates with the level of hyperglycemia and the presence of diabetic complications. Monoamine oxidase inhibitors (MAOIs) can induce hypoglycemia and weight gain. TCAs can produce hyperglycemia and carbohydrate craving. SSRIs, like MAOIs, may reduce fasting plasma glucose, but they are easier to use and may also improve dietary and medication compliance.

Depression may also occur with *hypothyroidism* or *hyperthyroidism*, in *neurologic disorders*, in *HIV*-positive individuals, and in *chronic hepatitis C infection* (depression worsens with interferon treatment). Some chronic disorders of uncertain etiology, such as *chronic fatigue syndrome* and *fibro-myalgia*, are strongly associated with depression.

| **TREATMENT** | Major Depression |

- Pts with suicidal ideation require treatment by a psychiatrist and may require hospitalization.
- Most other pts with an uncomplicated unipolar major depression (a major depression that is not part of a cyclical mood disorder, such as a bipolar disorder) can be successfully treated by a nonpsychiatric physician.
- Vigorous intervention and successful treatment appear to decrease the risk of future relapse.
- Pts who do not respond fully to standard treatment should be referred to a psychiatrist.
- Antidepressant medications are the mainstay of treatment, although combined treatment with psychotherapy improves outcome. Symptoms are ameliorated after 6–8 weeks at a therapeutic dose in 60–70% of pts.
- A guideline for the medical management of depression is shown in Fig. 208-1.
- Once remission is achieved, antidepressants should be continued for 6–9 months. Pts must be monitored carefully after termination of treatment since relapse is common.
- Pts with two or more episodes of depression should be considered for indefinite maintenance treatment.
- Electroconvulsive therapy is generally reserved for treatment-resistant depression unresponsive to medication or for pts in whom the use of antidepressants is medically contraindicated.
- Transcranial magnetic stimulation (TMS) is approved for treatment-resistant depression.
- Vagus nerve stimulation (VNS) has been approved for treatment-resistant depression as well, but its degree of efficacy is controversial.

Bipolar Disorder (Manic Depressive Illness)

Clinical Features A cyclical mood disorder in which episodes of major depression are interspersed with episodes of mania or hypomania; 1.5% of the population is affected. Most pts initially present with a manic episode in adolescence or young adulthood. Antidepressant therapy may provoke a manic episode; pts with a major depressive episode and a prior history of "highs" (mania or hypomania—which can be pleasant/euphoric or irritable/impulsive) and/or a family history of bipolar disorder should not be treated with antidepressants, but instead referred promptly to a psychiatrist.

With mania, an elevated, expansive mood, irritability, angry outbursts, and impulsivity are characteristic. Specific symptoms include: (1) unusual talkativeness; (2) flight of ideas and racing thoughts; (3) inflated self-esteem that can become delusional; (4) decreased need for sleep (often the

MEDICAL MANAGEMENT OF MAJOR DEPRESSIVE DISORDER ALGORITHM

Determine whether there is a history of good response to a medication in the patient or a first-degree relative; if yes, consider treatment with this agent if compatible with considerations in step 2.

↓

Evaluate patient characteristics and match to drug; consider health status, side effect profile, convenience, cost, patient preference, drug interaction risk, suicide potential, and medication compliance history.

↓

Begin new medication at 1/3 to 1/2 target dose if drug is a TCA, bupropion, venlafaxine, or mirtazapine, or full dose as tolerated if drug is an SSRI.

↓

If problem side effects occur, evaluate possibility of tolerance; consider temporary decrease in dose or adjunctive treatment.

↓

If unacceptable side effects continue, taper drug over 1 week and initiate new trial; consider potential drug interactions in choice.

↓

Evaluate response after 6 weeks at target dose; if response is inadequate, increase dose in stepwise fashion as tolerated.

↓

If inadequate response after maximal dose, consider tapering and switching to a new drug vs adjunctive treatment; if drug is a TCA, obtain plasma level to guide further treatment.

FIGURE 208-1 A guideline for the medical management of major depressive disorder. SSRI, selective serotonin reuptake inhibitor; TCA, tricyclic antidepressant.

first feature of an incipient manic episode); (5) increase in goal-directed activity or psychomotor agitation; (6) distractibility; (7) excessive involvement in risky activities (buying sprees, sexual indiscretions). Pts with full-blown mania can become psychotic. Hypomania is characterized by attenuated manic symptoms and is greatly underdiagnosed, as are "mixed episodes," where both depressive and manic or hypomanic symptoms coexist simultaneously.

Untreated, a manic or depressive episode typically lasts for several weeks but can last for 8–12 months. Variants of bipolar disorder include rapid and ultrarapid cycling (manic and depressed episodes occurring at cycles of weeks, days, or hours). In many pts, especially females, antidepressants trigger rapid cycling and worsen the course of illness. Pts with bipolar disorder are at risk for substance use, especially alcohol abuse, and for medical consequences of risky sexual behavior (STDs). Bipolar disorder has a strong genetic component; the concordance rate for monozygotic twins approaches 80%.

TREATMENT Bipolar Disorder

- Bipolar disorder is a serious, chronic illness that requires lifelong monitoring by a psychiatrist.
- Acutely manic pts often require hospitalization to reduce environmental stimulation and to protect themselves and others from the consequences of their reckless behavior.
- The recurrent nature of bipolar disorder necessitates maintenance treatment.
- Mood stabilizers (lithium, valproic acid, second-generation antipsychotic drugs, carbamazepine, lamotrigine) are effective for the resolution of acute episodes and for prophylaxis of future episodes.

■ SCHIZOPHRENIA AND OTHER PSYCHOTIC DISORDERS

Schizophrenia

Clinical Features Occurs in 0.85% of the population worldwide; lifetime prevalence is ~1–1.5%. Characterized by perturbations of language, perception, thinking, social activity, affect, and volition. Pts usually present in late adolescence, often after an insidious premorbid course of subtle psychosocial difficulties. Core psychotic features last ≥6 months and include positive symptoms (such as conceptual disorganization, delusions, or hallucinations) and negative symptoms (loss of function, anhedonia, decreased emotional expression, impaired concentration, and diminished social engagement). Negative symptoms predominate in one-third and are associated with a poor long-term outcome and poor response to treatment.

Prognosis depends not on symptom severity but on the response to antipsychotic medication. A permanent remission without recurrence does occasionally occur. About 10% of schizophrenic pts commit suicide. Comorbid substance abuse is common.

TREATMENT Schizophrenia

- Hospitalization is required for acutely psychotic pts who may be dangerous to themselves or others.
- Conventional antipsychotic medications are effective against hallucinations, delusions, and thought disorder.
- The novel antipsychotic medications—clozapine, risperidone, olanzapine, quetiapine, ziprasidone, and aripiprazole—are helpful in pts unresponsive to conventional neuroleptics and may also be more useful for negative and cognitive symptoms.
- Drug treatment by itself is insufficient, and educational efforts directed toward families and relevant community resources are necessary to maintain stability and optimize outcomes.

Other Psychotic Disorders

These include *schizoaffective disorder* (where symptoms of schizophrenia are interspersed with major mood episodes) and *schizophreniform* disorder (pts who meet the symptom requirements but not the duration requirements for schizophrenia).

■ ANXIETY DISORDERS

Characterized by severe, persistent anxiety or sense of dread or foreboding. Most prevalent group of psychiatric illnesses seen in the community; present in 15–20% of medical clinic pts.

Panic Disorder

Occurs in 1–3% of the population; familial aggregation may occur. Onset in late adolescence or early adulthood. Initial presentation is almost always to a nonpsychiatric physician, frequently in the ER, as a possible heart attack or serious respiratory problem. The disorder is often initially unrecognized or misdiagnosed. Three-quarters of pts with panic disorder will also satisfy criteria for major depression at some point.

Clinical Features Characterized by panic attacks, which are sudden, unexpected, overwhelming paroxysms of terror and apprehension with multiple associated somatic symptoms. Attacks usually reach a peak within 10 min, then slowly resolve spontaneously, occurring in an unexpected fashion. Diagnostic criteria for panic disorder include recurrent panic attacks and at least 1 month of concern or worry about the attacks or a change in behavior related to them. Panic attacks must be accompanied by at least four of the following: palpitations, sweating, trembling or shaking, dyspnea, choking, chest pain, nausea or abdominal distress, dizziness or faintness, derealization or depersonalization, fear of losing control, fear of death, paresthesias, and chills or hot flashes.

When the disorder goes unrecognized and untreated, pts often experience significant morbidity: they become afraid of leaving home and may develop anticipatory anxiety, agoraphobia, and other spreading phobias; many turn to self-medication with alcohol or benzodiazepines.

Panic disorder must be differentiated from cardiovascular and respiratory disorders. Conditions that may mimic or worsen panic attacks include hyperthyroidism, pheochromocytoma, hypoglycemia, drug ingestions (amphetamines, cocaine, caffeine, sympathomimetic nasal decongestants), and drug withdrawal (alcohol, barbiturates, opiates, minor tranquilizers).

TREATMENT | Panic Disorder

- The cornerstone of drug therapy is antidepressant medication.
- SSRIs benefit the majority of panic disorder pts and do not have the adverse effects of the TCAs.
- Benzodiazepines may be used in the short term while waiting for antidepressants to take effect.
- Early psychotherapeutic intervention and education aimed at symptom control enhances the effectiveness of drug treatment.
- Psychotherapy (identifying and aborting panic attacks through relaxation and breathing techniques) can be effective.

Generalized Anxiety Disorder (GAD)

Characterized by persistent, chronic anxiety; occurs in 5–6% of the population.

Clinical Features Pts experience persistent, excessive, and/or unrealistic worry associated with muscle tension, impaired concentration, autonomic arousal, feeling "on edge" or restless, and insomnia. Pts worry excessively over minor matters, with life-disrupting effects; unlike panic disorder, complaints of shortness of breath, palpitations, and tachycardia are relatively rare. Secondary depression is common, as is social phobia and comorbid substance abuse.

TREATMENT Generalized Anxiety Disorder

- A combination of pharmacologic and psychotherapeutic interventions is most effective; complete symptom relief is rare.
- Benzodiazepines are the initial agents of choice when generalized anxiety is severe and acute enough to warrant drug therapy; physicians must be alert to psychological and physical dependence on benzodiazepines.
- A subgroup of pts respond to buspirone, a nonbenzodiazepine anxiolytic.
- Some SSRIs also are effective at doses comparable to their efficacy in major depression.
- Anticonvulsants with GABA-ergic properties (gabapentin, oxcarbazepine, tiagabine, pregabalin, divalproex) may also be effective against anxiety.

Obsessive-Compulsive Disorder (OCD)

A severe disorder present in 2–3% of the population and characterized by recurrent obsessions (persistent intrusive thoughts) and compulsions (repetitive behaviors) that impair everyday functioning. Pts are often ashamed of their symptoms; physicians must ask specific questions to screen for this disorder including asking about recurrent thoughts and behaviors.

Clinical Features Common obsessive thoughts and compulsive behaviors include fears of germs or contamination, handwashing, counting behaviors, and having to check and recheck such actions as whether a door is locked.

Onset is usually in adolescence (childhood onset is not rare); more common in males and first-born children. Comorbid conditions are common, the most frequent being depression, other anxiety disorders, eating disorders, and tics. The course of OCD is usually episodic with periods of incomplete remission; some cases may show a steady deterioration in psychosocial functioning.

TREATMENT Obsessive-Compulsive Disorder

- Clomipramine and the SSRIs (fluoxetine, fluvoxamine, sertraline) are effective, but only 50–60% of pts show adequate improvement with pharmacotherapy alone.
- A combination of drug therapy and cognitive-behavioral psychotherapy is most effective for the majority of pts.

Posttraumatic Stress Disorder (PTSD)

Occurs in a subgroup of individuals exposed to a severe life-threatening trauma. If the reaction occurs shortly after the event, it is termed *acute stress disorder*, but if the reaction is delayed and subject to recurrence, PTSD is diagnosed. Predisposing factors include a past psychiatric history and personality characteristics of extroversion and high neuroticism.

Clinical Features Individuals experience associated symptoms of detachment and loss of emotional responsivity. The pt may feel depersonalized and unable to recall specific events of the trauma, although it is reexperienced through intrusions in thought, dreams, or flashbacks. Comorbid substance abuse and other mood and anxiety disorders are common. This disorder is extremely debilitating; most pts require referral to a psychiatrist for ongoing care.

> **TREATMENT** Posttraumatic Stress Disorder
>
> - TCAs, phenelzine (an MAOI), and the SSRIs all are somewhat effective.
> - Trazodone is frequently used at night to help with insomnia.
> - Psychotherapeutic strategies help the pt overcome avoidance behaviors and master fear of recurrence of the trauma.

Phobic Disorders

Clinical Features Recurring, irrational fears of specific objects, activities, or situations, with subsequent avoidance behavior of the phobic stimulus. Diagnosis is made only when the avoidance behavior interferes with social or occupational functioning. Affects ~10% of the population. Common phobias include fear of closed places, (claustrophobia), fear of blood, and fear of flying. Social phobia is distinguished by a specific fear of social or performance situations in which the individual is exposed to unfamiliar individuals or to possible examination and evaluation by others (e.g., having to converse at a party, use of public restrooms, meeting strangers).

> **TREATMENT** Phobic Disorders
>
> - Agoraphobia is treated as for panic disorder.
> - Beta blockers (e.g., propranolol, 20–40 mg PO 2 h before the event) are particularly effective in the treatment of "performance anxiety."
> - SSRIs are very helpful in treating social phobias. Social and simple phobias respond well to behaviorally focused psychotherapy.

Somatoform Disorders

Clinical Features

Pts with multiple somatic complaints that cannot be explained by a known medical condition or by the effects of substances; seen commonly in primary care practice (prevalence of 5%). In *somatization disorder*, the pt presents with multiple physical complaints referable to different organ systems.

Onset is before age 30, and the disorder is persistent; pts with somatization disorder can be impulsive and demanding. In *conversion disorder*, the symptoms involve voluntary motor or sensory function. In *hypochondriasis*, the pt believes there is a serious medical illness, despite reassurance and appropriate medical evaluation. As with somatization disorder, these pts have a history of poor relationships with physicians due to their sense that they have not received adequate evaluation. Hypochondriasis can be disabling and show a waxing and waning course. In *factitious illnesses*, the pt consciously and voluntarily produces physical symptoms; the sick role is gratifying. *Munchausen's syndrome* refers to individuals with dramatic, chronic, or severe factitious illness. A variety of signs, symptoms, and diseases have been simulated in factitious illnesses; most common are chronic diarrhea, fever of unknown origin, intestinal bleeding, hematuria, seizures, hypoglycemia. In *malingering*, the fabrication of illness derives from a desire for an external gain (narcotics, disability).

TREATMENT	Somatoform Disorders

- Pts with somatoform disorders are usually subjected to multiple diagnostic tests and exploratory surgeries in an attempt to find their "real" illness. This approach is doomed to failure.
- Successful treatment is achieved through behavior modification, in which access to the physician is adjusted to provide a consistent, sustained, and predictable level of support that is not contingent on the pt's level of presenting symptoms or distress.
- Visits are brief, supportive, and structured and are not associated with a need for diagnostic or treatment action.
- Pts may benefit from antidepressant treatment.
- Consultation with a psychiatrist is essential.

PERSONALITY DISORDERS (AXIS II DIAGNOSES)

Characteristic patterns of thinking, feeling, and interpersonal behavior that are relatively inflexible and cause significant functional impairment or subjective distress for the individual. Individuals with personality disorders are often regarded as "difficult pts."

DSM-IV describes three major categories of personality disorders; pts usually present with a combination of features.

■ CLUSTER A PERSONALITY DISORDERS

Includes individuals who are odd and eccentric and who maintain an emotional distance from others. The *paranoid* personality has pervasive mistrust and suspiciousness of others. The *schizoid* personality is interpersonally isolated, cold, and indifferent, while the *schizotypal* personality is eccentric and superstitious, with magical thinking and unusual perceptual experiences.

■ CLUSTER B PERSONALITY DISORDERS

Describes individuals whose behavior is impulsive, excessively emotional, and erratic. The *borderline* personality is impulsive and manipulative, with unpredictable and fluctuating intense moods and unstable relationships, a fear of abandonment, and occasional rage episodes. The *histrionic* pt is dramatic, engaging, seductive, and attention-seeking. The *narcissistic* pt is self-centered and has an inflated sense of self-importance combined with a tendency to devalue or de-mean others, while pts with *antisocial* personality disorder use other people to achieve their own ends and engage in exploitative and manipulative behavior with no sense of remorse.

■ CLUSTER C PERSONALITY DISORDERS

Enduring traits are anxiety and fear. The *dependent* pt fears separation, tries to engage others to assume responsibility, and often has a help-rejecting style. Pts with *compulsive* personality disorder are meticulous and perfectionistic but also inflexible and indecisive. *Avoidant* pts are anxious about social contact and have difficulty assuming responsibility for their isolation.

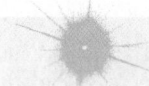

For a more detailed discussion, see Reus VI: Mental Disorders, Chap. 391, p. 3529, in HPIM-18.

CHAPTER **209**
Psychiatric Medications

Four major classes are commonly used in adults: (1) antidepressants, (2) anxiolytics, (3) antipsychotics, and (4) mood stabilizing agents. Nonpsychiatric physicians should become familiar with one or two drugs in each of the first three classes so that the indications, dose range, efficacy, potential side effects, and interactions with other medications are well known.

GENERAL PRINCIPLES OF USE

1. Most treatment failures are due to undermedication and impatience. For a proper medication trial to take place, an effective dose must be taken for an adequate amount of time. For antidepressants, antipsychotics, and mood stabilizers, full effects may take weeks or months to occur.

2. History of a positive response to a medication usually indicates that a response to the same drug will occur again. A family history of a positive response to a specific medication is also useful.

3. Pts who fail to respond to one drug will often respond to another in the same class; one should attempt another trial with a drug that has a different mechanism of action or a different chemical structure. Treatment failures should be referred to a psychiatrist, as should all pts with psychotic symptoms or who require mood stabilizers.

4. Avoid polypharmacy; a pt who is not responding to standard monotherapy requires referral to a psychiatrist.

5. Pharmacokinetics may be altered in the elderly, with smaller volumes of distribution, reduced renal and hepatic clearance, longer biologic half-lives, and greater potential for CNS toxicity. The rule with elderly pts is to "start low and go slow."

6. Never stop treatment abruptly; especially true for antidepressants and anxiolytics. In general, medications should be slowly tapered and discontinued over 2–4 weeks.

7. Review possible side effects each time a drug is prescribed; educate pts and family members about side effects and need for patience in awaiting a response.

ANTIDEPRESSANTS (ADs)

Useful to group according to known actions on CNS monoaminergic systems (Table 209-1). The selective serotonin reuptake inhibitors (SSRIs) have predominant effects on serotonergic neurotransmission, also reflected in side-effect profile. The TCAs, or tricyclic antidepressants, affect noradrenergic and, to a lesser extent, serotonergic neurotransmission but also have anticholinergic and antihistaminic effects. Venlafaxine, desvenlafaxine, duloxetine, and mirtazapine have mixed noradrenergic and serotonergic effects. Bupropion is a novel antidepressant that enhances noradrenergic function. Trazodone, nefazodone, and amoxapine have mixed effects on serotonin receptors and on other neurotransmitter systems. The MAOIs inhibit monoamine oxidase, the primary enzyme responsible for the degradation of monoamines in the synaptic cleft.

ADs are effective against major depression, particularly when neuro-vegetative symptoms and signs are present. Despite the widespread use of SSRIs, there is no convincing evidence that they are more efficacious than TCAs, although their safety profile in overdose is more favorable than that of the TCAs. ADs are also useful in treatment of panic disorder, post-traumatic stress disorder, chronic pain syndromes, and generalized anxiety disorder. The TCA clomipramine and the SSRIs successfully treat obsessive-compulsive disorder.

All ADs require at least 2 weeks at a therapeutic dose before clinical improvement is observed. All ADs also have the potential to trigger a manic episode or rapid cycling when given to a pt with bipolar disorder. The MAOIs must not be prescribed concurrently with other ADs or with narcotics, as potentially fatal reactions may occur. "Withdrawal syndromes" usually consisting of malaise can occur when ADs are stopped abruptly.

ANXIOLYTICS

Benzodiazepines bind to sites on the γ-aminobutyric acid receptor and are cross-tolerant with alcohol and with barbiturates. Four clinical properties: (1) sedative, (2) anxiolytic, (3) skeletal muscle relaxant, and (4) antiepileptic. Individual drugs differ in terms of potency, onset of action, duration of action (related to half-life and presence of active metabolites), and metabolism (Table 209-2). Benzodiazepines have additive effects with alcohol; like alcohol, they can produce tolerance and physiologic dependence, with serious withdrawal syndromes (tremors, seizures, delirium, and autonomic hyperactivity) if discontinued too quickly, especially for those with short half-lives.

TABLE 209-1 ANTIDEPRESSANTS

Name	Usual Daily Dose, mg	Side Effects	Comments
SSRIs			
Fluoxetine (Prozac)	10–80	Headache; nausea and other GI effects; jitteriness; insomnia; sexual dysfunction; can affect plasma levels of other medicines (except sertraline); akathisia rare	Once-daily dosing, usually in the morning; fluoxetine has very long half-life; must not be combined with MAOIs
Sertraline (Zoloft)	50–200		
Paroxetine (Paxil)	20–60		
Fluvoxamine (Luvox)	100–300		
Citalopram (Celexa)	20–60		
Escitalopram (Lexapro)	10–30		
TCAs			
Amitriptyline (Elavil)	150–300	Anticholinergic (dry mouth, tachycardia, constipation, urinary retention, blurred vision); sweating; tremor; postural hypotension; cardiac conduction delay; sedation; weight gain	Once-daily dosing, usually qhs; blood levels of most TCAs available; can be lethal in O.D. (lethal dose = 2 g); nortriptyline best tolerated, especially by elderly
Nortriptyline (Pamelor)	50–200		
Imipramine (Tofranil)	150–300		
Desipramine (Norpramin)	150–300		
Doxepin (Sinequan)	150–300		
Clomipramine (Anafranil)	150–300		
Mixed Norepinephrine/Serotonin reuptake inhibitors and receptor blockers			
Venlafaxine (Effexor)	75–375	Nausea; dizziness; dry mouth; headaches; increased blood pressure; anxiety and insomnia	Bid-tid dosing (extended release available); lower potential for drug interactions than SSRIs; contraindicated with MAOIs

Desvenlafaxine (Pristiq)	50–400	Nausea, dizziness, insomnia	Primary metabolite of venlafaxine. No increased efficacy with higher dosing
Duloxetine (Cymbalta)	40–60	Nausea, dizziness, headache, insomnia, constipation	May have utility in treatment of neuropathic pain and stress incontinence
Mirtazapine (Remeron)	15–45	Somnolence; weight gain; neutropenia rare	Once daily dosing
Mixed-action drugs			
Bupropion (Wellbutrin)	250–450	Jitteriness; flushing; seizures in at-risk pts; anorexia; tachycardia; psychosis	Tid dosing, but sustained release also available; fewer sexual side effects than SSRIs or TCAs; may be useful for adult ADD
Trazodone (Desyrel)	200–600	Sedation; dry mouth; ventricular irritability; postural hypotension; priapism rare	Useful in low doses for sleep because of sedating effects with no anticholinergic side effects
Nefazodone (Serzone)	300–600	Sedation; headache; dry mouth; nausea; constipation	Discontinued sale in United States and several other countries due to risk of liver failure
Amoxapine (Asendin)	200–600	Sexual dysfunction	Lethality in overdose; EPS possible
MAOIs			
Phenelzine (Nardil)	45–90	Insomnia; hypotension; anorgasmia; weight gain; hypertensive crisis; toxic reactions with SSRIs; narcotics	May be more effective in pts with atypical features or treatment-refractory depression
Tranylcypromine (Parnate)	20–50		
Isocarboxazid (Marplan)	20–60		
Transdermal selegiline (Emsam)	6–12	Local skin reaction hypertension	No dietary restrictions with 6 mg dose

Abbreviations: ADD, attention deficit disorder; EPS, extrapyramidal symptoms; MAOIs, monoamine oxidase inhibitors; SSRIs, selective serotonin reuptake inhibitors; TCAs, tricyclic antidepressants.

TABLE 209-2 ANXIOLYTICS

Name	Equivalent PO Dose, mg	Onset of Action	Half-Life, h	Comments
Benzodiazepines				
Diazepam (Valium)	5	Fast	20–70	Active metabolites; quite sedating
Flurazepam (Dalmane)	15	Fast	30–100	Flurazepam is a prodrug; metabolites are active; quite sedating
Triazolam (Halcion)	0.25	Intermediate	1.5–5	No active metabolites; can induce confusion and delirium, especially in elderly
Lorazepam (Ativan)	1	Intermediate	10–20	No active metabolites; direct hepatic glucuronide conjugation; quite sedating
Alprazolam (Xanax)	0.5	Intermediate	12–15	Active metabolites; not too sedating; may have specific antidepressant and antipanic activity; tolerance and dependence develop easily
Chlordiazepoxide (Librium)	10	Intermediate	5–30	Active metabolites; moderately sedating
Oxazepam (Serax)	15	Slow	5–15	No active metabolites; direct glucuronide conjugation; not too sedating
Temazepam (Restoril)	15	Slow	9–12	No active metabolites; moderately sedating
Clonazepam (Klonopin)	0.5	Slow	18–50	No active metabolites; moderately sedating
Nonbenzodiazepines				
Buspirone (BuSpar)	7.5	2 weeks	2–3	Active metabolites; tid dosing—usual daily dose 10–20 mg tid; nonsedating; no additive effects with alcohol; useful for controlling agitation in demented or brain-injured pts

Buspirone is a nonbenzodiazepine anxiolytic that is nonsedating, is not cross-tolerant with alcohol, and does not induce tolerance or dependence. It requires at least 2 weeks at therapeutic doses to achieve full effects.

ANTIPSYCHOTIC MEDICATIONS

These include the first-generation (typical) neuroleptics, which act by blocking dopamine D_2 receptors, and the second-generation (atypical) neuroleptics, which act on dopamine, serotonin, and other neurotransmitter systems. Some antipsychotic effect may occur within hours or days of initiating treatment, but full effects usually require 6 weeks to several months of daily, therapeutic dosing.

■ FIRST-GENERATION ANTIPSYCHOTICS

Useful to group into high-, mid-, and low-potency neuroleptics (Table 209-3). High-potency neuroleptics are least sedating, have almost no anticholinergic side effects, and have a strong tendency to induce extrapyramidal side effects (EPSEs). The EPSEs occur within several hours to several weeks of beginning treatment and include acute dystonias, akathisia, and pseudo-parkinsonism. Extrapyramidal symptoms respond well to trihexyphenidyl, 2 mg twice daily, or benztropine mesylate, 1 to 2 mg twice daily. Akathisia may respond to beta blockers. Low-potency neuroleptics are very sedating, may cause orthostatic hypotension, are anticholinergic, and tend not to induce EPSEs frequently.

Up to 20% of pts treated with conventional antipsychotic agents for >1 year develop tardive dyskinesia (probably due to dopamine receptor supersensitivity), an abnormal involuntary movement disorder most often observed in the face and distal extremities. Treatment includes gradual withdrawal of the neuroleptic, with possible switch to a novel neuroleptic; anticholinergic agents can worsen the disorder.

Rarely, pts exposed to neuroleptics develop neuroleptic malignant syndrome (NMS), a life-threatening complication with a mortality rate as high as 25%; hyperpyrexia, autonomic hyperactivity, muscle rigidity, obtundation, and agitation are characteristic, associated with increased WBC, increased creatine phosphokinase, and myoglobinuria. Treatment involves immediate discontinuation of neuroleptics, supportive care, and use of dantrolene and bromocriptine.

■ SECOND-GENERATION ANTIPSYCHOTICS

A new class of agents that has become the first line of treatment (Table 209-3); efficacious in treatment-resistant pts, tend not to induce EPSEs or tardive dyskinesia, and appear to have uniquely beneficial properties on negative symptoms and cognitive dysfunction. Main problem is side effect of weight gain (most prominent in clozapine and in olanzapine; can induce diabetes). The CATIE study, a large-scale investigation of antipsychotic agents in the "real world," revealed a high rate of discontinuation of all medications over 18 months; olanzapine was modestly more effective than other agents but with a higher discontinuation rate due to side effects.

MOOD-STABILIZING AGENTS

Four mood stabilizers in common use: lithium, valproic acid, carbamazepine/oxcarbazepine, and lamotrigine (Table 209-4). Lithium is the gold standard and the best studied, and along with carbamazepine and valproic

TABLE 209-3 ANTIPSYCHOTIC AGENTS

Name	Usual PO Daily Dose, mg	Side Effects	Sedation	Comments
First-generation antipsychotics				
Low potency				
Chlorpromazine (Thorazine)	100–1000	Anticholinergic effects; orthostasis; photosensitivity; cholestasis; QT prolongation	+++	EPSEs usually not prominent; can cause anticholinergic delirium in elderly pts
Thioridazine (Mellaril)	100–600			
Midpotency				
Trifluoperazine (Stelazine)	2–50	Fewer anticholinergic side effects	++	Well tolerated by most pts
Perphenazine (Trilafon)	4–64	Fewer EPSEs than with higher potency agents	++	
Loxapine (Loxitane)	30–100	Frequent EPSEs	++	
Molindone (Moban)	30–100	Frequent EPSEs	0	Little weight gain
High potency				
Haloperidol (Haldol)	5–20	No anticholinergic side effects; EPSEs often prominent	0/+	Often prescribed in doses that are too high; long-acting injectable forms of haloperidol and fluphenazine available
Fluphenazine (Prolixin)	1–20	Frequent EPSEs	0/+	
Thiothixene (Navane)	2–50	Frequent EPSEs	0/+	

Second-generation antipsychotics

Drug	Dose range	Side effects	Notes
Clozapine (Clozaril)	150–600	Agranulocytosis (1%); weight gain; seizures; drooling; hyperthermia	++	Requires weekly WBC count for first 6 months, then biweekly if stable
Risperidone (Risperdal)	2–8	Orthostasis	+	Requires slow titration; EPSEs observed with doses >6 mg qd
Olanzapine (Zyprexa)	10–30	Weight gain	++	Mild prolactin elevation
Quetiapine (Seroquel)	350–800	Sedation; weight gain; anxiety	+++	Bid dosing
Ziprasidone (Geodon)	120–200	Orthostatic hypotension	+/++	Minimal weight gain; increases QT interval
Aripiprazole (Abilify)	10–30	Nausea, anxiety, insomnia	0/+	Mixed agonist/antagonist
Paliperidone (Invega)	3–12	Restlessness, EPSEs	+	Active metabolite of risperidone
Iloperidone (Fanapt)	12–24	Dizziness, hypotension	0/+	Requires dose titration
Asenapine (Saphris)	10–20	Dizziness, EPSEs, weight gain	++	Sublingual tablets; bid dosing
Lurasidone (Latuda)	40–80	Nausea, EPSEs	++	Uses CYP3A4

Abbreviations: EPSEs, extrapyramidal side effects; WBC, white blood cell.

TABLE 209-4 CLINICAL PHARMACOLOGY OF MOOD STABILIZERS

Agent and Dosing	Side Effects and Other Effects
Lithium	**Common side effects**
Starting dose: 300 mg bid or tid Therapeutic blood level: 0.8–1.2 meq/L	Nausea/anorexia/diarrhea, fine tremor, thirst, polyuria, fatigue, weight gain, acne, folliculitis, neutrophilia, hypothyroidism
	Blood level is increased by thiazides, tetracyclines, and NSAIDs
	Blood level is decreased by bronchodilators, verapamil, and carbonic anhydrase inhibitors
	Rare side effects: Neurotoxicity, renal toxicity, hypercalcemia, ECG changes
Valproic acid	**Common side effects**
Starting dose: 250 mg tid Therapeutic blood level: 50–125 µg/mL	Nausea/anorexia, weight gain, sedation, tremor, rash, alopecia
	Inhibits hepatic metabolism of other medications
	Rare side effects: Pancreatitis, hepatotoxicity, Stevens-Johnson syndrome
Carbamazepine/ Oxcarbazepine	**Common side effects**
Starting dose: 200 mg bid for carbamazepine, 150 mg bid for oxcarbazepine	Nausea/anorexia, sedation, rash, dizziness/ataxia
Therapeutic blood level: 4–12 µg/mL for carbamazepine	Carbamazepine, but not oxcarbazepine, induces hepatic metabolism of other medications
	Rare side effects: Hyponatremia, agranulocytosis, Stevens-Johnson syndrome
Lamotrigine	**Common side effects**
Starting dose: 25 mg/d	Rash, dizziness, headache, tremor, sedation, nausea
	Rare side effect: Stevens-Johnson syndrome

Abbreviations: ECG, electrocardiogram; NSAIDs, nonsteroidal anti-inflammatory drugs.

acid, is used for treatment of acute manic episodes; 1–2 weeks to reach full effect. As prophylaxis, the mood stabilizers reduce frequency and severity of both manic and depressed episodes in cyclical mood disorders. In refractory bipolar disorder, combinations of mood stabilizers may be beneficial.

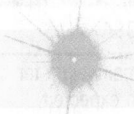

For a more detailed discussion, see Reus VI: Mental Disorders, Chap. 391, p. 3529, in HPIM-18.

CHAPTER **210**
Eating Disorders

■ DEFINITIONS AND EPIDEMIOLOGY

Anorexia nervosa is characterized by refusal to maintain normal body weight, resulting in a body weight <85% of the expected weight for age and height. *Bulimia nervosa* is characterized by recurrent episodes of binge eating followed by abnormal compensatory behaviors, such as self-induced vomiting, laxative abuse, or excessive exercise. Weight is in the normal range or above. *Binge eating disorder* is similar to bulimia nervosa but lacks the compensatory behavior element. As a result, binge eating disorder is typically associated with obesity.

Both anorexia nervosa and bulimia nervosa occur primarily among previously healthy young women who become overly concerned with body shape and weight. Binge eating and purging behavior may be present in both conditions, with the critical distinction between the two resting on the weight of the individual. The lifetime prevalence of anorexia nervosa is 1%, that of bulimia nervosa 1–3%, but mild forms of occasional bulimia may occur in up to 5–10% of women. Binge eating disorder has a 4% prevalence. There is a 10:1 female to male ratio for both conditions; binge eating disorder is more evenly divided between women and men (2:1). The typical time of onset of anorexia is mid-adolescence, that of bulimia in early adulthood. Both can occur later, but onset is uncommon after age 40.

Anorexia and bulimia nervosa are disorders of the affluent, well-educated societies in Western cultures. Affected pts frequently exhibit perfectionist and obsessional tendencies. Pursuit of activities that emphasize thinness (ballet, modeling, distance running) are prevalent, as is a drive for high scholastic achievement. Risk factors are a family history of mood disturbance, childhood obesity, and psychological or physical abuse during childhood.

The diagnostic features of anorexia and bulimia nervosa are shown in Tables 210-1 and 210-2.

■ CLINICAL FEATURES

Anorexia Nervosa

- General: feeling cold
- Skin, hair, nails: alopecia, lanugo hair, acrocyanosis, edema
- Cardiovascular: bradycardia, hypotension
- Gastrointestinal: salivary gland enlargement, slow gastric emptying, constipation, elevated liver enzymes

TABLE 210-1 DIAGNOSTIC FEATURES OF ANOREXIA NERVOSA

Refusal to maintain body weight at or above a minimally normal weight for age and height. (This includes a failure to achieve weight gain expected during a period of growth leading to an abnormally low body weight.)

Intense fear of weight gain or becoming fat.

Distortion of body image (e.g., feeling fat despite an objectively low weight or minimizing the seriousness of low weight).

Amenorrhea. (This criterion is met if menstrual periods occur only following hormone—e.g., estrogen—administration.)

- Hematopoietic: normochromic, normocytic anemia; leukopenia
- Fluid/electrolyte: increased blood urea nitrogen, increased creatinine, hyponatremia, hypokalemia. Hypokalemia can become life-threatening.
- Endocrine: low luteinizing hormone and follicle-stimulating hormone with secondary amenorrhea, hypoglycemia, normal thyroid-stimulating hormone with low normal thyroxine, increased plasma cortisol, osteopenia

Bulimia Nervosa
- Gastrointestinal: salivary gland enlargement, dental erosion from gastric acid exposure
- Fluid/electrolyte: hypokalemia, hypochloremia, alkalosis (from vomiting) or acidosis (from laxative abuse)
- Other: callus or scar on dorsum of hand (from repeated scraping against teeth during induced vomiting)

TREATMENT Eating Disorders

ANOREXIA NERVOSA Weight restoration to 90% of predicted weight (BMI >18.5 kg/m²) is the primary goal in the treatment of anorexia nervosa. The intensity of the initial treatment, including the need for hospitalization, is determined by the pt's current weight, the rapidity of recent weight loss, and the severity of medical and psychological complications (Fig. 210-1). Severe electrolyte imbalances should be identified and corrected. Nutritional restoration can almost always be successfully accomplished by oral feeding. For severely underweight pts, sufficient calories should be provided initially in divided meals as food or liquid supplements to maintain weight and to permit stabilization of fluid and electrolyte balance (1200–1800 kcal/d intake). Calories can be gradually increased to achieve a weight gain of 1–2 kg per week (3000–4000 kcal/d intake). Meals must be supervised. Intake of vitamin D (400 IU/d) and calcium (1500 mg/d) should be sufficient to minimize bone loss. The assistance of psychiatrists or psychologists experienced in the treatment of anorexia nervosa is usually necessary. No psychotropic medications are of established value in the treatment of anorexia nervosa. Medical complications occasionally occur during refeeding; most

TABLE 210-2 DIAGNOSTIC FEATURES OF BULIMIA NERVOSA

Recurrent episodes of binge eating, which is characterized by the consumption of a large amount of food in a short period of time and a feeling that the eating is out of control.

Recurrent inappropriate behavior to compensate for the binge eating, such as self-induced vomiting.

The occurrence of both the binge eating and the inappropriate compensatory behavior at least twice weekly, on average, for 3 months.

Overconcern with body shape and weight.

Note: If the diagnostic criteria for anorexia nervosa are simultaneously met, only the diagnosis of anorexia nervosa is given.

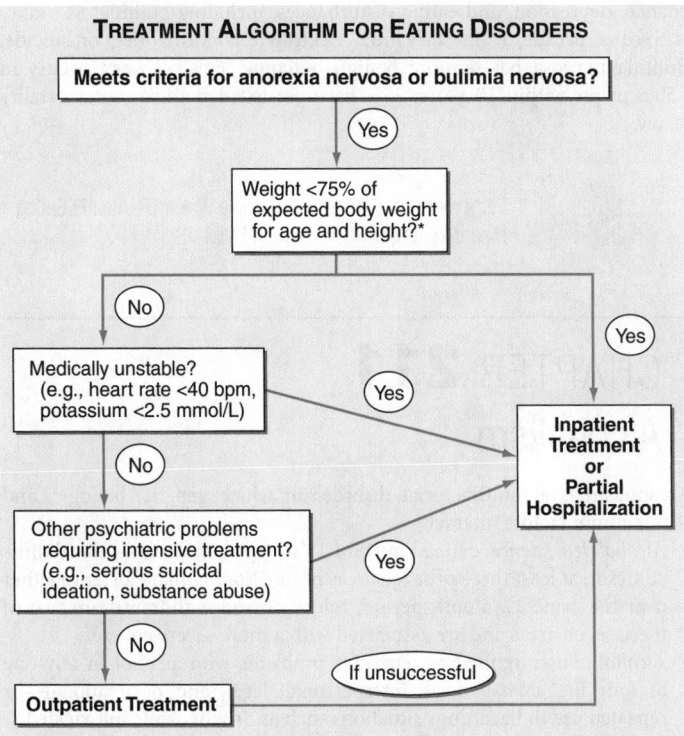

TREATMENT ALGORITHM FOR EATING DISORDERS

FIGURE 210-1 An algorithm for basic treatment decisions regarding pts with anorexia nervosa or bulimia nervosa. Based on the American Psychiatric Association practice guidelines for the treatment of pts with eating disorders. *Although outpatient management may be considered for pts with anorexia nervosa weighing more than 75% of expected, there should be a low threshold for using more intensive interventions if the weight loss has been rapid or if current weight is <80% of expected.

pts transiently retain excess fluid, occasionally resulting in peripheral edema. Congestive heart failure and acute gastric dilatation have been described when refeeding is rapid. Transient modest elevations in serum levels of liver enzymes occasionally occur. Low levels of magnesium and phosphate should be replaced. Mortality is 5% per decade, from either chronic starvation or suicide.

BULIMIA NERVOSA Bulimia nervosa can usually be treated on an out-patient basis (Fig. 210-1). Cognitive behavioral therapy and fluoxetine (Prozac) are first-line therapies. The recommended treatment dose for fluoxetine (60 mg/d) is higher than that typically used to treat depression.

◼ PROGNOSIS

The prognosis of anorexia nervosa is variable. Full recovery is seen in 25–50% of pts, but many have persistent difficulties with weight maintenance, depression, and eating disturbances, including bulimia. Mortality is 5% per decade, from starvation, electrolyte abnormalities, or suicide. Bulimia nervosa has a more benign outcome. Full recovery occurs in ~50% of pts within 10 years; 25% have persistent bulimia, but mortality is low.

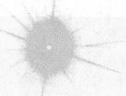

For a more detailed discussion, see Walsh TB, Attia E: Eating Disorders, Chap. 79, p. 636, in HPIM-18.

CHAPTER **211**
Alcoholism

Alcoholism is a multifactorial disorder in which genetic, biologic, and sociocultural factors interact.

- *Alcohol dependence*: defined in DSM-IV as repeated alcohol-related difficulties in at least three of seven areas of functioning that cluster together over the same 12-month period; tolerance and withdrawal are two of these seven areas and are associated with a more severe course.
- *Alcohol abuse*: defined as repetitive problems with alcohol in any one of four life areas—social, interpersonal, legal, and occupational—or repeated use in hazardous situations such as driving while intoxicated.

◼ CLINICAL FEATURES

Lifetime risk for alcohol dependence is 10–15% for men and 5–8% for women. Typically, the first major life problem from excessive alcohol use appears in early adulthood, followed by periods of exacerbation and remission. The course is not hopeless; following treatment, between half and two-thirds of pts maintain abstinence for years and often permanently. If the alcoholic continues to drink, life span is shortened by an average of 10 years due to increased risk of death from heart disease, cancer, accidents, or suicide.

Screening for alcoholism is important given its high prevalence. Probe for marital or job problems, legal difficulties, history of accidents, medical problems, and evidence of tolerance to alcohol. Standardized questionnaires can be helpful in busy clinical practices including the 10-item Alcohol Use Disorders Identification Test (AUDIT) (see Table 211-1).

Routine medical care requires attention to potential alcohol-related illness and to alcoholism itself:

1. Neurologic—blackouts, seizures, delirium tremens, cerebellar degeneration, neuropathy, myopathy
2. Gastrointestinal—esophagitis, gastritis, pancreatitis, hepatitis, cirrhosis, GI hemorrhage
3. Cardiovascular—hypertension, cardiomyopathy
4. Hematologic—macrocytosis, folate deficiency, thrombocytopenia, leukopenia
5. Endocrine—gynecomastia, testicular atrophy, amenorrhea, infertility
6. Skeletal—fractures, osteonecrosis
7. Cancer—breast cancer, oral and esophageal cancers, rectal cancers

Alcohol Intoxication

Alcohol is a CNS depressant that acts on receptors for γ-aminobutyric acid (GABA), the major inhibitory neurotransmitter in the nervous system. Behavioral, cognitive, and psychomotor changes can occur at blood alcohol levels as low as 0.02–0.03 g/dL, a level achieved after the ingestion of one or two typical drinks. "Legal intoxication" in most states requires a blood alcohol concentration of 0.08 g/dL; levels twice this can lead to deep but disturbed sleep. Incoordination, tremor, ataxia, confusion, stupor, coma, and even death occur at progressively higher blood alcohol levels.

Alcohol Withdrawal

Chronic alcohol use produces CNS dependence, and the earliest sign of alcohol withdrawal is tremulousness ("shakes" or "jitters"), occurring 5–10 h after decreasing ethanol intake. This may be followed by generalized seizures in the first 24–48 h; these do not require initiation of antiseizure medications. With severe withdrawal, autonomic hyperactivity ensues (sweating, hypertension, tachycardia, tachypnea, fever), accompanied by insomnia, nightmares, anxiety, and GI symptoms.

Delirium Tremens (DTs)

A very severe withdrawal syndrome characterized by profound autonomic hyperactivity, extreme confusion, agitation, vivid delusions, and hallucinations (often visual and tactile) that begins 3–5 days after the last drink. Mortality is 5–15%.

Wernicke's Encephalopathy

An alcohol-related syndrome characterized by ataxia, ophthalmoplegia, and confusion, often with associated nystagmus, peripheral neuropathy,

TABLE 211-1 THE ALCOHOL USE DISORDERS IDENTIFICATION TEST (AUDIT)[a]

Item	5-Point Scale (Least to Most)
1. How often do you have a drink containing alcohol?	Never (0) to 4+ per week (4)
2. How many drinks containing alcohol do you have on a typical day?	1 or 2 (0) to 10+ (4)
3. How often do you have six or more drinks on one occasion?	Never (0) to daily or almost daily (4)
4. How often during the last year have you found that you were not able to stop drinking once you had started?	Never (0) to daily or almost daily (4)
5. How often during the last year have you failed to do what was normally expected from you because of drinking?	Never (0) to daily or almost daily (4)
6. How often during the last year have you needed a first drink in the morning to get yourself going after a heavy drinking session?	Never (0) to daily or almost daily (4)
7. How often during the last year have you had a feeling of guilt or remorse after drinking?	Never (0) to daily or almost daily (4)
8. How often during the last year have you been unable to remember what happened the night before because you had been drinking?	Never (0) to daily or almost daily (4)
9. Have you or someone else been injured as a result of your drinking?	No (0) to yes, during the last year (4)
10. Has a relative, friend, doctor or other health worker been concerned about your drinking or suggested that you should cut down?	No (0) to yes, during the last year (4)

[a]Total score > 8 indicates harmful alcohol use and possible alcohol dependence.
Source: Adapted from DF Reinert, GP Allen: *Alcoholism: Clinical & Experimental Research* 26:272, 2002, and from MA Schuckit, *Drug and Alcohol Abuse: Clinical Guide to Diagnosis & Treatment*, 6th ed, New York: Springer, 2006.

cerebellar signs, and hypotension; there is impaired short-term memory, inattention, and emotional lability. Wernicke-Korsakoff's syndrome follows, characterized by anterograde and retrograde amnesia and confabulation. Wernicke-Korsakoff's syndrome is caused by chronic thiamine deficiency, resulting in damage to thalamic nuclei, mamillary bodies, and brainstem and cerebellar structures.

■ LABORATORY FINDINGS

Include mild anemia with macrocytosis, folate deficiency, thrombocytopenia, granulocytopenia, abnormal liver function tests, hyperuricemia, and elevated triglycerides. Two blood tests with ≥60% sensitivity and specificity are γ-glutamyl transferase (GGT) (>35 U) and carbohydrate-deficient transferrin (CDT) (>20 U/L or >2.6%); the combination of the two is likely to be more accurate than either alone. A variety of diagnostic studies may show evidence of alcohol-related organ dysfunction.

> **TREATMENT**   Alcoholism

ACUTE WITHDRAWAL

- Acute alcohol withdrawal is treated with multiple B vitamins including thiamine (50–100 mg IV or PO daily for ≥1 week) to replenish depleted stores; use the IV route if Wernicke-Korsakoff's syndrome is suspected since intestinal absorption is unreliable in alcoholics.
- CNS depressant drugs are used when seizures or autonomic hyperactivity is present to halt the rapid state of withdrawal in the CNS and allow for a slower, more controlled reduction of the substance. Low-potency benzodiazepines with long half-lives are the medication of choice (e.g., diazepam 10 mg PO q4–6 h, chlordiazepoxide 25–50 mg PO q 4–6 h) because they produce fairly steady blood levels of drug with a wide dose range within which to work. Risks include overmedication and oversedation, which occur less commonly with shorter-acting agents (e.g., oxazepam, lorazepam).
- In severe withdrawal or DTs, high doses of benzodiazepines are usually required. Fluid and electrolyte status and blood glucose levels should be closely followed. Cardiovascular and hemodynamic monitoring are crucial, as hemodynamic collapse and cardiac arrhythmia are not uncommon.
- Generalized withdrawal seizures rarely require aggressive pharmacologic intervention beyond that given to the usual pt undergoing withdrawal, i.e., adequate doses of benzodiazepines.

RECOVERY AND SOBRIETY
Counseling, Education, and Cognitive Approaches

- First, attempts should be made to help the alcoholic achieve and maintain a high level of motivation toward abstinence. These include education about alcoholism and instructing family and/or friends to stop protecting the person from the problems caused by alcohol.

- A second goal is to help the pt to readjust to life without alcohol and to reestablish a functional lifestyle through counseling, vocational rehabilitation, and self-help groups such as Alcoholics Anonymous (AA).
- A third component, called *relapse prevention*, helps the person to identify situations in which a return to drinking is likely, formulate ways of managing these risks, and develop coping strategies that increase the chances of a return to abstinence if a slip occurs.
- There is no convincing evidence that inpatient rehabilitation is more effective than outpatient care.

Drug Therapy Several medications may be useful in alcoholic rehabilitation; usually medications are continued for 6 months if a positive response is seen.

- The opioid-antagonist drug naltrexone, (50–150 mg/d PO or monthly 380 mg injection) decreases the probability of a return to drinking and shortens periods of relapse.
- A second medication, acamprosate (2 g/d divided into three oral doses), an *N*-methyl-D-aspartate receptor inhibitor, may be used; efficacy appears to be similar to naltrexone.
- A combination of naltrexone and acamprosate may be superior to either drug alone, although not all studies agree.
- Disulfiram (250 mg/d), an aldehyde dehydrogenase inhibitor, produces an unpleasant and potentially dangerous reaction in the presence of alcohol.

For a more detailed discussion, see Schuckit MA: Alcohol and Alcoholism, Chap. 392, p. 3546, in HPIM-18.

CHAPTER **212**
Narcotic Abuse

Narcotics, or opiates, bind to specific opioid receptors in the CNS and elsewhere in the body. These receptors mediate the opiate effects of analgesia, euphoria, respiratory depression, and constipation. Endogenous opiate peptides (enkephalins and endorphins) are natural ligands for the opioid receptors and play a role in analgesia, memory, learning, reward, mood regulation, and stress tolerance.

The prototypic opiates, morphine and codeine, are derived from the juice of the opium poppy. The semisynthetic drugs produced from morphine include hydromorphone (Dilaudid), diacetylmorphine (heroin), and oxycodone (OxyContin). The purely synthetic opioids and their cousins include meperidine, propoxyphene, diphenoxylate, fentanyl, buprenorphine, tramadol, methadone, and pentazocine. All of these substances produce analgesia and euphoria as well as physical dependence when taken in high enough doses for prolonged periods of time.

■ CLINICAL FEATURES

The 0.14% annual prevalence of heroin dependence in the United States is only about one-third the rate of prescription opiate abuse and is substantially lower than the 2% rate of morphine dependence in parts of Asia. Since 2007, prescription opiates have surpassed marijuana as the most common illicit drug that adolescents initially abuse.

Acute Effects

All opiates have the following CNS effects: sedation, euphoria, decreased pain perception, decreased respiratory drive, and vomiting. In larger doses, markedly decreased respirations, bradycardia, pupillary miosis, stupor, and coma ensue. Additionally, the adulterants used to "cut" street drugs (quinine, phenacetin, strychnine, antipyrine, caffeine, powdered milk) can produce permanent neurologic damage, including peripheral neuropathy, amblyopia, myelopathy, and leukoencephalopathy; adulterants can also produce an "allergic-like" reaction characterized by decreased alertness, frothy pulmonary edema, and an elevation in blood eosinophil count.

Chronic Effects

Tolerance and withdrawal commonly occur with chronic daily use after 6–8 weeks depending on the dose and frequency; the ever-increasing amounts of drug needed to sustain euphoriant effects and avoid discomfort of withdrawal strongly reinforce dependence once it has started.

Withdrawal

Withdrawal produces nausea and diarrhea, coughing, lacrimation, mydriasis, rhinorrhea, diaphoresis, twitching muscles, piloerection, fever, tachypnea, hypertension, diffuse body pain, insomnia, and yawning.

With shorter-acting opiates such as heroin, morphine, or oxycodone, withdrawal signs begin 8–16 h after the last dose, peak at 36–72 h, and subside over 5–8 days. With longer-acting opiates such as methadone, withdrawal begins several days after the last dose, peaks at 7–10 days in some cases, and lasts several weeks.

TREATMENT	Narcotic Abuse

OVERDOSE

- High doses of opiates, whether taken in a suicide attempt or accidentally when potency is misjudged, are potentially lethal. Toxicity occurs immediately after IV administration and with a variable delay after oral ingestion. Symptoms include miosis, shallow respirations, bradycardia, hypothermia, and stupor or coma.
- Managing overdose requires support of vital functions, including intubation if needed.

- The opiate antagonist naloxone is given at 0.4–2 mg IV or IM with an expected response within 1–2 min; repeated doses may be needed for 24–72 h depending on the opiate used in overdose

WITHDRAWAL

- Long-acting opiates such as methadone or buprenorphine can be used to treat withdrawal and achieve detoxification by slowly tapering the dose over weeks to months. Buprenorphine produces fewer withdrawal symptoms compared with methadone but does not appear to result in better outcomes.
- Several α-2-adrenergic agonists have relieved opioid withdrawal and achieved detoxification by suppressing central noradrenergic activity. Clonidine and lofexidine are commonly used orally in three to four doses per day. Completion rates of managed withdrawal are similar to methadone.
- Rapid opiate detoxification can be accomplished with naltrexone combined with an α-2-adrenergic agonist. Completion rates are high, but the approach is highly controversial due to the medical risks and even mortality associated with this approach.

OPIOID MAINTENANCE

- Methadone maintenance is a widely used treatment strategy in the management of opiate addiction. Methadone is a long-acting opioid optimally dosed at 80–150 mg/d (gradually increased over time).
- The partial agonist buprenorphine can also be used; it has several advantages, including low overdose danger, potentially easier detoxification than with methadone, and a probable ceiling effect in which higher doses do not increase euphoria. In the U.S. primary care physicians can prescribe buprenorphine; this may improve access and quality of treatment.

OPIATE ANTAGONISTS FOR OPIOID DEPENDENCE

- Rationale is that blocking the action of self-administered opioids should eventually extinguish the habit; poorly accepted by many pts.
- Naltrexone can be given three times a week (100- to 150-mg dose); a depot form for monthly injection is available and improves adherence, retention, and decreases opioid use.

DRUG-FREE PROGRAMS

- Medication-free treatments in inpatient, residential, or outpatient settings have poor 1- to 5-year outcomes compared with pharmacotherapy; exceptions are residential programs lasting 6–18 months, which require full immersion in a regimented system.

■ PREVENTION

Preventing opiate abuse is a critically important challenge for physicians. Sources of opiates for the 9000 adolescents in the United States that become abusers daily are most commonly family members, not drug dealers or the

Internet. Except for the terminally ill, physicians should carefully monitor opioid drug use in their pts, keeping doses as low as is practical and administering them over as short a period as the level of pain would warrant in the average person. Pts must dispose of any remaining opiates after treatment. Physicians must be vigilant regarding their own risk for opioid abuse and dependence, never prescribing these drugs for themselves.

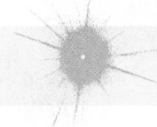

For a more detailed discussion, see Kosten TR: Opioid Drug Abuse and Dependence, Chap. 393, p. 3552, in HPIM-18.

CHAPTER **213**
Routine Disease Screening

A primary goal of health care is to prevent disease or to detect it early enough that interventions will be more effective. In general, screening is most effective when applied to relatively common disorders that carry a large disease burden and have a long latency period. Early detection of disease has the potential to reduce both morbidity and mortality; however, screening asymptomatic individuals carries some risk. False-positive results can lead to unnecessary lab tests and invasive procedures and can increase pt anxiety. Several measurements have been derived to better assess the potential gain from screening and prevention interventions:

- Number of subjects needed to be screened to alter the outcome in one individual
- Absolute impact of screening on disease (e.g., lives saved per thousand screened)
- Relative impact of screening on disease outcome (e.g., the % reduction in deaths)
- The cost per year of life saved
- The increase in average life expectancy for a population

Current recommendations include performance of a routine health care examination every 1–3 years before age 50 and every year thereafter. History should include medication use, allergies, vaccination history, dietary history, use of alcohol and tobacco, sexual practices, safety practices (seat belt and helmet use, gun possession), and a thorough family history. Routine measurements should include assessments of height, weight, body-mass index, and blood pressure. Screening should also be considered for domestic violence and depression.

Counseling by health care providers should be performed at health care visits. Tobacco and alcohol use, diet, and exercise represent the vast majority of factors that influence preventable deaths. While behavioral changes are frequently difficult to achieve, it should be emphasized that studies show even brief (<5 min) tobacco counseling by physicians results in a significant rate of long-term smoking cessation. Instruction about self-examination (e.g., skin, breast, testicular) should also be provided during preventative visits.

The top causes of age-specific mortality and corresponding preventative strategies are listed in Table 213-1. Formal recommendations from the U.S. Preventive Services Task Force are listed in Table 213-2.

In addition to the general recommendations applicable to all persons, screening for specific diseases and preventive measures need to be individualized based on family history, travel history, or occupational

TABLE 213-1 AGE-SPECIFIC CAUSES OF MORTALITY AND CORRESPONDING PREVENTATIVE OPTIONS

Age Group	Leading Causes of Age-Specific Mortality	Screening Prevention Interventions to Consider for Each Specific Population
15–24	1. Accident 2. Homicide 3. Suicide 4. Malignancy 5. Heart disease	• Counseling on routine seat belt use, bicycle/motorcycle/all terrain vehicle helmets (1) • Counseling on diet and exercise (5) • Discuss dangers of alcohol use while driving, swimming, boating (1) • Ask about vaccination status (tetanus, diphtheria, pertussis, hepatitis B, MMR, varicella, meningitis, HPV) • Ask about gun use and/or gun possession (2,3) • Assess for substance abuse history including alcohol (2,3) • Screen for domestic violence (2,3) • Screen for depression and/or suicidal/homicidal ideation (2,3) • Pap smear for cervical cancer screening, discuss STD prevention (4) • Recommend skin, breast, and testicular self-exams (4) • Recommend UV light avoidance and regular sun screen use (4) • Measurement of blood pressure, height, weight and body mass index (5) • Discuss health risks of tobacco use, consider emphasis of cosmetic and economic issues to improve quit rates for younger smokers (4,5) • *Chlamydia* screening and contraceptive counseling for sexually active females • HIV, hepatitis B, and syphilis testing if there is high-risk sexual behavior(s) or any prior history of sexually transmitted disease

TABLE 213-1 AGE-SPECIFIC CAUSES OF MORTALITY AND CORRESPONDING PREVENTATIVE OPTIONS (CONTINUED)

Age Group	Leading Causes of Age-Specific Mortality	Screening Prevention Interventions to Consider for Each Specific Population
25–44	1. Accident 2. Malignancy 3. Heart disease 4. Suicide 5. Homicide 6. HIV	*As above plus consider the following:* • Readdress smoking status, encourage cessation at every visit (2,3) • Obtain detailed family history of malignancies and begin early screening/prevention program if pt is at significant increased risk (2) • Assess all cardiac risk factors (including screening for diabetes and hyperlipidemia) and consider primary prevention with aspirin for pts at >3% 5-year risk of a vascular event (3) • Assess for chronic alcohol abuse, risk factors for viral hepatitis, or other risks for development of chronic liver disease • Begin breast cancer screening with mammography at age 40 (2)
45–64	1. Malignancy 2. Heart disease 3. Accident 4. Diabetes mellitus 5. Cerebrovascular disease 6. Chronic lower respiratory disease 7. Chronic liver disease and cirrhosis 8. Suicide	• Consider prostate cancer screen with annual PSA and digital rectal exam at age 50 (or possibly earlier in African Americans or pts with family history) (1) • Begin colorectal cancer screening at age 50 with either fecal occult blood testing, flexible sigmoidoscopy, or colonoscopy (1) • Reassess vaccination status at age 50 and give special consideration to vaccines against *Streptococcus pneumoniae*, influenza, tetanus, and viral hepatitis • Consider screening for coronary disease in higher risk pts (2,5)

(continued)

TABLE 213-1 AGE-SPECIFIC CAUSES OF MORTALITY AND CORRESPONDING PREVENTATIVE OPTIONS (CONTINUED)

Age Group	Leading Causes of Age-Specific Mortality	Screening Prevention Interventions to Consider for Each Specific Population
≥65	1. Heart disease 2. Malignancy 3. Cerebrovascular disease 4. Chronic lower respiratory disease 5. Alzheimer's disease 6. Influenza and pneumonia 7. Diabetes mellitus 8. Kidney disease 9. Accidents 10. Septicemia	*As above plus consider the following:* • Readdress smoking status, encourage cessation at every visit (1,2,3) • One-time ultrasound for AAA in men 65–75 who have ever smoked • Consider pulmonary function testing for all long-term smokers to assess for development of chronic obstructive pulmonary disease (4,6) • Vaccinate all smokers against influenza and *S. pneumoniae* at age 50 (6) • Screen all postmenopausal women (and all men with risk factors) for osteoporosis • Reassess vaccination status at age 65, emphasis on influenza and *S. pneumoniae* (4,6) • Screen for dementia and depression (5) • Screen for visual and hearing problems, home safety issues, and elder abuse (9)

Note: The numbers in parentheses refer to areas of risk in the mortality column affected by the specified intervention.
Abbreviations: AAA, abdominal aortic aneurysm; HPV, human papilloma virus; MMR, measles-mumps-rubella; PSA, prostate-specific antigen; STD, sexually transmitted disease; UV, ultraviolet.

history. For example, when there is a significant family history of breast, colon, or prostate cancer, it is prudent to initiate screening about 10 years before the age at which the youngest family member developed cancer.

Specific recommendations for disease prevention can also be found in subsequent chapters on "Immunization and Advice to Travelers" (Chap. 214), "Cardiovascular Disease Prevention" (Chap. 215), "Prevention and Early Detection of Cancer" (Chap. 216), "Smoking Cessation" (Chap. 217), and "Women's Health" (Chap. 218).

TABLE 213-2 CLINICAL PREVENTIVE SERVICES FOR NORMAL-RISK ADULTS RECOMMENDED BY THE U.S. PREVENTIVE SERVICES TASK FORCE

Test or Disorder	Population,[a] Years	Frequency
Blood pressure, height and weight	>18	Periodically
Cholesterol	Men >35	Every 5 years
	Women >45	Every 5 years
Depression	>18	Periodically[b]
Diabetes	>45 or earlier, if there are additional risk factors	Every 3 years
Pap smear[c]	Within 3 years of onset of sexual activity or 21–65	Every 1–3 years
Chlamydia	Women 18–25	Every 1–2 years
Mammography[a]	Women > 50[d]	Every 1–2 years
Colorectal cancer[a]	>50	
fecal occult blood and/or		Every year
sigmoidoscopy or		Every 5 years
colonoscopy		Every 10 years
Osteoporosis	Women >65; >60 at risk	Periodically
Abdominal aortic aneurysm (ultrasound)	Men 65–75 who have ever smoked	Once
Alcohol use	>18	Periodically
Vision, hearing	>65	Periodically
Adult immunization		
Tetanus-diphtheria (Td)	>18	Every 10 years
Varicella (VZV)	Susceptibles only, >18	Two doses
Zoster	>60	One dose
Measles, mumps, rubella (MMR)	Women, childbearing age	One dose
Pneumococcal	>65	One dose
Influenza	>50	Yearly
Human papillomavirus (HPV)	Up to age 26	If not done prior

[a]Screening is performed earlier and more frequently when there is a strong family history. Randomized, controlled trials have documented that fecal occult blood testing (FOBT) confers a 15–30% reduction in colon cancer mortality. Although randomized trials have not been performed for sigmoidoscopy or colonoscopy, well-designed case-control studies suggest similar or greater efficacy relative to FOBT.

[b]If staff support is available.

[d]In the future, Pap smear frequency may be influenced by HPV testing and the HPV vaccine.

^aSome authorities advocate starting mammography at age 40.

Note: Prostate-specific antigen (PSA) testing is capable of enhancing the detection of early-stage prostate cancer, but evidence is inconclusive that it improves health outcomes. PSA testing is recommended by several professional organizations and is widely used in clinical practice, but it is not currently recommended by the U.S. Preventive Services Task Force.

Source: Adapted from the U.S. Preventive Services Task Force, *Guide to Clinical Prevention Services*, 2010–2011. *www.ahrq.gov/clinic/pocketgd.htm.*

For a more detailed discussion, see Martin GJ: Screening and Prevention of Disease, Chap. 4, p. 29, in HPIM-18.

CHAPTER **214**
Immunization and Recommendations for Travelers

IMMUNIZATION

Few medical interventions of the past century can rival the effect that immunization has had on longevity, economic savings, and quality of life.

■ VACCINE IMPACT

- Vaccines have both a direct impact (protecting the vaccinated individual against infection) and indirect effects (reducing transmission of infectious agents from immunized people to others).
- Vaccine programs attempt to control, eliminate, or eradicate a disease.
  - *Control programs:* limit the disruptive impacts associated with outbreaks in a defined geographic area
  - *Elimination programs:* require a blockage in the indigenous sustained transmission of an infection in a defined geographic area, with possible importation of sporadic cases from other areas requiring ongoing interventions
  - *Eradication programs:* considered successful if elimination of a disease can be sustained without ongoing interventions. Smallpox is the only vaccine-preventable disease that has been globally eradicated; considerable effort is ongoing in attempts to eradicate polio.

■ IMMUNIZATION PRACTICE STANDARDS

- Figure 214-1 summarizes the adult immunization schedules for 2011.
- Before vaccination, pts must be screened for contraindications (conditions that substantially increase the risk of a serious adverse reaction) and precautions (conditions that may increase the risk of an adverse

event or that may compromise the ability of the vaccine to evoke immunity). Table 214-1 summarizes the contraindications and precautions for vaccines used commonly in adults.

- A vaccine information statement must be provided to all vaccine recipients; current VISs are available online at www.cdc.gov/vaccines *and* www.immunize.org/vis/. (The latter website includes translations.)
- Any adverse event that occurs after immunization and that may or may not be related to the vaccine should be reported to the Vaccine Adverse Event Reporting System (www.vaers.hhs.gov).

RECOMMENDATIONS FOR TRAVELERS

Travelers should be aware of various health risks that might be associated with given destinations. Information regarding country-specific risks can be obtained from the CDC publication *Health Information for International Travel*, which is available at www.cdc.gov/travel. Travelers should be encouraged to see a travel medicine practitioner before departure. Although infections contribute substantially to morbidity among travelers, they account for only ~1% of deaths; in contrast, injuries (e.g., motor vehicle, drowning, or aircraft accidents) account for 22% of deaths.

■ IMMUNIZATIONS FOR TRAVEL

There are three categories of immunization for travel.

- *Routine* immunizations (see Fig. 214-1) are needed regardless of travel. However, travelers from the United States should be certain that their routine immunizations are up to date because certain diseases (e.g., diphtheria, tetanus, polio, measles) are more likely to be acquired outside the United States than at home.
- *Required* immunizations (e.g., yellow fever vaccination) are mandated by international regulations for entry into certain areas.
- *Recommended* immunizations (e.g., hepatitis A, typhoid) are advisable because they protect travelers against illnesses for whose acquisition they are at increased risk. Table 214-2 lists vaccines required or recommended for travel.

■ PREVENTION OF MALARIA AND OTHER INSECT-BORNE DISEASES

- Chemoprophylaxis against malaria and other preventive measures are recommended for travel to malaria-endemic regions, particularly since fewer than 50% of travelers adhere to basic recommendations for malaria prevention.
- Chemoprophylactic regimens consist of chloroquine, doxycycline, atovaquone-proguanil, or mefloquine.
- In the United States, 90% of cases of *Plasmodium falciparum* infection occur in persons returning or immigrating from Africa and Oceania.
- The destination helps determine the particular medication chosen (e.g., whether chloroquine-resistant *P. falciparum* is present), as does the traveler's preference and medical history.
- Personal protective measures against mosquito bites [e.g., the use of DEET-containing insect repellents (25–50%), permethrin-impregnated bed nets, and screened sleeping areas], especially between dusk and dawn, can prevent malaria and other insect-borne diseases (e.g., dengue fever).

FIGURE 214-1 Recommended adult immunization schedules, United States, 2011. For complete statements by the Advisory Committee on Immunization Practices (ACIP), visit *www.cdc.gov/vaccines/pubs/ACIP-list.htm*.

Recommended Adult Immunization Schedule
UNITED STATES · 2011

Note: These recommendations *must* be read with the footnotes that follow containing number of doses, intervals between doses, and other important information.

Recommended adult immunization schedule, by vaccine and age group

VACCINE ▼ AGE GROUP▶	19–26 years	27–49 years	50–59 years	60–64 years	≥65 years
Influenza[1],*	1 dose annually				
Tetanus, diphtheria, pertussis (Td/Tdap)[2],*	Substitute 1-time dose of Tdap for Td booster; then boost with Td every 10 yrs				Td booster every 10 yrs
Varicella[3],*	2 doses				
Human papillomavirus (PHV)[4],*	3 doses (females)				
Zoster[5]				1 dose	1 dose
Measles, mumps, rubella (MMR)[6],*	1 or 2 doses		1 dose		
Pneumococcal (polysaccharide)[7,8]	1 or 2 doses				1 dose
Meningococcal[9],*	1 or more doses				
Hepatitis A[10],*	2 doses				
Hepatitis B[11],*	3 doses				

*Covered by the Vaccine Injury Compensation Program.

For all persons in this category who meet the age requirements and who lack evidence of immunity (e.g., lack documentation of vaccination or have no evidence of previous infection)	Recommended if some other risk factor is present (e.g., based on medical, occupational, lifestyle, or other indications)	No recommendation

Report all clinically significant postvaccination reactions to the Vaccine Adverse Event Reporting System (VAERS). Reporting forms and instructions on filing a VAERS report are available at http://www.vaers.hhs.gov or by telephone, 800-822-7967.

Information on how to file a Vaccine Injury Compensation Program claim is available at http://www.hrsa.gov/vaccinecompensation or by telephone, 800-338-2382. Information about filing a claim for vaccine injury is available through the U.S. Court of Federal Claims, 717 Madison Place, N.W., Washington, D.C. 20005; telephone, 202-357-6400.

Additional information about the vaccines in this schedule, extent of available data, and contraindications for vaccination also is available at http://www.cdc.gov/vaccines or from the CDC-INFO Contact Center at 800-CDC- INFO (800-232-4636) in English and Spanish, 24 hours a day, 7 days a week.

Vaccines that might be indicated for adults based on medical and other indications

INDICATION ▶ VACCINE ▼	Pregnancy	Immuno-compromising conditions (excluding human immunodeficiency virus [HIV])[3,5,6,13]	HIV infection[3,6,12,13] CD4 + T lympho - cyte count <200 cells/µL	HIV infection[3,6,12,13] CD4 + T lympho - cyte count ≥200 cells/µL	Diabetes, heart disease, chronic lung disease, chronic alcoholism	Asplenia[12] (including elective splenectomy) and persistent complement component deficiencies	Chronic liver disease	Kidney failure, end-stage renal disease, receipt of hemodialysis	Healthcare personnel
Influenza[1],*				1 dose TIV annually					1 dose TIV or LAIV annually
Tetanus, diphtheria, pertussis (Td/Tdap)[2],*	Td	Substitute 1-time dose of Tdap for Td booster; then boost with Td every 10 yrs							
Varicella[3],*	Contraindicated	Contraindicated		2 doses					
Human papillomavirus (HPV)[4],*		3 doses through age 26 yrs			3 doses through age 26 yrs				
Zoster[5]	Contraindicated	Contraindicated		1 dose			1 dose		
Measles, mumps, rubella (MMR)[6],*	Contraindicated	Contraindicated		1 or 2 doses			1 or 2 doses		
Pneumococcal (polysaccharide)[7,8]		1 or more doses				1 or 2 doses			
Meningococcal[9],*		2 doses				1 or 2 doses			
Hepatitis A[10],*									
Hepatitis B[11],*		3 doses							

*Covered by the Vaccine Injury Compensation Program.

For all persons in this category who meet the age requirements and who lack evidence of immunity (e.g., lack documentation of vaccination or have no evidence of previous infection)

Recommended if some other risk factor is present (e.g., on the basis of medical, occupational, lifestyle, or other indications)

No recommendation

These schedules indicate the recommended age groups and medical indications for which administration of currently licensed vaccines is commonly indicated for adults ages 19 years and older, as of February 4, 2011. For all vaccines being recommended on the adult immunization schedule, a vaccine series does not need to be restarted, regardless of the time that has elapsed between doses. Licensed combination vaccines may be used whenever any components of the combination are indicated and when the vaccine's other components are not contraindicated. For detailed recommendations on all vaccines, including those used primarily for travelers or that are issued during the year, consult the manufacturers' package inserts and the complete statements from the Advisory Committee on Immunization Practices (http://www.cdc.gov/vaccines/pubs/acip-list.htm).

The recommendations in this schedule were approved by the Centers for Disease Control and Prevention's (CDC) Advisory Committee on Immunization Practices (ACIP), the American Academy of Family Physicians (AAFP), the American College of Obstetricians and Gynecologists (ACOG), and the American College of Physicians (ACP).

U.S. DEPARTMENT OF HEALTH AND HUMAN SERVICES
CENTERS FOR DISEASE CONTROL AND PREVENTION **CDC**

1353

Footnotes
Recommended Adult Immunization Schedule—UNITED STATES · 2011
For complete statements by the Advisory Committee on Immunization Practices (ACIP), visit www.cdc.gov/vaccines/pubs/ACIP-list.htm.

1. Influenza vaccination
Annual vaccination against influenza is recommended for all persons aged 6 months and older, including all adults. Healthy, nonpregnant adults aged less than 50 years without high-risk medical conditions can receive either intranasally administered live, attenuated influenza vaccine (FluMist), or inactivated vaccine. Other persons should receive the inactivated vaccine. Adults aged 65 years and older can receive the standard influenza vaccine or the high-dose (Fluzone) influenza vaccine. Additional information about influenza vaccination is available at http://www.cdc.gov/vaccines/vpd-vac/flu/default.htm.

2. Tetanus, diphtheria, and acellular pertussis (Td/Tdap) vaccination
Administer a one-time dose of Tdap to adults aged less than 65 years who have not received Tdap previously or for whom vaccine status is unknown to replace one of the 10-year Td boosters, and as soon as feasible to all 1) postpartum women, 2) close contacts of infants younger than age 12 months (e.g., grandparents and child-care providers), and 3) healthcare personnel with direct patient contact. Adults aged 65 years and older who have not previously received Tdap and who have close contact with an infant aged less than 12 months also should be vaccinated. Other adults aged 65 years and older may receive Tdap. Tdap can be administered regardless of interval since the most recent tetanus or diphtheria-containing vaccine.

Adults with uncertain or incomplete history of completing a 3-dose primary vaccination series with Td-containing vaccines should begin or complete a primary vaccination series. For unvaccinated adults, administer the first 2 doses at least 4 weeks apart and the third dose 6–12 months after the second. If incompletely vaccinated (i.e., less than 3 doses), administer remaining doses. Substitute a one-time dose of Tdap for one of the doses of Td, either in the primary series or for the routine booster, whichever comes first.

If a woman is pregnant and received the most recent Td vaccination 10 or more years previously, administer Td during the second or third trimester. If the woman received the most recent Td vaccination less than 10 years previously, administer Tdap during the immediate postpartum period. At the clinician's discretion, Td may be deferred during pregnancy and Tdap substituted in the immediate postpartum period, or Tdap may be administered instead of Td to a pregnant woman after an informed discussion with the woman.

The ACIP statement for recommendations for administering Td as prophylaxis in wound management is available at http://www.cdc.gov/vaccines/pubs/acip-list.htm.

3. Varicella vaccination
All adults without evidence of immunity to varicella should receive 2 doses of single-antigen varicella vaccine if not previously vaccinated or a second dose if they have received only 1 dose, unless they have a medical contraindication. Special consideration should be given to those who 1) have close contact with persons at high risk for severe disease (e.g., healthcare personnel and family contacts of persons with immunocompromising conditions) or 2) are at high risk for exposure or transmission (e.g., teachers; child-care employees; residents and staff members of institutional settings, including correctional institutions; college students; military personnel; adolescents and adults living in households with children; nonpregnant women of childbearing age; and international travelers).

Evidence of immunity to varicella in adults includes any of the following: 1) documentation of 2 doses of varicella vaccine at least 4 weeks apart; 2) U.S.-born before 1980 (although for healthcare personnel and pregnant women, birth before 1980 should not be considered evidence of immunity); 3) history of varicella based on diagnosis or verification of varicella by a healthcare provider (for a patient reporting a history of or having an atypical case, a mild case, or both, healthcare providers should seek either an epidemiologic link with a typical varicella case or to a laboratory-confirmed case or evidence of laboratory confirmation, if it was performed at the time of acute disease); 4) history of herpes zoster based on diagnosis or verification of herpes zoster by a healthcare provider; or 5) laboratory evidence of immunity or laboratory confirmation of disease.

Pregnant women should be assessed for evidence of varicella immunity. Women who do not have evidence of immunity should receive the first dose of varicella vaccine upon completion or termination of pregnancy and before discharge from the healthcare facility. The second dose should be administered 4–8 weeks after the first dose.

4. Human papillomavirus (HPV) vaccination
HPV vaccination with either quadrivalent (HPV4) vaccine or bivalent vaccine (HPV2) is recommended for females at age 11 or 12 years and catch-up vaccination for females aged 13 through 26 years.

Ideally, vaccine should be administered before potential exposure to HPV through sexual activity; however, females who are sexually active should still be vaccinated consistent with age-based recommendations. Sexually active females who have not been infected with any of the four HPV vaccine types (types 6, 11, 16, and 18, all of which HPV4 prevents) or any of the two HPV vaccine types (types 16 and 18, both of which HPV2 prevents) receive the full benefit of the vaccination. Vaccination is less beneficial for females who have already been infected with one or more of the HPV vaccine types. HPV4 or HPV2 can be administered to persons with a history of genital warts, abnormal Papanicolaou test, or positive HPV DNA test, because these conditions are not evidence of previous infection with all vaccine HPV types.

HPV4 may be administered to males aged 9 through 26 years to reduce their likelihood of genital warts. HPV4 would be most effective when administered before exposure to HPV through sexual contact.

A complete series for either HPV4 or HPV2 consists of 3 doses. The second dose should be administered 1–2 months after the first dose; the third dose should be administered 6 months after the first dose.

Although HPV vaccination is not specifically recommended for persons with the medical indications described in Figure 2, "Vaccines that might be indicated for adults based on medical and other indications," it may be administered to these persons because the HPV vaccine is not a live-virus vaccine. However, the immune response and vaccine efficacy might be less for persons with the medical indications described in Figure 2 than in persons who do not have the medical indications described or who are immunocompetent.

5. Herpes zoster vaccination
A single dose of zoster vaccine is recommended for adults aged 60 years and older regardless of whether they report a previous episode of herpes zoster. Persons with chronic medical conditions may be vaccinated unless their condition constitutes a contraindication.

6. Measles, mumps, rubella (MMR) vaccination
Adults born before 1957 generally are considered immune to measles and mumps. All adults born in 1957 or later should have documentation of 1 or more doses of MMR vaccine unless they have a medical contraindication to the vaccine, laboratory evidence of immunity to each of the three diseases, or documentation of provider-diagnosed measles or mumps disease. For rubella, documentation of provider-diagnosed disease is not considered acceptable evidence of immunity.

Measles component: A second dose of MMR vaccine, administered a minimum of 28 days after the first dose, is recommended for adults who 1) have been recently exposed to measles or are in an outbreak setting; 2) are students in postsecondary educational institutions; 3) work in a healthcare facility; or 4) plan to travel internationally. Persons who received inactivated (killed) measles vaccine or measles vaccine of unknown type during 1963–1967 should be revaccinated with 2 doses of MMR vaccine.

Mumps component: A second dose of MMR vaccine, administered a minimum of 28 days after the first dose, is recommended for adults who 1) live in a community experiencing a mumps outbreak and are in an affected age group; 2) are students in postsecondary educational institutions; 3) work in a healthcare facility; or 4) plan to travel internationally. Persons vaccinated before 1979 with either killed mumps vaccine or mumps vaccine of unknown type who are at high risk for mumps infection (e.g. persons who are working in a healthcare facility) should be revaccinated with 2 doses of MMR vaccine.

Rubella component: For women of childbearing age, regardless of birth year, rubella immunity should be determined. If there is no evidence of immunity, women who are not pregnant should be vaccinated. Pregnant women who do not have evidence of immunity should receive MMR vaccine upon completion or termination of pregnancy and before discharge from the healthcare facility.

Healthcare personnel born before 1957: For unvaccinated healthcare personnel born before 1957 who lack laboratory evidence of measles, mumps, and/or rubella immunity or laboratory confirmation of disease, healthcare facilities should 1) consider routinely vaccinating personnel with 2 doses of MMR vaccine at the appropriate interval (for measles and mumps) and 1 dose of MMR vaccine (for rubella), and 2) recommend 2 doses of MMR vaccine at the appropriate interval during an outbreak of measles or mumps, and 1 dose during an outbreak of rubella. Complete information about evidence of immunity is available at http://www.cdc.gov/vaccines/recs/provisional/default.htm.

7. Pneumococcal polysaccharide (PPSV) vaccination

Vaccinate all persons with the following indications:

Medical: Chronic lung disease (including asthma); chronic cardiovascular diseases; diabetes mellitus; chronic liver diseases; cirrhosis; chronic alcoholism; functional or anatomic asplenia (e.g., sickle cell disease or splenectomy [if elective splenectomy is planned, vaccinate at least 2 weeks before surgery]); immunocompromising conditions (including chronic renal failure or nephrotic syndrome); and cochlear implants and cerebrospinal fluid leaks. Vaccinate as close to HIV diagnosis as possible.

Other: Residents of nursing homes or long-term care facilities and persons who smoke cigarettes. Routine use of PPSV is not recommended for American Indians/Alaska Natives or persons aged less than 65 years unless they have underlying medical conditions that are PPSV indications. However, public health authorities may consider recommending PPSV for American Indians/Alaska Natives and persons aged 50 through 64 years who are living in areas where the risk for invasive pneumococcal disease is increased

8. Revaccination with PPSV

One-time revaccination after 5 years is recommended for persons aged 19 through 64 years with chronic renal failure or nephrotic syndrome; functional or anatomic asplenia (e.g., sickle cell disease or splenectomy); and for persons with immunocompromising conditions. For persons aged 65 years and older, one-time revaccination is recommended if they were vaccinated 5 or more years previously and were aged less than 65 years at the time of primary vaccination.

9. Meningococcal vaccination

Meningococcal vaccine should be administered to persons with the following indications:

Medical: A 2-dose series of meningococcal conjugate vaccine is recommended for adults with anatomic or functional asplenia, or persistent complement component deficiencies. Adults with HIV infection who are vaccinated should also receive a routine 2-dose series. The 2 doses should be administered at 0 and 2 months.

Other: A single dose of meningococcal vaccine is recommended for unvaccinated first-year college students living in dormitories; microbiologists routinely exposed to isolates of *Neisseria meningitidis*; military recruits; and persons who travel to or live in countries in which meningococcal disease is hyperendemic or epidemic (e.g., the "meningitis belt" of sub-Saharan Africa during the dry season [December through June]), particularly if their contact with local populations will be prolonged. Vaccination is required by the government of Saudi Arabia for all travelers to Mecca during the annual Hajj.

Meningococcal conjugate vaccine, quadrivalent (MCV4) is preferred for adults with any of the preceding indications who are aged 55 years and younger; meningococcal polysaccharide vaccine (MPSV4) is preferred for adults aged 56 years and older. Revaccination with MCV4 every 5 years is recommended for adults previously vaccinated with MCV4 or MPSV4 who remain at increased risk for infection (e.g., adults with anatomic or functional asplenia, or persistent complement component deficiencies).

10. Hepatitis A vaccination

Vaccinate persons with any of the following indications and any person seeking protection from hepatitis A virus (HAV) infection:

Behavioral: Men who have sex with men and persons who use injection drugs.

Occupational: Persons working with HAV-infected primates or with HAV in a research laboratory setting.

Medical: Persons with chronic liver disease and persons who receive clotting factor concentrates.

Other: Persons traveling to or working in countries that have high or intermediate endemicity of hepatitis A (a list of countries is available at http://wwwn.cdc.gov/travel/contentdiseases.aspx).

Unvaccinated persons who anticipate close personal contact (e.g., household or regular babysitting) with an international adoptee during the first 60 days after arrival in the United States from a country with high or intermediate endemicity should be vaccinated. The first dose of the 2-dose hepatitis A vaccine series should be administered as soon as adoption is planned, ideally 2 or more weeks before the arrival of the adoptee.

Single-antigen vaccine formulations should be administered in a 2-dose schedule at either 0 and 6–12 months (Havrix), or 0 and 6–18 months (Vaqta). If the combined hepatitis A and hepatitis B vaccine (Twinrix) is used, administer 3 doses at 0, 1, and 6 months; alternatively, a 4-dose schedule may be used, administered on days 0, 7, and 21–30, followed by a booster dose at month 12.

11. Hepatitis B vaccination

Vaccinate persons with any of the following indications and any person seeking protection from hepatitis B virus (HBV) infection:

Behavioral: Sexually active persons who are not in a long-term, mutually monogamous relationship (e.g., persons with more than one sex partner during the previous 6 months); persons seeking evaluation or treatment for a sexually transmitted disease (STD); current or recent injection-drug users; and men who have sex with men.

Occupational: Healthcare personnel and public-safety workers who are exposed to blood or other potentially infectious body fluids.

Medical: Persons with end-stage renal disease, including patients receiving hemodialysis; persons with HIV infection; and persons with chronic liver disease.

Other: Household contacts and sex partners of persons with chronic HBV infection; clients and staff members of institutions for persons with developmental disabilities; and international travelers to countries with high or intermediate prevalence of chronic HBV infection (a list of countries is available at http://wwwn.cdc.gov/travel/contentdiseases.aspx).

Hepatitis B vaccination is recommended for all adults in the following settings: STD treatment facilities; HIV testing and treatment facilities; facilities providing drug-abuse treatment and prevention services; healthcare settings targeting services to injection-drug users or men who have sex with men; correctional facilities; end-stage renal disease programs and facilities for chronic hemodialysis patients; and institutions and nonresidential day-care facilities for persons with developmental disabilities.

Administer missing doses to complete a 3-dose series of hepatitis B vaccine to those persons not vaccinated or not completely vaccinated. The second dose should be administered 1 month after the first dose; the third dose should be given at least 2 months after the second dose (and at least 4 months after the first dose). If the combined hepatitis A and hepatitis B vaccine (Twinrix) is used, administer 3 doses at 0, 1, and 6 months; alternatively, a 4-dose Twinrix schedule, administered on days 0, 7, and 21 to 30, followed by a booster dose at month 12 may be used.

Adult patients receiving hemodialysis or with other immunocompromising conditions should receive 1 dose of 40 µg/mL (Recombivax HB) administered on a 3-dose schedule or 2 doses of 20 µg/mL (Engerix-B) administered simultaneously on a 4-dose schedule at 0, 1, 2, and 6 months.

12. Selected conditions for which Haemophilus influenzae type b (Hib) vaccine may be used

1 dose of Hib vaccine should be considered for persons who have sickle cell disease, leukemia, or HIV infection, or who have had a splenectomy, if they have not previously received Hib vaccine.

13. Immunocompromising conditions

Inactivated vaccines generally are acceptable (e.g., pneumococcal, meningococcal, influenza [inactivated influenza vaccine]) and live vaccines generally are avoided in persons with immune deficiencies or immunocompromising conditions. Information on specific conditions is available at http://www.cdc.gov/vaccines/pubs/acip-list.htm.

TABLE 214-1 CONTRAINDICATIONS AND PRECAUTIONS FOR COMMONLY USED VACCINES IN ADULTS

Vaccine Formulation	Contraindications and Precautions
All vaccines	**Contraindication** Severe allergic reaction (e.g., anaphylaxis) after a previous vaccine dose or to a vaccine component **Precaution** Moderate or severe acute illness with or without fever; defer vaccination until illness resolves
Td	**Precautions** GBS within 6 weeks after a previous dose of TT-containing vaccine History of Arthus-type hypersensitivity reactions after a previous dose of TT-containing vaccine; defer vaccination until at least 10 years have elapsed since the last dose
Tdap	**Contraindication** History of encephalopathy (e.g., coma or prolonged seizures) not attributable to another identifiable cause within 7 days of administration of a vaccine with pertussis components, such as DTaP or Tdap **Precautions** GBS within 6 weeks after a previous dose of TT-containing vaccine Unstable neurologic condition (e.g., cerebrovascular events and acute encephalopathic conditions) History of Arthus-type hypersensitivity reactions after a previous dose of TT-containing and/or DT-containing vaccine, including MCV4; defer vaccination until at least 10 years have elapsed since the last dose Pregnancy
HPV	**Contraindication** History of immediate hypersensitivity to yeast (for Gardasil) **Precaution** Pregnancy. If a woman is found to be pregnant after initiation of the vaccination series, the remainder of the 3-dose regimen should be delayed until after completion of the pregnancy. If a vaccine dose has been administered during pregnancy, no intervention is needed. A vaccine-in-pregnancy registry has been established for Gardasil; pts and health care providers should report any exposure to quadrivalent HPV vaccine during pregnancy (telephone: 800-986-8999).
MMR	**Contraindications** History of immediate hypersensitivity reaction to gelatin[a] or neomycin

TABLE 214-1 CONTRAINDICATIONS AND PRECAUTIONS FOR COMMONLY USED VACCINES IN ADULTS (CONTINUED)

Vaccine Formulation	Contraindications and Precautions
MMR (continued)	Pregnancy
	Known severe immunodeficiency (e.g., hematologic and solid tumors; chemotherapy; congenital immunodeficiency; long-term immunosuppressive therapy; severe immunocompromise due to HIV infection)
	Precaution
	Recent (within 11 months) receipt of antibody-containing blood product
Varicella	**Contraindications**
	Pregnancy
	Known severe immunodeficiency
	History of immediate hypersensitivity reaction to gelatin[a] or neomycin
	Precaution
	Recent (within 11 months) receipt of antibody-containing blood product
Influenza, injectable, trivalent	**Contraindication**
	History of immediate hypersensitivity reaction to eggs[b]
	Precautions
	History of GBS within 6 weeks after a previous influenza vaccine dose
	Pregnancy is *not* a contraindication or precaution. This vaccine is recommended for women who will be pregnant during the influenza season.
Influenza, live attenuated	**Contraindications**
	History of immediate hypersensitivity reaction to eggs[b]
	Age ≥50 years
	Pregnancy
	Immunosuppression, including that caused by medications or by HIV infection; known severe immunodeficiency (e.g., hematologic and solid tumors; chemotherapy; congenital immunodeficiency; long-term immunosuppressive therapy; severe immunocompromise due to HIV infection)
	Certain chronic medical conditions, such as diabetes mellitus; chronic pulmonary disease (including asthma); chronic cardiovascular disease (except hypertension); renal, hepatic, neurologic/neuromuscular, hematologic, or metabolic disorders
	Close contact with severely immunosuppressed persons who require a protected environment (e.g., isolation in a bone marrow transplantation unit)

(continued)

TABLE 214-1 CONTRAINDICATIONS AND PRECAUTIONS FOR COMMONLY USED VACCINES IN ADULTS (CONTINUED)

Vaccine Formulation	Contraindications and Precautions
Influenza, live attenuated (continued)	Close contact with persons with lesser degrees of immunosuppression (e.g., persons receiving chemotherapy or radiation therapy who are not being cared for in a protective environment; persons with HIV infection) is *not* a contraindication or precaution.
	Precaution
	History of GBS within 6 weeks of a previous influenza vaccine dose
Pneumococcal polysaccharide	None
Hepatitis A	**Precaution**
	Pregnancy
Hepatitis B	**Contraindication**
	History of immediate hypersensitivity to yeast
Meningococcal conjugate	**Contraindications**
	Age >55 years (licensed for use only among persons 2–55 years of age)
	History of severe allergic reaction to dry natural rubber (latex) or to DT-containing vaccines
	Precaution
	History of GBS
Meningococcal polysaccharide	**Contraindication**
	History of severe allergic reaction to dry natural rubber (latex)
Zoster	**Contraindications**
	Age <60 years
	Pregnancy
	Known severe immunodeficiency
	History of immediate hypersensitivity reaction to gelatin[a] or neomycin

[a]Extreme caution must be exercised in administering MMR, varicella, or zoster vaccine to persons with a history of an anaphylactic reaction to gelatin or gelatin-containing products. Before administration, skin testing for sensitivity to gelatin can be considered. However, no specific protocols for this purpose have been published.

[b]Protocols have been published for safely administering influenza vaccine to persons with egg allergies. See references 222–224 in Fiore AE et al: MMWR Recomm Rep 57:1, 2008.

Abbreviations: DT, diphtheria toxoid; DTaP, diphtheria, tetanus, and pertussis; GBS, Guillain-Barré syndrome; HPV, human papillomavirus; MMR, measles, mumps, and rubella; Td, tetanus and diphtheria toxoids; Tdap, tetanus and diphtheria toxoids and acellular pertussis; TT, tetanus toxoid.

TABLE 214-2 VACCINES COMMONLY USED FOR TRAVEL

Vaccine	Primary Series	Booster Interval
Cholera, live oral (CVD 103 HgR)	1 dose	6 months
Hepatitis A (Havrix), 1440 enzyme immunoassay U/mL	2 doses, 6–12 months apart, IM	None required
Hepatitis A (VAQTA, AVAXIM, EPAXAL)	2 doses, 6–12 months apart, IM	None required
Hepatitis A/B combined (Twinrix)	3 doses at 0, 1, and 6–12 months *or* 0, 7, and 21 days plus booster at 1 year, IM	None required *except* 12 months (once only, for accelerated schedule)
Hepatitis B (Engerix B): accelerated schedule	3 doses at 0, 1, and 2 months *or* 0, 7, and 21 days plus booster at 1 year, IM	12 months, once only
Hepatitis B (Engerix B or Recombivax): standard schedule	3 doses at 0, 1, and 6 months, IM	None required
Immune globulin (hepatitis A prevention)	1 dose IM	Intervals of 3–5 months, depending on initial dose
Japanese encephalitis (JE-VAX)	3 doses, 1 week apart, SC	12–18 months (first booster), then 4 years
Japanese encephalitis (Ixiaro)	2 doses, 1 month apart, SC	Optimal booster schedule not yet determined
Meningococcus, quadrivalent [Menimmune (polysaccharide), Menactra, Menveo (conjugate)]	1 dose SC	>3 years (optimal booster schedule not yet determined)
Rabies (HDCV), rabies vaccine absorbed (RVA), or purified chick embryo cell vaccine (PCEC)	3 doses at 0, 7, and 21 or 28 days, IM	None required except with exposure
Typhoid Ty21a, oral live attenuated (Vivotif)	1 capsule every other day × 4 doses	5 years
Typhoid Vi capsular polysaccharide, injectable (Typhim Vi)	1 dose IM	2 years
Yellow fever	1 dose SC	10 years

■ PREVENTION OF GASTROINTESTINAL ILLNESS

- Diarrhea, the leading cause of illness in travelers, is usually a short-lived, self-limited condition, although 20% of pts are confined to bed.
- Incidence rates per 2-week stay approach 55% in parts of Africa, Central and South America, and Southeast Asia.
- Travelers should eat only well-cooked hot foods, peeled or cooked fruits and vegetables, and bottled or boiled liquids (i.e., "boil it, cook it, peel it, or forget it!").
- The most common etiologies of travelers' diarrhea are toxigenic and enteroaggregative strains of *Escherichia coli*, although *Campylobacter* and norovirus are common in certain circumstances.
- Travelers should carry medications for self-treatment.
  – Mild to moderate diarrhea can be treated with loperamide and fluids.
  – Moderate to severe diarrhea should be treated with a 3-day course or a single double dose of a fluoroquinolone.
    • High rates of quinolone-resistant *Campylobacter* in Thailand make azithromycin a better choice for that country.
    • If fever and hematochezia are both absent, loperamide should be taken in combination with the antibiotic.
- Prophylaxis with bismuth subsalicylate is ~60% effective; for some pts (athletes, pts with repeated travelers' diarrhea, and persons with chronic diseases), a single daily dose of a quinolone, azithromycin, or rifaximin during travel of <1 month's duration is 75–90% effective.

■ PREVENTION OF OTHER TRAVEL-RELATED PROBLEMS

- Travelers are at high risk for sexually transmitted diseases preventable by condom use.
- Schistosomiasis can be prevented by avoidance of swimming or bathing in freshwater lakes, streams, or rivers in parts of northeastern South America, the Caribbean, Africa, and Southeast Asia.
- Travel-associated injury can be prevented with common-sense precautions: not riding on motorcycles and in overcrowded public vehicles, not traveling by road in rural areas of developing countries after dark, and not drinking excessive amounts of alcohol.
- Walking barefoot should be avoided given the risk of hookworm and *Strongyloides* infections and snakebites.

■ TRAVEL DURING PREGNANCY

- The safest part of pregnancy in which to travel is between 18 and 24 weeks, when the risk of spontaneous abortion or premature labor is low.
- Relative contraindications to international travel during pregnancy include a history of miscarriage, premature labor, incompetent cervix, or toxemia or the presence of other general medical problems (e.g., heart failure, severe anemia).
- Areas of excessive risk (e.g., where live virus vaccines are required for travel or where multidrug-resistant malaria is endemic) should be avoided throughout pregnancy.
- Malaria during pregnancy carries a significant risk of morbidity and death for both the mother and the fetus.

■ THE HIV-INFECTED TRAVELER

- HIV-seropositive persons with depressed CD4+ T cell counts should seek counseling from a travel medicine practitioner before departure, particularly when traveling to the developing world.
- Several countries routinely deny entry to HIV-positive persons for prolonged stay, even though these restrictions do not appear to decrease rates of transmission of the virus.
- Ensuring that HIV-infected pts' immunizations are up to date is critical, as many vaccine-preventable diseases are particularly severe in this population.
- Malaria is especially severe in pts with AIDS; the HIV load doubles during malaria, with subsidence in 8–9 weeks.

■ PROBLEMS AFTER RETURN FROM TRAVEL

- *Diarrhea:* After travelers' diarrhea, symptoms may persist because of the continued presence of pathogens (e.g., *Giardia lamblia*) or, more often, because of postinfectious sequelae such as lactose intolerance or irritable bowel syndrome. A trial of metronidazole for giardiasis, a lactose-free diet, or a several-week trial of high-dose hydrophilic mucilloid (plus an osmotic laxative such as lactulose or PEG 3350) may relieve symptoms.
- *Fever:* Malaria is the first diagnosis that should be considered when a traveler returns from an endemic area with fever. Malaria is acquired most often in Africa, dengue in Southeast Asia and the Caribbean, typhoid fever in southern Asia, and rickettsial infections in southern Africa.
- *Skin conditions:* Pyodermas, sunburn, insect bites, skin ulcers, and cutaneous larva migrans are the most common skin conditions in returning travelers; if persistent, a diagnosis of cutaneous leishmaniasis, mycobacterial infection, or fungal infection should be considered.

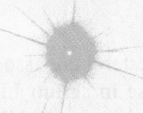

For a more detailed discussion, see Schuchat A, Jackson LA: Immunization Principles and Vaccine Use, Chap. 122, p. 1031; and Keystone JS, Kozarsky PE: Health Recommendations for International Travel, Chap. 123, p. 1042, in HPIM-18.

CHAPTER **215**
Cardiovascular Disease Prevention

Cardiovascular disease is the leading cause of death in developed nations; prevention is targeted at modifiable atherosclerosis risk factors (Table 215-1). Identification and control of these attributes reduce subsequent cardiovascular event rates.

TABLE 215-1 ESTABLISHED ATHEROSCLEROTIC RISK FACTORS

Modifiable Risk Factors

Cigarette smoking

Dyslipidemias (↑LDL or ↓HDL)

Hypertension

Diabetes mellitus

Obesity

Sedentary lifestyle

Unmodifiable Risk Factors

Premature coronary heart disease in first-degree relatives (age <55 in men, <65 in women)

Age (men ≥45 years; women ≥55 years)

Male sex

■ ESTABLISHED RISK FACTORS

Cigarette Smoking

Cigarette smoking increases the incidence of, and mortality associated with, coronary heart disease (CHD). Observational studies show that smoking cessation reduces excess risk of coronary events within months; after 3–5 years, the risk falls to that of individuals who never smoked. Pts should be asked regularly about tobacco use, followed by counseling and, as needed, antismoking pharmacologic therapy to assist cessation.

Lipid Disorders

(See Chap. 189) Both elevated LDL and low HDL cholesterol are associated with cardiovascular events. Each 1-mg/dL increase in serum LDL correlates with a 2–3% rise in CHD risk; each 1-mg/dL decrease in HDL heightens risk by 3–4%. ATP III guidelines advise a fasting lipid profile [total cholesterol, triglycerides, HDL, LDL (calculated or directly measured)] in all adults, repeated every 5 years. Recommended dietary and/or pharmacologic approach depends on presence or risk of coronary artery disease (CAD) and the LDL level (Table 215-2); treatment should be most aggressive in pts with established CAD and in those with "equivalent risk" (e.g., presence of peripheral arterial disease or diabetes mellitus). Drug therapy is indicated when LDL level exceeds goal in Table 215-2 by 30 mg/dL (0.8 mmol/L). If elevated triglyceride level [>200 mg/dL (> 2.6 mmol/L)] persists after control of LDL, secondary goal is to achieve non-HDL level (calculated as total cholesterol minus HDL) ≤30 mg/dL (0.8 mmol/L) above the target values listed in Table 215-2. In pts with isolated low HDL, encourage beneficial lifestyle measures: smoking cessation, weight loss, and increased physical activity. Consider addition of fibric acid derivative or niacin to raise HDL in pts with established CAD (see Chap. 189).

TABLE 215-2 LDL CHOLESTEROL GOALS AND CUTPOINTS FOR THERAPEUTIC LIFESTYLE CHANGES (TLC) AND DRUG THERAPY IN DIFFERENT RISK CATEGORIES

| Risk Category | LDL Level, mmol/L (mg/dL) | | |
	Goal	Initiate TLC	Consider Drug Therapy
Very high ACS, or CHD w/DM, or multiple CRF	<1.8 (<70)	≥1.8 (≥70)	≥1.8 (≥70)
High CHD or CHD risk equivalents (10-year risk > 20%)	<2.6 (<100) [optional goal: <1.8 (<70)]	≥2.6 (≥100)	≥2.6 (≥100) [<2.6 (<100): consider drug Rx]
If LDL < 2.6 (<100)	<1.8 (<70)		
Moderately high 2+ risk factors (10-year risk, 10–20%)	<2.6 (<100)	≥3.4 (≥130)	≥3.4 (≥130) [2.6–3.3 (100–129): consider drug Rx]
Moderate 2+ risk factors (risk < 10%)	<3.4 (<130)	≥3.4 (≥130)	≥4.1 (≥160)
Lower 0–1 risk factor	<4.1 (<160)	≥4.1 (≥160)	≥4.9 (≥190)

Abbreviations: ACS, acute coronary syndrome; CHD, coronary heart disease; DM, diabetes mellitus; CRF, coronary risk factors; LDL, low-density lipoprotein.
Source: Adapted from S Grundy et al: Circulation 110:227, 2004.

Hypertension

(See Chap. 126) Systolic or diastolic bp > "optimal" level of 115/75 mmHg is associated with increased risk of cardiovascular disease; each augmentation of 20 mmHg systolic, or 10 mmHg diastolic, above this value doubles the risk. Treatment of elevated blood pressure reduces the rate of stroke, congestive heart failure, and CHD events, with general goal of bp <140/85 mmHg or <130/80 in pts with diabetes or chronic kidney disease. Cardiovascular event rates in elderly pts with isolated systolic hypertension (systolic ≥140 but diastolic <90) are also reduced by antihypertensive therapy.

See Chap. 126 for antihypertensive treatment recommendations. Pts with "prehypertension" (systolic bp 120–139 mmHg or diastolic bp 80–89 mmHg) should receive counseling about beneficial lifestyle modifications such as those listed below (e.g., low-fat diet replete with vegetables and fruit, weight loss if overweight, increased physical activity, reduction of excessive alcohol consumption).

Diabetes Mellitus/Insulin Resistance/Metabolic Syndrome

(See Chaps. 127 and 184) Pts with diabetes most often succumb to cardiovascular disease. LDL levels are typically near average in diabetic pts, but LDL particles are smaller, denser, and more atherogenic; low HDL and elevated triglyceride levels are common. Tight control of serum glucose in type 2 diabetics reduces microvascular diabetic complications (retinopathy, renal disease), but a decrease in macrovascular events (CAD, stroke) has not been shown. Conversely, successful management of associated risk factors in diabetics (e.g., dyslipidemia and hypertension) *does* reduce cardiovascular events and should be vigorously pursued. Antilipidemic (i.e., statin) therapy should be used to lower LDL to <100 mg/dL in diabetics, even if pt has no symptoms of CAD.

Individuals without overt diabetes but who have "metabolic syndrome" (constellation of insulin resistance, central obesity, hypertension, hypertriglyceridemia, low HDL—see Chap. 127) are also at high risk of cardiovascular events. Dietary counseling, weight loss, and increased physical activity are important in reducing the prevalence of this syndrome.

Male Sex/Postmenopausal State

Coronary risk is greater in men compared to that of premenopausal women of same age, but female risk accelerates after menopause. Estrogen-replacement therapy lowers LDL and raises HDL in postmenopausal women and in observational studies has been associated with reduced coronary events. However, prospective clinical trials do not support such a benefit and hormone-replacement therapy should not be prescribed for the purpose of cardiovascular risk reduction, especially in older women.

■ EMERGING RISK FACTORS

May be assessed selectively in pts without above traditional risk factors who have premature vascular disease or strong family history of premature vascular disease.

Homocysteine

There is a graded correlation between serum homocysteine levels and risk of cardiovascular events and stroke. Supplemental folic acid and other B vitamins lower serum levels, but prospective clinical trials have not shown that such therapy reduces cardiac events.

Inflammation

Inflammatory serum markers, such as high-sensitivity C-reactive protein (CRP), correlate with the risk of coronary events. CRP prospectively predicts risk of MI and outcomes after acute coronary syndromes; its usefulness and role in prevention as an independent risk factor is currently being defined.

Potential benefits of assessing other emerging risk factors [e.g., lipoprotein(a), fibrinogen] remain unproven and controversial.

■ PREVENTION

Antithrombotic Therapy in Primary Prevention

Thrombosis at the site of disrupted atherosclerotic plaque is the most common cause of acute coronary events. In primary prevention trials, chronic low-dose aspirin therapy has reduced the risk of a first MI in men and the risk of stroke in women. The American Heart Association recommends aspirin (75–160 mg daily) for men and women who are at high cardiovascular risk (i.e., by Framingham Study criteria, for men with ≥10% 10-year risk, or women with ≥20% 10-year risk).

Lifestyle Modifications

Encourage beneficial exercise habits (>30 min moderate intensity physical activity daily) and sensible diet (low in saturated and trans fat; 2–3 servings of fish/week to ensure adequate intake of omega-3 fatty acids; balance caloric consumption with energy expenditure). Advise moderation in ethanol intake (no more than 1–2 drinks/day).

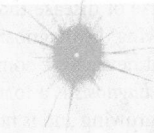

For a more detailed discussion, see Libby P: The Pathogenesis, Prevention, and Treatment of Atherosclerosis, Chap. 241, p. 1983; Gaziano TA and Gaziano JM: Epidemiology of Cardiovascular Disease, Chap. 225, p. 1811; and Martin GJ: Screening and Prevention of Disease, Chap. 4, p. 29; in HPIM-18.

CHAPTER **216**
Prevention and Early Detection of Cancer

One of the most important functions of medical care is to prevent disease or discover it early enough that treatment might be more effective. All risk factors for cancer have not yet been defined. However, a substantial number of factors that elevate risk are within a person's control. Some of these factors are listed in Table 216-1. Every physician visit is an opportunity to teach and reinforce the elements of a healthy lifestyle. Cancer screening in the asymptomatic population at average risk is a complex issue. To be of value, screening must detect disease at a stage that is more readily curable than disease that is treated after symptoms appear. For cervix cancer and colon cancer, screening has been shown to save lives. For other tumors, benefit is less clear. Screening can cause harm; complications may ensue from the screening test or the tests done to validate a positive screening test or from treatments for the underlying disease. Furthermore, quality of life can be adversely affected by false-positive tests. Evaluation of screening

TABLE 216-1 LIFESTYLE FACTORS THAT REDUCE CANCER RISK

Do not use any tobacco products
Maintain a healthy weight; eat a well-balanced diet[a]; maintain caloric balance
Exercise at least 3 times a week
Prevent sun exposure
Avoid excessive alcohol intake
Practice safe sex; use condoms

[a]Not precisely defined, but current recommendations include 5 servings of fruits and vegetables per day, 25 g fiber, and <30% of calories coming from fat.

tools can be biased and needs to rely on prospective randomized studies. *Lead-time bias* occurs when the natural history of disease is unaffected by the diagnosis, but the pt is diagnosed earlier in the course of disease than normal; thus, the pt spends more of his/her life span knowing the diagnosis. *Length bias* occurs when slow-growing cancers that might never have come to medical attention are detected during screening. *Overdiagnosis* is a form of length bias in which a cancer is detected when it is not growing and is not an influence on length of survival. *Selection bias* is the term for the fact that people who volunteer for screening trials may be different from the general population. Volunteers might have family history concerns that actually elevate their risk, or they may be generally more health-conscious, which can affect outcome.

The various groups that evaluate and recommend screening practice guidelines have used varying criteria to make their recommendations (Table 216-2). The absence of data on survival for a number of diseases has led to a lack of consensus. In particular, four areas are worth noting.

1. *Prostate cancer*: Prostate-specific antigen (PSA) levels are elevated in prostate cancer, but a substantial number of the cancers detected appear to be non-life-threatening. PSA screening has not been shown to improve survival. Efforts are underway to develop better tests (predominantly using bound vs. free and rate of increase of PSA) to distinguish lethal and nonlethal cancers.

2. *Breast cancer*: The data on annual mammography support its use in women age >50 years. However, the benefit for women age 40–49 years is quite small. One study shows some advantage for women who are screened starting at age 40 that appears 15 years later; however, it is unclear if this benefit would not have also been derived by starting screening at age 50 years. Women age 40–49 years have a much lower incidence of breast cancer and a higher false-positive rate on mammography. Nearly half of women screened during their forties will have a false-positive test. Refined methods of screening are in development.

3. *Colon cancer*: Annual fecal occult blood testing after age 50 years is felt to be useful. Colonoscopy is the gold standard in colorectal cancer

TABLE 216-2 SCREENING RECOMMENDATIONS FOR ASYMPTOMATIC NORMAL-RISK SUBJECTS[a]

Test or Procedure	USPSTF	ACS
Sigmoidoscopy	Adults 50–75 years: every 5 years ("A")[b] Adults 76–85 years: "C" Adults ≥85 years: "D"	Adults ≥50 years: Screen every 5 years
Fecal occult blood testing (FOBT)	Adults 50–75 years: Annually ("A") Adults 76–85 years: "C" Adults ≥85 years: "D"	Adults ≥50 years: Screen every year
Colonoscopy	Adults 50–75 years: every 10 years ("A") Adults 76–85 years: "C" Adults ≥85 years: "D"	Adults ≥50 years: Screen every 10 years
Fecal DNA testing	"I"	Adults ≥50 years: Screen, but interval uncertain
Fecal immunonochemical testing (FIT)	"I"	Adults ≥50 years: Screen every year
CT colonography	"I"	Adults ≥50 years: Screen every 5 years
Digital rectal examination (DRE)	No recommendation	Men ≥50 years, with a 10-year life expectancy; men ≥45 years, if African American, or men with a first-degree relative diagnosed with prostate cancer <65 years; ≥40, if has several relatives with prostate cancer <65 years: Discuss and offer (with PSA testing) annually
Prostate-specific antigen (PSA)	Men <75 years: "I" Men ≥75 years: "D"	As for DRE
Pap test	Women <65 years: Beginning 3 years after first intercourse or by age 21, screen at least every 3 years ("A") Women ≥65 years, with adequate, normal recent Pap screenings: "D"	Women <30 years: Beginning 3 years after first intercourse or by age 21. Yearly for standard Pap; every 2 years with liquid test. Women 30–70 years: Every 2–3 years if last 3 tests normal

(*continued*)

TABLE 216-2 SCREENING RECOMMENDATIONS FOR ASYMPTOMATIC NORMAL-RISK SUBJECTS[a] (CONTINUED)

Test or Procedure	USPSTF	ACS
	Women after total hysterectomy for noncancerous causes: "D"	Women ≥70 years: May stop screening if no abnormal Pap in past 10 years
		Women after total hysterectomy for noncancerous causes: Do not screen
Breast self-examination	"D"	Women ≥20 years: Breast self-exam is an option
Breast clinical examination	Women ≥40 years: "I" (as a stand-alone without mammography)	Women 20–40 years: Perform every 3 years
		Women ≥40 years: Perform annually
Mammography	Women 40–49 years: The decision should be an individual one, and take pt context into account ("C")	Women ≥40 years: Screen annually
	Women 50–74 years: every 2 years ("B")	
	Women ≥75 years: ("I")	
Magnetic resonance imaging (MRI)	"I"	Women >20% lifetime risk of breast cancer: Screen with MRI plus mammography annually
		Women 15–20% lifetime risk of breast cancer: Discuss option of MRI plus mammography annually
		Women <15% lifetime risk of breast cancer: Do not screen annually with MRI
Complete skin examination	"I"	Self-examination monthly; clinical exam as part of routine cancer-related checkup

[a]Summary of the screening procedures recommended for the general population by the U.S. Preventive Services Task Force and the American Cancer Society. These recommendations refer to asymptomatic persons who have no risk factors, other than age or gender, for the targeted condition.
[b]USPSTF lettered recommendations are defined as follows: "A": The USPSTF strongly recommends that clinicians provide (the service) to eligible pts; "B": The USPSTF recommends that clinicians provide (this service) to eligible pts; "C": The USPSTF makes no recommendation for or against routine provision of (the service); "D": The USPSTF recommends against routinely providing [the service] to asymptomatic pts; "I": The USPSTF concludes that the evidence is insufficient to recommend for or against routinely providing (the service).
Abbreviations: ACS, American Cancer Society; USPSTF, U.S. Preventive Services Task Force.

detection, but it is expensive and has not been shown to be cost-effective in asymptomatic people.

4. *Lung cancer*: Chest radiographs and sputum cytology in smokers appear to identify more early-stage tumors, but paradoxically, the screened pts do not have improved survival. Low-dose spiral CT scanning performed annually for 3 years reduces lung cancer death in older smokers by 20% compared with annual chest x-ray. However, 96% of the positive tests are false-positives and overall survival is improved by only 6.7%.

CANCER PREVENTION IN HIGH-RISK GROUPS

■ BREAST CANCER

Risk factors include age, early menarche, nulliparity or late first pregnancy, high body-mass index, radiation exposure before age 30 years, hormone-replacement therapy (HRT), alcohol consumption, family history, presence of mutations in *BRCA1* or *BRCA2*, and prior history of breast neoplasia. Risk assessment models have been developed to predict an individual's likelihood of developing breast cancer (see *www.cancer.gov/cancertopics/pdq/treatment/breast/healthprofessional#Section_627*).

Diagnosis

MRI scanning is a more effective screening tool than mammography in women with a familial breast cancer risk.

Interventions

Women whose risk exceeds 1.66% in the next 5 years have been shown to have a 50% reduction in breast cancer from taking tamoxifen or raloxifene. Aromatase inhibitors have generally been superior to tamoxifen in the adjuvant treatment of hormone-sensitive breast cancer, and one of them (exemestane) reduces the risk of breast cancer by 65% in postmenopausal women at increased risk. Women with strong family histories should undergo testing for mutations in *BRCA1* and *BRCA2*. Mutations in these genes carry a lifetime probability of >80% for developing breast cancer. Bilateral prophylactic mastectomy prevents at least 90% of these cancers but is a more radical prevention than the usual treatment for the disease. In addition, bilateral salpingo-oophorectomy reduces ovarian and fallopian tube cancer risk by about 96% in women with *BRCA1* or *BRCA2* mutations.

■ COLORECTAL CANCER

Risk factors include diets high in saturated fats and low in fruits and vegetables, smoking, and alcohol consumption. Stronger but less prevalent risk factors are the presence of inflammatory bowel disease or genetic disorders such as familial polyposis (autosomal dominant germline mutation in *APC*) and hereditary nonpolyposis colorectal cancer (mutations in DNA mismatch repair genes *hMSH2* and *hMLH1*).

Interventions

Pts with ulcerative colitis and familial polyposis generally undergo total colectomy. In familial polyposis, nonsteroidal anti-inflammatory drugs

(NSAIDs) reduce the number and size of polyps. Celecoxib, sulindac, and even aspirin appear to be effective, and celecoxib is approved by the U.S. Food and Drug Administration for this indication. Calcium supplementation can lead to a decrease in the recurrence of adenomas, but it is not yet clear that the risk of colorectal cancer is decreased and survival increased. The Women's Health Study noted a significant reduction in the risk of colorectal cancer in women taking HRT, but the increase in thrombotic events and breast cancers counterbalanced this benefit. Studies are underway to assess NSAIDs with and without inhibitors of the epidermal growth factor (EGF) receptor in other risk groups.

■ LUNG CANCER

Risk factors include smoking, exposure to radiation, asbestos, radon.

Interventions

Smoking cessation is the only effective prevention (Chap. 217). NSAIDs and EGF receptor inhibitors are being evaluated. Carotenoids, selenium, retinoids, and α-tocopherol do not work.

■ PROSTATE CANCER

Risk factors include age, family history, and possibly dietary fat intake. African Americans are at increased risk. The disease is highly prevalent, with autopsy studies finding prostate cancer in 70–80% of men over age 70.

Interventions

In a group of men age ≥55 years with normal rectal examinations and PSA levels <3 ng/mL, daily finasteride reduced the incidence of prostate cancer by 25%. Finasteride also prevents the progression of benign prostate hyperplasia. However, some men experience decreased libido as a side effect. The Gleason grade of tumors seen in men taking finasteride prevention was somewhat higher than the controls; however, androgen deprivation alters the morphology of the cells and it is not yet clear that the Gleason grade is a reliable indicator of tumor aggressiveness in the setting of androgen deprivation. Dutasteride, another 5α-reductase inhibitor, had similar effects. The FDA has reviewed the data and concluded that the reduction in risk is primarily in the group of pts with low-grade tumors whose risk from prostate cancer is unclear. One additional high-grade tumor emerges for every 3–4 low-grade tumors averted. More follow-up is necessary to see if higher-grade tumors emerging on preventive therapy have the same aggressive behavior as those occurring in the absence of preventive hormone blockade.

■ CERVICAL CANCER

Risk factors include early age at first intercourse, multiple sexual partners, smoking, and infection with human papillomavirus (HPV) types 16, 18, 45, and 56.

Interventions

Regular Pap testing can detect nearly all cases of the premalignant lesion called *cervical intraepithelial neoplasia*. Untreated, the lesion can progress to carcinoma in situ and invasive cervical cancer. Surgical removal, cryotherapy, or laser therapy is used to treat the disease and is effective in 80%. Risk of recurrence is highest in women over age 30, those with prior HPV infection, and those who have had prior treatment for the same condition. A vaccine (Gardasil) containing antigens of strains 6, 11, 16, and 18 has been shown to be 100% effective in preventing HPV infections from those strains. The vaccine is recommended for all females age 9–16 years and could prevent up to 70% of all cervical cancer. The vaccine is not effective after infection has been established.

■ HEAD AND NECK CANCER

Risk factors include smoking, alcohol consumption, and possibly HPV infection.

Interventions

Oral leukoplakia, white lesions of the oral mucosa, occur in 1–2 persons in 1000, and 2–3% of these pts go on to develop head and neck cancer. Spontaneous regression of oral leukoplakia is seen in 30–40% of pts. Retinoid treatment (13-*cis* retinoid acid) can increase the regression rate. Vitamin A induces complete remission in ~50% of pts. The use of retinoids in pts who have been diagnosed with head and neck cancer and received definitive local therapy has not produced consistent results. Initial studies claimed that retinoids prevented the development of second primary tumors, a common feature of head and neck cancer. However, large randomized studies did not confirm this benefit. Other studies are underway combining retinoids and NSAIDs with and without EGF receptor inhibitors.

PATIENT EDUCATION IN EARLY DETECTION

Pts can be taught to look for early warning signals. The American Cancer Society has identified seven major warning signs of cancer:

- A change in bowel or bladder habits
- A sore that does not heal
- Unusual bleeding or discharge
- A lump in the breast or other parts of the body
- Chronic indigestion or difficulty in swallowing
- Obvious changes in a wart or mole
- Persistent coughing or hoarseness

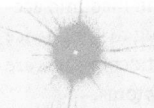

For a more detailed discussion, see Crosswell JM, Brawley OW, Kramer BS: Prevention and Early Detection of Cancer, Chap. 82, p. 655, in HPIM-18.

CHAPTER **217**
Smoking Cessation

Over 400,000 individuals die each year in the United States from cigarette use: one out of every five deaths nationwide. Approximately 40% of smokers will die prematurely unless they are able to quit; major diseases caused by cigarette smoking are listed in Table 217-1.

APPROACH TO THE PATIENT | Nicotine Addiction

All pts should be asked whether they smoke, their past experience with quitting, and whether they are currently interested in quitting; those who are not interested should be encouraged and motivated to quit. Provide a clear, strong, and personalized physician message that smoking is an important health concern. A quit date should be negotiated within a few weeks of the visit, and a follow-up contact by office staff around the time of the quit date should be provided. Incorporation of cessation assistance into a practice requires a change of the care delivery infrastructure. Simple changes include:

- Adding questions about smoking and interest in cessation on pt-intake questionnaires
- Asking pts whether they smoke as part of the initial vital sign measurements made by office staff
- Listing smoking as a problem in the medical record
- Automating follow-up contact with the pt on the quit date

TREATMENT | Nicotine Addiction

- Clinical practice guidelines suggest a variety of pharmacologic and nonpharmacologic interventions to aid in smoking cessation (Table 217-2).
- Numerous nicotine-replacement products exist, including over-the-counter nicotine patches, gum, and lozenges, as well as nicotine nasal and oral inhalers available by prescription; these products can be used for 3–6 months with a gradual step-down in dosage with increasing duration of abstinence.
- Prescription medications that have been shown to be effective include antidepressants such as bupropion (300 mg/d in divided doses for up to 6 months) and varenicline, a partial agonist for the nicotinic acetylcholine receptor (initial dose 0.5 mg daily increasing to 1 mg twice daily at day 8; treatment duration up to 6 months). Antidepressants are more effective in pts with a history of depressive symptoms.

TABLE 217-1 RELATIVE RISKS FOR CURRENT SMOKERS OF CIGARETTES

Disease or Condition	Current Smokers	
	Males	Females
Coronary heart disease		
Age 35–64	2.8	3.1
Age ≥65	1.5	1.6
Cerebrovascular disease		
Age 35–64	3.3	4
Age ≥65	1.6	1.5
Aortic aneurysm	6.2	7.1
Chronic airway obstruction	10.6	13.1
Cancer		
Lung	23.3	12.7
Larynx	14.6	13
Lip, oral cavity, pharynx	10.9	5.1
Esophagus	6.8	7.8
Bladder, other urinary organs	3.3	2.2
Kidney	2.7	1.3
Pancreas	2.3	2.3
Stomach	2	1.4
Cervix		1.6
Acute myeloid leukemia	1.4	1.4
Sudden infant death syndrome		2.3
Infant respiratory distress syndrome		1.3
Low birth weight at delivery		1.8

- Clonidine or nortriptyline may be useful for pts who have failed first-line therapies.
- Current recommendations are to offer pharmacologic treatment, usually with nicotine replacement therapy or varenicline, to all who will accept it and to provide counseling and other support as a part of the cessation attempt.

■ PREVENTION

Approximately 90% of individuals who will become cigarette smokers initiate the behavior during adolescence; prevention must begin early, preferably in the elementary school years. Physicians who treat adolescents should be sensitive to the prevalence of this problem and screen for tobacco use, reinforcing the fact that most adolescents and adults do not smoke, and explaining that all forms of tobacco are both addictive and harmful.

TABLE 217-2 CLINICAL PRACTICE GUIDELINES

Physician Actions

Ask: Systematically identify all tobacco users at every visit

Advise: Strongly urge all smokers to quit

Identify smokers willing to quit

Assist the pt in quitting

Arrange follow-up contact

Effective Pharmacologic Interventions[a]

First-line therapies

    Nicotine gum (1.5)

    Nicotine patch (1.9)

    Nicotine nasal inhaler (2.7)

    Nicotine oral inhaler (2.5)

    Nicotine lozenge (2.0)

    Bupropion (2.1)

    Varenicline (2.7)

Second-line therapies

    Clonidine (2.1)

    Nortriptyline (3.2)

Other Effective Interventions[a]

Physician or other medical personnel counseling (10 min) (1.3)

Intensive smoking cessation programs (at least 4–7 sessions of 20- to 30-min duration lasting at least 2 and preferably 8 weeks) (2.3)

Clinic-based smoking status identification system (3.1)

Counseling by nonclinicians and social support by family and friends

Telephone counseling (1.2)

[a]Numeric value following the intervention is the multiple for cessation success compared with no intervention.

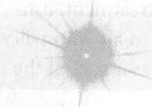

For a more detailed discussion, see Burns DM: Nicotine Addiction, Chap. 395, p. 3560, in HPIM-18.

CHAPTER **218**
Women's Health

The most common causes of death in both men and women are heart disease and cancer, with lung cancer the top cause of cancer death, despite common misperceptions that breast cancer is the most common cause of death in women. These misconceptions perpetuate inadequate attention to modifiable risk factors in women, such as dyslipidemia, hypertension, and cigarette smoking. Furthermore, since women in the Unites States live on average 5.1 years longer than men, the majority of the disease burden for many age-related disorders (e.g., hypertension, Alzheimer's disease) rests in women. For a discussion of the menopause transition and postmenopausal hormone therapy, see Chap. 186.

SEX DIFFERENCES IN HEALTH AND DISEASE

◼ ALZHEIMER'S DISEASE (SEE ALSO CHAP. 194)

Alzheimer's disease (AD) affects approximately twice as many women as men, due to larger numbers of women surviving to older ages and to sex differences in brain size, structure, and functional organization. Postmenopausal hormone therapy may worsen cognitive function and the development of AD.

◼ CORONARY HEART DISEASE (SEE ALSO CHAPS. 128–130)

Coronary heart disease (CHD) presents differently in women, who are usually 10–15 years older than men with CHD and are more likely to have comorbidities, such as hypertension, congestive heart failure, and diabetes. Women more often have atypical symptoms, such as nausea, vomiting, indigestion, and upper back pain. Physicians are less likely to suspect heart disease in women with chest pain and are less likely to perform diagnostic and therapeutic cardiac procedures in women. The conventional risk factors for CHD are the same in both men and women, though women receive fewer interventions for modifiable risk factors than do men. The marked increase in CHD occurring after menopause or oophorectomy suggests that endogenous estrogens are cardioprotective. However, hormone replacement therapy in postmenopausal women was not shown to be cardioprotective in controlled trials such as the Women's Health Initiative and other randomized trials. Therapy with estrogen plus progestin therapy was associated with *increased* cardiovascular events. The discrepancy between endogenous and exogenous estrogen effects is poorly understood but may be related to deleterious effects of late re-exposure to estrogen after a period of estrogen deficiency.

◼ DIABETES MELLITUS (SEE ALSO CHAP. 184)

The prevalence of type 2 diabetes mellitus (DM) is similar between men and women. Polycystic ovary syndrome and gestational diabetes mellitus are both common conditions in premenopausal women that carry an increased risk for type 2 DM. Premenopausal women with DM have identical rates of CHD to those of males.

■ HYPERTENSION (SEE ALSO CHAP. 126)

Hypertension, as an age-related disorder, is more common in women than in men after age 60. Antihypertensive drugs appear to be equally effective in women and men; however, women may experience more side effects.

■ AUTOIMMUNE DISORDERS (SEE ALSO CHAP. 169)

Most autoimmune disorders occur more commonly in women than in men; these include autoimmune thyroid and liver diseases, lupus, rheumatoid arthritis, scleroderma, multiple sclerosis, and idiopathic thrombocytopenic purpura. The mechanism for these sex differences remains obscure.

■ HIV INFECTION (SEE ALSO CHAP. 114)

Heterosexual contact with an at-risk partner is the fastest-growing transmission category of HIV, and women are more susceptible to HIV infection than men. Women with HIV have more rapid decreases in their CD4 cell counts than men do. Other sexually transmitted diseases, such as chlamydial infection and gonorrhea, are important causes of infertility in women, and papilloma virus infection predisposes to cervical cancer.

■ OBESITY (SEE ALSO CHAP. 183)

The prevalence of obesity is higher in women than in men, in part due to the unique risk factors of pregnancy and menopause. In addition, the distribution of body fat differs by sex, with a gluteal and femoral (gynoid) pattern in women and a central and upper body (android) pattern in men. The android distribution of fat carries a higher risk for metabolic syndrome, diabetes mellitus, and cardiovascular disease. Obesity increases a woman's risk for postmenopausal breast and endometrial cancer, in part because of adipose tissue aromatization of androgens to estrone.

■ OSTEOPOROSIS (SEE ALSO CHAP. 188)

Osteoporosis is much more prevalent in postmenopausal women than in age-matched men, since men accumulate more bone mass in their youth and lose bone more slowly than do women, in particular after age 50, when accelerated postmenopausal bone loss occurs in women. In addition, differences in calcium intake, vitamin D, and estrogen levels contribute to sex differences in bone formation and bone loss. Vitamin D insufficiency is present in a large proportion of elderly women living in Northern latitudes. Osteoporotic hip fracture is a major cause of morbidity and an important cause of mortality in elderly women.

■ PHARMACOLOGY

On average, women have lower body weights, smaller organs, higher percent body fat, and lower total-body water than men do. Gonadal steroids, menstrual cycle phase, and pregnancy can all affect drug metabolism and action. Women also take more medications than men do, including over-the-counter formulations and supplements. The greater use of medications, combined with biologic differences, may account for the reported higher frequency of adverse drug reactions in women.

■ PSYCHOLOGICAL DISORDERS (SEE ALSO CHAPS. 208 AND 210)

Depression, anxiety, and eating disorders (bulimia and anorexia nervosa) are more common in women than in men. Depression occurs in 10% of women during pregnancy and 10–15% of women during the postpartum period.

■ SLEEP DISORDERS (SEE ALSO CHAP. 62)

During sleep, women have an increased amount of slow-wave activity, differences in timing of delta activity, and an increase in the number of sleep spindles. They have a decreased prevalence of sleep apnea compared to men, a feature that may be related to lower androgen levels.

■ SUBSTANCE ABUSE AND TOBACCO (SEE ALSO CHAPS. 211 AND 217)

Substance abuse is more common in men than women. However, women alcoholics are less likely to be diagnosed than men and are less likely to seek help. When they do seek help, it is more likely to be from a physician than from a treatment facility. Alcoholic women drink less than alcoholic men but exhibit the same degree of impairment. Alcohol abuse poses special risks to a woman, adversely affecting fertility and the health of the baby (fetal alcohol syndrome). Even moderate alcohol use increases the risk of breast cancer, hypertension, and stroke in women. More men than women smoke tobacco, but the prevalence of smoking is declining faster in men than women. The effects of smoking on pulmonary disease (COPD and cancer) are more pronounced in women than in men.

■ VIOLENCE AGAINST WOMEN

Domestic violence is the most common cause of physical injury in women. Women may present with symptoms of chronic abdominal pain, headaches, substance abuse, and eating disorders, in addition to obvious manifestations such as trauma. Sexual assault is one of the most common crimes against women (reported by one in five women in the U.S.) and is more likely committed by a spouse, ex-spouse, or acquaintance than by a stranger.

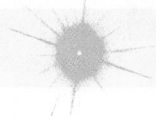

For a more detailed discussion, see Dunaif A: Women's Health, Chap. 6, p. 50, HPIM-18.

CHAPTER **219**
Adverse Drug Reactions

Adverse drug reactions are among the most frequent problems encountered clinically and represent a common cause for hospitalization. They occur most frequently in pts receiving multiple drugs and are caused by:

- Errors in self-administration of prescribed drugs (quite common in the elderly);
- Exaggeration of intended pharmacologic effect (e.g., hypotension in a pt given antihypertensive drugs);
- Concomitant administration of drugs with synergistic effects (e.g., aspirin and warfarin);
- Cytotoxic reactions (e.g., hepatic necrosis due to acetaminophen);
- Immunologic mechanisms (e.g., quinidine-induced thrombocytopenia, hydralazine-induced SLE);
- Genetically determined enzymatic defects (e.g., primaquine-induced hemolytic anemia in G6PD deficiency); or
- Idiosyncratic reactions (e.g., chloramphenicol-induced aplastic anemia).

Recognition

History is of prime importance. Consider the following:

- Nonprescription drugs and topical agents as potential offenders
- Previous reaction to identical drugs
- Temporal association between drug administration and development of clinical manifestations
- Subsidence of manifestations when the agent is discontinued or reduced in dose
- Recurrence of manifestations with cautious readministration (for less hazardous reactions)
- *Rare*: (1) biochemical abnormalities, e.g., red cell G6PD deficiency as cause of drug-induced hemolytic anemia; (2) abnormal serum antibody in pts with agranulocytosis, thrombocytopenia, or hemolytic anemia.

Table 219-1 lists a number of clinical manifestations of adverse effects of drugs. It is not designed to be complete or exhaustive.

TABLE 219-1 CLINICAL MANIFESTATIONS OF ADVERSE REACTIONS TO DRUGS

Multisystem manifestations

Anaphylaxis	**Angioedema**
Cephalosporins	ACE inhibitors
Dextran	**Drug-induced lupus erythematosus**
Insulin	Cephalosporins

(continued)

TABLE 219-1 CLINICAL MANIFESTATIONS OF ADVERSE REACTIONS TO DRUGS (CONTINUED)

Multisystem manifestations

Iodinated drugs or contrast media	Hydralazine
Lidocaine	Iodides
Penicillins	Isoniazid
Procaine	Methyldopa
Phenytoin	**Hyperpyrexia**
Procainamide	Antipsychotics
Quinidine	**Serum sickness**
Sulfonamides	Aspirin
Thiouracil	Penicillins
Fever	Propylthiouracil
Aminosalicylic acid	Sulfonamides
Amphotericin B	
Antihistamines	
Penicillins	

Endocrine manifestations

Addisonian-like syndrome	Guanethidine
Busulfan	Lithium
Ketoconazole	Major tranquilizers
Galactorrhea (may also cause amenorrhea)	Methyldopa
	Oral contraceptives
Methyldopa	Sedatives
Phenothiazines	**Thyroid function tests, disorders of**
Tricyclic antidepressants	Acetazolamide
Gynecomastia	Amiodarone
Calcium channel antagonists	Chlorpropamide
Digitalis	Clofibrate
Estrogens	Colestipol and nicotinic acid
Griseofulvin	Gold salts
Isoniazid	Iodides
Methyldopa	Lithium
Phenytoin	Oral contraceptives
Spironolactone	Phenothiazines
Testosterone	Phenylbutazone
Sexual dysfunction	Phenytoin
Beta blockers	Sulfonamides
Clonidine	Tolbutamide
Diuretics	

TABLE 219-1 CLINICAL MANIFESTATIONS OF ADVERSE REACTIONS TO DRUGS (CONTINUED)

Metabolic manifestations

Hyperbilirubinemia
Rifampin

Hypercalcemia
Antacids with absorbable alkali
Thiazides
Vitamin D

Hyperglycemia
Chlorthalidone
Diazoxide
Encainide
Ethacrynic acid
Furosemide
Glucocorticoids
Growth hormone
Potassium preparations including salt substitute
Potassium salts of drugs
Spironolactone
Succinylcholine
Triamterene

Hypokalemia
Alkali-induced alkalosis
Amphotericin B
Diuretics
Gentamicin
Insulin
Laxative abuse
Mineralocorticoids, some glucocorticoids
Osmotic diuretics
Sympathomimetics
Tetracycline
Theophylline
Vitamin B_{12}

Hyperuricemia
Aspirin
Cytotoxics

Oral contraceptives
Thiazides

Hypoglycemia
Insulin
Oral hypoglycemics
Quinine

Hyperkalemia
ACE inhibitors
Amiloride
Cytotoxics
Digitalis overdose
Heparin
Lithium
Ethacrynic acid
Furosemide
Hyperalimentation
Thiazides

Hyponatremia
1. Dilutional
    Carbamazepine
    Chlorpropamide
    Cyclophosphamide
    Diuretics
    Vincristine
2. Salt wasting
    Diuretics
    Enemas
    Mannitol

Metabolic acidosis
Acetazolamide
Paraldehyde
Salicylates
Spironolactone

(continued)

TABLE 219-1 CLINICAL MANIFESTATIONS OF ADVERSE REACTIONS TO DRUGS (CONTINUED)

Dermatologic manifestations

Acne

Anabolic and androgenic steroids

Bromides

Glucocorticoids

Iodides

Isoniazid

Oral contraceptives

Alopecia

Cytotoxics

Ethionamide

Heparin

Oral contraceptives (withdrawal)

Eczema

Captopril

Cream and lotion preservatives

Lanolin

Topical antihistamines

Topical antimicrobials

Topical local anesthetics

Erythema multiforme or Stevens-Johnson syndrome

Barbiturates

Chlorpropamide

Codeine

Penicillins

Phenylbutazone

Phenytoin

Chloroquine and other antimalarials

Corticotropin

Cyclophosphamide

Gold salts

Hypervitaminosis A

Oral contraceptives

Phenothiazines

Lichenoid eruptions

Aminosalicylic acid

Salicylates

Sulfonamides

Sulfones

Tetracyclines

Thiazides

Erythema nodosum

Oral contraceptives

Penicillins

Sulfonamides

Exfoliative dermatitis

Barbiturates

Gold salts

Penicillins

Phenylbutazone

Phenytoin

Quinidine

Sulfonamides

Fixed drug eruptions

Barbiturates

Captopril

Phenylbutazone

Quinine

Salicylates

Sulfonamides

Hyperpigmentation

Bleomycin

Busulfan

Aspirin

Glucocorticoids

Rashes (nonspecific)

Allopurinol

Ampicillin

Barbiturates

Indapamide

Methyldopa

Phenytoin

TABLE 219-1 CLINICAL MANIFESTATIONS OF ADVERSE REACTIONS TO DRUGS (CONTINUED)

Dermatologic manifestations

Antimalarials

Chlorpropamide

Gold salts

Methyldopa

Phenothiazines

Photodermatitis

Captopril

Chlordiazepoxide

Furosemide

Griseofulvin

Nalidixic acid

Oral contraceptives

Phenothiazines

Sulfonamides

Sulfonylureas

Tetracyclines, particularly demeclocycline

Thiazides

Purpura (see also **Thrombocytopenia**)

Allopurinol

Ampicillin

Skin necrosis

Warfarin

Toxic epidermal necrolysis (bullous)

Allopurinol

Barbiturates

Bromides

Iodides

Nalidixic acid

Penicillins

Phenylbutazone

Phenytoin

Sulfonamides

Urticaria

Aspirin

Barbiturates

Captopril

Enalapril

Penicillins

Sulfonamides

Hematologic manifestations

Agranulocytosis (see also **Pancytopenia**)

Captopril

Carbimazole

Chloramphenicol

Cytotoxics

Gold salts

Indomethacin

Methimazole

Oxyphenbutazone

Phenothiazines

Phenylbutazone

Propylthiouracil

Clotting abnormalities/ hypothrombinemia

Cefamandole

Cefoperazone

Moxalactam

Eosinophilia

Aminosalicylic acid

Chlorpropamide

Erythromycin estolate

Imipramine

L-Tryptophan

Methotrexate

(continued)

TABLE 219-1 CLINICAL MANIFESTATIONS OF ADVERSE REACTIONS TO DRUGS (CONTINUED)

Hematologic manifestations

Sulfonamides

Tolbutamide

Tricyclic antidepressants

Hemolytic anemia

Aminosalicylic acid

Cephalosporins

Chlorpromazine

Dapsone

Insulin

Isoniazid

Levodopa

Mefenamic acid

Melphalan

Methyldopa

Penicillins

Phenacetin

Procainamide

Quinidine

Rifampin

Sulfonamides

Hemolytic anemias in G6PD deficiency

See Table 68-3

Leukocytosis

Glucocorticoids

Lithium

Lymphadenopathy

Phenytoin

Primidone

Megaloblastic anemia

Folate antagonists

Nitrous oxide

Oral contraceptives

Phenobarbital

Phenytoin

Primidone

Nitrofurantoin

Procarbazine

Sulfonamides

Cytotoxics

Gold salts

Mephenytoin

Phenylbutazone

Phenytoin

Quinacrine

Sulfonamides

Trimethadione

Zidovudine (AZT)

Pure red cell aplasia

Azathioprine

Chlorpropamide

Isoniazid

Phenytoin

Thrombocytopenia (see also **Pancytopenia**)

Acetazolamine

Aspirin

Carbamazepine

Carbenicillin

Chlorpropamide

Chlorthalidone

Furosemide

Gold salts

Heparin

Indomethacin

Isoniazid

Methyldopa

Moxalactam

Phenylbutazone

Phenytoin and other hydantoins

Quinidine

TABLE 219-1 CLINICAL MANIFESTATIONS OF ADVERSE REACTIONS TO DRUGS (CONTINUED)

Hematologic manifestations

Triamterene	Quinine
Trimethroprim	Thiazides
Pancytopenia (aplastic anemia)	Ticarcillin
Carbamazepine	
Chloramphenicol	

Cardiovascular manifestations

Angina exacerbation

- Alpha blockers
- Beta blocker withdrawal
- Ergotamine
- Excessive thyroxine
- Hydralazine
- Methysergide
- Minoxidil
- Nifedipine
- Oxytocin
- Vasopressin
- Thyroid hormone
- Tricyclic antidepressants
- Verapamil

AV block

- Clonidine
- Methyldopa
- Verapamil

Cardiomyopathy

- Adriamycin
- Daunorubicin
- Emetine
- Lithium
- Phenothiazines
- Sulfonamides
- Sympathomimetics

Fluid retention or congestive heart failure

- Beta blockers
- Calcium antagonists

Arrhythmias

- Adriamycin
- Antiarrhythmic drugs
- Atropine
- Anticholinesterases
- Beta blockers
- Digitalis
- Emetine
- Lithium
- Phenothiazines
- Sympathomimetics
- Diuretics
- Levodopa
- Morphine
- Nitroglycerin
- Phenothiazines
- Protamine
- Quinidine

Hypertension

- Clonidine withdrawal
- Corticotropin
- Cyclosporine
- Glucocorticoids
- Monoamine oxidase inhibitors with sympathomimetics
- NSAIDs
- Oral contraceptives
- Sympathomimetics
- Tricyclic antidepressants with Sympathomimetics

(continued)

TABLE 219-1 CLINICAL MANIFESTATIONS OF ADVERSE REACTIONS TO DRUGS (CONTINUED)

Cardiovascular manifestations

Estrogens	**Pericarditis**
Indomethacin	Emetine
Mannitol	Hydralazine
Minoxidil	Methysergide
Phenylbutazone	Procainamide
Steroids	**Thromboembolism**
Hypotension	Oral contraceptives
Calcium antagonists	
Citrated blood	

Respiratory manifestations

Airway obstruction	**Pulmonary infiltrates**
Beta blockers	Acyclovir
Cephalosporins	Amiodarone
Cholinergic drugs	Azathioprine
NSAIDs	Bleomycin
Penicillins	Busulfan
Pentazocine	Carmustine (BCNU)
Streptomycin	Chlorambucil
Tartrazine (drugs with yellow dye)	Cyclophosphamide
Cough	Melphalan
ACE inhibitors	Methotrexate
Pulmonary edema	Methysergide
Contrast media	Mitomycin C
Heroin	Nitrofurantoin
Methadone	Procarbazine
Propoxyphene	Sulfonamides

Gastrointestinal manifestations

Cholestatic jaundice	Sodium valproate
Anabolic steroids	Sulfonamides
Androgens	Tetracyclines
Chlorpropamide	Verapamil
Erythromycin estolate	Zidovudine (AZT)
Gold salts	**Intestinal ulceration**
Methimazole	Solid KCl preparations

(continued)

TABLE 219-1 CLINICAL MANIFESTATIONS OF ADVERSE REACTIONS TO DRUGS (CONTINUED)

Gastrointestinal manifestations

Nitrofurantoin
Oral contraceptives
Phenothiazines

Constipation or ileus

Aluminum hydroxide
Barium sulfate
Calcium carbonate
Ferrous sulfate
Ion exchange resins
Opiates
Phenothiazines
Tricyclic antidepressants
Verapamil

Diarrhea or colitis

Antibiotics (broad-spectrum)
Colchicine
Digitalis
Magnesium in antacids
Methyldopa

Diffuse hepatocellular damage

Acetaminophen (paracetamol)
Allopurinol
Aminosalicylic acid
Dapsone
Erythromycin estolate
Ethionamide
Glyburide
Halothane
Isoniazid
Ketoconazole
Methimazole
Methotrexate
Methoxyflurane
Methyldopa
Monoamine oxidase inhibitors

Malabsorption

Aminosalicylic acid
Antibiotics (broad-spectrum)
Cholestyramine
Colchicine
Colestipol
Cytotoxics
Neomycin
Phenobarbital
Phenytoin

Nausea or vomiting

Digitalis
Estrogens
Ferrous sulfate
Levodopa
Opiates
Potassium chloride
Tetracyclines
Theophylline

Oral conditions

1. Gingival hyperplasia
   Calcium antagonists
   Cyclosporine
   Phenytoin
2. Salivary gland swelling
   Bretylium
   Clonidine
   Guanethidine
   Iodides
   Phenylbutazone
3. Taste disturbances
   Biguanides
   Captopril
   Griseofulvin
   Lithium

(continued)

TABLE 219-1 CLINICAL MANIFESTATIONS OF ADVERSE REACTIONS TO DRUGS (CONTINUED)

Gastrointestinal manifestations

- Niacin
- Nifedipine
- Nitrofurantoin
- Phenytoin
- Propoxyphene
- Propylthiouracil
- Pyridium
- Rifampin
- Salicylates

Pancreatitis

- Azathioprine
- Ethacrynic acid
- Furosemide
- Glucocorticoids
- Opiates
- Oral contraceptives

Renal/urinary manifestations

Bladder dysfunction

- Anticholinergics
- Disopyramide
- Monoamine oxidase inhibitors
- Tricyclic antidepressants

Calculi

- Acetazolamide
- Vitamin D

Concentrating defect with polyuria (or nephrogenic diabetes insipidus)

- Demeclocycline
- Lithium
- Methoxyflurane
- Vitamin D

Hemorrhagic cystitis

- Cyclophosphamide

Interstitial nephritis

- Allopurinol
- Furosemide
- Penicillins, esp. methicillin

- Metronidazole
- Penicillamine
- Rifampin

4. Ulceration
  - Aspirin
  - Cytotoxics
  - Gentian violet
  - Isoproterenol (sublingual)
  - Pancreatin
  - Sulfonamides
  - Thiazides

Peptic ulceration or hemorrhage

- Aspirin
- Ethacrynic acid
- Glucocorticoids
- NSAIDs

Nephrotic syndrome

- Captopril
- Gold salts
- Penicillamine
- Phenindione
- Probenecid

Obstructive uropathy

- Extrarenal: methysergide
- Intrarenal: cytotoxics

Renal dysfunction

- Cyclosporine
- NSAIDS
- Triamterene

Renal tubular acidosis

- Acetazolamide
- Amphotericin B
- Degraded tetracycline

Tubular necrosis

- Aminoglycosides
- Amphotericin B

TABLE 219-1 CLINICAL MANIFESTATIONS OF ADVERSE REACTIONS TO DRUGS (CONTINUED)

Renal/urinary manifestations

Phenindione

Sulfonamides

Thiazides

Nephropathies

Due to analgesics
(e.g., phenacetin)

Colistin

Cyclosporine

Methoxyflurane

Polymyxins

Radioiodinated contrast medium

Sulfonamides

Tetracyclines

Neurologic manifestations

Exacerbation of myasthenia

Aminoglycosides

Polymyxins

Extrapyramidal effects

Butyrophenones, e.g., haloperidol

Disopyramide

Ethambutol

Ethionamide

Glutethimide

Hydralazine

Isoniazid

Levodopa

Methyldopa

Methysergide

Metoclopramide

Metronidazole

Nalidixic acid

Nitrofurantoin

Oral contraceptives

Phenothiazines

Phenytoin

Polymyxin, colistin

Procarbazine

Streptomycin

Tolbutamide

Tricyclic antidepressants

Tricyclic antidepressants

Vincristine

Headache

Ergotamine (withdrawal)

Glyceryl trinitrate

Hydralazine

Indomethacin

Peripheral neuropathy

Amiodarone

Chloramphenicol

Chloroquine

Chlorpropamide

Clofibrate

Demeclocycline

Hypervitaminosis A

Oral contraceptives

Tetracyclines

Seizures

Amphetamines

Analeptics

Isoniazid

Lidocaine

Lithium

Nalidixic acid

Penicillins

Phenothiazines

Physostigmine

Theophylline

Tricyclic antidepressants

Vincristine

(*continued*)

TABLE 219-1 CLINICAL MANIFESTATIONS OF ADVERSE REACTIONS TO DRUGS (CONTINUED)

Neurologic manifestations

Pseudotumor cerebri (or intracranial hypertension)
Amiodarone
Glucocorticoids, mineralocorticoids

Stroke
Oral contraceptives

Ocular manifestations

Cataracts
Busulfan
Chlorambucil
Glucocorticoids
Phenothiazines

Glaucoma
Mydriatics
Sympathomimetics

Optic neuritis
Aminosalicylic acid
Chloramphenicol
Ethambutol
Isoniazid
Penicillamine
Phenothiazines
Phenylbutazone
Quinine
Streptomycin

Color vision alteration
Barbiturates
Digitalis
Methaqualone
Streptomycin
Thiazides

Corneal edema
Oral contraceptives

Corneal opacities
Chloroquine
Indomethacin
Vitamin D

Retinopathy
Chloroquine
Phenothiazines

Ear manifestations

Deafness
Aminoglycosides
Aspirin
Bleomycin
Chloroquine
Erythromycin
Ethacrynic acid

Furosemide
Nortriptyline
Quinine

Vestibular disorders
Aminoglycosides
Quinine

Musculoskeletal manifestations

Bone disorders
1. Osteoporosis
   Glucocorticoids
   Heparin

Chloroquine
Clofibrate
Glucocorticoids
Oral contraceptives

TABLE 219-1 CLINICAL MANIFESTATIONS OF ADVERSE REACTIONS TO DRUGS (CONTINUED)

Musculoskeletal manifestations

2. Osteomalacia
   Aluminum hydroxide
   Anticonvulsants
   Glutethimide

Myositis
Gemfibrozil
Lovastatin

Myopathy or myalgia
Amphotericin B

Psychiatric manifestations

Delirious or confusional states
Amantadine
Aminophylline
Anticholinergics
Antidepressants
Cimetidine
Digitalis
Glucocorticoids
Isoniazid
Levodopa
Methyldopa
Penicillins
Phenothiazines
Sedatives and hypnotics

Depression
Amphetamine withdrawal
Beta blockers
Centrally acting antihypertensives (reserpine, methyldopa, clonidine)
Glucocorticoids
Levodopa

Drowsiness
Antihistamines
Anxiolytic drugs
Clonidine
Major tranquilizers
Methyldopa
Tricyclic antidepressants

Hallucinatory states
Amantadine
Beta blockers
Levodopa
Meperidine
Narcotics
Pentazocine
Tricyclic antidepressants

Hypomania, mania, or excited reactions
Glucocorticoids
Levodopa
Monoamine oxidase inhibitors
Sympathomimetics
Tricyclic antidepressants

Schizophrenic-like or paranoid reactions
Amphetamines
Bromides
Glucocorticoids
Levodopa
Lysergic acid
Monoamine oxidase inhibitors
Tricyclic antidepressants

Sleep disturbances
Anorexiants
Levodopa
Monoamine oxidase inhibitors
Sympathomimetics

Source: Adapted from AJJ Wood: HPIM-15, pp. 432–436.

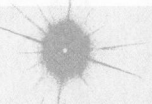

For a more detailed discussion, see Roden DM: Principles of Clinical Pharmacology, Chap. 5, p. 33, in HPIM-18; Wood AJJ: Adverse Reactions to Drugs, Chap. 71, p. 430, in HPIM-15.

CHAPTER **220**
Laboratory Values of Clinical Importance

INTRODUCTORY COMMENTS

In preparing for the Appendix, the authors have taken into account the fact that the system of international units (SI, système international d'unités) is used in most countries and in some medical journals. However, clinical laboratories may continue to report values in "conventional" units. Therefore, both systems are provided in the Appendix.

For many analytes, the reference ranges given here are meant as general guidelines rather than absolute normative ranges. Because of differences in methodology, assay reagents, and collection methods, reference values may differ among clinical laboratories. Therefore, for diagnostic pt management purposes, reference ranges provided by the laboratory performing the test should be used for interpretation of a given result.

REFERENCE VALUES FOR LABORATORY TESTS

(Tables 220-1 through 220-5)

TABLE 220-1 HEMATOLOGY AND COAGULATION

Analyte	Specimen	SI Units	Conventional Units
Activated clotting time	WB	70–180 s	70–180 s
Activated protein C resistance (factor V Leiden)	P	Not applicable	Ratio >2.1
ADAMTS13 activity	P	≥0.67	≥67%
ADAMTS13 inhibitor activity	P	Not applicable	≤0.4 U
ADAMTS13 antibody	P	Not applicable	≤18 U
Alpha₂ antiplasmin	P	0.87–1.55	87–155%
Antiphospholipid antibody panel			
PTT-LA (lupus anticoagulant screen)	P	Negative	Negative
Platelet neutralization procedure	P	Negative	Negative
Dilute viper venom screen	P	Negative	Negative
Anticardiolipin antibody	S		
IgG		0–15 arbitrary units	0–15 GPL
IgM		0–15 arbitrary units	0–15 MPL
Antithrombin III	P		
Antigenic		220–390 mg/L	22–39 mg/dL
Functional		0.7–1.30 U/L	70–130 %

Anti-Xa assay (heparin assay)	P	
Unfractionated heparin	0.3–0.7 kIU/L	0.3–0.7 IU/mL
Low-molecular-weight heparin	0.5–1.0 kIU/L	0.5–1.0 IU/mL
Danaparoid (Orgaran)	0.5–0.8 kIU/L	0.5–0.8 IU/mL
Autohemolysis test	WB	0.004–0.045	0.4–4.50%
Autohemolysis test with glucose	WB	0.003–0.007	0.3–0.7%
Bleeding time (adult)	<7.1 min	<7.1 min
Bone marrow: See Table 220-8		
Clot retraction	WB	0.50–1.00/2 h	50–100%/2 h
Cryofibrinogen	P	Negative	Negative
D-dimer	P	220–740 ng/mL FEU	220–740 ng/mL FEU
Differential blood count	WB		
Relative counts		
Neutrophils	0.40–0.70	40–70%
Bands	0.0–0.05	0–5%
Lymphocytes	0.20–0.50	20–50%
Monocytes	0.04–0.08	4–8%
Eosinophils	0.0–0.6	0–6%
Basophils	0.0–0.02	0–2%

(continued)

TABLE 220-1 HEMATOLOGY AND COAGULATION (CONTINUED)

Analyte	Specimen	SI Units	Conventional Units
Absolute counts			
Neutrophils		1.42–6.34×10^9/L	1420–6340/mm^3
Bands		0–0.45×10^9/L	0–450/mm^3
Lymphocytes		0.71–4.53×10^9/L	710–4530/mm^3
Monocytes		0.14–0.72×10^9/L	140–720/mm^3
Eosinophils		0–0.54×10^9/L	0–540/mm^3
Basophils		0–0.18×10^9/L	0–180/mm^3
Erythrocyte count	WB		
Adult males		4.30–5.60×10^{12}/L	4.30–5.60×10^6/mm^3
Adult females		4.00–5.20×10^{12}/L	4.00–5.20×10^6/mm^3
Erythrocyte life span	WB		
Normal survival		120 days	120 days
Chromium labeled, half-life ($t_{1/2}$)		25–35 days	25–35 days
Erythrocyte sedimentation rate	WB		
Females		0–20 mm/h	0–20 mm/h
Males		0–15 mm/h	0–15 mm/h
Euglobulin lysis time	P	7200–14,400 s	120–240 min
Factor II, prothrombin	P	0.50–1.50	50–150%

Factor V	P	0.50–1.50	50–150%
Factor VII	P	0.50–1.50	50–150%
Factor VIII	P	0.50–1.50	50–150%
Factor IX	P	0.50–1.50	50–150%
Factor X	P	0.50–1.50	50–150%
Factor XI	P	0.50–1.50	50–150%
Factor XII	P	0.50–1.50	50–150%
Factor XIII screen	P	Not applicable	Present
Factor inhibitor assay	P	<0.5 Bethesda Units	<0.5 Bethesda Units
Fibrin(ogen) degradation products	P	0–1 mg/L	0–1 µg/mL
Fibrinogen	P	2.33–4.96 g/L	233–496 mg/dL
Glucose-6-phosphate dehydrogenase (erythrocyte)	WB	<2400 s	<40 min
Ham's test (acid serum)	WB	Negative	Negative
Hematocrit	WB		
Adult males		0.388–0.464	38.8–46.4
Adult females		0.354–0.444	35.4–44.4
Hemoglobin			
Plasma	P	6–50 mg/L	0.6–5.0 mg/dL
Whole blood	WB		
Adult males		133–162 g/L	13.3–16.2 g/dL
Adult females		120–158 g/L	12.0–15.8 g/dL

(continued)

TABLE 220-1 HEMATOLOGY AND COAGULATION (CONTINUED)

Analyte	Specimen	SI Units	Conventional Units
Hemoglobin electrophoresis	WB		
Hemoglobin A		0.95–0.98	95–98%
Hemoglobin A_2		0.015–0.031	1.5–3.1%
Hemoglobin F		0–0.02	0–2.0%
Hemoglobins other than A, A_2, or F		Absent	Absent
Heparin-induced thrombocytopenia antibody	P	Negative	Negative
Immature platelet fraction (IPF)	WB	0.011–0.061	1.1–6.1%
Joint fluid crystal	JF	Not applicable	No crystals seen
Joint fluid mucin	JF	Not applicable	Only type I mucin present
Leukocytes			
Alkaline phosphatase (LAP)	WB	0.2–1.6 µkat/L	13–100 µL/L
Count (WBC)	WB	3.54–9.06×10^9/L	3.54–9.06×10^3/mm^3
Mean corpuscular hemoglobin (MCH)	WB	26.7–31.9 pg/cell	26.7–31.9 pg/cell
Mean corpuscular hemoglobin concentration (MCHC)	WB	323–359 g/L	32.3–35.9 g/dL
Mean corpuscular hemoglobin of reticulocytes (CH)	WB	24–36 pg	24–36 pg
Mean corpuscular volume (MCV)	WB	79–93.3 fL	79–93.3 µm^3
Mean platelet volume (MPV)	WB	9.00–12.95 fL	9.00–12.95 fL

Osmotic fragility of erythrocytes	WB		
Direct		0.0035–0.0045	0.35–0.45%
Indirect		0.0030–0.0065	0.30–0.65%
Partial thromboplastin time, activated	P	26.3–39.4 s	26.3–39.4 s
Plasminogen	P		
Antigen		84–140 mg/L	8.4–14.0 mg/dL
Functional		0.70–1.30	70–130%
Plasminogen activator inhibitor 1	P	4–43 µg/L	4–43 ng/mL
Platelet aggregation	PRP	Not applicable	>65% aggregation in response to adenosine diphosphate, epinephrine, collagen, ristocetin, and arachidonic acid
Platelet count	WB	165–415 × 10⁹/L	165–415 × 10³/mm³
Platelet, mean volume	WB	6.4–11 fL	6.4–11.0 µm³
Prekallikrein assay	P	0.50–1.5	50–150%
Prekallikrein screen	P	No deficiency detected	No deficiency detected
Protein C	P		
Total antigen		0.70–1.40	70–140%
Functional		0.70–1.30	70–130%

(continued)

1399

TABLE 220-1 HEMATOLOGY AND COAGULATION (CONTINUED)

Analyte	Specimen	SI Units	Conventional Units
Protein S	P		
Total antigen		0.70–1.40	70–140%
Functional		0.65–1.40	65–140%
Free antigen		0.70–1.40	70–140%
Prothrombin gene mutation G20210A	WB	Not applicable	Not present
Prothrombin time	P	12.7–15.4 s	12.7–15.4 s
Protoporphyrin, free erythrocyte	WB	0.28–0.64 μmol/L of red blood cells	16–36 μg/dL of red blood cells
Red cell distribution width	WB	<0.145	<14.5%
Reptilase time	P	16–23.6 s	16–23.6 s
Reticulocyte count	WB		
Adult males		0.008–0.023 red cells	0.8–2.3% red cells
Adult females		0.008–0.020 red cells	0.8–2.0% red cells
Reticulocyte hemoglobin content	WB	>26 pg/cell	>26 pg/cell
Ristocetin cofactor (functional von Willebrand factor)	P		
Blood group O		0.75 mean of normal	75% mean of normal
Blood group A		1.05 mean of normal	105% mean of normal
Blood group B		1.15 mean of normal	115% mean of normal
Blood group AB		1.25 mean of normal	125% mean of normal

Serotonin release assay	S	<0.2 release	<20% release
Sickle cell test	WB	Negative	Negative
Sucrose hemolysis	WB	<0.1	<10% hemolysis
Thrombin time	P	15.3–18.5 s	15.3–18.5 s
Total eosinophils	WB	150–300 × 10⁶/L	150–300/mm³
Transferrin receptor	S, P	9.6–29.6 nmol/L	9.6–29.6 nmol/L
Viscosity			
Plasma	P	1.7–2.1	1.7–2.1
Serum	S	1.4–1.8	1.4–1.8
von Willebrand factor (vWF) antigen (factor VIII:R antigen)	P		
Blood group 0		0.75 mean of normal	75% mean of normal
Blood group A		1.05 mean of normal	105% mean of normal
Blood group B		1.15 mean of normal	115% mean of normal
Blood group AB		1.25 mean of normal	125% mean of normal
von Willebrand factor multimers	P	Normal distribution	Normal distribution
White blood cells: see "Leukocytes"			

Abbreviations: JF, joint fluid; P, plasma; PRP, platelet-rich plasma; S, serum; WB, whole blood.

1401

TABLE 220-2 CLINICAL CHEMISTRY AND IMMUNOLOGY

Analyte	Specimen	SI Units	Conventional Units
Acetoacetate	P	49–294 µmol/L	0.5–3.0 mg/dL
Adrenocorticotropin (ACTH)	P	1.3–16.7 pmol/L	6.0–76.0 pg/mL
Alanine aminotransferase (ALT, SGPT)	S	0.12–0.70 µkat/L	7–41 U/L
Albumin	S	40–50 g/L	4.0–5.0 mg/dL
Aldolase	S	26–138 nkat/L	1.5–8.1 U/L
Aldosterone (adult)			
Supine, normal sodium diet	S, P	<443 pmol/L	<16 ng/dL
Upright, normal	S, P	111–858 pmol/L	4–31 ng/dL
Alpha fetoprotein (adult)	S	0–8.5 µg/L	0–8.5 ng/mL
Alpha$_1$ antitrypsin	S	1.0–2.0 g/L	100–200 mg/dL
Ammonia, as NH$_3$	P	11–35 µmol/L	19–60 µg/dL
Amylase (method dependent)	S	0.34–1.6 µkat/L	20–96 U/L
Androstenedione (adult)	S		
Males		0.81–3.1 nmol/L	23–89 ng/dL
Females			
Premenopausal		0.91–7.5 nmol/L	26–214 ng/dL
Postmenopausal		0.46–2.9 nmol/L	13–82 ng/dL
Angiotensin-converting enzyme (ACE)	S	0.15–1.1 µkat/L	9–67 U/L

Anion gap	S	7–16 mmol/L	7–16 mmol/L
Apolipoprotein A-1	S		
Male		0.94–1.78 g/L	94–178 mg/dL
Female		1.01–1.99 g/L	101–199 mg/dL
Apolipoprotein B	S		
Male		0.55–1.40 g/L	55–140 mg/dL
Female		0.55–1.25 g/L	55–125 mg/dL
Arterial blood gases	WB		
[HCO$_3^-$]		22–30 mmol/L	22–30 meq/L
P$_{CO_2}$		4.3–6.0 kPa	32–45 mmHg
pH		7.35–7.45	7.35–7.45
P$_{O_2}$		9.6–13.8 kPa	72–104 mmHg
Aspartate aminotransferase (AST, SGOT)	S	0.20–0.65 μkat/L	12–38 U/L
Autoantibodies	S		
Anticentromere antibody IgG		≤29 AU/mL	≤29 AU/mL
Anti-double-strand (native) DNA		<25 IU/L	<25 IU/L
Anti–glomerular basement membrane antibodies			
Qualitative IgG, IgA		Negative	Negative
Quantitative IgG antibody		≤19 AU/mL	≤19 AU/mL
Antihistone antibodies		<1.0 U	<1.0 U

(continued)

TABLE 220-2 CLINICAL CHEMISTRY AND IMMUNOLOGY (CONTINUED)

Analyte	Specimen	SI Units	Conventional Units
Anti-Jo-1 antibody		≤29 AU/mL	≤29 AU/mL
Antimitochondrial antibody		Not applicable	<20 Units
Antineutrophil cytoplasmic autoantibodies		Not applicable	<1:20
Serine proteinase 3 antibodies		≤19 AU/mL	≤19 AU/mL
Myeloperoxidase antibodies		≤19 AU/mL	≤19 AU/mL
Antinuclear antibody		Not applicable	Negative at 1:40
Anti-parietal cell antibody		Not applicable	None detected
Anti-RNP antibody		Not applicable	<1.0 U
Anti-Scl 70 antibody		Not applicable	<1.0 U
Anti-Smith antibody		Not applicable	<1.0 U
Anti-smooth muscle antibody		Not applicable	<1.0 U
Anti-SSA antibody		Not applicable	<1.0 U
Anti-SSB antibody		Not applicable	Negative
Antithyroglobulin antibody		<40 KIU/mL	<40 IU/mL
Anti-thyroid peroxidase antibody		<35 KIU/L	<35 IU/L
B-type natriuretic peptide (BNP)	P	Age and gender specific: <100 ng/L	Age and gender specific: <100 pg/mL
Bence Jones protein, serum qualitative	S	Not applicable	None detected

Bence Jones protein, serum quantitative	S	
Free kappa		3.3–19.4 mg/L	0.33–1.94 mg/dL
Free lambda		5.7–26.3 mg/L	0.57–2.63 mg/dL
K/L ratio		0.26–1.65	0.26–1.65
Beta-2-microglobulin	S	1.1–2.4 mg/L	1.1–2.4 mg/L
Bilirubin	S		
Total		5.1–22 μmol/L	0.3–1.3 mg/dL
Direct		1.7–6.8 μmol/L	0.1–0.4 mg/dL
Indirect		3.4–15.2 μmol/L	0.2–0.9 mg/dL
C peptide	S	0.27–1.19 nmol/L	0.8–3.5 ng/mL
C1-esterase-inhibitor protein	S	210–390 mg/L	21–39 mg/dL
CA 125	S	<35 kU/L	<35 U/mL
CA 19-9	S	<37 kU/L	<37 U/mL
CA 15-3	S	<33 kU/L	<33 U/mL
CA 27-29	S	0–40 kU/L	0–40 U/mL
Calcitonin	S		
Male		0–7.5 ng/L	0–7.5 pg/mL
Female		0–5.1 ng/L	0–5.1 pg/mL
Calcium	S	2.2–2.6 mmol/L	8.7–10.2 mg/dL

(continued)

TABLE 220-2 CLINICAL CHEMISTRY AND IMMUNOLOGY (CONTINUED)

Analyte	Specimen	SI Units	Conventional Units
Calcium, ionized	WB	1.12–1.32 mmol/L	4.5–5.3 mg/dL
Carbon dioxide content (TCO$_2$)	P (sea level)	22–30 mmol/L	22–30 meq/L
Carboxyhemoglobin (carbon monoxide content)	WB		
Nonsmokers		0.0–0.015	0–1.5%
Smokers		0.04–0.09	4–9%
Loss of consciousness and death		>0.50	>50%
Carcinoembryonic antigen (CEA)	S		
Nonsmokers		0.0–3.0 µg/L	0.0–3.0 ng/mL
Smokers		0.0–5.0 µg/L	0.0–5.0 ng/mL
Ceruloplasmin	S	250–630 mg/L	25–63 mg/dL
Chloride	S	102–109 mmol/L	102–109 meq/L
Cholesterol: see Table 220-5			
Cholinesterase	S	5–12 kU/L	5–12 U/mL
Chromogranin A	S	0–50 µg/L	0–50 ng/mL
Complement	S		
C3		0.83–1.77 g/L	83–177 mg/dL
C4		0.16–0.47 g/L	16–47 mg/dL
Complement total		60–144 CAE units	60–144 CAE units

Cortisol			
Fasting, 8 A.M.–12 noon	S	138–690 nmol/L	5–25 µg/dL
12 noon–8 P.M.		138–414 nmol/L	5–15 µg/dL
8 P.M.–8 A.M.		0–276 nmol/L	0–10 µg/dL
C-reactive protein	S	<10 mg/L	<10 mg/L
C-reactive protein, high sensitivity	S	Cardiac risk	Cardiac risk
		Low: <1.0 mg/L	Low: <1.0 mg/L
		Average: 1.0–3.0 mg/L	Average: 1.0–3.0 mg/L
		High: >3.0 mg/L	High: >3.0 mg/L
Creatine kinase (total)	S		
Females		0.66–4.0 µkat/L	39–238 U/L
Males		0.87–5.0 µkat/L	51–294 U/L
Creatine kinase-MB	S		
Mass		0.0–5.5 µg/L	0.0–5.5 ng/mL
Fraction of total activity (by electrophoresis)		0–0.04	0–4.0%
Creatinine	S		
Female		44–80 µmol/L	0.5–0.9 mg/dL
Male		53–106 µmol/L	0.6–1.2 mg/dL
Cryoglobulins	S	Not applicable	None detected

(continued)

TABLE 220-2 CLINICAL CHEMISTRY AND IMMUNOLOGY (CONTINUED)

Analyte	Specimen	SI Units	Conventional Units
Cystatin C	S	0.5–1.0 mg/L	0.5–1.0 mg/L
Dehydroepiandrosterone (DHEA) (adult)			
Male	S	6.2–43.4 nmol/L	180–1250 ng/dL
Female		4.5–34.0 nmol/L	130–980 ng/dL
Dehydroepiandrosterone (DHEA) sulfate	S		
Male (adult)		100–6190 μg/L	10–619 μg/dL
Female (adult, premenopausal)		120–5350 μg/L	12–535 μg/dL
Female (adult, postmenopausal)		300–2600 μg/L	30–260 μg/dL
11-Deoxycortisol (adult)(compound S)	S	0.34–4.56 nmol/L	12–158 ng/dL
Dihydrotestosterone	S, P		
Male		1.03–2.92 nmol/L	30–85 ng/dL
Female		0.14–0.76 nmol/L	4–22 ng/dL
Dopamine	P	0–130 pmol/L	0–20 pg/mL
Epinephrine	P		
Supine (30 min)		<273 pmol/L	<50 pg/mL
Sitting		328 pmol/L	<60 pg/mL
Standing (30 min)		491pmol/L	<90 pg/mL
Erythropoietin	S	4–27 U/L	4–27 U/L

Estradiol	S, P		
Female			
Menstruating			
Follicular phase		74–532 pmol/L	<20–145 pg/mL
Midcycle peak		411–1626 pmol/L	112–443 pg/mL
Luteal phase		74–885 pmol/L	<20–241 pg/mL
Postmenopausal		217 pmol/L	<59 pg/mL
Male		74 pmol/L	<20 pg/mL
Estrone	S, P		
Female			
Menstruating			
Follicular phase		<555 pmol/L	<150 pg/mL
Luteal phase		<740 pmol/L	<200 pg/mL
Postmenopausal		11–118 pmol/L	3–32 pg/mL
Male		33–133 pmol/L	9–36 pg/mL
Fatty acids, free (nonesterified)	P	0.1–0.6 mmol/L	2.8–16.8 mg/dL
Ferritin	S		
Female		10–150 µg/L	10–150 ng/mL
Male		29–248 µg/L	29–248 ng/mL

(continued)

1409

TABLE 220-2 CLINICAL CHEMISTRY AND IMMUNOLOGY (CONTINUED)

Analyte	Specimen	SI Units	Conventional Units
Follicle-stimulating hormone (FSH)	S, P		
Female			
Menstruating			
Follicular phase		3.0–20.0 IU/L	3.0–20.0 mIU/mL
Ovulatory phase		9.0–26.0 IU/L	9.0–26.0 mIU/mL
Luteal phase		1.0–12.0 IU/L	1.0–12.0 mIU/mL
Postmenopausal		18.0–153.0 IU/L	18.0–153.0 mIU/mL
Male		1.0–12.0 IU/L	1.0–12.0 mIU/mL
Fructosamine	S	<285 umol/L	<285 umol/L
Gamma glutamyltransferase	S	0.15–0.99 μkat/L	9–58 U/L
Gastrin	S	<100 ng/L	<100 pg/mL
Glucagon	P	40–130 ng/L	40–130 pg/mL
Glucose	WB	3.6–5.3 mmol/L	65–95 mg/dL
Glucose (fasting)	P		
Normal		4.2–5.6 mmol/L	75–100 mg/dL
Increased risk for diabetes		5.6–6.9 mmol/L	100–125 mg/dL

Diabetes mellitus		Fasting ≥7.0 mmol/L	Fasting ≥126 mg/dL
		A 2-hour level of ≥11.1 mmol/L during an oral glucose tolerance test	A 2-hour level of ≥200 mg/dL during an oral glucose tolerance test
		A random glucose level of ≥11.1 mmol/L in pts with symptoms of hyperglycemia	A random glucose level of ≥200 mg/dL in pts with symptoms of hyperglycemia
Growth hormone	S	0–5 µg/L	0–5 ng/mL
Hemoglobin A$_{1c}$	WB	0.04–0.06 Hgb fraction	4.0–5.6%
Pre-diabetes		0.057–0.064 Hgb fraction	5.7–6.4%
Diabetes mellitus		A hemoglobin A$_{1c}$ level of ≥0.065 Hgb fraction as suggested by the American Diabetes Association	A hemoglobin A$_{1c}$ level of ≥6.5% as suggested by the American Diabetes Association
Hemoglobin A$_{1c}$ with estimated average glucose (eAg)	WB	eAg mmol/L = 1.59 × HbA$_{1c}$ − 2.59	eAg (mg/dL) = 28.7 × HbA$_{1c}$ − 46.7
High-density lipoprotein (HDL) (see Table 220-5)			
Homocysteine	P	4.4–10.8 µmol/L	4.4–10.8 µmol/L
Human chorionic gonadotropin (HCG)	S		
Nonpregnant female		<5 IU/L	<5 mIU/mL
1–2 weeks postconception		9–130 IU/L	9–130 mIU/mL
2–3 weeks postconception		75–2600 IU/L	75–2600 mIU/mL

(continued)

TABLE 220-2 CLINICAL CHEMISTRY AND IMMUNOLOGY (CONTINUED)

Analyte	Specimen	SI Units	Conventional Units
3–4 weeks postconception		850–20,800 IU/L	850–20,800 mIU/mL
4–5 weeks postconception		4000–100,200 IU/L	4000–100,200 mIU/mL
5–10 weeks postconception		11,500–289,000 IU/L	11,500–289,000 mIU/mL
10–14 weeks post conception		18,300–137,000 IU/L	18,300–137,000 mIU/mL
Second trimester		1400–53,000 IU/L	1400–53,000 mIU/mL
Third trimester		940–60,000 IU/L	940–60,000 mIU/mL
β–Hydroxybutyrate	P	60–170 µmol/L	0.6–1.8 mg/dL
17-Hydroxyprogesterone (adult)	S		
Male		<4.17 nmol/L	<139 ng/dL
Female			
Follicular phase		0.45–2.1 nmol/L	15–70 ng/dL
Luteal phase		1.05–8.7 nmol/L	35–290 ng/dL
Immunofixation	S	Not applicable	No bands detected
Immunoglobulin, quantitation (adult)			
IgA	S	0.70–3.50 g/L	70–350 mg/dL
IgD	S	0–140 mg/L	0–14 mg/dL
IgE	S	1–87 KIU/L	1–87 IU/mL

IgG	S	7.0–17.0 g/L	700–1700 mg/dL
IgG_1	S	2.7–17.4 g/L	270–1740 mg/dL
IgG_2	S	0.3–6.3 g/L	30–630 mg/dL
IgG_3	S	0.13–3.2 g/L	13–320 mg/dL
IgG_4	S	0.11–6.2 g/L	11–620 mg/dL
IgM	S	0.50–3.0 g/L	50–300 mg/dL
Insulin	S, P	14.35–143.5 pmol/L	2–20 µU/mL
Iron	S	7–25 µmol/L	41–141 µg/dL
Iron-binding capacity	S	45–73 µmol/L	251–406 µg/dL
Iron-binding capacity saturation	S	0.16–0.35	16–35%
Ischemia modified albumin	S	<85 KU/L	<85 U/mL
Joint fluid crystal	JF	Not applicable	No crystals seen
Joint fluid mucin	JF	Not applicable	Only type I mucin present
Ketone (acetone)	S	Negative	Negative
Lactate	P, arterial	0.5–1.6 mmol/L	4.5–14.4 mg/dL
	P, venous	0.5–2.2 mmol/L	4.5–19.8 mg/dL
Lactate dehydrogenase	S	2.0–3.8 µkat/L	115–221 U/L
Lipase	S	0.51–0.73 µkat/L	3–43 U/L

(continued)

1413

TABLE 220-2 CLINICAL CHEMISTRY AND IMMUNOLOGY (CONTINUED)

Analyte	Specimen	SI Units	Conventional Units
Lipids: see Table 220-5			
Lipoprotein (a)	S	0–300 mg/L	0–30 mg/dL
Low-density lipoprotein (LDL) (see Table 220-5)			
Luteinizing hormone (LH)	S, P		
Female			
Menstruating			
Follicular phase		2.0–15.0 U/L	2.0–15.0 mIU/mL
Ovulatory phase		22.0–105.0 U/L	22.0–105.0 mIU/mL
Luteal phase		0.6–19.0 U/L	0.6–19.0 mIU/mL
Postmenopausal		16.0–64.0 U/L	16.0–64.0 mIU/mL
Male		2.0–12.0 U/L	2.0–12.0 mIU/mL
Magnesium	S	0.62–0.95 mmol/L	1.5–2.3 mg/dL
Metanephrine	P	<0.5 nmol/L	<100 pg/mL
Methemoglobin	WB	0.0–0.01	0–1%
Myoglobin	S		
Male		20–71 µg/L	20–71 µg/L
Female		25–58 µg/L	25–58 µg/L

Norepinephrine	P	
Supine (30 min)		650–2423 pmol/L	110–410 pg/mL
Sitting		709–4019 pmol/L	120–680 pg/mL
Standing (30 min)		739–4137 pmol/L	125–700 pg/mL
N-telopeptide (cross-linked), NTx	S		
Female, premenopausal		6.2–19.0 nmol BCE	6.2–19.0 nmol BCE
Male		5.4–24.2 nmol BCE	5.4–24.2 nmol BCE
BCE = bone collagen equivalent			
NT-Pro BNP	S, P	<125 ng/L up to 75 years	<125 pg/mL up to 75 years
		<450 ng/L >75 years	<450 pg/mL >75 years
5' Nucleotidase	S	0.00–0.19 μkat/L	0–11 U/L
Osmolality	P	275–295 mosmol/kg serum water	275–295 kg/kg serum water
Osteocalcin	S	11–50 μg/L	11–50 ng/mL
Oxygen content	WB		
Arterial (sea level)		17–21	17–21 vol%
Venous (sea level)		10–16	10–16 vol%
Oxygen saturation (sea level)	WB	Fraction:	Percent:
Arterial		0.94–1.0	94–100%
Venous, arm		0.60–0.85	60–85%
Parathyroid hormone (intact)	S	8–51 ng/L	8–51 pg/mL

(continued)

1415

TABLE 220-2 CLINICAL CHEMISTRY AND IMMUNOLOGY (CONTINUED)

Analyte	Specimen	SI Units	Conventional Units
Phosphatase, alkaline	S	0.56–1.63 μkat/L	33–96 U/L
Phosphorus, inorganic	S	0.81–1.4 mmol/L	2.5–4.3 mg/dL
Potassium	S	3.5–5.0 mmol/L	3.5–5.0 meq/L
Prealbumin	S	170–340 mg/L	17–34 mg/dL
Procalcitonin	S	<0.1 μg/L	<0.1 ng/mL
Progesterone	S, P		
Female: Follicular		<3.18 nmol/L	<1.0 ng/mL
Midluteal		9.54–63.6 nmol/L	3–20 ng/mL
Male		<3.18 nmol/L	<1.0 ng/mL
Prolactin	S		
Male		53–360 μg/L	2.5–17 ng/mL
Female		40–530 μg/L	1.9–25 ng/mL
Prostate-specific antigen (PSA)	S	0.0–4.0 μg/L	0.0–4.0 ng/mL
Prostate-specific antigen, free	S	With total PSA between 4 and 10 μg/L and when the free PSA is:	With total PSA between 4 and 10 ng/mL and when the free PSA is:
		>0.25 decreased risk of prostate cancer	>25% decreased risk of prostate cancer
		<0.10 increased risk of prostate cancer	<10% increased risk of prostate cancer

		SI units	Conventional units
Protein fractions:	S		
Albumin		35–55 g/L	3.5–5.5 g/dL (50–60%)
Globulin		20–35 g/L	2.0–3.5 g/dL (40–50%)
Alpha$_1$		2–4 g/L	0.2–0.4 g/dL (4.2–7.2%)
Alpha$_2$		5–9 g/L	0.5–0.9 g/dL (6.8–12%)
Beta		6–11 g/L	0.6–1.1 g/dL (9.3–15%)
Gamma		7–17 g/L	0.7–1.7 g/dL (13–23%)
Protein, total	S	67–86 g/L	6.7–8.6 g/dL
Pyruvate	P	40–130 µmol/L	0.35–1.14 mg/dL
Rheumatoid factor	S	<15 kIU/L	<15 IU/mL
Serotonin	WB	0.28–1.14 umol/L	50–200 ng/mL
Serum protein electrophoresis	S	Not applicable	Normal pattern
Sex hormone–binding globulin (adult)	S		
Male		11–80 nmol/L	11–80 nmol/L
Female		30–135 nmol/L	30–135 nmol/L
Sodium	S	136–146 mmol/L	136–146 meq/L
Somatomedin-C (IGF-1)(adult)	S		
16 years		226–903 µg/L	226–903 ng/mL
17 years		193–731 µg/L	193–731 ng/mL

(continued)

TABLE 220-2 CLINICAL CHEMISTRY AND IMMUNOLOGY (CONTINUED)

Analyte	Specimen	SI Units	Conventional Units
18 years		163–584 µg/L	163–584 ng/mL
19 years		141–483 µg/L	141–483 ng/mL
20 years		127–424 µg/L	127–424 ng/mL
21–25 years		116–358 µg/L	116–358 ng/mL
26–30 years		117–329 µg/L	117–329 ng/mL
31–35 years		115–307 µg/L	115–307 ng/mL
36–40 years		119–204 µg/L	119–204 ng/mL
41–45 years		101–267 µg/L	101–267 ng/mL
46–50 years		94–252 µg/L	94–252 ng/mL
51–55 years		87–238 µg/L	87–238 ng/mL
56–60 years		81–225 µg/L	81–225 ng/mL
61–65 years		75–212 µg/L	75–212 ng/mL
66–70 years		69–200 µg/L	69–200 ng/mL
71–75 years		64–188 µg/L	64–188 ng/mL
76–80 years		59–177 µg/L	59–177 ng/mL
81–85 years		55–166 µg/L	55–166 ng/mL

Analyte	Specimen	SI Units	Conventional Units
Somatostatin	P	<25 ng/L	<25 pg/mL
Testosterone, free	S		
Female, adult		10.4–65.9 pmol/L	3–19 pg/mL
Male, adult		312–1041 pmol/L	90–300 pg/mL
Testosterone, total	S		
Female		0.21–2.98 nmol/L	6–86 ng/dL
Male		9.36–37.10 nmol/L	270–1070 ng/dL
Thyroglobulin	S	13–318 µg/L	1.3–31.8 ng/mL
Thyroid-binding globulin	S	13–30 mg/L	1.3–3.0 mg/dL
Thyroid-stimulating hormone	S	0.34–4.25 mIU/L	0.34–4.25 µIU/mL
Thyroxine, free (fT4)	S	9.0–16 pmol/L	0.7–1.24 ng/dL
Thyroxine, total (T4)	S	70–151 nmol/L	5.4–11.7 µg/dL
Thyroxine index (free)	S	6.7–10.9	6.7–10.9
Transferrin	S	2.0–4.0 g/L	200–400 mg/dL
Triglycerides (see Table 220-5)	S	0.34–2.26 mmol/L	30–200 mg/dL
Triiodothyronine, free (fT3)	S	3.7–6.5 pmol/L	2.4–4.2 pg/mL
Triiodothyronine, total (T3)	S	1.2–2.1 nmol/L	77–135 ng/dL

(continued)

TABLE 220-2 CLINICAL CHEMISTRY AND IMMUNOLOGY (CONTINUED)

Analyte	Specimen	SI Units	Conventional Units
Troponin I (method dependent)	S,P		
99th percentile of a healthy population		0–0.04 μg/L	0–0.04 ng/mL
Troponin T	S,P		
99th percentile of a healthy population		0–0.01 μg/L	0–0.01 ng/mL
Urea nitrogen	S	2.5–7.1 mmol/L	7–20 mg/dL
Uric acid	S		
Females		0.15–0.33 mmol/L	2.5–5.6 mg/dL
Males		0.18–0.41 mmol/L	3.1–7.0 mg/dL
Vasoactive intestinal polypeptide	P	0–60 ng/L	0–60 pg/mL
Zinc protoporphyrin	WB	0–400 μg/L	0–40 μg/dL
Zinc protoporphyrin (ZPP)-to-heme ratio	WB	0–69 μmol ZPP/mol heme	0–69 μmol ZPP/mol heme

Abbreviations: P, plasma; S, serum; WB, whole blood.

TABLE 220-3 TOXICOLOGY AND THERAPEUTIC DRUG MONITORING

Drug	Therapeutic Range		Toxic Level	
	SI Units	Conventional Units	SI Units	Conventional Units
Acetaminophen	66–199 µmol/L	10–30 µg/mL	>1320 µmol/L	>200 µg/mL
Amikacin				
Peak	34–51 µmol/L	20–30 µg/mL	>60 µmol/L	>35 µg/mL
Trough	0–17 µmol/L	0–10 µg/mL	>17 µmol/L	>10 µg/mL
Amitriptyline/nortriptyline (total drug)	430–900 nmol/L	120–250 ng/mL	>1800 nmol/L	>500 ng/mL
Amphetamine	150–220 nmol/L	20–30 ng/mL	>1500 nmol/L	>200 ng/mL
Bromide	9.4–18.7 mmol/L	75–150 mg/dL	>18.8 mmol/L	>150 mg/dL
Mild toxicity			6.4–18.8 mmol/L	51–150 mg/dL
Severe toxicity			>18.8 mmol/L	>150 mg/dL
Lethal			>37.5 mmol/L	>300 mg/dL
Caffeine	25.8–103 µmol/L	5–20 µg/mL	>206 µmol/L	>40 µg/mL
Carbamazepine	17–42 µmol/L	4–10 µg/mL	>85 µmol/L	>20 µg/mL
Chloramphenicol				
Peak	31–62 µmol/L	10–20 µg/mL	>77 µmol/L	>25 µg/mL
Trough	15–31 µmol/L	5–10 µg/mL	>46 µmol/L	>15 µg/mL

(continued)

TABLE 220-3 TOXICOLOGY AND THERAPEUTIC DRUG MONITORING (CONTINUED)

Drug	Therapeutic Range		Toxic Level	
	SI Units	Conventional Units	SI Units	Conventional Units
Chlordiazepoxide	1.7–10 µmol/L	0.5–3.0 µg/mL	>17 µmol/L	>5.0 µg/mL
Clonazepam	32–240 nmol/L	10–75 ng/mL	>320 nmol/L	>100 ng/mL
Clozapine	0.6–2.1 µmol/L	200–700 ng/mL	>3.7 µmol/L	>1200 ng/mL
Cocaine			>3.3 µmol/L	>1.0 µg/mL
Codeine	43–110 nmol/mL	13–33 ng/mL	>3700 nmol/mL	>1100 ng/mL (lethal)
Cyclosporine				
Renal transplant				
0–6 months	208–312 nmol/L	250–375 ng/mL	>312 nmol/L	>375 ng/mL
6–12 months after transplant	166–250 nmol/L	200–300 ng/mL	>250 nmol/L	>300 ng/mL
>12 months	83–125 nmol/L	100–150 ng/mL	>125 nmol/L	>150 ng/mL
Cardiac transplant				
0–6 months	208–291 nmol/L	250–350 ng/mL	>291 nmol/L	>350 ng/mL
6–12 months after transplant	125–208 nmol/L	150–250 ng/mL	>208 nmol/L	>250 ng/mL
>12 months	83–125 nmol/L	100–150 ng/mL	>125 nmol/L	150 ng/mL
Lung transplant				
0–6 months	250–374 nmol/L	300–450 ng/mL	>374 nmol/L	>450 ng/mL

Liver transplant			
Initiation	208–291 nmol/L	250–350 ng/mL	>350 ng/mL
Maintenance	83–166 nmol/L	100–200 ng/mL	>200 ng/mL
Desipramine	375–1130 nmol/L	100–300 ng/mL	>500 ng/mL
Diazepam (and metabolite)			
Diazepam	0.7 –3.5 µmol/L	0.2–1.0 µg/mL	>2.0 µg/mL
Nordiazepam	0.4– 6.6 µmol/L	0.1–1.8 µg/mL	>2.5 µg/mL
Digoxin	0.64–2.6 nmol/L	0.5–2.0 ng/mL	>3.9 ng/mL
Disopyramide	5.3–14.7 µmol/L	2–5 µg/mL	>7 µg/mL
Doxepin and nordoxepin			
Doxepin	0.36–0.98 µmol/L	101–274 ng/mL	>503 ng/mL
Nordoxepin	0.38–1.04 µmol/L	106–291 ng/mL	>531 ng/mL
Ethanol			
Behavioral changes		>4.3 mmol/L	>20 mg/dL
Legal limit		≥17 mmol/L	≥80 mg/dL
Critical with acute exposure		>54 mmol/L	>250 mg/dL
Ethylene glycol			
Toxic		>2 mmol/L	>12 mg/dL
Lethal		>20 mmol/L	>120 mg/dL

(continued)

TABLE 220-3 TOXICOLOGY AND THERAPEUTIC DRUG MONITORING (CONTINUED)

Drug	Therapeutic Range		Toxic Level	
	SI Units	Conventional Units	SI Units	Conventional Units
Ethosuximide	280–700 µmol/L	40–100 µg/mL	>700 µmol/L	>100 µg/mL
Everolimus	3.13–8.35 nmol/L	3–8 ng/mL	>12.5 nmol/L	>12 ng/mL
Flecainide	0.5–2.4 µmol/L	0.2–1.0 µg/mL	>3.6 µmol/L	>1.5 µg/mL
Gentamicin				
Peak	10–21 µmol/mL	5–10 µg/mL	>25 µmol/mL	>12 µg/mL
Trough	0–4.2 µmol/mL	0–2 µg/mL	>42 µmol/mL	>2 µg/mL
Heroin (diacetyl morphine)			>700 µmol/L	>200 ng/mL (as morphine)
Ibuprofen	49–243 µmol/L	10–50 µg/mL	>970 µmol/L	>200 µg/mL
Imipramine (and metabolite)				
Desimipramine	375–1130 nmol/L	100–300 ng/mL	>1880 nmol/L	>500 ng/mL
Total imipramine + desimipramine	563–1130 nmol/L	150–300 ng/mL	>1880 nmol/L	>500 ng/mL
Lamotrigine	11.7–54.7 µmol/L	3–14 µg/mL	>58.7 µmol/L	>15 µg/mL
Lidocaine	5.1–21.3 µmol/L	1.2–5.0 µg/mL	>38.4 µmol/L	>9.0 µg/mL
Lithium	0.5–1.3 mmol/L	0.5–1.3 meq/L	>2 mmol/L	>2 meq/L
Methadone	1.0–3.2 µmol/L	0.3–1.0 µg/mL	>6.5 µmol/L	>2 µg/mL

Methamphetamine	0.07–0.34 µmol/L	0.01–0.05 µg/mL	>0.5 µg/mL
Methanol			>20 mg/dL
			>6 mmol/L
Methotrexate			
Low-dose	0.01–0.1 µmol/L	0.01–0.1 µmol/L	>0.1 mmol/L
High-dose (24h)	<5.0 µmol/L	<5.0 µmol/L	>5.0 µmol/L
High-dose (48h)	<0.50 µmol/L	<0.50 µmol/L	>0.5 µmol/L
High-dose (72h)	<0.10 µmol/L	<0.10 µmol/L	>0.1 µmol/L
Morphine	232–286 µmol/L	65–80 ng/mL	>720 µmol/L
			>200 ng/mL
Mycophenolic acid	3.1–10.9 µmol/L	1.0–3.5 ng/mL	>37 µmol/L
			>12 ng/mL
Nitroprusside (as thiocyanate)	103–499 µmol/L	6–29 µg/mL	860 µmol/L
			>50 µg/mL
Nortriptyline	190–569 nmol/L	50–150 ng/mL	>1900 nmol/L
			>500 ng/mL
Phenobarbital	65–172 µmol/L	15–40 µg/mL	>258 µmol/L
			>60 µg/mL
Phenytoin	40–79 µmol/L	10–20 µg/mL	>158 µmol/L
			>40 µg/mL
Phenytoin, free	4.0–7.9 µg/mL	1–2 µg/mL	>13.9 µg/mL
			>3.5 µg/mL
% Free	0.08–0.14	8–14%	
Primidone and metabolite			
Primidone	23–55 µmol/L	5–12 µg/mL	>69 µmol/L
			>15 µg/mL
Phenobarbital	65–172 µmol/L	15–40 µg/mL	>215 µmol/L
			>50 µg/mL

(continued)

1425

TABLE 220-3 TOXICOLOGY AND THERAPEUTIC DRUG MONITORING (CONTINUED)

Drug	Therapeutic Range		Toxic Level	
	SI Units	Conventional Units	SI Units	Conventional Units
Procainamide				
Procainamide	17–42 μmol/L	4–10 μg/mL	>43 μmol/L	>10 μg/mL
NAPA (*N*-acetylprocainamide)	22–72 μmol/L	6–20 μg/mL	>126 μmol/L	>35 μg/mL
Quinidine	6.2–15.4 μmol/L	2.0–5.0 μg/mL	>19 μmol/L	>6 μg/mL
Salicylates	145–2100 μmol/L	2–29 mg/dL	>2900 μmol/L	>40 mg/dL
Sirolimus (trough level)				
Kidney transplant	4.4–15.4 nmol/L	4–14 ng/mL	>16 nmol/L	>15 ng/mL
Tacrolimus (FK506) (trough)				
Kidney and liver				
Initiation	12–19 nmol/L	10–15 ng/mL	>25 nmol/L	>20 ng/mL
Maintenance	6–12 nmol/L	5–10 ng/mL	>25 nmol/L	>20 ng/mL
Heart				
Initiation	19–25 nmol/L	15–20 ng/mL		
Maintenance	6–12 nmol/L	5–10 ng/mL		

Theophylline	56–111 µg/mL	10–20 µg/mL	>168 µg/mL	>30 µg/mL
Thiocyanate				
After nitroprusside infusion	103–499 µmol/L	6–29 µg/mL	860 µmol/L	>50 µg/mL
Nonsmoker	17–69 µmol/L	1–4 µg/mL		
Smoker	52–206 µmol/L	3–12 µg/mL		
Tobramycin				
Peak	11–22 µg/L	5–10 µg/mL	>26 µg/L	>12 µg/mL
Trough	0–4.3 µg/L	0–2 µg/mL	>4.3 µg/L	>2 µg/mL
Valproic acid	346–693 µmol/L	50–100 µg/mL	>693 µmol/L	>100 µg/mL
Vancomycin				
Peak	14–28 µmol/L	20–40 µg/mL	>55 µmol/L	>80 µg/mL
Trough	3.5–10.4 µmol/L	5–15 µg/mL	>14 µmol/L	>20 µg/mL

TABLE 220-4 VITAMINS AND SELECTED TRACE MINERALS

Specimen	Analyte	Reference Range	
		SI Units	Conventional Units
Aluminum	S	<0.2 µmol/L	<5.41 µg/L
Arsenic	WB	0.03–0.31 µmol/L	2–23 µg/L
Cadmium	WB	<44.5 nmol/L	<5.0 µg/L
Coenzyme Q10 (ubiquinone)	P	433–1532 µg/L	433–1532 µg/L
β-Carotene	S	0.07–1.43 µmol/L	4–77 µg/dL
Copper	S	11–22 µmol/L	70–140 µg/dL
Folic acid	RC	340–1020 nmol/L cells	150–450 ng/mL cells
Folic acid	S	12.2–40.8 nmol/L	5.4–18.0 ng/mL
Lead (adult)	S	<0.5 µmol/L	<10 µg/dL
Mercury	WB	3.0–294 nmol/L	0.6–59 µg/L
Selenium	S	0.8–2.0 umol/L	63–160 µg/L
Vitamin A	S	0.7–3.5 µmol/L	20–100 µg/dL
Vitamin B_1 (thiamine)	S	0–75 nmol/L	0–2 µg/dL
Vitamin B_2 (riboflavin)	S	106–638 nmol/L	4–24 µg/dL
Vitamin B_6	P	20–121 nmol/L	5–30 ng/mL
Vitamin B_{12}	S	206–735 pmol/L	279–996 pg/mL
Vitamin C (ascorbic acid)	S	23–57 µmol/L	0.4–1.0 mg/dL
Vitamin D_3,1,25-dihydroxy, total	S, P	36–180 pmol/L	15–75 pg/mL
Vitamin D_3,25-hydroxy, total	P	75–250 nmol/L	30–100 ng/mL
Vitamin E	S	12–42 µmol/L	5–18 µg/mL
Vitamin K	S	0.29–2.64 nmol/L	0.13–1.19 ng/mL
Zinc	S	11.5–18.4 µmol/L	75–120 µg/dL

Abbreviations: P, plasma; RC, red cells; S, serum; WB, whole blood.

TABLE 220-5 CLASSIFICATION OF LDL, TOTAL, AND HDL CHOLESTEROL

LDL Cholesterol	
<70 mg/dL	Therapeutic option for very high-risk pts
<100 mg/dL	Optimal
100–129 mg/dL	Near optimal/above optimal
130–159 mg/dL	Borderline high
160–189 mg/dL	High
≥190 mg/dL	Very high
Total Cholesterol	
<200 mg/dL	Desirable
200–239 mg/dL	Borderline high
≥240 mg/dL	High
HDL Cholesterol	
<40 mg/dL	Low
≥60 mg/dL	High

Abbreviations: LDL, low-density lipoprotein; HDL, high-density lipoprotein.
Sources: Executive summary of the third report of the National Cholesterol Education Program (NCEP) expert panel on detection, evaluation, and treatment of high blood cholesterol in adults (adult treatment panel III). JAMA 2001; 285:2486–97. Implications of Recent Clinical Trials for the National Cholesterol Education Program Adult Treatment Panel III Guidelines. SM Grundy et al for the Coordinating Committee of the National Cholesterol Education Program: Circulation 110:227, 2004.

REFERENCE VALUES FOR SPECIFIC ANALYTES

(Tables 220-6 through 220-9)

TABLE 220-6 CEREBROSPINAL FLUID[a]

Constituent	Reference Range	
	SI Units	Conventional Units
Osmolarity	292–297 mmol/kg water	292–297 mosmol/L
Electrolytes		
Sodium	137–145 mmol/L	137–145 meq/L
Potassium	2.7–3.9 mmol/L	2.7–3.9 meq/L
Calcium	1.0–1.5 mmol/L	2.1–3.0 meq/L
Magnesium	1.0–1.2 mmol/L	2.0–2.5 meq/L
Chloride	116–122 mmol/L	116–122 meq/L
CO_2 content	20–24 mmol/L	20–24 meq/L
P_{CO_2}	6–7 kPa	45–49 mmHg
pH	7.31–7.34	
Glucose	2.22–3.89 mmol/L	40–70 mg/dL
Lactate	1–2 mmol/L	10–20 mg/dL
Total protein:		
Lumbar	0.15–0.5 g/L	15–50 mg/dL
Cisternal	0.15–0.25 g/L	15–25 mg/dL
Ventricular	0.06–0.15 g/L	6–15 mg/dL
Albumin	0.066–0.442 g/L	6.6–44.2 mg/dL
IgG	0.009–0.057 g/L	0.9–5.7 mg/dL
IgG index[b]	0.29–0.59	
Oligoclonal bands (OGB)	<2 bands not present in matched serum sample	
Ammonia	15–47 µmol/L	25–80 µg/dL
Creatinine	44–168 µmol/L	0.5–1.9 mg/dL
Myelin basic protein	<4 µg/L	
CSF pressure		50–180 mmH$_2$O
CSF volume (adult)	~150 mL	
Red blood cells	0	0
Leukocytes		
Total	0–5 mononuclear cells per µL	
Differential		
Lymphocytes	60–70%	
Monocytes	30–50%	
Neutrophils	None	

[a]Since cerebrospinal fluid concentrations are equilibrium values, measurements of the same parameters in blood plasma obtained at the same time are recommended. However, there is a time lag in attainment of equilibrium, and cerebrospinal levels of plasma constituents that can fluctuate rapidly (such as plasma glucose) may not achieve stable values until after a significant lag phase.
[b]IgG index = CSF IgG (mg/dL) × serum albumin (g/dL)/serum IgG (g/dL) × CSF albumin (mg/dL).

TABLE 220-7 URINE ANALYSIS AND RENAL FUNCTION TESTS

	Reference Range	
	SI Units	Conventional Units
Acidity, titratable	20–40 mmol/d	20–40 meq/d
Aldosterone	Normal diet: 6–25 µg/d	Normal diet: 6–25 µg/d
	Low-salt diet: 17–44 µg/d	Low-salt diet: 17–44 µg/d
	High-salt diet: 0–6 µg/d	High-salt diet: 0–6 µg/d
Aluminum	0.19–1.11 µmol/L	5–30 µg/L
Ammonia	30–50 mmol/d	30–50 meq/d
Amylase		4–400 U/L
Amylase/creatinine clearance ratio [(Cl$_{am}$/Cl$_{cr}$) × 100]	1–5	1–5
Arsenic	0.07–0.67 µmol/d	5–50 µg/d
Bence Jones protein, urine, qualitative	Not applicable	None detected
Bence Jones protein, urine, quantitative		
Free Kappa	1.4–24.2 mg/L	0.14–2.42 mg/dL
Free Lambda	0.2–6.7 mg/L	0.02–0.67 mg/dL
K/L ratio	2.04–10.37	2.04–10.37
Calcium (10 meq/d or 200 mg/d dietary calcium)	<7.5 mmol/d	<300 mg/d
Chloride	140–250 mmol/d	140–250 mmol/d
Citrate	320–1240 mg/d	320–1240 mg/d
Copper	<0.95 µmol/d	<60 µg/d
Coproporphyrins (types I and III)	0–20 µmol/mol creatinine	0–20 µmol/mol creatinine
Cortisol, free	55–193 nmol/d	20–70 µg/d
Creatine, as creatinine		
Female	<760 µmol/d	<100 mg/d
Male	<380 µmol/d	<50 mg/d
Creatinine	8.8–14 mmol/d	1.0–1.6 g/d
Dopamine	392–2876 nmol/d	60–440 µg/d
Eosinophils	<100 eosinophils/mL	<100 eosinophils/mL
Epinephrine	0–109 nmol/day	0–20 µg/day
Glomerular filtration rate	>60 mL/min/1.73 m^2	>60 mL/min/1.73 m^2
	For African Americans multiply the result by 1.21	For African Americans multiply the result by 1.21
Glucose (glucose oxidase method)	0.3–1.7 mmol/d	50–300 mg/d

(continued)

TABLE 220-7 URINE ANALYSIS AND RENAL FUNCTION TESTS (CONTINUED)

	Reference Range	
	SI Units	Conventional Units
5-Hydroindoleacetic acid [5-HIAA]	0–78.8 µmol/d	0–15 mg/d
Hydroxyproline	53–328 µmol/d	53–328 µmol/d
Iodine, spot urine		
WHO classification of iodine deficiency:		
Not iodine deficient	>100 µg/L	>100 µg/L
Mild iodine deficiency	50–100 µg/L	50–100 µg/L
Moderate iodine deficiency	20–49 µg/L	20–49 µg/L
Severe iodine deficiency	<20 µg/L	<20 µg/L
Ketone (acetone)	Negative	Negative
17 Ketosteroids	3–12 mg/d	3–12 mg/d
Metanephrines		
Metanephrine	30–350 µg/d	30–350 µg/d
Normetanephrine	50–650 µg/d	50–650 µg/d
Microalbumin		
Normal	0.0–0.03 g/d	0–30 mg/d
Microalbuminuria	0.03–0.30 g/d	30–300 mg/d
Clinical albuminuria	>0.3 g/d	>300 mg/d
Microalbumin/ creatinine ratio		
Normal	0–3.4 g/mol creatinine	0–30 µg/mg creatinine
Microalbuminuria	3.4–34 g/mol creatinine	30–300 µg/mg creatinine
Clinical albuminuria	>34 g/mol creatinine	>300 µg/mg creatinine
β_2-Microglobulin	0–160 µg/L	0–160 µg/L
Norepinephrine	89–473 nmol/d	15–80 µg/d
N-telopeptide (cross-linked), NTx		
Female, premenopausal	17–94 nmol BCE/mmol creatinine	17–94 nmol BCE/mmol creatinine
Female, postmenopausal	26–124 nmol BCE/mmol creatinine	26–124 nmol BCE/mmol creatinine
Male	21–83 nmol BCE/mmol creatinine	21–83 nmol BCE/mmol creatinine

TABLE 220-7 URINE ANALYSIS AND RENAL FUNCTION TESTS (CONTINUED)

	Reference Range	
	SI Units	Conventional Units
BCE = bone collagen equivalent		
Osmolality	500–800 kg/kg water	500–800 kg/kg water
Oxalate		
Male	80–500 µmol/d	7–44 mg/d
Female	45–350 µmol/d	4–31 mg/d
pH	5.0–9.0	5.0–9.0
Phosphate (phosphorus) (varies with intake)	12.9–42.0 mmol/d	400–1300 mg/d
Porphobilinogen	None	None
Potassium (varies with intake)	25–100 mmol/d	25–100 meq/d
Protein	<0.15 g/d	<150 mg/d
Protein/creatinine ratio	Male: 15–68 mg/g	Male: 15–68 mg/g
	Female: 10–107 mg/g	Female: 10–107 mg/g
Sediment		
Red blood cells	0–2/high-power field	
White blood cells	0–2/high-power field	
Bacteria	None	
Crystals	None	
Bladder cells	None	
Squamous cells	None	
Tubular cells	None	
Broad casts	None	
Epithelial cell casts	None	
Granular casts	None	
Hyaline casts	0–5/low-power field	
Red blood cell casts	None	
Waxy casts	None	
White cell casts	None	
Sodium (varies with intake)	100–260 mmol/d	100–260 meq/d
Specific gravity		
After 12-h fluid restriction	>1.025	>1.025
After 12-h deliberate water intake	≤1.003	≤1.003

(continued)

TABLE 220-7 URINE ANALYSIS AND RENAL FUNCTION TESTS (CONTINUED)

	Reference Range	
	SI Units	Conventional Units
Tubular reabsorption, phosphorus	0.79–0.94 of filtered load	79–94% of filtered load
Urea nitrogen	214–607 mmol/d	6–17 g/d
Uric acid (normal diet)	1.49–4.76 mmol/d	250–800 mg/d
Vanillylmandelic acid (VMA)	<30 µmol/d	<6 mg/d

TABLE 220-8A DIFFERENTIAL NUCLEATED CELL COUNTS OF BONE MARROW ASPIRATES[a] (SEE HPIM-18 **CHAPS.** 57, E17)

	Observed Range (%)	95% Range (%)	Mean (%)
Blast cells	0–3.2	0–3.0	1.4
Promyelocytes	3.6–13.2	3.2–12.4	7.8
Neutrophil myelocytes	4–21.4	3.7–10.0	7.6
Eosinophil myelocytes	0–5.0	0–2.8	1.3
Metamyelocytes	1–7.0	2.3–5.9	4.1
Neutrophils			
Males	21.0–45.6	21.9–42.3	32.1
Females	29.6–46.6	28.8–45.9	37.4
Eosinophils	0.4–4.2	0.3–4.2	2.2
Eosinophils plus eosinophil myelocytes	0.9–7.4	0.7–6.3	3.5
Basophils	0–0.8	0–0.4	0.1
Erythroblasts			
Male	18.0–39.4	16.2–40.1	28.1
Females	14.0–31.8	13.0–32.0	22.5
Lymphocytes	4.6–22.6	6.0–20.0	13.1
Plasma cells	0–1.4	0–1.2	0.6
Monocytes	0–3.2	0–2.6	1.3
Macrophages	0–1.8	0–1.3	0.4
M:E ratio			
Males	1.1–4.0	1.1–4.1	2.1
Females	1.6–5.4	1.6–5.2	2.8

[a]Based on bone marrow aspirate from 50 healthy volunteers (30 men, 20 women).
Abbreviation: M:E, myeloid to erythroid ratio.
Source: BJ Bain: Br J Haematol 94:206, 1996.

TABLE 220-8B BONE MARROW CELLULARITY

Age	Observed Range	95% Range	Mean
Under 10 years	59.0–95.1%	72.9–84.7%	78.8%
10–19 years	41.5–86.6%	59.2–69.4%	64.3%
20–29 years	32.0–83.7%	54.1–61.9%	58.0%
30–39 years	30.3–81.3%	41.1–54.1%	47.6%
40–49 years	16.3–75.1%	43.5–52.9%	48.2%
50–59 years	19.7–73.6%	41.2–51.4%	46.3%
60–69 years	16.3–65.7%	40.8–50.6%	45.7%
70–79 years	11.3–47.1%	22.6–35.2%	28.9%

Source: From RJ Hartsock et al: Am J Clin Pathol 1965; 43:326, 1965.

TABLE 220-9 STOOL ANALYSIS

	Reference Range	
	SI Units	Conventional Units
Alpha-1-antitrypsin	≤540 mg/L	≤54 mg/dL
Amount	0.1–0.2 kg/d	100–200 g/24 h
Coproporphyrin	611–1832 nmol/d	400–1200 µg/24 h
Fat		
Adult		<7 g/d
Adult on fat-free diet		<4 g/d
Fatty acids	0–21 mmol/d	0–6 g/24 h
Leukocytes	None	None
Nitrogen	<178 mmol/d	<2.5 g/24 h
pH	7.0–7.5	
Potassium	14–102 mmol/L	14–102 mmol/L
Occult blood	Negative	Negative
Osmolality	280–325 mosmol/kg	280–325 mosmol/kg
Sodium	7–72 mmol/L	7–72 mmol/L
Trypsin		20–95 U/g
Urobilinogen	85–510 µmol/d	50–300 mg/24 h
Uroporphyrins	12–48 nmol/d	10–40 µg/24 h
Water	<0.75	<75%

Source: Modified from: FT Fishbach, MB Dunning III: *A Manual of Laboratory and Diagnostic Tests,* 7th ed. Philadelphia, Lippincott Williams & Wilkins, 2004.

■ SPECIAL FUNCTION TESTS (TABLES 220-10 THROUGH 220-14)

TABLE 220-10 URINE ANALYSIS AND RENAL FUNCTION TESTS

	Reference Range	
	SI Units	Conventional Units
Acidity, titratable	20–40 mmol/d	20–40 meq/d
Aldosterone	Normal diet: 6–25 µg/d	Normal diet: 6–25 µg/d
	Low-salt diet: 17–44 µg/d	Low-salt diet: 17–44 µg/d
	High-salt diet: 0–6 µg/d	High-salt diet: 0–6 µg/d
Aluminum	0.19–1.11 µmol/L	5–30 µg/L
Ammonia	30–50 mmol/d	30–50 meq/d
Amylase		4–400 U/L
Amylase/creatinine clearance ratio [(Cl_{am}/Cl_{cr}) × 100]	1–5	1–5
Arsenic	0.07–0.67 µmol/d	5–50 µg/d
Bence Jones protein, urine, qualitative	Not applicable	None detected
Bence Jones protein, urine, quantitative		
Free Kappa	1.4–24.2 mg/L	0.14–2.42 mg/dL
Free Lambda	0.2–6.7 mg/L	0.02–0.67 mg/dL
K/L ratio	2.04–10.37	2.04–10.37
Calcium (10 meq/d or 200 mg/d dietary calcium)	<7.5 mmol/d	<300 mg/d
Chloride	140–250 mmol/d	140–250 mmol/d
Citrate	320–1240 mg/d	320–1240 mg/d
Copper	<0.95 µmol/d	<60 µg/d
Coproporphyrins (types I and III)	0–20 µmol/mol creatinine	0–20 µmol/mol creatinine
Cortisol, free	55–193 nmol/d	20–70 µg/d
Creatine, as creatinine		
Female	<760 µmol/d	<100 mg/d
Male	<380 µmol/d	<50 mg/d
Creatinine	8.8–14 mmol/d	1.0–1.6 g/d
Dopamine	392–2876 nmol/d	60–440 µg/d
Eosinophils	<100 eosinophils/mL	<100 eosinophils/mL

TABLE 220-10 URINE ANALYSIS AND RENAL FUNCTION TESTS (CONTINUED)

	Reference Range	
	SI Units	Conventional Units
Epinephrine	0–109 nmol/day	0–20 µg/day
Glomerular filtration rate	>60 mL/min/1.73 m^2	>60 mL/min/1.73 m^2
	For African Americans multiply the result by 1.21	For African Americans multiply the result by 1.21
Glucose (glucose oxidase method)	0.3–1.7 mmol/d	50–300 mg/d
5-Hydroindoleacetic acid [5-HIAA]	0–78.8 µmol/d	0–15 mg/d
Hydroxyproline	53–328 µmol/d	53–328 µmol/d
Iodine, spot urine		
WHO classification of iodine deficiency:		
Not iodine deficient	>100 µg/L	>100 µg/L
Mild iodine deficiency	50–100 µg/L	50–100 µg/L
Moderate iodine deficiency	20–49 µg/L	20–49 µg/L
Severe iodine deficiency	<20 µg/L	<20 µg/L
Ketone (acetone)	Negative	Negative
17 Ketosteroids	3–12 mg/d	3–12 mg/d
Metanephrines		
Metanephrine	30–350 µg/d	30–350 µg/d
Normetanephrine	50–650 µg/d	50–650 µg/d
Microalbumin		
Normal	0.0–0.03 g/d	0–30 mg/d
Microalbuminuria	0.03–0.30 g/d	30–300 mg/d
Clinical albuminuria	>0.3 g/d	>300 mg/d
Microalbumin/creatinine ratio		
Normal	0–3.4 g/mol creatinine	0–30 µg/mg creatinine
Microalbuminuria	3.4–34 g/mol creatinine	30–300 µg/mg creatinine
Clinical albuminuria	>34 g/mol creatinine	>300 µg/mg creatinine
β_2-Microglobulin	0–160 µg/L	0–160 µg/L
Norepinephrine	89–473 nmol/d	15–80 µg/d

(continued)

TABLE 220-10 URINE ANALYSIS AND RENAL FUNCTION TESTS (CONTINUED)

	Reference Range	
	SI Units	Conventional Units
N-telopeptide (cross-linked), NTx		
Female, premenopausal	17–94 nmol BCE/mmol creatinine	17–94 nmol BCE/mmol creatinine
Female, postmenopausal	26–124 nmol BCE/mmol creatinine	26–124 nmol BCE/mmol creatinine
Male	21–83 nmol BCE/mmol creatinine	21–83 nmol BCE/mmol creatinine
BCE = bone collagen equivalent		
Osmolality	100-800 mosm/kg	100-800 mosm/kg
Oxalate		
Male	80–500 μmol/d	7–44 mg/d
Female	45–350 μmol/d	4–31 mg/d
pH	5.0–9.0	5.0–9.0
Phosphate (phosphorus) (varies with intake)	12.9–42.0 mmol/d	400–1300 mg/d
Porphobilinogen	None	None
Potassium (varies with intake)	25–100 mmol/d	25–100 meq/d
Protein	<0.15 g/d	<150 mg/d
Protein/creatinine ratio	Male: 15–68 mg/g	Male: 15–68 mg/g
	Female: 10–107 mg/g	Female: 10–107 mg/g
Sediment		
Red blood cells	0–2/high-power field	
White blood cells	0–2/high-power field	
Bacteria	None	
Crystals	None	
Bladder cells	None	
Squamous cells	None	
Tubular cells	None	
Broad casts	None	
Epithelial cell casts	None	
Granular casts	None	
Hyaline casts	0–5/low-power field	
Red blood cell casts	None	
Waxy casts	None	

TABLE 220-10 URINE ANALYSIS AND RENAL FUNCTION TESTS (CONTINUED)

	Reference Range	
	SI Units	Conventional Units
White cell casts	None	
Sodium (varies with intake)	100–260 mmol/d	100–260 meq/d
Specific gravity		
After 12-h fluid restriction	>1.025	>1.025
After 12-h deliberate water intake	≤1.003	≤1.003
Tubular reabsorption, phosphorus	0.79–0.94 of filtered load	79–94% of filtered load
Urea nitrogen	214–607 mmol/d	6–17 g/d
Uric acid (normal diet)	1.49–4.76 mmol/d	250–800 mg/d
Vanillylmandelic acid (VMA)	<30 μmol/d	<6 mg/d

TABLE 220-11 CIRCULATORY FUNCTION TESTS

| Test | Results: Reference Range | |
	SI Units (Range)	Conventional Units (Range)
Arteriovenous oxygen difference	30–50 mL/L	30–50 mL/L
Cardiac output (Fick)	2.5–3.6 L/m² of body surface area per min	2.5–3.6 L/m² of body surface area per min
Contractility indexes		
Max. left ventricular *dp/dt* (*dp/dt*)	220 kPa/s (176–250 kPa/s)	1650 mmHg/s (1320–1880 mmHg/s)
DP when DP = 5.3 kPa	(37.6 ± 12.2)/s	(37.6 ± 12.2)/s
(40 mmHg) (DP, developed LV pressure)	3.32 ± 0.84 end-diastolic volumes per second	3.32 ± 0.84 end-diastolic volumes per second
Mean normalized systolic ejection rate (angiography)	1.83 ± 0.56 circumferences per second	1.83 ± 0.56 circumferences per second
Mean velocity of circumferential fiber shortening (angiography)		
Ejection fraction: stroke volume/end-diastolic volume (SV/EDV)	0.67 ± 0.08 (0.55–0.78)	0.67 ± 0.08 (0.55–0.78)
End-diastolic volume	70 ± 20.0 mL/m² (60–88 mL/m²)	70 ± 20.0 mL/m² (60–88 mL/m²)
End-systolic volume	25 ± 5.0 mL/m² (20–33 mL/m²)	25 ± 5.0 mL/m² (20–33 mL/m²)
Left ventricular work		
Stroke work index	50 ± 20.0 (g·m)/m² (30–110)	50 ± 20.0 (g·m)/m² (30–110)
Left ventricular minute work index	1.8–6.6 [(kg·m)/m²]/min	1.8–6.6 [(kg·m)/m²]/min
Oxygen consumption index	110–150 mL	110–150 mL
Maximum oxygen uptake	35 mL/min (20–60 mL/min)	35 mL/min (20–60 mL/min)
Pulmonary vascular resistance	2–12 (kPa·s)/L	20–130 (dyn·s)/cm⁵
Systemic vascular resistance	77–150 (kPa·s)/L	770–1600 (dyn·s)/cm⁵

Source: E Braunwald et al: *Heart Disease*, 6th ed. Philadelphia, W.B. Saunders Co., 2001.

TABLE 220-12 GASTROINTESTINAL TESTS

Test	Results SI Units	Conventional Units
Absorption tests		
D-Xylose: after overnight fast, 25 g xylose given in oral aqueous solution		
Urine, collected for following 5 h	25% of ingested dose	25% of ingested dose
Serum, 2 h after dose	2.0–3.5 mmol/L	30–52 mg/dL
Vitamin A: a fasting blood specimen is obtained and 200,000 units of vitamin A in oil is given orally	Serum level should rise to twice fasting level in 3–5 h	Serum level should rise to twice fasting level in 3–5 h
Plasma		>3.6 (±1.1) μg/mL at 90 min
Urine	>50% recovered in 6 h	>50% recovered in 6 h
Gastric juice		
Volume		
24 h	2–3 L	2–3 L
Nocturnal	600–700 mL	600–700 mL
Basal, fasting	30–70 mL/h	30–70 mL/h
Reaction		
pH	1.6–1.8	1.6–1.8
Titratable acidity of fasting juice	4–9 μmol/s	15–35 meq/h
Acid output		
Basal		
Females (mean ± 1 SD)	0.6 ± 0.5 μmol/s	2.0 ± 1.8 meq/h
Males (mean ± 1 SD)	0.8 ± 0.6 μmol/s	3.0 ± 2.0 meq/h
Maximal (after SC histamine acid phosphate, 0.004 mg/kg body weight, and preceded by 50 mg promethazine, or after betazole, 1.7 mg/kg body weight, or pentagastrin, 6 μg/kg body weight)		
Females (mean ± 1 SD)	4.4 ± 1.4 μmol/s	16 ± 5 meq/h
Males (mean ± 1 SD)	6.4 ± 1.4 μmol/s	23 ± 5 meq/h

(*continued*)

TABLE 220-12 GASTROINTESTINAL TESTS (CONTINUED)

Test	Results	
	SI Units	Conventional Units
Basal acid output/maximal acid output ratio	≤0.6	≤0.6
Gastrin, serum	0–200 μg/L	0–200 pg/mL
Secretin test (pancreatic exocrine function): 1 unit/kg body weight, IV		
Volume (pancreatic juice) in 80 min	>2.0 mL/kg	>2.0 mL/kg
Bicarbonate concentration	>80 mmol/L	>80 meq/L
Bicarbonate output in 30 min	>10 mmol	>10 meq

TABLE 220-13 NORMAL ECHOCARDIOGRAPHIC REFERENCE LIMITS AND PARTITION VALUES IN ADULTS

	Women Reference Range	Mildly Abnormal	Moderately Abnormal	Severely Abnormal	Men Reference Range	Mildly Abnormal	Moderately Abnormal	Severely Abnormal
Left ventricular dimensions								
Septal thickness, cm	0.6–0.9	1.0–1.2	1.3–1.5	≥1.6	0.6–1.0	1.1–1.3	1.4–1.6	≥1.7
Posterior wall thickness, cm	0.6–0.9	1.0–1.2	1.3–1.5	≥1.6	0.6–1.0	1.1–1.3	1.4–1.6	≥1.7
Diastolic diameter, cm	3.9–5.3	5.4–5.7	5.8–6.1	≥6.2	4.2–5.9	6.0–6.3	6.4–6.8	≥6.9
Diastolic diameter/BSA, cm/m²	2.4–3.2	3.3–3.4	3.5–3.7	≥3.8	2.2–3.1	3.2–3.4	3.5–3.6	≥3.7
Diastolic diameter/height, cm/m	2.5–3.2	3.3–3.4	3.5–3.6	≥3.7	2.4–3.3	3.4–3.5	3.6–3.7	≥3.8
Left ventricular volumes								
Diastolic, mL	56–104	105–117	118–130	≥131	67–155	156–178	179–201	≥202
Diastolic/BSA, mL/m²	35–75	76–86	87–96	≥97	35–75	76–86	87–96	≥97
Systolic, mL	19–49	50–59	60–69	≥70	22–58	59–70	71–82	≥83
Systolic/BSA, mL/m²	12–30	31–36	37–42	≥43	12–30	31–36	37–42	≥43
Left ventricular mass, 2D method								
Mass, g	66–150	151–171	172–182	≥183	96–200	201–227	228–254	≥255
Mass/BSA, g/m²	44–88	89–100	101–112	≥113	50–102	103–116	117–130	≥131
Left ventricular function								
Endocardial fractional shortening (%)	27–45	22–26	17–21	≤16	25–43	20–24	15–19	≤14

(continued)

TABLE 220-13 NORMAL ECHOCARDIOGRAPHIC REFERENCE LIMITS AND PARTITION VALUES IN ADULTS (CONTINUED)

	Women Reference Range	Mildly Abnormal	Moderately Abnormal	Severely Abnormal	Men Reference Range	Mildly Abnormal	Moderately Abnormal	Severely Abnormal
Midwall fractional shortening (%)	15–23	13–14	11–12	≤10	14–22	12–13	10–11	≤9
Ejection fraction, 2D method (%)	≥55	45–54	30–44	≤29	≥55	45–54	30–44	≤29
Right heart dimensions (cm)								
Basal RV diameter	2.0–2.8	2.9–3.3	3.4–3.8	≥3.9	2.0–2.8	2.9–3.3	3.4–3.8	≥3.9
Mid-RV diameter	2.7–3.3	3.4–3.7	3.8–4.1	≥4.2	2.7–3.3	3.4–3.7	3.8–4.1	≥4.2
Base-to-apex length	7.1–7.9	8.0–8.5	8.6–9.1	≥9.2	7.1–7.9	8.0–8.5	8.6–9.1	≥9.2
RVOT diameter above aortic valve	2.5–2.9	3.0–3.2	3.3–3.5	≥3.6	2.5–2.9	3.0–3.2	3.3–3.5	≥3.6
RVOT diameter above pulmonic valve	1.7–2.3	2.4–2.7	2.8–3.1	≥3.2	1.7–2.3	2.4–2.7	2.8–3.1	≥3.2
Pulmonary artery diameter below pulmonic valve	1.5–2.1	2.2–2.5	2.6–2.9	≥3.0	1.5–2.1	2.2–2.5	2.6–2.9	≥3.0
Right ventricular size and function in 4-chamber view								
Diastolic area, cm^2	11–28	29–32	33–37	≥38	11–28	29–32	33–37	≥38
Systolic area, cm^2	7.5–16	17–19	20–22	≥23	7.5–16	17–19	20–22	≥23
Fractional area change, %	32–60	25–31	18–24	≤17	32–60	25–31	18–24	≤17

Atrial sizes								
LA diameter, cm	2.7–3.8	3.9–4.2	4.3–4.6	≥4.7	3.0–4.0	4.1–4.6	4.7–5.2	≥5.3
LA diameter/BSA, cm/m²	1.5–2.3	2.4–2.6	2.7–2.9	≥3.0	1.5–2.3	2.4–2.6	2.7–2.9	≥3.0
RA minor axis, cm	2.9–4.5	4.6–4.9	5.0–5.4	≥5.5	2.9–4.5	4.6–4.9	5.0–5.4	≥5.5
RA minor axis/BSA, cm/m²	1.7–2.5	2.6–2.8	2.9–3.1	≥3.2	1.7–2.5	2.6–2.8	2.9–3.1	≥3.2
LA area, cm²	<20	20–30	30–40	≥41	<20	20–30	30–40	≥41
LA volume, mL	22–52	53–62	63–72	≥73	18–58	59–68	69–78	≥79
LA volume/BSA, mL/m²	16–28	29–33	34–39	≥40	16–28	29–33	34–39	≥40
Aortic stenosis, classification of severity								
Aortic jet velocity, m/s		2.6–2.9	3.0–4.0	>4.0		2.6–2.9	3.0–4.0	>4.0
Mean gradient, mmHg		<20	20–40	>40		<20	20–40	>40
Valve area, cm²		>1.5	1.0–1.5	<1.0		>1.5	1.0–1.5	<1.0
Indexed valve area, cm²/m²		>0.85	0.60–0.85	<0.6		>0.85	0.60–0.85	<0.6
Velocity ratio		>0.50	0.25–0.50	<0.25		>0.50	0.25–0.50	<0.25
Mitral stenosis, classification of severity								
Valve area, cm²		>1.5	1.0–1.5	<1.0		>1.5	1.0–1.5	<1.0
Mean gradient, mmHg		<5	5–10	>10		<5	5–10	>10
Pulmonary artery pressure, mmHg		<30	30–50	>50		<30	30–50	>50

(continued)

TABLE 220-13 NORMAL ECHOCARDIOGRAPHIC REFERENCE LIMITS AND PARTITION VALUES IN ADULTS (CONTINUED)

	Women Reference Range	Mildly Abnormal	Moderately Abnormal	Severely Abnormal	Men Reference Range	Mildly Abnormal	Moderately Abnormal	Severely Abnormal
Aortic regurgitation, indices of severity								
Vena contracta width, cm		<0.30	0.30–0.60	≥0.60		<0.30	0.30–0.60	≥0.60
Jet width/LVOT width, %		<25	25–64	≥65		<25	25–64	≥65
Jet CSA/LVOT CSA, %		<5	5–59	≥60		<5	5–59	≥60
Regurgitant volume, mL/beat		<30	30–59	≥60		<30	30–59	≥60
Regurgitant fraction, %		<30	30–49	≥50		<30	30–49	≥50
Effective regurgitant orifice area, cm²		<0.10	0.10–0.29	≥0.30		<0.10	0.10–0.29	≥0.30
Mitral regurgitation, indices of severity								
Vena contracta width, cm		<0.30	0.30–0.69	≥0.70		<0.30	0.30–0.69	≥0.70
Regurgitant volume, mL/beat		<30	30–59	≥60		<30	30–59	≥60
Regurgitant fraction, %		<30	30–49	≥50		<30	30–49	≥50
Effective regurgitant orifice area, cm²		<0.20	0.20–0.39	≥0.40		<0.20	0.20–0.39	≥0.40

Abbreviations: BSA, body surface area; CSA, cross-sectional area; LA, left atrium; LVOT, left ventricular outflow tract; RA, right atrium; RV, right ventricle; RVOT, right ventricular outflow tract; 2D, 2-dimensional.

Source: Values adapted from: American Society of Echocardiography, Guidelines and Standards. *www.asecho.org/i4a/pages/index.cfm?pageid=3317.* Accessed Feb 23, 2010.

TABLE 220-14 SUMMARY OF VALUES USEFUL IN PULMONARY PHYSIOLOGY

		Typical Values	
	Symbol	Man Age 40, 75 kg, 175 cm Tall	Woman Age 40, 60 kg, 160 cm Tall
Pulmonary mechanics			
Spirometry—volume-time curves			
Forced vital capacity	FVC	5.0 L	3.4 L
Forced expiratory volume in 1 s	FEV_1	4.0 L	2.8 L
FEV_1%	FEV_1%	80%	78%
Maximal midexpiratory flow rate	MMEF (FEF 25–75)	4.1 L/s	3.2 L/s
Maximal expiratory flow rate	MEFR (FEF 200–1200)	9.0 L/s	6.1 L/s
Spirometry—flow-volume curves			
Maximal expiratory flow at 50% of expired vital capacity	V_{max} 50 (FEF 50%)	5.0 L/s	4.0 L/s
Maximal expiratory flow at 75% of expired vital capacity	V_{max} 75 (FEF 75%)	2.1 L/s	2.0 L/s
Resistance to airflow			
Pulmonary resistance	RL (R_L)	<3.0 (cmH$_2$0/s)/L	
Airway resistance	Raw	<2.5 (cmH$_2$0/s)/L	
Specific conductance	SGaw	>0.13 cmH$_2$0/s	

(continued)

TABLE 220-14 SUMMARY OF VALUES USEFUL IN PULMONARY PHYSIOLOGY (CONTINUED)

| | Symbol | Typical Values | |
		Man Age 40, 75 kg, 175 cm Tall	Woman Age 40, 60 kg, 160 cm Tall
Pulmonary compliance			
Static recoil pressure at total lung capacity	Pst TLC	25 ± 5 cmH$_2$O	
Compliance of lungs (static)	CL	0.2 L cmH$_2$O	
Compliance of lungs and thorax	C(L + T)	0.1 L cmH$_2$O	
Dynamic compliance of 20 breaths per minute	C dyn 20	0.25 ± 0.05 L/cmH$_2$O	
Maximal static respiratory pressures			
Maximal inspiratory pressure	MIP	>110 cmH$_2$O	>70 cmH$_2$O
Maximal expiratory pressure	MEP	>200 cmH$_2$O	>140 cmH$_2$O
Lung volumes			
Total lung capacity	TLC	6.9 L	4.9 L
Functional residual capacity	FRC	3.3 L	2.6 L
Residual volume	RV	1.9 L	1.5 L
Inspiratory capacity	IC	3.7 L	2.3 L
Expiratory reserve volume	ERV	1.4 L	1.1 L
Vital capacity	VC	5.0 L	3.4 L

Gas exchange (sea level)

Arterial O$_2$ tension	Pao$_2$	12.7 ± 0.7 kPa (95 ± 5 mmHg)
Arterial CO$_2$ tension	Paco$_2$	5.3 ± 0.3 kPa (40 ± 2 mmHg)
Arterial O$_2$ saturation	Sao$_2$	0.97 ± 0.02 (97 ± 2%)
Arterial blood pH	pH	7.40 ± 0.02
Arterial bicarbonate	HCO$_3^-$	24 + 2 meq/L
Base excess	BE	0 ± 2 meq/L
Diffusing capacity for carbon monoxide (single breath)	D$_{LCO}$	37 mL CO/min/mmHg 27 mL CO/min/mmHg
Dead space volume	V$_D$	2 mL/kg body wt
Physiologic dead space; dead space–tidal volume ratio	V$_D$/V$_T$	
Rest		≤35% V$_T$
Exercise		≤20% V$_T$
Alveolar-arterial difference for O$_2$	P(A − a)A0$_2$	≤2.7 kPa ≤20 kPa (≤24 mmHg)

Source: Based on: AH Morris et al: *Clinical Pulmonary Function Testing. A Manual of Uniform Laboratory Procedures*, 2nd ed. Salt Lake City, Utah, Intermountain Thoracic Society, 1984.

■ **MISCELLANEOUS** (TABLE 220-15)

TABLE 220-15 BODY FLUIDS AND OTHER MASS DATA

	Reference Range	
	SI Units	Conventional Units
Ascitic fluid: See Chap. 49		
Body fluid		
Total volume (lean) of body weight	50% (in obese) to 70%	
Intracellular	30–40% of body weight	
Extracellular	20–30% of body weight	
Blood		
Total volume		
Males	69 mL/kg body weight	
Females	65 mL/kg body weight	
Plasma volume		
Males	39 mL/kg body weight	
Females	40 mL/kg body weight	
Red blood cell volume		
Males	30 mL/kg body weight	1.15–1.21 L/m² of body surface area
Females	25 mL/kg body weight	0.95–1.00 L/m² of body surface area
Body mass index	18.5–24.9 kg/m²	18.5–24.9 kg/m²

INDEX